Contents

T0290515

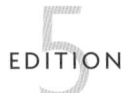

EDITION 5

Edmunds'
PHARMACOLOGY
for the PRIMARY CARE
PROVIDER

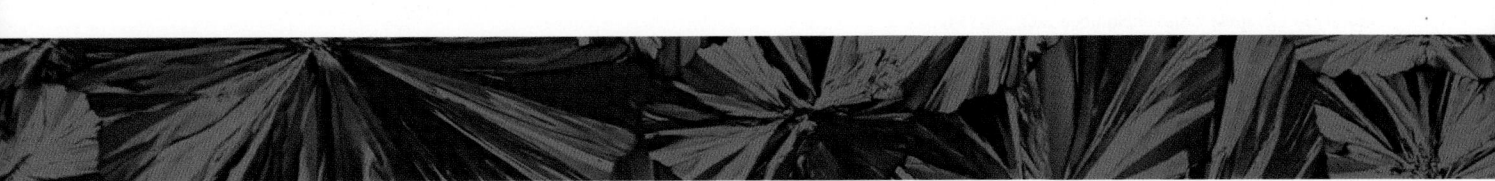

Constance G. Visovsky, PhD, RN, ACNP, FAAN
Professor and Lewis & Leona Hughes Endowed Chair in Nursing Science
College of Nursing
University of South Florida
Tampa, Florida

Cheryl H. Zambroski, PhD, RN
Associate Professor
College of Nursing
University of South Florida
Tampa, Florida

Rebecca M. Lutz, DNP, APRN, FNP-BC
Assistant Professor
College of Nursing
University of South Florida
Tampa, Florida

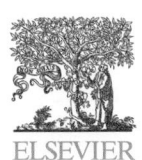

ELSEVIER

Elsevier
3251 Riverport Lane
St. Louis, Missouri 63043

EDMUNDS' PHARMACOLOGY FOR THE PRIMARY CARE PROVIDER,
FIFTH EDITION

ISBN: 978-0-323-66117-1

Previous editions copyrighted 2014, 2009, 2004, 1999

Library of Congress Control Number: 2021940334

Executive Content Strategist: Lee Henderson
Senior Content Development Specialist: Laura Goodrich
Publishing Services Manager: Julie Eddy
Senior Project Manager: Jodi Willard
Design Direction: Bridget Hoette

Printed in India

Last digit is the print number: 9 8 7 6 5 4 3 2 1

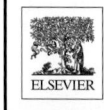

Working together
to grow libraries in
developing countries

www.elsevier.com • www.bookaid.org

Contributors

Deborah Adell, PhD, ARNP, FNP-C
Professor
Nursing
Purdue University Global
Indianapolis, Indiana;
Professor
Princess Noura Bint Abdul Rahman University
Riyadh, Saudi Arabia;
Consultant
Nursing
Dublin City University
Dublin, Ireland

Jaclyn Cole, PharmD, BCPS
Associate Professor
Pharmacotherapeutics & Clinical Research
University of South Florida Taneja College of Pharmacy
Tampa, Florida

Melanie Combs, MSN, PMHNP-BC
Adjunct Faculty
College of Nursing
University of South Florida
Tampa, Florida

Abigail L. Crouch, DNP, AGACNP-BC
Clinician Educator
College of Nursing
University of South Florida
Tampa, Florida;
Assistant Professor
University of South Florida Morsani College of Medicine
Tampa, Florida

Andrea J. Efre, DNP, APRN, FNP-C
Assistant Professor
College of Nursing, Graduate Nursing
University of South Florida
Tampa, Florida

Brenda Gilmore, DNP, CNM, FNP-BC, CNE, NCMP
Assistant Professor
Nursing
University of South Florida
Tampa, Florida

Juan Manuel Gonzalez, DNP, APRN, AGACNP-BC, ENP-C, FNP-BC, CEN, CNE
Associate Professor of Clinical
School of Nursing and Health Studies
University of Miami
Coral Gables, Florida

Teresa Gore, PhD, DNP, APRN, FNP-BC, CHSE-A, FSSH, FAAN
Professor
Ron and Kathy Assaf College of Nursing
Tampa Regional Campus
Tampa, Florida

Umesh Kumar Jinwal, PhD
Associate Professor
Department of Pharmaceutical Sciences
University of South Florida Taneja College of Pharmacy
Tampa, Florida

Marcia Johansson, DNP, APRN, ACNP-BC, FCCM, FAANP
Associate Professor
Director of Clinical Affairs
Adult-Gerontology Acute Care Concentration Director
Advanced Practice Provider Fellowship Director
College of Nursing
University of South Florida
Tampa, Florida

Karla L. Maldonado, DrAP, CRNA, APRN
Assistant Program Director
Nurse Anesthesia Program
University of South Florida
Tampa, Florida

Stephen McGhee, DNP, MSc, PGCE, RNT, RN, VR, FAAN
Associate Professor of Clinical Nursing
Director of Assessment and Evaluation
College of Nursing
The Ohio State University
Columbus, Ohio

Aimon C. Miranda, PharmD, BCPS
Associate Professor and Coordinator of Clinical Informatics
Pharmacotherapeutics and Clinical Research
University of South Florida Taneja College of Pharmacy
Tampa, Florida

Eleanor Rawson, DNP, CRNA, CHSE
Assistant Professor
Nurse Anesthesia Program Simulation Coordinator
University of South Florida
Tampa, Florida

Elizabeth Remo, BSHSE, MS, DNP, APRN, FNP-BC
Assistant Professor
College of Nursing
University of South Florida
Tampa, Florida

Janet Roman, DNP, APRN, ACNP-BC, CHFN, ACHPN
Associate Professor
Director DNP Program
College of Nursing
University of South Florida
Tampa, Florida

Melissa Ruble, PharmD, BCPS
Assistant Professor
Pharmacotherapeutics and Clinical Research
University of South Florida Taneja College of Pharmacy
Tampa, Florida

Maria Russ, PhD, MSN, BSN, APRN, RN, CPNP
Supervisor of School Health Services
School Health Services
Hillsborough County Public Schools
Tampa, Florida;
Visiting Professor
College of Nursing
Chamberlain University
Chicago, Illinois;
Advanced Practice Registered Nurse
Evening Pediatrics Urgent Care
Tampa, Florida

Erini Serag-Bolos, PharmD
Associate Professor
Pharmacotherapeutics & Clinical Research
University of South Florida Taneja College of Pharmacy
Tampa, Florida

Kristy M. Shaeer, PharmD, MPH, BCIDP, AAHIVP
Assistant Professor
Department of Pharmacotherapeutics & Clinical
   Research
University of South Florida Taneja College of Pharmacy
Tampa, Florida;
Clinical Pharmacy Specialist
Tampa General Hospital
Tampa, Florida

Tracey L. Taylor, DNP, APRN, ACNP-BC
Senior Associate Dean of Academic Affairs and
   Educational Innovation
College of Nursing
University of South Florida
Tampa, Florida

Beatriz Valdes, PhD, RN, CHSE
Assistant Professor of Clinical
School of Nursing & Health Studies
University of Miami
Miami, Florida

Reviewers

Tiffanie C. Bourgeois, MSN, FNP-C
Hospice and Palliative Nurse
LaPlace, Louisiana

Sarah Cantrell, MSN, AGACNP-BC
Advanced Practice Provider
Indianapolis, Indiana

Crystal Fortuna, PA-C
At Your Door: Visiting Healthcare Services, LLC
Dayton, Ohio

Shannon Gerow, MSN, RN, FNP-BC
Family Nurse Practitioner
Indiana Wesleyan University
Marion, Indiana

Aleko Kimbouris, MPH, MSHS, PA-C
Assistant Professor
Johnson & Wales University
Providence, Rhode Island

Senthilkumaran Lakshmanan, BS, MD, PA-C
NCCPA Certification
Assistant Professor of Instruction
University of Texas Medical Branch
Galveston, Texas

LeAnne Martinelli, RPh, MMSc, DHS
Academic Director and Associate Professor
Mercer University
College of Health Professions
Atlanta, Georgia

Heidi Medina, MSPAS, PA-C
Emergency Medicine Physician Assistant
Wellspan Ephrata Community Hospital
Ephrata, Pennsylvania

Ana Lisa Nardin, MHS, PA-C
Physician Assistant
Duke University Hospital
Durham, North Carolina

Robert M. Poutré, BS, MPAS, PA-C
Idaho State University
Pocatello, Idaho

Jennifer Sass, MSN, RN, FNP-C, CRN-MNN, BS
Family Nurse Practitioner
Cabarrus Rowan Community Health Centers
Concord, North Carolina

Peggy Soper, DNP, CNE, RN-BC
Core Faculty DNP Capella
Strayer University
Herndon, Virginia;
Capella School of Nursing
Minneapolis, Minnesota

Rebecca Joy Stam, RN, MSN, APRN
Adult Nurse Practitioner
Vanderbilt University
Grand Rapids, Michigan

Jessica Tuczapski, BS, MSPAS, PA-C
Physician Assistant
Naugatuck Valley Gastroenterology Consultants
Waterbury Hospital, St. Mary's Hospital
Prospect, Connecticut

Preface

As its title suggests, *Edmunds' Pharmacology for the Primary Care Provider* is intended for primary care providers, but it is written with a special emphasis on nurse practitioners and physician assistants practicing in a community-based primary care setting. Our goals are to assist prescribers to master the essential information necessary for making pharmacological treatment decisions and to present updated information for medications prescribed in a primary care practice.

As in the previous four editions of *Pharmacology for the Primary Care Provider,* this fifth edition assumes that the reader has a strong grasp of basic pharmacology and its application to clinical practice. Unlike many pharmacology textbooks that have extensive text for each drug classification, presenting only one drug exemplar per classification, we have combined the best of a traditional pharmacology text and a drug handbook to permit the learner to see a multitude of medications within the classification and how they may be similar or differ in action, adverse effects, and monitoring. In addition, we used the World Health Organization's (WHO) Process for Rational Prescribing that considers pharmacogenetics, life span, gender, comorbidities, and patient and family counseling. With the advances in research and the many changes in drug availability, new drug findings, U.S. Food and Drug Administration (FDA) regulations, and official warnings posted online, it is extremely difficult to keep a pharmacology textbook current. Thus this book focuses instead on assisting clinicians to learn how to evaluate drug information, presenting the most updated clinical guidelines and practice pearls to best assist the new prescriber.

Edmunds' Pharmacology for the Primary Care Provider is a unique textbook that mirrors how clinicians really practice. It consistently focuses on the condition or disease to be treated, with a brief explanation of the relevant pathophysiology. Research has indicated that most clinicians have a small and basic list of medications that they prescribe; this text expands on this by providing a more comprehensive medication classification index for the prescriber to reference when making treatment decisions. The rational prescribing focus assists the clinician in a step-by-step method to use when making treatment decisions. This text compares mechanisms of action, treatment principles, adverse effects, and monitoring requirements. This helps the prescriber develop a depth of knowledge in how to think about prescribing the medications. The format used is especially useful for graduate students and new prescribers.

New and Special Features

Edmunds' Pharmacology for the Primary Care Provider includes a number of features designed to aid the practitioner in decision making and practice:

- An overview of the pathophysiology of the disease processes is addressed within each chapter, as opposed to drug classes or drug type.
- A new organizational format uses a systems-based approach to address medications prescribed for common health problems occurring within the specific body systems as they apply to primary care practice.
- Updated medication information and clinical practice guidelines are incorporated and addressed, with a "Bookmark This" feature to highlight websites where updated clinical guidelines can be found for beginning prescribers.
- Pharmacogenetic considerations that influence prescribing are incorporated in both a separate introductory chapter and within appropriate chapters.
- Medication dosages in tables are addressed using dose ranges, maintenance doses and, where appropriate, plans for dose escalation and de-escalation.
- Practice Pearls boxes for prescribing practices, safety measures, follow-up recommendations, and serum blood level monitoring are included in individual chapters.
- The six-step process for rational prescribing is included at the end of each chapter to reinforce the principles of medication selection through patient and family counseling.

Organization

Edmunds' Pharmacology for the Primary Care Provider is divided into units beginning with pharmacological principles and then delves into medications by body system.

- Unit 1 contains the principles of pharmacology, including pharmacokinetics, pharmacodynamics, and pharmacogenomics.
- Units 2 through 13 are focused on individual medication categories for the treatment of specific conditions or symptoms.
- Unit 14 addresses health promotion, including immunizations, weight management, and smoking cessation.
- Unit 15 focuses on prescribing considerations, medication adherence, and issues of cost containment and prescription writing.

Ancillary Resources

Of additional interest to the instructor, the Evolve Resources website also contains valuable faculty-only resources. A collection of more than 800 PowerPoint lecture slides has been thoroughly updated to help faculty to teach each chapter. The Evolve Resources website also provides a 575-question Test Bank that features an enhanced emphasis on application-level questions in formats that match those of certification exams. An Electronic Image Collection includes all illustrations from the textbook.

Contents

Unit 13: Antiinfective Medications

Unit 14: Health Promotion

Unit 15: Prescribing Considerations

1

Pharmacokinetics and Pharmacodynamics

CONSTANCE G. VISOVSKY

Overview

To understand the pharmacokinetic and pharmacodynamic principles of medication, primary care providers must first understand several important definitions and concepts.

Pharmacokinetics (PK) is the analysis of the processes of absorption, distribution, metabolism, and elimination of medication, or the concentration of a medication in the body over time. PK information is used to determine the dose and frequency of medication prescribed to a patient.

An important concept in understanding PK is how the pharmacokinetic properties of medication are affected by the administration route and the dose delivered. When medication is administered intravenously (IV), only distribution and elimination occur; absorption is immediate, and 100% of the medication is bioavailable. When medication is administered orally, absorption occurs over time and is followed by distribution and elimination. Also, absorption occurs more quickly than elimination. Absorption can be affected by several factors, such as the condition of gastrointestinal (GI) mucosa, GI transit time, and gastric pH.

Another important concept in understanding PK is the half-life of a medication. A medication's half-life is calculated using a formula that includes volume of distribution (Vd), or the components of the body (blood serum, tissue, or plasma) that contain the medication; and clearance, expressed as the elimination rate constant (Ke). Vd is considered when determining the peak and trough levels when medication is at a steady state, as this affects the medication's half-life. The formula for discerning the half-life of a medication is Half-Life = 0.693 / Ke.

A commonly accepted assumption is that it takes about 5.5 half-lives to clear a medication completely from the body. *Metabolism* is the process of converting a medication from one chemical into another, primarily in the liver or gut. In *elimination*, the medication or its metabolite is lost in the bile, urine, sweat, or lungs (Loucks et al., 2015). Another important concept in understanding pharmacokinetics is *clearance*, which refers to the rate of medication removal from the plasma, not the amount eliminated.

Pharmacodynamics (PD) refers to the biochemical and physiologic action or effect of a medication on the body (Loucks et al., 2015). PD includes the dose–response relationship between a medication's concentration and its subsequent effect. Some examples of medication actions or effects include binding, stimulating, or blocking receptors and interacting with enzymes, proteins, or ions. A drug's PD can be affected by physiologic changes due to disease or disorder (e.g., genetic mutation), aging (e.g., alterations in receptor binding), and medication interactions (e.g., competition for receptor binding sites).

Pharmacokinetics

Recall that pharmacokinetics is concerned with absorption, distribution, metabolism, and elimination of medication, or the concentration of a medication in the body over time (Fig. 1.1).

Absorption

Absorption is the transportation of a medication from the administration site to the bloodstream (Currie, 2018). The *rate* of absorption determines the time it takes for the medication's expected effect to be achieved, while the *amount* of absorption determines the intensity of the medication's effect. *Bioavailability* refers to the amount of medication that reaches the systemic circulation after administration. The fraction of the drug that reaches the systemic circulation is called the *f value*. While IV medications have 100% bioavailability, any medication that requires metabolism naturally would have less than 100% bioavailability. The oral route is the most common route for administering medication and can have highly variable bioavailability due to several factors.

One of these factors is first-pass metabolism. *First-pass metabolism* is the process in which an orally administered medication is first absorbed from the GI tract and then transported to the liver via the portal vein, where metabolism takes place (Currie, 2018). First-pass metabolism can affect the bioavailability of some medications by inactivating

	Absorption	Distribution	Biotransformation	Elimination
SITES	Gut ⟶ Plasma	Plasma ⟶ Tissue	Liver	Kidney
CONCEPTS	Bioavailability	Volume of distribution	Enzyme inhibition/ induction First-pass effect	Clearance Half-life Steady state Linear/nonlinear kinetics
	Factors: Drug characteristics Blood flow Cell membrane	Phases: 1. Blood flow from site of administration 2. Delivery of drug into tissues at site of drug action	Phase 1: Oxidation Cytochrome P450 Phase 2: Glucuronidation	

• **Fig. 1.1** The process of pharmacokinetics.

a percentage of the active medication. In contrast, the oral mucosa is highly vascular, permitting the medication to rapidly enter the systemic circulation as it avoids first-pass metabolism.

Factors Affecting Absorption

Four factors affect medication absorption: blood flow, cell membrane characteristics, medication characteristics, and route of administration.

Blood Flow

Circulation at the site of medication administration is important in the absorption process. Any condition that decreases circulation at the administration point will result in decreased drug absorption. For example, insulin injected subcutaneously into a thigh muscle, followed by exercise, will produce more rapid absorption of the insulin than occurs without exercise. It is important to remember that in orally administered medications, the blood supply from the gut passes through the liver before reaching the systemic circulation. This is known as the *first-pass effect*, and it refers to the metabolism of a medication at a specific location in the body that results in a reduced concentration of the active drug when the site of action or circulation is reached. The first-pass effect is typically associated with the liver as the major site of drug metabolism.

Cell Membrane Characteristics

The cell membrane is composed of a semipermeable, two-molecule layer of lipids that contains specialized membrane transport protein molecules in between them and carbohydrate molecules attached to the outer membrane surface. Medications cross the cell membrane in three ways: through channels or pores, through a transport system, or by direct

penetration. The structure of the cell membrane influences this process (Fig. 1.2).

Only small molecules (e.g., potassium and sodium) can pass through channels or pores. Transport proteins are critical to medication transit from one side of the cell membrane to the other. These transport proteins can be *integral* (intrinsic) or *peripheral* (McCance & Huether, 2019). Integral proteins act as structural channels for the transportation of water-soluble substances (ions) or as carrier proteins in *active transport*. Peripheral proteins are active molecules that can attach to or detach from the cell membrane and move substances within or outside the cell. One transport protein, P-glycoprotein (PGP), present in the liver, kidneys, placenta, intestines, and capillaries of the brain, is responsible for transporting a variety of medications *out* of the cell. For example, in the kidneys, PGP assists in the excretion of medications into the urine. For most drugs, direct membrane penetration is dependent upon the medication being lipid soluble, or *lipophilic*.

Medications can also pass through the cell membrane using *passive diffusion*. In passive diffusion, medications cross the cell membrane from areas of high medication concentration to areas of low drug concentration (Fig. 1.3). This process (unlike active transport) does not require energy in the form of adenosine triphosphate (ATP). The pH of a drug also affects diffusion. Nonionized drugs are more lipid soluble and may readily diffuse across cell membranes. Ionized drugs are lipid insoluble and nondiffusible.

Medication Characteristics

Several general medication components affect absorption and are relevant to all routes of administration. For example, *medication formulation* influences the dissolution rate of the solid form of a drug. *Dissolution* is the process by which a medication enters a solution and is used to predict bioavailability.

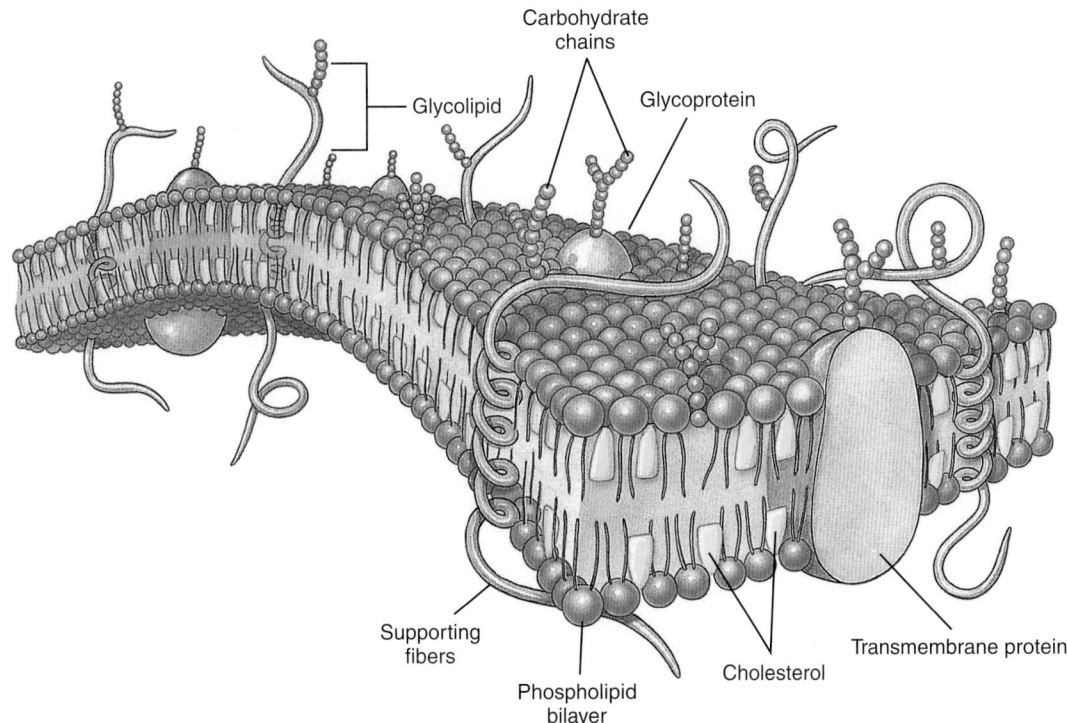

• **Fig. 1.2 Cell membrane structure.** The lipid bilayer provides the basic structure and serves as a relatively impermeable barrier to most water-soluble molecules. (Modified from Thibodeau, G. A., & Patton, K. I. (2008). *Structure and function of the body* (13th ed.). St. Louis: Mosby.)

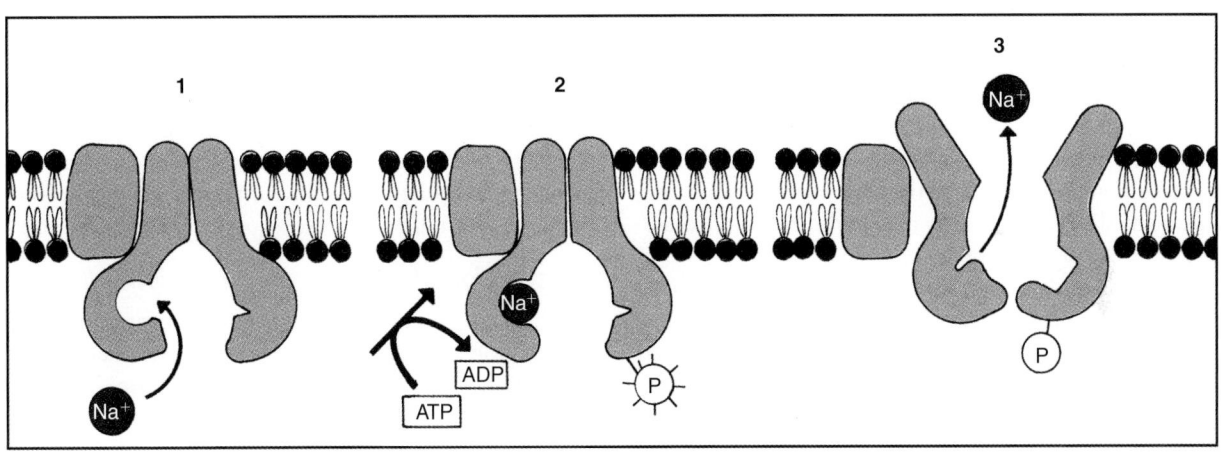

• **Fig. 1.3** Passive diffusion.

Lipophilic medication formulations are more readily absorbable. Acidic medications become nonionized in the acidity of the stomach and then diffuse across membranes. Ionized medications are lipid insoluble and, therefore, nondiffusible.

Medication concentration refers to the amount of medication present in a given volume of blood plasma measured in micrograms per milliliter. The higher the concentration, the more quickly the medication is absorbed.

Routes of Administration

The most common routes for administering medications are oral, sublingual, percutaneous/transdermal, rectal, inhalation, intraocular, otic, nasal (for cold relief), and parenteral.

Absorption of Oral Medications

Delivering medication orally is the most common method of administration and is considered the most convenient, safest, and most economical route. Oral medication formulations are available in the following variations (listed in order from fastest to slowest absorption rate): liquids, elixirs, syrups, suspensions, solutions, powders, capsules, tablets, coated tablets, enteric-coated tablets, and controlled-release formulations (Brunton et al, 2017; Currie, 2018). Controlled-release preparations are designed to provide slow, uniform absorption of the medication (usually with a short half-life) over a long period, usually from 8 to 12 hours.

In terms of medication absorption, the following factors are considered limitations of the oral route:
- Variable bioavailability may occur because of the molecular size of the medication and first-pass effect.
- Bioavailability can be affected by changes in the gut caused by vomiting, diarrhea, or constipation.
- There is a slower onset of action using the oral route.
- The medication form may interact with gastric juices, limiting absorption.
- Interactions may occur between medication and food in the GI tract.

Absorption of Sublingual Medications

Sublingually administered medications can provide the following benefits over the oral route in terms of medication administration and absorption:
- Medications administered sublingually avoid the first-pass effect, thereby increasing bioavailability.
- The sublingual route allows the medication to reach the site of action quickly and with a more immediate effect. Sublingual nitroglycerin is an example of a sublingually administered medication that needs to work quickly for episodes of angina.
- The sublingual route permits easy and convenient medication delivery.
- Changes in absorption can occur if the medication is swallowed, chewed, or taken following an episode of emesis.

Absorption of Percutaneous/Transdermal Medications

Percutaneous or transdermal medications are administered by application to areas of the body such as the skin or mucous membranes and include those that can be applied directly to other surfaces such as the lung. Examples include inhalation medications used to treat asthma and medications to treat eye or ear disorders.
- Percutaneous medications are available in different preparations, including creams, foams, gels, lotions, and ointments.
- Depending on the type of formulation, the strength of percutaneous medications varies. For example, the potency of a medication increases when moving from a cream to an ointment.
- The absorption of lipid-soluble transdermal or percutaneous medications may be impeded to some degree, as the skin acts as a lipid barrier. Mucous membranes are highly vascular, and thus medications applied topically to mucous membranes are more readily absorbed.
- Application of topical medications has the advantage of avoiding the first-pass metabolism of the drug through the liver.
- Pharmacodynamically, percutaneous or transdermal medications can exert their effects locally and systemically. Examples include creams for the treatment of localized skin lesions, transdermal preparations for hormone replacement therapy, and birth control.
- Transdermal application permits slow, prolonged medication delivery (e.g., transdermal fentanyl).
- Local skin reactions are possible.

Absorption of Rectal Medications

Medications that cannot be given orally often can be administered rectally. The rectal route is most useful when patients experience a disease or disorder of the GI tract that affects motility, such as dysphagia, ileus, or a bowel obstruction. This route is often used to administer medications at the end of life, as the rectal route is a safe and lower-cost alternative to injectable medications (Lowry, 2016).
- Rectal medications are absorbed by the blood vessels of the rectum into the body's circulatory system, which then distributes the medication to the body tissues.
- Medications administered rectally will generally have a faster onset, better bioavailability, and a shorter duration of action as compared to orally administered medications. Rectal medications avoid much of first-pass metabolism, as the venous drainage of the rectum is mostly systemic, with only one-third metabolized via the portal vein.

Absorption of Inhalation Medications

Drugs can be given via a nasal spray for local topical absorption through mucous membranes or via an inhaler or nebulizer for pulmonary absorption.
- Inhalation rapidly delivers the medication directly to the desired site of action.
- Inhalation of medication avoids first-pass metabolism in the liver and has high bioavailability.
- Inhaled pulmonary medications (e.g., albuterol) target a large surface area of the lung, which allows for rapid absorption.
- The disadvantages of inhalation therapy include problems associated with regulating the exact dosage and the fact that patients may have difficulty self-administering a drug via an inhaler, decreasing medication efficacy.

Absorption of Ophthalmic and Otic Medications

Ophthalmic or otic drops or ointments are prescribed for instillation into the eye or ear for the treatment of specific conditions or infections. These medications may be prescribed for short- or long-term use. Most ophthalmic medications are administered topically. Topical administration of medication into the eye has several advantages, including increased localized drug effects and avoidance of the first-pass effect. Topical ophthalmic medication can be formulated in a suspension or in a solution. An instilled eyedrop is diluted by tears and blinking, and most of the medication's active ingredient will be transferred to the systemic circulation through the nasolacrimal duct within a few minutes. Otic medications are typically administered into the ear canal or applied externally to the outer ear.
- For ophthalmic medications, the cornea, conjunctiva, and sclera serve as the primary routes of topical absorption.
- Absorption of a drug from the middle ear to the perilymph of the inner ear can occur through diffusion into the round window membrane, through the perilymph of the vestibule of the oval window, and perhaps by the perilymph into the bony otic capsule (Salt & Plontke, 2009).

- Topical administration, however, still results in low bio-availability to intraocular tissues due to physiologic barriers that exist to protect the eye. Consequently, only 1% to 7% of a topically applied drug dose reaches the aqueous humor.
- Excess amounts of eye or ear medications can sometimes cause unwanted systemic bioavailability if the amount applied exceeds the amount absorbed.
- Children are subject to a much higher risk of systemic side effects because ocular dosing is not weight adjusted.

PRACTICE PEARLS

Medication Delivery in Infants and Children

- By 4 months of age, pancreatic enzyme activity increases, and by 6 to 8 months of age, gastric emptying accelerates.
- If a sustained-release medication passes too quickly, absorption is insufficient and a subtherapeutic dose is delivered.
- Avoid rectal suppositories, as the medication may not be able to be retained to achieve the correct dose.
- Children have the potential for increased medication absorption through the skin because the skin is thinner, allowing for greater penetration.

Absorption of Parenteral Administration

Parenteral medication administration can occur through the intradermal, subcutaneous, intramuscular (IM), and IV routes. Under special conditions, clinical specialists can deliver medications parenterally through the intrathecal, intraspinal, or intraepidural route.

- Parenteral medications have the distinct advantage of having rapid absorption and distribution, high bioavailability, and avoidance of the first-pass effect.
- IV medications have immediate and complete absorption because of their direct deposit into the bloodstream.
- Because they are immediately and completely absorbed, IV medications pose a certain risk to patients. Once they are administered, any error (wrong medication, wrong dose) may result in patient harm.

Distribution

Distribution is the transport of a medication from the bloodstream (at the site of absorption) to various tissues in the body. Medications need to be distributed to the site of action within the body in concentrations that can produce the desired therapeutic effect. Medications vary in their ability to move into various body compartments (e.g., brain, fat, lung, or eye). Standard reference texts can be consulted to determine the distribution of specific medications into the target body compartment. Several factors can influence medication distribution, including diffusion rate, the relationship of the medication to the target tissue, tissue perfusion, and plasma protein binding (Currie, 2018).

Unless given intravenously, a medication must cross several semipermeable cell membranes before it reaches the systemic circulation. Cell membranes are composed of a lipid matrix that determines membrane permeability characteristics. Medications may cross cell membranes by passive diffusion, facilitated passive diffusion, active transport, or pinocytosis. In passive diffusion, a medication diffuses from areas of high concentration to areas of low concentration, while in facilitated passive diffusion, a carrier molecule from within the cell membrane combines with a molecule outside the cell membrane to facilitate diffusion. Active transport requires energy expenditure to carry a medication against a concentration gradient to the target tissue (Fig. 1.4). Pinocytosis involves the engulfment of the medication by the cell membrane. The cell membrane folds back on itself and encloses the medication particles, forming a vesicle that later detaches and moves to the cell interior.

Tissue perfusion at the site of a medication's action will affect the dose required. When body tissues are poorly perfused, plasma concentrations of medication are decreased. Since tissue concentration of a medication is difficult to measure, blood plasma concentrations are used as an estimate of tissue concentration. The dose-related effects of a drug are then correlated with a given blood concentration or range of concentration. Once a relationship has been established, blood concentrations can be used to monitor therapy. Some medications bind to certain plasma proteins, namely albumin and glycoproteins. Medications that are highly bound to plasma proteins can have significant clinical implications. The majority of protein binding is reversible and can release free drug as medication concentrations

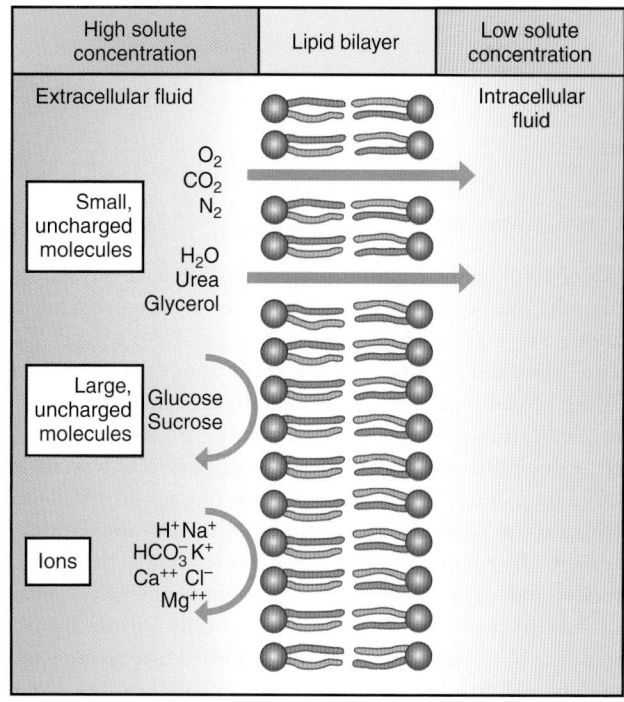

High solute concentration	Lipid bilayer	Low solute concentration

Extracellular fluid — Intracellular fluid

Small, uncharged molecules: O_2 CO_2 N_2 H_2O Urea Glycerol

Large, uncharged molecules: Glucose Sucrose

Ions: H^+ Na^+ HCO_3^- K^+ Ca^{++} Cl^- Mg^{++}

• **Fig. 1.4** Active mediated transport.

decline. An irreversibly bound medication is not released in response to low plasma or tissue concentrations.

Some medications, such as ibuprofen, have a great deal of protein binding and exert a longer effect through sustained release. Medications such as aspirin and warfarin compete for the same plasma protein binding sites, so administration results in potentiation of the effects. Box 1.1 lists some medications that have significant protein binding, which may result in greater free concentrations when albumin is significantly reduced.

Generally, drugs that are highly protein bound to albumin should be prescribed in reduced doses for patients with low serum albumin values. Other protein changes also may have an influence on drug therapy. The level of albumin declines with age; however, alpha1-acid glycoprotein levels are not affected by age, but by hepatic, renal, or cardiovascular disease states resulting in altered protein binding. Understanding the relationships between aging, disease states, and protein binding is necessary for effective therapeutic monitoring (Grandison & Boudinot, 2000).

As noted earlier, volume of distribution (Vd) is a concept that is useful when one seeks to understand where a drug goes once it is absorbed. Vd is the amount of medication administered divided by plasma concentration. More specifically, it is the calculated volume or size of a compartment necessary to account for the total amount of drug in the body if it were present throughout the body at the same concentration found in the plasma (Brunton et al., 2017). A high Vd is reflective of low medication plasma concentration, little protein binding, and extensive distribution in the body tissues. If a medication has a low Vd, it stays in the central compartment and is not widely distributed. The Vd may be calculated by examining the following relationships:
If

$$\text{Concentration of drug in blood} = \frac{\text{Dose}}{\text{Vd}}$$

then

$$\text{Vd} = \frac{\text{Dose}}{\text{Concentration}}$$

Water-soluble medications have a Vd that is similar to plasma volume. The plasma volume for an average adult is about 3 to 5 liters. Lipophilic medications have a larger Vd. The total fluid volume in the body is about 40 liters for a 70-kg (154-lb) person. We are able to measure the amount of medication in the bloodstream only through serum levels; calculation of the volume of distribution allows us to estimate or predict the concentration of drug in the tissue (Brunton et al., 2017). Because most medications are not equally distributed, this concept represents a theoretical model and does not represent real volume. It is, however, useful in predicting medication concentrations, understanding how well a medication is absorbed into tissues, and understanding whether it will be accumulated in the tissues. Other factors that affect the volume of distribution include

cachexia, obesity, dehydration, and edema. Therefore the Vd for a given medication can change as a function of the patient's age, gender, disease, and body composition.

Older adult patients often have relatively less muscle and more fat, placing them at risk for accumulation of lipophilic drugs in the adipose tissue. If these patients lose weight without adjusting their medication dosages, they could experience toxicity. Medication toxicity can be a problem with benzodiazepines because they are lipophilic. In patients, water-soluble drugs have a smaller Vd, resulting in increased blood concentrations. This effect is even greater if the patient is dehydrated. An example of a medication that may cause this problem is gentamicin. In addition, excess fluid in the interstitial spaces, as seen with edema, for example, will affect the distribution of water-soluble medications.

Any alteration in the normal muscle-to-fat ratio will change the Vd of a medication. In obesity, lipophilic medications are distributed into adipose tissue and tend to accumulate. Thus little drug is available elsewhere to produce an effect. For example, phenobarbital is fat soluble. The drug may become trapped in the fatty tissue, causing low blood levels of phenobarbital and potentially increasing seizure activity. Fat-soluble drugs are slowly released from the fat into the bloodstream, so they have a longer duration of action. This factor also may prolong the duration of side effects or may affect dosing schedules. It is not generally necessary to calculate Vd when drugs are used. However, it is an important concept to understand when one is administering a drug, and it may influence the dosage or choice of a drug. Always consider where the drug will go and how much will get to the target organ or tissue.

The distribution of drugs from the bloodstream to the central nervous system is different from the distribution of drugs through other cell membranes. The endothelial cells of the brain capillaries do not have intercellular pores and vesicles. Therefore passive distribution of hydrophilic drugs is restricted. However, lipophilic drugs will easily pass the blood–brain barrier and are limited only by cerebral blood flow (Brunton et al., 2017). Highly fat-soluble drugs also cross the blood–brain barrier easily and are likely to cause central nervous system side effects such as confusion and drowsiness.

Metabolism

Metabolism is the biotransformation of medications so that they can be excreted from the body. Metabolism occurs primarily in the liver, but may occur in the kidneys, lungs, skin, and GI tract. The term *biotransformation* is synonymous with metabolism and refers to a chemical alteration of medication in the body. Metabolism involves two major phases of enzyme activity. Phase I of metabolism is called *preconjugation*. During this phase, the drug becomes more hydrophilic (water soluble) through oxidation, reduction, or hydrolysis so that it can be more easily excreted. The cytochrome P450 enzyme system is part of phase I. Phase II of metabolism is called *glucuronidation*. This phase involves *conjugation,* or attachment of the medication to a polar molecule, making it a highly water-soluble substance with little or no pharmacologic activity (Brunton et al., 2017). Glucuronidation occurs in the liver and serves to make medications more water soluble, with elimination occurring through urine or feces (via bile from the liver). The metabolism of lipid-soluble medications to a water-soluble form is needed for renal elimination. Lipophilic medications pass easily through membranes, including renal tubules, making them difficult to excrete. Biotransformation changes a lipophilic medication that is active and transforms it into a hydrophilic inactive compound that is readily excreted. However, metabolites occasionally have biologic activity or toxic properties. Liver disease can have an effect on the metabolism of medications. If blood flow to the liver is decreased, drugs will be metabolized more slowly, leading to a longer duration of action (Fig. 1.5).

Cytochrome P450

The most extensively studied pathway in medication metabolism is the family of enzymes known as cytochrome (CYP) P450 mixed-function oxidase reaction. The cytochrome P450 enzyme system operates throughout the body but is concentrated in the liver, intestines, and lungs. The P450 enzyme system resides in the ribosomes, which are sacs in the endoplasmic reticulum. Chemically, the enzyme is a glycoprotein or a sugar plus a protein. As many as 50 different human CYP P450 enzymes have been characterized and are organized and numbered based upon their function. The major groups named 1, 2, 3, and 4 are known to be involved in drug interactions. These major groups are further divided into groups by their chemical structure, named A, B, and C. The A, B, and C groups are then divided into subgroups named 1, 2, 3, and so on. The groups that are most important in human drug interactions are CYP 2D6, CYP 3A3/4, CYP 1A2, CYP 2C9/10, and CYP 2C19 (Manikandan & Nagini, 2018).

Each type of enzyme is responsible for one type of metabolic reaction, and each medication can undergo several types of biotransformation before being excreted. The CYP 3A4 subfamily is a major medication-metabolizing enzyme that is necessary for the metabolism of many drugs, such as antihistamines, antibiotics, lipid-lowering drugs, antihypertensives, protease inhibitors, and azole antifungals. The essential facts to master about the P450 enzyme system are that six primary enzymes account for the metabolism of

nearly all clinically important drugs, and two of these systems are critically important for drug metabolism.

The CYP 2D6 enzyme looks different and is different. It metabolizes selective serotonin reuptake inhibitors (SSRIs), pain relievers, β-blockers, and other drugs. Other characteristics of this enzyme are that it metabolizes about 30% of all clinically useful medications, it is the second most abundant enzyme, and it participates in converting codeine to morphine.

Knowledge of the substrates, inhibitors, and inducers of these enzymes assists primary care providers in predicting clinically significant drug interactions. The P450 metabolizing enzyme system can differ in each individual. Minor genetic mutations in the CYP enzyme system, known as *single nucleotide polymorphisms* (SNPs), can incur changes in the metabolic activity of medications in individuals and populations. These genetic variations explain why patients react differently to medications or have certain drug–drug interactions. For example, some patients metabolize codeine (CYP 2D6) quickly and need larger doses, whereas other patients metabolize it slowly and need smaller doses.

Following are the most notable features of the other four CYP enzymes:
- CYP 2C19—metabolizes proton pump inhibitors, nonsteroidal antiinflammatory drugs (NSAIDs), and β-blockers
- CYP 2C9—metabolizes sulfonylureas, NSAIDs, (S)-warfarin, and sildenafil citrate (Viagra)
- CYP 1A2—metabolizes acetaminophen, (R)-warfarin, theophylline, caffeine, diazepam (Valium), and verapamil
- CYP 2E1—metabolizes acetaminophen, ethanol, inactivation of toxins, and dextromethorphan

A medication can act as a *substrate* affected by alteration of its enzyme metabolism. A medication can also cause the alteration in the enzyme metabolism of another drug by being an inhibitor or an inducer. The CYP P450 enzyme system may speed up a reaction because it causes the drug to change to a more hydrophilic substance. An *inhibitor* is any drug that causes the enzyme to metabolize more slowly or decreases the capacity of the enzyme pathway. For example, if a patient on fluoxetine (Prozac) takes warfarin, the fluoxetine inhibits the P450 enzyme system from metabolizing warfarin and may produce adverse effects such as bleeding. An *inducer* is any medication that causes the enzymes to metabolize the substrate more quickly. These types of medications increase enzyme activity by increasing the number

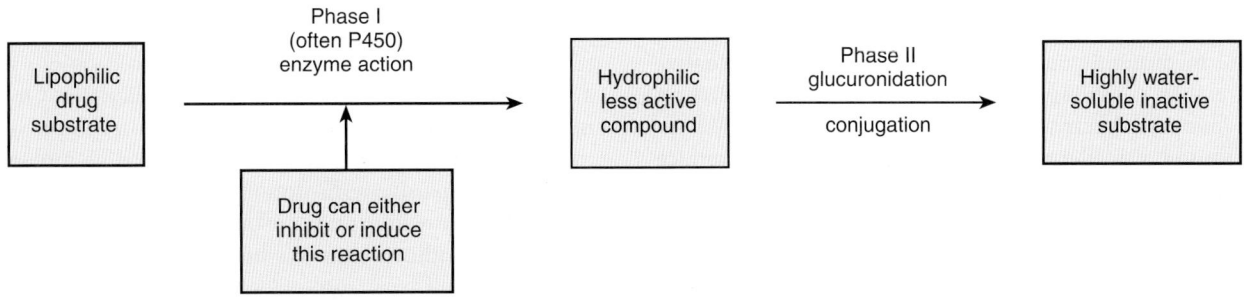

• **Fig. 1.5** Process of biotransformation.

of CYP 450 enzymes. The same drug can be both a substrate and an inducer or inhibitor (Brunton et al., 2017). For example, carbamazepine is an auto inducer—it induces its own metabolism. It is the enzyme system and *not* the medication that is being induced or inhibited.

A medication can inhibit an enzyme pathway through two mechanisms. The first is competition. *Competition* occurs when two different medications are metabolized by the same enzyme, and one medication may be metabolized first, delaying the metabolism of the second medication and increasing its half-life. In *inhibition*, the medication decreases the production of the enzyme needed for metabolism. It may take anywhere from 24 hours to 7 days to see the effect, depending on the half-life of the drug (Brunton et al., 2017). From a pharmacokinetic standpoint, the major effects of drug–drug interactions are understood in terms of causing a high or low plasma and tissue level of the medication. Enzyme induction is much less common than inhibition. Medications causing enzyme induction make the metabolic pathway work quickly, causing the substrate drug to be deactivated more rapidly. This will lower the level of the medication in the body. Anticonvulsant medications are clinically important inducers. Evaluation of anticonvulsants is particularly important when they are being added to a patient's existing medication regimen.

In addition to CYP P450, oxidation of medications can be mediated by non-P450 enzymes, the most significant of which are flavin monooxygenase, monoamine oxidase, alcohol dehydrogenase, aldehyde dehydrogenase, aldehyde oxidase, and xanthine oxidase. The oxidation of medications catalyzed by some of these enzymes can produce the same metabolites as those generated by P450; thus drug interactions may be difficult to predict without clear knowledge of the underlying enzymology. Although oxidation catalyzed by non-P450 enzymes can lead to drug inactivation, oxidation may be essential for the generation of active metabolites that create drug action (Brunton et al., 2017).

First-Pass Effect

The first-pass effect in metabolism refers to the amount of medication lost during the process of absorption. Recall that when a medication is taken orally, it is absorbed by the GI system and then enters the hepatic portal system to the liver before reaching the rest of the body. The liver can extensively metabolize some medications, so little of it is left over to enter the circulation. This *first pass* through the liver thus greatly reduces the *bioavailability* of the medication (Drozdzik et al., 2017). Due to the first-pass effect, some medications may be administered via an alternative route, such as sublingually or topically, to avoid the liver on the first pass. Alternative-route dosing makes it possible to administer a smaller amount of the medication to produce the desired therapeutic effect.

Prodrug

A *prodrug* is a biologically inactive medication precursor that is biotransformed (activated) following administration, with the aim of improving the pharmacokinetic properties of the original compound. It is estimated that from 10% to 12% of all marketed medications are prodrugs (Rautio et al., 2018). A prodrug can be made to be susceptible to many enzymes, and then can be split to produce the active form of the drug. The inactive oral prodrug can be stable in the GI tract and only be biotransformed by CYP 450 in the liver, plasma, or GI tract. Sulfasalazine used in the treatment of Crohn's disease is one of the earliest prodrugs. Sulfasalazine reaches the colon and is metabolized by bacteria into two active metabolites: sulfapyridine and 5-aminosalicylic acid (5-ASA). The angiotensin-converting enzyme inhibitor enalapril is an example of a medication that must be transformed from a prodrug to a biologically active metabolite (Brunton et al., 2017). Prodrugs are also used to increase the duration of action of medications in a chemical-sustained release form. Targeted prodrugs are being used in oncology to minimize side effects and improve the tolerability of chemotherapy.

Elimination

Elimination is the process by which medications and their metabolites leave the body. Elimination primarily occurs through excretion by the kidneys. The processes involved in renal elimination consist of glomerular filtration, tubular secretion, and partial reabsorption. The nephron is considered the functional unit of the kidney, with the glomerulus using the process of ultrafiltration to allow substances in the plasma to pass through relatively small pores in the glomerular capillary membrane.

Glomerular filtration is the first step in producing the urine that will ultimately contain the excreted medication. The process of filtration removes free drug and other waste products from the plasma. Medications bound to plasma proteins remain in the bloodstream. Some factors that can influence filtration are the molecular size of the drug and the medication charge. Large-sized medications will have a slower filtration rate due to the size of the pores in the glomerulus at the site of filtration. The glomerular pores have a negative charge, so nonionized or uncharged forms of the medication diffuse more readily. The nephron also uses secretion to move medications from the plasma to the nephron lumen. The transport system secretes and actively transports anions or cations into the cells to facilitate passive transport into the lumen of the nephron (Fig. 1.6). Two drugs may compete for the same active transport carriers, causing their excretion rate to decrease (Brunton et al., 2017). Tubular secretion is helpful to renal elimination of medications with a short half-life, such as penicillin G and salicylates. Once a medication is excreted via active transport in the proximal tubule of the nephron, weakly acidic or alkaline molecules may undergo passive reabsorption. The pH of the urine can impact tubular reabsorption. Alkaline urine will increase the excretion of acidic molecules, while acidic urine will increase the excretion of basic molecules. Clinical alteration of the pH of urine will hasten the excretion of some medications,

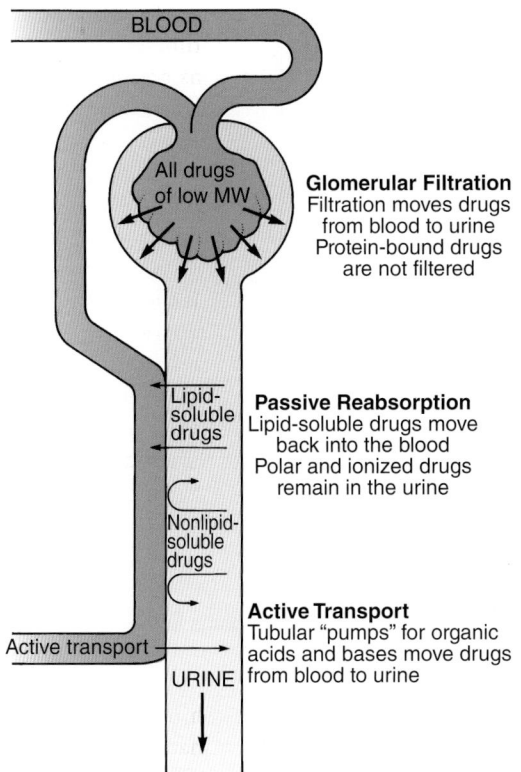

BLOOD

All drugs of low MW

Glomerular Filtration
Filtration moves drugs
from blood to urine
Protein-bound drugs
are not filtered

Lipid-soluble drugs

Passive Reabsorption
Lipid-soluble drugs move
back into the blood
Polar and ionized drugs
remain in the urine

Nonlipid-soluble drugs

Active transport

Active Transport
Tubular "pumps" for organic
acids and bases move drugs
from blood to urine

URINE

• **Fig. 1.6** Drug elimination by the kidney. (From Burchum, J. R., & Rosenthal, L. D. [2019]. *Lehne's pharmacology for nursing care* [10th ed.]. St. Louis: Elsevier.)

as in the case of drug poisoning or drug toxicity. If the glomerular filtration rate in the kidneys is reduced, medications remain in the blood for longer periods. In patients with renal failure, it is necessary to calculate an estimated creatinine clearance to modify the dosage of medication necessary. This is calculated with the following formula:

$$\text{Creatinine clearance} = \frac{\text{Weight}^a \, (\text{kg}) \times (140 - \text{Age [in years]})}{72 \times \text{Serum creatinine} \, (\text{mg/dL}) (\times 0.85)^b}$$

Medications and their metabolites may be eliminated by other routes, such as the fecal and respiratory routes, through breast milk, and through the skin. Medications that are metabolized in the liver can have metabolites that are excreted in the bile. These metabolites are reabsorbed into the blood and then are excreted in the urine or, less commonly, in the feces. Excretion from the liver into the bile is accomplished by active transport systems, which are limited in the quantity of metabolites they can excrete (Ayrton & Morgan, 2001). The respiratory route is an important route of excretion in anesthetic gases. Excretion in breast milk is also important, not for the quantity excreted but because of the effect it may have on a nursing infant. Other routes such as perspiration, saliva, tears, hair, and skin are not usually clinically significant.

---

[a]Lean body weight may reflect creatinine in production more accurately.
[b]In women, multiply the value × 0.85.

Half-Life and Steady State

The concept of *half-life* is important to understand. The half-life of a medication is the amount of time required for the amount of medication in the body to decrease by one-half and is a significant factor in accumulation and elimination of medications in the body. The half-life is dependent upon clearance and volume of distribution. When a patient is given a medication on a regular schedule, the medication will continue to accumulate until steady state is achieved (Fig. 1.7). You may recall that the term *steady state* refers to the equilibrium of medication intake with elimination. Half-life is useful for estimating the amount of time it takes to reach the steady state of a drug after a dosage regimen is started. The half-life of a drug found in reference books is based upon an approximation in normal, healthy adults. However, much individual variation that can occur is based on factors that affect volume of distribution and elimination.

Steady state is reached after four to five half-lives, which represents 94% to 97% of the eventual steady state. Half-life also can be used to estimate the amount of time it takes to eliminate a drug from the body after it has been discontinued. Again, after four to five half-lives, about 94% to 97% of the drug will have been eliminated from the body (Brunton et al., 2017). Of course, there is always a difference between the absolute (or theoretical) steady state and what is seen in specific patients.

Medications with short half-lives include ibuprofen and the benzodiazepine lorazepam. Examples of medications with long half-lives are diazepam, digoxin, and fluoxetine (Prozac). Medications with long half-lives must be closely monitored because any toxic or adverse effects last for a longer period. In linear or first-order kinetics, medication

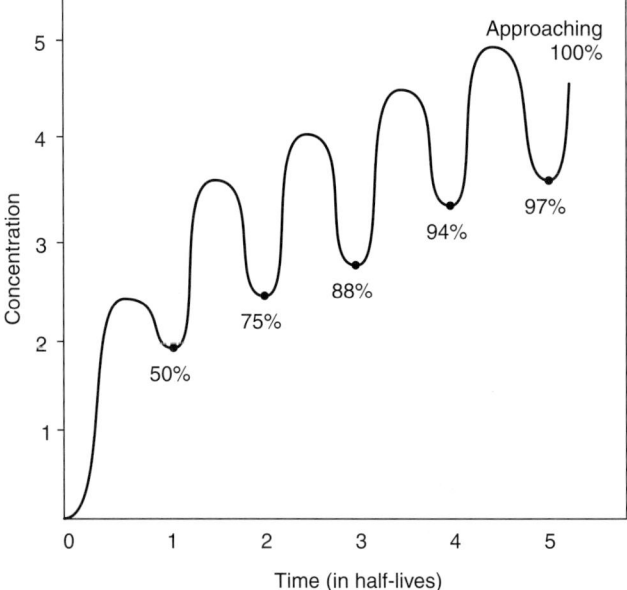

• **Fig. 1.7** Drug accumulation time to steady state. The line shows concentrations of drugs in the body. (Modified from Brunton, L. L., Chabner, B., & Knollman, B. [Eds.], [2010]. *Goodman & Gilman's pharmacological basis of therapeutics* [12th ed.]. New York: McGraw-Hill.)

concentration is increased or decreased in a linear fashion, depending upon dosage, clearance, volume of distribution, and half-life. Average concentration when the steady state is attained during intermittent drug administration may be calculated as follows:

$$\text{Concentration} = \frac{\text{Drug availability} \times \text{Dose}}{\text{Clearance} \times \text{Time}}$$

Clearance

Clearance is the measure of the rate at which a medication is removed from the plasma per minute, and is expressed as mL/min (Alsanosi et al., 2014). Specifically, clearance is defined as the volume of plasma from which all drug is removed in a given time. It is measured as volume divided by time:

$$\text{Clearance} = \frac{\text{Rate of removal of drug (mg/mL)}}{\text{Plasma concentration of drug (mg/mL)}}$$

Drug clearance helps determine how much drug should be administered and how frequently to dose the patient. Several factors can affect medication clearance, including the presence of any disease process, such as liver or renal disease; impaired blood flow to the clearing organ; and the volume of distribution. For example, liver disease impairs metabolism. Additionally, blood flow to the kidney is dependent upon having adequate cardiac output. In conditions of decreased cardiac output, medications that rely on renal elimination can be adversely affected by poor blood flow to the kidney, placing the patient at risk for toxicity. If a medication is stored in adipose tissue, it cannot be cleared from the body. Thus volume of distribution affects medication clearance and hence the half-life. *Total body clearance* is the sum of clearances from the various metabolizing and eliminating organs.

Pharmacokinetics

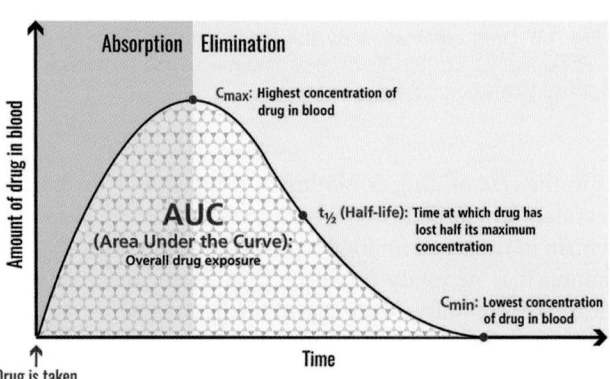

• **Fig. 1.8** Area under the curve. (From U.S. Department of Health and Human Services, AIDSinfo, https://clinicalinfo.hiv.gov/en/glossary/area-under-curve-auc.)

Area Under the Curve

The area under the curve (AUC), also known as the plasma concentration–time curve (Fig. 1.8), illustrates how the concentration of a drug changes in the body over time. The AUC is influenced by the rate of medication elimination from the body and the amount of dose administered. The AUC is also inversely related to medication clearance. In other words, the higher the clearance, the less time a medication would spend in the systemic circulation and the faster the decline in plasma drug concentration. Therefore the body's exposure to the medication and the area under the concentration–time curve is smaller. The AUC can be estimated by measuring the plasma concentration of a medication at several time points.

- Absorption of medication is altered in infants due to prolonged GI tract emptying time, variable peristalsis, and decreased gastric pH. Also, infants and children have differing blood flow to tissues that decrease medication absorption.
- Distribution is altered by body composition of increased total body water and decreased body fat in newborns and infants. Decreased levels of plasma proteins in infants alter medication binding that affects medication dosage.
- Metabolism of medications in newborns and infants is affected by delays in drug-metabolizing enzymes that can result in toxicity.
- Excretion by the renal system is reduced in newborns and infants due to a lower glomerular filtration rate and decreased renal blood flow. Liver immaturity can prolong medication half-life.

First-Order/Linear Pharmacokinetics

In clinical pharmacology, first-order linear kinetics occurs when a constant proportion of a medication is eliminated over a specified unit of time. The rate of elimination is proportional to the amount of medication in the body; therefore higher concentrations of medication result in greater amounts of medication eliminated over time. Because of the relationship to medication concentration, first-order kinetics is considered a linear process.

Zero-Order/Nonlinear Pharmacokinetics

Nonlinear pharmacokinetics, or zero-order kinetics, occurs due to protein binding (limiting the amount of protein available for binding), hepatic metabolism (limiting the amount of enzyme-causing metabolism), or active renal transport of a medication (limiting the number of carriers). Typically, as the dose of a medication increases, the plasma concentration of that medication in steady state will also increase in direct proportion to the dose. In some cases, the plasma drug concentration changes are not in proportion to the dose, but can be either more or less than would be expected. This is known as *nonlinear pharmacokinetics* and can cause problems when adjusting doses. The medication is removed by saturation of a function, such as protein binding, hepatic metabolism, or active renal transport (Stein & Peletier, 2018).

Phenytoin is a clinically important example of nonlinear kinetics because of both protein binding and hepatic metabolism. As phenytoin is absorbed, it is bound to plasma protein. Therefore when a regimen is started, most of the medication is bound to protein, leaving little free drug. However, as the proteins reach saturation, suddenly a much greater percentage of the absorbed medication is not protein bound and is now free drug (medication). When the proteins are saturated, suddenly the free medication, measured as a serum level, rises rapidly. A narrow therapeutic window makes medication toxicity a frequent problem. When the amount of medication concentration exceeds the ability of the liver to metabolize the medication, nonlinear kinetics occurs (Stein & Peletier, 2018).

Again, the body has a finite ability to produce enzymes that metabolize medication. Once the body is working at capacity, any additional medication will accumulate and cause toxicity. Drugs that follow nonlinear kinetics are far more difficult to maintain in the therapeutic range and must be monitored closely for toxicity.

- Pregnant women take a variety of over-the-counter (OTC) and prescription medications.
- Changes in pharmacokinetics are the result of physiologic and anatomical changes occurring during pregnancy, such as increases in drug-metabolizing enzymes, altered body composition, organ blood flow, and increased glomerular filtration rate.
- Increased elimination results in decreased drug exposure.
- For medications that require therapeutic monitoring regarding dose alterations, pregnancy can produce decreased medication levels despite adherence to the prescribed regimen.
- There are a lack of studies outlining the clinical consequences of these changes during pregnancy.

Pharmacodynamics

Pharmacodynamics (PD) is the study of the biochemical and physiologic effects of medication on the body, and the mechanisms responsible for producing those effects (Brunton et al., 2017).

Mechanisms of Action

The term *mechanism of action* refers to the specific biochemical interaction through which a medication produces its pharmacologic effect, and usually includes the specific molecular target(s), such as an enzyme or receptor, that the medication binds to (Prichard et al., 2013).

Receptors

Receptors that mediate the action of medications are made up of proteins located inside the cell or on the cell surface. Receptors can be "turned on" or "turned off" through interaction with medications. Receptors respond to specific neurotransmitters, hormones, antigens, and other chemical substances. Substances that interact with receptors are known as *ligands.* A ligand may activate or inactivate a receptor (Fig. 1.9). So when a specific medication binds to a receptor, there will be either an increase or a decrease in

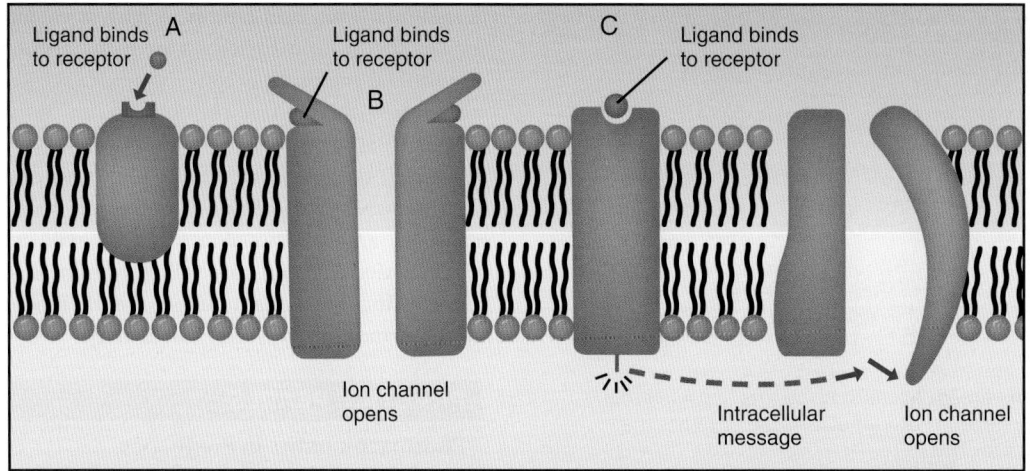

• **Fig. 1.9 Cellular receptors.** A, Plasma membrane receptor for a ligand on the surface of an integral protein. B and C, A neurotransmitter can exert its effect on a postsynaptic cell by means of two fundamentally different types of receptor proteins: channel-linked receptors and non–channel-linked receptors. Channel-linked receptors are also known as ligand-gated channels. (A from Huether, S. E. et al. [2008]. *Understanding pathophysiology* [4th ed.]. St Louis: Mosby. B and C modified from Alberts, B., Johnson, A. D., Lewis, J., Morgan, D., Raff, M., Roberts, K., & Walter, P. (Eds.), [1994]. *Molecular biology of the cell* [3rd ed.]. New York: Garland.

Agonist: Chemical fits receptor site well; chemical response is usually good.

Antagonist: Drug attaches at drug receptor site but then remains chemically inactive: no chemical drug response is produced.

Partial agonist: Drug attaches at drug receptor site but only a slight chemical action is produced.

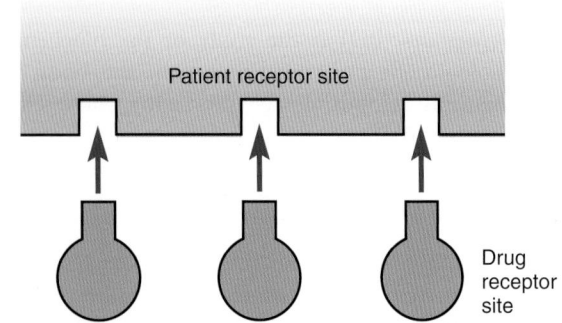

• **Fig. 1.10 Drug receptor sites.** (From Edmunds, M. W. [2013]. *Introduction to clinical pharmacology* [7th ed.]. St Louis: Mosby.)

the rate of physiologic activity regulated by that receptor. In general, drugs produce their effects by interacting with a receptor. The lock-and-key model of drug–receptor interaction states that the drug molecule must fit into a receptor like key fits into a lock (Fig. 1.10). The site at which a medication acts depends upon the location of the specific receptors (McCance & Huether, 2019).

The strength and type of chemical bonds (covalent, ionic, hydrogen, hydrophobic) determine the degree of affinity of a ligand to a receptor. *Affinity* is the strength of attraction of a medication to its receptor site. Medications with high

affinity are strongly attracted to their receptors, while those with low affinity are only weakly attracted. Medications with high affinity are also more effective at lower doses as compared to low-affinity medications that need high concentrations in order to bind to their receptors. Medications that are attracted to receptors are classified as agonists or antagonists. *Agonists* are molecules that activate the biological response as a result of receptor–ligand binding. *Antagonists* are drugs that inhibit or counteract effects produced by other medications. An antagonist may work competitively, with an affinity for the same receptor site as an agonist, or noncompetitively, in which case it inactivates the receptor so that the agonist cannot be effective at any concentration. An example of an agonist is dobutamine, which mimics the action of norepinephrine in the heart, increasing heart rate and contraction force. Medications that are antagonists produce their effects by blocking receptor activity. For example, naloxone blocks the receptors for opioids, preventing activation of opioid receptors and reversing opioid overdose.

Medications can also be classified as partial agonists, or agonist-antagonists, having only moderate agonist properties that limit the degree of response. For example, tramadol is considered a partial agonist at μ opioid receptors. While tramadol is less efficacious than morphine for the management of severe pain, the risk of respiratory depression is minimal.

Quantifying Medication–Receptor Interaction

Attempts to quantify medication–receptor interaction involve calculating the concentration of dose–response relationships. The dose–response relationship determines the minimal dose of a medication given that can elicit the desired response, the maximum medication response expected, and the amount of dose increase that produces the desired increase in response. Generally, as the dose of a medication increases, the effect increases. A medication dose, therefore can be adjusted upward or downward until the desired response is achieved.

Adverse Medication Reactions

Adverse medication reactions, commonly referred to as adverse drug reactions (ADRs) or adverse drug events (ADEs), are defined as "an appreciably harmful or unpleasant reaction, resulting from an intervention related to the use of a medicinal product, which predicts hazard from future administration and warrants prevention or specific treatment, or alteration of the dosage regimen, or withdrawal of the product" (Edwards & Aaronson, 2000, p. 1255). The World Health Organization's Adverse Reaction Terminology, which is a subset of the International Classification of Diseases, classifies ADRs into six types (with mnemonics): dose-related (Augmented), non–dose-related (Bizarre), dose-related and time-related (Chronic), time-related (Delayed), withdrawal (End of use), and failure of therapy (Failure) (Edwards & Aronson, 2000). Table 1.1 lists some behaviors of primary care providers, pharmacists, and patients that may result in ADRs. Serious ADEs are defined by the U.S. Food and Drug Administration (FDA) as events, caused by a drug, that result in a patient's death, hospitalization, or disability; cause a congenital abnormality or a life-threatening event; or require intervention to prevent permanent damage. This is different from a *side effect,* which is an additional effect, desirable or undesirable, of a drug that is not the primary purpose of giving the drug. For example, an adverse reaction could be the development of a pancytopenia from taking chloramphenicol. A side effect might include photosensitivity caused by tetracycline taken for acne.

An 11-year national analysis of ADEs found that patient visits to outpatient clinics due to ADEs increased over the study period from nine to 17 per 1000 persons. Factors associated with ADE visits included the patient's age (≥ 65 years), number of medications taken (≥ five medications), and sex. Overall, outpatient ADEs resulted in 107,468 hospital admissions annually, with older patients at highest risk for hospitalization (Bourgeois et al., 2010). The annual costs of national hospital expenses to treat patients who experience ADEs during hospitalization are estimated to be between $1.56 billion and $5.6 billion.

Most ADEs occur as a result of extension of the desired pharmacologic effects of a medication, often due to variability in the pharmacokinetics and pharmacodynamics seen among patients. Medications such as warfarin and digoxin are at higher risk for causing ADEs, particularly because of their narrow therapeutic index when toxicity can occur at concentrations at or near the upper end of the therapeutic range.

If a suspected ADE occurs, it is important to confirm and document the reaction. Following are the key questions that should be answered (Seagrave & Bamba, 2017):
- Has the reaction been previously documented when the medication was taken by the patient?

TABLE 1.1	Risk Factors for Developing Adverse Drug Reactions	
	Activities That Increase Risk of Drug Reactions
Primary Care Provider	Duplication of medications
	Unclear directions and patient education
	Incomplete medication history
	Failure to adjust dosage for age and comorbid conditions
	Lack of follow-up
Pharmacist	Automatic refills
	Prescription filling errors
	Failure to review medication profile
	Lack of patient education
Patient	Use of OTC medications and nutraceuticals
	Incomplete medication history to provider
	Use of alcohol with medications
	Use of multiple pharmacies
	Use of multiple providers
	Poor compliance: drug overuse or underuse

- Is the time course of the reaction consistent with the time(s) of medication administration?
- Could this reaction be due to another clinical condition in the patient?
- Did the reaction improve when the medication was discontinued?
- If the medication was not discontinued, did the reaction resolve?
- If the dose was reduced but not discontinued, did the reaction resolve?
- If an antidote was given, did the patient's condition improve?
- Did the reaction recur when (if) the medication was administered again?
- Was the dose appropriate for the patient in terms of age or organ function?

For a primary care provider to conclude that a patient is having an adverse reaction to a medication, causality must be demonstrated and confirmed. This process may be done sequentially by (1) evaluating the relationship chronologically between the adverse reaction and medication administration, (2) confirming resolution of the adverse reaction once the medication dosage has been decreased or the medication has been discontinued (dechallenge), and (3) evaluating recurrence of the same symptoms after readministration of the agent (rechallenge). Nurse practitioners should work in consultation with a specialist on this problem if a decision is made to rechallenge the medication in the patient to confirm causality and only when it is imperative to use that medication.

Adverse reactions are classified by severity. With mild reactions, the patient may have some signs or symptoms, but these may be responses the patient is willing to tolerate and often do not require treatment. Moderate reactions produce more discomfort and may interfere with the patient's activities; these reactions often require some form of treatment. Severe adverse reactions may incapacitate the patient, be life threatening, or interfere with the patient's ability to work or complete activities of daily living. Severe drug reactions often require hospitalization, intensive medical care, and longer than 15 days for recovery.

Serious adverse reactions should be voluntarily reported to MedWatch, the FDA's medical product safety reporting program. The FDA compiles a quarterly report of medication adverse reactions based on data from the Adverse Event Reporting System (AERS). The appearance of a medication on the FDA list is an indication that the FDA requires additional study to determine whether there is a causal link between the medication and the reported AED. If a link is established, the FDA may consider a variety of options: taking regulatory action, such as revising the drug's label; requiring a risk evaluation and mitigation strategy; or gathering more data to better characterize the risk.

If a serious warning to prescribers is required to ensure the continued safe use of a product, the FDA may require the manufacturer to print a warning to be displayed in heavy type and boxed text at the beginning of the package insert (i.e., the "black box"). Finally, the FDA can require a manufacturer to recall or withdraw a product because of a serious problem.

Medication Interactions

A medication (drug) interaction is defined as two or more medications that interact in such a way that either the effectiveness or the toxicity of one or more of the medications taken is modified (Sánchez-Fidalgo et al., 2017). These are preventable medication errors associated with serious adverse events and death. When an interaction between medications is suspected, the primary care provider will need to consider several important factors in determining a course of action. The first consideration is the potential seriousness of the reaction and whether the reaction is reversible with discontinuance or a recommended antidote. There are specific risk factors for medication interactions that warrant the prescriber's attention. A medication with a narrow therapeutic index, such as warfarin and lithium, pose a higher risk for medication interactions. A medication with a long half-life will consequently result in a longer adverse reaction as compared to a medication with a short half-life. Extremes of age involving patients that are very young or very old are known risk factors for adverse medication reactions. Coexisting morbidity is also an important risk factor for medication interactions. Patients with a seizure disorder, cardiovascular or liver disease, human immunodeficiency virus (HIV), or other infection are at risk for drug interactions. Patients with cardiovascular or liver disease are at risk for medication interactions

due to polypharmacy, poor organ perfusion, and liver dysfunction that can impede P450 interactions and metabolism of medications.

> ### PRACTICE PEARLS
> #### Medication Interactions
>
> - When adding a drug to a patient's regimen, the primary care provider should always consult a comprehensive drug reference for any known drug–drug interactions.
> - The primary care provider should review the profile of all new medications for additive side effects or adverse effects that can result from existing therapy, with consideration of CYP 450 enzyme metabolism, organ function, and other patient-specific factors.

When monitoring drug therapy, it is essential for the primary care provider to counsel the patient regarding specific signs and symptoms that might accompany medication interactions, side effects, and the adverse effects to report. Occasionally, the dosage of one medication may have to be adjusted when another medication is added (Brunton, et al., 2017).

The effects of medication interactions can be cumulative, as in the case of an angiotensin-converting enzyme inhibitor (ACE-I) plus a potassium-sparing diuretic leading to hyperkalemia; additive, as in hypotension caused by an ACE-I and a loop diuretic; synergistic, as is seen when alcohol is taken with a sedative; or antagonistic, as when NSAIDs result in a reduced effect of ACE-I on blood pressure (Currie, 2018).

Medications and Food Interactions

Food effect, also known as food–medication interaction, is defined as changes in absorption rate or absorption extent when medications are orally administered (Deng et al., 2017). Food–medication interactions can be clinically relevant either to prevent undesirable effects or to optimize medication therapy. Some of these interactions may result from activation of the P450 enzyme system or from competition with receptor sites. Monoamine oxidase inhibitors (MAOIs) are some of the drugs most noted for food–medication interactions because they cannot be taken with aged cheese or many processed foods.

Interactions between the bioactive components of certain foods and medications are well known. An example is the interactive effect of grapefruit juice with various medications. Grapefruit juice is known to affect an isoenzyme of cytochrome P450, CYP3A4, which is responsible for the metabolism of various medications into their metabolites. When grapefruit juice is consumed, the enzyme CYP3A4 is inhibited, leading to higher blood plasma concentrations of the nonmetabolized portion of the medication, which in turn can lead either to overdosing when a medication is not metabolized to its inactive form, or to a highly reduced dose when the active form of the medication must be metabolized to be activated (Pirmohamed, 2013). Because prescription and OTC medications can interact with food, certain principles are important to consider for each patient. See Table 1.2 for specific information concerning

TABLE 1.2   Common Food–Medication Interactions

Food	Medication Category	Interaction
Grapefruit Juice	Calcium channel blockers	All calcium channel blockers interact with grapefruit juice, with felodipine (Plendil) having as much as a 200% increase in AUC when taken with grapefruit juice.
	HMG-CoA reductase inhibitors (statins)	Inhibits cytochrome P450, increasing blood levels, predisposing patients to statin-related adverse effects such as muscle toxicity, myopathy, and rhabdomyolysis. Atorvastatin (Lipitor), simvastatin (Zocor), and lovastatin (Mevacor) are most affected.
	Phosphodiesterase inhibitors	Increased serum levels with co-administration of grapefruit juice, leading to a potential for adverse effects such as priapism, hypotension, and vision disturbances.
	Estrogen-containing oral contraceptives	Modest increase in serum levels when taken with grapefruit juice.
	Tricyclic antidepressants	Clomipramine (Anafranil) interactions with grapefruit juice are well documented.
	Benzodiazepines	Diazepam (Valium) and temazepam (Restoril) have increased serum levels when taken with grapefruit juice. Lorazepam and oxazepam appear unaffected by grapefruit juice ingestion.
	Corticosteroids	Grapefruit juice can double the systemic effects of corticosteroids.
	Antiarrhythmics	When grapefruit juice is given with amiodarone, the AUC can increase or decrease, making the clinical effect unpredictable.
	Immunosuppressants	Grapefruit juice inhibits tacrolimus (Prograf) metabolism and should be avoided.
Caffeine	Fluoroquinolones	Ciprofloxacin inhibits caffeine metabolism, increasing caffeine's effects. Other fluoroquinolones do not appear to be affected by caffeine and can be used as alternatives for patients ingesting larger quantities of caffeine throughout the day.
	H_2 antagonists	Cimetidine increases caffeine levels, so an alternative H_2 antagonist (such as ranitidine or famotidine) should be used for patients ingesting larger quantities of caffeine throughout the day.
	Oral contraceptives	Oral contraceptives increase caffeine levels.
	Corticosteroids	Prednisone increases caffeine levels.
	Xanthines	Theophylline-related side effects (jitteriness, insomnia, arrhythmias) increase when taken with caffeine.
Dairy Products and Calcium-Enriched Foods	Fluoroquinolones	Ciprofloxacin and levofloxacin may be made ineffective when taken with dairy products or calcium-containing foods.
	Antibiotics	Calcium binds with tetracycline and prevents absorption of the antibiotic in the gut. For cephalosporin antibiotics, such as cefuroxime, levels become decreased when taken with dairy products.
	Bisphosphonates	Alendronate, risedronate, and ibandronate have low bioavailability with little medication absorption when taken with dairy products.
	Antimetabolites	Oral methotrexate levels decrease when taken with dairy products.
Fiber-Rich Foods	Biguanides	Metformin blood levels decrease when taken with fiber-rich foods (e.g., oatmeal).
	Thyroid hormones	Levothyroxine absorption can decrease when taken with calcium-rich foods. This medication should be taken on an empty stomach.
Tyramine-Containing Foods	MAOIs	A very dangerous, potentially fatal interaction can occur when MAOIs are taken with foods that contain tyramine. Examples include foods and beverages such as beer, red and aged wines (port, sherry), cheeses (blue, brie, cheddar, Swiss), caffeine (chocolate, coffee, tea), beef or chicken livers, sour cream, yogurt, smoked meats (sausage or salami), bananas, avocados, fermented products (soy sauce, miso, tofu, tempeh), pickled foods (sauerkraut), sourdough breads, and some beans (fava, broad beans). Patients may develop severe hypertension with hypertensive crisis.

Continued

TABLE 1.2	Common Food–Medication Interactions–cont'd	
Food	**Medication Category**	**Interaction**
Green, Leafy Vegetables	Anticoagulants	Warfarin (Coumadin) interferes with synthesis of vitamin K–derived clotting factors. Consuming quantities of green, leafy vegetables such as spinach, Swiss chard, and Brussels sprouts will reduce warfarin efficacy.
Alcohol	Anticoagulants	Acute alcohol use enhances the availability of warfarin, increasing the risk of life-threatening hemorrhage. Chronic alcohol consumption reduces the availability of warfarin, thereby lessening protection in blood-clotting disorders.
	Antidepressants	Alcohol increases the sedative effect of tricyclic antidepressants, such as amitriptyline. Alcohol consumption increases the availability of some antidepressants, increasing the risk for motor impairment, ataxia, falls, somnolence, and respiratory depression. MAOIs taken with alcohol can result in dangerously high blood pressure.
	Analgesics	Excessive acetaminophen use, especially with regular alcohol consumption, increases the risk for hepatotoxicity. NSAIDs taken in conjunction with alcohol increase the risk for severe GI bleeding.
	Antihistamines	Alcohol can intensify sedation from antihistamines and result in excessive dizziness in older patients.
	Antiepileptics	Alcohol increases serum levels of phenytoin (Dilantin) and the risk of side effects. Daily alcohol consumption actually decreases serum levels of phenytoin, significantly increasing seizure risk.
	Antipsychotics	Alcohol use increases the sedative effect of these medications and may result in respiratory distress and liver damage.
	Antidiabetics	When taken with alcohol, antidiabetic agents can induce abnormally low blood pressure, rapid heart rate, sudden changes in blood pressure, nausea, vomiting, and headache.
	Antihypertensives	Drinking alcohol while taking antihypertensive medications can result in dizziness, fainting, and irregular heart rate. Garlic-containing foods can exacerbate antihypertensive effects of medication.

Adapted from Hulisz, D., & Jakab, J. (2007). Food–drug interactions: Which ones really matter? *U.S. Pharmacist, 32*(3), 93–98; and Bushra, R., et al. (2011). Food–drug interactions. *Oman Medical Journal, 26*(2), 77–83.

food–medication interactions that should be incorporated into the patient education plan.

Medication and Alcohol Interactions

Alcohol is one of the most widely utilized legal substances. Thus it is important to understand how alcohol is metabolized in the body (Chan & Anderson, 2014). The major enzyme system responsible for the oxidation of ethanol is alcohol dehydrogenase, and to a lesser extent, the cytochrome P450–dependent ethanol-oxidizing system. Both of these systems are present in the liver. Short- and long-term ethanol use can cause changes to many physiologic responses in different organ systems that result in both pharmacokinetic and pharmacodynamic interactions. Evaluating medication interactions with long-term use of ethanol is difficult. First, there is not a standard definition of what comprises chronic alcohol use, and second, there is difficulty in distinguishing between the effects of long-term ethanol use on liver disease and chronic malnutrition. Liver damage lowers the rate of alcohol oxidation and elimination and results in decreased activity of hepatic metabolic enzymes and

changes in protein binding. In addition, some medications affect the metabolism of alcohol, thus altering its potential for intoxication and the adverse effects associated with alcohol consumption (Table 1.2).

Over-the-Counter and Prescription Medication Interactions

The use of OTC preparations is extremely common among adult patients for the self-treatment of many minor ills. The interaction effects between prescription medications and OTC preparations can become problematic without appropriate counseling and patient education from the primary care provider. Medications to treat GI motility disorders, diarrhea, constipation, and gastroesophageal reflux disease (GERD) all affect the absorption and bioavailability of prescription medications and alter the GI microbiome. These OTC preparations can change the pharmacokinetics of some prescription medications when they are co-administered, leading to treatment failure or serious adverse events. Specific medications should always be evaluated for their potential OTC interactions. Several drug-interaction checklist tools are available online and can be utilized for investigating such interactions before the medication is prescribed. Patients should be taught to always read the labels of OTC products because common medication interactions are listed in the "warning" section on the label. Patients who experience a side effect after taking an OTC medicine for a common ailment should discontinue the product at once and consult a health care provider for guidance.

Herbal Preparations and Prescription Medication Interactions

The use of herbal preparations and nutritional supplements by the general population has increased significantly over the past few years. The scientific literature reports that the use of herbal preparations, including those from traditional Chinese medicine for increasing breast milk supply and for the self-treatment of hypertension, diabetes, anxiety, and cancer, is rising. The significance of the interaction between the herbal product and prescription medication varies, but it is essential to recognize the potential for harm. The prescription medications that are of greatest concern for adverse interactions with herbal preparations are anticoagulants or antiplatelet agents and any medication with a narrow therapeutic index. Popular herbal drugs such as St. John's wort, ginkgo, ginseng, and garlic are known to interact with anticoagulants or antiplatelet medications and should be strictly avoided. Chinese herbal preparations such as Dong quai, Danshen, and ginger also may adversely interact with medications. In a recent scientific review, curcumin (turmeric), which is used for its antiinflammatory effect, can induce pharmacokinetic alterations when concomitantly used with prescription cardiovascular medications, antidepressants, anticoagulants, antibiotics, chemotherapeutic agents, and antihistamines (Bahramsoltani et al., 2017; Amadi & Mgbahurike, 2018). The underlying mechanisms of these interactions include inhibition of CYP isoenzymes and P-glycoprotein.

Of concern to the primary care provider is that patients who are taking both herbal preparations and prescription medications typically do not report this during their appointments or hospitalizations, so it is of utmost importance to ask specific questions during medication reconciliation. The NIH National Center for Complementary and Alternative Medicine has a list of herbal products and their potential interactions with common medications that may be consulted when primary care providers do learn that patients are using herbal preparations.

Therapeutic Monitoring

Therapeutic monitoring involves measuring the serum levels in patients receiving medications with a narrow therapeutic index, to maximize efficacy and minimize toxicity (Brunton et al., 2017). Some of the most commonly administered medications that are closely monitored through serum blood levels include lithium citrate, theophylline, valproic acid, phenytoin, and digoxin. When monitoring serum

levels for therapeutic purposes, it is important to consider the time of sampling of the medication. If intermittent dosing is used, the sample can be obtained at any time during the dosing interval to provide information to support clinical findings suggestive of drug toxicity. Serum medication levels obtained for the purpose of adjusting the dosing regimen must be taken at specified intervals to reflect accurate levels.

The trough level is often used in medication monitoring and refers to the lowest concentration reached by a medication before the next dose is administered. When the goal of determining the serum medication level is adjustment of dosage, a blood sample should be taken just before the next planned dose, when the concentration is at its minimum level. For individuals with renal failure, in whom concerns about drug accumulation are high, determination of both maximum and minimum concentrations is recommended.

Before taking a serum sample, it is also important to consider whether the patient has reached steady-state concentrations. Steady state usually is achieved after four to five half-lives have passed. A sample obtained too soon after a dose will not accurately reflect clearance. For medications with a narrow therapeutic index, it is unwise to wait for a steady state to be reached, as the serum level may already be within a toxic range. Taking the first serum sample after two half-lives is recommended for such medications. If the serum result shows a concentration exceeding 90% of the expected mean steady-state concentration, the dose should be halved and another sample should be obtained after two half-lives have passed. This strategy may be repeated if the target value is still exceeded (Table 1.3).

Practical Application of Pharmacokinetics and Pharmacodynamics to Prescription Medication

When the underlying scientific principles inherent in pharmacokinetics and pharmacodynamics are applied, some very practical suggestions can be made for rational drug therapy:

- Use a medication only when clearly indicated for a specific purpose. It may be difficult for a provider to resist prescribing a medication for every symptom that annoys the patient, particularly when the patient is demanding resolution or relief. Well-directed advice, sound instructions, and specific lifestyle changes are occasionally required in lieu of medication.
- Use as few medications as possible. Many patients with chronic disease take numerous medications that require the primary care provider to perform medication reconciliation at each office or clinic visit to maintain an accurate accounting of medications prescribed by the primary care provider and other specialists caring for the patient.
- Use the lowest effective dose. If the medication dosage was increased but no additional benefit was derived, titrate the medication to the original prescribed dosage. Adverse medication reactions are often dose related.

TABLE 1.3	Therapeutic Ranges for Serum Drug Concentrations	
Drug	**Serum Concentration**	**Time to Draw Blood Samples (Hours After Last Dose)**
Antibiotics		
amikacin (Amikin)	15–25 mcg/mL	Obtain peak and trough levels: draw peak 15-30 min after intravenous (IV) dose or 1 hour after intramuscular (IM) dose; trough 5 min before next dose.
gentamicin (Garamycin)	4–10 mcg/mL	
netilmicin (Netromycin)	6–10 mcg/mL	
tobramycin (Nebcin)	4–10 mcg/mL	
Anticonvulsants		
carbamazepine (Tegretol)	4–12 mcg/mL	Steady state 1–2 weeks
ethosuximide	10–100 mcg/mL	Steady state 10–30 days
phenobarbital	10-40 mcg/mL	Steady state 1–2 weeks
phenytoin (Dilantin)	10–20 mcg/mL	Steady state 2–3 days
primidone (Mysoline)	5–12 mcg/mL	Steady state 1–2 days
valproic acid (Depakene, Depakote)	50–100 mcg/mL	Steady state 1–2 days; then draw sample before next dose
Antidepressants		
lithium	0.6–1.4 mEq/L	Steady state 3 weeks; draw before next dose
Cardiovascular		
digoxin (Lanoxin)	0.9–2 ng/nL	Steady state 1 week; draw before next dose, at least 6 hours after last dose
lidocaine (Xylocaine)	1.5–5 mcg/mL	Steady state 6–12 hours; draw any time during infusion
procainamide (Pronestyl)	4–10 mcg/mL	Steady state 12–24 hours; draw before next dose
quinidine (various)	3–6 mcg/mL	Steady state 1.5 days; draw before next dose
Respiratory		
theophylline (various)	10–20 mcg/mL	Steady state in 1–2 days in adults; up to 1 week in neonates; IV: draw any time; oral: draw before next dose

Modified from McKenry, L. M., et al. (2005). *Mosby's pharmacology in nursing* (22nd ed.). St. Louis: Mosby; and DiPiro, J. T., et al. (2011). *Pharmacotherapy: A pathophysiologic approach* (8th ed.). Norwalk, CT: McGraw-Hill.

- Start low and go slow. If an increased medication dose is required, change the dosage by no more than 50% and no more frequently than every three to four half-lives. This means that, in practice, there may be no change for 1 to 2 weeks after an increase in dosage is begun.
- Simplify the regimen whenever possible. Give the fewest number of doses and at the most convenient hours of the day to assist with regimen compliance.
- Occasionally, the side-effect profile of one medication can treat other symptoms. For example, if a patient has both depression and insomnia, prescribe trazodone or mirtazapine, which may be sedating, instead of sertraline (Zoloft) or fluoxetine (Prozac), which are most commonly associated with insomnia.
- Monitor the patient closely for therapeutic and adverse effects. Although medication levels are evaluated as appropriate, also consider your assessment and the patient's report in addition to the clinical medication level. For example, the therapeutic level of phenytoin is usually between 10 and 20 mcg/mL. However, older adult patients tolerate this medication best at a level of 8 mcg/mL. Medications given over prolonged periods are more apt to produce adverse reactions; thus the patient's response to the dose must be carefully monitored and reduced as appropriate.
- Keep accurate and complete patient records. In prescribing medications, it is important for the primary care provider to consider any history of medication allergy, liver or renal dysfunction, or other comorbidity that places the patient at greater risk for developing adverse or medication interactions.
- Closely monitor patients taking medications highly associated with adverse effects. Medications such as insulin, steroids, lithium, and anticoagulants require close monitoring. When prescribing such medications, the primary care provider has the additional responsibility of providing extensive education to the patient and the family to ensure patient safety.

- Always keep drug interactions and adverse effects in mind when evaluating the patient. This principle is undertaken to avoid serious adverse medication effects. For example, pancytopenia need not occur if leukopenia is detected early; deafness will not result if signs of eighth nerve impairment are promptly investigated.
- Maintain current knowledge of clinical guidelines and prescribing practices. Reading the latest journal articles related to your patient population and practice area helps maintain current knowledge. New research findings should constantly be consulted and evaluated; valid findings should be incorporated into practice. In this age of electronic information dissemination, the standards of practice may be expected to shift to incorporate more new knowledge than was ever available before. Thus it is imperative for primary care providers to find ways to update their knowledge on a regular basis.

Many publishers of pharmaceutical information have realized that information about new products and new recommendations must reach health care providers in a timely manner. Clinical Pharmacology Gold Standard Drug Database (https://www.elsevier.com/solutions/drug-database) is an electronic drug information reference for health care professionals that can be accessed online.

Selected Bibliography

Alsanosi, SM, Skiffington, C., & Padmanabhan, S. (2014). Pharmacokinetic Pharmacogenomics. *Handbook of Handbook of Pharmacogenomics and Stratified Medicine.* Philadelphia: Elsevier.

Amadi, CN, & Mgbahurike, AA. (2018). Selected food/herb-drug interactions: Mechanisms and clinical relevance. *Am J Ther, 25*(4) 2018;25(4):e423–e433. doi:10.1097/MJT.0000000000000705.

Anas, N, & Rafik, K (2019). The prodrug approach in the era of drug design. *Expert Opinion on Drug Delivery, 16*(1), 1–5. doi:10.10 80/17425247.2019.1553954.

Ayrton, A, & Morgan, P (2001). Role of transport proteins in drug absorption, distribution and excretion. *Xenobiotica, 31*:8–9, 469-497, doi:10.1080/00498250110060969.

Bahramsoltani, R, Rahimi, R, & Farzaei, MH (2017). Pharmacokinetic interactions of curcuminoids with conventional drugs: A review. *J Ethnopharmacol, 209*, 1–12. doi:10.1016/j.jep.2017.07.022.

Bourgeois, F, Shannon, MW, Valim, C, & Mandl, KD (2010). Adverse drug events in the outpatient setting: An 11-year national analysis. *Pharmacoepidemiology & Drug Safety, 19*(9), 901–910.

Brunton, LL, Chabner, B, & Knollman, B (2017). *Goodman and Gilman's The Pharmacological Basis of Therapeutics* (13th Edition): Mcgraw-Hill Medical.

Byers, JP, & Sarver, JG (2009). Pharmacokinetic modeling. In M Hacker, W Messer, & K Bachman (Eds.), *Pharmacology Principles and Practice* (pp. 201–277): Academic Press.

Chan, LN, & Anderson, GD (2014). Pharmacokinetic and pharmacodynamic drug interactions with ethanol (alcohol). *Clin Pharmacokinet, 53*(12), 1115–1136. doi:10.1007/s40262-014-0190-x.

Currie, G. M. (2018). Pharmacology, Part 2: Introduction to Pharmacokinetics. *J Nucl Med Technol, 46*, 221–230.

Deng, J, Zhu, X, Chen, Z, Fan, CH, Kwan, HS, Wong, CH, Shek, KY, Zuo, Z, & Lam, TN (2017). A review of food–drug interactions on oral drug absorption. *Drugs, 77*(17), 1833–1855.

Drozdzik, M, Busch, D, Lapczuk, J, Muller, J, Ostrowski, M, Kurzawski, M, & Oswald, S. (2017). Protein abundance of clinically relevant drug-metabolizing enzymes in the human liver and intestine: A comparative analysis in paired tissue specimens. *Clin Pharm & Therap, 104*(3), 515–524.

Edwards, RE, & Aaronson, JK (2000). Adverse drug reactions: Definitions, diagnosis, and management. *The Lancet, 356*(9237), 1212-.

Grandison, MK, & Boudinot, FD (2000). Age-related changes in protein binding of drugs: Implications for therapy. *Clin Pharmacokinet, 38*(3), 271–290.

Hobbs, AL, Shea, KM, Roberts, KM, & Daley, MJ (2015). Implications of Augmented Renal clearance on drug dosing in critically ill patients: A focus on antibiotics. *Pharmacotherapy, 35*(11), 1063–1075. doi:10.1002/phar.1653.

Hughes, G. (2016). Friendly pharmacokinetics: A simple introduction. *Nurse Prescribing, 14*(1), 34–43.

Litou, C, Effinger, A, Kostewicz, ES, Box, KJ, Fotaki, N, & Dressman, JB (2019). Effects of medicines used to treat gastrointestinal diseases on the pharmacokinetics of coadministered drugs: a PEARRL Review. *J Pharm Pharmacol, 71*(4), 643–673. doi:10.1111/jphp.12983.

Loucks, J., Yost, S., & Kaplan, B. (2015). An introduction to pharmacokinetics. *Transplantation, 99*(5), 903–907.

Lowry, M. (2016). Rectal drug administration in adults: How, when, why. *Nursing Times, 112*(8), 12–14.

Manikandan, P, & Nagini, S. (2018). Cytochrome P450 structure, function and clinical significance: A review. *Curr Drug Targets, 19*(1), 38–54. doi:10.2174/1389450118666170125144557.

Masereeuw, R, & Russel, FG (2001). Mechanisms and clinical implications of renal drug excretion. *Drug Metab Rev, 33*(3-4), 299–351.

McCance, KL, & Huether, SE (2019). *Pathophysiology: The biological basis for disease in adults and children* (8th Ed.). St Louis, Mo: Elsevier.

Pirmohamed, M. (2013). Drug-grapefruit juice interactions. *BMJ Br. Med. J., 346.* http://dx.doi.org/10.1136/bmj.f1.

Pritchard, JR, Bruno, PM, Gilbert, LA, Kelsey, LC, Lauffenburger, & Hemann, MT (2013). Defining principles of combination drug mechanisms of action. *PNAS, 110*(2), E179. E170. https://doi.org/10.1073/pnas.1210419110.

Rautio, J, Meanwell, NA, Di, L, et al. (2018). The expanding role of prodrugs in contemporary drug design and development. *Nat Rev Drug Discov, 17*(8), 559–587.

Salt, AN, & Plontke, SK (2009). Principles of drug delivery to the inner ear. *Audiol Neurootol, 14*(6), 350–360. doi:10.1159/000241892.

Sánchez-Fidalgo, S, Guzmán-Ramos, MI, Galván-Banqueri, M, Bernabeu-Wittel, M, & Santos Ramos, B. (2017). Prevalence of drug interactions in elderly patients with multimorbidity in primary care. *Int J Clin Pharm, 39*(2), 343–353. doi:10.1007/s11096-017-0439-1.

Seagrave, Z, & Bamba, S. (2017). Adverse drug reactions. *Dis Mon, 63*(2), 49–53. doi:10.1016/j.disamonth.2016.09.006.

Stein, AM, & Peletier, LA (2018). Predicting the Onset of Nonlinear Pharmacokinetics. *CPT Pharmacometrics Syst Pharmacol, 7*(10), 670–677.

Zhou, SF (2008). Drugs behave as substrates, inhibitors and inducers of human cytochrome P450 3A4. *Curr Drug Metab, 9*(4), 310–322.

2
Pharmacogenomics

CONSTANCE G. VISOVSKY

Overview

Pharmacogenomics is the science of deoxyribonucleic acid (DNA) analysis for the purpose of identifying gene variations that impact medication response (Mele & Goldschmidt, 2014). To achieve the desired outcome from pharmacologic therapies and avoidance of adverse effects, pharmacogenomics considers variations in medication response that are the result of genetic influences. Variable responses to medications can result from both individual and inherited alterations that affect populations, such as those found among specific ethnicities and races. There are many reasons for variations in medication response; medication interactions, disease states that can alter medication concentrations or responsiveness, and poor compliance have been commonly cited. Pharmacogenomics refers to genetic polymorphisms found in specific patient populations and considers individual differences in medication response. Additionally, genetic differences in metabolizing enzymes and protein receptors account for variations in therapeutic responses that can range from no response to dangerous adverse drug reactions (ADEs). Other factors, including age, gender, and preexisting comorbid conditions, can also affect medication response. The *clinical relevance* of pharmacogenomics is underscored by family genetics showing racial differences in medication metabolism (Box 2.1).

Genetics and Pharmacogenomics

The term *genome* refers to the genetic material of an organism. An organism's genetic material consists of *genes* comprising protein-coding DNA (1%) and noncoding DNA (99%; controls gene activity). Mitochondrial DNA is essential for carrying out the function of the mitochondria. The Human Genome Project mapped approximately 95% of the human genome and proposes that humans have from 20,000 to 25,000 genes. The human genome is composed of 23 base pairs of chromosomes that are made up of DNA. DNA provides the genetic "blueprint" for producing all proteins made in the body to support the body's structure and function. Through the processes of transcription and translation, information from genes is used to make proteins.

DNA consists of two strands of polynucleotides formed into a double helix resembling a ladder. Adenine, guanine, thymine, and cytosine compose the bases of DNA. Each strand of polynucleotides consists of a sequential string of these bases, known as a base pair (Howland, 2012). In arrangement, the base pairs are called a *DNA sequence* or *codon* (Fig. 2.1). These nucleotide bases appear in differing arrangements to form the body's necessary proteins. If the normal sequence of the nucleotide bases is altered, substituting one base for another, the function changes and is known as a genetic or single nucleotide polymorphism (SNP). Because everyone inherits from their parents two copies of each gene, the SNP can present as a single copy (homozygous) or in both copies (heterozygous). Thus an individual's genetic makeup or genotype is a result of genes inherited from both parents. The effect of the SNP on the function of the gene is dependent upon whether one or both copies of the gene are altered.

Single nucleotide polymorphisms account for individual genetic differences and variations in medication metabolism and response. By understanding how genetics can influence pharmacologic treatment, primary care providers can identify which medications will result in optimal outcomes for their patients. All genetic variations result from a change in DNA sequence. The differing sequences are known as *alleles*. Individual differences in genetic makeup can alter the structure or function of proteins involved in pharmacokinetics and pharmacodynamics (Fig. 2.2). These individual genetic differences are implicated in the variability of a patient's response to different medications. Inherited differences in medication metabolism due to genetic polymorphisms may have an even greater influence on medication efficacy and toxicities experienced. As a result, a patient can be a poor metabolizer (lack of a working enzyme), an intermediate metabolizer (one functioning and one mutated allele), an extensive metabolizer (two normally functioning alleles), or an ultrarapid metabolizer (more than one functioning allele copy). Other factors such as age, body mass index, and comorbidities can also influence the therapeutic effects of medications.

• Box 2.1 Definitions of Terms

Term	Definition
Pharmacogenomics	The study of genetic factors influencing the effectiveness, toxicity, and metabolism of medication.
Pharmacogenetics	The study of hereditary factors on individual responses to medications.
Genetic Polymorphism	Differences in DNA sequencing found at a rate of at least 1% in the population.
Single Nucleotide Polymorphism	A variation in a single base pair in a DNA sequence.
Allele	Variation or differences in DNA sequences.

Genes and Medication Metabolism

Differences in metabolism resulting in either low or high concentrations of a medication were found in some patients despite having been administered the same medication type and dose. Evidence has shown that a common single-gene variant can affect pharmacokinetics to varying degrees. The bioactivation pathways needed for some medications involve a single drug-metabolizing enzyme, and genetic variants can result in loss of function of this enzyme, which results in a decrease of pharmacologic action. When a patient fails to respond to treatment, in individuals homozygous for the variant, increasing the dose of a medication does not elicit a response because they completely lack the enzyme needed for the activity. However, some variants result in a function gain as opposed to a function loss and can be associated with excess drug response (Roden et al., 2019).

The cytochrome (CYP) P450 enzyme system located in the liver is responsible for the metabolism of many medications. Each enzyme is associated with a gene and uses the nomenclature "CYP" followed by a mix of numbers and letters. In some cases, more than one gene can be identified as a pharmacogenomic target. For example, warfarin is affected by both CYP2C19 and VKORCI while tricyclic antidepressants are affected by CYP2C19 and CYP2D6, demonstrating that one gene can affect multiple medications. Pharmacogeneticists have adopted a star nomenclature (e.g., CYP2C19*2) to describe gene variants responsible for variability in drug response.

The CYP2D6 enzyme accounts for 30% of metabolism of many prescription medications, including antidepressants, antipsychotics, opioids, and β-blockers (Beery & Workman, 2018). Examples of genetically induced variability in drug response usually involve single DNA variants that are commonly present in a population. Ethnic makeup can also influence how CYP enzymes work in the metabolism of medications. For example, the CYP3A5 gene is expressed in 50% of African Americans but not in most Caucasians (Belle & Singh, 2008). Individuals with CYP3A5 metabolize some CYP3A substrates more rapidly

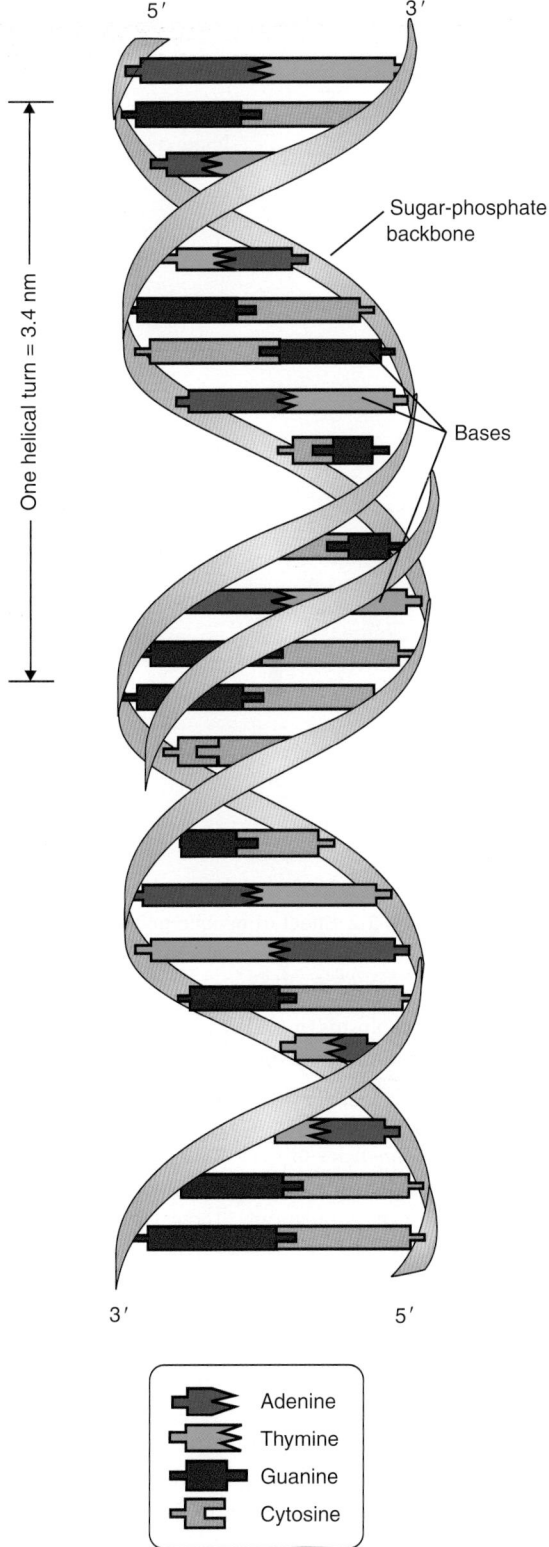

• **Fig. 2.1** DNA sequence. (From Jorde, C. B., Carey, J .C., Bamshead, M. J., et al. [Eds.], [2006]. *Medical genetics* [3rd ed.]. St. Louis: Mosby.)

than those who do not possess the gene. CYP3A5 has been implicated as a genetic determinant of differences in lipid-lowering response to statin drugs, but results have been inconsistent.

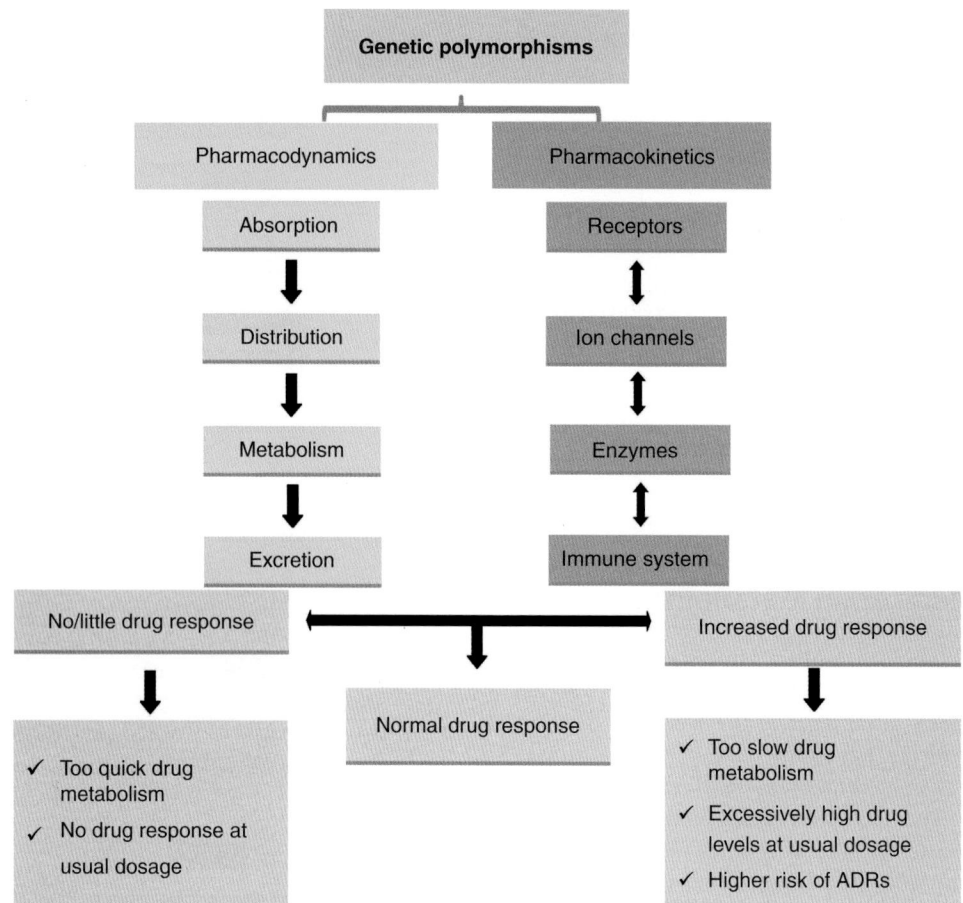

• **Fig. 2.2** Effect of genetic polymorphism on pharmacokinetics and pharmacodynamics. (From Ahmed, S., et al. (2016). Pharmacogenomics: A key component of precision medicine 299. *Genomics, Proteomics & Bioinformatics 14*, 298–313.)

Genetic polymorphisms in CYP2C19 expression can occur in different populations. Approximately 3% to 5% of Europeans and 15% to 20% of Asians have genetic polymorphisms in CYP2C19 and are poor metabolizers who lack CYP2C19 function. The allele frequencies of CYP2C19*2 and CYP2C19*3 are significantly higher in Chinese populations as opposed to European or African populations. These types of polymorphisms are clinically relevant, as they may reduce the efficacy of the antiplatelet clopidogrel. Clopidogrel is administered as a *prodrug*, or a medication that is inactive when taken and only becomes activated through the action of a specific enzyme. In patients who have a gene associated with reduced activity, clopidogrel may not be metabolized to its active form and therefore may not achieve the desired pharmacologic effect. The relative risk of major cardiac events among patients treated with clopidogrel is 1.53 to 3.69 times higher for carriers of loss-of-function alleles CYP2C19*2, CYP2C19*3, and CYP2C19*17 compared with noncarriers. Another consequence of variation in drug response is the occurrence of adverse events (Table 2.1).

Clinical Diagnostic Testing

To be useful in delivering patient care, pharmacogenomic testing must be reliable and valid in clinical utility. Clinical utility involves the assessment of pharmacogenomics testing

that leads to improved outcomes for the patient as well as the healthcare system. The validity of testing will depend largely upon the data quality from genomic tests performed and the predictive value of the tests.

Once testing is concluded, alternative therapies are needed in order for providers to be able to act on gene–drug interactions. Providing an alternative therapy will require scientific evidence for efficacy with consideration of toxicity. However, taking an alternative action may not be possible. There may not be an adequate medication substitution, or there may be absent or conflicting evidence for any alternative therapy. At present, only 17 of approximately 18,000 genes are considered actionable as they relate to pharmacogenomics. There is increasing evidence that testing multiple genes concurrently is more cost-effective and proactive than single-gene testing.

For pharmacogenomics testing to be more widely available and useful to primary care providers, more efficient and accurate testing procedures, a cost and reimbursement structure, and computational approaches to identify and interpret genome variants are necessary. An additional barrier to pharmacogenomics testing is the lack of gold-standard clinical guidelines for translating genomic information into prescribing recommendations. Several professional societies are working on standardized genomic

TABLE 2.1 Drugs and Genes With Guidelines From the Clinical Pharmacogenetics Implementation Consortium for Use in Clinical Practice

Gene	Drug
Pharmacokinetic Mechanisms	
CYP2B6	Efavirenz
CYP2C19	Clopidogrel, SSRIs, TCAs, voriconazole, proton pump inhibitors[a], celecoxib,[a] phenytoin, warfarin, codeine, oxycodone, tramadol, SSRIs, TCAs, ondansetron, tamoxifen,
CYP2C9	Atomoxetine
CYP2D6	Tacrolimus, 5-fluorouracil, capecitabine, tegafur, azathioprine, mercaptopurine
CYP3A5 DPYD	Thioguanine, simvastatin
TPMT and NUDT15	Atazanavir
Pharmacodynamic Mechanisms	
CFTR	Ivacaftor
CYP4F2 G6PD	Warfarin, rasburicase
HLA-B	Abacavir, allopurinol, carbamazepine, phenytoin, interferon
IFNL3 (IL28B)	Inhaled anesthetics, succinylcholine
RYR1 and CACNA1S	Warfarin

[a]Guidelines in progress.

SSRI, Selective serotonin reuptake inhibitor; *TCA,* tricyclic antidepressant.

From Roden, D. M., McLeod, H. L., Relling, M. V., Williams, M. S., Mensah, G. A., Peterson, J. F., & Van Driest, S. L. (2019). Pharmacogenomics. *The Lancet, Genomic Medicine series: Vol. 394, Issue 10197:* 521–532.

testing terminology to be used with electronic health record (EHR) systems.

BOOKMARK THIS!

- Clinical Pharmacogenetics Implementation Consortium (CPIC): https://cpicpgx.org/
- European Pharmacogenetics Implementation Consortium: www.eu-pic.net
- NIH Pharmacogenomics Research Network: www.nigms.nih.gov/maps/Pages/Pharmacogenomics-Research-Network-Members.aspx)
- Electronic Medical Records and Genomics (eMERGE) Network: www.genome.gov/Funded-Programs-Projects/Electronic-Medical-Records-and-Genomics-Network-eMERGE
- Implementing Genomics in Practice (IGNITE): www.genome.gov/Funded-Programs-Projects/Implementing-Genomics-in-Practice-IGNITE
- List of FDA-Approved Companion Diagnostic Devices: https://www.fda.gov/medical-devices/vitro-diagnostics/list-cleared-or-approved-companion-diagnostic-devices-vitro-and-imaging-tools

Clinical Implementation of Pharmacogenomics

As the amount of pharmacogenomic information continues to increase, making such information available in a practical manner that is useful to primary care providers is an important consideration. Objective, evidence-based guidelines and timely genetic information is needed for providers to take pharmacogenomics into account when prescribing medication for patients. Fortunately, the advent of the EHR system means that genetic information is already being stored in a place that providers access frequently. To assist in these efforts, some institutions have created automatic computer alerts that are triggered when a medication is prescribed that has known pharmacogenomics information that can help guide treatment decisions for specific patients. For example, the Clinical Pharmacogenetics Implementation Consortium (CPIC) has established guidelines for human leukocyte antigen (HLA) genotype testing in the use of carbamazepine or oxcarbazepine (Phillips et al., 2018).

The U.S. Food and Drug Administration (FDA) also has a role in pharmacogenomic testing (Box 2.2). The FDA

Recommendations for Patients

- Do not change or stop taking any medications based on a report from a direct-to-consumer genetic test. Discuss the results of the genetic test with your primary care provider. Medications should always be taken as prescribed by your primary care provider.

- Many genetic tests make claims about the effects of specific medications that are not supported by scientific evidence.

Recommendations for Health Care Providers

- If you are considering using a genetic test to predict a patient's response to a specific medication, be aware that the relationship between DNA variations and the medication's effects may not have strong scientific evidence. Check the FDA-approved drug label or approved genetic test for information regarding whether genetic information should be used for determining therapeutic treatment.

- If a patient brings you a report from a direct-to-consumer genetic test, seek guidance from the FDA regarding whether genetic information should be used for determining therapeutic treatment.

- Be aware that there are some FDA-approved drug and genetic test labels and labels of FDA-cleared genetic tests that provide general information about the impact of DNA variations on drug levels, but they do not describe how that genetic information can be used for determining therapeutic treatment. These labels are intended to be informational and should not be used in making treatment decisions.

- Information regarding therapeutic treatment recommendations for patients with certain genetic variations can be found in the warnings (Boxed Warning, or Warnings and Precautions), Indications and Usage, Dosage and Administration, and Use in Specific Populations sections of FDA-approved drug labels.

has classified direct-to-consumer pharmacogenomics tests as medical devices; however, they are reviewed by the FDA only if they are being used for moderate- to high-risk prescribing purposes, or if the results of the testing may have a high impact on care. The FDA reviews test accuracy and reliability and examines company-provided information to ensure that it is easy to understand. In 2018, the FDA issued a statement regarding individual, direct-to-consumer genetic testing. In the statement, agency officials expressed concerns with pharmacogenetic tests whose claims have not been reviewed by the FDA and are not supported by prescribing recommendations in the FDA-approved drug label, may not be supported by scientific and clinical evidence, and may not be accurate. Therefore it is important for primary care providers to understand and educate their patients about pharmacogenetic testing to avoid inappropriately selecting or changing drug treatments based on the results from insufficiently substantiated genetic tests, which could lead to potentially serious health consequences

for patients. For example, there are available genetic tests that claim their results can be used to help primary care providers determine which antidepressant medications would have increased effectiveness or adverse effects as compared to other antidepressant medications. However, the relationship between DNA variations and the effectiveness of antidepressant medication has never been established. This example drives home the point that no prescribing decisions should be made that are not supported by scientific evidence.

Clinical Impact of Pharmacogenomics

Increasingly, primary care providers are bombarded with an explosion of pharmacogenomic information that can impact prescribing practices. Over the past decade, the understanding of medication variability in medication response has advanced the notion that we can influence the efficacy of some medications and decrease adverse events in our patient populations. The potential impact is substantial, considering the costs due to either ineffective therapies or hospitalizations related to adverse effects of prescribed medications. To date, although the effects of pharmacogenomic variants are well established, there remains a varied spectrum of pharmacogenomic effects that influence the clinical utility of testing. Some examples of the potential influence of genetic variations on prescribing practices are discussed in the following sections.

Warfarin

Warfarin is a commonly prescribed medication, with approximately 2 million patients beginning warfarin therapy each year. However, warfarin has a narrow therapeutic index that predisposes patients to bleeding-related adverse events. In the first 6 months of therapy, 20% of patients will be hospitalized for bleeding related to excessive anticoagulation (Elias & Topol, 2008; Epstein et al., 2010). Warfarin is an example of a medication that has variable actions determined by both pharmacokinetic and pharmacodynamic gene variants. Pharmacogenomic studies suggest that genotyping for patients on warfarin therapy could potentially decrease hospitalizations for patients on warfarin by 30% (Epstein et al., 2010). Studies also suggest that there is a direct relationship between the warfarin dose and the genetic status of CYP2C9, a major drug-metabolizing enzyme. Patients who have copies of the wild type of the CYP2C9 gene, CYP2C9*1, metabolize warfarin well and are considered "extensive warfarin metabolizers." Patients who possess the variants CYP2C9*2 and CYP2C9*3 have decreased ability to metabolize warfarin. The CYP2C9 genotype accounted for 12% of the interindividual variability of warfarin dose requirements (Au & Rettie, 2008).

Warfarin decreases the synthesis of vitamin-K–dependent clotting factors by inhibiting vitamin K 2,3–epoxide reductase (VKOR), which in turn influences dose requirements. Patients with a specific guanine-to-adenine SNP will require a lower warfarin dose, as a VKORC1 polymorphism accounts for 25% of the interindividual variation in warfarin dose. Currently, there are pharmacogenetic tests to guide warfarin use for CYP2C9 and VKORC1 polymorphisms, but there remains some difficulty in obtaining third-party payment, as it is not considered the standard of care.

Clopidogrel

Like warfarin, clopidogrel is a commonly prescribed platelet inhibitor that is activated by CYP2C19 and is used to prevent cardiac events and stent thrombosis. However, unlike warfarin, clopidogrel is a prodrug, so it must be transformed to a more active metabolite in order to achieve the desired result. As CYP2C19 is responsible for activating clopidogrel, the loss of function in the CYP2C19 alleles is associated with a diminished response to clopidogrel, accounting for increased cardiovascular events and 12% of the variation in drug response. At least one loss-of-function allele is carried by 18% of Mexicans, 24% of Whites (non-Hispanics), 33% of African Americans, and 50% of Asians. So, in patients heterozygous for CYP2C19*2, an increased dose of clopidogrel would result in an antiplatelet effect, since they still have some CYP2C19 activity. However, a similar increase in dose for patients who are homozygous for the variant would not generate an antiplatelet effect, because they completely lack CYP2C19 activity. Most variants that were studied confer either a partial or a complete loss of function. However, there are also gain-of-function variants associated with excess drug response, including CYP2C19*17, which has been associated with bleeding during clopidogrel therapy.

PRACTICE PEARLS

Pharmacogenomics

- Studies have shown that testing for genetic markers is associated with the safety and efficacy of clopidogrel and warfarin.
- The FDA has updated clopidogrel and warfarin labels with genetic information.
- Guidelines have been established to assist in determining dosage requirements for clopidogrel and warfarin based on genotype. However, clinical utility is still limited.
- Large, randomized clinical trials are underway to define the role of clopidogrel and warfarin pharmacogenetics in clinical practice.

The FDA includes pharmacogenomic information on more than 100 drug labels, as well as black-box warnings against the use of certain medications or dosages in genetically mediated variances. For example, the label for simvastatin limits doses to no more than 40 mg daily because higher doses increase the risk of myopathy, although this risk is nearly completely confined to patients with the SLCO1B1 variant. Ultrarapid metabolizers of codeine have a risk of respiratory depression when this medication is used post-tonsillectomy, and thus the label now recommends against the use of codeine in this setting.

Scientific trials reported in the literature have used both a point-of-care and a preemptive strategy for the implementation of pharmacogenomic testing. Point-of-care testing utilizes rapid genetic testing to uncover a small number of individual variants when a target medication such as clopidogrel is prescribed. Preemptive genetic testing provides data for multiple variants; then these data are made part of the EHR and are available before prescribing any medication. Several studies of pharmacogenomic testing across multiple medication–gene pairs have demonstrated variants considered to be important if specific target medications are prescribed. In the United States, CPID is addressing barriers to pharmacogenomic testing, such as adequate pharmacogenomic evidence, clinical expertise regarding prescribing the target agent or alternatives, and development of guidelines.

Selected Bibliography

Au N, & Rettie AE. (2008). Pharmacogenomics of 4-hydroxycoumarin anticoagulants *Drug Metab Rev. 40*:355–375.

Beery, T, Workman, ML, & Eggert, J (2018). *Genetics and Genomics in Nursing and Health Care* (2nd Edition). FA Davis, Philadelphia, PA.

Belle, DJ & Singh, H (2008). Genetic factors in drug metabolism. *American Family Physician, 77*(11), 1553–1560.

Elias DJ, Elias DJ, Topol EJ. Warfarin pharmacogenomics: a big step forward for individualized medicine: Enlightened dosing of warfarin. *Eur J Hum Genet. 16*:532–534.

Epstein RS, Moyer TP, Aubert RE, et al. Warfarin genotyping reduces hospitalization rates results from the MM-WES (Medco-Mayo Warfarin Effectiveness study). *J Am Coll Cardiol. 55*:2804–2812.

Howland, R. (2012). Future prospects for pharmacogenetics in the quest for personalized medicine. *Journal of Psychosocial Nursing, 50*: 13–60.

Mele, C & Goldschmidt, K (2014). Pharmacogenomics in pediatrics: Personalized medicine showing eminent promise. *J. Pediatric Nursing, 29*, 378–382.

Phillips, EJ, Sukasem, C, Whirl-Carrillo, M, Muller, DJ, Dunnernberger, HM, Chantratita, Goldspiel, B, Chen, YT, Carleton, BC, George, AL, Mushiroda, T, Klein, T, Gammal, RS, & Pirohamed, M (2018). Clinical pharmacogenetics implementation consortium (CPIC) guideline for HLA genotype and use of carbamazepine and oxcarbazepine. *Clin Pharmacol Ther. 103*(4), 574–581.

Relling, MV & Evans, WE (2015). Pharmacogenomics in the clinic. Nature, 526(75730: 343-50. Volpe, S et al (2018). Research directions in the clinical implementation of pharmacogenomics-An overview of US programs and projects. *Clin Pharmacol Ther, 103*(5): 778–786.

Roden, DM, McLeod, HL, Relling, MV, Williams, MS, Mensah, GA, Peterson, JF, Van Driest, SL (2019). Pharmacogenomics. *Lancet, 394*: 521–532.

Weinshilboum, R & Wang, L (2017). Pharmacogenomics: Precision, medicine and drug response. *Mayo Clinic Proc. 92*(11): 1711–1722.

3

Integumentary System Medications

REBECCA M. LUTZ

Overview

The integumentary system is composed of the skin, hair, nails, and glands. The skin is the largest and most visible organ of the body. Life-threatening diseases of the skin are uncommon, though the appearance of skin disease may represent the presence of systemic disease. Skin diseases affect a large portion of the population; approximately 27% of people in the United States have a dermatologic condition (Lim et al., 2017). All ages may develop skin disease, though the highest prevalence is among adults 65 years and older. Alterations in normal skin physiology are common. Multiple factors can affect the skin barrier, including age, genetics, race and ethnicity, risk-taking behaviors, trauma, infections, chemicals, sun exposure, and skin care practices.

Relevant Physiology

The skin is the largest organ of the body in terms of surface area and weight. Skin surface size is relative to body size, and skin comprises approximately 15% to 20% of total body weight. The skin is composed of three distinct layers. The epidermis is the outermost layer, the dermis is the middle layer, and the hypodermis (subcutaneous layer) is the innermost layer (Fig. 3.1). Primary functions of the integumentary system include barrier protection (physical and biological), sensation, metabolism, and thermoregulation.

The epidermis is composed of five layers of varying thickness. The stratum corneum is made up of keratinocytes and is the outermost barrier. The three middle layers are composed of keratinocytes that change as they migrate to eventually form the stratum corneum. These layers are the stratum lucidum (found on the soles and palms), stratum granulosum (the site of keratin production), and stratum spinosum (provides strength and structure to the skin). The innermost layer is the stratum basale, where the basal cells divide to form keratinocytes. This layer also contains melanin, which provides pigment and ultraviolet protection to the skin. The thinnest skin on the body is on the eyelids and the thickest is on the soles of the feet and palms.

The dermis is composed of connective tissue and varies in thickness. The dermis provides support (binds the dermis to the epidermis) and flexibility. The dermis contains nerves, blood vessels, hair follicles, sweat glands, and sebaceous glands.

The hypodermis is the innermost layer. This layer contains macrophages, fibroblasts, adipose cells, nerves, fine muscles, blood vessels, lymphatic capillaries, and hair follicle roots. This layer provides protection, cushioning, and insulation.

Relevant Pathophysiology

Understanding the presentations of skin diseases is crucial to a diagnosis. A comprehensive patient assessment and complete physical examination lead to the underlying pathophysiology. The patient assessment includes a review of personal and familial history, health status, medications, and allergies. The physical examination identifies lesions, texture or color changes, and the location and distribution of lesions.

Lesions are classified as primary or secondary. Primary lesions arise from healthy skin and have specific characteristics. They may be congenital or acquired over time and may indicate a disease process. Secondary lesions result from a primary lesion and may be due to disease progression, damage (such as excoriation from scratching), or infection.

The pathophysiology of acne, dermatitis, infections (bacterial, viral, and fungal), infestations, and psoriasis will be discussed briefly in the following sections. Topical mediations will be reviewed by category rather than by disease because therapeutic interventions may overlap.

Acne

Acne vulgaris is caused by multiple factors including *Cutibacterium acnes* (formerly *Propionibacterium acnes*) and the balance of the skin microbiome, the proliferation of keratinocytes in the follicle, androgen-mediated increases in sebum production, and inflammation (Masterson, 2018). Acne commonly affects adolescents and young adults but

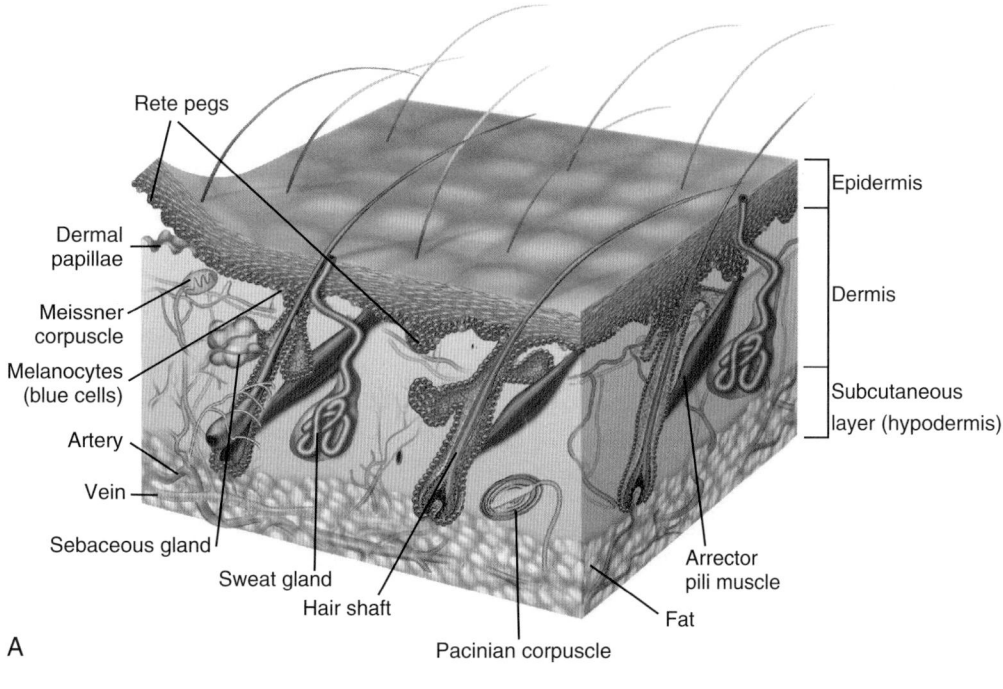

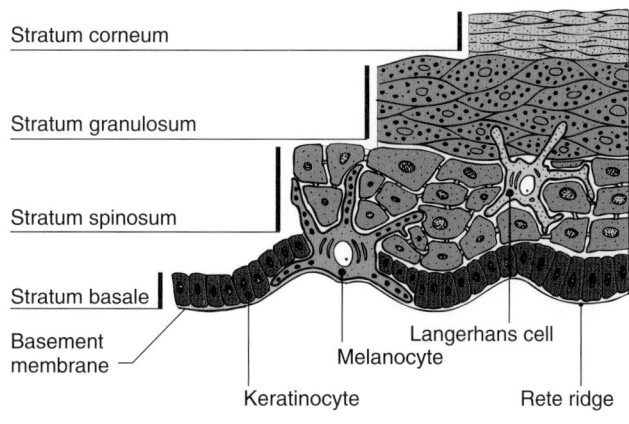

• **Fig. 3.1** Structure of the skin. **(A)** Cross section showing major skin structures. **(B)** Layers of the epidermis. (A from Kumar, V., et al. [2012]. *Robbins & Cotran: Pathologic basis of disease* [9th ed.]. St. Louis: Saunders; B from Gawkrodger D., & Ardern-Jones, M. R. [2012]. *Dermatology* [5th ed.]. Philadelphia: Churchill Livingstone.)

can occur in adulthood. The prevalence of acne is similar in males and females, though the presentation in males is often more severe.

The goal of treatment is to decrease symptoms and prevent scarring to minimize the psychological effects of acne. The topical therapy of acne vulgaris includes over-the-counter (OTC) or prescription products. Pharmacologic treatment of acne includes topical therapies, systemic antibiotics, hormonal therapy, and isotretinoin. Agents may be used as monotherapy or combination therapy. Health care providers should consider the patient's age, location and severity of the disease, and patient preference when choosing a treatment. This chapter will review one exemplar from each therapeutic category: antibacterial agents, topical retinoids, and antibacterial-retinoid combination therapy. Oral contraceptives and some oral antibiotics are effective for the

treatment of acne. These will be covered in Chapter 20 and Unit 13, respectively.

Atopic Dermatitis/Eczema

Atopic dermatitis is a broad term that is used interchangeably with *eczema*. Atopic dermatitis results from an inflammatory response to irritants, allergens, autoimmune factors, genetics, or a combination of many causes. This condition affects children (15%), with higher rates noted among females and those identifying as Black (McKenzie & Silverberg, 2019). Children with atopic dermatitis have higher rates of asthma and decreased quality-of-life indicators compared to their peers. The prevalence rate in adults is 7%, with females having a higher prevalence than males (Chiesa Fuxench et al., 2019; Perrone et al., 2017). Adults with atopic dermatitis reported decreased quality of life and increased anxiety or depression (Chiesa Fuxench et al., 2019; Perrone et al., 2017).

Atopic dermatitis is classified as mild, moderate, or severe and may be chronic or acute. Acute lesions are characterized by defined borders of inflammation with erythema, pustules, crusts, scales, erosions, pruritus, and pain. Chronic changes occur gradually with less-defined borders, erythema, scaling, patches and plaques, dry skin, lichenification, and desquamation. Initial treatment focuses on removing or avoiding irritants or allergens. Therapeutic options include emollients, topical corticosteroids, antibiotics if infected, and topical calcineurin inhibitors.

Infections

Skin and soft tissue infections are common in both the outpatient and inpatient settings. Infections include bacterial, viral, and fungal pathogens. Treatment of these infections includes topical as well as systemic therapeutics.

Bacterial Infections

The most common causes of bacterial skin infections are *Staphylococcus aureus*, *Streptococcus* spp., gram-negative organisms, and mixed pathogens (both gram-negative and gram-positive bacteria). Adults older than 18 years have higher incidence rates than children and adolescents younger than 18 years. Cellulitis and abscesses are the most common bacterial infections, followed by folliculitis and impetigo (Ray et al., 2013).

Viral Infections

Four common viral infections include herpes simplex virus (HSV-1 and HSV-2), herpes zoster (shingles), varicella-zoster (chickenpox), and human papillomavirus (warts). Viral infections may be transmitted by contact with skin, mucous membranes, or saliva. Chapter 48 includes information on the use of oral antiviral medications.

Fungal Infections

Fungal infections are common and are caused by dermatophytes (*Epidermophyton*, *Microsporum*, and *Trichophyton*). Dermatophyte infections are limited to the stratum corneum layer of the skin (nails and hair) because they require keratin. Dermatophytes are classified depending on their location: tinea capitis (head), tinea corporis (body), tinea cruris (groin), or tinea pedis (foot). Candidiasis is predominately caused by the yeast *Candida albicans*. Tinea versicolor is caused by the yeast *Malassezia furfur*. Tinea versicolor results in discolored and hypopigmented patches or lesions on the skin.

The most common sites of fungal infection include the skin, nails, skin folds of the groin, mucosal areas of the mouth, throat, esophagus, and vulvovaginal area. Yeast is a normal part of the body's flora, but overgrowth can be precipitated by an imbalance caused by drugs, disease, or obesity. Individuals with compromised immune systems are the most vulnerable to fungal infections. Additional information on antifungals can be found in Chapter 47.

Infestations

Scabies and pediculosis are the most common skin and hair infestations. They cause pruritis and secondary lesions, and infections are common.

Scabies

Scabies is the infestation of the stratum corneum by the *Sarcoptes scabiei* mite. The female mite burrows into the stratum corneum to lay eggs. A hypersensitivity reaction produces intense pruritus and urticaria. Scabies affects people of all ages, sexes, and socioeconomic classes. It is more prevalent in overcrowded conditions and hot, humid environments. Transmission is by direct, prolonged skin-to-skin contact with an infected person.

Pediculosis

Pediculosis results from an infestation of pediculi (lice). Head lice (*pediculosis capitis*) infestations are common in all ages but are most common in school-age children. Crab lice (*pthirus pubis*) are transmitted primarily by sexual contact. Body lice (*pediculosis corporis*) are often associated with poor hygiene and transmit diseases such as typhus, relapsing fever, and trench fever.

Psoriasis

Psoriasis is a chronic, inflammatory disorder of the skin and is characterized by the presence of papules, scales, plaques, and erythema. Manifestations of psoriasis also occur on the nails. There are several types of psoriasis, but the most common is plaque psoriasis. A family history of psoriasis is common, with onset occurring before age 40. Late onset is usually due to comorbidities such as obesity, smoking, hypertension, or diabetes rather than a familial relationship.

Pharmacologic treatment of mild psoriasis includes the use of emollients (moisturization), keratolytic agents (scaling), corticosteroids (inflammation), and vitamin D analogs (epidermal proliferation). Moderate to severe psoriasis treatments include cyclosporine, methotrexate, acitretin, and biologics. Nontopical pharmacologic treatments of psoriasis are not included in this chapter.

General Prescribing Principles

Several factors affect treatment outcomes, and health care providers should consider these variables before prescribing topical therapeutics. Effective topical therapy depends on the site of application, delivery method (vehicle), dosing, and potency.

Site of Application

The thickness and integrity of the epidermis affect penetration and absorption. When the stratum corneum is thin, broken, inflamed, or irritated, drug absorption is increased. Areas with thick epidermis, such as the soles of the feet, or intact epidermis have decreased penetration and absorption.

Drug Delivery Method (Vehicle)

Absorption of the drug depends on the delivery method (the vehicle), the base, and the active medication concentration. Vehicles include ointments, creams, lotions, solutions, suspensions, gels, foams, and sprays. Ointments and creams are useful as lubricants but may be difficult to apply. Ointments and creams are usually used for the treatment of dry, scaly lesions. Lotions, gels, foams, and sprays are useful drying agents and are convenient to apply. Table 3.1 provides a summary of common vehicles available for topical preparations.

Dosing

Health care providers should consider the size of the treatment area and the frequency of application when determining the quantity of medication to dispense. Topical medications are commonly dispensed in 15-gm, 30-gm, 45-gm, and 60-gm containers. Factors influencing the amount include body

PRACTICE PEARLS

Guidelines to Determine Vehicle of Delivery

All Populations

- Use only until control is achieved; use beyond 2 weeks should be reevaluated.

Geriatrics

- Start at the low end of the dosing range.

Pediatrics

- Limit dosage to smallest clinically effective amount due to potential for corticosteroid-induced hypothalamic–pituitary–adrenal (HPA) axis suppression and Cushing's syndrome.
- Parents of pediatric patients should be advised not to use tight-fitting diapers or plastic pants on a child being treated in the diaper area, as these garments may constitute occlusive dressings.

TABLE 3.1 Common Vehicles for Topical Preparations

Vehicle	Characteristics	Areas of Application
Ointments	Useful for treating dry or thick, hyperkeratotic lesions Translucent in color Poor patient satisfaction: • Thick and greasy with oil or petroleum jelly base • Difficult to wash off • Not easily spreadable	Skin, palms, soles of feet Do not use on intertriginous areas
Creams: Mixes of Water Suspended in Oil	Less potent than ointments but more potent than lotions Vehicle most frequently prescribed White in color Easy to apply and remove: less greasy than ointments Preservatives may cause irritation, stinging, burning	Skin with short or sparse hair Intertriginous areas
Lotions	Contain alcohol: drying effect Least greasy and occlusive Easy to apply and remove	Intertriginous areas Hairy areas Easily covers large areas
Solutions and Suspensions	Spread easily Cooling and soothing sensation Aid in drying of lesions If alcohol-based, may cause stinging, dryness, or irritation	All areas including hair-bearing areas
Gels	Become nongreasy liquids during application Easy to apply and remove Cooling sensation, but if alcohol-based, may cause stinging, dryness, or irritation	Face, scalp Hair-bearing areas
Foams	Easy to apply and remove Low residue Increased absorption Stinging and burning sensation	All areas including large areas and hair-bearing areas
Sprays	Treat large areas easily Ability to apply thin layers Generally cooling sensation Depending on base: stinging and burning	Caution in intertriginous areas due to increased absorption

TABLE 3.2	Fingertip Units (FTUs) Needed to Treat Different Body Parts		
Body Part	FTUs for One Application	Weight of Ointment Required for One Application	Tube Size to Dispense for Complete Coverage of Area for Twice-Daily Application Over 10 Days
Face and neck	2.5	1.25 Gm	30 Gm
Trunk (front or back)	7	3.5 Gm	60 Gm
One arm	3	1.5 Gm	30 Gm
One hand (both sides)	1	0.5 Gm	15 Gm
One leg	6	3 Gm	60 Gm
One foot	2	1 Gm	30 Gm

Modified from Habif, T. P. (2009). *Clinical dermatology* (5th ed.). St. Louis: Mosby.

size (height and weight), age, delivery method, and thickness of application. A commonly used method of measurement is the fingertip unit (FTU). An FTU is the amount of ointment from a tube with a standard 5-mm nozzle tip that covers from the tip of the finger to the distal crease. In adults, one FTU is approximately 0.5 Gm and is equal to the area covered by two hands. Topical ointment and creams are dispensed in 15-Gm, 30-Gm, and 60-Gm tubes. Table 3.2 provides a summary of FTUs needed for treatment depending on body part.

Medication Classifications

Topical Corticosteroids

Corticosteroids are steroid hormones produced by the adrenal gland (endogenous) or are synthetic analogs. Glucocorticoids and mineralocorticoids are the two main classes of corticosteroids. Topical corticosteroids have antiinflammatory, vasoconstrictive, immunomodulatory, gluconeogenic, and antimitotic properties. Topical corticosteroids are useful in managing acute, chronic, and relapsing dermatologic processes in adults and children. Therapeutic uses of topical corticosteroids include dermatitis, pruritis, eczema, psoriasis, rash, and similar noninfectious skin conditions. The selection of topical corticosteroids is based on the age of the patient, disease and type of lesion, location of lesion, size of the area requiring treatment, quantity of steroid required, frequency of application, and duration of therapy.

Potency is an important variable when considering topical corticosteroid therapy. Topical corticosteroids are grouped based on their potency, ranging from Group I (super-high potency) to Group VII (lowest potency). The potency of a steroid is determined using the skin-blanching assay (also known as the vasoconstrictor assay). Once applied to the skin, topical corticosteroids cause a superficial blanching (or vasoconstriction) of the skin which is used as a measurement of potency or absorption. Table 3.3 provides a summary of the medications in each group based on equivalent potency. Table 3.4 provides a summary of indications and dosing. Health care providers should note that certain drugs cross the group thresholds. Numerous drug–drug interactions may occur with the use of corticosteroids, and health care providers should review potential interactions when prescribing.

PRACTICE PEARLS

Prescribing Tips for Topical Corticosteroids

- Penetration of the drug varies by individual, vehicle, degree of damage to the skin barrier, and use of occlusive dressings.
- The use of topical corticosteroids in intertriginous, flexor, and facial areas increases the risk of adverse effects.
- The topical application of corticosteroids to the genitourinary tract for prolonged periods may produce systemic effects.
- Localized adverse effects increase with the use of an occlusive dressing, extended treatment periods, and use in young children with diapers which act as an occlusive dressing.
- Systemic effects may occur when corticosteroids are used over large areas of the body, for a prolonged period, in areas with high permeability or poor integrity, under an occlusive dressing, in infants and children, or when Group I agents are used.
- Topical corticosteroids are contraindicated when primary infection is suspected or with altered skin integrity.

PRACTICE PEARLS

Topical Corticosteroid Use During Pregnancy and Lactation

- Topical corticosteroids should be used during pregnancy in small amounts for short periods, and only when need outweighs risk.
- Mild/moderate topical corticosteroids are preferred to potent/very potent preparations in pregnancy.
- High-potency and ultrahigh-potency preparations are contraindicated in preconception and the first trimester.
- Restrictions in fetal growth with maternal exposure to potent/very potent topical corticosteroids have been reported.
- The effects on lactation are not known. Corticosteroids absorbed systemically can be detected in breast milk, but quantities are not likely to affect the infant.

TABLE 3.3 **Potency Ranking of Topical Corticosteroids**

Potency	Generic	Strength	Vehicle	U.S. Brand
Group I: Super-High Potency	Betamethasone dipropionate, augmented	0.05%	Gel, lotion, ointment (optimized)	Diprolene
	Clobetasol propionate	0.05%	Cream, gel, ointment, solution (scalp)	Temovate
		0.05%	Cream, emollient base	Temovate E
		0.05%	Lotion, shampoo, spray aerosol	Clobex
		0.05%	Foam aerosol	Olux-E, Tovet
		0.05%	Solution (scalp)	Cormax
	Fluocinonide	0.1%	Cream	Vanos
	Flurandrenolide	4 mcg/cm^2	Tape (roll)	Cordran
	Halobetasol propionate	0.05%	Cream, lotion, ointment	Ultravate
Group II: High Potency	Amcinonide	0.1%	Ointment	Amcinonide
	Betamethasone dipropionate	0.05%	Ointment	— [a]
		0.05%	Cream, AF	Diprolene AF
	Clobetasol propionate	0.025%	Cream	Impoyz
	Desoximetasone	0.25%	Cream, ointment, spray	Topicort
		0.05%	Gel	Topicort
	Diflorasone diacetate	0.05%	Ointment	— [a]
		0.05%	Cream, emollient	ApexiCon E
	Fluocinonide	0.05%	Cream, gel, ointment, solution	Lidex
	Halcinonide	0.1%	Cream, ointment, solution	Halog
	Halobetasol propionate	0.01%	Lotion	Bryhali
Group III: Medium-High Potency	Amcinonide	0.1%	Cream, lotion	Amcinonide
	Betamethasone dipropionate	0.05%	Cream, hydrophilic emollient	— [a]
	Betamethasone valerate	0.1%	Ointment	Beta-Val
		0.12%	Foam	Luxiq
	Desoximetasone	0.05%	Cream	Topicort
	Diflorasone diacetate	0.05%	Cream	— [a]
	Fluocinonide	0.05%	Cream, aqueous emollient	— [a]
	Fluticasone propionate	0.005%	Ointment	Cutivate
	Mometasone furoate	0.1%	Ointment	Elocon
	Triamcinolone acetonide	0.5%	Cream, ointment	Triderm
Group IV: Medium Potency	Betamethasone dipropionate	0.05%	Spray	Sernivo
	Clocortolone pivalate	0.1%	Cream	Cloderm
	Fluocinolone acetonide	0.025%	Ointment	Synalar
	Flurandrenolide	0.05%	Ointment	Cordran
	Hydrocortisone valerate	0.2%	Ointment	Westcort
	Mometasone furoate	0.1%	Cream, lotion, ointment, solution	Elecon

Continued

TABLE 3.3	**Potency Ranking of Topical Corticosteroids—cont'd**				

Potency	Generic	Strength	Vehicle	U.S. Brand
	Triamcinolone acetonide	0.1%	Cream	Triderm
		0.1%	Ointment	— [a]
		0.05%	Ointment	Trianex
		0.2 mg per 2 sec spray	Aerosol spray	Kenalog
		0.1%	Dental paste	Oralone
Group V: Lower-Mid Potency	Betamethasone dipropionate	0.05%	Lotion	— [a]
	Betamethasone valerate	0.1%	Cream	Beta-Val
	Desonide	0.05%	Ointment	Des Owen
		0.05%	Gel	Desonate
	Fluocinolone acetonide	0.025%	Cream	Synalar
	Flurandrenolide	0.05%	Cream, lotion	Cordran
	Fluticasone propionate	0.05%	Cream, lotion	Cutivate
	Hydrocortisone butyrate	0.1%	Cream, lotion, ointment, solution	Locoid, Locoid Lipocream
	Hydrocortisone probutate	0.1%	Cream	Pandel
	Hydrocortisone valerate	0.2%	Cream	— [a]
	Prednicarbate	0.1%	Cream (emollient), ointment	— [a]
	Triamcinolone acetonide	0.1%	Lotion	— [a]
		0.025%	Ointment	— [a]
Group VI: Low Potency	Alclometasone dipropionate	0.05%	Cream, ointment	Aclovate
	Betamethasone valerate	0.1%	Lotion	— [a]
	Desonide	0.05%	Cream	DesOwen,
		0.05%	Lotion	DesOwen, LoKara
		0.05%	Foam	Verdeso
	Fluocinolone acetonide	0.01%	Cream, solution	Synalar
		0.01%	Shampoo	Capex
		0.01%	Oil (48% refined peanut oil)	Derma-Smoothe/FS Body, Derma-Smoothe/FS Scalp
	Triamcinolone acetonide	0.025%	Cream, lotion	Triderm (cream)
Group VII: Least Potent	Hydrocortisone (base, ≥2%)	2.5%	Cream, ointment	Hytone
		2.0%	Lotion	Hytone, Ala Scalp, Scalacort
		2.5%	Solution	Texacort
	Hydrocortisone (base, <2%)	1.0%	Ointment	Cortaid, Cortizone 10, Hytone, Nutracort
		1.0%	Cream	Cortizone 10, Hytone, Synacort
		1.0%	Gel	Cortizone 10

TABLE 3.3   Potency Ranking of Topical Corticosteroids—cont'd

Potency	Generic	Strength	Vehicle	U.S. Brand
		1.0%	Lotion	Aquanil HC, Sarnol-HC, Cortizone 10
		1.0%	Spray	Cortaid
		1.0%	Solution	Cortaid, Noble, Scalp Relief
		0.5%	Cream, ointment	Cortaid
	Hydrocortisone acetate	2.5%	Cream	MiCort-HC
		2.0%	Lotion	Nucort

ªKey: — Generic may be available; *AF*: augmented formulation

Data from Comparison of representative topical corticosteroid preparations (classified according to the US system), Up-To-Date, 2020 (accessed November 29, 2020); Comparison of representative topical corticosteroid preparations (classified according to the US system) (Lexi-Drugs), Lexicomp Online, Copyright © 1978–2020 Lexicomp, Inc. (accessed November 29, 2020); U.S. Food & Drug Administration. (n. d.), Orange book: Approved drug products with therapeutic equivalence evaluations (accessed November 29, 2020), https://www.accessdata.fda.gov/scripts/cder/ob/search_product.cfm.

TABLE 3.4   Topical Corticosteroids Dosing Recommendations

Potency	Medication	Indications	Dosage	Considerations and Monitoring
Group I: Super-High Potency	Betamethasone dipropionate, augmented	Moderate-to-severe inflammation and pruritus due to corticosteroid-responsive dermatologic disorders Plaque psoriasis Seborrheic dermatitis	**0.05% Cream, gel, lotion, ointment:** *Adults and children >12 yr:* Apply thin layer to affected area once or twice daily. Cream, gel, ointment: Maximum dosage: 50 Gm/wk. Lotion: Maximum dosage: 50 mL/wk.	Limit treatment to 2 consecutive weeks.
	Clobetasol propionate	Corticosteroid responsive dermatoses Moderate to severe plaque psoriasis	**0.05% Non-emollient cream, foam, gel, ointment, scalp solution, spray:** *Adults, adolescents, and children ≥12 yr:* Apply thin layer to affected areas twice daily. Maximum dosage: 50 Gm/wk or 50 mL/wk. **0.05% Lotion:** *Adults:* Apply a thin layer to affected areas twice daily. Moderate to severe plaque psoriasis: Do not exceed 10% body surface area. Maximum dosage: 50 Gm/wk. **0.05% Emollient cream (psoriasis):** *Adults and adolescents ≥16 yr:* Apply a thin layer to affected area twice daily. Maximum dosage: 50 g/wk. Body surface area >10%: Limit treatment to 2 consecutive weeks. Body surface area 5%-10%: treatment can be extended to 4 consecutive weeks. **0.05% Shampoo (Psoriasis):** *Adults:* Apply to dry affected areas once daily, leave in place 15 min, then lather and rinse. Maximum dosage: 50 mL/wk.	Limit treatment to 2 consecutive weeks.

Continued

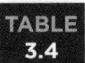

TABLE 3.4   Topical Corticosteroids Dosing Recommendations—cont'd

Potency	Medication	Indications	Dosage	Considerations and Monitoring
	Halobetasol propionate	Corticosteroid-responsive dermatoses Moderate to severe plaque psoriasis	**0.05% Cream, lotion, ointment** *Adults:* Apply thin layer to affected area once or twice daily. Maximum dosage: 50 Gm/wk. *Adolescents and children >12 yr:* Apply a thin layer to affected area twice daily. Maximum dosage: 50 Gm/wk. **0.05% Topical foam:** *Adults:* Apply a thin layer to affected area twice daily. Maximum dosage: 50 Gm/wk. **0.01% Lotion (Bryhali lotion):** *Adults:* Apply a thin layer to affected area once daily. Limit treatment to 8 consecutive weeks. Maximum dosage: 50 Gm/wk.	FDA not recommended for children <12 yr; safety and efficacy have not been established.
Group II: High Potency	Amcinonide	Corticosteroid-responsive dermatoses Psoriasis	**0.1% Cream, lotion, ointment:** *Adults, adolescents, and children:* Apply topically and sparingly to affected area two to three times daily. Maximum dosage: Three times daily.	Infants and neonates: safety and efficacy have not been established.
	Desoximetasone	Moderate to severe inflammatory manifestations, including pruritus, of corticosteroid responsive dermatoses	**0.25% Cream, ointment; 0.5% Cream, gel, ointment:** *Adults, adolescents, and children ≥10 yr:* Apply sparingly to affected areas twice daily. Rub in gently. **0.25% Spray (plaque psoriasis only):** *Adults:* Apply sparingly to affected areas twice daily. Rub in gently. Do not use if atrophy present. Discontinue after 4 weeks of treatment.	Limit treatment to 2 consecutive weeks. Safety and efficacy not established in children <10 yr.
	Diflorasone diacetate	Corticosteroid-responsive dermatoses Psoriasis Inflammatory hyperkeratotic dermatosis Severe chronic plaque-type psoriasis	**0.05% Non-emollient cream, ointment:** *Adults, adolescents, and children:* Apply thin layer to affected area one to four times daily. Maximum dosage: Adults and adolescents: 50 Gm/wk. Maximum dosage: Children: 10 Gm/wk. **0.05% Emollient cream, ointment:** *Adults:* Apply thin layer to affected area one to three times daily. Maximum dosage: Adults: 50 Gm/wk.	Limit treatment to 2 consecutive weeks.
	Fluocinonide	Corticosteroid-responsive dermatoses Psoriasis	**0.05% Cream, gel, ointment, solution:** *Adults, adolescents, and children:* Apply a thin layer to affected areas two to four times daily. Maximum dosage: 4 times daily.	
			0.1% Cream: *Adults, adolescents, and children ≥12 yr:* Apply a thin layer to affected area once or twice daily up to 2 weeks. Maximum dosage: 60 Gm/wk.	If no response is seen within 2 weeks, reassess treatment options.
		Atopic dermatitis	**0.05% Cream, gel, ointment, solution:** *Adults, adolescents, and children:* Apply a thin layer to affected areas two to four times daily. Maximum dosage: 4 times daily.	
			0.1% Cream: *Adults, adolescents, and children ≥12 yr:* Apply a thin layer to affected area once daily up to 2 weeks. Maximum dosage: 60 Gm/wk.	If no response is seen within 2 weeks, reassess treatment options.

TABLE 3.4   Topical Corticosteroids Dosing Recommendations—cont'd

Potency	Medication	Indications	Dosage	Considerations and Monitoring
	Halcinonide (Halog)	Corticosteroid-responsive dermatoses	**0.1% Cream, ointment, solution:** *Adults, adolescents, and children:* Apply sparingly to affected area two to three times daily.	
Group III: Medium to High Potency	Betamethasone dipropionate, nonaugmented	Inflammatory and pruritic dermatoses	**0.05% Cream, ointment:** *Adults and children >13 yr:* Apply thin film to affected skin area once or twice daily. Maximum dosage: 50 Gm/wk or 50 mL/wk.	Do not use on the face, groin, axilla, or other intertriginous areas.
	Betamethasone valerate	Inflammatory and pruritic dermatoses of skin and scalp	**0.1%, Cream, ointment:** *Adults, adolescents, and children:* Apply to affected area one to three times daily. **0.1% Lotion:** *Adults, adolescents, and children:* Apply a few drops twice daily morning and night. Decrease to once daily following improvement. **0.12% Foam:** *Adults:* Apply to scalp twice daily morning and night. If no improvement within 2 wk, discontinue and reassess.	Occlusive dressing may be applied if no infection present.
	Fluticasone propionate	Corticosteroid-responsive dermatoses	**0.05% Ointment:** *Adults:* Apply thin layer to affected areas twice daily up to 2 weeks. **0.05% Cream:** *Adolescents, children, infants ≥3 months:* Apply thin layer twice daily up to 4 weeks.	Do not use occlusive dressings. Maximum dosage: *Adults, adolescents, and children >5 yr:* Cream/ointment: Twice daily; Lotion: Once daily *Children ≥3 months:* Cream: Twice daily; Lotion: Once daily
		Atopic dermatitis	**0.05% Ointment:** *Adults:* Apply thin layer to affected areas twice daily up to 2 weeks. **0.05% Cream:** *Adults:* Apply thin layer to affected area once or twice daily up to 2 weeks. *Adolescents, children, infants ≥3 months:* Apply thin layer once or twice daily up to 4 weeks. **0.05% Lotion:** *Adults, adolescents, and children:* Apply thin layer to affected area once daily up to 4 weeks.	
Group IV: Medium Potency	Flurandrenolide	Corticosteroid-responsive dermatoses Mild to moderate pruritus Corticosteroid-responsive dermatitis	**0.025 %–0.05% Cream; 0.05% lotion, ointment:** *Adults, adolescents, and children:* Apply thin layer to affected area two to three times daily. Maximum dosage: 3 applications daily. **Cordran tape:** *Adults, adolescents, and children:* Apply to affected area every 12–24 hr.	
	Hydrocortisone valerate	Corticosteroid-responsive disorders	**0.2% Cream, ointment:** *Adults:* Apply thin layer to affected area two to three times daily.	

Continued

TABLE 3.4   Topical Corticosteroids Dosing Recommendations—cont'd

Potency	Medication	Indications	Dosage	Considerations and Monitoring
	Mometasone furoate	Corticosteroid-responsive dermatoses Psoriasis	**0.1% Cream, ointment:** *Adults, adolescents, and children >2 yr:* Apply thin layer to affected area once daily. Maxiumum dosage: Once daily. **0.1% Lotion:** *Adults and adolescents ≥12 yr:* Apply a few drops topically to affected area once daily. Maxiumum dosage: Once daily.	Safety and efficacy of treatment for more than 3 weeks in pediatric patients have not been established; limit treatment to 2 consecutive weeks.
Group V: Lower-Mid Potency	Desonide	Corticosteroid-responsive dermatoses	**0.05% Cream, lotion, ointment:** *Adults:* Apply thin layer two to three times daily for up to 2 weeks. Maximum dosage: Cream, ointment: Four applications daily; Lotion: Three applications daily. **0.05% Foam, gel:** *Adults, adolescents, children, infants ≥3 mo:* Apply thin layer to affected area twice daily for up to 4 weeks. Maximum dosage: 2 applications daily.	
	Prednicarbate	Inflammatory and pruritic manifestations of corticosteroid-responsive dermatoses	**0.1% Ointment:** *Adults and children ≥10 yr:* Apply to affected area twice daily. **0.1% Emollient cream:** *Adults and adolescents:* Apply to affected area twice daily. *Children:* Apply to affected area twice daily for not more than 3 weeks.	Safety and efficacy in neonates and infants have not been established.
	Triamcinolone acetonide	Corticosteroid-responsive dermatoses	**0.025%–0.05% Cream, lotion, ointment:** *Adults, adolescents, and children:* Apply thin layer to affected areas two to four times daily. **0.1%–0.5% Cream, lotion, ointment:** *Adults, adolescents, and children:* Apply thin layer to affected areas two to three times daily. **Aerosol:** *Adults, adolescents, and children:* Apply topically to affected areas three to four times daily.	
Group VI: Low Potency	Alclometasone dipropionate	Corticosteroid-responsive dermatoses	**0.05% Cream, ointment:** *Adults, adolescents, and children:* Apply thin layer two to three times daily for up to 2 weeks.	Safety and efficacy in infants have not been established.
Group VII: Least Potent	Hydrocortisone (base, <2%)	Mild to moderate corticosteroid-responsive dermatoses	**0.05% Cream, ointment:** *Adults, adolescents, and children ≥2 yr:* Apply thin layer three to four times daily. **1% Cream, gel, lotion, ointment, spray:** *Adults and children 2–17 yr:* Apply thin layer three to four times daily.	

Life Span Considerations With Topical Corticosteroid Use

Geriatrics

- Increased susceptibility to secondary infections.
- Increased systemic effects due to thinner skin.
- Start at the lowest possible dose.

Pediatrics

- Increased susceptibility to topical corticosteroid-induced hypothalamic-pituitary-adrenal axis suppression and Cushing's syndrome.
- In general, children younger than 12 years should not be treated with Group I or Group II topical corticosteroids without referral to a specialist.

(Hajar et al., 2015)

Group I: Super-High Potency

Clobetasol Propionate 0.05% Cream, Emollient, Foam, Gel, Lotion, Ointment, Shampoo, Solution (Scalp), Spray

Pharmacokinetics. Clobetasol binds to protein at varying rates and is metabolized by the liver. Primary excretion occurs through the renal system with some biliary excretion.

Indications. Clobetasol propionate is a synthetic fluorinated topical corticosteroid. Indications include mild to moderate and moderate to severe plaque psoriasis as well as moderate to severe scalp psoriasis. Treatment of psoriasis may require up to 4 weeks. It is also indicated for the short-term treatment of corticosteroid-responsive dermatoses of the skin.

Adverse Effects. As with other topical corticosteroids, local adverse effects may include atrophy, striae, telangiectasias, folliculitis, acneiform eruptions, hypopigmentation, perioral dermatitis, secondary infection, and milia. Adverse systemic effects include endocrine and metabolic disorders such as hyperglycemia, Cushing's syndrome, hypothalamic-pituitary-adrenal axis, worsening liver failure, glaucoma, and posterior subcapsular cataracts.

Contraindications. Vehicle affects the administration. In children younger than 12 years, the safety and efficacy of the use of the cream, emollient, gel, foam, ointment, and scalp solutions have not been established. In children younger than 18 years, the safety and efficacy of the use of the spray, lotion, and shampoo solutions have not been established. Avoid in the event of primary scalp infections and avoid the use of occlusive dressing or clothing. Avoid application to eyes, lips, face, groin, or axillae. Avoid ophthalmic, oral, or intravaginal use.

Monitoring. Monitor use of the medication and advise patients not to exceed a maximum dosage of 50 Gm/week or 50 mL/week with a maximum duration of 2 consecutive weeks. If the desired response is not achieved after 2 weeks, reassess for alternate diagnosis or treatment plan. Monitor the hypothalamic-pituitary-adrenal axis and adjust dose

using an adrenocorticotropic hormone stimulation test or urine-free cortisol test.

Clobetasol Propionate Foam

- Clobetasol propionate foam is flammable.
- Avoid exposure to flames or smoking during and immediately after application.

Group II: High Potency

Desoximetasone 0.25% Cream, Ointment, Spray

Pharmacokinetics. Desoximetasone is metabolized in the liver. Systemic absorption from intact skin may be increased using an occlusive dressing or with inflammation of the skin. Absorption also varies by application site. Elimination half-life is about 15 hours. Excretion occurs primarily through the kidneys, with less excretion through the bile.

Indications. Desoximetasone is indicated for the treatment of inflammatory hyperkeratotic dermatosis and plaque psoriasis in adults. In the pediatric population, desoximetasone is approved for the treatment of inflammatory hyperkeratotic dermatosis. Desoximetasone is available in a cream, gel, ointment, and spray. No renal or hepatic dose adjustments are required.

Adverse Effects. Local adverse effects may include allergic contact dermatitis, atrophy, blistering, burning and stinging sensations, erythema, folliculitis, periorbital dermatitis, photosensitivity, pruritus, striae, hypopigmentation, and secondary infection. Adverse systemic effects include endocrine and metabolic disorders such as hyperglycemia, adrenal suppression, Cushing's syndrome, hypothalamic-pituitary-adrenal axis dysfunction, intracranial hypertension in pediatric patients, and glaucoma.

Contraindications. Avoid in patients with hypersensitivity to any component of the preparation. Desoximetasone preparations should not be applied to the face, groin, or axillae. Apply with caution around the eyes to decrease risk of visual impairment, ocular hypertension, worsening cataracts, or glaucoma. The spray formulation is contraindicated in children. Use with caution in pediatrics, geriatrics, and altered skin integrity.

Desoximetasone Spray

- Desoximetasone spray formulation is flammable.
- Avoid exposure to flames or smoking during and immediately after application.

Monitoring. Monitor for improvement in symptoms. After 2 weeks, assess for improvement; if there is no improvement, reconsider diagnosis or treatment plan. Monitor for hypothalamic-pituitary-adrenal axis suppression in pediatric patients, and if used over extensive areas, over prolonged periods, under occlusion, or with nonintact skin.

Group III: Medium to High Potency

Betamethasone Dipropionate 0.05% Cream, Hydrophilic Emollient

Pharmacokinetics. Systemic absorption from intact skin may be increased using an occlusive dressing or with inflammation of the skin. Absorption also varies by application site. Betamethasone dipropionate is metabolized in the liver by CYP3A4 to inactive metabolites. Elimination half-life is approximately 5.5 hours. Excretion occurs primarily through the kidneys, with less excretion through the bile.

Indications. Betamethasone dipropionate 0.05% cream is indicated to treat corticosteroid-responsive dermatoses in adults and children. The topical cream should be applied sparingly. In adults, betamethasone dipropionate 0.05% spray is indicated in the treatment of mild to moderate plaque psoriasis. After application, rub in gently and then wash hands.

Adverse Effects. Adverse effects may include bruised skin, erythema, folliculitis, pruritus, skin atrophy, stinging sensations, and unwanted hair growth. Serious adverse systemic effects include allergic contact dermatitis, hyperglycemia, glucosuria, Cushing's syndrome, hypothalamic-pituitary-adrenal axis dysfunction, glaucoma, and posterior subcapsular cataract formation.

Contraindications. Avoid in patients with hypersensitivity to betamethasone dipropionate, other corticosteroids, or any component of the product. In adults and pediatrics, avoid dosages over 50 Gm/week or 50 mL/week. Do not use for longer than 2 weeks. Use with caution for patients with endocrine, immunologic, metabolic, or ophthalmic diseases.

Monitoring. As with other topical corticosteroids, monitor for adverse effects including hypothalamic-pituitary-adrenal axis suppression, visual impairment, ocular hypertension, worsening cataracts, or glaucoma. Laboratory monitoring recommendations include blood glucose and serum potassium. Monitor for improvement in symptoms after 2 weeks. Reassess diagnosis and treatment plan as indicated.

Group IV: Medium Potency

Mometasone Furoate 0.1% Cream, Lotion, Ointment, Solution

Pharmacokinetics. Following topical application, the patient can expect to see an initial response in 3 days to 3 weeks. Excretion is primarily through the kidneys, with a smaller amount through the bile.

Indications. Mometasone furoate is indicated in the treatment of inflammatory hyperkeratotic dermatosis. No dose adjustments are required for patients with renal or hepatic impairment. Discontinue use when control is achieved.

Adverse Effects. Itching, burning, and stinging at the application site are common adverse effects. Other adverse effects include acneiform eruption, skin atrophy, paresthesia, and folliculitis. More serious adverse systemic effects common to other corticosteroids include endocrine and metabolic disorders such as hyperglycemia, adrenal suppression,

Cushing's syndrome, hypothalamic-pituitary-adrenal axis dysfunction, intracranial hypertension in pediatric patients, and glaucoma.

Contraindications. Use in patients with hypersensitivity to mometasone furoate or when any component of the formulation is contraindicated. Use with caution for patients with endocrine, immunologic, metabolic, or ophthalmic diseases.

Monitoring. Monitor for adverse effects including hypothalamic-pituitary-adrenal axis suppression, visual impairment, ocular hypertension, worsening cataracts, or glaucoma. Monitor for improvement of symptoms. If there is no improvement within 2 weeks, reassess the patient.

Group V: Lower to Medium Potency

Fluocinolone acetonide 0.025% cream

Pharmacokinetics. Following topical application, systemic absorption is minimal. Metabolism occurs primarily in the liver. Half-life is between 1 and 2 hours. Excretion is by the kidneys.

Indications. Fluocinolone acetonide 0.025% cream is indicated for the relief of inflammatory and pruritic manifestations of corticosteroid-responsive dermatoses of the skin in adults and children. In adults, fluocinolone acetonide 0.025% cream may also be prescribed for anal and genital pruritus. Difficult-to-manage conditions may be covered by an occlusive dressing.

Adverse Effects. The most common adverse effects include acneiform rash/eruptions, burning, erythema, hypopigmentation, skin atrophy, and telangiectasia. In pediatric patients with a history of atopic dermatitis, a cough, nasal discharge, and nasopharyngitis have been reported. Other adverse effects are those seen with corticosteroids, including endocrine and metabolic disorders such as hyperglycemia, adrenal suppression, Cushing's syndrome, hypothalamic-pituitary-adrenal axis dysfunction, intracranial hypertension in pediatric patients, and glaucoma.

Contraindications. There are few specific contraindications with the use of topical fluocinolone acetonide 0.025% cream. It is contraindicated in patients with hypersensitivity to fluocinolone or any component of the formulation. Use with caution for patients with endocrine, immunologic, metabolic, or ophthalmic diseases.

Monitoring. Monitor for improvement of skin conditions, relief of pruritus, and/or healing of lesions. Reevaluate if there is no improvement after 2 weeks. Monitor for adverse effects including hypothalamic-pituitary-adrenal axis suppression, visual impairment, ocular hypertension, worsening cataracts, or glaucoma.

Group VI: Low Potency

Alclometasone dipropionate 0.05% cream, ointment

Pharmacokinetics. An initial response to eczema or psoriasis occurs in 5 to 7 days. Peak responses are seen in about 14 days. Following topical application, about 3% of the medication is absorbed systemically. Metabolism occurs extensively through the liver. Alclometasone dipropionate metabolites are excreted through the kidneys.

Indications. Alclometasone dipropionate is a low-potency topical corticosteroid effective for a variety of corticosteroid-responsive dermatoses (e.g., eczema, anogenital or senilis pruritus, psoriasis of the facial or genital area). The safety and efficacy of use for infants younger than 1 year have not been established. Dose adjustments are not required for the older adult or for any age patient with renal or hepatic impairment.

Adverse Effects. Common adverse reactions include burning, pruritus, dry skin, folliculitis, acneiform rash/eruption, and hypopigmentation. Skin atrophy usually occurs after prolonged use but may occur if applied to intertriginous or flexor areas, or to the face. Visual impairment, ocular hypertension, worsening cataracts, or glaucoma have been reported. Systemic absorption may result in reversible hypothalamic-pituitary-adrenal axis suppression, Cushing's syndrome, hypertension, hyperglycemia, or glycosuria.

Contraindications. The use of alclometasone dipropionate is contraindicated in patients with hypersensitivity to the medication or any component of the preparation. Use with caution for patients with endocrine, immunologic, metabolic, or ophthalmic diseases.

Monitoring. Routine laboratory monitoring is not required. Monitor for adverse effects including hypothalamic-pituitary-adrenal axis suppression, visual impairment, ocular hypertension, worsening cataracts, or glaucoma. Monitor for improvement of symptoms. If there is no improvement within 2 weeks, reassess for accuracy of diagnosis.

Group VII: Least Potent

Hydrocortisone (base, ≥ 2%), 2.5% cream, ointment
Pharmacokinetics. Topical preparations are absorbed at the area of application. They are minimally absorbed into the circulation. Topical hydrocortisone is metabolized in the skin.

Indications. Low-potency hydrocortisone is available in prescription and OTC formulations. Indications for use include anal and genital pruritus, hemorrhoids, and corticosteroid-responsive dermatoses (e.g., atopic and seborrheic dermatitis, contact dermatitis, vulvar dermatitis, and psoriasis).

Adverse Effects. Few adverse effects have been reported with the use of the lowest-potency hydrocortisone when used as directed. Topical application of hydrocortisone 2.5% may result in acneiform eruption, atrophy, burning, pruritis, skin irritation, or xeroderma at the application site. Following application of hydrocortisone 2.5% cream or ointment, absorption is increased in neonates, infants, and young children.

Contraindications. Avoid use in patients with hypersensitivity to hydrocortisone or any of its components.

Monitoring. Monitor patients for adverse effects including skin atrophy. Though risk is less due to decreased systemic absorption, monitor patients on prolonged therapy for hypothalamic pituitary axis suppression, visual impairment, ocular hypertension, worsening cataracts, or glaucoma. Monitor for potential for overuse.

Calcineurin Inhibitors

The calcineurin inhibitors, tacrolimus and pimecrolimus, are topical immunosuppressants approved for treatment of atopic dermatitis in patients who have not responded to glucocorticoids. Calcineurin inhibitors suppress calcineurin, which affects T-helper cell activity. The resultant decrease in inflammatory mediators (mast cells and neutrophils) results in decreased inflammation. Table 3.5 provides a summary of dosing recommendations.

> **BLACK BOX WARNING!**
>
> **Topical Calcineurin Inhibitors**
> - Long-term safety of topical calcineurin inhibitors has not been established.
> - Skin malignancy and lymphoma have been reported.
> - Avoid long-term, continuous use.
> - Limit application to the affected area only.

TABLE 3.5 Dosing Recommendations: Calcineurin Inhibitors

Medication	Indication	Dose	Considerations and Monitoring
Tacrolimus	Short-term or intermittent long-term treatment of moderate to severe atopic dermatitis	**Ointment 0.03%:** *Adults and children ≥2 yr:* Apply thin layer twice daily for 3 weeks, then once daily until lesions disappear. Maximum dosage: 2 applications/day. **Ointment 0.1%:** *Adults and children ≥16 yr:* Apply thin layer twice daily for 3 weeks, then once daily until lesions disappear. Maximum dosage: 2 applications/day.	Do not use under occlusive dressing. Discontinue when symptoms clear. Reassess diagnosis if no improvement in 6 weeks.
Pimecrolimus	Short-term and intermittent long-term treatment of mild to moderate atopic dermatitis in nonimmunocompromised patients	**Cream 1%:** *Adults and children ≥2 yr:* Apply thin layer twice daily until lesions disappear. Maximum dosage: 2 applications/day.	

Calcineurin Inhibitor Use During Pregnancy and Lactation

- Tacrolimus and pimecrolimus: Fetal abnormalities have been observed in animal studies.
- Tacrolimus and pimecrolimus: Breastfeeding is not recommended.

Tacrolimus 0.1% and 0.03% Ointment

Pharmacokinetics. Topical application of tacrolimus results in minimal systemic absorption or accumulation. Pharmacokinetic studies concluded that blood concentrations of tacrolimus are minimal in adults and children.

Indications. Treatment indications include moderate to severe atopic dermatitis, prevention of relapses, and extending the time between recurrences in patients with frequent exacerbations. Tacrolimus is approved in adults and children older than 2 years (potency is dose dependent). Tacrolimus 0.03% is indicated in children 2 to 16 years. Tacrolimus 0.1% is indicated for children older than 16 years.

Adverse Effects. The most common local symptoms include skin burning sensations and pruritus. Other adverse effects include erythema, flu-like symptoms, headache, allergic reaction, and skin infection. Adults treated with tacrolimus 0.1% reported slightly higher incidence of reported adverse effects when compared with the incidence of adverse effects reported with the use of tacrolimus 0.03%. There have been reports of skin cancer or lymphoma with therapy.

Contraindications. Tacrolimus is contraindicated in the presence of hypersensitivity to tacrolimus or any component of the product. Avoid if bacterial or viral cutaneous infections are present. Infections should be resolved before tacrolimus is initiated. Exposure to ultraviolet light (sunlight) should be avoided.

Monitoring. No laboratory monitoring is required for use of tacrolimus topical preparations. Monitor for signs of toxicity, hypersensitivity, worsening of condition, or adverse effects. Monitor for improvement in the appearance of lesions after 6 weeks of treatment. If there is no improvement, discontinue and reassess diagnosis. Monitor for development of skin cancer or lymphoma.

Pimecrolimus 1% Cream

Pharmacokinetics. A significant response to treatment usually occurs within 8 days. Blood-level concentrations and systemic absorption are minimal in adults and children. Topical application results in minimal metabolism. Patients with renal or hepatic insufficiency do not require dose adjustments.

Indications. Pimecrolimus is indicated as second-line therapy in the treatment of mild to moderate atopic dermatitis when topical corticosteroids are contraindicated or not tolerated. The treatment of relapses or recurrences has not been approved. Indicated for use in adults and children older than 2 years.

Adverse Effects. Application site irritation, including burning, stinging, or soreness, is the most commonly reported reaction in adults and children. Other adverse effects include headache, fever, upper respiratory tract infections, nasopharyngitis, cough, and bronchitis. These effects were more common in children and adolescents than in adults. Post-marketing reports of anaphylactic reactions, ocular irritation after application of the cream to the eyelids or near the eyes, angioneurotic edema, facial edema, and skin flushing have infrequently been reported. Skin cancer or lymphoma have been reported.

Contraindications. Pimecrolimus is contraindicated in individuals with a history of hypersensitivity to pimecrolimus or any of the components of the cream. Avoid in immunocompromised patients, those with bacterial or viral skin infections, and patients with malignant or premalignant skin conditions. Skin infections should be resolved before pimecrolimus is initiated. Exposure to ultraviolet light should be avoided. Safety of noncontinuous use for longer than 1 year has not been established.

Monitoring. No laboratory monitoring is required. Monitor for signs of toxicity, hypersensitivity, worsening of condition, or adverse effects. Monitor for development of skin cancer or lymphoma. Monitor for improvement in the appearance of lesions after 6 weeks of treatment. If there is no improvement, discontinue and reassess diagnosis.

Retinoids

Retinoids are a mainstay of acne therapy. Retinoids are derivatives of vitamin A with comedolytic and antiinflammatory properties. As comedolytics, retinoids normalize desquamation which decreases clogging of comedones. The antiinflammatory properties inhibit inflammation by decreasing the release of cytokines and nitric oxide. Table 3.6 provides a summary of dosing recommendations.

Retinoid Use During Pregnancy and Lactation

- Retinoids are teratogenic.
- Establish negative pregnancy prior to therapy.
- The effects of these medications during lactation are not known.

Tretinoin

Topical retinoids are vitamin A derivatives. They decrease visible comedones, inhibit microcomedones, stimulate mitotic activity, and increase the turnover of follicular epithelial cells causing extrusion of the comedones.

Pharmacokinetics. The onset of action is 2 to 7 weeks. Systemic absorption is minimal and is dependent upon skin integrity and the length of treatment. Metabolism is within the liver and excretion occurs through the urine and feces.

TABLE 3.6   Dosing Recommendations: Retinoids

Medication	Indications	Dosage	Considerations and Monitoring
Adapalene	Acne vulgaris	**0.1% Cream, gel, lotion, solution; 0.3% gel:** *Adults and children ≥12 yr:* Apply thin film to affected areas once daily. Use cream and gel at bedtime. May take 8 to 12 weeks for benefits to appear. *Children <12 yr:* Efficacy and safety not established.	There are no adequate and well controlled studies in pregnant women.
Tazarotene	Acne vulgaris	**0.1% Cream, gel:** *Adults and children ≥12 yr:* Clean and dry face. Apply thin layer once daily in evening at bedtime to lesions for up to 12 weeks. **Lotion 0.045%:** *Adults, adolescents, and children ≥9 yr:* Apply thin layer to affected area once daily.	Contraindicated in pregnancy or in women who may become pregnant. Initiate therapy during menstrual cycle.
	Plaque psoriasis	**0.05% or 1% Cream:** *Adults:* Apply in evening at bedtime to clean, dry lesions. **0.5% or 1% Gel:** *Adults, adolescents and children ≥12 yr:* Apply in the evening at bedtime. Apply thin film to no more than 20% of body surface area. Begin with 0.5% and increase to 1% if necessary.	
	Adjunct therapy: fine facial wrinkles, facial hyperpigmentation or hypopigmentation	**0.1% Cream:** *Adults and adolescents ≥17 yr:* Apply pea-sized amount to clean, dry facial skin at bedtime.	
Tretinoin	Acne vulgaris	**0.025% or 0.05% or 0.1% Cream; 0.025% or 0.01% or 0.05% gel:** *Adults, adolescents, and children ≥12 yr:* Apply thin layer to affected areas at bedtime. Up to 7 weeks of therapy may be required before improvement is evident. **Atralin 0.05% Gel:** *Adults, adolescents, and children ≥10 yr:* Apply a thin layer to affected areas at bedtime. Up to 6 weeks of therapy may be required before improvement is evident. **Altreno 0.05% Lotion:** *Adults, adolescents, and children ≥9 yr:* Apply thin layer to affected areas once daily.	Avoid use over large areas of skin or for prolonged periods. Avoid sunlight (UV) exposure. Avoid in areas of eczema. Use with caution during breastfeeding. Do not apply to nipple area.
	Adjunct therapy: fine facial wrinkles, hyperpigmentation of skin, roughness of facial skin	**Renova 0.02% and 0.05% or Refissa 0.05%:** *Adults:* Apply pea-sized amount to cover affected area at bedtime for 24 to 48 weeks.	

Indications. Topical treatment of acne vulgaris in adults and children, product choice, and dosing vary by age. Tretinoin is also approved as adjunct therapy in adults for the treatment of fine facial wrinkles, hyperpigmentation, mottling, and roughness of facial skin.

Adverse Effects. Adverse effects of topical tretinoin are usually localized to the area of application. The severity of the effects varies by dose and concentration. The most common adverse effects include dryness, erythema, scaling, pruritus, and stinging and burning sensations. Less common effects include facial edema, alopecia, cellulitis, photosensitivity, and skin hypo- and/or hyperpigmentation. Tretinoin increases the risk of sunburn. Do not apply to areas already affected by a sunburn.

Contraindications. Tretinoin is contraindicated in patients who experience retinoid hypersensitivity reactions to vitamin A, aniline dye allergies, paraben hypersensitivity, and sensitivity to other retinoids, because cross-sensitivity between agents is possible. Some product formulas contain soluble fish proteins and should be used with caution in patients with fish allergies. Keep away from eyes, mouth, nasal creases, and mucous membranes.

Monitoring. Laboratory monitoring with topical tretinoin is not necessary. Efficacy is indicated by improvement in the severity of acne lesions. Improvement may take from 2 to 6 weeks. Monitor closely for adverse effects when vehicle, concentration, or frequency of application changes. Monitor for discontinuation of therapy due to adverse effects.

Antibiotics

The prescriptive use of topical antibiotics will be reviewed here. Topical antibiotics are useful for treatment of localized areas of impetigo and superficial bacterial skin infections. Antibiotics are available both as a prescription and OTC. There is an increased risk of allergic contact dermatitis when using OTC antibiotics. Oral antibiotic therapies are reviewed in this book in Unit 13, Antiinfective Medications. Table 3.7 provides a summary of dosing recommendations for select topical antibiotics.

Benzoyl peroxide

Benzoyl peroxide is an antibacterial agent that improves both inflammatory and noninflammatory lesions. The keratolytic effect decreases comedones, and the effects of drying and desquamation contribute to its efficacy.

Pharmacokinetics. Benzoyl peroxide is absorbed through the skin. Excretion occurs through the urine as the metabolite benzoate.

Indications. Benzoyl peroxide is indicated for the treatment of mild to moderate acne in adults and adolescents. Benzoyl peroxide is an antibiotic (suppresses *P. acnes* without promoting resistance) and keratolytic agent (promotes keratolysis). Safety and effectiveness have not been established in children younger than 12 years of age. Clinically visible improvements will normally occur by the third week of therapy.

Adverse Effects. The most common adverse effects include drying of the skin, which is manifested by peeling, erythema, and skin irritation at the application site. Other, less common effects include contact dermatitis, pruritus, blistering, and swelling. Anaphylactic hypersensitivity

TABLE 3.7   Dosing Recommendations: Antibiotics

Medication	Indications	Dosage	Considerations and Monitoring
Bacitracin	Susceptible skin infection *Staphylococcus aureus* (MSSA), *Streptococcus* sp.	**500 unit/g Ointment:** *Adults, adolescents, and children:* Apply thin film to affected areas two to three times daily for up to 7 days. Maximum dosage: Five times daily.	Reassess after 7 days.
Benzoyl peroxide	Acne vulgaris	**2.5% to 10% Concentrations: cream, gel, lotion, solution:** *Adults and adolescents:* Apply to affected area once daily and gradually increase to four times daily. **Foam:** *Adults and adolescents:* Facial acne: Apply marble-sized amount once daily. Back/chest acne: Apply walnut-sized amount once daily. **Cleansing lotion, foam cloths, cleansing bars, liquid:** *Adults and adolescents:* Apply one to three times daily following product label. **Facial mask:** *Adults and adolescents:* Apply to affected area once weekly to once daily.	Start with lowest dosage. Maximum effects seen in 8 to 12 weeks. If used with Dapsone, may turn skin orange.
Clindamycin	Acne vulgaris	**1% Gel, lotion, solution:** *Adults, adolescents, and children ≥12 yr:* Apply thin layer to affected area twice daily. **1% Foam:** *Adults, adolescents, and children ≥12 yr:* Apply to affected area once daily for up to 6 to 8 weeks. **Medicated pledget:** *Adults, adolescents, and children ≥12 yr:* Apply thin film to affected area twice daily.	Combine with benzoyl peroxide to decrease clindamycin resistance if long-term (more than a few weeks) topical therapy required.

TABLE 3.7   Dosing Recommendations: Antibiotics—cont'd

Medication	Indications	Dosage	Considerations and Monitoring
Dapsone	Acne vulgaris	**5% Gel:** *Adults, adolescents, and children ≥12 yr:* Apply thin layer to affected area twice daily for up to 12 weeks. **7.5% Gel:** *Adults, adolescents, and children ≥9 yr:* Apply thin layer once daily for up to 12 weeks.	Risk for hemolytic anemia in G6PD deficiency. If used with benzoyl peroxide, may turn skin orange.
Erythromycin	Acne vulgaris	**1.5% to 2% Gel, ointment, pledget, solution:** *Adults:* Apply to affected area twice daily.	Combine with benzoyl peroxide to decrease erythromycin resistance.
Gentamicin	Minor bacterial skin infection	**0.1% Cream, ointment:** *Adults, adolescents, and children:* Remove crusts. Apply to affected area three to four times daily.	
Mupirocin	Impetigo	**2% Ointment:** *Adults and children 2 mo to 15 yr:* Remove crusts. Apply to affected area three times daily for up to 10 days.	
	Skin and skin structure infections due to susceptible strains of *Staphylococcus aureus* or *Streptococcus pyogenes*	**2% Cream:** *Adults, adolescents, and children ≥3 mo:* Apply small amount to affected area three times daily for up to 10 days.	
Retapamulin	Impetigo due to susceptible strains of *Staphylococcus aureus* or *Streptococcus pyogenes*	**1% Ointment:** *Adults:* Apply thin layer to affected area up to 100 cm^2 twice daily for 5 days. *Adolescents, children, infants ≥9 mo:* Apply thin layer to affected area up to 2% of body surface area twice daily for 5 days.	

reactions have been reported with the use of OTC products that also contain salicylic acid.

PRACTICE PEARLS

Benzoyl Peroxide Use During Pregnancy and Lactation

- There are no adequate and well-controlled studies in pregnant women. Animal studies have shown adverse effects on fetuses. Weigh potential benefits to the mother against potential risk to the fetus.
- The effects during lactation are unknown.

Contraindications. Benzoyl peroxide should not be used in patients who have shown hypersensitivity to benzoyl peroxide or to any of the other ingredients in the product. Benzoyl peroxide may cause serious hypersensitivity reaction in patients with asthma. Safety and effectiveness have not been established in children younger than 12 years of age. Avoid contact with eyes or mucous membranes. Use caution when the product contains salicylic acid.

Monitoring. Monitor for improvement in lesions. Maximum improvement occurs after approximately 8 to

12 weeks of drug use. Advise patients that continuing use of the drug is normally required to maintain a satisfactory clinical response. Monitor for hypersensitivity reactions and advise patient to discontinue if hypersensitivity occurs.

Mupirocin 2%

Pharmacokinetics. Mupirocin inhibits bacterial protein and ribonucleic acid synthesis. Initial therapeutic response begins within days of topical use. The drug is rapidly metabolized and excreted through the kidneys. No renal or hepatic dose adjustments are required.

Indications. Mupirocin is a naturally occurring antibiotic that is structurally different from other topical antibiotics. Mupirocin is approved for the treatment of bullous and nonbullous impetigo in children older than 2 years of age and in adult patients. The use of mupirocin calcium for the treatment of nasal colonization of methicillin-resistant *Staphylococcus aureus* (MRSA) is approved in children older than 12 years of age and in adults. Mupirocin calcium cream is indicated in the treatment of secondary infections of traumatic skin lesions due to susceptible strains of methicillin-resistant *Staphylococcus* and *streptococcus pyogenes* in children older than 3 months of age and in adult patients.

Adverse Effects. The use of ointment or cream preparations results in infrequent and generally mild adverse effects. Localized burning, stinging, pain, and pruritus are the most common effects. Other reactions include dermatitis, erythema, increased exudate, and dryness. While rare, systemic allergic reactions, including anaphylaxis/anaphylactic reactions, urticaria, and angioedema, have been reported. Adverse effects related to intranasal mupirocin calcium include rhinitis, nasal congestion and irritation, pharyngitis, and dysgeusia. The possibility of antibiotic-associated colitis and associated *Clostridium difficile* diarrhea exists.

PRACTICE PEARLS

Mupirocin Use During Pregnancy and Lactation

- In animal studies, no risk to the fetus was demonstrated. There are no adequate and well-controlled studies in pregnant women.
- It is unknown whether mupirocin is present in breast milk. Remove cream from breast or nipple area prior to breastfeeding.

Contraindications. Long-term use is contraindicated due to the risk of resistant organisms and overgrowth of fungi which may lead to a superinfection. Mupirocin ointment should not be used on extensive burns, large open wounds, or other damaged skin due to the risk of polyethylene glycol absorption. Mupirocin is considered a low risk to nursing infants, although health care providers should consider the benefits of breastfeeding along with the mother's clinical need.

Monitoring. Laboratory monitoring is not required. Monitor for antibiotic-associated colitis and associated *Clostridium difficile* diarrhea. Reevaluate patients if there is no response within 3 to 5 days. Because polyethylene glycol is excreted via the kidneys, the product should not be used over large areas in patients with renal failure.

Retapamulin 1%

Pharmacokinetics. Bacteriostatic properties result from the inhibition of normal bacterial protein biosynthesis. Topical application results in low systemic absorption when applied to intact skin. Absorption is greater in infants and young children and those with areas of abraded skin. Hepatic metabolism occurs through CYP3A4 and substrates.

Indications. Retapamulin is indicated in the treatment of impetigo resulting from methicillin-susceptible *Staphylococcus aureus* (MSSA) or *streptococcus pyogenes (Group A beta-hemolytic streptococci).* Retapamulin is recommended for external use only. It is not recommended for intranasal, intravaginal, ophthalmic, oral, or mucosal application. It has been approved for use in infants older than 9 months, children, adolescents, and adults. No dose adjustment is indicated for renal or hepatic impairment.

PRACTICE PEARLS

Retapamulin Use During Pregnancy and Lactation

- There are no available data on retapamulin use in pregnant women.
- There are no available data on the presence of retapamulin in breast milk. Health care providers should consider the benefits of breastfeeding along with the mother's clinical need.

Adverse Effects. The most common adverse effects include headache, diarrhea, and nausea. Topical application may result in site irritation, pruritus, site pain, and erythema. More serious adverse effects include contact dermatitis, allergic reactions, and angioedema.

Contraindications. CYP3A4 inhibitors may increase the serum concentration of retapamulin. Avoid concomitant use in patients younger than 2 years of age.

Monitoring. Laboratory monitoring is not required. Monitor for use of CYP3A4 inhibitors. Reevaluate in 3 to 5 days. If there is no improvement, change treatment.

Antivirals

Acyclovir 5%

Pharmacokinetics. Systemic absorption is minimal following topical application. Excretion occurs through the renal system.

Indications. Topical therapy is approved for the treatment of:

- Recurrent herpes labialis (perioral herpes, cold sores, fever blisters) in immunocompetent adults and children 12 years and older
- Initial episodes of genital herpes in immunocompromised or immunocompetent adults
- Non–life-threatening, nongenital mucocutaneous herpes simplex virus infections in immunocompromised adults
- Acute herpetic keratitis caused by HSV-1 and HSV-2 in adults and children 2 years and older
- Herpes zoster (shingles) in adults
- Varicella in adults and children 2 years and older

Adverse Effects. Topical cream application may result in contact dermatitis. Follicular conjunctivitis, superficial punctate keratitis, eye pain, or eye stinging may follow application of ophthalmic ointment.

PRACTICE PEARLS

Acyclovir Use During Pregnancy and Lactation

- In animal studies, no risk to the fetus was demonstrated. There are no adequate and well-controlled studies in pregnant women.
- The American Academy of Pediatrics considers acyclovir topical to be compatible with breastfeeding. Consideration to continuing breastfeeding should be given if lesions do not involve the breast/nipple.

Contraindications. Avoid if patient exhibits hypersensitivity to acyclovir, valacyclovir, or any component of the product with the topical cream or ophthalmic ointment. Avoid use of topical ointment or cream near the eyes. Avoid topical cream in the mouth or nose.

Monitoring. Topical use requires no laboratory monitoring. Monitor for the healing of lesions and decrease of associated pain. Monitor for adherence to recommended dosage, frequency, and duration of therapy. Table 3.8 provides a summary of dosing recommendations for select antiviral medications.

Penciclovir 1%

Pharmacokinetics. Drug absorption was not detectable in plasma or urine following topical application.

Indications. Penciclovir is approved by the U.S. Food and Drug Administration (FDA) for the treatment of recurrent herpes labialis in adults and children 12 years and older. Treatment should be initiated as early as possible. Advise patients to apply to lips and face only.

Adverse Effects. The most-reported adverse effect is headache. The incidence of an application site reaction occurring is rare. Other reported effects include discoloration of the skin, localized edema at the application site, erythematous rash, urticaria, and oral and pharyngeal edema.

Contraindications. Avoid in the event of hypersensitivity to penciclovir or any component of the product. Avoid contact with mucous membranes and eyes.

Monitoring. Monitor for symptom improvement.

Antifungals

Dermatophyte and *Candida* infections are treated with antifungals. Fungicides inhibit the biosynthesis of ergosterol leading to alterations of the fungal cell membrane. Some preparations are available only by prescription while others are OTC. This chapter includes an exemplar drug of each class, though health care providers should consider the severity and extent of the infection, prior treatment history, onset of action, treatment duration, and drug cost when initiating treatment (Lanier et al., 2018). Table 3.9 provides a summary of dosing recommendations.

Imidazoles

Miconazole

Pharmacokinetics. Method of delivery affects peak action and absorption. When it is applied topically, systemic absorption has not been reported. Metabolism is within the liver. Excretion is primarily through the gastrointestinal (GI) tract, with minimal excretion through the renal system.

Indications. Miconazole is indicated in the treatment of uncomplicated vulvovaginal candidiasis (for children 12 years and older), superficial tinea, and cutaneous candidiasis

---

PRACTICE PEARLS

Miconazole Use During Pregnancy and Lactation

- There are no adequate and well-controlled studies in pregnant women. Animal studies have shown adverse effects on the fetus. Weigh potential benefits to the mother against potential risk to the fetus.
- The use of miconazole for the treatment of vaginal candidiasis has not been associated with fetal harm. Miconazole is only recommended for use during pregnancy when there are no alternatives and the benefit outweighs the risk.
- Miconazole cream may be applied to the nipples following breastfeeding. Remove cream prior to breastfeeding.

TABLE 3.8 Dosing Recommendations: Antivirals

Medication	Indications	Dosage	Considerations and Monitoring
Acyclovir	Herpes labialis caused by herpes simplex virus	**5% Ointment:** *Immunocompromised adults: Initial therapy:* Apply to lesions every 3 hours (six times daily) for 7 days in sufficient quantities to adequately cover lesion. **5% Cream:** *Immunocompetent adults, adolescents, and children ≥12 yr:* Apply to lesions five times daily for 4 days.	Initiate at the first sign of symptoms or lesions. The CDC discourages topical dosing, although it is FDA approved.
	Herpes genitalis infection caused by herpes simplex virus	**Ointment 5%:** *Immunocompromised adults: Initial therapy:* Apply ointment topically to lesions every 3 hours (six times daily) for 7 days in sufficient quantities to adequately cover lesion.	
Penciclovir	Recurrent herpes labialis	**1% Cream:** *Adults, adolescents, and children ≥12 yr:* Apply every 2 hours, while awake, for 4 days.	Initiate treatment as early as possible.
Acyclovir/ hydrocortisone	Recurrent herpes labialis	**5%/1% Cream:** *Adults, adolescents, and children ≥6 yr:* Apply to affected areas five times daily for 5 days.	Initiate treatment as early as possible.

(topical only for children 2 years and older). Treatment of oropharyngeal candidiasis is only recommended in those 16 years and older.

Adverse Effects. Though not common, adverse effects include reaction after topical application. Generalized, pruritic, maculopapular contact dermatitis may occur. Following vaginal application, abdominal cramps, burning, irritation, and pruritus were reported. Adverse effects after oral therapy include headache, diarrhea, nausea, vomiting, and cough. As with other antifungal medications, hematological effects of anemia, lymphocytopenia, and neutropenia have been reported.

Contraindications. Miconazole contraindications include hypersensitivity to miconazole or any component of the product. The buccal tablets are contraindicated in patients with milk protein hypersensitivity. Use oral tablets with caution in patients with hepatic disease.

Monitoring. Extensive laboratory monitoring is not required. In the event of prolonged oral treatment, monitor complete blood count (CBC) with differential, liver function, and prothrombin level.

Allylamines

Terbinafine

Pharmacokinetics. Terbinafine is an analog derivative of naftifine available both topically and orally. Absorption begins within 24 hours and may last up to 3 months in the skin and 1 month in the nails after discontinuation of therapy. Metabolism of the oral form occurs in the liver. Excretion is primarily renal for both topical and oral forms.

Indications. Terbinafine is labeled for use in treating dermal mycosis, onychomycosis, and various other forms of tinea. Topical formulations include cream, lotion, gel,

> ### PRACTICE PEARLS
>
> **Terbinafine Use During Pregnancy and Lactation**
>
> - There are no adequate and well-controlled studies in pregnant women. Animal studies have shown adverse effects on the fetus. Use only after weighing the potential benefits to the mother against potential risk to the fetus.
> - Terbinafine is present in breast milk. Weigh the potential benefit of breastfeeding against the risk to the infant.
> - Topical cream: Avoid topical application to the breast.

solution, and spray. Initiation of therapy in older adults should begin at the lower end of the dosing range.

Adverse Effects. Topical adverse effects are uncommon but include localized skin irritation, burning, pruritus, and dryness. Oral use of terbinafine has more adverse effects. Dermatologic effects include rash, urticaria, pruritus, and more severe effects such as Stevens-Johnson syndrome, erythema multiforme, and cutaneous or systemic lupus erythematosus. GI disturbances include alteration in taste and smell, dyspepsia, nausea, and diarrhea. Hematologic effects of lymphocytopenia, severe neutropenia, and liver failure in patients with and without preexisting disease have been reported.

Contraindications. Terbinafine use is contradicted in patients with a history of an allergic reaction to any component. Oral terbinafine is contraindicated in patients with chronic or active hepatic impairment, renal impairment, or renal failure (creatinine clearance ≤50 mL/min). Use with caution in patients with known or suspected immunodeficiency syndromes or immunosuppression.

Monitoring. Obtain baseline complete blood count with differential prior to initiation of therapy. Repeat if treatment extends past 6 weeks. Monitor liver function.

TABLE 3.9 **Dosing Recommendations: Antifungals**

Medication	Indication	Dosing	Considerations and Monitoring
Imidazoles			
Miconazole	Tinea pedis and tinea corporis	**2% cream, ointment, powder, solution, spray:** *Adults, adolescents, and children ≥2 yr:* Apply to clean, dry affected areas twice daily for 4 weeks.	
	Tinea cruris	**2% cream, ointment, powder, solution, spray:** *Adults, adolescents, and children ≥2 yr:* Apply to clean, dry affected areas twice daily for 2 weeks.	
	Tinea versicolor Cutaneous candidiasis	**2% Skin cream:** *Adults, adolescents, and children ≥2 yr:* Apply to clean, dry affected areas twice daily for up to 2 weeks.	
Clotrimazole	Cutaneous candidiasis Tinea versicolor	**1% Cream, ointment, solution:** *Adults, adolescents, and children:* Apply to affected skin and surrounding area twice daily, morning and evening.	
	Tinea corporis, tinea cruris, tinea pedis	**1% Cream, ointment, solution:** *Adults, adolescents, and children ≥2 yr:* Apply thin layer to affected skin and surrounding area twice daily, morning and evening.	

TABLE 3.9 **Dosing Recommendations: Antifungals—cont'd**

Medication	Indication	Dosing	Considerations and Monitoring
Ketoconazole	Tinea corporis, tinea cruris, tinea versicolor	**2% Cream:** *Adults:* Apply to affected area and surrounding skin once daily for 2 weeks.	
	Tinea pedis	**2% Cream:** *Adults:* Apply to affected area and surrounding skin once daily for 6 weeks.	
	Tinea versicolor	**2% Shampoo:** *Adults:* Apply to damp skin/hair and surrounding area; lather, leave on for 5 minutes, rinse.	
	Seborrheic dermatitis	**2% Cream:** *Adults:* Apply twice daily for 4 weeks or until clear. **2% Foam:** *Adults, adolescents, and children ≥12 yr:* Apply to affected area twice daily for 4 weeks. **Gel 2%:** *Adults, adolescents, and children ≥12 yr:* Apply to affected area twice daily for 2 weeks.	
	Dandruff	**2% Shampoo:** *Adults:* Apply to damp skin/hair and surrounding area; lather, leave on for 5 minutes, rinse. **1% OTC shampoo:** *Adults, adolescents, and children ≥12 yr:* Apply to wet hair; lather, rinse, repeat. Apply every 3 to 4 days for up to 8 weeks, if needed, or as directed.	
Allylamines			
Terbinafine	Tinea corporis Tinea cruris	**1% Prescription gel:** *Adults:* Apply once daily for 7 days. **1% OTC cream, gel, solution, spray:** *Adults and children ≥12 yr:* Apply once daily for 7 days.	
	Tinea pedis	**1% Prescription gel:** *Adults:* Apply once daily for 7 days. **1% OTC gel, cream:** *Adults and children ≥12 yr:* Interdigital: apply twice daily for 1 week. Plantar: apply twice daily for 2 weeks.	
	Tinea versicolor	**1% Prescription gel, solution:** Apply to affected area once daily for 7 days. **1% OTC spray, solution:** *Adults and children ≥12 yr:* Interdigital: use twice daily for 1 week.	
Naftifine	Tinea cruris	**2% Cream:** *Adults and children ≥12 yr:* Apply once daily for 2 weeks. **1% Cream:** *Adults:* Apply to affected area once daily for 4 weeks. **1% Gel:** *Adults:* Apply to affected area morning and night for up to 4 weeks.	
	Tinea pedis	**2% Cream, gel:** *Adults and children ≥12 yr:* Apply once daily for 2 weeks. **1% Cream:** *Adults:* Apply to affected area once daily for 4 weeks. **1% Gel:** *Adults:* Apply to affected area morning and evening for 4 weeks.	
	Tinea corporis	**2% Cream:** *Adults and children ≥12 yr:* Apply once daily for 2 weeks. **1% Cream:** *Adults:* Apply to affected area once daily for 4 weeks. **1% Gel:** Apply to affected area morning and evening for 4 weeks.	

Continued

			Considerations
Medication	Indication	Dosing	and Monitoring

TABLE 3.9 Dosing Recommendations: Antifungals—cont'd

Polyenes

Nystatin	Cutaneous candidiasis	**Cream, ointment:** *Adults, adolescents, children, infants, neonates:* Apply to affected area twice daily until healed.	Prefer cream in intertriginous areas
		Topical powder: *Adults, adolescents, children, infants, neonates:* Apply to affected area two to three times daily until healed.	Prefer powder for moist lesions

Miscellaneous

Tolnaftate	Tinea barbae, tinea capitis, tinea corporis, tinea cruris, tinea manuum, tinea pedis	**1% Cream, gel, powder spray, solution, spray:** *Adults and children ≥ 2 yr:* Apply to affected area morning and evening for 2 to 4 weeks.	
Ciclopirox	Mild to moderate onychomycosis in immunocompetent patients	**Nail lacquer 8% solution:** *Adults and children ≥12 yr:* Apply once daily at bedtime to affected nails. Leave on 8 hours. Remove every 7 days.	
	Seborrheic dermatitis of scalp	**0.77% Gel:** *Adults and children ≥16 yr:* Apply to affected scalp twice daily for 4 weeks. **1% Shampoo:** *Adults and children ≥16 yr:* Apply 5 mL to wet hair; lather and leave for 3 minutes, then rinse. Use twice a week at least 3 days apart for up to 4 weeks.	
	Tinea corporis, tinea cruris, tinea pedis, tinea versicolor Cutaneous candidiasis	**0.77% Gel:** *Adults and children ≥16 yr:* Apply to affected areas twice daily for 4 weeks. **0.77% Cream, lotion, topical suspension:** *Adults and children ≥10 yr:* Apply sparingly to affected area morning and night for 2 to 4 weeks.	

Polyenes

Nystatin
Pharmacokinetics. Topical preparations result in poor systemic absorption.

Indications. Clinical uses include superficial cutaneous fungal infections, oral and pharyngeal candidiasis, and vaginal candidiasis. Topical preparations are available in creams, ointments, and powders. In pediatrics, topical preparations are available to treat candidal diaper dermatitis.

PRACTICE PEARLS

Nystatin Use During Pregnancy and Lactation

- There are no adequate and well-controlled studies in pregnant women. Animal studies have shown adverse effects on the fetus. Weigh potential benefits to the mother against potential risk to the fetus.
- Nystatin cream may be applied to the nipples following breastfeeding. Remove cream prior to breastfeeding.

Adverse Effects. Rare instances of urticaria and Stevens-Johnson syndrome have occurred. Topical adverse effects include burning, pruritus, pain, and rash.

Contraindications. Use of nystatin is contraindicated with hypersensitivity to nystatin products or components. Some preparations contain methylparaben and propylparaben; caution is advised in patients with paraben hypersensitivity.

Monitoring. Laboratory monitoring is not required. Monitor for resolution of infection and adverse effects.

Thiocarbamates

Tolnaftate
Pharmacokinetics. Tolnaftate mechanisms of action include distortion of the hyphae, stunting of mycelial growth, and possible inhibition of ergosterol biosynthesis. Pharmacokinetic data are limited. Onset of action is approximately 24 to 72 hours. Tolnaftate is considered less effective than other antimycotic therapies.

Indications. Tolnaftate is a nonprescription topical antifungal agent approved for the treatment of mild to moderate superficial dermatophyte infections. It is not indicated for candida or for use in patients younger than 2 years.

Adverse Effects. Allergic contact dermatitis is possible. Presentation includes erythema, irritation, inflammation, and pruritus. The use of sprays, gels, or liquid formulations may cause stinging and drying of skin due to alcohol content.

Tolnaftate Use During Pregnancy and Lactation

- Tolnaftate has not been assigned a specific FDA pregnancy risk category rating.
- Advise pregnant women not to self-medicate during pregnancy.
- Data are limited regarding use of tolnaftate during breastfeeding, and its excretion in breast milk is unknown. Consider the benefits of breastfeeding against risks to the infant. Avoid topical application to the breast.

Contraindications. Tolnaftate should not be used in patients with known tolnaftate hypersensitivity, or sensitivity to any components of the specific formulation. Limited data are available regarding pregnancy and lactation considerations. Data suggest a low risk since the product is available OTC, but consideration is always recommended.

Monitoring. Laboratory monitoring is not required. Monitor for resolution of infection. Monitor for adverse effects.

Benzoxaboroles

Tavaborole

Pharmacokinetics. An oxaborole antifungal agent, tavaborole inhibits synthesis of fungal proteins. Excretion is from the kidney.

Indications. Tavaborole is approved for the treatment of onychomycosis due to *Trichophyton rubrum* or *Trichophyton mentagrophytes* in adults and children 6 years and older. Due to the slow growth of the toenail, treatment should continue for 48 weeks.

Tavaborole Use During Pregnancy and Lactation

- There are no adequate and well-controlled studies in pregnant women. Animal studies have shown adverse effects on the fetus. Weigh potential benefits to the mother against potential risk to the fetus.
- Data are limited regarding use of tavaborole during breastfeeding, and its excretion in breast milk is unknown. Consider the benefits of breastfeeding against risks to the infant.

Adverse Effects. The most common adverse effects are limited to the area around the application site and include dermatitis, peeling skin, and an ingrown nail.

Contraindications. No specific contraindications or warnings have been identified. No dose adjustments are recommended. Avoid use near open flame or excessive heat as product is flammable.

Monitoring. No laboratory monitoring is required. Monitor for continuation of therapy and signs of ingrown nail.

Hydroxypyridones

Ciclopirox

Pharmacokinetics. Ciclopirox distributes to the stratum corneum, hair follicles, sebaceous glands, dermis, and nails. Systemic absorption is minimal. The primary method of excretion is through the renal system.

Indications. Ciclopirox is a broad-spectrum antifungal effective against dermatophytes, yeasts, and molds commonly found on the skin and nails. It also has mild antiinflammatory effects. Ciclopirox is available in a cream, gel, nail lacquer, shampoo, and topical suspension.

Ciclopirox Use During Pregnancy and Lactation

- There are no adequate and well-controlled studies in pregnant women. Animal studies have demonstrated no adverse effects on the fetus. Weigh potential benefits to the mother against potential risk to the fetus.
- Data are limited regarding use of ciclopirox during breastfeeding, and its excretion in breast milk is unknown. Topical application is not expected to result in significant maternal absorption, and thus should not be of great risk to a breastfeeding infant.

Adverse Effects. Adverse effects include application site reactions such as erythema, burning, blistering, swelling, oozing, and itching. Patients may also report a burning sensation, pain, rash, or pruritis. Other adverse effects reported include eye pain, facial edema, ventricular tachycardia (with use of shampoo), headache, alopecia, and change in nail shape or color (with nail lacquer).

Contraindications. Ciclopirox is contraindicated in patients with sensitivities to the product. Previous hypersensitivity to the product is a contraindication to repeating therapy.

Monitoring. Laboratory monitoring is not necessary. Monitor for resolution of symptoms. Advise patients to report no improvement or worsening conditions and/or signs of adverse effects at the application site.

Scabicides/Pediculocides

Scabicides are available only with a prescription. Pediculocides are available in nonprescription formulations. Table 3.10 provides dosing recommendations for select medications.

Permethrin

Pharmacokinetics. Permethrin disrupts the sodium channel current that regulates the polarization of the membrane and leads to paralysis of the louse or mite. Minimal amounts are topically absorbed. Permethrin is undetectable in plasma and is metabolized by the liver. The primary route of excretion is the renal system.

Indications. Permethrin 5% cream is approved for the treatment of scabies, crab lice, and body lice in adults and children 2 months and older. It is considered a first-line treatment for scabies. Permethrin 1% cream is approved for

Permethrin and Lindane Use During Pregnancy and Lactation

Permethrin

- Reproductive studies in animals revealed no evidence of impaired fertility or harm to the fetus. There are no adequate and well-controlled studies in pregnant women. Thus permethrin should be used during pregnancy only if clearly needed.
- It is unknown whether permethrin is present in breast milk. Consider benefit of breastfeeding against risk to the infant.

Lindane

- There are no adequate and well-controlled studies in pregnant women. Animal studies have shown adverse effects on the fetus. Weigh potential benefits to the mother against potential risk to the fetus.
- Pregnant caregivers should avoid exposure through the application of lindane to another person.
- Lindane is not recommended for use while breastfeeding. Lindane is present in breast milk.

the treatment of head lice and crab lice in adults and children 2 months and older. Permethrin 1% cream kills live lice but not nits.

Adverse Effects. Treatment with permethrin may temporarily exacerbate the symptoms of pruritus, edema, and erythema caused by scabies and pediculosis. Topical application to the scalp may result in pruritus, burning, and stinging. Less common were reports of pain, numbness, tingling, edema, erythema, and rash.

Contraindications. Use with caution in patients with hypersensitivity to other synthetic pyrethroids or pyrethrins. Avoid if allergic to chrysanthemums or ragweed.

Monitoring. After treatment, monitor for the presence of live pediculus. Retreat if live pediculus are present 14 days after the initial application of permethrin. Laboratory monitoring is not necessary. Monitor for resistance, treatment failures, and secondary infections resulting from scratching.

Lindane 1% shampoo

Pharmacokinetics. Absorption increases when in contact with nonintact scalp or skin. Lindane is metabolized through the liver and excreted through urine and feces.

Indications. Lindane is indicated as a second-line therapy for pediculosis. Limit use to patients weighing over 110 lb (50 kg) and nongeriatric in age who cannot tolerate or have failed treatment with other approved therapies.

Adverse Effects. In addition to the black box warnings of seizure and death, lindane may cause ataxia, dizziness, neurotoxicity, and restlessness. Dermatologic side effects include pruritus, burning sensation, dry skin, contact dermatitis, and eczematous rash.

Contraindications. Use with caution in infants, children, patients weighing less than 110 lb (50 kg), and older adults due to toxicity. Re-treatment is contraindicated, and no time frame was suggested by manufacturers as the risk of toxicity is unknown after the first treatment. Avoid contact in individuals with skin conditions or nonintact scalp or skin. Do not use in or near the mouth. Do not use in patients who are immunocompromised, have previously used lindane, have a history of reaction to lindane or any ingredient, or are taking sedatives, as this may increase the risk of seizures.

TABLE 3.10 Dosing Recommendations: Scabicides/Pediculicides

Medication	Indications	Dosage	Considerations and Monitoring
Permethrin	Scabies	**5% Cream:** *Adults, adolescents, children, and infants ≥2 mo:* (30 Gm for average adult) Apply from the head to soles of feet. Leave on for 8 to 14 hours and then wash off.	Apply once to affected area; do not repeat for ≥7 days.
	Pediculosis capitis	**1% Lotion:** *Adults, adolescents, children, and infants ≥2 mo:* Shampoo hair with regular shampoo, rinse, and towel dry. Saturate the hair and scalp (usually 25 to 30 mL). Leave on hair for 10 minutes, then rinse thoroughly with water.	
Crotamiton	Scabies	**10% Cream, lotion:** *Adults:* Apply topically over the entire body from chin to toes. Repeat in 24 hours. Patient may take a cleansing bath 48 hours after second dose.	Not recommended by CDC for treatment of scabies.
	Pruritus	**10% Cream, lotion:** *Adults:* Apply to affected area and massage in until completely absorbed. Repeat if needed.	
Lindane	Pediculosis	**1% Shampoo:** *Adults, adolescents, and children:* Apply 1 ounce (do not use more than 2 ounces) to dry hair. Leave on for 4 minutes maximum, then add small amounts of water to lather, then rinse immediately. Apply only once. Do not repeat.	Use only if other treatments are unavailable or have failed. Use with caution if <110 lb (50 kg) and in older adults.

Lindane

- Risk of seizures and death
- Do not use:
  - In infants, children, older adults, and/or patients weighing less than 110 lb (50 kg)
  - In immunocompromised patients
  - In patients with a history of any seizure, in conjunction with sedatives, a previous reaction, or nonintact scalp/skin

Monitoring. Educate patients on risk potential and application. Monitor for adverse effects and evidence of toxicity. Monitor for the presence of lice after 7 days.

Analgesics

Topical, local anesthetics discussed in this chapter are indicated for relief of mild to moderate pain resulting from injuries (sprains, strains), minor wounds (abrasions, scraps, burns), osteoarthritis, postherpetic neuralgia, anorectal disorders, and/or hemorrhoids. They may be applied as an ointment, cream, gel, lotion, liquid, aerosol spray, or viscous solution. Local anesthetics provide relief of pain and are a treatment option for chronic pain. Table 3.11 provides a summary of dosing recommendations for select topical analgesics.

Diclofenac epolamine 1.3%

Pharmacokinetics. Diclofenac epolamine may inhibit cyclooxygenase (COX-1 and COX-2). It is metabolized in the liver. Excretion occurs in the renal and biliary systems. Half-life is approximately 12 hours.

Indications. Diclofenac epolamine topical has analgesic, antiinflammatory, and antipyretic properties. It is indicated for the relief of mild to moderate joint pain from osteoarthritis or acute pain associated with minor sprains, strains, and contusions. It is approved for use in children older than 6 years of age and in adults. Application instructions are to apply twice daily to the most painful area.

Adverse Effects. The most common adverse effects include pruritus, contact dermatitis, site reaction, headache, nausea, and indigestion. Less common but more

BLACK BOX WARNING

Diclofenac Topical

- Risk of cardiovascular thrombotic events (myocardial infarction and stroke)
- Risk of serious GI adverse effects (bleeding, ulceration, perforation)
- Contraindicated:
  - Coronary artery bypass graft surgery
- Extreme caution:
  - Older adults
  - History of peptic ulcer disease and/or GI bleed

severe adverse effects included myocardial infarction, erythroderma, hyperkalemia, GI ulcer, hemorrhage or perforation, liver disease/failure, anaphylaxis, kidney injury, and asthma.

Contraindications. Black Box and Beers Criteria warnings exist for this drug. It is contraindicated in patients with renal impairment or patients with a history of asthma, urticaria, or allergic-type reactions following the use of nonsteroidal antiinflammatory drugs or aspirin products. Avoid in patients with hypersensitivity to diclofenac or any component. Avoid long-term use or use on nonintact or damaged skin.

PRACTICE PEARLS

Diclofenac Use During Pregnancy and Lactation

- Pregnancy: avoid beginning at 30 weeks' gestation, as premature closure of ductus arteriosus may occur.
- Discontinue in event of infertility: chronic use may cause reversible infertility.
- Breastfeeding: unknown if detectable following topical application. Consider risk to infant versus benefit to mother.

Monitoring. Monitor for toxicity. Measure transaminase levels at baseline, within 4 to 8 weeks of initiation of therapy, and periodically thereafter. Monitor renal function, CBC, and chemistry profiles if on long-term therapy. Monitor blood pressure at baseline and throughout. Monitor for adverse events: cardiovascular, GI, respiratory, and renal.

PRACTICE PEARLS

Life Span Considerations With Diclofenac: Beers Criteria

- Increased risk of bleeding, elevated blood pressure, kidney injury
- Avoid chronic use
- Recommend: proton-pump inhibitor or Misoprostol

Benzocaine

Pharmacokinetics. Benzocaine is poorly absorbed through intact skin. Metabolism occurs in the blood by plasma esterases. Metabolism results in inactivation. Absorption increases with application to mucous membranes or nonintact skin. Benzocaine spray results in an anesthetic effect within seconds of application.

Indications. Topical application of benzocaine is indicated for the temporary relief of pain. Use is approved for skin irritation, oral pain due to ulcerations, stomatitis, dental procedures or toothache, and ear pain when no perforation is present. Benzocaine is approved for use in children older than 2 years and in adults. It is available in a variety of vehicles.

TABLE 3.11	Dosing Recommendations: Analgesics		
Medication	Indications	Dosage	Considerations and Monitoring
Nonsteroidal Antiinflammatory Drugs (NSAIDs)			
Diclofenac	Osteoarthritis (excluding spine, hip, shoulder)	**1% Gel:** *Knee, ankle, foot:* Adult: Apply 4 Gm (4.5 inches) four times daily. Maximum dosage: 16 Gm daily. *Elbow, wrist, hand:* Adult: Apply 2 Gm (2.25 inches) four times daily. Maximum dosage: 8 Gm daily. **1.5% Topical solution:** *Knee:* Adult: Apply 10 drops to affected area and rub in. Repeat until 40 drops applied. Repeat four times daily. **2% Topical solution:** *Knee:* Adult: Apply 40 mg (2 pumps) to affected area twice daily.	Black Box Beers Criteria Renal impairment: Not recommended.
	Acute, localized joint/muscle injuries	**1.3% Patch:** *Adults, adolescents, and children ≥6 yr:* Apply one patch twice daily to the most painful area. **1.3% Topical system:** *Adults:* Apply one topical system once daily to the most painful area.	
Botanical irritant: Chili peppers			
Capsaicin	Rheumatoid arthritis Osteoarthritis Myalgia Arthralgias	**OTC Cream, lotion, solution:** *Adults:* Apply thin film to affected areas three to four times daily. **0.025% Patch:** *Adults, adolescents, and children ≥12 yr:* Apply one patch to affected area three to four times daily for up to 7 days. Remove patch within 8 hours.	
	Diabetic neuropathy	**8% Dermal patch:** *Adults:* Apply up to 4 patches for 30 minutes, then remove. Repeat every 3 months. **0.25% cream:** *Adults, adolescents, and children ≥10 yr:* Apply to affected area two to four times daily. **0.075% Cream:** *Adults:* Apply to affected areas four times daily.	
	Postherpetic neuralgia	**8% Dermal patch:** *Adults:* Apply up to 4 patches for 30 minutes, then remove. Repeat every 3 months. **0.25% cream:** *Adults:* Apply to affected area two to four times daily.	
Lidocaine	Pressure ulcer (stage 1 to 4) Venous statis and diabetic ulcers Burns (1st and 2nd degree) Cuts/abrasions	**LDO Plus 4% Hydrogel wound dressing:** *Adults, adolescents, and children ≥2 yr:* Apply to wound surface and surrounding area three to four times daily.	
	Postherpetic neuralgia	**Lidocaine patch 5% equivalent to lidocaine topical system 1.8%:** *Adults:* Apply up to three patches or topical systems to most painful area for up to 12 hours in a 24-hr period.	

TABLE 3.11	Dosing Recommendations: Analgesics—cont'd		
Medication	**Indications**	**Dosage**	**Considerations and Monitoring**
	Skin anesthesia for relief of minor burns, scrapes, irritations, bites	**Gel, jelly, lotion, ointment, solution:** *Adults, adolescents, children and infants:* Apply up to affected area as needed to control symptoms. Maximum dosage: 4.5 mg/kg (300 mg), three patches to affected area for up to 12 hr. **GEN7T 3.5% lotion:** *Adults, adolescents, and children ≥12 yr:* Apply to affected area up to four times daily. **OTC cream, gel, spray, solution:** *Adults, adolescents, and children ≥2 yr:* Apply to affected area up to three to four times daily. **Lidocare 4% pain relief patch back/ shoulder:** *Adults and adolescents:* Apply to affected area. Leave on 8–12 hr. **Alocane emergency burn pads:** *Adults, adolescents, and children ≥2 yr:* Apply to burn or wound and cover with gauze or adhesive tape.	

Adverse Effects. Contact dermatitis may result at the application site. Presentation includes pruritus, erythema, edema, pain, rash, and urticaria. It is rare for central nervous system and cardiovascular effects to occur, since the drug is poorly absorbed. Another rare adverse effect is methemoglobinemia, which results from high levels of methemoglobin production. Methemoglobinemia presents as respiratory distress or cyanosis due to decreased blood oxygenation.

Contraindications. In 2018 the FDA issued a warning that OTC oral drug products containing benzocaine should not be used to treat infants and children younger than 2 years due to a high-risk/poor-benefit ratio. It is contraindicated in patients with hypersensitivities to benzocaine or any component of the product, including aniline dye allergies. Avoid otic use if patient has a known or suspected perforated tympanic membrane. Avoid in patients at risk for breathing problems, including asthma, bronchitis, and emphysema, or at increased risk for complications related to methemoglobinemia.

Monitoring. Monitor patients for signs and symptoms of methemoglobinemia such as cyanosis, dyspnea, weakness, or tachycardia. Monitor for effective pain relief. Advise patients not to cover the application site, as this may increase the risk of adverse effects.

Lidocaine

BLACK BOX WARNING!

2% Xylocaine Viscous (Lidocaine HCl) Solution

- Do not use in children younger than 3 years of age.
- Do not use for teething pain.
- Adhere to application and dosing regimen.

Data from U.S. Food and Drug Administration (2018). Risk of serious and potentially fatal blood disorder prompts FDA action on oral over-the-counter benzocaine products used for teething and mouth pain and prescription local anesthetics. Drug Safety Communications.https://www.fda.gov/media/113261/download; and Fresenius Kabi USA, LLC. (2014). 2% viscousvLidocaine. https://www.accessdata.fda.gov/drugsatfda_docs/label/2014/009470s025lbl.pdf.

PRACTICE PEARLS

Benzocaine Use During Pregnancy and Lactation

- There are no controlled data in human pregnancy. Benzocaine topical is only recommended for use during pregnancy when benefit outweighs risk.
- Benzocaine has not been studied during breastfeeding. Weigh benefits to mother against risk to infant during breastfeeding. If determined necessary to the mother, apply away from the breast or nipple.

Pharmacokinetics. Metabolism occurs in the liver and results in inactivation. The rate and extent of absorption after topical administration are dependent upon the concentration, total dose, site of application, and duration of exposure. Topical administration of ointment or jelly results in peak effects typically within 3 to 5 minutes. Transdermal absorption of lidocaine is related to the duration of application and the surface area over which the patch is applied. When the dermal patch (Lidoderm) is used as directed, very little is systemically absorbed. The lidocaine concentration does not increase with daily use in patients with normal renal function.

Indications. Lidocaine is a topical anesthetic for use in children older than 3 years and in adults. Indications include the treatment of irritated or inflamed oral mucous membranes of the oropharynx, insect bites (pruritus and eczemas), minor burns/sunburns, and skin abrasions. Lidocaine also relieves discomfort due to pruritus ani, pruritus vulvae, hemorrhoids, and anal fissures. Lidocaine patches are approved for pain associated with postherpetic neuralgia and minor localized pain.

Adverse Effects. The risk of adverse effects varies with formulation, absorption, and the age of the patient. The most common adverse effects in adults and children are related to the use of intradermal powders and present as erythema or petechial. Less frequent effects are edema, pruritus, nausea, and vomiting. Caution is advised in patients with aniline dye allergies, as this increases the risk of adverse events. Applying dermal, transdermal, or oromucosal lidocaine preparations to severely traumatized skin, large surface areas, or warm skin can increase its absorption, possibly increasing the risk of systemic toxicity. To avoid risk of toxicity, do not apply large amounts, do not use an occlusive dressing, and do not leave on large body areas for longer than 2 hours.

PRACTICE PEARLS

Lidocaine Topical Use During Pregnancy and Lactation

- Topical application is not expected to result in systemic exposure. However, there are no adequate and well-controlled studies in pregnant women. Animal studies have not demonstrated adverse effects on the fetus. Weigh potential benefits to the mother against potential risk to the fetus.
- Lidocaine is present in breast milk. Consider benefit of breastfeeding against risk to the infant.

Contraindications. Contraindicated with hypersensitivity to lidocaine or any component of the formulation, hypersensitivity to another local anesthetic of the amide type, traumatized mucosa, or bacterial infection at the site of application, as this may increase toxicity. Oral formulations are contraindicated within 1 hour of eating due to increased risk of aspiration. Lidocaine is contraindicated in patients with amide local anesthetic hypersensitivity.

Monitoring. Laboratory monitoring with topical application is not necessary. Monitor for signs of hypersensitivity and systemic toxicity. Monitor for signs and symptoms of methemoglobinemia. Monitor patients with glucose-6-phosphate dehydrogenase deficiency, preexisting methemoglobinemia, cardiac or pulmonary compromise, those younger than 6 months, and concurrent exposure to oxidizing agents or their metabolites, as these patients are more susceptible to developing methemoglobinemia.

Prescriber Considerations for Integumentary System Medications

Clinical Practice Guidelines

At some point, almost every primary care provider can expect to care for a patient presenting for an evaluation of a skin disorder. Topical medications are the first-line treatment for many of these diseases. Clinical practice guidelines offer providers evidence for practice and multiple agencies offer practice guidelines.

Clinical Reasoning for Topical Integumentary Medications

Consider the individual patient's health problem requiring topical therapy. Health care providers must consider the diagnosis and comorbid conditions, severity of the disease, distribution of lesions, available resources, and patient preferences prior to prescribing topical medications (Perrone et al., 2017). Chronic skin diseases may also cause a psychological burden that must be addressed. Definitive diagnosis is obtained through microscopic examinations of scrapings, potassium hydroxide (KOH) preparation, calcofluor white stain, fungal culture, and susceptibility testing. Key points to consider include:

- Prescribing the least-potent corticosteroid that is compatible with effective treatment
- Prescribing low-potency topical corticosteroids for long-term use, on large areas, on thin skin, and in children
- Prescribing high-potency or ultra-high-potency topical corticosteroids on areas with thicker skin such as the palms and soles, and for short-term therapy
- Avoiding high-potency or super-high-potency topical corticosteroids on the intertriginous areas such as the face, groin, axilla, or under occlusion

Determine the desired therapeutic outcome based on the patient's health problem. Health care providers must advise their patients of expected outcomes. In some instances, the outcome will be curative. In other instances, the chronic and recurrent nature of some diseases such as atopic dermatitis and psoriasis limits the complete resolution of symptoms with topical medications. The development and implementation of treatment goals in patients with psoriasis improved overall patient satisfaction and adherence to recommended therapies.

Assess the selected therapy for its appropriateness for an individual patient by considering the patient's age, race/ethnicity, comorbidities, side effects of medications, and genetic factors. Incorporating evidence-based practice guidelines in conjunction with FDA guidelines offers providers and patients a starting point to discuss treatment options.

Initiate the treatment plan with the selected medication by first providing adequate patient education to ensure the patient's understanding and promote full participation in the therapy. The chronic, recurrent nature of some skin disorders may decrease patients' adherence to their treatment plan. One study found that dermatologists are concerned with the overuse (dependence) and underuse of topical corticosteroids resulting in poor control of the disease (Lee et al., 2019). Education and counseling on the disease process, proper use of medications, and expected outcomes may improve adherence (Burroni et al., 2015). Topical

---

• Box 3.1	TCS Addiction and Withdrawal

Key Points

- Caused by prolonged, frequent, inappropriate use (face and genital areas) of moderate- to high-potency TCS.
- Occurs primarily in females.
- Begins within days to weeks of discontinuing steroid.

Presentation

Burning, pain, stinging, itching, peeling or exfoliating skin, oozing, edema, papules, pustules, hives, excessive sweating, confluent erythema, depression, and insomnia.

Treatment

- Discontinue steroid (taper dosing).
- Offer supportive care (ice or cool compresses), consider antihistamines for itching, sleep aids, monitor for secondary infections, and psychological support.

---

corticosteroids can cause dependence and withdrawal in some eczema patients with a history of moderate- to high-potency TCS use, especially to the face or genital area. Health care providers have an essential role in supporting patients as they withdraw from TCS (Box 3.1).

Ensure complete patient and family understanding of the medication prescribed for therapy using a variety of education strategies. Education of the patient and family takes many different forms. Rathod et al. (2013) determined that topical corticosteroids were prescribed in 28% of all prescriptions. In addition, prescriptions lacked clear information regarding the frequency, site, and duration. Prescribing principles (see Chapter 54) cover the importance of including the medication name, dose, frequency, administration details (such as how to apply topical creams), adverse effects, and when to seek further treatment. Extended office visits, multidisciplinary visits, structured counseling, and motivational interviewing can assist the provider in recognizing and addressing the patient's educational needs.

Conduct follow-up and monitoring of patient responses to therapy. Response to therapy should be addressed at each office visit. If possible, consider scheduling the first follow-up visit shortly after the initial visit. In addition, the use of phone calls, text messages, interactive voice response systems, and video conferencing improves communication between scheduled office visits. The use of more than one method is beneficial.

Teaching Points for the Use of Topical Medications

Health Promotion Strategies

- Individualize care for each patient. Assess access to medications and reference resources to obtain medications.
- Demonstrate proper administration or application and necessity of completing full therapy.

- Establish follow-up visits at each visit.
- Monitor for signs of medication effectiveness or adverse effects.

Patient Education for Medication Safety

Topical medications come in ointments, creams, lotions, gels, shampoos, foams, sprays, and powders.

- Do not use the medication for longer than prescribed.
- Use the medication dosage as prescribed. Do not use more or less of the medication than prescribed.
- Avoid applying to the face, axillae, groin, or diaper area unless directed by the health care provider.
- Clean the skin with soap and water or debride the tissue of old medication and encrustation before applying new medication.
- If the condition does not improve in 3 to 5 days, call the health care provider.
- If the condition worsens or if a reaction develops, discontinue use. Wash the affected area and call the health care provider.
- Avoid contact with the eyes and mucous membranes (such as the skin inside the nose, mouth, and genitals).
- The affected skin should not be bandaged, covered, or wrapped unless specifically directed to do so by the health care provider.
- Do not apply topical pain relievers onto damaged or irritated skin.
- Certain medications may cause severe birth defects or death. Use contraceptives to prevent pregnancy.
- Tretinoin: apply sunscreen with sun protection factor of 15 or more. Wear protective clothing. Do not apply to areas already affected by a sunburn.
  Tell your provider:
- If you are allergic to this medication, any other medications, foods, dyes, or preservatives
- If you develop depression, anxiety, thoughts of suicide, or other mental health concerns
- If you develop any response that would suggest an allergic reaction
- If you are pregnant or thinking of becoming pregnant and/or breastfeeding

Application Questions for Discussion

1. What are two common adverse effects related to topical corticosteroid use?
2. What are the goals of treatment for acne therapy?
3. Identify three factors that affect the absorption of topical medications.

Selected Bibliography

Burroni, A. G., Fassino, M., Torti, A., & Visentin, E. (2015). How do disease perception, treatment features, and dermatologist-patient relationship impact on patients assuming topical treatment? An Italian survey. *Patient Related Outcome Measures, 6,* 9–17. doi:10.2147/PROM.S76551.

Chiesa Fuxench, Z. C., Block, J. K., Boguniewicz, M., Boyle, J., Fonacier, L., Gelfand, J. M., Grayson, M. H., Margolis, D. J., Mitchell, L., Silverberg, J. I., Schwartz, L., Simpson, E. L., & Ong, P. Y. (2019). Atopic dermatitis in America study: A cross-sectional study examining the prevalence and disease burden of atopic dermatitis in the US adult population. *Journal of Investigative Dermatology, 139*(3), 583–590. doi.org/10.1016/j.jid.2018.08.028.

Ellis, K. K., & Colcher, K. R. (2017). Principles of dermatologic therapy. In T. M Buttaro, J. Trybulski, P. Polgar-Bailey, & J. Sandberg-Cook (Eds.), *Primary Care: A Collaborative Practice.* (5th ed.). St. Louis: Elsevier.

Fresenius Kabi USA, LLC. (2014). *2% Viscous Lidocaine.* https://www.accessdata.fda.gov/drugsatfda_docs/label/2014/009470s025lbl.pdf.

Hajar, T., Leshem, Y. A., Hanifin, J. M., Nedorost, S. T., Lio, P. A., Paller, A. S., Block, J., & Simpson, E. L. the National Eczema Task Force. (2015). A systematic review of topical corticosteroid withdrawal ("steroid addiction") in patients with atopic dermatitis and other dermatoses. *Journal of the American Academy of Dermatology, 72*(3), 541–549.e2. http://dx.doi.org/10.1016/j.jaad.2014.11.024.

Lanier, C., Laurent, D., & Kelly, K. (2018). Topical treatment of dermatophytes and candida in the hospital setting. *U. S. Pharmacist, 43*(6), HS-9–HS-12. https://www.uspharmacist.com/article/topical-treatment-of-dermatophytes-and-candida-in-the-hospital-setting.

Lee, L., El-Den, S., Horne, R., Carter, S. R. (2019). Patient satisfaction with information, concerns, beliefs and adherence to topical corticosteroids. *Patient Education & Counseling, 102*(6), 1203-1209. http://dx.doi.org.ezproxy.hsc.usf.edu/10.1016/j.pec.2019.01.019.

Lexicomp. (2020, November 29). *Comparison of representative topical corticosteroid preparations (classified according to the US system) (Lexi-Drugs).* https://online-lexi-com.ezproxy.hsc.usf.edu/lco/action/doc/retrieve/docid/patch_f/3674386.

Lim, H. W., Collins, S. A. B., Resneck, J. S., Bolognia, J. L., Hodge, J. A., Rohrer, T. A., Van Beck, M. J., Margolis, D. J., Sober, A. J., Weinstok, M. A., Nerenz, D. R., Begolka, W. S., & Moyano, J. V. (2017). The burden of skin disease in the United States. *American Academy of Dermatology, 76*(5), 958–972.e2. http://dx.doi.org/10.1016/j.jaad.2016.12.043.

Masterson, K. N. (2018). Acne basics: pathophysiology, assessment, and standard treatment options. *Dermatology Nurses' Association, 10*(1S), S1–S10. https://journals.lww.com/jdnaonline/fulltext/2018/01001/Acne_Basics__Pathophysiology,_Assessment,_and.2.aspx.

McKenzie, C. & Silverberg, J. I. (2019). The prevalence and persistence of atopic dermatitis in urban United States children. *Annals of Allergy, 123*(2), 173–178.e1. https://doi.org/10.1016/j.anai.2019.05.014.

Perrone, V., Sangiorgi, D., Buda, S., & Esposti, L. D. (2017). Topical medication utilization and health resources consumption in adult patients affected by psoriasis: Findings from the analysis of administrative databases of local health units. *ClinicoEconomics and Outcomes Research, 9,* 181–188. https://doi.org/10.2147/CEOR.S126975.

Rathod, S. S., Motghare, V. M., Deshmukh, V. S., Deshpande, R. P., Bhamare, C. G., & Patil, J. R. (2013). Prescribing practices of topical corticosteroids in the outpatient dermatology department of a rural tertiary care teaching hospital. *Indian Journal of Dermatology, 58*(5), 342–345. https://doi.org/10.4103/0019-5154.117293.

Ray, G. T., Suaya, J. A., & Baxter, R. (2013). Incidence, microbiology, and patient characteristics of skin and soft-tissue infections in a U.S. population: A retrospective population-based study. *BMC Infectious Disease, 13*(252), 1–11. https://doi.org/10.1186/1471-2334-13-252.

Up-To-Date. (2020, November 29). *Comparison of representative topical corticosteroid preparations (classified according to the US system).* https://www.uptodate.com/contents/image?imageKey=DERM%2F62402&topicKey=DERM%2F1730&source=see_link.

U. S. Food & Drug Administration. (n. d.). *Orange book: Approved drug products with therapeutic equivalence evaluations.* (Accessed November 29, 2020). https://www.accessdata.fda.gov/scripts/cder/ob/search_product.cfm.

U. S. Food and Drug Administration. (2018). Risk of serious and potentially fatal blood disorder prompts FDA action on oral over-the-counter benzocaine products used for teething and mouth pain and prescription local anesthetics. *Drug Safety Communications.* https://www.fda.gov/media/113261/download.

4

Eye and Ear Medications

CHERYL H. ZAMBROSKI

Overview

The primary care provider may serve as the first line of defense in the prevention of chronic vision and hearing loss through careful assessment, proper management, and appropriate referral to specialty providers. According to the Centers for Disease Control and Prevention (CDC), approximately 61 million adults are at risk for serious vision loss, with hearing loss ranking as the third most chronic physical condition in the United States (CDC, 2018). In addition, more than 45 million contact lens wearers engage in behaviors that increase their risk for serious eye infection (Konne et al., 2019). Furthermore, nearly 15% of children have some degree of hearing impairment and nearly 85% experience ear infections before the age of 3 (National Institute on Deafness and Other Communication Disorders [NIDCD], 2016). These statistics illustrate the importance of screening and early intervention and referral for problems of the eye and ear in both children and adults.

This chapter reviews common disorders associated with vision and hearing that are amenable to pharmacologic management in primary care. Selected disorders include conditions commonly treated in primary care and those that may be managed by ophthalmologists but are often seen in primary care patients. Given that many ophthalmic and otic medications are commonly prescribed at primary care visits, a goal of this chapter is to help the provider reduce the risk of medication interactions, reinforce ophthalmology recommendations, and recognize complications requiring referral.

Relevant Physiology

The eyes are globe-shaped sense organs located within bony orbits that surround and protect the eyes. Extraocular muscles innervated by cranial nerves III (*oculomotor*), IV (*trochlear*), and VI (*abducens*) allow the eyes to focus on single objects through coordinated movements. Cranial nerve V (*trigeminal*) stimulates the blink reflex, while cranial nerve VII (*facial*) innervates the muscles for lid closure and tearing. The external part of the eye includes the eyelids, conjunctiva, and lacrimal apparatus. The *eyelids* protect the eye from foreign bodies and help control the amount of light reaching the eye. The *conjunctiva* are thin, translucent membranes that line the anterior part of the sclera and the eyelids. The *bulbar conjunctiva* begins at the edge of the cornea and covers the visible part of the sclera while the *palpebral conjunctiva* lines the inside of the eyelids (Fig. 4.1). Lacrimal glands are located at the upper outer corners of the orbit and produce tears that lubricate and protect the cornea (Fig. 4.2). Tears can also protect the eye from irritants such as smoke, fumes from onions, and foreign bodies. Tears are evenly distributed over the lens by blinking. Tears drain through the puncta at the lid margins into the lacrimal ducts and sac, then to the nasolacrimal duct and the nose.

Fig. 4.3 shows the basic internal anatomy of the eye. Light enters the eye through the cornea. The iris is a thin, circular structure that is responsible for adjusting the diameter of the pupil. It controls the amount of light that is focused on the retina by the lens. The lens and cornea are nourished by the aqueous humor, a clear, watery fluid secreted by the ciliary body. The fluid drains through the canal of Schlemm and into the spongelike trabecular meshwork where it is reabsorbed. This free flow of aqueous humor and reabsorption through the canal of Schlemm helps maintain consistent intraocular pressure (IOP).

The vitreous chamber is filled with *vitreous humor*, a gel-like substance that is behind the lens. The *retina* is the innermost layer of the eye that contains photoreceptors, rods, and cones that convert light into nerve impulses. These nerve impulses pass through the optic nerve.

The ear is composed of three major sections: external, middle, and internal. The external ear consists of the pinna and the external auditory canal. The external auditory canal secretes *cerumen* (earwax) that serves to reduce or block penetration of water and helps prevent bacterial or fungal infection. The external auditory canal also directs sound waves to the tympanic membrane. The tympanic membrane separates the external ear from the middle ear. The middle ear houses the malleus, incus, and stapes that transmit sound vibrations from the tympanic membrane to the inner ear. The eustachian tube connects the middle ear to the *nasopharynx*, a tube that allows air to enter the middle ear, helps maintain equal air pressure on both sides of the tympanic membrane, and prevents fluid from accumulating in the middle ear. The inner ear then transduces the sound into nerve impulses.

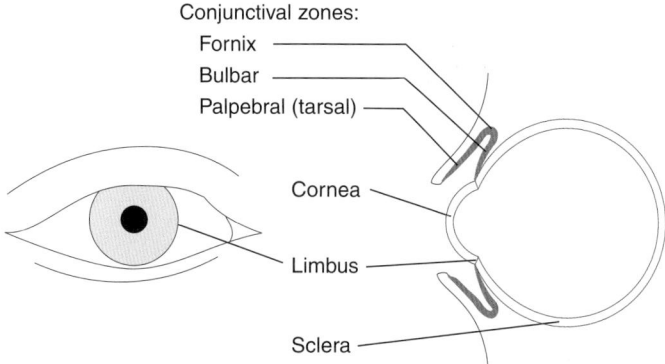

• **Fig. 4.1 Normal conjunctival anatomy.** The conjunctiva is a thin membrane covering the sclera (bulbar conjunctiva, labeled with blue) and the inside of the eyelids (palpebral conjunctiva, labeled with blue). (From McGee, S. [2018]. *Evidence-based physical diagnosis* [4th ed.]. St. Louis: Elsevier.)

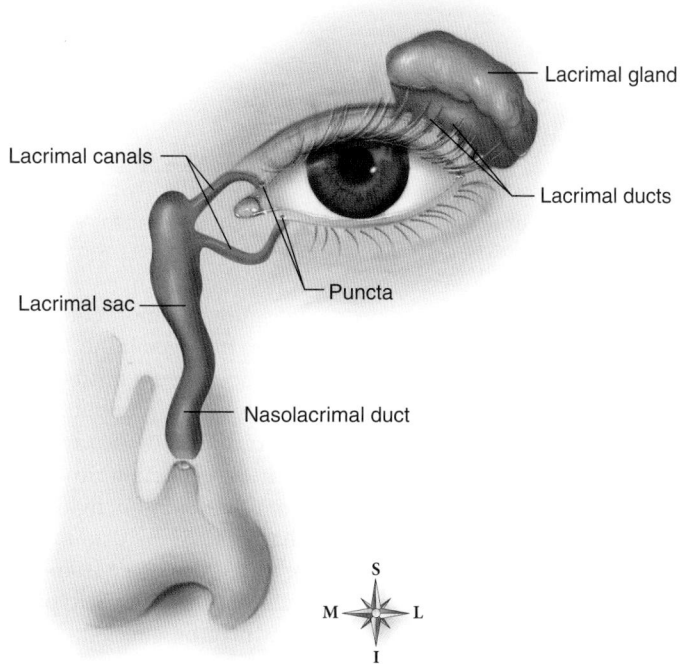

• **Fig. 4.2 Lacrimal apparatus.** Fluid produced by lacrimal glands (tears) streams across the eye surface, enters the canals, and then passes through the lacrimal sac and nasolacrimal duct to enter the nose. (From Patton, K., Thibodeau, G., & Douglas, M. [2011]. *Essentials of anatomy & physiology*. St. Louis: Mosby.)

Pathophysiology

Eye Disorders Commonly Seen in Primary Care

This section covers common eye disorders that are amenable to medication therapy in primary care, including conjunctivitis (bacterial and allergic), blepharitis, chalazion, hordeolum, dacrocystitis, keratoconjunctivitis sicca, and corneal abrasion. This section also covers medications for glaucoma, a chronic eye condition frequently seen in older adults.

The most common ophthalmic condition treated by primary care providers is *conjunctivitis* (also known as *pink eye*). Conjunctivitis is an inflammatory disorder characterized by dilation of the blood vessels nourishing the conjunctiva, which results in redness, swelling, and irritation. Vison can become blurry and the eye may release watery or purulent discharge, depending on the etiology. Patients may also experience itchiness or burning of the eye and mild pain. Some patients may feel as though they have grit or sand in their eye, even with no evidence of a foreign body.

Inflammation of the conjunctiva can be of infectious or noninfectious origin. *Infectious conjunctivitis* is caused by a virus or bacteria; *noninfectious conjunctivitis* can be caused by a wide variety of factors, including allergens, a foreign body, a subconjunctival hemorrhage, or a chemical burn. Viruses are the most common cause of infectious conjunctivitis

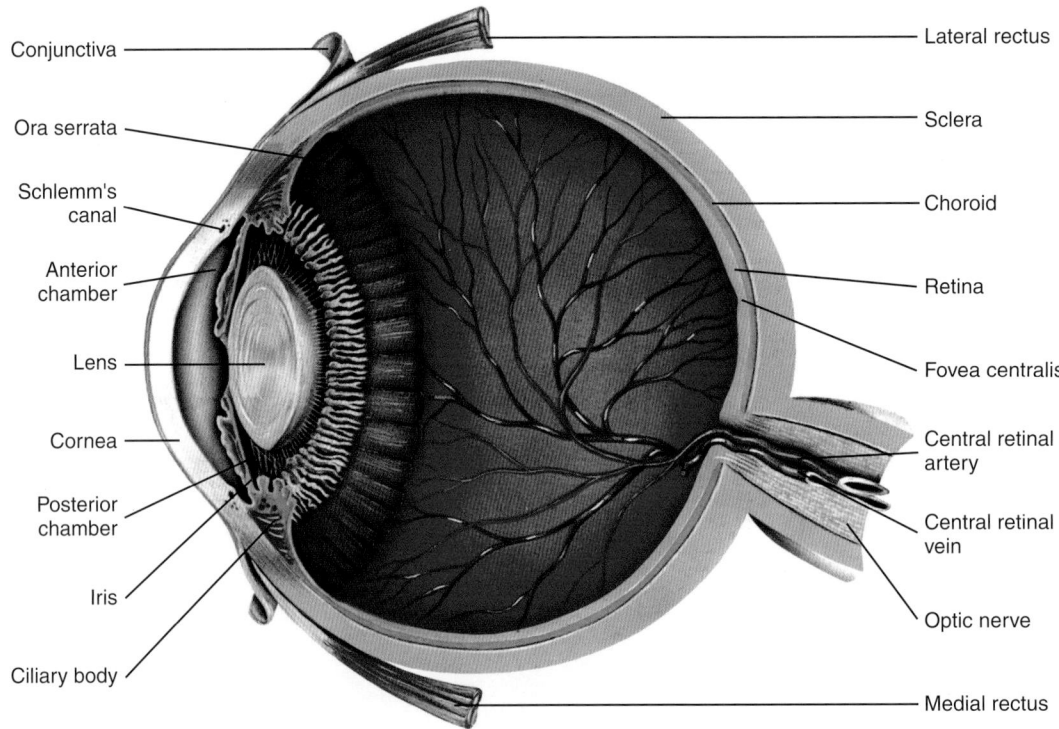

Conjunctiva

Ora serrata

Schlemm's canal

Anterior chamber

Lens

Cornea

Posterior chamber

Iris

Ciliary body

Lateral rectus

Sclera

Choroid

Retina

Fovea centralis

Central retinal artery

Central retinal vein

Optic nerve

Medial rectus

• **Fig. 4.3** Internal anatomy of the eye. (From Thibodeau, G. A., & Patton, K. T. [2009]. *Anatomy & physiology* [7th ed.]. St Louis: Mosby.)

overall (Azari & Barney, 2013), predominantly due to adenoviruses. Other examples of viral causes include herpes simplex virus (HSV), herpes zoster, enterovirus, and coxsackievirus. Herpes zoster conjunctivitis usually affects one eye, is accompanied by a vesicular rash distributed along the ophthalmic division of the trigeminal cranial nerve, and is often associated with severe eye pain.

Bacterial conjunctivitis is most commonly caused by *Streptococcus pneumoniae, Haemophilus influenzae, Staphylococcus aureus,* or *Moraxella* species. *Haemophilus influenzae* and *Streptococcus pneumoniae* are common in children. Symptoms include conjunctival redness, tearing, mild pain, and itchiness or a gritty feeling in the eye. Discharge from the eye is typically purulent but may be watery or mucopurulent. Patients may awaken with crusting and stickiness of the eyelids. Mild bacterial conjunctivitis may be self-limiting and may clear within 10 days. Nevertheless, antibiotics may reduce the duration and severity of symptoms.

PRACTICE PEARLS

Culturing Eye Discharge

Culture of eye discharge in routine cases of conjunctivitis is rarely helpful in determining treatment in children and adults. It may be helpful in patients with recurrent, severe, or chronic purulent conjunctivitis or in cases in which patients did not respond to treatment (Varu et al., 2019).

Adult inclusion conjunctivitis, an acute infection associated with *Chlamydia trachomatis*, is a sexually transmitted infection. It is more common in female patients and typically results from genital-to-hand-to-eye transmission. Symptoms include redness, mucopurulent discharge, tearing, swollen eyelids, and photophobia. The patient may also have enlarged preauricular lymph nodes.

It is important to distinguish bacterial conjunctivitis from viral conjunctivitis (Fig. 4.4). Viral conjunctivitis is characterized by conjunctival redness with diffuse, watery, or serous discharge from the eye as well as mild burning or itching of the eye. It typically begins in one eye, but both eyes may be affected. Viral conjunctivitis is often associated with symptoms of upper respiratory infection such as sore throat, fever, and preauricular lymphadenopathy. It is easily transmitted to others, so hand hygiene is essential. In addition, patients should avoid wearing contact lenses and sharing personal care items (Box 4.1). If symptoms do not resolve in 10 days or if there is involvement of the cornea, the patient should be referred to an ophthalmologist (Box 4.2).

A major cause of noninfectious conjunctivitis is allergies. *Allergic conjunctivitis* occurs upon exposure to specific allergens, typically molds and pollens. It is often seasonal but may occur year-round in patients allergic to dust or molds. It presents with itching and tearing and is characterized by cobblestone papillae on the upper tarsal conjunctiva.

Blepharitis is a chronic inflammatory condition of the eyelids. It is often associated with *Staphylococcus* infection as well as seborrheic dermatitis. Blepharitis is typically classified as anterior and/or posterior. *Anterior blepharitis* involves inflammation of the eyelash follicles and skin on the eyelids, causing the rims of the eyelids to appear red.

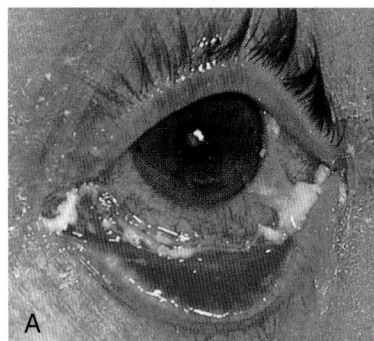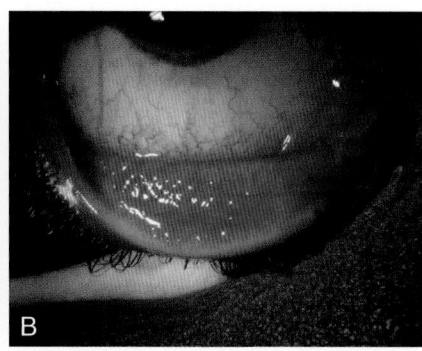

• **Fig. 4.4** Characteristic appearance of bacterial and viral conjunctivitis. **(A)** Bacterial conjunctivitis characterized by mucopurulent discharge and conjunctival hyperemia. **(B)** Intensely hyperemic response with thin, watery discharge characteristic of viral conjunctivitis. (A from Buttaro, T.M., Polgar-Bailey, P., Sandberg-Cook, J., & Trybulski, J. [2021]. *Primary care* [6th ed.]. St. Louis: Elsevier. B from Chabner, D. [2021]. *The language of medicine* [12th ed.]. St. Louis: Elsevier.)

• Box 4.1   Patient Teaching for Contact Lens Wearers

- Avoid wearing contact lenses while sleeping or napping.
- Only use re-wetting drops that are preservative free and in single-use packaging.
- Wash and dry hands before and after inserting or removing contact lenses.
- Use recommended products for cleaning and storing contact lenses.
- Replace contact lenses according to manufacturer's recommendations.
- Remove contact lenses before swimming or entering a hot tub.
- Avoid washing or storing contact lenses in water.
- Replace contact lens cases every three months or as recommended by manufacturer.
- Avoid showering while wearing contact lenses.
- If you wear makeup/cosmetics:
  - Use only cosmetics that are designed to be used around the eyes.
  - Choose nonallergenic makeup.
  - Make sure to insert the contact lenses before applying makeup.
  - Apply makeup outside the lash line to avoid blocking oil glands of the upper and lower eyelids.
  - Avoid keeping eye makeup for longer than three months.
  - Water-based cream shadows are preferred over powder.
  - If your makeup causes irritation, wash it off and contact your provider.
  - If you develop conjunctivitis, discard all eye makeup.
  - Do not share eye makeup or other cosmetics.
  - Remove all makeup before bedtime.

Adapted from Gudgel, D. (2019). American Academy of Ophthalmology: How to use cosmetics safely around your eyes (retrieved from https://www.aao.org/eye-health/tips-prevention/eye-makeup); and Konne, N. M., et al. (2019). Healthy contact lens behaviors communicated by eye care providers and recalled by patients — United States, 2018, *Morbidity and Mortality Weekly Report* (68), 693–697, doi: http://dx.doi.org/10.15585/mmwr.mm6832a2.

• Box 4.2   Conditions of Conjunctivitis Recommended for Referral to Ophthalmology Specialty

- Vision loss
- Moderate or severe pain
- Patients with corneal involvement
- Evidence of conjunctival scarring
- Lack of response to therapy
- Recurrent episodes
- History of HSV eye disease
- Patient who is immunocompromised

Adapted from Varu, D. M., et al. (2019). Conjunctivitis preferred practice pattern. *Ophthalmology, 126* (1), P94–P169. doi:10.1016/j.ophtha.2018.10.020.

Posterior blepharitis is inflammation of the *meibomian glands* (located on the rims of the eyelids). These glands normally produce oils that help prevent evaporation of tears. Both types of blepharitis may be associated with recurrent conjunctivitis. Symptoms include swollen, itchy eyelids; matting of eyelashes upon awakening; excessive tearing; and sensitivity to light. While excellent eye hygiene is imperative for treatment of blepharitis, some patients may require medication.

A *chalazion* is a chronic, lipogranulomatous inflammation of a meibomian gland. It is typically slow growing and painless. The nodule is pea-like at the margin of the eyelid. Symptoms may include mild tenderness, tearing, and the sensation of a foreign body in the eye. If infection is present, the entire eyelid may be swollen.

A *hordeolum* (stye) is an acute bacterial infection located near the root of the eyelashes and is usually caused by *Staphylococcus aureus*. An *external hordeolum* is caused by a blockage of the glands of Zeis (sebaceous) or glands of Moll (sweat) of the eye. The blocked glands become painful and swollen and form a pustule on the external surface of the eye. An *internal hordeolum* is the result of blocked meibomian glands. In this case, the pustule forms on the internal surface of the eyelid. Treatment for hordeolum typically consists of an eyelid scrub and warm compresses. If draining is present or if the hordeolum occurs with blepharoconjunctivitis, topical antibiotic ointment can be used.

Dacryocystitis is an infection of the lacrimal sac that typically occurs as a result of an obstruction of the nasolacrimal duct. Organisms commonly associated with dacryocystitis are *Staphylococcus* and *Streptococcus* species, *Haemophilus influenza*, and *Pseudomonas aeruginosa*. Symptoms include redness, swelling, and pain around the lacrimal sac. In addition, gentle pressure over the lacrimal sac may express purulent drainage. Tearing of the eyes and a fever are common. Oral antibiotics such as dicloxacillin or erythromycin may be prescribed; see Chapter 41, Cephalosporins, and Chapter 44, Fluoroquinolones.

Keratoconjunctivitis sicca (KCS), often called *dry eye*, is a chronic condition associated with insufficient lubrication of the eye. Etiology can be from insufficient production of tears or from loss of tears due to rapid evaporation. The rapid evaporation can be due to lack of oils produced by the meibomian glands. KCS is more common in older patients and postmenopausal patients. It is commonly associated with autoimmune disorders such as rheumatoid arthritis and Sjögren's syndrome. In addition, several common medications can result in symptoms of KCS, including beta-blockers, antihistamines, anticholinergics, and certain antidepressants such as sertraline and paroxetine.

Corneal abrasions result from direct trauma to the eye caused by a foreign object such as a fingernail, a tree branch, a pet, metal shavings, or a contact lens. Even sand or dust in the eye, if the eye is rubbed, can cause an abrasion to the cornea. Symptoms include pain, tearing, photophobia, redness, and, at times, the sensation of a foreign body in the eye. Corneal abrasions are extremely painful to the sufferer, so they often present to the primary care provider on an urgent basis.

Glaucoma is a group of eye diseases characterized by increased IOP resulting in damage to the optic nerve with diminished peripheral vision and ultimately blindness. The most common type of glaucoma is *primary open-angle glaucoma* (POAG). POAG results from an obstruction to the outflow of aqueous humor at the trabecular meshwork or canal of Schlemm (Fig. 4.5). POAG typically has no symptoms, so the increase in IOP and decrease in peripheral vision is gradual and may be undetected until significant vision loss has occurred. Box 4.3 lists risk factors for glaucoma. *Normal-tension glaucoma* results in optic nerve damage, even with normal IOPs. While the exact cause is unknown, normal-tension glaucoma is more common in patients of Japanese ancestry or those with a history of systemic heart disease. For all patients who have a history of glaucoma or are at risk for glaucoma, it is important to recognize that a variety of medications can increase IOP (Box 4.4). *Acute angle-closure glaucoma* results in a sudden decrease in outflow of aqueous humor with a rapid increase in IOP, eye pain, and loss of visual acuity. Acute angle-closure glaucoma is a medical emergency, and the patient must be referred to an ophthalmologist for pharmacologic treatment.

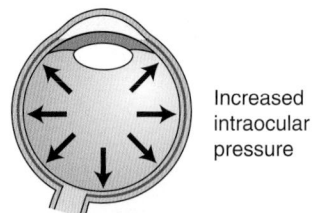

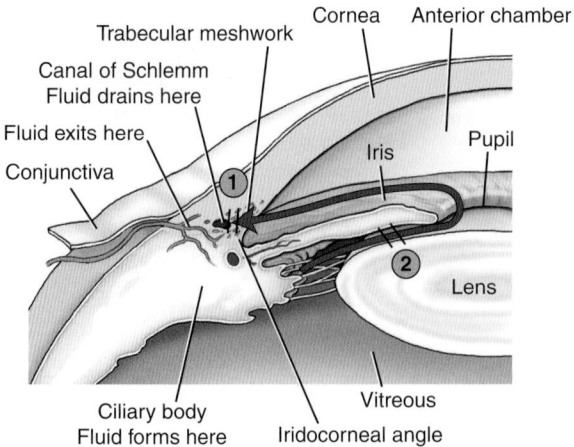

• **Fig. 4.5** Glaucoma. *1*, Open-angle glaucoma. The obstruction to aqueous flow lies in the trabecular meshwork. *2*, Closed-angle glaucoma. The iris presses against the lens, blocking aqueous flow into the anterior chamber and raising IOP. (From McCance, K., & Huether, S. [2019]. *Pathophysiology* [8th ed.]. St. Louis: Elsevier.)

• **Box 4.3** **Risk Factors for Glaucoma**

- African Americans >40 years of age
- Hispanic descent
- Asian descent
- All adults >60 years of age
- Family history of glaucoma
- People with diabetes
- Obstructive sleep apnea
- People with history of eye injury

• **Box 4.4** **Examples of Medications That May Increase Intraocular Pressure**

- Corticosteroids (systemic, nasal, inhaled, ophthalmic)
- Ophthalmic anticholinergics
- Vasodilators
- Antihistamines
- Venlafaxine
- Serotonin-selective reuptake inhibitors (SSRIs)
- Ipratropium
- Antipsychotics
- Sulfa drugs
- Epinephrine
- Topiramate
- Tricyclic antidepressants
- Monoamine oxidase inhibitors (MAOIs)

aMany other medications can increase IOP. Primary care providers should check medications before prescribing to patients with glaucoma.

Ear Disorders Commonly Seen in Primary Care

This section covers common ear disorders that are amenable to medication therapy in primary care, including acute otitis media, otitis externa, and cerumen impaction. While tinnitus may be seen in primary care, there are no specific pharmacologic interventions that are routinely used, and the provider may choose to refer the patient to a specialist in the area.

Acute otitis media is one of the most common conditions seen in primary care globally (Finley et al., 2018). While it is more common in children, adults can also be diagnosed with acute otitis media. It is an inflammatory condition of the middle ear associated with an acute bacterial infection. Bacteria and fluid accumulate in the middle ear, often due to eustachian tube dysfunction. The most common organisms associated with acute otitis media are *Streptococcus pneumoniae*, *Haemophilus influenzae*, and *Moraxella catarrhalis*. Symptoms include ear pain, fever, nausea, sleeplessness, and in some cases, diarrhea. Acute otitis media may follow an upper respiratory infection. *Recurrent otitis media* is defined as acute otitis media that occurs three or more times within 6 months or four or more times within 12 months. These patients may require longer-term antibiotics and/or referral to a specialist. Oral antibiotic therapies are discussed in Unit 13, Antiinfective Medications.

Otitis externa is an acute inflammatory condition of the external auditory canal and auricle generally caused by bacteria. Symptoms include pain (particularly with manipulation or gentle pressure on the tragus), redness and swelling of the external canal, purulent drainage from the ear, and possibly reduction or loss of hearing. Common causes include water remaining in the ear after swimming, trauma from removal of cerumen, use of hearing aids, and skin conditions such as seborrhea and eczema. Organisms that are often associated with otitis externa include *Pseudomonas aeruginosa*, *Staphylococcus aureus*, *Staphylococcus epidermidis*, and *Microbacterium otitis*.

PRACTICE PEARLS

Prevention of Swimmer's Ear

To prevent otitis externa in swimmers (also known as swimmer's ear), encourage patients to keep ears as dry as possible (through use of a swim cap or ear plugs, for example), and to dry ears thoroughly after swimming and then tilt the head down to let water drain freely. If ears are still wet, patients can use a hair dryer, running on the lowest setting and held several inches from the ears, to dry them.

Cerumen impaction results from a buildup of the cerumen in the external ear canal. It most commonly occurs in older patients, when cilia lining the ear canal become stiff and cerumen becomes trapped. Additionally, improper use of cotton swabs as well as use of paper clips and hair pins in the ear canal can push cerumen into the canal, causing impaction. Patients who use hearing aids may also be at higher risk. Symptoms include hearing loss, dizziness, ear pain, and dryness or itching of the ear canal.

Common Eye and Ear Therapy

Once an assessment has been completed and diagnosis has been determined, the primary care provider will select appropriate pharmacologic therapies. Categories of medications discussed in this section include antibiotics, antivirals, nonsteroidal antiinflammatories, medications for allergic conjunctivitis, medications for glaucoma, lubricants, immunomodulators, topical anesthetics, diagnostic agents, and medications to treat cerumen impaction (Table 4.1).

Fluoroquinolones

Fluoroquinolones are broad-spectrum antibiotics used to treat a number of infectious diseases including those affecting the eyes. They inhibit deoxyribonucleic acid (DNA) gyrase and topoisomerase IV, thereby interfering with DNA replication, repair, and transcription. Fluoroquinolones are active against a number of gram-positive and gram-negative organisms including *Streptococcus pneumonia*, *Staphylococcus aureus*, *Chlamydia* species, and *Haemophilus influenza*. Fluoroquinolones are available in ophthalmic and otic forms. Chapter 44 provides a review of oral and parenteral forms of fluoroquinolone antibiotics.

Ofloxacin

Pharmacokinetics. There is minimal systemic absorption of ophthalmic ofloxacin. Serum concentrations of ofloxacin otic solution have been detected in patients with perforated tympanic membranes but are highly variable.

Indications. Ofloxacin is indicated for treatment of ophthalmic bacterial infections including conjunctivitis and corneal ulcers. It can also be used for treatment of otitis externa and otitis media. Olfoxacin is effective in treating organisms including *Escherichia coli*, *Haemophilus influenzae*, *Moraxella catarrhalis*, *Neisseria gonorrhoeae*, *Pseudomonas aeruginosa*, *Staphylococcus aureus*, *Staphylococcus epidermidis*, *Streptococcus pneumoniae*, and *Chlamydia trachomatis*.

Adverse Effects. Ophthalmic preparations of ofloxacin can cause temporary burning or stinging upon application of the eye drops. Rarely, patients may experience itching, sensation of a foreign body, mild eye pain, photophobia, or tearing. Otic solutions may cause irritation to the site of application, mild ear pain, or tinnitus.

Contraindications. Ofloxacin is contraindicated in patients with quinolone hypersensitivity. Patients with symptoms of bacterial conjunctivitis should not use contact lenses while being treated with ofloxacin ophthalmic preparations.

Monitoring. Remind patients of the importance of proper dosing and proper technique when administering eye drops to minimize risk of secondary infection. Teach patients to report to the primary care provider any increase in purulent discharge from the eye or increased inflammation and pain. Teach patients to report any increase in discharge from the ear or increase in ear pain when using otic preparations.

TABLE 4.1   **Eye and Ear Medications**

Category	Medication	Indication	Dosage	Considerations
Fluoroquinolones	Ciprofloxacin ophthalmic	Bacterial conjunctivitis	**Solution:** *Adults, adolescents, children, and infants:* Instill 1–2 drops into affected eye(s) every 2 hr, while awake, for the first 2 days and then every 4 hr, while awake, for the next 5 days. **Ointment:** *Adults, adolescents, and children >2 yr:* Apply ½-inch ribbon to conjunctival sac three times daily for the first 2 days, then ½-inch ribbon twice daily for the next 5 days.	Use only solutions labeled "For Ophthalmic Use Only." Apply topically, avoiding contamination. Teach proper technique. Do not touch tip of the eyedropper to the eye, fingertips, or other surfaces.
	Besifloxacin ophthalmic		**0.6% Solution:** *Adults, adolescents, and children:* Instill 1 drop into affected eye(s) three times daily, 4–12 hr apart, for 7 days.	
	Ofloxacin ophthalmic		**0.3% Solution:** *Adults, adolescents, and children:* Instill 1–2 drops into affected eye(s) every 2–4 hr for the first 2 days, then 1–2 drops four times daily for the next 5 days.	
	Levofloxacin		**0.5% Solution:** *Adults, adolescents, and children:* Instill 1–2 drops into affected eye(s) every 2 hr while awake, up to eight times daily for the first 2 days, then 1–2 drops every 4 hr while awake, up to four times daily for the next 5 days.	
	Moxifloxacin	Bacterial conjunctivitis, including chlamydial conjunctivitis	**0.5% Solution:** *Adults, adolescents, children, and infants:* Instill 1 drop into affected eye(s) three times daily for 7 days.	
	Ciprofloxacin otic	Otitis externa	**Solution:** *Adults, adolescents, and children:* Instill 0.5 mg (one 0.25 mL single-use container) into affected ear(s) every 12 hr for 7 days. **Suspension:** *Adults, adolescents, children, and infants 6-11 mo:* Instill 12 mg (0.2 mL) into external ear canal of affected ear(s) as a single dose.	For otic use only. Teach proper technique for otic administration.

TABLE 4.1   **Eye and Ear Medications—cont'd**

Category	Medication	Indication	Dosage	Considerations
Aminoglycosides	Gentamicin sulfate	Bacterial conjunctivitis, blepharitis, blepharoconjunctivitis, dacryocystitis, keratoconjunctivitis, and acute meibomianitis	**0.3% Solution:** *Adults, adolescents, children, and infants:* Instill 1–2 drops into affected eye(s) every 4 hr. For severe infections, instill up to 2 drops hourly. **0.3% Ointment:** *Adults, adolescents, children, and infants:* Apply small amount (approximately ½-inch ribbon) to affected eye(s) two or three times daily.	Instruct patient on proper instillation of eye ointment and/or solution. Do not touch the tip of the dropper to the eye, fingertips, or other surfaces. Avoid activities requiring visual acuity until vison clears, particularly after use of ointment.
	Tobramycin ophthalmic		**0.3% Solution:** *Adults, adolescents, children, and infants ≥2 mo:* Instill 1–2 drops into affected eye(s) every 4 hr. For severe infections, instill 2 drops hourly until improvement, then reduce to less frequent intervals. **0.3% Ointment:** *Adults, adolescents, children, and infants ≥2 mo:* Apply thin strip (about ½ inch) to conjunctiva every 8–12 hr. For severe infections, apply every 3–4 hr until improvement, then reduce to less frequent intervals.	
Macrolides	Azithromycin ophthalmic	Bacterial conjunctivitis	**1% Solution:** *Adults, adolescents, and children ≥1 yr:* Instill 1 drop into affected eye(s) twice daily (8–12 hr apart) for the first 2 days, followed by 1 drop into affected eye(s) once daily for the next 5 days.	Instruct patient on proper instillation of eye ointment and/or solution. Do not touch the tip of the dropper to the eye, fingertips, or other surfaces. Avoid activities requiring visual acuity until vison clears, particularly after use of ointment forms.
	Erythromycin ophthalmic	Superficial ophthalmic infection involving the conjunctiva and/or cornea	**0.5% Ointment:** *Adults, adolescents, children, and infants:* Apply a ribbon approximately 1 cm in length to infected structure of the eye up to six times daily, depending on severity of infection.	

Continued

TABLE 4.1 Eye and Ear Medications—cont'd

Category	Medication	Indication	Dosage	Considerations
Sulfonamides	Sulfacetamide sodium ophthalmic	Bacterial conjunctivitis, corneal ulcer, and other superficial ophthalmic infections, and as adjunctive treatment in systemic sulfonamide therapy of chlamydial conjunctivitis, including trachoma and inclusion conjunctivitis	**10% Solution:** *Adults, adolescents, children, and infants >2 mo:* Instill 1–2 drops into affected eye(s) every 1–3 hr during the day, less frequently at night. Dosage frequency depends on severity of infection. **10% Ointment:** *Adults, adolescents, children, and infants >2 months:* Apply small amount to affected eye(s) four times daily and at bedtime. May be used adjunctively with sulfacetamide solutions.	Instruct patient on proper instillation of eye ointment or solution into the lower conjunctival sac. Do not touch the tip of the dropper or tube to the eye, fingertips, or other surfaces. The ointment may be applied at night in combination with daytime use of the solution or before application of an eye patch. Do not share eye products between patients.
Combination	Polymyxin B sulfate/trimethoprim sulfate 10,000 units/1 mg/mL ophthalmic	Ocular infections, including bacterial conjunctivitis and blepharoconjunctivitis	**Solution:** *Adults, adolescents, children, and infants ≥2 months:* Instill 1 drop into affected eye(s) every 3 hr up to six times daily for 7–10 days.	Instruct patient on proper instillation of eye ointment and/or solution. Do not touch the tip of the dropper to the eye, fingertips, or other surfaces. Avoid activities requiring visual acuity until vison clears, particularly after use of ointment forms.
	Bacitracin, neomycin, polymyxin B ophthalmic	Superficial ophthalmic infection (e.g., bacterial conjunctivitis, keratitis, keratoconjunctivitis, blepharitis, and blepharoconjunctivitis)	**Ointment:** *Adults only:* Apply thin strip (approximately ½ inch) to affected eye(s) every 3–4 hr for 7–10 days, depending on severity of infection.	
	Bacitracin, hydrocortisone, neomycin, polymyxin B ophthalmic	Corticosteroid-responsive inflammatory ocular conditions in which a bacterial ophthalmic infection or risk of bacterial ophthalmic infection exists	**Ointment:** *Adults only:* Apply thin strip into affected eye(s) every 3–4 hr, depending on severity of infection. Do not use more than 8 g or for longer than 10 days initially; prescription should not be refilled without further evaluation.	
Antivirals	Trifluridine ophthalmic	Herpes simplex keratitis (dendritic keratitis), including primary keratoconjunctivitis and recurrent epithelial keratitis due to HSV types 1 and 2	**1% Solution:** *Adults, adolescents and children ≥6 years:* Instill 1 drop into affected eye(s) every 2 hr during waking hours, for a maximum daily dosage of 9 drops. Continue until corneal ulcer has completely re-epithelialized, then treat for an additional 7 days with 1 drop every 4 hr during waking hours, for a minimum daily dosage of 5 drops.	These patients should be referred to ophthalmology.

TABLE 4.1   **Eye and Ear Medications—cont'd**

Category	Medication	Indication	Dosage	Considerations
NSAIDs	Ketorolac ophthalmic	Reduction of ocular pruritis due to seasonal allergic conjunctivitis	**0.5% Solution:** *Adults, adolescents, and children >2 yr:* Instill 1 drop into affected eye(s) four times daily.	
Histamine H1 Blockers	Azelastine HCl ophthalmic	Ocular pruritus associated with allergic conjunctivitis	**0.05% Solution:** *Adults, adolescents, and children ≥3 yr:* Instill 1 drop into affected eye(s) twice daily.	
	Emedastine difumarate ophthalmic	Temporary relief of signs and symptoms on allergic conjunctivitis, including ocular pruritus	**0.05% Solution:** *Adults, adolescents, and children ≥3 yr:* Instill 1 drop into affected eye(s) four times daily.	
	Olopatadine HCl ophthalmic	Ocular pruritis associated with allergic conjunctivitis	**0.1% Solution:** *Adults, adolescents, and children ≥3 yr:* Instill 1 drop into affected eye(s) twice daily at intervals of 6–8 hr. **0.2% and 0.7% Solutions:** *Adults, adolescents, and children ≥2 yr:* Instill 1 drop into affected eye(s) once daily.	
Mast Cell Stabilizers	Lodoxamide tromethamine ophthalmic	Ocular inflammatory states such as vernal conjunctivitis, vernal keratitis, and vernal keratoconjunctivitis	**0.1% Solution:** *Adults, adolescents, and children ≥ 2 yr:* Instill 1–2 drops into affected eye(s) four times daily; not to be used for longer than 3 months.	
	Nedocromil ophthalmic	Ocular pruritis related to allergic ocular disorders, including allergic conjunctivitis	**2% Solution:** *Adults, adolescents, and children ≥3 yr:* Instill 1–2 drops into affected eye(s) twice daily at regular intervals.	
Corticosteroids	Dexamethasone ophthalmic	Allergic conjunctivitis; may also be used with caution in patients with viral infection secondary to herpes zoster or in patients with corneal abrasion	**0.1% Solution:** *Adults, adolescents, and children:* Instill 1 or 2 drops into affected eye(s) hourly during the day and every 2 hr at night. Reduce application to every 4 hr (while awake) once a favorable response occurs. Later, further reduction in dosage to 1 drop three or four times daily may suffice to control symptoms. **0.1% Suspension:** *Adults, adolescents, and children:* Instill 1 or 2 drops into affected eye(s). In mild disease, drops may be used up to six times daily.	Most viral infections resolve without pharmacologic treatment. For patients with viral infection secondary to herpes zoster, referral to ophthalmology is recommended.

Continued

TABLE 4.1 **Eye and Ear Medications—cont'd**

Category	Medication	Indication	Dosage	Considerations
Corticosteroids—cont'd	Prednisolone ophthalmic	Allergic conjunctivitis; may also be used in some cases of bacterial conjunctivitis	**1% Solution:** *Adults only:* 01 or 2 drops into affected eye(s) every hour while awake, and every 2 hours at night. When a favorable response is observed, reduce dosage to 1 drop every 4 hours. Thereafter, 1 drop given three or four times daily may suffice to control symptoms. Dosage and duration of treatment will vary with the condition treated and may extend from a few days to several weeks, according to therapeutic response. Relapses, more common in chronic active lesions than in self-limited conditions, usually respond to retreatment. In chronic conditions, withdrawal of treatment should be carried out by gradually decreasing the frequency of applications. **0.12%, 0.125%, or 1% Suspension:** *Adults only:* Instill 1–2 drops into affected eye(s) two to four times daily or 2 drops into affected eye(s) four times daily. During the first 24–48 hr, dose frequency may be increased if necessary. If signs and symptoms fail to improve after 2 days, reevaluate. Once the patient is responding, a lower dosage may be used, but care should be taken not to discontinue therapy prematurely.	
	Loteprednol etabonate ophthalmic	Signs and symptoms of seasonal allergic conjunctivitis	**0.2% Suspension:** *Adults only:* Instill 1 drop into conjunctival sac of affected eye(s) four times daily.	
Selective alpha-2 adrenergic agonist	Brimonidine ophthalmic	Elevated IOP in patients with ocular hypertension or open-angle glaucoma	**0.1%, 0.15%, 0.2% Ophthalmic solution:** *Adults, adolescents, and children ≥2 yr:* Instill 1 drop into affected eye(s) three times daily, approximately every 8 hr.	
		Eye redness due to minor ocular pain or irritation	**0.025% Solution:** *Adults, adolescents, and children ≥5 yr:* Instill 1 drop into the affected eye(s) every 6 to 8 hours as needed. Do not use more than four times daily.	

TABLE 4.1 **Eye and Ear Medications—cont'd**

Category	Medication	Indication	Dosage	Considerations
Beta-blockers	Timolol ophthalmic	Elevated IOP in patients with ocular hypertension or open-angle glaucoma	**0.25% Solution:** *Adults, adolescents, and children ≥ 2 yr:* Instill 1 drop into affected eye(s) twice daily. Dosage may be increased to 1 drop of a 0.5% solution twice daily, if necessary, for adequate reduction of IOP. Dosage may be reduced to 1 drop, once daily, of effective strength to maintain reduced pressure.	In some patients, the IOP-lowering effects may require a few weeks to stabilize. If the IOP is not controlled on this regimen, concomitant therapy with alternative agents may be considered. Nasolacrimal occlusion or eyelid closure is recommended for at least 2–3 minutes after administration.
	Betaxolol ophthalmic		**0.5% Solution:** *Adults:* Instill 1–2 drops into affected eye(s) twice daily. If the IOP is not controlled on this regimen, concomitant therapy with other agent(s) for lowering IOP can be instituted.	
	Carteolol ophthalmic	Chronic open-angle glaucoma and ocular hypertension, either alone or in combination with other intraocular pressure–lowering agents	**1% Solution:** *Adults:* Apply 1 drop to conjunctiva of affected eye(s) twice daily. If the patient's intraocular pressure is not controlled on this regimen, concomitant therapy with alternative agents may be considered.	
Anticholinergic	Pilocarpine ophthalmic	Elevated IOP in patients with ocular hypertension or open-angle glaucoma	**1%, 2%, or 4% Solution:** *Adults, adolescents, and children ≥2 yr:* Instill 1 drop into affected eye(s) up to four times daily. Pilocarpine-naive patients should be started on the lowest available concentration as higher concentrations are often not tolerated initially.	Can be used in acute angle-closure glaucoma. To limit systemic exposure to pilocarpine, patients may be instructed to perform nasolacrimal occlusion or eyelid closure for 2-3 minutes after administration.
Carbonic anhydrase inhibitors	Dorzolamide ophthalmic	Elevated IOP in patients with ocular hypertension or open-angle glaucoma	**2% Solution:** *Adults, adolescents, children, infants, and neonates ≥1 week:* Instill 1 drop into affected eye(s) three times daily.	The safety and efficacy of treatment durations longer than 3 months has not been established in pediatric patients.
	Brinzolamide ophthalmic		**1% Suspension:** *Adults only:* Instill 1 drop into affected eye(s) three times daily.	May be used concomitantly with other topical ophthalmic agents to lower IOP.
Prostaglandins	Latanoprost ophthalmic	Increased IOP in patients with open-angle glaucoma or ocular hypertension	**0.005% Solution and emulsion:** *Adults:* Instill 1 drop into affected eye(s) once daily in the evening.	More frequent administration may decrease the IOP-lowering effect or cause paradoxical elevations in IOP.

Continued

TABLE 4.1 **Eye and Ear Medications—cont'd**

Category	Medication	Indication	Dosage	Considerations
Prostaglandins—cont'd	Travoprost ophthalmic		**0.004% Solution:** *Adults and adolescents ≥16 yr:* Instill 1 drop into affected eye(s) once daily in the evening.	
	Bimatoprost ophthalmic		**0.01%, 0.03% Solution:** *Adults and adolescents ≥16 yr:* Instill 1 drop into affected eye(s) once daily in the evening.	
Decongestants	Naphazoline hydrochloride ophthalmic	Use as a topical ocular vasoconstrictor in treatment of conjunctival hyperemia	**0.1% Solution:** *Adults:* Instill 1–2 drops into conjunctival sac(s) every 3–4 hr as needed.	Avoid in patients with glaucoma.
	Phenylephrine hydrochloride nasal spray and nasal drops	Sinus and nasal congestion and eustachian tube congestion due to the common cold, allergic rhinitis, or sinusitis	**1% Nasal drops or 0.5%, 1% nasal spray:** *Adults, adolescents, and children ≥12 yr:* Administer 2–3 sprays to each nostril every 4 hr as needed. **0.25% Nasal spray:** *Adults, adolescents, and children ≥6 yr:* Administer 2 to 3 sprays to each nostril every 4 hr as needed. **Nasal drops 0.125% solution:** *Children 2–5 yr:* Administer 2–3 drops to each nostril every 4 hr as needed.	Spray is available in multiple concentrations including 0.25%, 0.5%, and 1%. Use beyond 3 days is not recommended. Avoid in patients with glaucoma
Lubricants	Artificial tears	Temporary relief of xerophthalmia and minor ocular irritation	**Solution and gel** *Adults, adolescents, and children ≥6 yr:* Instill 1–2 drops into affected eye(s) two to four times daily as needed, adjusting frequency of application as needed. *Children <6 yr and infants:* Instill 1–2 drops into the affected eye(s) one or more times per day as needed to relieve symptoms. **Ointment** *Adults, adolescents, and children ≥6 yr:* Apply a small amount of ointment, roughly 6 mm or ¼ inch, to the inside of the lower eyelid. Apply one to four times per day as needed, adjusting frequency of application as needed. It is common to apply the ointment just once daily at bedtime. *Children <6 yr and infants:* Apply a small amount of ointment, roughly 6 mm or ¼ inch, to the inside of the lower eyelid. Apply one or more times per day as needed, adjusting frequency of application as needed.	Discontinue use of a nonprescription (OTC) product if ocular pain, ocular pruritus, or other ocular irritation symptoms occur or worsen, or if the condition has not improved within 72 hours of use of the product. Remove contact lenses prior to use unless product packaging specifies it may be used with contact lenses.

TABLE 4.1   Eye and Ear Medications—cont'd

Category	Medication	Indication	Dosage	Considerations
Immunomodulator	Cyclosporine ophthalmic	Xerophthalmia due to ocular inflammation associated with keratoconjunctivitis sicca	**0.05% Emulsion:** *Adults and adolescents ≥16 yr:* Instill 1 drop into affected eye(s) twice daily approximately 12 hr apart. **0.09% Solution:** *Adults only:* Instill 1 drop into affected eye(s) twice daily, approximately 12 hr apart.	Artificial tears may be used concurrently, allowing a 15-minute interval between administration of products. Patients with decreased tear production should not wear contact lenses.
Diagnostics	Fluorescein sodium ophthalmic	For staining the anterior segment of the eye for diagnosis of eye trauma such as corneal abrasion	**Strip** *Adults:* Use 1 strip per eye; either touch tip of strip to bulbar conjunctiva of anesthetized eye until adequate amount of stain is available or moisten strip with sterile water and place at fornix in lower cul-de-sac close to punctum, then have patient close eyes tightly and blink several times after strip is removed. *Children:* Dose is the same "off label use."	Remove soft contact lenses prior to use as staining may occur. Following application, flush the eye(s) with sterile normal saline solution. Patient should wait at least 1 hour before replacing contact lenses.
Ophthalmic anesthetics	Tetracaine ophthalmic	Ophthalmic anesthesia	**0.5% Solution:** *Adults, adolescents, and children:* Instill 1 drop into affected eye(s) as needed.	Must be used with great caution, as accidental injury may occur while eye is anesthetized. Instruct patient to avoid touching, rubbing, or wiping the eyes for at least 10–20 minutes after administration. Contact lenses should not be reinserted for at least 20 minutes to ensure anesthesia has faded completely to avoid injury to the eye. Prolonged use may result in permanent corneal damage.
Cerumenolytics	Carbamide peroxide otic (otic use only)	Cerumen removal	**6.5% Solution:** *Adults and children ≥12 yr:* Instill 5–10 drops twice daily in the affected ear(s) for up to 4 days. After the drops are instilled, remain lying with the affected ear upward for 5 minutes to facilitate penetration of the drops into the ear canal. A cotton pledget may be gently inserted at the ear opening for no longer than 5–10 minutes to ensure retention.	The solution may be warmed by holding the bottle in the hand for 1–2 minutes Any wax remaining after treatment may be removed by gently flushing the ear with warm water, using a soft rubber bulb ear syringe. Do not irrigate the ear if the tympanic membrane is perforated.

Levofloxacin

Pharmacokinetics. Following administration of levofloxacin ophthalmic, a small amount is systemically absorbed. Of the amount absorbed, levofloxacin undergoes limited metabolism, and nearly 90% is excreted unchanged in the urine.

Indications. Levofloxacin is indicated in treatment of bacterial conjunctivitis. It is effective against common bacteria including *Haemophilus influenzae, Pseudomonas aeruginosa, Staphylococcus aureus, Staphylococcus epidermidis*, and *Streptococcus sp.*

Adverse Effects. Patients taking ophthalmic levofloxacin may experience transient visual impairment, sensation of a foreign body in the eye, or ocular irritation. Some patients may experience mild eye pain or discomfort as well as photophobia. Rarely, patients may experience allergic reactions, edema of the eyelids, dry eyes, or ocular pruritus.

Contraindications. Levofloxacin is contraindicated in patients with quinolone hypersensitivity. Patients should not wear contact lenses while being treated for bacterial conjunctivitis.

Monitoring. Remind patients that proper technique is essential to decrease risk of contamination of the dropper. Teach patients to report any increase in purulent drainage from the eye or significant eye pain.

Aminoglycosides

Aminoglycosides are broad-spectrum antibiotics typically used to treat infections caused by aerobic gram-negative bacteria such as *Pseudomonas* and *Haemophilus sp.* as well as some gram-positive cocci such as *staphylococci*. Aminoglycosides act by interfering with protein synthesis in the bacteria, and they may be bacteriostatic or bactericidal, depending on the concentration. They may be used as topical agents to treat bacterial infections of the eye including conjunctivitis, blepharitis, and keratoconjunctivitis. These agents are not commonly used for ear infections. For more information about the use of aminoglycosides, refer to Chapter 48, Antiviral and Antiretroviral Medications.

Gentamicin Sulfate

Pharmacokinetics. Gentamicin is administered topically as either a solution or an ointment. Systemic absorption through either route is negligible.

Indications. Gentamicin can be used to treat conditions including bacterial conjunctivitis, blepharitis, dacryocystitis, and keratoconjunctivitis. It has been shown to be effective against organisms including *Haemophilus influenza, Pseudomonas aeruginosa, Staphylococcus aureus, Staphylococcus epidermidis, Staphylococcus sp.*, and *Streptococcus pneumonia*.

Adverse Effects. The most frequent side effect of the ophthalmic preparation is burning and stinging of the eye with instillation. Ophthalmic administration of gentamicin can cause conjunctival hyperemia. Rarely, use has resulted in formation of bacterial and fungal corneal ulcers. Ophthalmic ointment may result in impaired wound healing of a corneal lesion or abrasion.

Contraindications. Gentamicin sulfate ophthalmic is contraindicated in patients with known hypersensitivity to gentamicin or other aminoglycosides.

Monitoring. Remind patients of the importance of proper dosing and proper technique when administering eye drops to minimize risk of secondary infection. Patients who receive the ointment form must be reminded to avoid driving until vision clears after the ointment has been administered. Teach patients to report to the primary care provider any increase in purulent discharge from the eye or increased inflammation and pain.

Tobramycin

Pharmacokinetics. The pharmacokinetics of tobramycin ophthalmic drops and ointment are not well known. Tobramycin is not available in otic forms.

Indications. Tobramycin ophthalmic preparations may be used in treatment of external eye infections including bacterial conjunctivitis, blepharitis, dacryocystitis, and keratoconjunctivitis. They have been shown to be effective in treating common causative organisms including *Haemophilus influenza, Pseudomonas aeruginosa, Staphylococcus aureus, Staphylococcus epidermidis*, and *Streptococcus pneumoniae*.

Adverse Effects. Patients may experience mild ocular itching or irritation as well as conjunctival erythema. Some patients may experience mild swelling or itching of the eyelids.

Contraindications. Avoid prescription of tobramycin to patients with known hypersensitivity to aminoglycosides.

Monitoring. Teach patients to use the prescribed dose of eye drops for best effect and to take the full course of the medication. Remind patients of the importance of proper dosing and proper technique when administering eye drops to minimize risk of secondary infection. Patients who receive the ointment form must be reminded to avoid driving until vision clears after the ointment has been administered. Teach patients to report to the primary care provider any increase in purulent discharge from the eye or increased inflammation and pain.

Macrolides

Macrolides are protein synthesis inhibitors effective against a variety of aerobic and anaerobic gram-positive cocci as well as some gram-negative organisms such as *Neisseria*. Select macrolides can be used to treat mycobacteria and chlamydia as well as a number of common organisms found in bacterial conjunctivitis. These are not preferred agents to be used in otitis media and are not available in otic form.

Azithromycin

Pharmacokinetics. After administration of azithromycin ophthalmic solution to the eye, systemic concentration of the medication is not detectable.

Indications. Azithromycin is effective in treating bacterial conjunctivitis caused by organisms including *Haemophilus influenza, Staphylococcus aureus, Streptococcus mitis* group, and *Streptococcus pneumonia*. While it has been used for treatment of otitis media, it is no longer recommended by the American Academy of Pediatrics for treatment of otitis media in children due to organism resistance.

Adverse Effects. Ocular irritation is the most common adverse reaction occurring in 1% to 2% of patients. Rarely, patients may experience blurred vision, corneal erosion, mild ocular pain, itching, or dry eyes. Patients taking ophthalmic azithromycin may also experience a change in taste (*dysguesia*).

Contraindications. Azithromycin is contraindicated in patients with macrolide hypersensitivity. Patients should avoid wearing contact lenses while being treated with azithromycin ophthalmic solution.

Monitoring. Teach patients proper dosing and proper technique when administering azithromycin ophthalmic solution. Instruct patients to report any increase in purulent drainage from the eye or significant ocular pain.

Sulfonamides

Sulfonamides are broad-spectrum bacteriostatic agents that act by inhibiting synthesis of folic acid required for biosynthesis of ribonucleic acid (RNA), DNA, and proteins essential for bacterial growth. They are effective for treating susceptible strains of common eye pathogens including *Staphylococcus aureus, Streptococcus pneumoniae*, and *Haemophilus influenza*. Oral doses of sulfonamides are available for use in otitis media and will be discussed in Chapter 45.

Sulfacetamide Sodium

Pharmacokinetics. Sulfacetamide sodium is available as an ophthalmic solution or ointment. It penetrates ocular fluid, although it does not produce significant systemic absorption. Caution should still be taken, however, as enough is absorbed to cause sensitization upon readministration.

Indications. Sulfacetamide sodium has been shown to be effective for treating a variety of infections including *Chlamydia trachomatis, Enterobacter sp., Escherichia coli, Haemophilus influenzae, Klebsiella sp., Staphylococcus aureus, Streptococcus pneumoniae*, and *Viridans streptococci*. It is most commonly prescribed for conjunctivitis, corneal ulcers, and other superficial ophthalmic infections. It may also be used as an adjunct to systemic sulfonamide therapy for chlamydial conjunctivitis.

Adverse Effects. Patients may experience localized stinging and burning with application of the drops. Rarely, patients may experience nonspecific conjunctivitis, conjunctival hyperemia, and allergic reactions. Irritation to the skin is uncommon and typically transient. Superinfection with nonsusceptible organisms is rare but may occur with prolonged use. Hypersensitivity reactions are rare in patients with previously demonstrated sulfonamide hypersensitivity.

Contraindications. Sulfacetamide sodium is contraindicated in patients with renal disease and those with sulfonamide hypersensitivity. Because of structural similarity, sulfonamide preparations should be used with caution in patients with a history of allergic reactions to oral sulfonylureas, thiazide diuretics, or carbonic anhydrase inhibitors. It is not known whether topical sulfonamides can cause fetal harm during pregnancy, however sulfonamides are not recommended for use by patients who are breastfeeding.

Monitoring. Remind patients of the importance of proper dosing and proper technique when administering eye drops to minimize risk of secondary infection. Teach patients to report to the primary care provider any increase in purulent discharge from the eye or increased inflammation and pain.

Combination Agents

Polymyxin B/Trimethoprim

Pharmacokinetics. When applied via the ophthalmic route, polymyxin B does not penetrate significantly into the aqueous humor. Blood samples following instillation of 2 drops of ophthalmic polymyxin B 10,000 units/mL and trimethoprim 1 mg/mL yielded peak plasma concentrations of polymyxin B and trimethoprim of 1 unit/mL and 0.03 mcg/mL, respectively.

Indications. Polymyxin B/trimethoprim has been shown to be effective in the treatment of ocular infections including bacterial conjunctivitis and blepharoconjunctivitis. Examples of organisms that are sensitive to polymyxin B/trimethoprim include *Haemophilus influenza, Pseudomonas aeruginosa, Staphylococcus aureus, Staphylococcus epidermidis,* and *Streptococcus pneumoniae.*

Adverse Effects. Signs and symptoms of ocular irritation including redness, burning, stinging, and/or itching are the most common adverse effects associated with polymyxin B/trimethoprim. Other adverse effects include swelling of the eyelids, as well as tearing and rash. Rarely, polymyxin B/trimethoprim can cause overgrowth of nonsusceptible organisms, especially fungi, resulting in superinfection.

Contraindications. Polymyxin B/trimethoprim is contraindicated in patients who have hypersensitivity to either ingredient. It can cause the overgrowth of nonsusceptible organisms, resulting in superinfection. It has not been studied in pregnant patients and it is not known whether it is excreted in breast milk.

Monitoring. Laboratory testing is not necessary. Monitor patients for increased purulent discharge from the eye that may indicate superinfection. Instruct patients to avoid wearing contact lenses while undergoing therapy.

Antivirals

Most viral infections of the eye resolve without pharmacologic treatment. Antivirals may be used for treatment of HSV types 1 and 2. Patients diagnosed with herpes zoster ophthalmicus are typically treated with oral antiviral medications and should be referred to an ophthalmologist.

Trifluridine Ophthalmic Solution

Pharmacokinetics. Trifluridine ophthalmic solution has a half-life of approximately 12 minutes, so it requires frequent dosing. Following therapeutic doses, systemic absorption of trifluridine ophthalmic is negligible.

Indications. Trifluridine ophthalmic solution has been shown to be effective against HSV types 1 and 2. It is also used to treat herpes simplex keratitis, including primary keratoconjunctivitis and recurrent epithelial keratitis.

Adverse Effects. The most common adverse effects are transient burning and stinging upon instillation and mild blepharedema. Contact dermatitis, keratitis, and ocular hypertension are rare.

Contraindications. Trifluridine is contraindicated in patients who develop a hypersensitivity reaction to the medication. It should not be administered for periods greater than 21 days due to the risk of ocular toxicity.

Monitoring. Remind patients to remove contact lenses prior to and during treatment. There are no known drug interactions associated with trifluridine.

Nonsteroidal Antiinflammatories

Nonsteroidal antiinflammatories are used to reduce ocular pain and inflammation after ocular surgery, eye trauma, or other ophthalmic conditions. Topical ophthalmic nonsteroidal antiinflammatory drugs (NSAIDs) can provide both antiinflammatory and analgesic effects without the risks of the systemic route.

Ketorolac Tromethamine Ophthalmic

Pharmacokinetics. Low serum concentrations were detectable after ophthalmic administration in fewer than 20% of patients after 10 days at usual doses. If absorbed, it is primarily metabolized by the liver and excreted via the urine.

Indications. Ketorolac tromethamine can be used to treat ocular pruritis due to seasonal allergic conjunctivitis. It is also used after ophthalmic surgery to reduce ocular pain and inflammation.

Adverse Effects. The most common adverse effects are burning and stinging upon instillation of the eye drops. Allergic reactions, ocular irritation, corneal edema, and superficial ocular infection occur in fewer than 10% of patients. Impaired wound healing of the eye and keratitis may occur with ophthalmic administration of ketorolac.

Contraindications. Ketorolac is contraindicated in patients with known ketorolac or other NSAID hypersensitivity. It should be used cautiously in patients with complicated or repeated eye surgeries, because of increased risk for adverse effects. Patients must remove contact lenses prior to instillation of ketorolac ophthalmic drops to enhance penetration of the medication into the eye. In addition, the preservative commonly used may be absorbed by soft contact lenses.

Monitoring. Laboratory monitoring is not necessary unless the patient shows signs and symptoms of complications. Monitor wound healing if the patient is taking ketorolac to address post-surgery ocular inflammation and pain.

Antihistamines

Over-the-counter (OTC) topical antihistamines in combination with vasoconstrictor agents may be used to reduce mild allergic conjunctivitis. In general, second-generation histamine$_1$ receptor antagonists, applied via the ophthalmic route, are effective in reducing symptoms of allergic conjunctivitis. Many of the antihistamine agents are combined with mast cell stabilizers for maximum effect. Oral antihistamines are not recommended for allergic conjunctivitis as they can cause dry eyes and impair tear formation.

Azelastine HCl

Pharmacokinetics. Absorption is minimal following azelastine ophthalmic administration. Onset of action is rapid (within 3 minutes) with a duration of action of approximately 8 hours.

Indications. Azelastine ophthalmic solution can be used for the treatment of ocular pruritis associated with allergic conjunctivitis. It may be applied in patients older than 3 years of age.

Adverse Effects. Common adverse effects associated with ophthalmic formulations of azelastine include dysgeusia, headache, dyspnea, and fatigue. Ocular symptoms include temporary blurred vision, burning and stinging upon application, and conjunctivitis. Fewer than 10% of patients will experience ocular pain.

Contraindications. Azelastine should not be used to treat irritation caused by contact lenses. Patients who wear soft contact lenses should wait at least 10 minutes after instilling the ophthalmic solution before inserting the lenses.

PRACTICE PEARLS

Eye Drop Administration

Teach patients to wait at least 5 minutes before adding a second drop or a second drug to decrease the washout effect.

Monitoring. Patients should be advised to use caution when driving or operating machinery until vision is clear and symptoms of fatigue are not present. No laboratory tests are needed.

Olopatadine HCl

Pharmacokinetics. After administration of ophthalmic preparations of olopatadine, plasma concentrations were in the range of 0.5–1.3 ng/mL within 2 hours of dosing. Olopatadine is not extensively metabolized, and excretion is primarily via the kidneys.

Indications. Olopatadine HCl is used for the treatment of allergic conjunctivitis, including ocular pruritis. It can be prescribed in varying concentrations and is available for use by adults, adolescents, and children older than 2 years of age. Of note, olopatadine has both antihistamine and mast cell stabilizing effects.

Adverse Effects. Ocular symptoms associated with olopatadine ophthalmic drops include burning or stinging of the eye, foreign-body sensation, redness of the eye, blurred vision, and dry eyes. Severe keratitis has been reported in fewer than 5% of patients.

Contraindications. Olopatadine ophthalmic is formulated with a preservative, benzalkonium chloride, which may be absorbed by soft contact lenses. Contact lenses may be inserted 10 minutes following instillation.

Monitoring. Monitor for adverse effects of the medication. Laboratory monitoring is not necessary.

Mast Cell Stabilizers

Mast cell stabilizers inhibit type 1 immediate hypersensitivity reactions. Therefore they inhibit the increased cutaneous vascular permeability that is associated with reagin or immunoglobulin (Ig)E and antigen-mediated reactions. This prevents antigen-stimulated release of histamine and other mast cell inflammatory mediators and inhibits eosinophil chemotaxis. The exact mechanism of action is unknown, but these medications have been reported to prevent calcium influx into the mast cell upon antigen stimulation. They have no intrinsic vasoconstrictor or other antiinflammatory activity.

Lodoxamide Ophthalmic

Pharmacokinetics. Lodoxamide is administered in solution form via the ophthalmic route. Ophthalmic administration in healthy adults did not result in any measurable plasma concentration.

Indications. Lodoxamide is used for the treatment of ocular inflammatory conditions including vernal conjunctivitis, vernal keratitis, and vernal keratoconjunctivitis.

Adverse Effects. The most common adverse effects include transient burning, stinging, and mild discomfort upon instillation of the eye drops. Rarely, patients experience ocular pain, blurred vision, or foreign-body sensation.

Contraindications. Lodoxamide is contraindicated in patients with known lodoxamide hypersensitivity. Patients who wear soft contact lenses must remove them prior to instillation of the ophthalmic drops as the preservative used may affect the lenses.

Monitoring. Laboratory monitoring is not necessary for patients using ophthalmic lodoxamide. Reinforce patient teaching regarding proper dosing of eye medications.

Nedocromil Ophthalmic

Pharmacokinetics. Absorption of nedocromil after ocular administration is minimal (less than 4% of the total dose of a 2% solution). Absorption occurs mainly via the nasolacrimal duct. If absorbed, the solution is not metabolized and is excreted through the kidney (64%) and feces (36%).

Indications. Nedocromil ophthalmic is recommended for the treatment of pruritis related to allergic ocular disorders including allergic conjunctivitis.

Adverse Effects. The most common adverse effect associated with nedocromil ophthalmic solution is mild headache, occurring in approximately 40% of patients. Other adverse effects include ocular burning, stinging, and irritation. Between 10% and 30% of patients experience nasal congestion and dysgeusia. Fewer than 10% of patients experience conjunctivitis, eye redness, or photophobia.

Contraindications. Patients should be advised that the ophthalmic solution contains a preservative that may affect soft contact lenses. Safety and efficacy have not been established in children younger than 3 years of age.

Monitoring. Laboratory monitoring is not needed while patients are taking nedocromil ophthalmic solution. Teach patients proper dosing of eye medications to avoid adverse effects.

Corticosteroid Antiinflammatory Drugs

Topical corticosteroids are used to reduce inflammation in a variety of ocular conditions. For example, ophthalmic corticosteroids are used to manage inflammatory conditions of the conjunctiva and cornea including allergic conjunctivitis. In addition, topical corticosteroids may be used in combination with antibiotics to alleviate symptoms in patients with bacterial conjunctivitis or in patients with adenoviral conjunctivitis (Holland et al., 2019). While the American Academy of Ophthalmology (2018) recommends cautious use of topical corticosteroids in patients with conjunctivitis, recent evidence suggests that perceived risk of increased IOP, viral shedding, and HSV reactivation from corticosteroids has not been supported in the literature with short-term use (Holland et al., 2019).

Dexamethasone

Pharmacokinetics. Dexamethasone is available in ophthalmic solution, suspension, and ointment forms. It is absorbed through the aqueous humor and into local tissue with minimal systemic absorption. The medication is metabolized locally.

Indications. Dexamethasone ophthalmic can be used in a variety of inflammatory conditions of the conjunctiva and cornea including allergic conjunctivitis. It may be used cautiously in patients with certain types of viral conjunctivitis such as herpes zoster ocular infection and corneal abrasion.

Adverse Effects. Patients taking ophthalmic preparations of dexamethasone may experience temporary stinging, burning, or tearing upon installation of the medication. Allergic reactions and ocular pruritus may also occur. Mild eye discomfort occurs in fewer than 10% of patients. Dexamethasone may cause an increased IOP or ocular hypertension. This can occur within 1 to 6 weeks of topical ophthalmic therapy (and is reversible after discontinuation of the medication). Prolonged use of dexamethasone by any route may result in open-angle glaucoma.

Contraindications. Ophthalmic dexamethasone should not be used in patients with any *acute* purulent bacterial, viral, or fungal ocular infection or periocular infection, nor should it be used to treat patients with dacryocystitis. Dexamethasone also should not be used to treat most viral diseases of the cornea and conjunctiva, including active *herpes simplex,* keratitis, varicella, mycobacterial infections, and fungal infection. Because ophthalmic dexamethasone is more likely than other ophthalmic agents to increase IOP, it is contraindicated in patients with glaucoma.

Monitoring. For patients requiring chronic administration of dexamethasone ophthalmic medications, IOP should be measured every 2 to 4 weeks for the first two months of therapy. Should IOP remain within normal limits, it can then be measured every one to two months thereafter.

Prednisolone

Pharmacokinetics. Prednisolone ophthalmic is absorbed through the aqueous humor. There is only minimal systemic absorption. It is available in ophthalmic suspension and solution forms.

Indications. Prednisolone ophthalmic is indicated in the treatment of a variety of corticosteroid-responsive eye disorders including allergic conjunctivitis, bacterial conjunctivitis, and certain corneal injuries such as from thermal or chemical burns or penetration of foreign bodies.

Adverse Effects. Prolonged use of ophthalmic prednisolone may result in ocular hypertension, open-angle glaucoma, ocular nerve damage, and visual defects. While ocular hypertension typically reverses after discontinuation of the drug, it should be used with caution. Other adverse effects include ocular irritation, conjunctival redness, conjunctivitis, and ocular pain or discomfort.

> **PRACTICE PEARLS**
>
> **Ophthalmic Corticosteroids**
>
> Refer to or consult with an ophthalmologist if considering ophthalmic corticosteroids for patients in primary care.

Contraindications. Ophthalmic preparations of prednisolone are contraindicated in most forms of conjunctival and corneal viral infections as well as any fungal infections of the eye. While it may be used in herpes viral infections, it should be used with caution. Ophthalmic preparations of prednisolone should also be used with caution in patients with corneal abrasion and in those with preexisting ophthalmic disorders, particularly due to the possibility of increased IOP.

Monitoring. Monitor patients carefully as length of therapy varies with the condition treated. In fact, medication therapy may vary between a few days to several weeks based on clinical response. If using for chronic conditions, withdrawal of treatment should be carried out by gradually decreasing the frequency of applications.

Prostaglandin Analogues

Prostaglandin analogues were introduced in the late 1990s to reduce IOP in patients with glaucoma. They act by stimulating drainage of the aqueous humor through uveoscleral and trabecular meshwork outflow. A recent systematic review concluded that prostaglandin analogues were the most efficacious of first-line drugs (including beta-blockers, carbonic anhydrase inhibitors, and alpha-2 adrenergic agonists) for primary open-angle glaucoma (Li et al., 2016). Of note, while they are typically administered at night, they are most likely as effective if given during the day (Fiscella et al., 2017).

Latanoprost

Pharmacokinetics. Latanoprost is absorbed through the cornea and metabolized by the liver. Peak aqueous humor concentration occurs approximately 2 hours after instillation of the eye drops with onset of action (reduction of IOP). Peak effect occurs after 8 to 12 hours. It is primarily excreted through the kidney.

Indications. Latanoprost is used to reduce elevated intraocular hypertension in patients with open-angle glaucoma. It may also be used to reduce ocular hypertension, a risk factor for glaucoma.

Adverse Effects. As many as 50% of patients may experience mild ocular discomfort and irritation with administration of latanoprost ophthalmic preparation. Other common adverse effects include conjunctival redness, tearing, ocular pruritis, and keratitis (which may be severe). Of note, approximately 7% of patients experience increased brown pigment in the iris due to increased melanosomes in melanocytes. This change in pigment may not be noticed for several months or even years, though it may be permanent. Eyelashes in the affected eye may increase in length, thickness, and number (a condition known as *hypertrichosis*). Darkening of the eyelid has been reported.

Contraindications. Latanoprost should not be used in patients with closed-angle glaucoma. Reactivation of herpes simplex keratitis has also been reported during latanoprost use. Any inflammatory condition of the eye or any damage to the ocular surface should be reported to an ophthalmologist.

Monitoring. Monitor patients with ocular hypertension carefully as it is a risk factor for open-angle glaucoma. Reinforce to patients the importance of removing contact lenses before administration of the eye drops. Lenses may be reinserted 15 minutes after medication administration. Remind patients of the possibility of discoloration of the iris and eyelid as well as the potential for eyelash changes.

Travoprost

Pharmacokinetics. Travoprost is administered topically to the eye and is primarily absorbed through the cornea. Peak blood concentrations are achieved within 30 minutes and are undetectable after 1 hour. Reduction of IOP occurs approximately 2 hours after instillation; travoprost achieves maximum effect at approximately 12 hours after administration.

Indications. Travoprost is used to reduce elevated IOP in patients with open-angle glaucoma. Like latanoprost, travoprost can be used to treat patients with ocular hypertension.

Adverse Effects. The most common adverse effect associated with travoprost ophthalmic drops is conjunctival hyperemia, occurring in 30% to 50% of patients. Additional adverse effects occurring in 5% to 10% of patients include ocular irritation, pain, and itching as well as sensation of a foreign body in the eye. Fewer than 5% of patients experience discoloration of the iris on the affected side. This may occur slowly and may not be noticeable for months to years, but it may be permanent. In addition, travoprost may cause changes in eyelash length, thickness, and number. Rarely, patients may experience cardiovascular, neurological, and gastrointestinal side effects.

Contraindications. Travoprost should not be used in patients with closed-angle glaucoma. It should be used with caution in patients with active intraocular inflammation (such as iritis or uveitis). Some patients may experience photophobia and sensitivity to UV exposure.

Monitoring. Remind patients to remove contact lenses prior to instillation of ophthalmic drops and to wait at least 15 minutes before reinserting the lenses. Promote regular evaluation of IOP as recommended by the patient's ophthalmologist.

PRACTICE PEARLS

Quality and Safety

To avoid systemic absorption, no more than one drop of eye medication should be applied to each eye. Apply eye drops into the conjunctival sac. To reduce systemic absorption of eye drops after administration, lasolacrimal occlusion for at least 3 minutes or eyelid closure for at least 2 minutes is recommended (Farkouh, Frigo, & Czejka, 2016).

Alpha-2 Adrenergic Agonists

Alpha-2 adrenergic agonists decrease IOP by slowing the rate of aqueous humor production. In addition, they may increase uveoscleral outflow. Used alone, they can reduce IOP by 18% to 27% at peak (2–5 hours) and 10% at 8 to 12 hours (Fiscella et al., 2017). Combining alpha-2 adrenergic agonists with other first-line glaucoma agents may decrease IOP further.

Brimonidine

Pharmacokinetics. After ophthalmic administration of brimonidine, maximum plasma concentration occurs within 30 minutes to 4 hours. The time to peak effect on IOP is approximately 2 hours. Brimonidine is metabolized by the liver and excreted by the kidneys.

Indications. Brimonidine is used in the treatment of increased IOP in patients with open-angle glaucoma or ocular hypertension. It can also be used for the treatment of eye redness due to minor ocular irritation or pain.

Adverse Effects. The most common adverse effects associated with ophthalmic administration of brimonidine are blurred vision, stinging, drowsiness, fatigue, and conjunctival redness. In addition, patients may experience mild headache, ocular pruritis, xerostomia, and a foreign-body sensation in the eye. Cardiovascular effects include hypertension (≤9%), hypotension (≤4%), palpitations or arrhythmias (3%), and bradycardia (<1%).

Contraindications. Brimonidine is contraindicated in children younger than 2 years of age. While it has minimal effects on blood pressure and cardiopulmonary hemodynamics, it should be avoided in patients with advanced coronary or cerebral artery disease.

Monitoring. Remind patients that contact lenses should be removed prior to instillation and can be reinserted 15 minutes later. Patients should avoid driving if blurred vision, drowsiness, or fatigue after administration of the eye drops occurs.

Beta-Adrenergic Blocking Agents

Beta-adrenergic blocking agents reduce IOP by decreasing the production of aqueous humor by the ciliary body. Visual acuity, pupil size, and accommodation are not affected by the ophthalmic beta-blocking agents. These medications are often used in combination with other agents to reduce IOP.

Timolol
Pharmacokinetics. Ophthalmic timolol decreases IOP within approximately 30 minutes after instillation, peaks 1 to 2 hours later, and lasts approximately 24 hours. Some systemic absorption may occur, but data are limited. If absorbed, it is metabolized by the liver and excreted by the kidneys.

Indications. Ophthalmic preparations are used to treat increased IOP in patients with open-angle glaucoma. They may also be used for ocular hypertension.

Adverse Effects. Patients may experience transient blurred vision, burning, and stinging after instillation of ophthalmic timolol. Ocular pain, discharge or crusting of the eye, foreign-body sensation, and ocular pruritis may occur in up to 5% of patients. While systemic reactions are generally low, cardiovascular effects are possible as a result of beta-blockade.

Contraindications. Do not use timolol in patients with known hypersensitivity to beta-blockers. Older adults receiving ophthalmic timolol may be more likely to experience adverse systemic effects following ophthalmic application. Avoid use in patients with advanced cardiovascular or cerebrovascular disease. Patients wearing soft contact lenses should not use timolol while wearing the lenses but may reinsert them 15 minutes after using the eye drops.

Monitoring. Older adults should be monitored for systemic effects. To reduce systematic absorption, the primary care provider should demonstrate nasolacrimal occlusion or eyelid closure techniques to the patient.

Betaxolol
Pharmacokinetics. Systemic absorption of betaxolol ophthalmic preparations is minimal but does occur. Following administration, IOP is reduced within 30 to 60 minutes and peaks at about 2 hours. Maximum effects are usually evident after 1 to 2 weeks of therapy.

Indications. Betaxolol is used to treat chronic open-angle glaucoma and ocular hypertension. It is less effective for angle-closure glaucoma.

Adverse Effects. Systemic effects are rare with ophthalmic preparations of betaxolol. After application of the eye drops, some patients experience ocular irritation, discomfort, and blurred vision, but these are typically resolved within several minutes. Other ocular adverse effects include foreign-body sensation, ocular discharge, photophobia, and crusty lashes.

Contraindications. Ophthalmic drops are formulated with a specific preservative that may be absorbed into soft contact lenses. Therefore lenses should be removed prior to application of the drops and may be reinserted after approximately 15 minutes.

Monitoring. While systemic effects are rare, bradycardia has been reported in a small number of patients. Older adults are at greatest risk of adverse effects.

Cholinergic Agonists

Cholinergic agonists directly stimulate cholinergic receptors, resulting in contraction of the iris sphincter (causing *miosis*), the ciliary muscle, and the trabecular network and leading to increased outflow of aqueous humor. In open-angle glaucoma, increased outflow of aqueous humor is accomplished by contraction of the ciliary muscle. In closed-angle glaucoma, stimulation of cholinergic receptors causes miosis, which opens the angle of the anterior chamber of the eye and leads to increased aqueous humor outflow.

Pilocarpine
Pharmacokinetics. Onset of action usually occurs within approximately 1 hour and persists for 4 to 14 hours for the 1% solution of pilocarpine. Duration of action varies by 0.5% to 4% depending on the strength of the solution used. Ophthalmic gel can be used once daily with duration of approximately 18 to 24 hours.

Indications. Pilocarpine is considered a second-line drug used in the treatment of open-angle glaucoma or ocular hypertension. It may also be used in acute angle-closure glaucoma under the direction of an ophthalmologist.

Adverse Effects. Adverse effects from ophthalmic pilocarpine include myopia, decreased night vision, ocular pain, ocular irritation, and photophobia. In rare cases, ciliary spasms can lead to retinal detachment. Older adults are at greatest risk for adverse effects. Systemic adverse effects of pilocarpine are rare but possible.

Contraindications. Pilocarpine ophthalmic gel is contraindicated in situations in which miosis is undesirable, such as in patients with iritis. Patients should remove contact lenses prior to application and may reinsert lenses about 10 minutes after instillation.

Monitoring. Glaucoma patients who are treated with pilocarpine ophthalmic should have regular ophthalmologic exams to ensure that IOP goals are being met and optic nerve damage is avoided. Reinforce proper techniques for administration of eye drops to avoid infection.

Carbonic Anhydrase Inhibitors

Ophthalmic carbonic anhydrase inhibitors decrease production of aqueous humor from the ciliary body of the eye by inhibiting carbonic anhydrase II (CA-II). This leads to decreased IOP. Ophthalmic carbonic anhydrase inhibitors are frequently used in combination with other glaucoma medications.

Brinzolamide

Pharmacokinetics. Brinzolamide is administered as an ophthalmic suspension. It is absorbed systemically and distributed into erythrocytes. Half-life is 111 days in whole blood due to its affinity for CA-II. It is eliminated virtually unchanged in the urine.

Indications. Brinzolamide is indicated for the treatment of elevated IOP in patients with open-angle glaucoma or ocular hypertension. It is often used as part of combination therapy.

Adverse Effects. Mild changes in taste are possible with ophthalmic brinzolamide. From 5% to 10% of patients may experience blurred vision. Other adverse reactions (1%–5%) include blepharitis, mild headache, ocular discharge, mild ocular pain, ocular pruritis, and xerophthalmia. Rarely, patients may experience conjunctivitis, keratoconjunctivitis, ocular fatigue, or diplopia.

Contraindications. Brinzolamide is a chemical sulfonamide, so it should be used cautiously in patients with a history of sulfonamide hypersensitivity. It should also be used cautiously in patients with renal or liver disease. There are no adequate studies in pregnant or breastfeeding patients. Patients should remove contact lenses before instillation of drops and may reinsert lenses after about 15 minutes.

Monitoring. Reinforce proper techniques for instillation of eye medications to ensure safe practices. Patients should maintain regular appointments for ophthalmologic evaluation to prevent or reduce progression of glaucoma.

Lubricants

Artificial tears are used for the relief of *xerophthalmia* (dry eyes) and ocular irritation. They are available in solution and ointment forms and act to maintain moisture by stabilizing tear film and increasing tear viscosity. Artificial tears generally produce few side effects other than transient stinging or blurred vision with application. Artificial tears should not be used in patients with symptoms of corneal abrasion, conjunctivitis, presence of a foreign body, or ocular trauma. If the tear solutions are formulated with preservatives, patients should remove soft contact lenses prior to instillation. Patients should discontinue use of the product if ocular pain or itching or other symptoms of ocular irritation occur. Most artificial tears are available without a prescription.

Immunomodulators

Immunomodulators such as cyclosporine ophthalmic are typically prescribed by ophthalmologists for patients with xerophthalmia associated with keratoconjunctivitis sicca who are not responsive to artificial tears. When they are administered through the ophthalmic route, no detectable drug accumulation in the blood was detected after 12 months of use. The most common adverse effects associated with immunomodulators are ocular pain, ocular irritation, and conjunctival hyperemia.

Decongestants/Sympathomimetics

Decongestants are sympathomimetic agents that typically act on alpha-1 adrenergic receptors, resulting in vasoconstriction. Ophthalmic decongestants can be used in combination with antihistamines to reduce symptoms associated with seasonal allergic conjunctivitis. Decongestants are also available in nasal spray and nasal drop forms for use in patients with eustachian tube congestion secondary to the common cold, allergic rhinitis, or sinusitis. Nasally administered agents that affect blood pressure, such as phenylephrine, should be used cautiously in patients with a history of cardiovascular disease or hypertension. Tolerance to the decongestant effects of these medications can occur within 3 days of use. Chronic use of sympathomimetic agents can result in rebound vasodilation after the medication is stopped.

Diagnostic Agents

A commonly used diagnostic agent in primary care for patients with eye disorders is fluorescein. Fluorescein is a *fluorescent*, which is a water-soluble dye applied topically to the eye to detect abrasions or lesions of the corneal epithelium. Once available in multidose vials, fluorescein is now typically applied using impregnated ophthalmic strips to avoid contamination related to multiple-use droppers. To use a fluorescein strip, moisten the strip with sterile water and then place it at the fornix in the lower cul-de-sac close to the punctum of the eye. Instruct the patient to blink several times and allow a few seconds for the staining to occur. A blue light with magnification is then used to enhance the fluorescence. Intact areas of the cornea remain without color while abrasions or foreign bodies appear bright green. Following the exam, rinse the eye with sterile irrigating solution. Adverse reactions are rare from topical use, however severe allergic reaction may occur. Patients should remove contact lenses prior to application of the dye.

Anesthetics

Ophthalmic analgesics are used only when eye pain makes it impossible for the primary care practitioner to examine the eye and only for temporary pain relief. Following ophthalmic preparations of tetracaine or a comparable ophthalmic anesthetic, maximum anesthesia is typically achieved within 10 to 20 seconds of administration, with the effect lasting for 10 to 20 minutes. Caution must be used to prevent injury to the eye while the patient's eye is anesthetized. Contact lenses should not be inserted until the anesthetic effects of tetracaine have completely waned.

QUALITY AND SAFETY

Topical Anesthetics for the Eye

Topical anesthetics should be used only when eye pain makes it impossible for the practitioner to examine the eye. Following discharge from the clinic or hospital, use of topical anesthetics for pain management should only be prescribed in consultation with an ophthalmologist.

Cerumenolytics

Cerumenolytics are used to soften hardened cerumen in order to facilitate easy removal from the ear. A variety of OTC medications are available, typically as carbamide peroxide. *Cerumen impaction* is an accumulation of cerumen that causes symptoms or prevents assessment of the ear canal, tympanic membrane, or audiovestibular system. Patients with nonimpacted cerumen who are asymptomatic do not require intervention, but rather, watchful waiting and surveillance. Cerumenolytic agents (including water and saline solution), irrigation, or manual removal requiring instrumentation may be used. If unsuccessful or if perforation of the tympanic membrane is suspected, refer the patient to a provider who has special equipment and training to clean and evaluate ear canals.

PRACTICE PEARLS

Use of Hearing Aids

Patients with hearing aids, particularly older adults, are at greater risk for buildup of cerumen in the ear, so they should be evaluated frequently.

Prescriber Considerations for Eye and Ear Therapy

Clinical Reasoning for Eye and Ear Therapy

Clinical practice guidelines are available through several organizations to inform pharmacologic management of a variety of eye and ear conditions. Examples include the American Academy of Ophthalmology, American Academy of Pediatrics, and American Academy of Otolaryngology–Head and Neck Surgery.

BOOKMARK THIS!

Clinical Guidelines for Eye Therapy

The American Academy of Ophthalmology provides preferred practice patterns and clinical practice guidelines on a variety of topics discussed in this chapter: https://www.aao.org/guidelines-browse?filter=Preferred%20Practice%20Patterns&sub=AllPreferredPracticePatterns.

Consider the individual patient's health problem requiring eye and ear medications. Is the problem amenable to management within primary care or does it require specialty referral? Is the conjunctivitis infectious or noninfectious? For patients with infectious conjunctivitis, differentiation between viral and bacterial causes is essential. Viral conjunctivitis is the most common and typically resolves without medication. Mild cases of bacterial conjunctivitis may be self-limiting, and as such, no treatment may be needed. On the other hand, conjunctivitis secondary to sexually transmitted infections, including *Neisseria gonorrhea* and *Chlamydia trachomatis*, require systemic antibiotic therapy. In children older than 2 years of age who are diagnosed with uncomplicated otitis media, pain management is typically used in the early phase (48–72 hours) rather than immediate antibiotic therapy.

Determine the desired therapeutic outcome for the patient's health problem. For all patients with infectious conjunctivitis, it is important to teach strategies to avoid the spread of infection. Bacterial infections are typically contagious until 24 to 48 hours after treatment is initiated, while viral infections are considered contagious during the entire course of the infection. For patients with otitis media, relief of pain is essential while monitoring the patient for a sufficient period to avoid unnecessary antibiotic treatment if the otitis is of viral etiology. Patients with otitis externa require adequate pain management while recommending strategies to prevent reoccurrence.

Assess the eye and ear medications selected for their appropriateness to the patient by considering the medication's side effects and the patient's age, race/ethnicity, comorbidities, and genetic factors. Thorough assessment of health history, risk factors, and signs and symptoms is essential for reducing complications associated with eye and ear disorders. For example, patients with previous or recurrent episodes of conjunctivitis may require referral to ophthalmology. Patients who are being treated for glaucoma should have all medications carefully reviewed to reduce the risk of drug interactions and increased IOP. Older adults may be more sensitive to systemic absorption of medications, so they should be taught nasolacrimal occlusion techniques.

Initiate the treatment plan with the selected medication by first providing adequate patient education to ensure the patient's understanding and promote full participation in the therapy. Depending on the condition to be treated and the goal of treatment, a thorough explanation to the patient and family is important. Emphasize the importance of using proper technique to minimize risk of infection and provide for adequate medication absorption. For example, using excellent hand hygiene in the administration of eye drops prevents the spread of infection. In cases of suspected adenovirus as the cause of conjunctivitis, reassure patients that these are typically self-limiting and do not require medication therapy. For patients with glaucoma, reinforce the need for long-term management and working closely with an ophthalmologist to prevent vision loss.

BOOKMARK THIS!

The Glaucoma Research Foundation

The Glaucoma Research Foundation provides a list of tips for administration of eye medication that may be useful for any patient requiring eye drops: https://www.glaucoma.org/treatment/eyedrop-tips.php.

Ensure complete patient and family understanding of the medication prescribed for therapy using a variety of education strategies. Use of proper technique for eye and ear medication administration cannot be understated. A variety of websites provide written and video instructions for administering eye and ear medications. In addition, patients can practice instilling eye drops using OTC saline solutions specifically created for ophthalmic use. This will help them develop the technique without using the actual medication.

Conduct follow-up and monitoring of patient responses to eye and ear medication therapy. Recommend follow-up as appropriate for the patient's condition to evaluate the effectiveness of the therapy. Consider referring the patient to a specialist if the therapy is not progressing as expected based on sufficient dosing and adherence. In cases involving corneal abrasion, reevaluate the patient after 24 hours to ensure progress in healing. For patients with otitis media, follow up in 48 to 72 hours to determine effectiveness of pain management as well as need for antibiotic therapy.

Teaching Points for Eye and Ear Therapy

Health Promotion Strategies

- Teach patients proper techniques for administration of eye and ear medications to ensure optimal adherence and optimal effectiveness of therapy.
- Recommend strategies to prevent spread of infectious conjunctivitis, including frequent hand hygiene (soap and water), use of separate towels, and avoiding contact with the contagion during the course of the infection (American Academy of Ophthalmology, 2022).
- Recommend recombinant herpes zoster vaccine for adults 50 years of age and older using CDC guidelines.
- For patients at risk of adult inclusion conjunctivitis, treatment of concurrent genital infection is essential in addition to treatment of sexual partners.
- Teach patients to avoid contact lens use while on therapy to resolve conjunctivitis. If lenses are disposable, discard the contact lenses and cases to avoid reinfection.
- Instruct patients who use eye makeup (including eye shadow, eye cream, liners, and mascaras) to discard these products to prevent reinfection of ocular infections.
- Teach patients to blot excess medications from under the eye or eyelid after eye drop administration to avoid absorption through the skin.
- To reduce the risk of otitis media in infants and children, encourage breastfeeding in infants, avoid bottle-feeding infants in supine position, reduce exposure to second-hand smoke, avoid pacifier use for infants older than 10 months, and use careful handwashing before handling children.

Patient Education for Medication Safety

- Always wash your hands before and after instilling eye or ear medication.
- Do not share medications designed for the eye or the ear to avoid contamination of the medication dispensers.
- Use the precise dosage as prescribed. Using more or less medication can increase the risk of adverse effects, promote waste, and/or decrease medication effectiveness.
- Wait at least 5 minutes between administration of each eye drop to enhance absorption and avoid the washout effect.
- If the medication is in suspension form, mix it gently to ensure equal distribution of the drug in the solution.
- Wait until vision is fully cleared after instilling eye drops or ointment before participating in any activity requiring visual acuity.
- Immediately report to your primary care provider any significant changes in pain, burning, or redness or increases in drainage from the eye.
- Avoid taking OTC medications or herbal medications without contacting your primary care provider to decrease risk of adverse effects.

Application Questions for Discussion

1. As a primary care provider, what are the patient and safety factors that should be considered before prescribing antibiotics for the eye? Before prescribing steroids for the eye?

2. What strategies should be used to determine the best therapy for patients with infectious or noninfectious conjunctivitis? Which conditions should be immediately referred to ophthalmology and which should be managed in primary care and then referred if there is a resistance to treatment?

3. What clinical practice guidelines will be most useful in caring for patients with eye and ear disorders?

Selected Bibliography

American Academy of Opthamology (2022). *Conjunctivitis: what is pink eye,* https://www.aao.org/eye-health/diseases/pink-eye-conjunctivitis.

Azari, A. A., & Barney, N. P. (2013). Conjunctivitis: A systematic review of diagnosis and treatment. *JAMA, 310*(16), 1721–1730. http://doi.org/10.1001/jama.2013.280318.

Beauduy, C. E., & Winston, L. G. (2017). Tetracyclines, macrolides, clindamycin, chloramphenicol, streptogramins, & oxazolidinones. In B. G. Katzung (Ed.), *Basic & Clinical Pharmacology* (14th ed.). New York: McGraw-Hill Education.

Carlisle, R. T., & Digiovanni, J. (2015). Differential diagnosis of the swollen red eyelid. *American Family Physician, 92*(2), 106–112.

Castillo, M., Scott, N. W., Mustafa, M. Z., Mustafa, M. S., & Azuara-Blanco, A (2015). Topical antihistamines and mast cell stabilisers for treating seasonal and perennial allergic conjunctivitis. *Cochrane Database of Systemic Reviews* (6), Article Cd009566. http://doi.org/10.1002/14651858.CD009566.pub2.

Centers for Disease Control and Prevention (CDC). (2018). *CDC launches the nation's first vision and eye health surveillance system.* https://www.cdc.gov/media/releases/2018/a0726-vision-health.html.

Duncan, J. L., Parikh, N. B., Seitzman, G. D., & Riordan-Eva, P. (2020). Disorders of the lids & lacrimal apparatus. In M. A. Papadakis, S. J. McPhee, & M. W. Rabow (Eds.), *Current Medical Diagnosis & Treatment 2020.* New York: McGraw-Hill Education.

Farkouh, A., Frigo, P., & Czejka, M. (2016). Systemic side effects of eye drops: A pharmacokinetic perspective. *Clinical Ophthalmology (Auckland, N.Z.), 10*, 2433–2441. http://doi.org/10.2147/OPTH.S118409.

Finley, C. R., Chan, D. S., Garrison, S., Korownyk, C., Kolber, M. R., Campbell, S., & Allan, G. M. (2018). What are the most common conditions in primary care? Systematic review. *Canadian Family Physician, 64*(11), 832–840.

Fiscella, R. G., Lesar, T. S., Owaidhah, O. A., & Edward, D. P. (2017). Glaucoma. In J. T. DiPiro, R. L. Talbert, G. C. Yee, G. R. Matzke, B. G. Wells, & L. M. Posey (Eds.), *Pharmacotherapy: A Pathophysiologic Approach* (10th ed.). New York: McGraw-Hill Education.

Flach, A. J. (2008). The importance of eyelid closure and nasolacrimal occlusion following the ocular instillation of topical glaucoma medications, and the need for the universal inclusion of one of these techniques in all patient treatments and clinical studies. *Transactions of the American Ophthalmological Society, 106*, 138–148.

Greco, A., Rizzo, M. I., De Virgilio, A., Gallo, A., Fusconi, M., & de Vincentiis, M. (2016). Emerging concepts in glaucoma and review of the literature. *American Journal of Medicine, 129*(9), 1000. e1007–1000.e1013. https://doi.org/10.1016/j.amjmed.2016.03.038.

Gudgel, D. (2019). American Academy of Ophthalmology: How to Use Cosmetics Safely Around Your Eyes. Retrieved from https://www.aao.org/eye-health/tips-prevention/eye-makeup.

Gupta, P., Zhao, D., Guallar, E., Ko, F., Boland, M. V., & Friedman, D. S. (2016). Prevalence of glaucoma in the United States: The 2005–2008 National Health and Nutrition Examination Survey. *Investigative Ophthalmology & Visual Science, 57*(6), 2905–2913. http://doi.org/10.1167/iovs.15-18469.

Henderer, J. D., & Rapuano, C. J. (2017). Ocular pharmacology. In L. L. Brunton, R. Hilal-Dandan, & B. C. Knollmann (Eds.), *Goodman & Gilman's: The Pharmacological Basis of Therapeutics* (13th ed.). New York: McGraw-Hill Education.

Holland, E. J., Fingeret, M., & Mah, F. S. (2019). Use of topical steroids in conjunctivitis: A review of the evidence. *Cornea, 38*(8), 1062–1067. http://doi.org/10.1097/ico.0000000000001982.

Horton, J. C. (2018). Disorders of the eye. In J. L. Jameson, A. S. Fauci, D. L. Kasper, S. L. Hauser, D. L. Longo, & J. Loscalzo (Eds.), *Harrison's Principles of Internal Medicine* (20th ed.). New York: McGraw-Hill Education.

Konne, N. M., Collier, S. A., Spangler, J., & Cope, J. R. (2019). Healthy contact lens behaviors communicated by eye care providers and recalled by patients — United States, 2018. *Morbidity and Mortality Weekly Report, 68*, 693–697. http://dx.doi.org/10.15585/mmwr.mm6832a2.

Lambert, L. (2019). Diagnosing a red eye: An allergy or an infection? *Professional Nursing Today, 23*(1), 27–34.

Li, T., Lindsley, K., Rouse, B., Hong, H., Shi, Q., Friedman, D. S., Wormald, R., Dickersin, K. (2016). Comparative effectiveness of first-line medications for primary open-angle glaucoma: a systematic review and network meta-analysis. *Ophthalmology. 123*(1), 129–140. doi:10.1016/j.ophtha.2015.09.005.

McMonnies, C. W. (2017). Glaucoma history and risk factors. *Journal of Optometry, 10*(2), 71–78. http://doi.org/10.1016/j.optom.2016.02.003.

Mounsey, A. L., & Gray, R. E. (2016). Topical antihistamines and mast cell stabilizers for treating allergic conjunctivitis. *American Family Physician, 93*(11), 915–916.

National Institute on Deafness and Other Communication Disorders. (2016). Quick statistics about hearing. Retrieved from https://www.nidcd.nih.gov/health/statistics/quick-statistics-hearing#11.

Ossorio, A. (2015). Red eye emergencies in primary care. *Nurse Practitioner, 40*(12), 46–53. quiz 53-44. http://doi.org/10.1097/01.Npr.0000473384.55251.25.

Pflipsen, M., Massaquoi, M., & Wolf, S. (2016). Evaluation of the painful eye. *American Family Physician, 93*(12), 991–998.

Rosenfeld, R. M., Shin, J. J., Schwartz, S. R., Coggins, R., Gagnon, L., Hackell, J. M., & Corrigan, M. D. (2016). Clinical practice guideline: Otitis media with effusion (update). *Otolaryngology–Head and Neck Surgery, 154*, S1–S41. http://doi.org/10.1177/0194599815623467.

Schwartz, S. R., Magit, A. E., Rosenfeld, R. M., Ballachanda, B. B., Hackell, J. M., Krouse, H. J., & Cunningham, E. R. (2017). Clinical practice guideline (update): Earwax (cerumen impaction). *Otolaryngology–Head and Neck Surgery, 156*(1_suppl), S1–S29. http://doi.org/10.1177/0194599816671491.

Teweldemedhin, M., Gebreyesus, H., Atsbaha, A. H., Asgedom, S. W., & Saravanan, M. (2017). Bacterial profile of ocular infections: A systematic review. *BMC Ophthalmology, 17*(1), 212–220. http://doi.org/10.1186/s12886-017-0612-2.

van Eyk, A. D. (2019). Pharmacotherapeutic options for ophthalmic conjunctivitis. *Professional Nursing Today, 23*(2), 8–13.

Varu, D. M., Rhee, M. K., Akpek, E. K., Amescua, G., Farid, M., Garcia-Ferrer, F. J., & Dunn, S. P. (2019). Conjunctivitis preferred practice pattern®. *Ophthalmology, 126*(1), P94–P169. http://doi.org/10.1016/j.ophtha.2018.10.020.

5

Allergy and Respiratory Medications

REBECCA M. LUTZ

Overview

Allergy and upper respiratory symptoms generate 12 million office visits per year (Centers for Disease Control and Prevention [CDC] National Health Interview Survey, 2016). This chapter will discuss allergy and respiratory medications commonly used in the primary care setting. Medications in this chapter may also be useful in treating asthma (discussed in Chapter 6, Asthma Medications) and chronic obstructive pulmonary disease (COPD) (discussed in Chapter 7, Chronic Obstructive Pulmonary Disease Medications). Bacterial infections related to the respiratory system are covered in Unit 13, Antiinfective Medications.

Relevant Physiology

The respiratory system is composed of the upper and lower structures working together to transport air, exchange gases, and eliminate waste products, thus maintaining homeostasis. The upper structures are composed of the nasal cavity, sinus passages, pharynx, and larynx. The lower respiratory structures include the trachea, bronchi, and lungs. The dividing anatomical landmark is the epiglottic flap.

The nasal passages are composed of a mucosal epithelial layer that contains goblet cells and cilia. The goblet cells secrete mucous to form a protective barrier that traps foreign particles. Receptors interact with the cilia to trigger sneeze and cough reflexes to remove the foreign particles from the airways.

The trachea divides into the primary bronchi, which further divide into smaller segments within each lung. The primary bronchi divide into the secondary bronchi, which further divide into the tertiary bronchi and then the terminal bronchioles, alveolar ducts, and alveoli. Within the alveoli, gas exchange occurs as oxygen enters the blood and CO_2 is removed.

Pathophysiology

Allergic Rhinitis

Allergic rhinitis (AR) is a common problem affecting 19 million people in the United States (CDC National Health Interview Survey, 2018). AR occurs as an immune response to an allergen and is often classified as seasonal AR or perennial AR. Seasonal AR typically occurs in the fall and spring and is triggered by pollen from trees, grasses, and weeds. Perennial AR occurs year-round and can be attributed to mold, dust mites, and animals. The following evidence-based guidelines aid in classifying AR (Bousquet et al., 2020):
• The frequency (intermittent or persistent) of symptoms
• The severity (mild or moderate to severe) of symptoms
• The effect of frequency and severity on quality of life

Nonallergic (Vasomotor) Rhinitis

Nonallergic rhinitis, also called *vasomotor rhinitis*, commonly presents after the age of 20, has no hereditary pattern, and affects females more commonly than males (Kushnir & Kaliner, 2015). Symptoms include nasal congestion, sneezing, rhinorrhea, and postnasal drip. Symptoms are not immune-mediated responses but may result from drinking alcohol, environmental changes in weather, irritants such as smoke and odors, medical conditions, and medications (Papadopoulos & Guibas, 2016). The over-the-counter (OTC) availability and thus overuse of topical (intranasal) decongestants is known to cause rhinitis medicamentosa, also known as rebound congestion.

Rhinosinusitis (Sinusitis)

Rhinosinusitis is an inflammation of the nasal mucosa and sinuses. It may be classified by the duration of symptoms: acute (less than 4 weeks), subacute (4–12 weeks), recurrent acute (four or more episodes per year, each lasting at least 7 days), or chronic (12 weeks or longer). Symptoms include nasal inflammation, nasal discharge, postnasal drip, nasal obstruction, nasal congestion, facial pain, cough, fever, and fatigue.

Viral rhinosinusitis is caused by a viral infection such as *rhinovirus*, *adenovirus*, *influenza virus*, or *parainfluenza virus*. Symptoms typically resolve within 10 days but may last up to 12 weeks. Treatment is targeted to relieve symptoms and many OTC medications are available.

Chronic rhinosinusitis (CRS) is classified by the absence or presence of nasal polyps: chronic rhinosinusitis without nasal polyps (CRSsNPs) and chronic rhinosinusitis with nasal polyps (CRSwNPs). Treatment goals include avoiding allergens, decreasing inflammation, and treating underlying diseases or conditions. Adequate treatment and control of CRS is also important considering that CRS is an associated comorbidity in patients with asthma (Jarvis et al., 2012). CRS increases risk of sinusitis, which itself impacts asthma.

Bacterial rhinosinusitis is an inflammation of the nasal mucosa and sinuses caused by bacteria. The bacterial organisms most commonly attributed to bacterial rhinosinusitis are *Streptococcus pneumoniae*, *Haemophilus influenzae*, *Staphylococcus aureus*, and *Moraxella catarrhalis*.

Pharyngitis

Pharyngitis may be acute or chronic, noninfectious or infectious. Noninfectious causes include irritants such as allergens, smoke, dust, and trauma. Infectious pharyngitis can be viral or bacterial. Causes of viral pharyngitis include a variety of coronaviruses, Epstein-Barr virus, influenza, and rhinovirus. Symptoms include cough, fatigue, fever, headache, myalgias, rhinitis, and sore throat. Treatment focuses on symptom management. The most common cause of bacterial pharyngitis is *Streptococcus pyogenes* including groups A, C, and G *β-hemolytic streptococci*. Symptoms include a sudden onset of chills, high fever, headache, and sore throat with painful swallowing.

Bronchitis

Acute bronchitis is an acute inflammation of the bronchi caused primarily by viruses. Symptoms include a paroxysmal cough with or without mucus production, wheezing, dyspnea, fever, and chest pain resulting from frequent coughing. The cough associated with bronchitis may last up to 6 weeks. In acute, uncomplicated bronchitis, treatment goals are directed to the relief of symptoms with antitussive medications and beta2-agonists. The use of antibiotics in cases of acute, uncomplicated bronchitis is *not* recommended. Clinical differentiation between bronchitis and pneumonia is important. Bronchitis does not result in consolidation or infiltrates on radiographs.

Chronic bronchitis, often referred to as *chronic obstructive lung disease*, manifests as a recurring, mucus-producing cough lasting longer than 3 months to over 2 years. Multiple factors cause bronchitis, including cigarette smoking, secondhand smoke, dust, pollution, fumes, exhaust, and smoke. Chapter 7, Chronic Obstructive Pulmonary Disease Medications, provides further information.

Pneumonia

Bacterial community-acquired pneumonia is commonly caused by *Streptococcus pneumoniae*, *Haemophilus influenzae*, *Mycoplasma pneumoniae*, *Staphylococcus aureus*, *Legionella species*, *Chlamydia pneumoniae*, and *Moraxella catarrhalis*. Viral community-acquired pneumonia is commonly caused by influenza and rhinovirus (Burk et al., 2016). Other potential viral causes include a variety of coronaviruses, respiratory syncytial virus, human metapneumovirus, adenovirus, and parainfluenza virus (Burk et al., 2016; Mandell et al., 2007). Symptoms of pneumonia include tachycardia, tachypnea, fever, cough with mucous production, chest pain, abnormal physical examination findings (rales, egophony, or tactile fremitus), and a chest X-ray revealing infiltrates and consolidation.

Allergy and Respiratory Therapy

A wide array of medications are available to treat symptoms associated with allergy and respiratory conditions. Medications may be by prescription or OTC; intranasal or oral; and as a mono-therapeutic medication or a combination of medications. Despite the abundance of medications, the American College of Chest Physicians (CHEST®) recommends against the use of OTC antitussive agents, expectorants, mucolytic agents, antihistamines, or combination products for reducing cough in adult and pediatric patients due to limited efficacy (Malesker et al., 2017).

Intranasal Corticosteroids

In 2017, updated clinical guidelines recommended the use of intranasal corticosteroids (INSs) as a first-line treatment (Dykewicz et al., 2017; Seidman et al., 2015). INSs (Table 5.1) are the most effective agents for AR symptom management. INSs decrease inflammation, rhinorrhea, sneezing, and nasal pruritus by inhibiting the infiltration of inflammatory cells and inhibiting the maturation and release of cytokines. Daily or seasonal steroid use is more effective than intermittent use. Therapeutic effects usually begin in less than 12 hours.

General contraindications and precautions with INS use include disorders of the endocrine, immunologic, metabolic, or musculoskeletal systems; hypersensitivity reactions; and immunosuppression. Monitor patients with pulmonary tuberculosis for systemic fungal, bacterial, viral, or parasitic infections or ocular herpes simplex.

PRACTICE PEARLS

Life Span Considerations with INS

Geriatrics

- INSs are considered safer than antihistamines and more effective than leukotriene receptor antagonists (LTRAs).

Pediatrics

- Assess risk of disease exacerbation/symptom management compared to potential decrease in growth velocity, but not overall growth delay, associated with corticosteroid use.

All Ages

- Do not exceed recommended dosing levels.

TABLE 5.1   Intranasal Corticosteroids

Medication	Indication	Dosage	Considerations and Monitoring
Beclomethasone dipropionate	Vasomotor (nonallergic) rhinitis Prevention of nasal polyps following surgical removal	**42 mcg/spray (suspension):** *Adults, adolescents, and children ≥12 yr:* 1 or 2 sprays in each nostril twice daily. Maximum dosage: 168–336 mcg/day. *Children 6-11 yr:* 1 spray in each nostril twice daily. May increase to 2 sprays each nostril twice daily for severe symptoms. Maximum dosage: 168–336 mcg/day.	Discontinue if no improvement after 3 weeks of use.
	Seasonal or perennial allergies	**80 mcg/spray (aerosol):** *Adults and children ≥12 yr:* 2 sprays in each nostril once daily. Maximum dosage: 320 mcg/day. **40 mcg/spray (aerosol):** *Children 4-11 yr:* 1 spray in each nostril once daily. Maximum dosage: 80 mcg/day.	
Budesonide	Seasonal or perennial allergies	**32 mcg/spray:** *Adults, adolescents, and children ≥12 yr:* 2 sprays in each nostril once daily. Decrease to 1 spray after desired response obtained. Maximum dosage: for adolescents and children ≥12 yr: 256 mcg/day. *Children 6-11 yr:* 1 spray in each nostril once daily. If inadequate response, may use up to 2 sprays in each nostril. Maximum dosage: 128 mcg/day.	
Ciclesonide	Seasonal allergies	**50 mcg/spray:** *Adults, adolescents, and children ≥6 yr:* 2 sprays in each nostril once daily. Maximum dosage: 200 mcg/day. **37 mcg/spray:** *Adults and adolescents ≥12 yr:* 1 spray in each nostril once daily. Maximum dosage: 74 mcg/day.	
	Perennial allergies	**50 mcg/spray:** *Adults, adolescents, and children ≥12 yr:* 2 sprays in each nostril once daily. Maximum dosage: 200 mcg/day. **37 mcg aerosol spray:** *Adults, adolescents, and children ≥12 yr:* 2 sprays in each nostril once daily. Maximum dosage: 74 mcg/day.	
Flunisolide	Seasonal or perennial allergies	**0.025% spray:** *Adults and adolescents: ≥15 yr:* 2 sprays (25 mcg/spray) in each nostril twice daily. May increase to 2 sprays three times daily. Maximum dosage: 400 mcg/day. *Children ≥6–14 yr:* 1 spray (25 mcg/spray) in each nostril three times daily or 2 sprays in each nostril twice daily. Maximum dosage: 200 mcg/day.	Maintenance dose: smallest amount necessary to control the symptoms.
Fluticasone furoate	Seasonal or perennial allergies Allergic rhinitis Allergic conjunctivitis	**27.5 mcg/spray:** *Adults, adolescents, and children ≥12 yr:* 2 sprays in each nostril once daily for 1 week. Maintenance:1 to 2 sprays in each nostril once daily. Maximum dosage: 110 mcg/day. *Children 2-11 yr:* 1 spray in each nostril once daily. Maintenance:1 spray in each nostril once daily. Maximum dosage: 55 mcg/day.	

TABLE 5.1 Intranasal Corticosteroids—cont'd

Medication	Indication	Dosage	Considerations and Monitoring
Fluticasone propionate	Seasonal or perennial allergies Vasomotor (nonallergic) rhinitis	**50 mcg/spray:** *Adults, adolescents, and children ≥12 yr:* 2 sprays in each nostril once daily for 1 week. Then 1 to 2 sprays in each nostril once daily. Maximum dosage: 200 mcg/day. *Children 4-11 yr:* 1 spray in each nostril once daily. May titrate up to 2 sprays in each nostril once daily until symptoms are controlled, then decrease to 1 spray again. Use for shortest time possible. Maximum dosage: 200 mcg/day.	
	Treatment of nasal polyps	**93 mcg/spray:** *Adults:* 1 to 2 sprays in each nostril twice daily. Maximum dosage: 744 mcg/day.	
Mometasone furoate	Seasonal or perennial allergies	**50 mcg/spray:** *Adults, adolescents, and children ≥12 yr:* 2 sprays in each nostril once daily. Maximum dosage: 200 mcg/day. *Children 2–11 yr:* 1 spray in each nostril once daily. Maximum dosage: 100 mcg/day.	
	Seasonal allergic rhinitis prophylaxis	**50 mcg/spray:** *Adults and adolescents ≥12 yr:* 2 sprays in each nostril once daily. Maximum dosage: 200 mcg/day.	Begin 2 to 4 weeks prior to start of allergy season.
Triamcinolone acetonide	Seasonal or perennial allergies	**55 mcg/spray:** *Adults, adolescents, and children ≥12 yr:* 2 sprays in each nostril once daily. Maintenance: 1 spray in each nostril once daily. Maximum dosage: 220 mcg/day. *Children 6-11 yr:* 1 spray in each nostril once daily. May increase to 2 sprays in each nostril once daily until symptoms are controlled, then decrease to 1 spray again. Maintenance: 1 spray in each nostril once daily. Maximum dosage: 220 mcg/day. *Children 2–5 yr:* 1 spray in each nostril once daily. Maximum dosage: 110 mcg/day.	

PRACTICE PEARLS

INS Use in Pregnancy and Lactation

- Weigh potential benefits to the mother against potential risk to the fetus.
- Breastfeeding is not recommended. Weigh potential benefits to the mother against potential adverse effects on the infant.

Fluticasone Propionate

Pharmacokinetics. Fluticasone propionate nasal spray is an aqueous suspension that delivers 50 mcg of the medication. Following administration of the nasal spray, the initial response occurs within 12 hours. Peak response requires several days and lasts several days after therapy is discontinued. Fluticasone propionate is metabolized in the liver by cytochrome (CYP) 3A4. Excretion is primarily through the feces (95%).

Indications. Fluticasone propionate is a corticosteroid nasal spray available with or without a prescription. Fluticasone propionate is indicated for the management of nasal symptoms in adults and children age 4 and older with rhinitis. Advise patients that medication effectiveness (symptom relief) may take several days. Administration at regular intervals increases effectiveness.

Adverse effects. Local effects of fluticasone propionate nasal spray include epistaxis, nasal burning, nasal ulcerations, *candida* infections, and nasal septal perforation. Other adverse effects include headache, pharyngitis, nausea/vomiting, cough, and asthmatic symptoms (3%–16%). Patients with a history of nasal ulcers, surgery, or trauma may experience delayed healing and should avoid using fluticasone propionate nasal spray until healing occurs. Glaucoma and cataracts have been reported.

Contraindications. Avoid use in patients with hypersensitivities to fluticasone propionate or any portion of the product. Advise parents not to use fluticasone propionate nasal sprays in children younger than 4 years of age. Precautions include the risk of increased systemic corticosteroid effects. Drug–drug interactions include desmopressin and CYP 3A4 inhibitors. In addition, food–drug interactions are known to exist with grapefruit juice.

Monitoring. Monitor for improvement in symptoms of rhinitis and for development of adverse effects. No routine laboratory testing is recommended. Though the systemic response is low with the intranasal route, routine monitoring of growth velocity in pediatric patients is advised. Refer patients to ophthalmology for additional monitoring. Reassess patients after 6 months of daily use to assess efficacy.

Mometasone Furoate

Pharmacokinetics Onset of action with mometasone nasal spray is usually within 12 hours to 2 days. The intranasal spray formula has limited bioavailability (<1%). The medication is metabolized via the liver. Excretion is in the urine. Estimated half-life by the intravenous (IV) route is 5 hours.

Indications. Mometasone is a medium-potency corticosteroid intranasal spray. Mometasone is approved for the treatment of perennial and seasonal AR, the prophylaxis of seasonal AR, and nasal polyps. Mometasone nasal spray does not carry a black box warning associated with other formulations.

Adverse effects. The adverse effects reported most often in adults and children age 12 and older include headache, viral infection, pharyngitis, and epistaxis. Less common side effects (in 2%–10% of patients) include symptoms associated with the musculoskeletal, upper respiratory, gastrointestinal (GI), and reproductive systems. Adverse effects reported by children younger than 12 years of age include upper respiratory infections (URIs), vomiting, and skin trauma (5%–7%), followed by diarrhea, nasal irritation, otitis media, and wheezing (2%–5%). In children, there is an increased risk of toxicity.

Contraindications. Absolute contraindications include patients with known hypersensitivity and cross-sensitivity reactions to steroids. Use with caution in patients with known endocrine, metabolic, immunologic, musculoskeletal, ophthalmic, or pulmonary diseases.

Monitoring. Monitor patients during the concomitant use of mometasone with CYP 3A4 inhibitors due to the possible increased risk of systemic corticosteroid adverse effects. Impaired liver function increases peak plasma concentrations. Monitor growth velocity in pediatric patients at each visit. Monitor patient for adverse ocular effects and refer patient to ophthalmology if necessary.

Antihistamines

Antihistamines are available by prescription or OTC as oral or intranasal formulations (Table 5.2). Patients may be self-medicating when they present for evaluation of symptoms. Evaluate patient for history of self-medication and for any perceived improvement of symptoms.

Oral Antihistamines

Chlorpheniramine, diphenhydramine, and hydroxyzine are first-generation oral antihistamines with antiinflammatory and antimuscarinic effects. Sedation, dry mouth and eyes, and urinary retention are common adverse effects of this classification. Second-generation oral antihistamines include cetirizine, fexofenadine, desloratadine levocetirizine, and loratadine. Second-generation antihistamines are preferred over first-generation antihistamines because the former have fewer adverse effects. However, INSs are still recommended before the use of any oral antihistamines.

> **PRACTICE PEARLS**
>
> **Life Span Considerations With Antihistamine Use in Older Adults**
>
> In older adults, the use of antihistamines has resulted in an increased incidence of:
> - Adverse effects
> - Drug–drug interactions
> - Risks related to comorbidities

Diphenhydramine

Pharmacokinetics. The initial antihistamine effects of diphenhydramine begin within 15 minutes following an oral dose. Peak concentrations occur between 2 and 4 hours and continue for 4 to 6 hours. Half-life is extended in older adults compared with young adults and children. Diphenhydramine is widely distributed. Metabolism is via the liver and excretion is via the urine.

Indications. Diphenhydramine is approved to treat reactions caused by the release of histamine. Diphenhydramine is available in oral, topical, and injectable formulations. The antihistamine effects relieve symptoms such as rhinorrhea, nasal and ocular pruritus and conjunctivitis, dermatologic urticaria, and pruritis. Oral and parenteral diphenhydramine are considered adjunctive therapy in the treatment of anaphylaxis. Additional indications not discussed in this chapter include insomnia, dystonia, kinetosis, and Parkinson's disease.

> **PRACTICE PEARLS**
>
> **Diphenhydramine Use in Pregnancy and Lactation**
>
> - Diphenhydramine crosses the placenta. Weigh potential benefits to the mother against potential risk to the fetus. Limit to short-term use.
> - Breastfeeding is not recommended. Weigh potential benefits to the mother against potential adverse effects on the infant.

TABLE 5.2 **Antihistamines**

Drug Category/ Medication	Indication	Dosage	Considerations and Monitoring
First-Generation Oral Antihistamines			
Brompheniramine	Perennial or seasonal allergic rhinitis	**Extended-release tablet (6 mg):** *Adults, adolescents, and children ≥12 yr:* 6–12 mg orally every 12 hr. Maximum dosage: 24 mg/24 hr. *Children 6–11 yr:* 6 mg orally every 12 hr. Maximum dosage: 12 mg/24 hr. **Extended-release tablet (11 mg):** *Adults, adolescents, and children ≥12 yr:* 11 mg orally every 12 hr. Maximum dosage: 2 doses/24 hr. **Solution (1 mg/1 mL):** *Children 6–12 yr:* 2 mL (2 mg) orally four times daily. Maximum dosage: 4 doses/24 hr.	Beers Criteria (American Geriatrics Society Beers Criteria, 2019). FDA warns against use in children younger than 2 years of age.
Chlorpheniramine maleate	Allergic rhinitis, seasonal allergies, and other histamine-mediated allergic symptoms	**Immediate-release tablet, lozenge, solution (2 mg/5 mL):** *Adults, adolescents, and children ≥12 yr:* 4 mg orally every 4–6 hr. Maximum dosage: 24 mg/day. *Children 6–11 yr:* 2 mg orally every 4–6 hr. Maximum dosage: 12 mg/day. **Extended-release capsule or tablet:** *Adults, adolescents, and children ≥12 yr:* 8–12 mg orally two times daily. Maximum dosage: 24 mg/24 hr. **Immediate-release 2 mg/mL solution:** *Children 6 to 11 yr:* 2 mg orally every 4–6 hr. Maximum dosage: 12 mg/24 hr. *Children 2–5 yr:* 1 mg orally every 4–6 hr. Maximum dosage: 6 mg/24 hr.	Beers Criteria (American Geriatrics Society Beers Criteria, 2019).
Diphenhydramine	Allergic rhinitis and common cold symptoms Cough caused by minor throat and bronchial irritation	**Oral:** *Adults:* 25–50 mg orally every 4–6 hr as needed. Maximum dosage: 300 mg/day. *Infants, children, and adolescents:* 1–1.5 mg/kg/dose to 5 mg/kg/day orally three to four times daily. Maximum dosage: 25–50 mg/dose or 300 mg/24 hr.	Beers Criteria (American Geriatrics Society Beers Criteria, 2019).
	Nonprescription treatment of allergic rhinitis or common cold	**Tablet, capsule, liquid:** *Adults and adolescents ≥13 yr:* 25–50 mg orally every 4–6 hr. Maximum dosage: 300 mg/24 hr. *Children 6–12 yr:* 12.5–25 mg orally every 4–6 hr as needed. Maximum dosage: 150 mg/24 hr.	
	Nonprescription treatment of cough caused by minor throat or bronchial irritation	*Adults and adolescents ≥13 yr:* 25 mg orally every 4–6 hr. Maximum dosage: 150 mg/24 hr. *Children 6–12 yr:* 12.5 mg orally every 4–6 hr as needed. Maximum dosage: 75 mg/24 hr.	
Second-Generation Oral Antihistamines			
Cetirizine	Seasonal allergies or perennial allergies Allergic rhinitis Chronic idiopathic urticaria	**Tablets, orally disintegrating tablets, liquid-gels, chewable tablets, syrup, and solution:** *Adults ≥77 yr:* 5 mg orally once daily. *Adults to 76 yr, adolescents, and children ≥6 yr:* 5–10 mg orally once daily. Maximum dosage: 10 mg/day. **Chewable tablet, syrup, solution:** *Children 2–5 yr:* 2.5 mg orally once or twice daily. **Syrup and solution:** *Children ≤2 yr:* 2.5 mg orally once or twice daily.	For patients with moderate or severe renal impairment, on dialysis, or with chronic liver disease: dose adjustment required. Dose dependent on severity of symptoms.
	Perennial allergies.	**Syrup and solution:** *Infants >6 months:* 2.5 mg orally once daily.	

Continued

TABLE 5.2   **Antihistamines—cont'd**

Drug Category/ Medication	Indication	Dosage	Considerations and Monitoring
Desloratadine	Seasonal allergies or perennial allergies Allergic rhinitis Chronic idiopathic urticaria	**Tablets, orally disintegrating tablets:** *Adults, adolescents, and children ≥12 yr:* 5 mg orally once daily. Maximum dosage: 5 mg/day. **Orally disintegrating tablets, solution:** *Children 6–11 yr:* 2.5 mg orally once daily. Maximum dosage: 2.5 mg/day. *Children 1–5 yr:* 1.25 mg orally once daily. Maximum dosage: 1.25 mg/day. *Infants ≥6 months:* 1 mg orally once daily. Maximum dosage: 1 mg/day.	**Note:** Desloratadine not FDA approved to treat allergic rhinitis in children <2 yr.
Loratadine	Seasonal allergies or perennial allergies Allergic rhinitis Chronic idiopathic urticaria	**Tablets, capsules, orally disintegrating tablets:** *Adults, adolescents, and children ≥6 yr:* 10 mg orally once daily. Maximum dosage: 10 mg orally/day. **Chewable tablet, solution:** *Adults, adolescents, and children ≥6 yr:* 10 mg orally once daily. Maximum dosage: 10 mg orally/day. *Children 2–5 yr:* 5 mg orally once daily. Maximum dosage: 5 mg orally/day.	
Fexofenadine	Seasonal allergies or perennial allergies Allergic rhinitis	**Tablets, capsules:** *Adults, adolescents, and children ≥12 yr:* 60 mg orally twice daily or 180 mg orally once daily. Maximum dosage: 120 mg/day for twice-daily dose and 180 mg/day for once-daily dosage. *Children 6–11 yr:* 30 mg orally twice daily. Maximum dosage: 60 mg/day. **Orally disintegrating tablets and oral suspension (5 mg/5 mL):** *Adults, adolescents, and children ≥12 yr:* 60 mg orally twice daily. Maximum dosage: 120 mg/day. *Children 6–11 yr:* 30 mg orally twice daily. Maximum dosage: 60 mg/day.	Renal impairment: adjust dose
	Chronic idiopathic urticaria	**Tablets, capsules:** *Adults, adolescents, and children ≥12 yr:* 60 mg orally twice daily or 180 mg orally once daily. Maximum dosage: 120 mg/day for twice-daily dose and 180 mg/day for once-daily dose. *Children 6–11 yr:* 30 mg orally twice daily. Maximum dosage: 60 mg/day. **Orally disintegrating tablets:** *Children 6–11 yr:* 30 mg orally twice daily. Maximum dosage: 60 mg/day. **Oral suspension (5 mg/5 mL):** *Children 2–11 yr:* 60 mg daily. Maximum dosage: 60 mg/day. *Children 6–23 months:* 15 mg orally twice daily. Maximum dosage: 30 mg/day	
Levocetirizine	Seasonal allergies or perennial allergies Allergic rhinitis Chronic idiopathic urticaria	**Tablet, solution:** *Adults, adolescents, and children ≥12 yr:* 2.5–5 mg orally once daily in the evening. *Children 6–11 yr:* 2.5 mg orally once daily in the evening. **Solution:** *Children 6 months–5 yr:* 1.25 mg orally once daily in the evening.	*Older adults:* Use lowest dose. Renal impairment: Adjust dose.

TABLE 5.2   Antihistamines—cont'd

Drug Category/ Medication	Indication	Dosage	Considerations and Monitoring
Intranasal Antihistamines			
Azelastine	Perineal allergic rhinitis	**OTC Dosing: Astepro spray: 0.15% (205.5 mcg/spray):**	May cause sedation. Do not drive or operate machinery until effects known.
		Adults, adolescents, and children ≥12 yr: 1 or 2 sprays in each nostril twice daily, or 2 sprays in each nostril once daily.	
		Children 6–11 yr: 1 spray in each nostril twice daily.	
		Prescription Dosing: Astepro spray: 0.15% (205.5 mcg/spray):	
		Adults, adolescents, and children ≥12 yr: 2 sprays each nostril twice daily.	
		Children 6 months–5 yr: 1 spray each nostril twice daily.	
	Seasonal allergic rhinitis	**Astelin spray 0.1% (137 mcg/spray):**	
		Adults, adolescents, and children ≥12 yr: 1 or 2 sprays in each nostril twice daily.	
		Children 5–11 yr: 1 spray in each nostril twice daily.	
		Astepro spray 0.1% (137 mcg/spray) or 0.15% (205.5 mcg/spray):	
		Adults, adolescents, and children ≥12 yr: 1 or 2 sprays in each nostril twice daily.	
		Children 6–11 yr: 1 spray in each nostril twice daily.	
		Astepro spray 0.1% (137 mcg/spray): *Children 2–5 yr:* 1 spray in each nostril twice daily.	
	Vasomotor rhinitis	**Astelin spray 0.1% (137 mcg/spray):**	
		Adults, adolescents, and children ≥12 yr: 2 sprays in each nostril twice daily.	
Olopatadine	Seasonal allergies Seasonal allergic rhinitis	**Nasal spray (665 mcg/spray):**	
		Adults, adolescents, and children ≥12 yr: 2 sprays in each nostril twice daily.	
		Children 6–11 yr: 1 spray in each nostril twice daily.	

Adverse effects. The most frequently reported adverse effects include those related to the central nervous system (CNS), respiratory system, and GI system. Older adults are at risk for dizziness, sedation, and hypotension.

Contraindications. The Beers Criteria for Potentially Inappropriate Medication Use in Older Adults identify diphenhydramine as a drug to avoid in older adults due to anticholinergic effects and reduced clearance (American Geriatrics Society, 2019). Use with caution with other anti-histamines and other mediations that may increase CNS effects or anticholinergic effects, such as alcohol, opioids, sedatives, antidepressants, quinidine, disopyramide, and monoamine oxidase inhibitors (MAOIs).

Monitoring. Laboratory testing is not routinely recommended. Consider monitoring renal status in older adults or in those with renal impairment. Monitor for adverse effects. Therapeutic effects are noted with the improvement in symptoms.

PRACTICE PEARLS

Life Span Considerations With Diphenhydramine

Geriatrics

- Beers Criteria for Potentially Inappropriate Medication Use in Older Adults

Pediatrics

- Patients may experience paradoxical CNS stimulation, excitation, and mental alertness.

Cetirizine

Pharmacokinetics. Cetirizine is rapidly absorbed and binds well to proteins. Half-life is 6 to 8 hours. Half-life and clearance are prolonged in older adults and in patients with chronic liver disease, so health care providers should consider obtaining a baseline serum creatinine level. Excretion is via the kidneys and is about 70% in healthy adults.

Indications. Cetirizine, a metabolite of hydroxyzine, is available in several oral formulations, including tablets, orally disintegrating tablets, and liquid-filled capsules. Cetirizine is approved for the treatment of seasonal and perennial AR. It is available OTC and by prescription.

Adverse effects. Adults and adolescents age 12 and older reported somnolence as the primary adverse effect, followed by fatigue, dry mouth, pharyngitis, dizziness, headache, and nausea. Children 6 to 11 years of age were more likely to report dose-dependent headache as the primary adverse effect, followed by abdominal pain, coughing, pharyngitis, and somnolence. Caregivers of children 6 months to 2 years of age reported irritability, fussiness, insomnia, fatigue, and malaise.

PRACTICE PEARLS
Cetirizine Use in Pregnancy and Lactation

- Clinical animal studies have shown no risk to the fetus. However, there are no adequate and well-controlled studies in pregnant women. Weigh potential benefits to the mother against potential risk to the fetus, and limit to short-term use.
- Breastfeeding is not recommended. Weigh potential benefits to the mother against potential risk to the infant.

Contraindications. Cetirizine is contraindicated in patients with known hypersensitivities to cetirizine, levocetirizine, and hydroxyzine. Use with caution in older adults. Adjust the dose in pediatric and adult patients with hepatic or renal impairment or those who are on dialysis (Table 5.3). Sedative effects may decrease mental alertness; therefore advise patients to avoid use if operating machinery or driving.

Monitoring. Monitor renal and hepatic function at baseline and periodically, especially in older adults. Adjust dose as recommended. Monitor for adverse effects. Monitor for improvement of AR symptoms.

Fexofenadine
Pharmacokinetics. Peak concentration levels of fexofenadine are reached in approximately 2 hours. In patients

TABLE 5.3	Cetirizine Dosing Adjustment Based on Creatinine Clearance or Hepatic Impairment	
Patient Criteria	Dose Recommendations	
Adults and Children ≥12 Years of Age		
Creatinine clearance >11–31 mL/min	5 mg orally once daily	
On hemodialysis		
Hepatic impairment		
Pediatric 6–11 Years of Age		
Impaired renal or hepatic function	5 mg orally once daily	

with normal renal function, the half-life is 14 hours. Renal impairment extends the half-life by 59% to 72% depending on the severity of impairment. Fexofenadine binds to protein. Fexofenadine is excreted unchanged through the GI and renal systems. Though fexofenadine is a metabolite of terfenadine, there have been no reports of associated lengthening between ventricular depolarization and repolarization (known as long QT) or of ventricular tachycardia.

Indications. Fexofenadine is approved for the treatment of seasonal AR in adults and children 2 years of age and older. Fexofenadine is available by prescription or OTC in both generic and brand products.

Adverse effects. Adverse effects related to the CNS include headache, drowsiness and fatigue, dizziness, fever, and pain, including myalgias and extremity pain. The most common adverse effects on the GI system include vomiting, diarrhea, nausea, and dyspepsia. Rare adverse effects include chronic idiopathic urticaria, insomnia, nervousness, pruritis, sleep disorders, and hypersensitivity reactions.

PRACTICE PEARLS
Fexofenadine Use in Pregnancy and Lactation

- Weigh potential benefits to the mother against potential risk to the fetus.
- Breastfeeding is not recommended. Weigh potential benefits to the mother against adverse effects on the infant.

Contraindications. Avoid administration of fexofenadine in patients with hypersensitivity to the drug or any of its components. Fexofenadine oral disintegrating tablets (Allegra) contain phenylalanine. Avoid use in patients with phenylketonuria. Dose adjustments are required in patients with renal disease.

Monitoring. Monitor renal function. Monitor for improvement of symptoms.

Intranasal Antihistamines
Intranasal antihistamines direct therapeutic action to the nasal passages and have decreased adverse and systemic effects, which makes them beneficial in the treatment of seasonal, allergic, and episodic AR. Azelastine hydrochloride and olopatadine hydrochloride are second-generation antihistamine nasal sprays that reduce the symptoms of AR. They are expensive compared to oral antihistamines

PRACTICE PEARLS
Intranasal Antihistamine Use in Pregnancy and Lactation

- Weigh potential benefits to the mother against potential risk to the fetus.
- Breastfeeding is not recommended. Weigh potential benefits to the mother against adverse effects on the infant.

and may be cost prohibitive for some patients. Common side effects of intranasal antihistamines include a bad taste in the mouth, epistaxis, headache, and sedation.

Azelastine

Pharmacokinetics. Following administration, the onset of action occurs within minutes. The duration of action is about 12 to 24 hours. Half-life varies with formulation. Elimination is through the GI tract. No age-related, renal, or hepatic dose adjustments are required.

Indications. Azelastine is a topical antihistamine (H_1-receptor blocking agent). Azelastine is approved for the treatment of perennial and seasonal AR and vasomotor rhinitis. Several formulations are available. Health care providers should review dosing recommendations and current guidelines prior to prescribing.

Adverse effects. The most frequently reported adverse effects include somnolence, headache, and a bitter taste in the mouth. Other, less common adverse effects include nasal discomfort, weight gain, epistaxis, dizziness, fatigue, rhinitis, nausea, dry mouth, paroxysmal sneezing, pharyngitis, and nasal burning. Formulations varied in frequency of reported effects.

Contraindications. There are no absolute contraindications. Caution is advised when used by patients operating machinery or driving. Avoid concurrent use with CNS depressants such as alcohol. Patients should be instructed to avoid getting the spray into their eyes.

Monitoring. No laboratory monitoring is required. Monitor for response to therapy and adverse effects.

Olopatadine

Pharmacokinetics. Peak plasma concentrations of olopatadine occur from 15 minutes to 2 hours after dosing. The drug primarily binds to albumin. Half-life is 8 to 12 hours. Excretion occurs through the renal system, with 86% of the drug unchanged in the urine.

Indications. Olopatadine is an H_1-blocker approved for the treatment of seasonal allergies. Olopatadine relieves allergy-related symptoms in adults and children 6 years of age and older. The metered-dose spray delivers 0.6% (335 mcg/spray), with dosage varying by age. No dose adjustments are required in patients with hepatic or renal impairment.

Adverse effects. In adults, the most frequently reported adverse effect was a bitter taste in the mouth. Other adverse effects included headache, epistaxis, and pharyngolaryngeal

pain. Infrequent adverse effects included upper respiratory symptoms, dry mouth, fatigue, somnolence, and creatine phosphokinase (CPK) elevations. In children, there were fewer reports of adverse effects, with epistaxis being the most common.

Contraindications. Treatment with olopatadine is contraindicated in patients with hypersensitivity to any component of the product. Patients experiencing somnolence are advised to use caution when driving or operating machinery. Advise patients to avoid the use of alcohol and other CNS depressants. Patients should be instructed to avoid getting the spray into their eyes.

Monitoring. Prior to prescribing and on subsequent visits, evaluate nasal passages for mucosal ulcerations, trauma, and septal defect. No laboratory monitoring is required.

Intranasal Mast Cell Stabilizers

Cromolyn

Pharmacokinetics. Cromolyn is poorly absorbed via the intranasal route. The onset of action takes about 1 to 2 weeks. Half-life is 80 to 90 minutes. Excretion is through the feces and urine.

Indications. Cromolyn nasal spray is an OTC mast cell stabilizer with antiinflammatory properties approved for use in adults and children over age 2 (Table 5.4). Cromolyn nasal spray acts directly on nasal mucosal tissue by inhibiting histamine release from mast cells. Cromolyn is most effective if treatment begins prior to an exposure to antigens. It has a limited duration of effectiveness, and repeat dosing throughout the day is required for maximum benefit.

Adverse effects. Adverse effects are limited and generally related to the route of administration. The most common adverse effects include upper respiratory symptoms of nasal burning and stinging, mucosal irritation, and sneezing. Less common adverse effects include headache, cough, hoarseness, post-nasal drip, epistaxis, and an unpleasant taste in the mouth.

The most common adverse effects of the nebulizer solution include diarrhea, headache, pharyngitis, dyspnea, hoarseness, and an unpleasant taste in the mouth. Other, less common adverse effects include throat irritation, cough, nasal congestion, nasal itching, and nosebleed. Significant adverse effects are rare but may include bronchospasm, laryngeal edema, swollen parotid gland, angioedema, and pulmonary infiltrates with eosinophilia.

TABLE 5.4	**Intranasal Mast Cell Stabilizer**			
Medication	Indication	Dosage		Considerations and Monitoring
Cromolyn sodium	Seasonal and perennial allergies	**Spray (5.2 mg/spray):** *Adults, adolescents, and children ≥2 yr: 1* spray in each nostril three to four times daily. Maximum dose: 6 times/day		Must be used prophylactically.

Contraindications. Avoid use in patients with hypersensitivities to cromolyn or any of its components. The use of cromolyn nasal spray is not recommended as a treatment for asthma or URIs.

Monitoring. Routine laboratory monitoring is not required. Monitor for improvement in symptoms. Monitor for appropriate initiation of cromolyn in relation to expected allergy season.

Intranasal Anticholinergics

Ipratropium Bromide Nasal Spray

Pharmacokinetics. Onset of action occurs within 15 minutes. Absorption rates of ipratropium are poor, with mucosal absorption <20% and systemic absorption 2% to 3%. Excretion is via the urine. In pediatric populations, excretion is higher than in adults (11% and 5%, respectively).

Indications. Ipratropium nasal spray is used to relieve symptoms of allergic and nonallergic perennial rhinitis in adults and children 6 years of age and older (Table 5.5). Ipratropium improves rhinorrhea; however it does not improve symptoms of sneezing or congestion. Ipratropium nasal spray is currently available in two strengths: 0.03% and 0.06%.

Adverse effects. The most commonly reported adverse effects include headache, epistaxis, pharyngitis, nasal dryness, and URIs. Less common adverse effects include dryness of the mouth/throat, dizziness, eye irritations, hoarseness, cough, or a bitter taste in the mouth. The use of intranasal ipratropium rarely results in serious adverse effects such as palpitations, tachycardia, nervousness, insomnia, or tremor.

Contraindications. Avoid use in patients with hypersensitivities to any component of ipratropium and to ipratropium bromide-containing products. Though ipratropium has low absorption rates, health care providers should be alert to its anticholinergic effects. Consider using with caution in patients with closed-angle glaucoma, bladder or urinary obstructions, cardiac arrhythmias, older adults, and patients who operate machinery or drive.

Monitoring. Monitor for the relief of symptoms associated with rhinorrhea. If there is no improvement, reassess patient's technique using the nasal spray. If there is still no improvement in rhinorrhea, consider an alternate therapy. Monitor for adverse effects. Monitor for vision changes, urinary retention, and cardiac arrhythmias. If used during lactation, monitor for potential adverse effects on the nursing infant and reduction in milk production.

Leukotriene Modifiers

Leukotriene Receptor Antagonists

Leukotriene receptor antagonists (LTRAs) inhibit the cysteinyl leukotriene CysLT1 receptor, which decreases the inflammatory response seen in AR. LTRAs are equivalent to oral antihistamines but are not as effective as intranasal steroids in treating symptoms. Montelukast sodium is the only LTRA approved to treat AR; however, the U.S. Food and Drug Administration (FDA) has provided restrictions and recommendations for the use of montelukast for AR (Table 5.6).

Montelukast Sodium

Pharmacokinetics. Montelukast sodium is rapidly absorbed. Distribution is minimal across the blood–brain barrier. Metabolism results in undetectable metabolites in adults and children. Excretion occurs via the liver via CYP 3A4, 2C8, and 2C9. Mild to moderate liver impairment extends half-life elimination from a maximum of 5.5 hours to 7.4 hours.

TABLE 5.5	Intranasal Anticholinergics	
Medication	**Indication**	**Dosage**
Ipratropium bromide	Perennial allergies	**0.03% Nasal spray:** *Adults, adolescents, and children ≥6 yr:* 2 sprays (42 mcg) in each nostril two to three times daily.
	Seasonal allergies Rhinorrhea due to common cold	**0.06% Nasal spray:** *Adults, adolescents, and children ≥5 yr:* 2 sprays (84 mcg) in each nostril four times daily up to 3 weeks.

TABLE 5.6	Leukotriene Receptor Antagonists (LTRAs)			
Medication	**Indication**	**Dosage**		**Considerations and Monitoring**
Montelukast	Seasonal and perennial AR	**Tablet:** *Adults and children ≥15 yr:* 10 mg orally once daily. **Chewable tablet, granules:** *Children and adolescents 6–14 yr:* 5 mg orally once daily. *Children 2–5 yr:* 4 mg once daily. **Granules (4 mg) packet:** *Children 6 months–2 yr:* 4 mg orally once daily.		Reserve use for patients who are not treated effectively with or cannot tolerate other allergy medications.

Indications. Montelukast is an LTRA approved for the treatment of AR in adults and children over 2 years of age. In March 2020, the FDA issued a black box warning regarding its use.

BLACK BOX WARNING!

Montelukast

- Use montelukast only for patients who have an inadequate response to or are unable to tolerate other allergy treatments.
- Montelukast increases the risk of serious neuropsychiatric events including agitation, aggression, depression, sleep disturbances, and suicidal thoughts and behaviors (including suicide).

PRACTICE PEARLS

Montelukast Use in Pregnancy and Lactation

- Animal trials reveal no demonstratable risk to the fetus. However, there are no adequate and well-controlled studies in pregnant women.
- Montelukast is excreted in breast milk at ranges below the therapeutic index. Weigh the benefits of breastfeeding to the mother and infant against adverse effects on the infant.

Adverse effects. The most common adverse reactions are URI, fever, headache, pharyngitis, cough, abdominal pain, diarrhea, otitis media, influenza, rhinorrhea, sinusitis, and otitis. Other adverse effects reported post-marketing include thrombocytopenia, hypersensitivity reactions, psychiatric disorders, and multiple system disorders including those of the nervous, cardiovascular, respiratory, GI, hepatobiliary, skin and subcutaneous tissue, muscle, and renal systems.

Contraindications. Avoid the use of montelukast sodium in patients with hypersensitivity to any component of this product. Montelukast chewable tablets contain phenylalanine and should be avoided or used with caution in patients with phenylketonuria. Do not use in patients with a known history of psychiatric and/or neurologic disease.

Monitoring. Monitor patients for behavior changes consistent with psychiatric and/or neurologic disease. Monitor patients with severe hepatic impairment, jaundice, or hepatitis, though no dosing adjustments are recommended by the manufacturer. No routine laboratory monitoring is required.

Decongestants

Decongestants stimulate alpha-adrenergic receptors resulting in vasoconstriction, which leads to nasal decongestion and increased nasal drainage. Oral and topical decongestants are available OTC and many patients self-treat prior to visiting their primary care provider (Table 5.7). Oral decongestants relieve symptoms but have adverse systemic effects. Topical nasal decongestants provide direct therapy to nasal membranes and have less frequent systemic effects. Overuse of topical nasal decongestants may cause rebound congestion; therefore they are recommended only in acute conditions and only for a limited time.

The use of decongestants has long been controversial due to the risk of serious adverse effects and limited benefits, particularly in children under 4 years of age. As a result, OTC cough and cold products intended for use in children under 2 years of age were removed from the market,

PRACTICE PEARLS

Contraindications to Decongestants

- Benign prostatic hyperplasia or urinary obstruction
- Diabetes mellitus
- Heart disease
- Increased intraocular pressure or angle-closure glaucoma
- Renal failure
- Seizure disorder
- Severe or uncontrolled hypertension
- Thyroid disease

TABLE 5.7   Decongestants

Drug Category/ Medication	Indication	Dosage	Considerations and Monitoring
Oral Decongestants			
Pseudoephedrine hydrochloride	Sinus and nasal congestion	**Immediate-release tablets, liquid-filled capsules, solution 15 mg/5 mL or 30 mg/5 mL:** *Adults, adolescents, and children ≥12 yr:* 60 mg orally every 4–6 hr. Maximum dosage: 240 mg daily. *Children 6–11 yr:* 30 mg orally every 4–6 hr. Maximum dosage: 120 mg daily. **12-Hour extended-release tablet:** *Adults, adolescents, and children ≥12 yr:* 120 mg orally every 12 hr. Maximum dosage: 240 mg/day. **24-Hour extended-release tablet:** *Adults, adolescents, and children ≥12 yr:* 240 mg every 24 hr. Maximum dosage: 240 mg/day. **Solution 15 mg/5 mL:** *Children 4–5 yr:* 15 mg orally every 4–6 hr. Maximum dosage: 60 mg daily.	Decrease dose in patients with renal impairment.
Phenylephrine	Nasal congestion	*Adults, adolescents, and children ≥12 yr:* 10–20 mg orally every 4–6 hr. Maximum dosage: 60 mg daily. *Children 6–11 yr:* 5 mg orally every 4–6 hr. Maximum dosage: 30 mg daily. *Children 4–5 yr:* 2.5 mg orally every 4 hr. Maximum dosage: 15 mg daily.	Pediatric renal impairment: use lower initial dosing.
Intranasal Decongestants			
Oxymetazoline	Non-FDA use: nasal congestion	**0.05% Solution:** *Adults and children ≥6 yr:* 2–3 drops or sprays in each nostril twice daily for up to 3 days. Maximum dosage: 2 doses/24 hr. **0.025% Solution:** *Children 2–5 yr:* 2–5 drops in each nostril twice daily for up to 3 days. Maximum dosage: 2 doses/24 hr.	
Phenylephrine hydrochloride	Nasal congestion	**Solution 0.25%–1.0%, Nasal drops 1%:** *Adults, adolescents, and children ≥12 yr:* 2 or 3 drops or sprays in each nostril every 4 hr as needed. *Children 6–11 yr:* 2 or 3 drops or sprays in each nostril every 4 hr as needed. **0.125% Solution:** *Children 2–5 yr:* 2 or 3 drops or sprays in each nostril every 4 hr as needed.	Do not use for more than 3 days.

and warning labels were added to available products to limit use to children over 4 years of age (U.S. Food and Drug Administration, n.d.). In response to concerns, the Combat Methamphetamine Epidemic Act of 2005 was established. This act limits the number of decongestant medications a patient can purchase each month, requires photo identification for purchase, and requires retail stores to keep records of purchases (U. S. Department of Justice, 2005.

Oral Decongestants

Pseudoephedrine Hydrochloride

Pharmacokinetics. The onset of action is 30 minutes. Peak effect occurs in approximately 1 to 2 hours and duration is 4 to 6 hours. Pseudoephedrine is metabolized in the liver and excreted in the kidneys.

PRACTICE PEARLS

Pseudoephedrine Use in Pregnancy and Lactation

- Avoid use in the first trimester. Weigh potential benefits to the mother against potential risk to the fetus.
- Pseudoephedrine hydrochloride is excreted in breast milk. Adverse effects include irritability in nursing infants and a decrease in milk production. Consider the risk to the infant versus the benefits of breastfeeding.

Indications. Pseudoephedrine hydrochloride is approved for the treatment of nasal congestion due to AR or the common cold in adults and children 2 years of age and older, though product labels recommend use in children over age 4.

Adverse effects. Reports of multiple systemic adverse effects are noted with the use of pseudoephedrine and include anxiety, nervousness, restlessness, insomnia, and tachycardia. Taking the medications at night may result in impaired sleep. Older adults may be more sensitive to these adverse effects.

Contraindications. Do not use in patients taking MAOIs or within 14 days of stopping MAOIs. Do not use in patients with a hypersensitivity to pseudoephedrine, sympathomimetics, or any component of the product. Avoid use in patients with severe coronary artery disease or hypertension. Evaluate concomitant medications due to numerous drug–drug interactions with pseudoephedrine.

Monitoring. Routine laboratory monitoring is not required. Monitor patients with a history of renal impairment and adjust dosage or discontinue use. Monitor for adverse effects and discontinue medication if they occur.

Intranasal Decongestants

Intranasal decongestants cause vasoconstriction, providing symptomatic relief of nasal congestion and improved patency (Kushnir, 2011). They do not improve nasal itching, sneezing, or rhinorrhea. These medications should only be used for 3 to 5 days due to rebound congestion.

Oxymetazoline
Pharmacokinetics. Vasoconstriction of the nasal mucosa contributes to the relief of rhinitis symptoms. Relief occurs within 5 to 10 minutes and lasts 6 to 7 hours. Drug metabolism by the liver is minimal. Excretion occurs primarily through the renal system.

Indications. Oxymetazoline is available OTC. Oxymetazoline is used routinely, though off-label for the treatment of nasal congestion in adults and children. Oxymetazoline is available in a solution (drops, mist, and spray). Advise patients that rebound congestion may occur if treatment continues for more than 5 consecutive days.

Adverse effects. The most frequently reported adverse effects include dryness and burning of the nasal mucosa,

sneezing, rebound congestion, agitation, nervousness, headache, seizure, and insomnia. Serious adverse effects may include dysrhythmias, hypertension, and tachycardia. In children age 5 and younger, accidental ingestion caused serious cardiopulmonary and neurological effects.

Contraindications. Use oxymetazoline with caution in patients with cardiovascular disease, hypotension, orthostatic hypotension, or hypertension due to its vasoconstrictive properties. Use with caution in patients with diabetes mellitus, thyroid disease, prostatic hyperplasia, vascular disease, or autoimmune disease. Patients taking MAOIs may experience increased vasoconstrictive effects. There is an increased risk of angle-closure glaucoma in patients with closed-angle glaucoma.

Monitoring. No routine laboratory monitoring is required. Monitor for relief of symptoms. Monitor children for accidental ingestion and advise caregivers to seek immediate assistance. Instruct patients on correct use of nasal sprays.

Combination Medications

A variety of combination medications to treat the symptoms of AR and upper respiratory illnesses are available. This section will review the combination of intranasal antihistamines with intranasal steroids in depth due to the proven efficacy of the combination (Table 5.8). A brief description of commonly available OTC combinations will follow. Refer to each medication classification's dosing recommendations, adverse effects, and contraindications. Primary care providers may expect that their patients will use one of these combinations to self-treat. Patients will benefit when primary care providers explain the efficacy and risks of these medications.

Intranasal Antihistamine/Intranasal Corticosteroid

Azelastine and Fluticasone Propionate
Pharmacokinetics. Peak concentration levels of azelastine were reached in 30 minutes. Bioavailability is 40% and the medication binds well to protein (88%). Hepatic metabolism is by CYP 450. Excretion is through the feces, and half-life is 25 hours. Peak concentration levels of fluticasone propionate were reached in 1 hour. Bioavailability is 44% to 61% greater than with monotherapy and the medication binds well to protein (91%). Hepatic metabolism is by CYP 3A4. Excretion is through the feces, and half-life is about 8 hours.

TABLE 5.8	Combination Medications: Intranasal Antihistamines/Intranasal Corticosteroids			
Medication	**Indication**	**Dosage**		**Considerations and Monitoring**
Azelastine and fluticasone propionate	Seasonal allergic rhinitis	**Azelastine 137 mcg/Fluticasone 50 mcg/spray:** *Adults, adolescents, and children ≥6 yr:* 1 spray in each nostril twice daily (every 12 hr). Maximum dosage: 2 sprays/day.		May cause sedation. Do not drive or operate machinery until effects known.

Indications. Azelastine (an antihistamine) and fluticasone propionate (a corticosteroid) is a combination intranasal spray. Treatment with a combination of an intranasal antihistamine and an INS provides better relief of symptoms than monotherapy with an INS or an intranasal antihistamine (Dykewicz et al., 2017). No dose adjustment is required in the older-adult population or in patients with renal or hepatic impairment.

Adverse effects. Common adverse effects include headache, epistaxis, cough, sore throat, and a change in taste. Drowsiness, fatigue, or sleepiness may occur as a result of the antihistamine effect. Refer to individual medication classifications for adverse effects.

Contraindications. Alcohol and other CNS depressants may increase adverse CNS effects. This medication is not recommended if patients require mental alertness or must operate machinery. Refer to individual medication classifications for additional contraindications.

Monitoring. Monitor for improvement of symptoms. Monitor for adverse reactions. Assess for appropriate technique. Refer to individual medication classifications for specific monitoring guidelines.

Other Combination Medications

- *Oral antihistamines and oral decongestants:* Oral antihistamines and oral decongestant combinations are numerous. Combination therapy provides improved symptom relief over monotherapy. The combination of medications also increases the risk of adverse effects.
- *Intranasal steroids and oral antihistamines:* The addition of oral antihistamines offers no improvement for patients reporting an inadequate response to intranasal steroids.
- *Intranasal steroids and intranasal oxymetazoline:* This combination of intranasal steroids and oxymetazoline is effective for AR symptom relief. However there is a risk of rebound nasal congestion as an effect of the oxymetazoline. Therapy should be limited to no more than 3 days.
- *Oral antihistamines and LTRAs:* Evidence does not support recommendations for the use of oral antihistamines with LTRAs (Seidman et al., 2015).
- *Intranasal steroids and LTRAs:* Evidence does not support recommendations for the use of intranasal steroids with LTRAs (Seidman et al., 2015).

Cough Therapy

Pharmacologic therapeutic options for cough include antitussives and expectorants as monotherapy or combination therapy (Table 5.9). Antitussives and/or expectorants may also be found in combination with antihistamines and decongestants. Antitussive and expectorant therapies are available by prescription and OTC and in non-narcotic (nonopioid) and narcotic (opioid) formulations. Despite their popularity, evidence regarding the efficacy of antitussive and expectorant therapy does not support widespread use.

Antitussives

The goal of antitussive (cough suppressant) therapy is reduction in the frequency and intensity of the cough. CHEST® recommends against the use of codeine-containing medications in patients younger than 18 years of age for cough due to the common cold. CHEST® noted the potential for serious side effects including respiratory distress and the lack of efficacy as support for this recommendation (Maleskar et al., 2017). Based on the lack of evidence and efficacy supporting the use of codeine or codeine-containing medications for the treatment of cough, these medications are not included in this chapter. Primary care providers are advised to consider these concerns prior to prescribing medications or recommending OTC medications.

BLACK BOX WARNING!

Codeine and Hydrocodone

The FDA has required changes in the labels on all cough and cold medicines containing opioids. The labels must:

- Limit the use of these products to adults 18 years of age and older, and state that the risks of these medicines outweigh their benefits in children younger than 18
- Include a boxed warning regarding the risks of misuse, abuse, addiction, overdose, death, and slowed or difficult breathing (FDA, 2018)

Benzonatate

Pharmacokinetics. Limited information regarding the pharmacokinetics of benzonatate is available. The onset of action is within 15 to 20 minutes. The effects continue for 3 to 8 hours.

Indications. Benzonatate is approved for the relief of coughs in adults and children age 10 and older. Benzonatate temporarily relieves the cough by anesthetizing cough receptors in the respiratory passages, lungs, and pleura. Benzonatate is an ester anesthetic. Advise patients not to chew, crush, or dissolve capsules as this may cause topical anesthetizing effects.

Adverse effects. Benzonatate adverse effects include hypersensitivity and anesthesia-type reactions (numbness or tingling of the tongue, mouth, throat, or face). CNS effects include sedation, headache, dizziness, mental confusion, and visual hallucinations. Other adverse effects may include constipation, nausea, pruritus, skin eruptions, nasal congestion, or a sensation of burning eyes or generalized chills or numbness. The risk of overdose, especially in children, results in seizures, arrhythmias, coma, and death.

Contraindications. Benzonatate is contraindicated in patients with ester local anesthetic hypersensitivity or a previous history of reaction to benzonatate. Avoid in patients with paraben hypersensitivity.

TABLE 5.9 **Cough: Antitussives and Expectorants**

Drug Category/ Medication	Indication	Dosage	Considerations and Monitoring
Antitussive			
Benzonatate	Cough	*Adults, adolescents, and children ≥10 yr:* 100–200 mg orally three times daily. Maximum dosage: 600 mg daily.	Benzonatate should be swallowed whole.
Dextromethorphan	Cough	**Immediate-release oral films, capsules, solutions, suspensions, and syrups:** *Adults, adolescents, and children ≥12 yr:* 10–20 mg orally every 4 hr OR 20–30 mg orally every 6–8 hr. Maximum dosage: 120 mg daily. *Children 6–11 yr:* 5–10 mg orally every 4 hr as needed OR 15 mg every 6–8 hr as needed. Maximum dosage: 60 mg/day. *Children 2–5 yr:* 2.5–5 mg orally every 4 hr as needed OR 7.5 mg orally every 6–8 hr as needed. Maximum dosage: 30 mg/day. **Extended-release (30 mg/5 mL):** *Adults, adolescents, and children ≥12 yr:* 60 mg (10 mL) orally every 12 hr as needed. Maximum dosage: 120 mg/day. *Children 6–11 yr:* 30 mg (5 mL) orally every 12 hr as needed. Maximum dosage: 60 mg/day. *Children 4–5 yr:* 15 mg (2.5 mL) orally every 12 hr as needed. Maximum dosage: 30 mg/day.	Renal and hepatic impairment: no dose adjustment required. **NOTE:** Use with caution in pediatrics. The American Academy of Pediatrics and the FDA recommend against use in children.
Expectorant			
Guaifenesin	Cough, phlegm and bronchial secretions	**Immediate-release capsules or tablets, solutions, and syrup:** *Adults, adolescents, and children ≥12 yr:* 200–400 mg orally every 4 hr as needed. Maximum dosage: 2400 mg daily. **Extended-release or biphasic capsules or tablets:** *Adults and children ≥12 yr:* 600–1200 mg orally every 4 hr as needed. Maximum dosage: 2400 mg daily. **Solutions and syrup:** *Children 6–11 yr:* 100–200 mg orally every 4 hr as needed. Maximum dosage: 1200 mg daily. *Children 2–5 yr:* 50–100 mg orally every 4 hr as needed. Maximum dosage: 600 mg daily. **Granule (100 mg) packet:** *Adults, adolescents, and children ≥12 yr:* 2–4 packets orally every 4 hr as needed. Maximum dosage: 24 packets/day. *Children 6–11 yr:* 1–2 packets orally every 4 hr as needed. Maximum dosage: 12 packets/day. *Children 2–5 yr:* 1 packet orally every 4 hr as needed. Maximum dosage: 6 packets/day.	

Monitoring. No routine laboratory monitoring is required. Monitor for appropriate therapeutic dosing. Monitor for numbness or tingling of the tongue, mouth, throat, or face. Advise patients to seek medical care if symptoms worsen or persist.

Dextromethorphan

Pharmacokinetics. The initial onset of cough relief is 15 to 30 minutes. Cough relief lasts 5 to 6 hours. Dextromethorphan binds to protein and is metabolized in the liver via CYP 2D6 and CYP 3A enzymes. Individual metabolism of dextromethorphan may increase the potential for abuse due to the metabolite dextrorphan. Dextrorphan produces neurobehavioral effects such as dissociative experiences, hypertension, tachycardia, and diaphoresis. Excretion occurs via the renal system.

Indications. Dextromethorphan is approved for suppression of cough due to irritants or the common cold. The antitussive effects of dextromethorphan and codeine are similar. Dextromethorphan has no analgesic effects.

Adverse effects. Adverse effects when administered at the recommended dosage are generally mild and include drowsiness, dizziness, restlessness, nervousness, and fatigue. Rare adverse effects include rash and anaphylaxis.

Contraindications. Dextromethorphan is contraindicated:
- With concurrent use or within 14 days of MAOI use
- In the treatment of coughs related to comorbid disease process, tobacco use, and symptoms that possibly signify a more serious illness, such as fever, nausea/vomiting, rash, or headache

Use with caution in patients with hepatic impairment. The use of dextromethorphan in children younger than 2 years of age is contraindicated and may result in fatal adverse effects and overdose.

Monitoring. No routine laboratory monitoring is required. Primary care providers are advised to monitor hepatic function and for toxic effects in patients with hepatic impairment. Monitor patient medications for use of MAOIs.

Expectorants

Guaifenesin

Pharmacokinetics. Guaifenesin is readily absorbed from the GI tract. Half-life is approximately 1 hour. It is excreted by the renal system.

Indications. Guaifenesin loosens and thins bronchial secretions, making coughs associated with colds and URIs more productive and potentially less irritating to the patient. Guaifenesin should not be used in children younger than age 2 due to serious and life-threatening effects. Guaifenesin is available in immediate-release, in extended-release, and in a combination immediate–extended-release formulation. Guaifenesin is administered as monotherapy or in conjunction with other OTC cold products.

Adverse effects. Patients report few adverse effects with the use of guaifenesin at recommended doses. Adverse effects include GI distress, nausea, vomiting, rash, dizziness, and headache. Overdose of guaifenesin may result in urolithiasis.

Contraindications. Guaifenesin is contraindicated for the treatment of a cough resulting from the use of angiotensin-converting enzyme (ACE) inhibitors or as a result of heart failure. Avoid use in patients with known hypersensitivity.

Monitoring. Monitor for reports of symptom improvement. Reevaluate if symptoms have not improved in 2 weeks. No routine lab monitoring is required. Guaifenesin may alter urine specimen results. Discontinue use 48 hours prior to collecting specimen.

Antiviral Therapy (Neuraminidase Inhibitors)

Neuraminidase inhibitors (NAIs) inhibit neuraminidase and disrupt viral replication associated with influenza type A and influenza type B (Table 5.10). The FDA has approved four medications for the treatment of acute, uncomplicated influenza: oseltamivir phosphate (Tamiflu), zanamivir (Relenza), peramivir (Rapivab), and baloxavir marboxil (Xofluza). Additionally, oseltamivir phosphate (Tamiflu)

Antiviral Medications (Neuraminidase Inhibitors)

Medication	Indication	Dosage	Considerations and Monitoring
Oseltamivir phosphate	Treatment of influenza types A and B	*Adults and adolescents ≥13 yr:* 75 mg orally twice daily for 5 days. *Children 1–12 yr based on body weight:* ≥40.1 kg: 75 mg orally once daily for 5 days. 23.1–40 kg: 60 mg orally twice daily for 5 days. 15.1–23 kg: 45 mg orally twice daily for 5 days. ≤15 kg: 30 mg orally twice daily for 5 days *Children 2 weeks–11 months:* 3 mg/kg/dose orally twice daily for five days	Initiate treatment within 48 hours of symptom onset. Adult renal impairment: dose adjustments required (Table 5.11).
	Prophylaxis of influenza types A and B	*Adults and adolescents ≥13 yr:* 75 mg orally once daily for at least 10 days OR up to 6 weeks during community outbreak. *Children 1–12 yr based on body weight:* ≥40.1 kg: 75 mg orally once daily for 10 days OR up to 6 weeks during community outbreak. 23.1–40 kg: 60 mg orally once daily for at least 10 days OR up to 6 weeks during community outbreak. 15.1–23 kg: 45 mg orally once daily for at least 10 days OR up to 6 weeks during community outbreak. ≤15 kg: 30 mg orally once daily for at least 10 days OR up to 6 weeks during community outbreak.	
Zanamivir	Treatment of influenza types A and B	**Inhalation:** *Adults, adolescents, and children ≥7 yr:* 10 mg orally every 12 hours for 5 days.	Initiate treatment within 48 hours of symptom onset. Oral inhalation does not require renal or hepatic dose adjustments.
	Prophylaxis of influenza types A and B	**Inhalation:** *Adults, adolescents, and children ≥5 yr:* 10 mg orally once daily for 10 days for household exposure OR 10 mg once daily for 28 days for community outbreak.	
Peramivir	Acute, uncomplicated influenza types A and B in nonhospitalized patients	*Adults and adolescents ≥13 yr:* 600 mg intravenously as a single dose *Infants and children 6 months–12 yr:* 12 mg/kg/dose intravenously as a single dose. Maximum 600 mg/dose .	Initiate treatment within 48 hours of symptom onset. Adult renal impairment: dose adjustments required (Table 5.12)
Baloxavir marboxil	Acute, uncomplicated influenza types A and B	*Adults, adolescents, and children ≥12 yr AND ≥ 80 kg:* 80 mg as a single dose. *Adults, adolescents, and children ≥12 yr AND <80 kg:* 40 mg as a single dose.	Initiate treatment within 48 hours of symptom onset.
	Postexposure seasonal influenza prophylaxis	*Adults, adolescents, and children ≥12 yr AND ≥80 kg:* 80 mg as a single dose. *Adults, adolescents, and children ≥12 yr AND <80 kg:* 40 mg as a single dose.	Initiate treatment as soon as possible after exposure to contact with influenza.

TABLE 5.10

and zanamivir (Relenza) are approved for prophylaxis in the event of a confirmed or suspected exposure to influenza types A and B. NAI therapy should begin within 48 hours of symptom onset for the greatest reduction in symptom severity and risk of complications. Oseltamivir phosphate will be discussed as an exemplar of the NAIs.

Oseltamivir

Pharmacokinetics. Oral administration results in absorption by the GI tract. Metabolism occurs in the liver. Half-life ranges from 1 to 4 hours. Excretion (>99%) occurs via the urine.

Indications. Oseltamivir is approved for the treatment of influenza types A and B in patients 2 weeks of age and older within 48 hours of the onset of symptoms. Dose recommendations are determined by age or by weight. Prophylactic treatment of influenza types A and B is approved in patients age 1 and older. Prophylactic treatment should be 10 days for a close-contact exposure and up to 6 weeks during a community outbreak.

Adverse effects. The most common adverse effects during treatment of adults and adolescents older than 13 years of age include nausea, vomiting, headache, and pain. Pediatric patients 1 to 12 years of age were most likely to experience vomiting. In patients younger than age 1, vomiting, diarrhea, and diaper rash were the most common adverse effects. Serious but rare adverse effects include anaphylactic reactions, allergic reactions, toxic epidermal necrolysis, Stevens-Johnson syndrome, and neuropsychiatric disorders.

Contraindications. Oseltamivir is contraindicated in patients with known serious hypersensitivity to oseltamivir or any component of the product. Avoid administering oseltamivir phosphate 2 days before or 2 weeks after the administration of the intranasal live attenuated influenza vaccine (LAIV).

PRACTICE PEARLS

Oseltamivir Use in Pregnancy and Lactation

- Clinical trials on animals have demonstrated fetal harm. Clinical trials on pregnant women lack data to address fetal risk. Weigh potential benefits to the mother against potential risk to the fetus.
- Low levels of oseltamivir phosphate have been reported in breast milk. Low levels are unlikely to lead to toxicity in infants. Weigh potential benefits to the mother against potential risk to the infant.

Monitoring. Prior to prescribing, assess patient history for onset of symptoms. Monitor for adverse effects. Monitor patients with known or suspected renal impairment. Adjust dosing during treatment and prophylaxis (Table 5.11)

TABLE 5.11	Oseltamivir Phosphate for Adult Dosing Adjustment Based on Creatinine Clearance	
Creatinine Clearance	**Dose Recommendations**	
Treatment of Influenza		
>60 mL/min	No dosage adjustment necessary	
>31–60 mL/min	30 mg orally twice daily for 5 days	
>11–30 mL/min	30 mg orally once daily for 5 days	
10 mL/min or less not on hemodialysis	Oseltamivir not recommended	
Prophylaxis of Influenza		
>60 mL/min	No dosage adjustment necessary	
>31–60 mL/min	30 mg orally once daily	
>11–30 mL/min	30 mg orally every other day	
10 mL/min or less not on hemodialysis	Oseltamivir not recommended	

TABLE 5.12	Peramivir Dosing Adjustment Based on Creatinine Clearance
Creatinine Clearance	**Dose Recommendations**
Adults and Adolescents	
>50 mL/min	No dosage adjustment necessary
>30–49 mL/min	200 mg intravenously as a single dose
>10–29 mL/min	100 mg intravenously as a single dose
Children 2 to 12 years	
>50 mL/min	No dosage adjustment necessary
>30–49 mL/min	4 mg/kg intravenously as a single dose (Maximum dose: 200 mg)
>10–29 mL/min	2 mg/kg intravenously as a single dose (Maximum dose: 100 mg)

Children 2 to 12 years: Emergency Authorization Use only; not FDA approved

Allergy Immunotherapy: Implications for Primary Care

Allergy immunotherapy (AIT) has proven to be efficacious and safe as an adjunct treatment of respiratory allergens. It is important for primary care providers to have knowledge of AIT therapies as they will most likely have patients who would benefit from AIT or who are currently on therapy. Initially only available as a subcutaneous injection (subcutaneous immunotherapy or SCIT), AIT is now available as sublingual immunotherapy (SLIT). Advantages of SLIT therapy are convenience and ability to self-administer.

The FDA has approved four SLIT tablets: Odactra (dust mite), Grastek (northern grass), Oralair (timothy grass), and Ragwitek (ragweed). Under current approvals, the FDA has included a black box warning for all SLIT tablets. FDA and manufacturer recommendations advise the initiation of SLIT under the supervision of health care providers experienced in the diagnosis and treatment of allergic diseases. Contraindications for therapy include patients with a hypersensitivity to any inactive ingredient (gelatin, mannitol, and sodium hydroxide); severe, unstable, or uncontrolled asthma; history of any severe systemic allergic reaction; history of any severe local reaction after taking any SLIT; and history of eosinophilic esophagitis.

BLACK BOX WARNING!

SLIT

- Life-threatening allergic reactions, including anaphylaxis and severe laryngopharyngeal restrictions, may occur.
- Do not administer to patients with severe, unstable, or uncontrolled asthma.
- Auto-injectable epinephrine should be prescribed to patients; instruct patients on appropriate use and to obtain immediate medical care upon use.
- Use may not be suitable for patients with conditions that may reduce their ability to survive a serious allergic reaction.
- Use may not be suitable for patients who may be unresponsive to epinephrine or inhaled bronchodilators due to concomitant drug therapy.
- Monitor all patients for at least 30 minutes after initial dose in a health-care setting.

Prescriber Considerations for Allergy and Respiratory Therapy

Clinical Reasoning for Allergy and Respiratory Therapy

The overall prevalence of allergies and viral URIs makes it likely that primary care providers will encounter patients seeking relief of aggravating symptoms. The presenting symptoms of allergies and URIs may mimic or disguise the symptoms of more serious disease processes. Primary care providers must determine the appropriate diagnosis, provide education, initiate treatment, monitor health outcomes, and if required, refer the patient for specialty care. Clinical practice guidelines provide assessment and treatment algorithms based on classification of symptoms in terms of course and severity.

Consider the patient's health problem. Medication selection is based on efficacy, symptoms, symptom frequency and severity, patient preference, drug availability, and cost. Key points to consider include:
- Comorbid health conditions

BOOKMARK THIS!

Clinical Practice Guidelines

- AAO-HNSF Clinical Practice Guideline: Allergic Rhinitis https://journals.sagepub.com/doi/full/10.1177/0194599814561600
- Diagnosis and Treatment of Respiratory Illness in Children and Adults: https://www.icsi.org/wp-content/uploads/2019/01/RespIllness.pdf
- IDSA Clinical Practice Guideline for Acute Bacterial Rhinosinusitis in Children and Adults: https://academic.oup.com/cid/article/54/8/e72/367144
- Treatment of seasonal allergic rhinitis: An evidence-based focused 2017 guideline update: https://www.aaaai.org/Aaaai/media/MediaLibrary/PDF%20Documents/Practice%20and%20Parameters/2017-Rhinitis-Guideline-Updates.pdf

Note: This is not an exhaustive list of guidelines.

- The onset of symptoms (acute versus chronic; recurrent versus continuous)
- The severity of symptoms as perceived by the patient
- Prior or present treatment

Determine the desired therapeutic outcome based on the patient's health problem. Determine the patient's reason and goal in seeking treatment. Patient concerns may center on relief of symptoms such as sneezing, congestion, rhinorrhea, cough, fatigue, or malaise. Decreased quality of life may result from poor sleep or adverse drug effects related to current or lack of treatment.

Assess the selected pharmacotherapy for its appropriateness for the patient by considering the medication's side effects as well as the patient's age, race/ethnicity, comorbidities, and genetic factors. Due to the widespread availability of OTC medications, it is important that health care providers ask what medications the patient has already tried. The selection of pharmacotherapeutic options includes:
- Identifying and targeting symptoms that are most important to the patient and evaluating the duration and severity of symptoms
- The patient's age, comorbid conditions, and concomitant drug use
- Consideration of the efficacy of the medication and the potential for adverse effects
- Patient preference (oral versus intranasal formulations)
- Cost

Initiate the treatment plan with the selected medication by first providing adequate patient education to ensure the patient's understanding and to promote full participation in the therapy. Patients with allergic diseases should be educated in the disease process. For example, seasonal AR regularly occurs at about the same season/time each year. Encourage patients to keep a symptoms chart. With continued use, they can identify when they might notice the onset of symptoms. This enables them to initiate early, preventive treatment that might alleviate the worst of their symptoms. Similarly, patients with viral URIs may expect antibiotic therapy in hopes of decreasing their symptoms. Primary care providers can also educate patients on the current recommendations (selected medication, route, dose, and frequency) and expected results of therapy, which may prevent overdose and/or overuse of the medications. Primary care providers should also include health promotion education such as recommending yearly vaccinations. Patients may also question the need for additional testing, SLIT, or immunomodulator medications. Dependent of the practice setting, a referral to an allergist/immunologist might be considered for allergy testing or intensive therapy.

Ensure complete patient and family understanding of the medication using a variety of education strategies. Written materials, printed handouts, and electronic resources provide reinforcement of information verbally when given during an office visit. Encourage questions at the end of each new concept, at the end of the visit, and between visits. Electronic patient portals offer a convenient method of communication that some patients prefer over voicemail. For patients interested in accurate internet resources, the Asthma and Allergy Foundation of America (n.d.) and the American Academy of Allergy, Asthma & Immunology (n.d.) websites include patient information such as definitions, diagnoses, treatments, and prevention tips.

Conduct follow-up and monitoring of patient responses to pharmacotherapies. At each visit, review the patient history with attention to changes that may have occurred since the last visit. The use of visual analogue scales (VASs) to document the severity of AR-related symptoms is well validated and is part of the 2020 Allergic Rhinitis and its Impact on Asthma (ARIA) guidelines (Bousquet et al., 2020). Review current medications, taking care to review OTC medications. Review any adverse effects patients may have experienced since their last visit. Discuss improvement or lack of improvement in symptoms (severity and frequency), the method of medication administration, and the level of satisfaction with the therapy.

Teaching Points for Allergy and Respiratory Therapy

Health Promotion Strategies

The avoidance of allergens is often the first strategy recommended to patients. Avoidance requires a multipronged approach to:
- Evaluate the physical environment (inside and outside). School, home, and work environments are unavoidable. Patients may not have the ability to exercise any control over their environment.
- Identify allergen triggers. Common environmental triggers are pollen, pets, dust mites, molds, and pests.
- Determine whether work, school, or home interventions are feasible and whether patients are willing to perform the interventions. Interventions include acaricides, protective barriers, humidity control, hand sanitizers, cleaning and the use of vacuum filters, and laminar airflow systems.

Recognize that efficacy varies and evidence strongly supporting effectiveness varies (Cipriani et al., 2017).
- Avoid irritants such as smoke (tobacco, woodburning fires), odors, cold air, common colds and infections, and exhaust fumes.

Patient Education for Medication Safety

- Use intranasal sprays as directed. Use saline spray and expel spray and mucus prior to administering medicated spray. Avoid spraying in eyes or mouth. Avoid spraying directly on the septum (center) of the nose. Follow manufacturers' recommendations for administration and cleaning of the device.
- The use of topical (intranasal) decongestants may lead to rhinitis medicamentosia, also called rebound congestion, which produces symptoms of nasal congestion from overuse of topical decongestants. Do not take topical decongestants longer than prescribed.
- Take prescription medications as directed by your primary care provider. Do not take more/less or use longer than instructed.
- Notify your health-care provider if you develop a fever, rash, shortness of breath, change in cough, increasing fatigue, or persistent headache or if symptoms do not improve within 7 days.
- If changes in mood or behavior occur, or if suicidal thoughts develop, stop taking the medication and contact your primary care provider immediately.
- Talk to your primary care provider about all prescription and nonprescription (OTC) medicines, vitamins, and herbal supplements you are taking.
- Talk to your primary care provider about any medical conditions you have; if you are pregnant or plan to become pregnant; or if you are breastfeeding or plan to breastfeed.
- Do not use alcohol, sleeping pills, sedatives, or tranquilizers (MAOIs) without consulting your primary care provider.
- Avoid driving a car, operating heavy machinery, or performing hazardous tasks until the effects of the medication are known. Some medications may cause sedation or dizziness.

Application Questions for Discussion

1. Which medication class is the considered first-line therapy in managing AR symptoms?
2. Discuss the implication of newly instituted FDA black box warnings in relation to LTRAs.
3. Discuss the role of the primary care provider in relation to AIT.

Selected Bibliography

American Academy of Allergy, Asthma & Immunology. (n.d.). https://www.aaaai.org/.

American Geriatrics Society. (2019). American geriatrics society 2019 updated AGS Beers Criteria® for potentially inappropriate medication use in older adults. *Journal of the American Geriatrics Society, 67*(4), 674–694. http://doi.org/10.1111/jgs.15767 .

Asthma and Allergy Foundation of America. (n.d.). https://www.aafa.org/.

Bousquet, J., Schunemann, H. J., Togias, A., Bachert, C., Erhola, M., Hellings, P. W., Klimek, L., Pfaar, O., Wallace, D., Ansotegui, I., Agache, I., Bedbrook, A., Bergmann, K-C., Bewick, M., Bonniaud, P., Bosnic-Anticevich, S., Bosse, I., Bouchard, J., Boulet, L-P., & Zubervier, T. (2020). Next-generation allergic rhinitis and its impact on asthma (ARIA) guidelines for allergic rhinitis based on Grading of Recommendations Assessment, Development and Evaluation (GRADE) and real-world evidence. *Journal of Allergy and Clinical Immunology, 145*(1), 70–80. https://doi.org/10.1016/j.jaci.2019.06.049.

Burk, M., El-Kersh, K., Saad, M., Wiemken, T., Ramirez, J., & Cavallazzi, R. (2016). Viral infection in community-acquired pneumonia: A systematic review and meta-analysis. *European Respiratory Review, 25*, 178–188. https://doi.org/10.1183/16000617.0076-2015.

Centers for Disease Control and Prevention, National Health Interview Survey. (2016). National Ambulatory Medical Care Survey: 2016 National Summary Tables. https://www.cdc.gov/nchs/data/ahcd/namcs_summary/2016_namcs_web_tables.pdf.

Centers for Disease Control and Prevention, National Health Interview Survey. (2018). Summary Health Statistics: National Health Interview Survey, 2018. https://ftp.cdc.gov/pub/Health_Statistics/NCHS/NHIS/SHS/2018_SHS_Table_A-2.pdf.

Chow, A. W., Benninger, M. S., Brook, I., Brozek, J. L., Goldstein, E. J. C., Hicks, L. A., Pankey, G. A., Seleznick, M., Volturo, G., Wald, E. R., & File, T. M. (2012). ISDA clinical practice guideline for acute bacterial rhinosinusitis in children and adults. *Clinical Infectious Diseases, 54*(8), e72–112. https://doi.org/10.1093/cid/cis370.

Cipriani, F., Calamelli, E., & Ricci, G. (2017). Allergen avoidance in allergic asthma. *Frontiers in Pediatrics, 5*(103). http://doi.org/10.3389/fped.2017.00103.

Dykewicz, M. S., Wallace, D. V., Baroody, F., Bernstein, J., Craig, T., Finegold, I., Huang, F., Larenas-Linnemann, D., Meltzer, E., Steven, G., Bernstein, D. I., Blessing-Moore, J., Dinakar, C., Greenhawt, M., Horner, C. C., Khan, D. A., Lang, D., Oppenheimer, J., Portnoy, J. M., & Rank, M. A. (2017). Treatment of seasonal allergic rhinitis: An evidence-based focused 2017 guideline update. *Annuls of Allergy, Asthma & Immunology, 119*(6), 489–511. e41. https://doi.org/10.1016/j.anai.2017.08.012.

Jarvis, D., Newson, R., Lotvall, J., Hastan, D., Tomassen, P., Keil, T., Gjomarkaj, M., Forsberg, B., Gunnbjornsdottir, M., Minov, J., Brozek, G., Dahlen, S. E., Toskala, E., Kowalski, M. L., Olze, H., Howarth, P., Krämer, U., Baelum, J., Loureiro, C., & Burney, P. (2012). Asthma in adults and its association with chronic rhinosinusitis: The GA²LEN survey in Europe. *Allergy, 67*(1), 91–98. https://doi.org/10.1111/j.1398-9995.2011.02709.x.

Kushnir, N. M. (2011). The role of decongestants, cromolyn, guafenesin, saline washes, capsaicin, leukotriene antagonists, and other treatments on rhinitis. *Immunology and Allergy Clinics of North America, 31*, 601–617. https://doi.org/10.1016/j.iac.2011.05.008.

Kushnir, N. M., & Kaliner, M. A. (2015). In-depth review of allergic rhinitis. World Allergy Organization. Retrieved June 22, 2020, from https://www.worldallergy.org/education-and-programs/education/allergic-disease-resource-center/professionals/in-depth-review-of-allergic-rhinitis#.

Malesker, M. A, Callahan-Lyon, P., Ireland, B., & Irwin, R. S. (2017). Pharmacologic and nonpharmacologic treatment for acute cough associated with the common cold. CHEST expert panel report. *CHEST Journal, 152*(5), 1021–1037. https://doi.org/10.1016/j.chest.2017.08.009.

Mandell, L. A., Wunderink, R. G., Anzueto, A., Bartlett, J. G., Campbell, G. D., Dean, N. C., Dowell, S. F., File, T. M., Jr., Musher, D. M., Niederman, M. S., Torres, A., & Whitney, C. G.Infectious Diseases Society of America; American Thoracic Society. (2007). Infectious Diseases Society of America/American Thoracic Society consensus guidelines on the management of community-acquired pneumonia in adults. *Clinical Infectious Diseases, 1*(44), Suppl 2, S27–S72. https://doi.org/10.1086/511159.

Papadopoulos, N. G., & Guibas, G. V. (2016). Rhinitis subtypes, endotypes, and definitions. *Immunology and Allergy Clinics of North America, 36*, 215–233. http://dx.doi.org/10.1016/j.iac.2015.12.001.

Seidman, M. D., Gurgel, R. K., Lin, S. Y., Schwartz, S. R., Baroody, F. M., Bonner, J. R., Dawson, D. E., Dykewicz, M. S., Hackell, J. M., Han, J. K., Ishman, S. L., Krouse, H. J., Malekzadeh, S., Mims, J. W., Omole, F. S., Reddy, W. D., Wallace, D. V., Walsh, S. A., Warren, B. E., Wilson, M. N., & Nnacheta, L. C. (2015). AAO-HNSF Clinical practice guideline: Allergic rhinitis. *Otolaryngology–Head and Neck Surgery, 52*(1S), S1–S43. https://journals.sagepub.com/doi/pdf/10.1177/0194599814561600.

Short, S., Bashir, H., Marshall, P., Miller, N., Olmschenk, D., Prigge, K., & Solyntjes, L (2017). Institute for Clinical Systems Improvement. Diagnosis and Treatment of Respiratory Illness in Children and Adults. Updated September 2017. https://www.icsi.org/wp-content/uploads/2019/01/RespIllness.pdf.

U. S. Department of Justice, Drug Enforcement Administration, Diversion Control Division (2005). Title VII of Public Law 109-177, The Combat Methamphetamine Epidemic Act of 2005. https://www.deadiversion.usdoj.gov/meth/.

U. S. Food and Drug Administration. (n.d.). Use caution when giving cough and cold products to kids. Retrieved July 7, 2020, from https://www.fda.gov/drugs/special-features/use-caution-when-giving-cough-and-cold-products-kids.

U. S. Food and Drug Administration. (2018). FDA Drug Safety Communication: FDA requires labeling changes for prescription opioid cough and cold medicines to limit their use to adults 18 years and older. https://www.fda.gov/drugs/drug-safety-and-availability/fda-drug-safety-communication-fda-requires-labeling-changes-prescription-opioid-cough-and-cold#:~:text=%5B1%2D11%2D2018%5D,benefits%20in%20children%20younger%20than.

U. S. Food and Drug Administration. (2020). FDA requires Boxed Warning about serious mental health side effects for asthma and allergy drug montelukast (Singulair); Advises restricting use for allergic rhinitis. https://www.fda.gov/drugs/drug-safety-and-availability/fda-requires-boxed-warning-about-serious-mental-health-side-effects-asthma-and-allergy-drug.

6

Asthma Medications

REBECCA M. LUTZ AND MARIA RUSS

Overview

Asthma is a common chronic inflammatory disease resulting in bronchial hyperresponsiveness and airway obstruction. Uncontrolled asthma leads to a decrease in lung functioning. Asthma is a complex disease with multiple clinical presentations, known as *phenotypes*. Due to its complexity, asthma requires multiple treatment approaches to improve health outcomes in children, adolescents, adults, and older adults.

The Global Asthma Report 2018 revealed an increased prevalence of asthma (3.6%) since 2006. Asthma affects approximately 339 million people worldwide and is the 23rd leading cause of death globally (The Global Asthma Network, 2018). Asthma rates are more common among children and adolescents younger than 14 years of age and adults older than 75 years of age (The Global Asthma Network, 2018).

In the United States, asthma affects about 19 million adults 18 years of age and older. In addition, about 6 million children under the age of 18 are affected by asthma (Centers for Disease Control and Prevention [CDC], n.d.). When children and adolescents younger than 18 were asked if they ever had asthma or still have asthma, a higher percentage of males (13.1% and 8.4%, respectively) reported asthma than females (10% and 6.6%, respectively) (CDC, n.d.). When adults were asked if they ever had asthma or still have asthma, a higher percentage of females (15.3% and 9.6%, respectively) reported asthma than males (11.7% and 5.5%, respectively) (CDC, n.d.). Multiracial/non-Hispanic populations had the highest prevalence rates of asthma, followed by Black/non-Hispanic, American Indian/Alaskan Native, and Caucasian populations, respectively (CDC, n.d.).

Relevant Physiology

The primary role of the pulmonary system is to ensure adequate gas exchange. This is a multistep process of ventilation, diffusion, and perfusion and requires synchrony between the pulmonary and cardiac systems. *Ventilation* is the process of air movement in and out of the lungs. *Diffusion* involves the exchange of oxygen and carbon dioxide between the lungs and the blood. *Perfusion* is the movement of blood in and out of lung capillaries and into the body tissue. Gas exchange occurs when oxygen enters the blood and carbon dioxide (CO_2) is removed (Fig. 6.1).

The pulmonary system includes the thorax, diaphragm, upper respiratory tract, lungs, lower respiratory tract, and blood vessels. The right lung is divided into the superior, middle, and inferior lobes. The left lung is divided into the superior and inferior lobes. The upper respiratory tract is composed of the nasopharynx, the oropharynx, and their related structures. The lower respiratory tract begins at the left and right mainstem bronchi. These bronchi gradually branch into the smaller bronchioles. The bronchioles lead to alveolar ducts, smaller alveolar sacs, and ultimately the alveoli. The alveoli are the primary site of gas exchange within the lungs.

The alveoli contain two main types of epithelial cells. Type I provide structural support to the alveoli. Type II produce *surfactant*, which decreases surface tension and allows for alveolar expansion. Surfactant has bacteriostatic properties that bind it to pathogens. This promotes phagocytosis, releases proinflammatory mediators, prevents oxidative injuries, and aids in airway remodeling.

A disruption of the ventilation, diffusion, and perfusion process results in inadequate oxygenation. This disruption can be obstructive (blocking) or restrictive (reducing chest wall movement). Asthma is one type of obstructive lung disease. Characteristics of obstructive lung disease include increased expiratory force along with the use of accessory muscles, airway damage, and increased mucous production caused by the infiltration of inflammatory cells and cytokine release.

Pathophysiology: Asthma

Chronic pulmonary inflammation is a physiologic response occurring after an exposure to risk factors. It results in narrowing, obstruction, and hyperresponsiveness of the

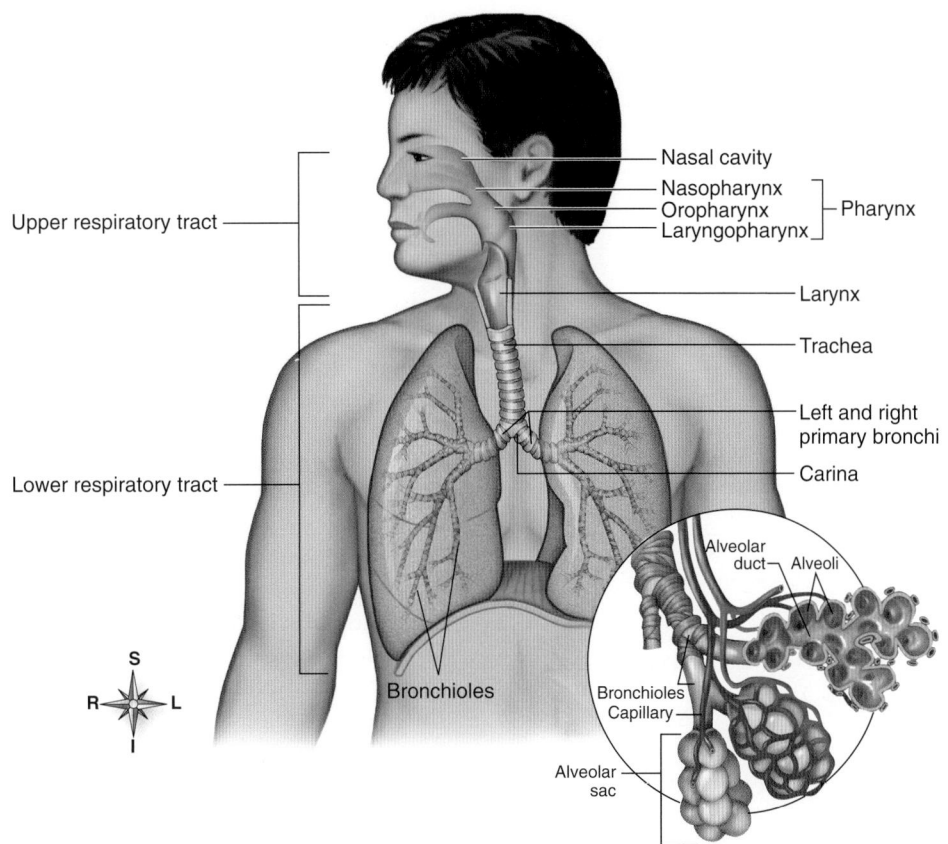

• **Fig. 6.1** Structural plan of the respiratory system. (From Patton, K. T., & Thibodeau, G.A. [2018]. *The human body in health & disease* [7th ed.]. St Louis: Mosby.)

airway. Airway narrowing and hyperresponsiveness lead to the classic symptoms of wheezing, chest tightness, cough, and dyspnea.

Overview of Cellular Response to Inflammation

An in-depth review of the cellular response to inflammation is beyond the scope of this text. However, it is important for the primary care provider to understand cellular response when considering the type of asthma and appropriate pharmacologic therapies (Table 6.1).

Asthma Phenotypes and Endotypes

Until recently, clinicians did not differentiate between asthma patients and provided the same medication regimen to all. Researchers and clinicians now recognize the different asthma phenotypes defined by the patient's age, gender, ethnicity, smoking history, and obesity as well as the clinical presentation of atopy and lung function (Kuruvilla et al., 2019; Bates et al., 2017; Blaiss et al., 2017). In addition, the classification of asthma by endotype (underlying cellular and molecular changes) has emerged through research. Endotypes are classified by blood biomarkers (IgE, eosinophils, periostin, and cytokines), sputum biomarkers (eosinophils, neutrophils, and cytokines), and laboratory findings (fractional exhaled nitric oxide [FeNO]). By evaluating phenotypes and targeting endotypes, researchers are continuing to develop new medications to improve asthma symptoms and patient outcomes (Kuruvilla et al., 2019; Bates et al., 2017; Blaiss et al., 2017).

While the use of phenotyping or endotyping seems to be straightforward on the surface, there are overlaps. A phenotype may have multiple endotypes and an endotype may have multiple phenotypes. This has led to many classifications of asthma. It is beyond the scope of this book to delve into these overlaps. The types of asthma highlighted here include allergic asthma, nonallergic asthma, obesity-related asthma, occupational asthma (OA), aspirin-sensitive

TABLE 6.1	Cellular Response to Inflammation
Cell Type	**Response to Inflammation**
Immunoglobulin E (IgE)	Binds to the allergen. Results in chronic inflammation. Also binds to basophils, lymphocytes, and mast cells.
Inflammatory mediator cells	Promotes an inflammatory response.
Mast cells	Activated by allergens and high-affinity IgE receptors, resulting in bronchoconstriction.
Eosinophils	Release proteins that damage epithelial cells. Produce cysteinyl leukotrienes and growth hormones.
Lymphocytes	Regulate eosinophilia inflammation, the production of mucus, and IgE production. Helper T-lymphocyte (Th0) cells trigger either a helper T-lymphocyte 1 (Th1) response or a helper T-lymphocyte 2 (Th2) response.
Macrophages	Release inflammatory mediators and cytokines, which increase the inflammatory response.
Neutrophils	Neutrophils and secretion of proteins lead to processing and release of cytokines IL-1β and IL-18.
Dendritic cells	Interact with allergens to stimulate Th2 cell production.

asthma/aspirin-exacerbated respiratory disease (AERD), and exercise-induced bronchoconstriction (EIB)/exercise-induced asthma (EIA).

Allergic (Eosinophilic) Asthma

This phenotype of asthma is the most common. Allergic (*eosinophilic*) asthma is also referenced in the literature as extrinsic, atopic, and early-onset asthma. Allergic asthma is characterized by two major endotypes: a type 2 high (T2-high) endotype featuring increased eosinophilic airway inflammation and a T2-low endotype presenting with neutrophilic inflammation (Stokes & Casale, 2016). Out of all the phenotypes, this one is the most most easily identified and diagnosed. Allergic asthma usually begins during childhood. Common environmental triggers include pollen, food, and dust mites. Approximately 40% of patients diagnosed with allergic asthma have a history of seasonal or perennial allergic rhinitis (AR) (Asthma and Allergy Foundation of America, 2015). Patients with this type of asthma tend to respond predictably and positively to targeted treatment with lifestyle changes (avoidance of allergens and risk factors), corticosteroids, bronchodilators, leukotriene modifiers, and immunomodulator therapy.

Nonallergic (Noneosinophilic) Asthma

Nonallergic asthma is also known as intrinsic, adult-onset, noneosinophilic, and nonatopic asthma. Onset often begins in mid-adulthood and affects females more than males. Patients are less responsive to standard therapy. Adults tend to have more frequent and severe symptoms while children tend to have less severe symptoms. Effects on the lungs include bronchial hyperresponsiveness, increased mucus secretion, and airway obstruction. This leads to symptoms of coughing, wheezing, shortness of breath or rapid breathing, and chest tightness.

Diagnosis includes a review of the patient's history with attention to allergen sensitivity, control and severity of symptoms, risk factors and comorbidities, and response to previous treatment. Skin testing does not demonstrate evidence of allergic sensitivity. Biomarkers reveal low levels of sputum eosinophils, high levels of sputum neutrophils, and an FeNO less than 30 ppb (Esteban-Gorgojo et al., 2018). In addition to reducing risk factors and comorbid conditions, medication treatment options include beta-agonists, muscarinic receptors, antibiotics, and immunomodulators (Rogalini et al., 2020). Bronchial thermoplasty (BT), another form of treatment, will not be discussed in this text.

Obesity-Related Asthma

Obesity affects both eosinophilic and noneosinophilic asthmatic patients. In eosinophilic (allergic) asthma, increased adipose tissue results in cytokines and adipokines that affect the airways (Mohanan et al., 2014). In noneosinophilic (nonallergic) asthma, restriction of lung function (decreased tidal volume) results from the obesity, especially when the thorax and abdominal areas are obese (Mohanan et al., 2014). Patients with obesity-related asthma may be less responsive to inhaled corticosteroids (ICSs) and bronchodilators. Weight loss therapy may improve health outcomes (Chapter 51, Weight Management Medications).

Work-Related Asthma

Work-related asthma is divided into occupational asthma and work-exacerbated asthma (Jolly et al., 2015). Occupational asthma (OA) results from the inhalation of chemicals or exposure to irritants. OA may include hypersensitivity reactions to a specific agent or an inflammatory response to an irritant. Diagnosis is based on history and testing. Patient history may include reports of worsening symptoms during work hours. Standard testing includes skin-prick testing, bronchial provocation testing, PFTs, FeNO testing, immunologic testing, and inhalation challenge testing (Jolly et al., 2015). Work-exacerbated asthma (WEA) is not actually caused by the workplace, but the workplace exacerbates the symptoms (Friedman-Jimenez et al., 2015).

Aspirin-Sensitive Asthma/Aspirin-Exacerbated Respiratory Disease

Aspirin-sensitive asthma is also known as aspirin-exacerbated respiratory disease (AERD). This type of asthma affects about 7% of adult asthmatics (Rajan et al., 2015). On clinical presentation, patients report a history of asthma, chronic rhinitis with nasal polyps, and an increase in asthmatic symptoms with the use of aspirin or nonsteroidal antiinflammatory drugs (NSAIDs).

Exercise-Induced Bronchoconstriction/ Exercise-Induced Asthma

Exercise-induced asthma (EIA) is induced by vigorous physical activity. Symptoms begin within minutes of exercise or exposure. Common symptoms include cough, shortness of breath, and tightness in the chest. Diagnosis includes a review of the patient's history with attention to exercise or exposure history and pulmonary function tests (PFTs) pre- and post-exercise. Treatment includes the use of beta2-agonists, ICSs, and leukotriene modifiers (American College of Allergy, Asthma & Immunology [ACAAI], n.d.).

Asthma Therapy

Management of asthma is directed at improving symptoms, lung function, and quality of life and decreasing exacerbations and mortality. Medication therapy requires a stepwise approach based on the level of symptom control and severity. An overview of the standard medication therapies in asthma care will be covered in this section. Drug-drug interactions associated with corticosteroids, leukotriene receptor antagonists, beta2-agonists, and anticholinergics (antimuscarinic) are listed in Table 6.2.

Inhaled Delivery

The primary delivery method of most antiasthmatic drugs is inhalation. There are three advantages to this route: (1) the drug is delivered directly to the site of action, (2) systemic effects are minimized, and (3) patients experience rapid relief during acute attacks. Three types of inhalation devices are usually employed: metered-dose inhalers, dry-powder inhalers, and nebulizers.

- **Metered-Dose Inhalers (MDIs):** MDIs deliver a measured dose of medication with each inhalation. They are relatively inexpensive compared to other methods. MDIs offer convenience in dosing and carrying. They require hand–breath coordination. The patient must begin inhaling prior to activating the inhaler, which may be difficult for some patients. Even with optimal use, only about 10% of the dose reaches the lungs. Much of the medication remains in the mouth and is swallowed. A spacer attached to the MDI can help patients take slow, deep breaths, increasing the amount of medication getting into the lungs.

TABLE 6.2 Drug-Drug Interactions[a]

Classification	Medication	Interaction
Corticosteroids	CYP 3A4 inhibitors	Increased corticosteroid systemic levels and cardiovascular adverse effects
	Desmopressin	Increased risk of severe hyponatremia
	Fluoroquinolones (select)	Increased risk of tendon rupture
Leukotriene Receptor Antagonists	Aspirin	Increased risk of zafirlukast adverse effects
	Astemizole, pimozide	Use with Zileuton may result in prolonged QT, torsades de pointes, cardiac arrest
	Beta-blockers	Use with Zileuton may increase beta-adrenergic blockage
	Ergot derivatives	Use with Zileuton increases ergot concentrations that may result in nausea, vomiting, and vasospastic ischemia
	Loxapine	Increased toxic effects of loxapine
	Terfenadine, erythromycin	Decreased zafirlukast efficacy
	Theophylline	Increased theophylline concentrations / Decreased zafirlukast efficacy
	Warfarin	Increased risk of bleeding
Beta2-Agonists	Atomoxetine	Increases cardiovascular effects
	Tricyclic antidepressants	Increased cardiovascular effects
Anticholinergics (Antimuscarinic)	Anticholinergic	Concomitant use increased risk of anticholinergic side effects
	Methacholine	Inhibits airway response

[a]There are many other drug–drug interactions. The health care provider should check all drug interactions among the patient's medications before prescribing any new medications.

- **Dry-Powder Inhalers (DPIs):** DPIs are also used to deliver a measured dose of dry, powdered medication directly to the lungs. DPIs do not require hand–breath coordination and they deliver more medication to the lungs compared to MDIs. DPIs require the patient to complete a powerful inhalation. Due to this, DPIs may not be suitable for older adults or those with nerve or muscle weakness.
- **Nebulizers:** A nebulizer converts a solution into a mist for easy inhalation. Nebulizers deliver higher concentrations of the medication to the lungs. They do not require physical coordination to use. Nebulizers can be expensive to purchase or rent. There is a risk of contamination if the equipment is not cleaned properly.

Long-Term Control Asthma Therapy

Inhaled Corticosteroids

Inhaled corticosteroids (ICSs) are considered first-line therapy for any patient with continuous symptoms, severe airflow obstruction, or a history of asthma exacerbations. ICSs reduce exacerbations, improve symptom control and lung function, and reduce airway hyperresponsiveness. In general, all ICSs exhibit similarities in adverse reactions. At low to moderate doses, ICSs are usually well tolerated by most patients. Table 6.3 provides an overview of the most common adverse effects. The Global Initiative for Asthma (GINA) recommends that all adults and adolescents age 12 and older with asthma should receive low-dose ICS treatment (GINA, 2020) (Table 6.4). The maximum benefit of ICSs may take up to several weeks. Because of this delayed response, ICSs are not suitable for use as a rescue inhaler in acute asthma attacks or during acute exacerbations of asthma.

PRACTICE PEARLS

ICS Use in Pregnancy and Lactation

- ICSs are not contraindicated for use during pregnancy or while breastfeeding based on the specific needs of the patient and consideration of the potential benefits or risks to the fetus (GINA, 2020).
- The National Heart Lung and Blood Institute/National Asthma Education Prevention Program (NHLBI/NAEPP) recommends the use of inhaled budesonide over other ICSs because more data are available describing its use in human pregnancy.
- ICSs are distributed into breast milk in low concentrations but are not a contraindication to breastfeeding.

Beclomethasone Dipropionate

Pharmacokinetics. After beclomethasone DPI administration, 25% to 60% of the medication reaches the airways. Onset of action is within 24 hours. Maximum benefit may take 1 to 4 weeks. Hepatic metabolism is via cytochrome (CYP) 3A4. Half-life is about 3 hours. Excretion is predominantly fecal.

TABLE 6.3   Adverse Effects of Inhaled Corticosteroids

Most Common	Least Common
Acne vulgaris	Cataracts
Arthralgia	Cough and bronchospasm
Candidiasis	Decreased bone mineral density (BMD)
Cushing's syndrome	Delayed growth in pediatric patients
Dysphonia	Glaucoma
Epistaxis	Hypersensitivity to ingredients (e.g., milk proteins)
Fatigue	Hypothalamus-pituitary-adrenal (HPA) suppression
Headache	Impaired glucose metabolism
Hoarseness	Skin changes, particularly in older adults
Infection	
Insomnia	
Malaise	
Musculoskeletal pain	
Nasal congestion	
Nausea	
Pharyngitis	
Rhinitis	
Sinusitis	
Throat irritation	
Vomiting	

Indications. Beclomethasone is ICS approved for the long-term treatment of asthma in patients 4 years of age and older. Beclomethasone may be used in the treatment of exercise-induced bronchospasms. Beclomethasone is not intended for treatment of acute exacerbations, status asthmaticus, or acute bronchospasms.

Adverse Effects. The most common adverse effects (>5%) include headache, pharyngitis, upper respiratory tract infections, and rhinitis. Less frequent adverse effects include cough, nausea, oral candidiasis, sinusitis, and dysmenorrhea. Post-marketing reports include aggression, depression, sleep disorders, psychomotor hyperactivity, and suicidal ideation, primarily in children.

Contraindications. The use of beclomethasone dipropionate is contraindicated in patients with known hypersensitivity to the medication or any of its components. Avoid in patients with hypersensitivity reactions such as urticaria, angioedema, rash, and bronchospasm. If hypersensitivities are present, be alert for cross-hypersensitivity to other corticosteroids.

Monitoring. Monitor for signs of adverse effects including alterations in blood sugar, growth, and vision. Assess for improvement in asthma symptoms and a decrease in frequency of exacerbations. Monitor PFTs.

TABLE 6.4   **Corticosteroids**

Drug Category/ Medication	Indication	Dosage	Considerations and Monitoring
Inhaled Corticosteroids (GINA and NAEPP Guidelines May Vary)			
Beclomethasone	Asthma maintenance, not currently on an ICS	**Aerosol: 40–80 mcg/actuation:** *Adults, adolescents & children ≥12 yr*: Initial dose: 1 or 2 inhalations twice daily every 12 hr. Maximum dosage: 320 mcg twice daily.	If inadequate response after 2 weeks, may increase dose.
	Asthma maintenance, switching from another ICS	*Adults, adolescents, and children ≥12 yr*: 40–320 mcg twice daily every 12 hr. Select dose depending on previous dosing and disease severity. Maximum dosage: 320 mcg twice daily.	
	Asthma maintenance, based on previous therapy and asthma severity	**40 mcg/actuation:** *Children 4–11 yr*: Initial dose: 1 inhalation twice daily every 12 hr. If inadequate response after 2 weeks, may increase to 80 mcg twice daily every 12 hr. Maximum dosage: 80 mcg twice daily.	May see improvement within 24 hours. Expect improvement within first or second week.
Ciclesonide	Asthma maintenance, previously on bronchodilators alone	**Inhalation aerosol: 80 mcg/actuation:** *Adults, adolescents, and children ≥12 yr*: 1 oral inhalation twice daily. Maximum dosage: 160 mcg twice daily.	Titrate up after four weeks if inadequate response
	Asthma maintenance, previously on ICS	**80 mcg/actuation:** *Adults, adolescents, and children ≥12 yr:* 1 oral inhalation twice daily. Maximum dosage: 160 mcg twice daily.	
	Asthma maintenance, previously on oral corticosteroids	**160 mcg/actuation:** *Adults and adolescents ≥12 yr:* 2 oral inhalations twice daily. Maximum dosage: 320 mcg twice daily.	
Fluticasone furoate	Asthma maintenance, not on ICS	**Inhalation powder:** **100 mcg/actuation:** *Adults, adolescents, and children ≥12 yr:* 1 oral inhalation once daily at same time each day. Maximum dosage: 200 mcg daily. **50 mcg/actuation:** *Children 5–11 yr:* 1 oral inhalation once daily at same time each day. Maximum dosage: 50 mcg daily.	Consider larger initial dose if poorly controlled asthma or if on previous high-dose ICS. If inadequate response after 2 weeks, may increase dose.
Fluticasone propionate	Asthma maintenance, not on ICS	**Inhalation aerosol: 44 mcg/actuation:** *Adults, adolescents, and children ≥12 yr:* 2 oral inhalations twice daily every 12 hr. Maximum dosage: 880 mcg twice daily. **Inhalation powder:** **55 mcg/actuation:** *Adults, adolescents, and children ≥12 yr:* 1 oral inhalation twice daily. Maximum dosage: 232 mcg twice daily. **30 mcg/actuation:** *Children 4–11 yr:* 1 oral inhalation twice daily. Maximum dosage: 55 mcg twice daily.	Adults, adolescents, and children ≥12 yr: if inadequate response, titrate after 2 weeks. Use lowest effective level.
	Asthma maintenance	**Inhalation aerosol: 44 mcg/actuation:** *Children 4–11 yr:* Initial dose: 2 oral inhalations twice daily every 12 hr. Maximum dosage: 88 mcg/day. **Inhalation powder:** **100 mcg/actuation:** *Adults, adolescents, and children ≥12 yr:* 1 oral inhalation twice daily every 12 hr. Maximum dosage: 1000 mcg twice daily. **50 mcg/actuation:** *Children 4–11 yr:* 1 oral inhalation twice daily every 12 hr. Maximum dosage: 100 mcg twice daily.	If inadequate control, reassess and consider additional therapeutic options. All ages: Consider larger initial dose if poorly controlled asthma or if on previous high-dose ICS. If inadequate response after 2 weeks, may increase dose.

Continued

TABLE 6.4   Corticosteroids—cont'd

Drug Category/ Medication	Indication	Dosage	Considerations and Monitoring
Mometasone furoate	Asthma maintenance, previously on bronchodilators	**Inhalation powder:** **220 mcg/actuation:** *Adults, adolescents, and children ≥12 yr:* 1 oral inhalation once daily in the evening. Maximum dosage: 1 oral inhalation of 220 mcg/actuation twice daily or 2 oral inhalations of 220 mcg/actuation once daily in the evening (440 mcg/day). **110 mcg/actuation:** *Children 4–11 yr:* 1 oral inhalation once daily in the evening. Maximum dosage: 110 mcg/day.	Titrate after 2 weeks if needed for control.
		Inhalation aerosol: **100 mcg/actuation or 200 mcg/actuation:** *Adults, adolescents, and children ≥12 yr:* 2 inhalations twice daily. Maximum dosage: 400 mcg twice daily. **50 mcg/actuation:** *Children 5–11 yr:* 2 oral inhalations twice daily. Maximum dosage: 100 mcg twice daily.	Titrate after 2 weeks if needed for control.
	Asthma maintenance, previously on oral corticosteroids	**Inhalation powder:** **220 mcg/actuation:** *Adults, adolescents, and children ≥12 yr:* 2 oral inhalations twice daily. Maximum dosage: 440 mcg twice daily. **110 mcg/actuation:** *Children 4-11 yr:* 1 oral inhalation once daily in evening. Maximum dosage: 110 mcg once daily. **Inhalation aerosol:** **200 mcg/actuation:** *Adults, adolescents, and children ≥12 yr:* 2 inhalations twice daily. Maximum dosage: 400 mcg twice daily. **50 mcg/actuation:** *Children 5–11 yr:* 2 oral inhalations twice daily. Maximum dosage: 100 mcg twice daily.	*Adults, adolescents, and children ≥12 yr:* One week after therapy initiation, begin titration of oral corticosteroids (maximum reduction: 2.5 mg/day on weekly basis), then titrate oral inhalation to lowest dose. *Children 5–11 yr:* After at least 1 week of inhaled therapy, consider slow reduction of the oral corticosteroid.
Oral Corticosteroids			
Prednisone	Asthma exacerbation in outpatient setting	*Adults, adolescents, and children ≥12 yr:* 40–60 mg orally in 1 or 2 divided doses for 3–10 days or until peak expiratory flow 80% of personal best or until symptoms resolve. Maximum dosage: 60 mg/day. *Infants and children <12 yr:* 1–2 mg/kg/day in divided doses once or twice daily for 3–10 days or until peak expiratory flow 80% of personal best or until symptoms resolve. Maximum dosage: 60 mg/day.	The Beers Criteria for Potentially Inappropriate Medication Use in Older Adults Confused name alert: Prednisolone
	Asthma maintenance, with severe, persistent asthma	*Adults, adolescents, and children ≥12 yr:* 7.5–60 mg daily given as 1 dose in the morning or every other day as needed for control of asthma. Maximum dosage: 60 mg/day. *Infants and children <12 yr:* 0.25–2 mg/kg orally daily in the morning or every other day as needed for control of asthma. Maximum dosage: 60 mg/day.	Adults with nocturnal asthma: Consider dose at 3 p.m. if no adrenal suppression

TABLE 6.4 Corticosteroids—cont'd

Drug Category/ Medication	Indication	Dosage	Considerations and Monitoring
Prednisolone	Asthma exacerbation in outpatient setting	*Adults, adolescents, and children ≥12 yr:* 40–60 mg orally in 1 or 2 divided doses for 3–10 days or until peak expiratory flow 80% of personal best or until symptoms resolve. Maximum dosage: 60 mg/day.	The Beers Criteria for Potentially Inappropriate Medication Use in Older Adults
		Infants and children <12 yr: 1–2 mg/kg/day in divided doses one or two times daily for 3–10 days or until peak expiratory flow 80% of personal best or until symptoms resolve. Maximum dosage: 60 mg/day.	Confused name alert: Prednisone In pediatric patients, limit oral corticosteroids to a few weeks until symptoms are controlled and patient is stabilized on other therapies.
	Asthma maintenance, with severe, persistent asthma	*Adults, adolescents, and children ≥12 yr:* 7.5–60 mg daily given as 1 dose in the morning or every other day as needed for control of asthma. Maximum dosage: 60 mg/day.	
		Infants and children <12 yr: 0.25–2 mg/kg orally daily in the morning or every other day as needed for control of asthma. Maximum dosage: 60 mg/day.	
Methylprednisolone	Asthma exacerbation in outpatient setting	*Adults:* 40–60 mg/day orally in 1–2 divided doses for 5–10 days. Maximum dosage: 60 mg/day.	In pediatric patients, limit oral corticosteroids to a few weeks until symptoms are controlled and patient is stabilized on other therapies
		Children 12–17 yr: 40–80 mg/day orally in 1–2 divided doses for 3–10 days and continue until peak expiratory flow 70% of personal best. Maximum dosage: 80 mg/day.	
		Infants and children 1 month–11 yr: 1–2 mg/kg/day orally in 1–2 divided doses for 3–10 days (usually 5 days). Continue until peak expiratory flow is 70% of predicted or personal best or symptoms resolve. Maximum dosage: 60 mg/day.	
	Asthma exacerbation in outpatient setting with nausea/vomiting or compliance concern	*Adults, adolescents, and children ≥5 yr:* 240 mg IM once.	
		Infants and children 1 month–4 yr: 7.5 mg/kg IM once.	
	Asthma maintenance, with severe, persistent asthma	*Adults, adolescents, and children ≥12 yr:* 7.5–60 mg/day orally once daily in morning or as alternate-day therapy as needed for symptom control. Maximum dosage: 60 mg/day.	
		Infants and children <12 yr: 0.25–2 mg/kg/day orally daily in the morning or as alternate-day therapy as needed for symptom control. Maximum dosage: 60 mg/day.	

Oral Corticosteroids

Corticosteroids reduce airway inflammation. Oral corticosteroids are used for short bursts during asthma exacerbations (see Table 6.4). Patients with severe asthma may be on long-term therapy with monitoring of risk profile.

Oral Corticosteroids

Prednisone

Pharmacokinetics. Pharmacokinetics provided in this section are based on oral regular-release tablets. Peak concentration is reached in 2 hours and half-life is 2 to 3 hours. Extensive liver metabolism of prednisone by 11-β-HSD liver enzymes produces prednisolone and is eliminated by the kidneys. No dosing adjustments are required for older patients or those with renal or kidney impairment.

Indications. Prednisone is approved to treat asthma and disorders of the respiratory system. Prepackaged, tapered-dose packs are the more common method of delivery when short bursts of corticosteroids are recommended. Prior to prescribing, consider the minimum effective dose and duration to improve the patient's status.

Adverse Effects. Similar to other corticosteroids, the frequency and seriousness of adverse effects is dependent on patient comorbidities, dosage, and duration of therapy. Common adverse effects include hypertension, fluid retention, increased appetite, osteoporosis, and mood disturbances. A few of the more serious effects are extensive and include the cardiovascular (congestive heart failure, cardiac arrest, syncope), endocrine (Cushing's syndrome, hyperglycemia, hypocalcemia), ophthalmic (glaucoma), GI (pancreatitis), hematologic (thrombolytic disorders), immunologic (anaphylaxis, angioedema), musculoskeletal (fracture), and neurologic (seizure) systems.

Contraindications. Use is contraindicated in patients with hypersensitivity to corticosteroids or any component of the product. Common drug–drug interactions include NSAIDs, antiinfectives, immune suppressants, diuretics, and anticoagulants. As with other corticosteroids, observe for increased adverse effects in patients with immune and adrenocortical dysfunction, recent myocardial infarction or cardiovascular disease, endocrine disorders, thyroid disease, or ocular disease. Corticosteroids can mask or increase the severity of fungal, viral, or bacterial infections.

Monitoring. Monitor for adverse effects including abnormal glucose levels or changes in intraocular pressure. This is particularly important for patients receiving long-term therapy. Monitor for improvement in symptoms, frequency of SABA use, and PFTs. Monitor patients for stability or alterations with comorbidities. For patients on long-term or frequent prednisone therapy, the administration of live vaccines may result in an increased risk of infection. Monitor drug–drug interactions.

Combination Therapy: Inhaled Corticosteroids/ Long-Acting Beta2-Adrenergics

The use of inhaled corticosteroids/long-acting beta2-adrenergics is recommended for patients uncontrolled on previous ICSs (GINA, 2020).

PRACTICE PEARLS

ICS/LABA Therapy in Asthma

In 2017, the U. S. Food and Drug Administration (FDA) removed the black box warnings against LABA in combination with ICSs in asthmatic patients after studies revealed no increase in deaths when the medications were used in combination (U.S. Food and Drug Administration, 2018).

This combination is referred to as ICS/LABA or LABA/ICS depending on the resource (Table 6.5). For the purposes of this section, we will refer to the combination order as ICS/LABA. Primary care providers should consider the individual properties of each medication and the amount of each medication in the selected combination. Fluticasone/salmeterol is an example of one of the ICS/LABA combinations available.

Fluticasone/Salmeterol

Pharmacokinetics. Pharmacokinetic properties discussed here are for individual medications.

Fluticasone Propionate. Peak concentration levels are reached in 30 to 60 minutes with a half-life of 8 to 11 hours, depending on the product. Extensive hepatic metabolism is via CYP 3A4 to 17β-carboxylic acid. Excretion is primarily fecal.

Salmeterol. Onset of action is 30 to 48 minutes. Peak concentration levels are reached in 3 hours with a half-life of about 5 to 12 hours, depending on the product. Extensive hepatic metabolism is via CYP 3A4. Excretion is primarily fecal.

Indications. The combination medication contains fluticasone (an ICS) and salmeterol (a LABA) and is approved as a maintenance therapy for uncontrolled asthmatics. DPI or inhaled aerosol products provide treatment options for adults and children over 4 years of age. No dose adjustments are required in patients with renal or hepatic impairment.

Adverse Effects. The most common adverse reactions resulting from the combination of fluticasone/salmeterol are bronchitis, hoarseness, pharyngitis, throat irritation, and upper respiratory infections. Adverse effects primarily related to salmeterol include headaches and pain. Adverse effects resulting from fluticasone are similar to those commonly noted with all corticosteroids.

Contraindications. Contraindications to fluticasone/salmeterol result from the individual medication classifications. Consider each medication classification prior to prescribing. Avoid use in patients with hypersensitivity to any component of the product. Avoid use of the inhalation powder formulations in patients with milk allergies. Evaluate benefit versus risk when used in patients currently under monoamine oxidase inhibitor (MAOI) or tricyclic therapy and in patients taking beta-blockers, non–potassium-sparing diuretics, or corrected QT interval (QTc) interval-prolonging medications. Use with caution in patients with metabolic disorders, narrow-angle glaucoma, urinary retention, prostatic hyperplasia, bladder-neck obstruction, seizure disorders, or thyrotoxicosis or those who are unusually responsive to sympathomimetic amines.

Monitoring. Monitor for improvement in symptoms, frequency and severity of exacerbations, and adverse effects. Monitor PFTs. Observe for systemic corticosteroid adverse effects. Monitor patients with hepatic impairment.

Leukotriene Modifiers

Leukotriene modifiers decrease bronchoconstriction and inflammatory responses such as edema and mucus secretion

TABLE 6.5	**Combination Therapy: Inhaled Corticosteroids/Long-Acting Beta2-Adrenergics**		
Medication	Indication	Dosage	Considerations and Monitoring
Budesonide/ formoterol	Asthma mainte- nance	**Inhalation aerosol:** **80 mcg/4.5 mcg or 160 mcg/4.5 mcg, depending on severity:** *Adults, adolescents, and children ≥12 yr:* 2 oral inhalations twice daily at same time each day. Maximum dosage: 2 oral inhalations of 160 mcg/4.5 mcg twice daily. **80 mcg/4.5 mcg:** *Children 6–11 yr:* 2 oral inhalations twice daily at same time each day. Maximum dosage: 2 oral inhalations of 80 mcg/4.5 mcg twice daily.	GINA and NAEPP recommendations may vary from FDA recommenda- tions. Dosage based on severity of asthma and previous therapy. Not indicated for relief of acute bron- chospasm.
Mometasone/ formoterol	Asthma mainte- nance	**Inhalation aerosol:** **100 mcg/5 mcg or 200 mcg/5 mcg:** *Adults, adoles- cents, and children ≥12 yr:* 2 oral inhalations twice daily every 12 hr. Maximum dosage: 2 oral inhalations of 200 mcg/5 mcg twice daily. **50 mcg/5 mcg:** *Children 5–11 yr:* 2 inhalations twice daily every 12 hr. Maximum dosage: 2 oral inhalations of 50 mcg/5 mcg twice daily.	Choose initial dose based on severity of disease and previous therapy. Titrate to lowest effective dose.
Fluticasone/ salmeterol	Asthma mainte- nance	**Inhalation aerosol: HFA 45 mcg/21 mcg, or HFA 115 mcg/21 mcg, or HFA 230 mcg/21 mcg:** *Adults, adolescents, children ≥12 yr:* 2 inhalations daily every 12 hr. Maximum dosage: 2 oral inhalations 230 mcg/ 21 mcg twice daily. **Inhalation powder: 55 mcg/14 mcg or 113 mcg/ 14 mcg or 232 mcg/14 mcg:** *Adults, adolescents, and children ≥12 yr:* 1 oral inhalation twice daily 12 hr apart.	No spacer device or volume cham- ber use. If previously on another ICS, select dose based on previous therapy. Wean slowly from systemic cortico- steroids.
		Inhalation powder diskus: 100 mcg/50 mcg, 250 mcg/ 50 mcg, and 500 mcg/50 mcg: *Adults, adolescents, and children ≥12 yr:* 1 inhalation twice daily every 12 hr. Maximum dosage: 1 oral inhalation of 500 mcg/50 mcg twice daily.	If previously on another ICS, select dose based on previous therapy and control of symptoms or risk of exacerbations. Wean slowly from systemic cortico- steroids.
		Inhalation powder diskus: 100 mcg/50 mcg: *Children 4–11 yr:* 1 oral inhalation twice daily every 12 hr. Maximum dosage: 1 oral inhalation of 100 mcg/50 mcg twice daily.	Approved only for those not con- trolled on ICS.
Fluticasone/ vilanterol	Asthma mainte- nance	**Inhalation Powder: 100 mcg/25 mcg or 200 mcg/ 25 mcg:** *Adults:* 1 inhalation once daily at the same time every day. Maximum dosage: 200 mcg/25 mcg: 1 inhalation once daily.	Dosage based on disease severity and previous therapy.

(Table 6.6). Though not as effective as ICSs, they can be used as an alternate therapy in place of an ICS. Leukotriene modifiers in combination with ICSs increase asthma control and allow for decreasing dosages of the ICS.

Leukotriene Receptor Antagonists

Zafirlukast

Pharmacokinetics. Initial onset of action occurs within 30 minutes, with a peak response in about 3 hours. Food decreases absorption by about 40%, so it should be taken either 1 hour before or 2 hours after meals. Extensive hepatic metabolism is via CYP 2C9. The half-life is about 10 hours but may be up to 20 hours in older adults. Excretion is primarily fecal.

Indications. Zafirlukast is approved for use in children over 5 years of age and adults. Zafirlukast is an add-on therapy for patients with chronic uncontrolled asthma or for patients unable to use ICSs. Zafirlukast is not recom- mended as a first-line therapy.

Adverse Effects. The most common side effects are head- ache, infection, gastrointestinal (GI) issues (stomach pain, nausea, diarrhea), and generalized pain. Liver impairment or disease may result. Although generally well tolerated, all leu- kotriene modifiers can cause adverse neuropsychiatric effects, including depression, suicidal thinking, and suicidal behav- ior. The rare but serious Churg-Strauss syndrome, also known as eosinophilic granulomatosis with polyangiitis, is character- ized by blood vessel inflammation resulting in the restriction

TABLE 6.6	Leukotriene Modifiers			
Drug Category/Medication	**Indication**	**Dosage**		**Considerations and Monitoring**
Leukotriene Receptor Antagonists (LTRAs)				
Montelukast	Asthma maintenance	**Oral 10-mg tablet:** *Adults and adolescents ≥15 yr:* 10 mg orally once every evening.		FDA black box warning
		Chewable tablet (4 mg): *Children 2–5 yr:* 4 mg orally once every evening.		
		Chewable tablet (5 mg): *Children 6–14 yr:* 5 mg orally once every evening.		
		Granules packet (4 mg): *Children: 1–5 yr:* 4 mg orally once every evening.		
	Exercise-induced asthma	**Oral 10-mg tablet:** *Adults and adolescents ≥15 yr:* 1 dose at least 2 hr before exercise. Maximum dosage: 10 mg/24 hr.		
		Chewable tablet (5 mg): *Children 6–14 yr:* 1 dose at least 2 hr before exercise. Maximum dosage: 10 mg/24 hr.		
Zafirlukast	Asthma maintenance	**Tablet 20 mg:** *Adults, adolescents, and children ≥12 yr:* 20 mg orally twice daily. Maximum dosage: 40 mg/day.		
		Tablet 10 mg: *Children 5–11 yr:* 10 mg orally twice daily. Maximum dosage: 20 mg/day.		
Leukotriene Synthesis Inhibitor				
Zileuton	Asthma maintenance	**Immediate-release tablet (600 mg):** *Adults, adolescents, and children ≥12 yr:* 600 mg orally four times daily with meals and at bedtime.		
		Extended-release tablet (600 mg): *Adults, adolescents, and children ≥12 yr:* 1200 mg orally twice daily 1 hour after meal.		

of blood flow. Churg-Strauss syndrome can develop when glucocorticoid dosage is adjusted or withdrawn, suggesting that glucocorticoid withdrawal may be a contributing factor.

Contraindications. Zafirlukast is contraindicated in patients with known hypersensitivity to any of its components and in patients with hepatic impairment, including cirrhosis. It is not for use during exercise-induced bronchospasms, acute asthma attacks, or bronchospasms.

PRACTICE PEARLS

Zafirlukast Use in Pregnancy and Lactation

- There are no adequate, well-controlled studies in pregnant women, and fetal risk is unknown. Evaluate risks to the mother and the fetus associated with poorly controlled asthma during pregnancy.
- Zafirlukast is excreted in breast milk; breastfeeding is contraindicated.

Monitoring. Monitor liver function tests and PFTs. Monitor for decrease in severity and frequency of asthma symptoms.

Leukotriene Synthesis Inhibitors

Zileuton

Pharmacokinetics. Following oral administration, peak response occurs in 1 to 5 hours. Zileuton immediate-release tablets may be taken with or without food. Zileuton extended-release tablets should be taken with food. Hepatic metabolism is via CYP 1A2, CYP 2C9, and CYP 3A4. Half-life varies between 2 and 3 hours. Excretion is primarily through the kidneys.

Indications. Zileuton is FDA approved for use in patients with chronic asthma. Practice guidelines include the off-label use of zileuton for AERD and EIA (Laidlaw, 2019). GINA (2020) guidelines recommend zileuton as controller therapy particularly in children 12 years of age and older. Zileuton is not an effective monotherapy when compared to monotherapy with ICSs nor is it as effective as combination therapy with ICS/LABA.

Adverse Effects. Headaches are a common adverse effect reported by patients. Other adverse effects include nose and throat irritation, sinusitis, upper respiratory infection, throat pain, muscle aches, nausea, and diarrhea. Neuropsychiatric events have been reported in adult and adolescent patients.

PRACTICE PEARLS

Life Span Considerations With Zileuton

- **Children:** Not recommended for children younger than 12 years of age due to risk of hepatoxicity.
- **Older adults:** Females over age 65 are at increased risk of alanine transaminase (ALT) elevations.

Contraindications. Drug–drug interactions mentioned in product labeling include theophylline (increase theophylline level), warfarin (increase prothrombin times), and propranolol (decreased heart rate). Avoid in patients with liver impairment since elevated liver function tests may occur. Avoid in patients with hypersensitivity reactions to zileuton or any of its components.

PRACTICE PEARLS

Zileuton Use in Pregnancy and Lactation

- **Pregnancy:** There are no adequate, well-controlled studies in pregnant women, and fetal risk is unknown. Evaluate risks to the mother and the fetus associated with poorly controlled asthma during pregnancy.
- **Lactation:** Zileuton is excreted in breast milk; breastfeeding is contraindicated.

Monitoring. Monitor liver function studies and signs and symptoms of liver dysfunction. Monitor PFTs for improvement in asthma symptoms. Patients and primary care providers should be alert for neuropsychiatric changes.

Muscarinic Receptors

Long-Acting Muscarinic Antagonists (LAMAs)

Tiotropium

Pharmacokinetics. Tiotropium is available as a soft-mist inhaled solution for the treatment of asthma. After inhalation, about 33% of the medication is available. Maximum plasma concentrations are reached in 5 to 7 minutes. Half-life elimination is about 44 hours. Hepatic metabolism occurs via CYP 2D6 and CYP 3A4 and excretion is through the kidneys.

Indications. Tiotropium (as Spiriva, Respimat) is a LAMA approved for once-daily maintenance treatment of asthma (Table 6.7). Tiotropium improves lung function and decreases exacerbations. Tiotropium is not used to treat acute symptoms or bronchospasms. GINA guidelines recommend tiotropium as an add-on therapy in patients 6 years of age and older who

are not well controlled on an ICS/LABA (Global Initiative for Asthma, 2020). NHLBI guidelines do not currently make any recommendations regarding the role of LAMAs in the treatment of patients with asthma (NHLBI/NAEPP, 2007).

Adverse Effects. The most common adverse effects are pharyngitis, headache, bronchitis, and sinusitis. Less common adverse effects include palpitations, gastroesophageal reflux, oral candidiasis, dysphonia, pruritis, and rash. Adverse effects resulting from tiotropium's anticholinergic properties include constipation, dizziness, and cognitive problems. Serious adverse effects include paradoxical bronchospasms and hypersensitivity reactions.

Contraindications. Avoid in patients with hypersensitivity to tiotropium, ipratropium, or any component of the product. This medication should be used with caution in patients with narrow-angle glaucoma, urinary retention, and severe renal impairment. Avoid administration with other anticholinergic-containing drugs.

Monitoring. Primary care providers and patients should be alert for signs and symptoms of acute narrow-angle glaucoma, such as severe headache, eye pain or redness, blurred vision or halos, nausea, or vomiting. Monitor patients with moderate to severe renal impairment for potential anticholinergic side effects. Monitor for improvement in PFTs, symptoms, and pulmonary status.

Immunomodulators

Immunomodulators change the immune system and thus decrease the inflammation caused by asthma (Table 6.8).

Anti-IL5

Reslizumab

Pharmacokinetics. Peak concentration levels were reached by the end of the infusion. Clearance was approximately 7 mL/hr. Half-life is about 24 days. Metabolism is by proteolytic degradation via enzymes.

Indications. Reslizumab is intended for patients with severe asthma and as add-on therapy for patients 18 years of age and older with eosinophilic-type asthma. Reslizumab

BLACK BOX WARNING!

Reslizumab

- Anaphylaxis may occur during or within 20 minutes of reslizumab infusions.
- Administer only in health care settings that can manage anaphylaxis and provide emergency care.

TABLE 6.7 Long-Acting Muscarinic Antagonists (LAMA)

Medication	Indication	Dosage	Considerations and Monitoring
Tiotropium bromide	Asthma maintenance	Inhalation spray 1.25 mcg/actuation: *Adults, adolescents, and children ≥6 yr:* 2 oral inhalations once daily. Maximum dosage: 2 inhalations/day.	

TABLE 6.8   **Immunomodulators**

Category	Medication	Indication	Dosage	Considerations and Monitoring
Anti-IL5	Mepolizumab	Add-on maintenance treatment for severe eosinophilic asthma	*Adults, adolescents, and children ≥12 yr:* 100 mg subcutaneous injection once every 4 weeks. Maximum dosage: Dosage listed is usual and maximum dosage.	Injection site: upper arm, thigh, or abdomen.
			Children 6–11 yr: 40 mg subcutaneous injection once every 4 weeks. Maximum dosage: Dosage listed is usual and maximum dosage.	
	Reslizumab	Add-on maintenance treatment for severe eosinophilic asthma	*Adults:* 3 mg/kg intravenously every 4 weeks. Maximum dosage: Dosage listed is usual and maximum dosage.	Discontinue intravenous infusion for severe, systemic reaction, anaphylaxis
Anti-IL5R	Benralizumab	Add-on treatment for severe asthma and eosinophilic asthma	*Adults, adolescents, and children ≥12 yr:* 30 mg subcutaneous injection once every 4 weeks for 3 doses, then once every 8 weeks. Maximum dosage: Dosage listed is usual and maximum dosage.	
Anti-IL4R	Dupilumab	Add-on treatment for moderate to severe eosinophilic asthma	**Subcutaneous injection:** *Adults, adolescents, and children ≥12 yr:* 400 mg subcutaneous loading dose (administer as two 200-mg injections), then 200 mg subcutaneously every other week OR 600 mg subcutaneous loading dose (administer as two 300-mg injections), then 300 mg every other week.	
			Children 6–11 yr weighing ≥30 kg: 200 mg subcutaneously every other week.	
			Children 6–11 yr weighing 15–29 kg: 100 mg subcutaneously every other week OR 300 mg subcutaneously every 4 weeks.	
		Oral corticosteroid-dependent asthma	*Adults, adolescents, and children ≥12 yr:* 600 mg subcutaneous loading dose (administer as two 300-mg injections), then 300 mg every other week.	
			Children 6–11 yr weighing ≥30 kg: 200 mg subcutaneously every other week.	
			Children 6–11 yr weighing 15–29 kg: 100 mg subcutaneously every other week OR 300 mg subcutaneously every 4 weeks.	
		Asthma with moderate to severe atopic dermatitis	*Adults, adolescents, and children ≥12 yr:* 600 mg subcutaneous loading dose (administer as two 300-mg injections), then 300 mg every other week.	
			Children 6–11 yr weighing ≥60 kg: 600 mg subcutaneous loading dose (administer as two 300-mg injections), then 300 mg every other week.	
			Children 6–11 yr weighing 30–59 kg: 400 mg subcutaneously loading dose (administer as two 200-mg injections), then 200 mg every other week.	
			Children 6–11 yr weighing 15–29 kg: 600 mg subcutaneous loading dose (administer as two 300-mg injections), then 300 mg every other week.	
		Asthma in adults with chronic rhinosinusitis with nasal polyps	*Adults:* 600 mg subcutaneous loading dose (administer as two 300-mg injections), then 300 mg every other week.	

				Considerations and
TABLE 6.8	**Immunomodulators—cont'd**			
Category	Medication	Indication	Dosage	Considerations and Monitoring
Anti-IgE	Omalizumab	Add-on treatment for moderate to severe persistent allergic asthma	Dosing highly variable. Dosing based on age, weight, and baseline serum IgE Refer directly to product insert for accurate dosing.	Black box warning for hypersensitivity to omalizumab. Monitor weight and adjust dose. Do not administer more than 150 mg per injection site.

blocks IL5 from binding to eosinophils. Reslizumab is administered by intravenous infusion in a setting able to provide emergency care. Primary care providers may have patients taking reslizumab within their practice, so knowledge of the medication may be helpful.

Adverse Effects. The most serious adverse effect is anaphylaxis (see Black Box Warning: Reslizumab). More common adverse effects include those of the immunologic, musculoskeletal, and respiratory systems, such as myalgia, throat pain, sinusitis, headache, worsening of asthma, nasopharyngitis, upper respiratory tract infection, antibody development, and increased creatine kinase levels. Patients have experienced a slight increase in the diagnosis of malignancies (0.6% in a treatment group compared to 0.3% in a placebo group) within 6 months of receiving reslizumab, with 5 of the 15 patients reporting a history of prior malignancy (Murphy et al., 2017). Malignancies included basal-cell carcinoma, malignant melanoma, and breast, prostate, anal, and ovarian/ovarian epithelial cancer.

Contraindications. Reslizumab should not be used to treat acute asthma symptoms, acute exacerbations, acute bronchospasms, or status asthmaticus. Reslizumab is contraindicated in patients who have known hypersensitivity to reslizumab or any component of the product. No results are available for drug–drug interactions. Reslizumab is not expected to affect CYP 1A2, CYP 2B6, or CYP 3A4 enzyme activity.

PRACTICE PEARLS

Reslizumab Use in Pregnancy and Lactation

- Limited data exist regarding reslizumab and pregnancy risk. Consider the mother's clinical status and level of asthma control. Consider the long half-life of reslizumab prior to prescribing.
- No information is available regarding reslizumab in breast milk or risks to the fetus. Consider developmental and health benefits to infants with breastfeeding as well as the mother's clinical status and level of asthma control.

Monitoring. Monitor for improvement in asthma symptoms and in PFTs. Monitor for development of common adverse reactions and parasitic infections. Treat patients with parasitic infections prior to initiating therapy. If a parasitic infection develops while under treatment with reslizumab and fails to respond to antiparasitic therapy, discontinue reslizumab.

Anti-IL5R

Benralizumab

Pharmacokinetics. After subcutaneous administration of benralizumab, bioavailability was about 60%. Injection site location did not affect bioavailability. The absorption half-life was 3.5 days. Benralizumab is metabolized by proteolytic enzymes distributed throughout the body. Elimination half-life was 15.5 days.

Indications. Benralizumab was approved in 2017. It is an add-on medication administered as a subcutaneous injectable medication for patients 12 years of age and older with severe asthma and eosinophilic phenotype asthma. Benralizumab is a humanized monoclonal antibody (IgG1 kappa) targeting interleukin-5 (IL-5). By inhibiting IL-5, benralizumab decreases eosinophil production and survival.

Adverse Effects. The most common adverse effects include headache and pharyngitis. Hypersensitivity reactions include urticaria, urticaria popular, and rash. Injection site reactions of pain, erythema, pruritis, and papule were at comparable rates to those from placebo injections.

Contraindications. Benralizumab is not intended for the treatment of acute bronchospasms, status asthmaticus, or other eosinophilic conditions. Benralizumab is contraindicated in patients with known hypersensitivity to benralizumab or any of its components. When initiating benralizumab, taper instead of abruptly discontinuing corticosteroids due to the risk of secondary adrenal insufficiency, symptoms of steroid withdrawal, and relapse of asthma.

Monitoring. Monitor for improvement of asthma symptoms and PFTs. Patients with renal or hepatic impairment should be monitored since no clinical studies evaluating risk have been conducted. Monitor for adverse reactions related to drug–drug interaction studies as no clinical studies have been conducted.

Anti-IL4R

Dupilumab

Pharmacokinetics. Following subcutaneous injection, the time to peak concentration was about 1 week. Bioavailability ranged between 60% and 65%. The half-life in animal studies is 4 to 20 days but is unknown in humans. The process of metabolism is unclear, but dupilumab is degraded into small peptides and amino acids.

Indications. Dupilumab is a human monoclonal IgG4 antibody. Dupilumab is approved as an adjunct medication in patients with eosinophilic or oral corticosteroid–dependent asthma. Dupilumab is shown to decrease the frequency of asthma exacerbations and improve lung function. Dupilumab is an add-on maintenance treatment in adult patients with inadequately controlled chronic rhinosinusitis with nasal polyposis. Dupilumab is approved for patients 12 years of age and older. No dosage adjustments are required in patients with renal or hepatic impairment.

Adverse Effects. For patients with asthma, the most common adverse effects include injection site reactions, oropharyngeal pain, and eosinophilia. Injection site reactions include pain, erythema, bruising, edema, swelling, pruritus, and inflammation. Injection site reactions occurred most often with the initial loading dose. For patients with chronic rhinosinusitis with nasal polyposis, the most common adverse effects include injection site reactions, eosinophilia, insomnia, toothache, gastritis, arthralgia, and conjunctivitis.

Contraindications. Dupilumab is contraindicated in patients with known hypersensitivity to dupilumab or any of its components. Dupilumab may enhance the adverse or toxic effect of live vaccines. Avoid concomitant administration of live vaccines in patients treated with dupilumab.

Monitoring. Monitor for hypersensitivity reactions, signs of infection, and adverse effects. Monitor PFTs in asthma patients.

Anti-IgE

Omalizumab

Pharmacokinetics. Omalizumab reaches peak serum concentrations within 7 to 8 days. Within 12 weeks of injection, the majority of patients had a response to the medication. Elimination half-life was about 24 to 26 days. Excretion is via hepatic degradation.

Indications. Omalizumab is indicated for patients with IgE-mediated moderate to severe persistent allergic asthma. Omalizumab is for patients 6 years of age and older who demonstrate a positive skin test or in vitro reactivity and whose asthma symptoms are not controlled by ICSs. In these patients, omalizumab decreases the incidence of asthma exacerbations. Omalizumab is administered by subcutaneous injection.

Adverse Effects. The most common adverse reactions reported by adolescents and adults included arthralgia, generalized pain, leg pain, fatigue, dizziness, fracture, pruritus, dermatitis, and earache. By comparison, children more commonly reported nasopharyngitis, headache, pyrexia, upper abdominal pain, streptococcal pharyngitis, otitis media, viral gastroenteritis, arthropod bites, and epistaxis. Malignancies were reported at slightly higher rates in clinical trial patients than in control groups. Serious adverse effects included angina, thrombosis, anaphylaxis, pulmonary hypertension, pulmonary embolism, Helminth infection (parasitic infections), and serum sickness.

Contraindications. Do not abruptly discontinue corticosteroids when beginning omalizumab therapy due to the risk of secondary adrenal insufficiency, symptoms of steroid withdrawal, and relapse of asthma. Avoid in patients with known hypersensitivity to omalizumab or any component of the product. No drug–drug interaction studies have been completed. The use of omalizumab with allergen immunotherapy has not been studied.

BLACK BOX WARNING!

Omalizumab and Anaphylaxis

- Anaphylaxis (bronchospasm, hypotension, syncope, urticaria, and/or angioedema) has occurred after injection.
- Administration in a health care setting equipped to handle anaphylaxis is recommended. See prescribing guidelines if considering administration in an alternate setting.
- Monitor patient for up to 120 minutes after administration.

PRACTICE PEARLS

Omalizumab Use in Pregnancy and Lactation

- Omalizumab crosses the placenta during the second and third trimesters. Clinical trials lack data to address risk, though fetal risk is potentially higher in the third trimester. Consider the mother's clinical status and level of asthma control.
- No information is available regarding omalizumab in breast milk or risks to the fetus. Consider developmental and health benefits to infants with breastfeeding as well as the mother's clinical status and level of asthma control.

Monitoring. Monitor baseline serum IgE levels in patients with allergic asthma. Retesting of serum IgE levels during therapy does not impact dosing. Monitor patient weight at each visit and adjust omalizumab dose according to weight. Monitor for improvement in symptoms and PFTs. Reevaluate if response is insufficient. For patients at risk for Helminth infection, examine stool for parasites.

Mast Cell Stabilizers

Mast cell stabilizers prevent the release of mast cell mediators, block mast cell degranulation, and stabilize the mast cell membrane (Table 6.9).

Cromolyn

Pharmacokinetics. After nebulizer inhalation, about 8% of the medication reaches the lungs. Peak response is about 15 minutes. Elimination half-life is 80 to 90 minutes. Excretion is through the kidneys and fecal route.

Indications. Cromolyn is FDA approved for asthma maintenance and for patients with exercise-induced bronchospasms unresponsive to short-acting beta-agonists (SABAs) or ICS with SABAs. However, it is not recommended by GINA as an effective maintenance therapy for asthma (GINA, 2020; NHLBI/NAEPP, 2007). According to the manufacturer, cromolyn inhibits bronchoconstrictive reactions, though the medication has no intrinsic bronchodilator or antihistamine effects.

Adverse Effects. After nebulizer inhalation, commonly reported adverse effects include cough and wheezing. General adverse effects of cromolyn also include nasal congestion, nausea, sneezing, drowsiness, nasal itching, nose bleed, nose burning, serum sickness, and upset stomach. Significant adverse effects are rare but may include bronchospasms, laryngeal edema, swollen parotid gland, angioedema, and pulmonary infiltrates with eosinophilia.

Contraindications. Avoid in patients with hypersensitivities to cromolyn or any component of the product. Cromolyn is not intended for the treatment of acute bronchospasm or status asthmaticus.

PRACTICE PEARLS

Cromolyn Use in Pregnancy and Lactation

- Animal trials reveal no evidence of fetal harm. Clinical trials on pregnant women lack data to address fetal risk. Consider use during pregnancy only if clearly needed.
- It is unknown whether cromolyn is excreted in breast milk. Use caution and consider the potential benefit of treatment to the potential adverse effects on the infant.

Monitoring. Routine laboratory monitoring is not required. Consider monitoring patients with hepatic and renal impairment. Monitor for improvement in symptoms.

Methylxanthines

Theophylline is the most well known methylxanthine. Theophylline use has declined as medications with improved

TABLE 6.9 Mast Cell Stabilizers

Medication	Indication	Dosage	Considerations and Monitoring
Cromolyn	Adjunct asthma maintenance	**Nebulizer solution 20 mg/2 mL vial:** *Adults, adolescents, and children ≥2 yr:* 20-mg ampule via nebulizer four times daily. Maximum dosage: 20 mg inhaled via nebulization four times daily	FDA approved, though use not recommended by current clinical guidelines.
	Bronchospasm, exercise-induced or other precipitating factor	*Adults, adolescents, and children ≥2 yr:* 20 mg ampule via nebulizer 1 hr before exercise.	

profiles and fewer adverse effects have been introduced. Theophylline is not a first-line therapy for asthma.

The use of theophylline to treat asthma is not included in the GINA 2020 report. The NHLBI/NAEPP (2007) includes the use of sustained-release theophylline as an adjunct therapy beginning in Step 2. Theophylline with ICS is also recommended as adjunctive therapy in Steps 3 and 4. The FDA does not recommend theophylline for the treatment of acute bronchospasm due to status asthmaticus. Primary care providers considering the use of theophylline are directed to current practice guidelines.

Medication Classification: Quick Relief Medications
Inhaled Beta2-Adrenergic Agonists

Short-acting inhaled beta2-adrenergic agonists are listed in Table 6.10.

Albuterol

Pharmacokinetics. Pharmacokinetic properties of inhalation preparations differ by formulation. Onset of action is less than 8 minutes. Duration of action varies from 2 to 6 hours. Half-life is 4 to 7 hours. Albuterol is excreted through the kidneys. Onset of action of oral preparations is less than 30 minutes. Duration of action varies from 6 to 12 hours with extended-release tablets. Half-life is 9 hours. Excretion is through the kidneys.

Indications. Albuterol is a short-acting bronchodilator approved for the treatment of asthma and the prophylaxis of EIA. It is available in a variety of formats. Routine use of SABAs is not recommended. SABAs may be used as intermittent monotherapy with careful monitoring of frequency of use, which will indicate the need to adjust medications (GINA, 2020).

Adverse Effects. The frequency and severity of adverse effects are age, dose, and route dependent. Common adverse effects include bronchitis, headache, hypersensitivity reactions, nausea, nervousness, palpitations, tachycardia, throat pain, vomiting, pharyngitis, rhinitis, tremors, and upper respiratory infections. Serious side effects include anaphylaxis, angioedema, cardiac tachyarrhythmias, diabetic ketoacidosis, hyperglycemia, and paradoxical bronchospasm.

Contraindications. Avoid in patients with hypersensitivity to albuterol, levalbuterol, or milk proteins. Patients with a history of cardiovascular disease may experience alterations in blood pressure, heart rate, electrocardiogram changes, and central nervous system (CNS) stimulation. Use with caution in patients with diabetes, glaucoma, hyperthyroidism, hypokalemia, or renal impairment.

Monitoring. Monitor for relief or improvement in asthma symptoms, PFTs, and laboratory studies (blood chemistries and renal function). Observe for adverse effects and changes in cardiovascular status. Observe for hypersensitivity reactions.

Prescriber Considerations for Asthma Therapy

The 2020 GINA Report outlines the five-step approach to asthma therapy in adults and adolescents 12 years of age and older and for children 6 to 11 years of age.

> ### BOOKMARK THIS!
> - Clinical Guidelines
> - Global Initiative for Asthma (2020). *Global strategy for asthma management and prevention. 2020 Update.* https://ginasthma.org/wp-content/uploads/2020/06/GINA-2020-report_20_06_04-1-wms.pdf
> - National Heart, Lung, and Blood Institute. National Asthma Education and Prevention Program. (2007). *Expert panel report 3: Guidelines for the diagnosis and management of asthma.* https://www.nhlbi.nih.gov/sites/default/files/media/docs/EPR-3_Asthma_Full_Report_2007.pdf

Clinical Reasoning for Asthma Therapy

Consider the individual patient's pulmonary status. Initial evaluation begins with a symptom assessment, a comprehensive history, and a physical exam. If spirometry testing confirms a diagnosis of asthma, treatment should be initiated following current guidelines. Treatment goals include controlling symptoms, maintaining pulmonary function, improving and maintaining normal activities of daily living, preventing exacerbations, and decreasing asthma mortality. Consider differential diagnoses if the evaluation (symptom assessment, a comprehensive history, and a physical exam) do not point to a diagnosis of asthma (GINA, 2020).

Determine the desired therapeutic outcome based on the degree of control and severity of asthma symptoms. GINA recommendations include a step-by-step control assessment guide for adults, adolescents, and children 6 to 11 years of age (GINA, 2020). Determination of control and severity guides the primary care provider in selecting the appropriate medication and dosage (GINA, 2020; NHLBI/NAEPP, 2007). Asthma control is based on symptom control and the potential risk of adverse outcomes in relation to ongoing therapeutic interventions. Asthma control is categorized as well controlled, partly controlled, or uncontrolled. Control of symptoms can be estimated by asking about the frequency of daytime and nighttime symptoms, the frequency of SABAs, risk factors, and any activity limitations (GINA, 2020). Severity assesses the intensity of the disease in relation to treatment. Severity is categorized as intermittent, mild persistent, moderate persistent, or severe persistent. Severity of symptoms is the level of treatment (Step 1 to Step 5) required to control symptoms and exacerbations (GINA, 2020). Health care providers should refer to current clinical practice guidelines.

Assess the medication therapy selected for its appropriateness for an individual patient by considering the medication's side effects and the patient's age, race/ethnicity, comorbidities, and genetic factors. Primary care providers must consider multiple medications when determining a treatment plan. Individual patient characteristics may affect medication efficacy (Blaiss et al., 2017). In addition, these characteristics should be considered when evaluating the potential risk for adverse effects and contraindications. Phenotype

TABLE 6.10 Short-Acting Beta2-Adrenergic Agonist (SABA)

Medication	Indication	Dosage	Considerations and Monitoring
Albuterol Multiple prescription and generic formulations available	Asthma reliever therapy for transient bronchospasm	**Inhalation aerosol or powder 90 mcg/actuation:** *Adults, adolescents, and children ≥4 yr:* 1 or 2 oral inhalations every 4–6 hr as needed. Maximum dosage: 12 oral inhalations/day.	Renal impairment: creatinine clearance may be reduced. Older adults: usually start at the low end of the dosing range.
		Nebulized inhalation: *Adults, adolescents and children ≥15 kg:* 2.5 mg (3 mL) via oral inhalation three or four times daily as needed. Maximum dosage: 4 doses (10 mg) daily. *Children 2–12 yr and <15 kg:* 0.63–1.25 mg dose at 0.1–0.15 mg/kg albuterol base per nebulizer three or four times daily as needed. Maximum dosage: 4 doses (5 mg) daily.	
		Immediate-release tablets *Adults and adolescents ≥13 yr:* 2–4 mg orally three or four times daily. If inadequate response, may give up to 8 mg orally four times daily. Maximum dosage: 32 mg/day. *Children 6–12 yr:* 2 mg orally three or four times daily. Maximum dosage: 24 mg/day.	Dosage dependent on response. Unless specified, may cautiously increase to achieve response. Do not exceed maximum dosage.
		Extended-release tablets: *Adults and adolescents ≥13 yr:* 4–8 mg orally every 12 hr. Maximum dosage: 32 mg/day. *Children 6–12 yr:* 4 mg orally every 12 hr. Maximum dosage: 24 mg/day.	
		Solution or syrup *Adults and adolescents ≥15 yr:* 2–4 mg orally three or four times daily. If inadequate response, may give up to 8 mg orally four times daily Maximum dosage: 32 mg/day. *Children 6–14 yr:* 2 mg orally three or four times daily. Maximum dosage: 24 mg/day. *Children 2–5 yr:* 0.1 mg/kg/dose orally three times daily. If inadequate response, may give up to 0.2 mg/kg/dose orally three times daily. Maximum dosage: 12 mg/day.	
	Exercise-induced bronchospasm	**Inhalation aerosol or powder, 90 mcg/actuation:** *Adults and children ≥4 yr:* 2 oral inhalations 15–30 minutes before exercise.	
	Primary care or acute care management of mild to moderate exacerbation of asthma	**Inhalation aerosol or powder 90 mcg/actuation:** *Adults, adolescents, and children ≥6 yr:* First hour: 4–10 oral inhalations every 20 minutes; then dose may vary: 4–10 oral inhalations every 3–4 hr up to 6–10 oral inhalations every 1–2 hr. *Infants and children up to 5 yr:* First hour: 2–6 oral inhalations every 20 minutes; then 2 or 3 oral inhalations every hour as needed.	*Infants and children up to 5 yr:* Use a spacer and a mask.
		Nebulizer: *Adults, adolescents, and children ≥6 yr and weight >15 kg:* First hour: 2.5 mg via nebulizer every 20 minutes; then dose may vary: 2.5 mg via nebulizer every 3–4 hours up to 2.5 mg via nebulizer every 1–2 hr. *Children 6–12 yr and weight <15 kg:* First hour: 2.5 mg via nebulizer every 20 minutes; then dose may vary: 2.5 mg via nebulizer every 3–4 hours up to 2.5 mg via nebulizer every 1–2 hr. Dosing varies 0.63 mg–1.25 mg via nebulizer three to four times daily. *Children 2–5 yr:* First hour: 2.5 mg via nebulizer every 20 minutes; then reassess for response. Expected dosing varies 0.63 mg–1.25 mg via nebulizer three to four times daily.	

Continued

TABLE 6.10   **Short-Acting Beta2-Adrenergic Agonist (SABA)—cont'd**

Medication	Indication	Dosage	Considerations and Monitoring
Levalbuterol	Treatment and prevention of asthma	**Inhalation aerosol, 45 mcg/actuation:** *Adults and children ≥4 yr:* 1–2 oral inhalations every 4–6 hr. Maximum dosage: 12 inhalations/daily.	
		Nebulized inhalation: *Adults and adolescents ≥12 yr:* 0.63–1.25 mg via oral inhalation three times daily (every 6–8 hr). Maximum dosage: 3 doses/day. *Children 6–11 yr:* 0.31–0.63 mg via oral inhalation three times daily (every 6–8 hr). Maximum dosage: 3 doses/day.	

and endotype classifications may overlap, adding another layer of complexity to the selection of medication.

Initiate the treatment plan with the selected medication by first providing adequate patient education to ensure the patient's understanding and promote full participation in the therapy. Patient education includes the normal function and structure of the lung compared to the abnormal lung function due to asthma; medication options and side effects; how to assess and manage changes in condition, including when to seek attention; and the need to manage comorbid conditions. In addition, the patient's ability to use inhalers should be evaluated before they leave the office. MDIs, DPIs, soft-mist inhalers, and nebulizers all involve multiple steps to deliver the medication. Unintentional medication errors can result from technique errors. The use of multiple medications and/or multiple delivery systems can compound the errors. Prior to prescribing a medication, evaluate the patient for barriers to medication adherence by assessing physical limitations such as arthritis, literacy barriers, and medication cost.

Ensure complete patient and family understanding about the medication prescribed for asthma management using a variety of education strategies. Patient education on decreasing modifiable risk factors includes information about routine vaccinations, increasing exercise, following a healthy diet and losing weight, eliminating smoking and avoiding secondhand smoke, managing or eliminating allergen and environmental exposures, and managing comorbid conditions such as AR, sleep apnea, gastroesophageal reflux disease (GERD), and cardiac disease. Include education on maintenance and emergency medications (dose, frequency, route, and side effects) and how to properly use and care for inhalers and nebulizers.

The avoidance of allergens is often the first strategy recommended to patients. Avoidance requires a multi-pronged approach to:
- Evaluate the physical environment (inside and outside). School, home, and work environments are unavoidable. Patients may not have the ability to exercise any control over their environment.
- Identify allergen triggers. Common environmental triggers are pollen, pets, dust mites, molds, and pests.
- Determine whether interventions are feasible and whether patients are willing to perform the interventions. Interventions include acaricides, protective barriers, humidity control, cleaning and the use of vacuum filters, and laminar airflow systems (Cipriani et al., 2017).

Providing written instructions, demonstrating with a task-trainer or placebo inhaler, and watching the patient demonstrate how they use the inhaler are all methods for increasing patient success. The National Asthma Education and Prevention Program (NAEPP) and the American Lung Association offer numerous asthma-related resources available to patients.

Conduct follow-up and monitoring of patient responses to anticoagulant therapy. Once therapy is initiated, evidence-based tools (Box 6.1) provide continuing assessments for asthma severity and control.

• Box 6.1   Evidence-Based Asthma Control Tools[a]

- 30 Second Asthma Test™
- Asthma APGAR Tool
- Asthma Control Test™
- Asthma Control Questionnaire (ACQ)
- Asthma Therapy Assessment Questionnaire (ATAQ)
- Childhood Asthma Control Test (c-ACT)
- TRACK™ Test for Respiratory and Asthma Control in Kids

[a]Not an exhaustive list of established screening tools. Data from Alzahrani, Y. A. & Becker, E. A. (2016). Asthma control assessment tools. *Respiratory Care, 61*(1), 106-116. DOI: https://doi.org/10.4187/respcare.04341; Dinakar, C., Chipps, B. E., AAP SECTION ON ALLERGY AND IMMUNOLOGY, AAP SECTION ON PEDIATRIC PULMONOLOGY AND SLEEP MEDICINE. (2017). Clinical tools to assess asthma control in children. *Pediatrics, 139*(1):e20163438. https://doi.org/10.1542/peds.2016-3438; Yawn, B. P., Wollan, P. C., Rank, M. A., Bertram, S. L., Juhn, Y., & Pace, W. (2018). Use of asthma APGAR tools in primary care practices: A cluster-randomized controlled trial. *The Annals of Family Medicine, 16*(2), 100-110. https://doi.org/10.1370/afm.2179.

Teaching Points for Asthma Therapy

Health Promotion Strategies

Primary Care Provider

At each visit:
- Incorporate the use of an asthma control tool to assess symptoms.
- Evaluate the use of an inhaler or nebulizer and correct the technique as needed.
- Evaluate comorbidities and concurrent over-the-counter (OTC) and prescription medications for potential confounding triggers.
  - Certain medications (NSAIDs, aspirin) may make asthma symptoms worse.
- Develop an asthma action plan.
- Counsel patients on nonpharmacologic strategies to improve health outcomes, such as smoking cessation, avoidance of environmental and occupational triggers, avoidance of indoor and outdoor allergens, physical activity, weight reduction and a healthy diet, and psychological responses to stress (emotional or physical).
  - Refer to Chapter 52, Smoking Cessation Medications.
- Consider teaching or referring the patient for breathing or relaxation techniques.
- Consider referring the patient for expert advice under the following circumstances: when the diagnosis is uncertain, the symptoms are due to occupational-related asthma, there are persistent or severe uncontrolled asthma exacerbations, exacerbations require frequent or long-term oral corticosteroid use, or there is a risk of asthma-related death (admission to intensive care units, mechanical ventilation, anaphylaxis or food allergies in an asthma patient, or significant adverse effects from therapy).

Patient
- Keep all appointments with health care providers and seek medical care as appropriate for any change in status.
- Always carry your rescue inhaler.
- Recognize early signs and symptoms of worsening asthma such as wheezing, shortness of breath, coughing, or yellow, green, gray, bloody, or thicker-than-usual sputum.
- Initiate your asthma treatment plan and seek help if you recognize the early signs and symptoms of worsening asthma: shortness of breath, coughing, or yellow, green, gray, bloody, or thicker-than-usual sputum.
- Tell your provider about all prescription and OTC medications.
- Take your medications correctly; use the appropriate type of inhaler and spacer with the proper technique.
- Identify and avoid asthma triggers.
- Self-monitor your level of asthma control. Use a peak flow meter as instructed.
- Follow your asthma treatment plan. Initiate emergency medication therapy and contact your primary care provider for changes in status.

- Caregivers of children: Communicate asthma information to school, child care center, and other caregivers.

Patient Education for Medication Safety

1. Use all medications as directed. Do not use asthma medications more often than ordered. Use rescue inhalers only as ordered. If you feel your symptoms are not under control or you are using the rescue inhaler more than ordered, contact your health care provider.
2. Use medication reminders for missing or late dosages.
3. Refer to specific delivery methods for instructions on use and care of equipment. Follow manufacturers' recommendations.
4. Check your inhaler or nebulizer technique periodically to ensure that you are using the equipment correctly. Refer to videos or ask your primary care provider for guidance.
5. After use of a nebulizer or inhaler, rinse your mouth and then spit to remove residual medication. This may help reduce the risk of adverse effects.

Application Questions for Discussion

1. What benefits do phenotype and endotype determinations have on patient therapy?
2. What should be included in the education plan for a patient who has been prescribed a SABA?
3. What criteria are used in determining step-up or step-down therapy in adults, adolescents, and children?

Selected Bibliography

American College of Allergy, Asthma & Immunology (n.d.). Exercise-Induced Bronchoconstriction (EIB). https://acaai.org/asthma/types-asthma/exercise-induced-bronchoconstriction-eib. Accessed August 23, 2020.

American Lung Association. (n.d.). *Asthma patient resources and videos.*https://www.lung.org/lung-health-diseases/lung-disease-lookup/asthma/patient-resources-and-videos.

Asthma and Allergy Foundation of America. (2015). *Allergens and allergic asthma.* Retrieved Sept. 14, 2019 from https://www.aafa.org/allergic-asthma/.

Bates, J. H. T., Poynter, M. E., Frodella, C. M., Peters, U., Dixon, A. E., & Suratt, B. T (2017). Pathophysiology to phenotype in the asthma of obesity. *Annals of the American Thoracic Society, 14*(S5), S395–S398. https://doi.org/10.1513/AnnalsATS.201702-122AW.

Blaiss, M. S., Castro, M., Chipps, B. E., Zitt, M., Panettieri, R. A., & Foggs, M. B. (2017). Guiding principles for use of newer biologics and bronchial thermoplasty for patients with severe asthma. *Annals of Allergy, Asthma & Immunology, 119*(6), 533–540. https://doi.org/10.1016/j.anai.2017.09.058.

Cipriani, F., Calamelli, E., & Ricci, G. (2017). Allergen avoidance in allergic asthma. *Frontiers in Pediatrics, 5*(103). https://doi.org/10.3389/fped.2017.00103.

Centers for Disease Control and Prevention, National Center for Health Statistics (n.d.) *Asthma.* https://www.cdc.gov/nchs/fastats/asthma.htm. Accessed August 22, 2020.

Esteban-Gorfojo, I., Antolin-Amerigo, D., Dominguez-Ortega, J., & Quirce, S. (2018). Non-eosinophilic asthma: Current perspectives. *Journal of Asthma and Allergy, 11*, 267–281. https://doi.org/10.2147/JAA.S153097.

Friedman-Jimenez, G., Harrison, D., & Luo, H. (2015). Occupational asthma and work-exacerbated asthma. *Seminars in Respiratory and Critical Care Medicine, 36*(3), 388–407. https://doi.org/10.1055/s-0035-1550157.

Global Initiative for Asthma. (2020). *Global strategy for asthma management and prevention.* https://ginasthma.org/wp-content/uploads/2020/06/GINA-2020-report_20_06_04-1-wms.pdf.

Jolly, A. T., Klees, J. E., Pucheco, K. A., Guidotti, T. L., Kipen, H. M., Biggs, J. J., Hyman, M. H., Bohnker, B. K., Thiese, M. S., Hegmann, K. T., & Harber, P. (2015). ACOEM practice guidelines: Work-related asthma. *Journal of Occupational and Environmental Medicine, 57*(10), e121–e129. https://doi.org/10.1097/jom.0000000000000572.

Kuruvilla, M. E., Lee, F. E., & Lee, G. B. (2019). Understanding asthma phenotypes, endotypes, and mechanisms of disease. *Clinical Reviews in Allergy & Immunology, 56*(2), 219–233. https://doi.org/10.1007/s12016-018-8712-1.

Laidlaw, T. M. (2019). Clinical updates in aspirin-exacerbated respiratory disease. *Allergy and Asthma Proceedings, 40*(1), 4–6. https://doi.org/10.2500/aap.2019.40.4188.

Mohanan, S., Tapp, H., McWilliams, A., & Dulin, M. (2014). Obesity and asthma: Pathophysiology and implications for diagnosis and management in primary care. *Experimental Biology and Medicine (239)*, 1531–1540. https://doi.org/10.1177/1535370214525302.

Murphy, K., Jacobs, J., Bjermer, L., Fahrenholz, J. M., Shalit, Y., Garin, M., Zangrilli, J., & Castro, M. (2017). Long-term safety and efficacy of reslizumab in patients with eosinophilic asthma. *The Journal of Allergy and Clinical Immunology: In Practice, 5*(6), 1572–1581. https://doi.org/10.1016/j.jaip.2017.08.024.

National Asthma Education and Prevention Program. (n.d.). *All NHLBI Publications and Resources.* https://www.nhlbi.nih.gov/health-topics/all-publications-and-resources?title=asthma&items_per_page=10.

National Heart, Lung, and Blood Institute. National Asthma Education and Prevention Program. (2007) (NHLBI/NAEPP). *Expert panel report 3: Guidelines for the diagnosis and management of asthma.* https://www.nhlbi.nih.gov/sites/default/files/media/docs/EPR-3_Asthma_Full_Report_2007.pdf.

Rajan, J. P., Wineinger, N. E., Stevenson, D. D., & White, A. A. (2015). Prevalence of aspirin-exacerbated respiratory disease among asthmatic patients: A meta-analysis of the literature. *The Journal of Allergy and Clinical Immunology, 135*(3), P676–P681. E1. https://doi.org/10.1016/j.jaci.2014.08.020.

Ray, A., & Kolls, J. K. (2017). Neutrophilic inflammation in asthma and association with disease severity. *Trends in Immunology, 38*(12), 942–954. https://doi.org/10.1016/j.it.2017.07.003.

Rogalini, P., Calzetta, L., Matera, M. G., Laitano, R., Ritondo, B. L., Hanania, N. A., & Cazzola, M. (2020). Severe asthma and biological therapy: When, which, and for whom. *Pulmonary Therapy, 6*, 47–66. https://doi.org/10.1007/s41030-019-00109-1.

Stokes, J. R., & Casale, T. B. (2016). Characterization of asthma endotypes: Implications for therapy. *Annals of Allergy, Asthma & Immunology, 117*(2), 121–125. https://doi.org/10.1016/j.anai.2016.05.016.

The Global Asthma Network. (2018). *The Global Asthma Report 2018.* http://www.globalasthmareport.org/.

U. S. Food & Drug Administration. (2018). *FDA Drug Safety Communication: FDA review finds no significant increase in risk of serious asthma outcomes with long-acting beta agonists (LABAs) used in combination with inhaled corticosteroids (ICS).* https://www.fda.gov/drugs/drug-safety-and-availability/fda-drug-safety-communication-fda-review-finds-no-significant-increase-risk-serious-asthma-outcomes.

7

Chronic Obstructive Pulmonary Disease Medications

ANDREA J. EFRE AND REBECCA M. LUTZ

Overview

Chronic obstructive pulmonary disease (COPD) is a common respiratory condition treated in primary care that is characterized by progressive airflow limitation that is not fully reversible. This obstructive lung condition is currently the fourth leading cause of death in the world and is expected to increase in future decades due to the aging population and continued exposure to risk factors (Global Initiative for Chronic Obstructive Lung Disease [GOLD], 2020). Smoking tobacco is by far the leading risk factor for COPD. The severity of the disease process is largely dependent on the patient's comorbidities and frequency of exacerbations. Reduction of risk factors (e.g., smoking cessation) and effective pharmacologic management can help reduce exacerbations.

PRACTICE PEARLS

Risk Factors for Developing COPD

- Tobacco smoking (includes exposure to secondhand smoke)
- Occupational exposures (such as coal mining, textile dust, or exposure to toxins)
- Air pollution (indoor or outdoor)
- Recurrent lung infections or other respiratory diseases (e.g., airway hyperreactivity, asthma, bronchitis, childhood respiratory infections)
- Low socioeconomic status
- Age (65 and older), gender (females rate higher), and race (American Indians/Alaska Natives and multiracial non-Hispanics)
- Alpha-1 antitrypsin (AAT) deficiency

Data from Global Initiative for Chronic Obstructive Lung Disease. (2020). *Global strategy for the diagnosis, management, and prevention of chronic obstructive pulmonary disease. 2020 Report.* Available at https://goldcopd. org/; and Centers for Disease Control and Prevention. (2019). *Basics about COPD.* Available at https://www.cdc.gov/copd/basics-about.html.

COPD encompasses several chronic lung diseases, but the two main conditions are chronic bronchitis and emphysema. Three cardinal symptoms of COPD are dyspnea, chronic cough, and sputum production. Other symptoms of COPD include wheezing and chest tightness, which are emphasized during exacerbations. These symptoms are also found in asthma, which can make differentiating between asthma and COPD difficult. Although both COPD and asthma are obstructive lung diseases, asthma is *reversible* (symptoms can come and go) and COPD is *progressive* (symptoms are constant). Also, sputum production is not a typical finding in asthma, but it can be with COPD. COPD and asthma may be combined in an overlapping syndrome, which is more likely to increase exacerbations and symptom severity (review Chapter 6 for more specific information).

The Global Initiative for Chronic Obstructive Lung Disease, or GOLD, guides the diagnosis, management, and prevention of COPD. GOLD directs pharmacologic treatment, recommending medications for maintenance therapy and exacerbation of symptom control. This chapter is based on the recommendations of GOLD.

Pathophysiology

With COPD, long-term exposure to airway irritants disturbs the epithelial cells and cilia cells, causing inflammation. Chronic irritation causes small airway disease and parenchymal destruction and constriction of the bronchial tree. Airway inflammation, airflow limitations, and damage to terminal bronchioles and alveoli are common factors in both types of COPD. As the disease progresses, abnormalities in gas exchange cause low levels of blood oxygen, known as *hypoxemia*, and elevated levels of carbon dioxide, known as *hypercapnia*. Chronic bronchitis and emphysema both result in ventilation and perfusion deficits that cause dyspnea.

Normal ventilation (V) and perfusion (Q) occur as the alveoli allow oxygen to enter the vasculature and carbon dioxide to exit as the alveoli recoil. The VQ ratio equates to a normal gas exchange. A ventilation mismatch occurs if ventilation is inadequate or blood flow is inhibited. In the lungs of a person with COPD, inflammation throughout the airways and lungs causes disruption of the normal VQ ratio.

Chronic Bronchitis

In chronic bronchitis, inflammation causes fibrosis and thickening of the bronchiolar walls, causing bronchoconstriction, in addition to mucus hypersecretion and airway edema. The hypersecretion of mucus triggers a productive cough, and the bronchoconstriction leads to airway obstruction and expiratory wheezing. Airway obstruction causes alveolar hypoxia, which can lead to a *VQ mismatch*, causing hypoxemia and hypercapnia (leading to *respiratory acidosis*). In a response to hypoxia, the body produces additional red blood cells (*polycythemia*). The hypoxemia and polycythemia produce the physical presentation of cyanosis (hence the nickname "blue bloaters" for chronic bronchitis).

Alveolar hypoxia causes pulmonary vessel constriction, and shunting occurs to push the blood to healthier alveoli. The pulmonary vasoconstriction can lead to pulmonary hypertension, consequently inducing right-sided heart failure, cor pulmonale, and increased jugular venous pressure. Pulmonary hypertension can also decrease left ventricular output, which activates the renin-angiotensin-aldosterone system (RAAS) and increases systemic fluid retention.

Emphysema

In emphysema, inflammation from chronic irritants causes an immune response that triggers neutrophils to secrete protease elastase. This breaks down the elastin fibers responsible for the alveolar recoil, causing a decrease in ventilation. The protease also leads to destruction of the alveolar walls and capillary beds, which leads to a decrease in perfusion. The result decreases both ventilation and perfusion, resulting in a *matched VQ* deficit. This causes hypoxemia and hypercapnia (leading to respiratory acidosis). The loss of alveolar elasticity causes air trapping, meaning oxygen and carbon dioxide remain in the alveoli sac after expiration. This increasing end expiratory volume results in the barrel-chested appearance of the classic emphysema patient. The destruction of the alveolar walls increases the work of breathing, and the patient presents with symptoms of dyspnea and cachexia (hence the nickname "pink puffers" for emphysema).

Alpha-1 antitrypsin (AAT) is a protease inhibitor that protects the lungs from inflammation. Deficiency of AAT leads to destruction of the elastin fibers in the alveolar walls and the development of emphysema, generally at an early age. This is a genetic condition in which low levels of AAT reduce the ability of the lungs to protect themselves from inflammation caused by infection or irritants. If a nonsmoker younger than age 65 presents with a history of dyspnea, and COPD is suspected, a serum AAT test may be helpful in the diagnosis.

Diagnosis, Staging, and Intermittent Assessment

The reduced inspirational reserve volume (from air trapping) caused by COPD makes activities of daily living problematic, and tasks such as stair climbing may not be possible. People with a history of smoking (past or present), or those who have progressive difficulty breathing, a productive cough, and frequent upper respiratory infections should be suspected of having COPD. A pulmonary function test (PFT), often called *spirometry*, measures airflow over time and is used to confirm the diagnosis and classify the disease severity. There are two measurements of spirometry that are especially important in COPD diagnosis and staging. The forced vital capacity (FVC) is the total amount of air that a person can exhale after taking a deep breath; and the forced expiratory volume in 1 second (FEV1) gauges the amount of air that can be forced out of the lungs in the first second of expiration.

The PFT is useful in making a diagnosis of COPD by calculating the FEV1/FVC ratio. The obstructive nature of COPD reduces the FEV1 and the diagnosis is confirmed by an FEV1/FVC ratio of less than 0.7, or 70%. Staging of the disease severity compares the FEV1 measurement to a normal expected result. The FEV1 values of healthy individuals with the same age, gender, height, and race are calculated to provide the normal predicted value, and the patient's reading is rated in the form of a percentage. This measurement of airflow limitation is illustrated in the GOLD classification of airflow limitation severity following bronchodilator therapy (Fig. 7.1).

The stages of severity are based on spirometry measurements following administration of albuterol, a short-acting bronchodilator, in a metered-dose inhaler (MDI) of 100 mcg (1 puff). The albuterol inhalation is performed four times (this can be reduced to two times if significant side effects occur). The PFT measurement is performed 10 to 20 minutes following the last albuterol inhalation (Sim et al., 2017). Response to the bronchodilator helps to differentiate the underlying presence of persistent airflow obstruction indicating COPD. This is different from the obstructive findings of asthma, which are reversible and typically improve following albuterol bronchodilation.

Following diagnosis, it is advisable to intermittently assess symptoms that interfere with activities of daily living. The COPD Assessment Test (CAT) is a questionnaire the patient completes assessing the impact of COPD on their health (GlaxoSmithKline, n.d.). The CAT does not replace spirometry and does not diagnose or confirm a diagnosis. The CAT does offer a forum for shared decision-making discussions during the office visit. Additionally, the Modified Medical Research Council (mMRC) Dyspnea Scale may be used to assess symptom severity and functional limitations of daily activities due to dyspnea (MD+Calc, n.d.). These questionnaires provide a numeric value for the patient's self-assessment of their symptoms of breathlessness and help to quantify dyspnea levels in patients with COPD.

CLASSIFICATION OF AIRFLOW LIMITATION SEVERITY IN COPD (BASED ON POST-BRONCHODILATOR FEV₁)

In patients with FEV1/FVC < 0.70:

GOLD 1:	Mild	$FEV_1 \geq 80\%$ predicted
GOLD 2:	Moderate	$50\% \leq FEV_1 < 80\%$ predicted
GOLD 3:	Severe	$30\% \leq FEV_1 < 50\%$ predicted
GOLD 4:	Very Severe	$FEV_1 < 30\%$ predicted

• **Fig. 7.1** Classification of airflow limitation severity in COPD. (From Global Initiative for Chronic Obstructive Lung Disease [2020]. *Global strategy for the diagnosis, management, and prevention of chronic obstructive pulmonary disease [2020 Report]*. https://goldcopd.org/wp-content/uploads/2019/12/GOLD-2020-FINAL-ver1.2-03Dec19_WMV.pdf.)

COPD THERAPY

The goal of medication therapy is to improve the quality of life for patients by relieving and controlling symptoms, decreasing the frequency and severity of exacerbations, and improving tolerance of daily activities. Medications are classified by their primary action. Primary care providers must consider the benefits against the risk ratio, the cost, and the patient's ability to use the medication appropriately. Throughout this chapter, medications will focus on generic names rather than brands. Primary care providers should refer to manufacturer labeling regarding the pharmacokinetics, adverse effects, and contraindications of specific brands or delivery methods.

Bronchodilators

Bronchodilators relax smooth muscles, resulting in dilation of the airways. Types of bronchodilators include beta2-agonist, anticholinergic, and methylxanthine. Each medication has a different action, onset, and duration.

Beta2-Agonist Medications

Beta2-agonists can be short-acting or long-acting and stimulate the beta2-adrenergic receptors, which relax airway smooth muscle. Short-acting beta2-agonists are for intermittent or emergency use for bronchospasms, wheezing, or exacerbation symptoms. Long-acting beta2-agonists are used once or twice daily for control but are not useful for intermittent or emergency use due to their slow onset of action. Short-acting beta2-agonists are recommended as combination therapy, but not as monotherapy in COPD.

Short-Acting Beta2-Agonists (SABAs)

Albuterol Sulfate

Pharmacokinetics. Pharmacokinetic properties differ by formulation. In all forms, albuterol is excreted by the kidneys. No specific dose adjustments are required in patients with renal or hepatic impairment (Table 7.1). Administration with inhalation results in a half-life of about 4 to 6 hours.

Aerosol inhalation. Delivery is via an MDI. The onset of action is 5 to 10 minutes. The peak effect is reached in about 50 minutes. Duration is 3 to 6 hours.

Nebulizer inhalation. Delivery is via a nebulizer machine, tubing of desired length, and a mask or T-piece. The onset of action is less than 5 minutes. Peak effects occur between 60 and 120 minutes. Duration is 3 to 6 hours. Absorption rates are less than 20%.

Indications. As a bronchodilator, albuterol relieves bronchospasms and COPD exacerbations. Albuterol is not indicated as maintenance therapy.

Adverse Effects. Adverse effects are age, dose, and route dependent. Serious side effects include cardiac tachyarrhythmias, cardiac ischemia, palpitations, and paradoxical bronchospasm. Common adverse effects include nervousness, excitement, tremors, pharyngitis, and upper respiratory infections. Less common adverse effects include throat irritation, headache, tachycardia, dizziness, nausea, and vomiting. Hypersensitivity reactions including anaphylaxis have been reported.

Contraindications. Use caution in patients with a history of cardiovascular disease as they may experience arrythmias and electrocardiogram (ECG) changes (flattening of the T wave, prolongation of the QTc interval, ST-segment depression) and cause elevation in blood pressure, heart rate, and

TABLE 7.1   Beta2-Agonists

Category/ Medication	Indication	Dosage	Considerations and Monitoring
Short-Acting Beta2-Agonists (SABAs)			
Albuterol	Bronchospasm associated with COPD	**Inhalation aerosol 90 mcg/actuation:** *Adults:* 1–2 inhalations every 4–6 hr as needed. Maximum dosage: 12 actuations/day **Nebulized inhalation (various concentrations available):** *Adults:* 2.5 mg via oral inhalation delivered over 5–15 minutes every 6–8 hr as needed. Maximum dosage: 4 doses/day or 10 mg/day. **Immediate-release tablets, oral solution, or syrup:** *Adults:* 2–4 mg orally every 6–8 hr. Maximum dosage: 32 mg/day. **Extended-release tablets:** *Adults:* 4–8 mg orally every 12 hr. Maximum dosage: 32 mg/day.	Older adults: Monitor for cardiac symptoms and dysrhythmias. Optimal dosing during acute exacerbation not established: adjust based on clinical symptoms or development of adverse effects.
Levalbuterol	Bronchospasm associated with COPD	**Inhalation aerosol: 45 mcg/actuation:** *Adults:* 1–2 actuations (90 mcg) every 4–6 hr. **Nebulized inhalation: (various concentrations available):** *Adults:* 0.63–1.25 mg orally via nebulization three times daily every 6–8 hr.	Optimal dosage for the treatment of an acute COPD exacerbation is not established; adjust dosage based on clinical symptoms or the development of adverse effects.
Long-Acting Beta2-Agonists (LABAs)			
Salmeterol xinafoate	Maintenance treatment of COPD	**Inhalation 50 mcg/actuation:** *Adults:* 1 oral inhalation twice daily 12 hr apart. Maximum dosage: 1 inhalation every 12 hr.	Not indicated for acute bronchospasm or acute symptoms of COPD.
Formoterol fumarate	Maintenance treatment of COPD	**Nebulizer solution 20 mcg/2 mL:** *Adults:* 20 mcg inhaled by nebulizer in the morning and evening. Maximum dosage: 40 mcg/day.	
Indacaterol maleate	Maintenance treatment of COPD	**Inhalation: 75 mcg/1 capsule:** *Adults:* 75 mcg (1 capsule) oral inhalation once daily at the same time each day. Maximum dosage: 1 dose (75 mcg)/24 hr.	
Olodaterol	Maintenance treatment of COPD	**Inhalation: 2.5 mcg/actuation solution:** *Adults:* 2 oral inhalations (5 mcg) once daily at the same time each day.	

central nervous system (CNS) stimulation. Use with caution in patients with diabetes, glaucoma, hyperthyroidism, hypokalemia, renal impairment, and seizures. Avoid in patients with hypersensitivity to albuterol or levalbuterol. Avoid dry-powder inhalers (DPIs) in patients with milk protein allergies.

Monitoring. Monitor for symptom relief, PFTs, and laboratory studies (including glucose, potassium, and renal function). Observe for adverse effects and changes in cardiovascular status evidenced by tachyarrhythmias and blood pressure alterations. Observe for hypersensitivity reactions (anaphylaxis).

Long-Acting Beta2-Agonists (LABAs)

Salmeterol Xinafoate

Pharmacokinetics. Salmeterol acts within the lungs, resulting in low system levels of the medication. Salmeterol is extensively metabolized in the liver by hydroxylation to α-hydroxysalmeterol. After inhalation, initial bronchodilation begins within 1 hour. The peak bronchodilation effect (increase in PEFR and FEV1) occurs in 2 to 5 hours and lasts about 12 hours. The half-life is about 5 hours. Excretion is primarily in the feces.

Indications. Salmeterol is approved for the twice-daily maintenance and prevention of bronchospasms associated with COPD (see Table 7.1). Salmeterol is not recommended to treat acute bronchospasm. Salmeterol improves lung volume (FEV1) and relieves associated symptoms of COPD. Salmeterol (as Serevent Diskus) has not been shown to increase the risk of death in patients with mild to moderate COPD, as was noted with asthma. In patients with very severe COPD, a LABA in combination with inhaled corticosteroids (ICSs) and/or long-acting muscarinic antagonists (LAMAs) is recommended (GOLD, 2020).

Adverse Effects. The most common adverse effects are headache, musculoskeletal pain, nasal congestion, throat irritation, pharyngitis, cough, and rhinitis. The LABA medications have the potential for serious adverse effects similar to SABAs. These include cardiovascular effects, prolonged QT interval, hypersensitivity reactions, tremors, paradoxical bronchospasm, and death.

Contraindications. Avoid in patients with severe hypersensitivity to milk proteins, salmeterol, or any of the components of the product. Salmeterol use with cytochrome (CYP) 3A4 inhibitors may increase risk of cardiovascular effects. Evaluate risk versus benefit in patients on monoamine oxidase inhibitors (MAOIs) or tricyclics (wait at least 14 days before starting LABA). Use with caution in patients taking beta blockers, non–potassium-sparing diuretics, or QTc interval-prolonging medications. Patients with congenital long QT syndrome or cardiovascular disease may experience arrhythmias or ECG changes (flattening of the T wave, prolongation of the QT interval, or ST-segment depression). Salmeterol may cause elevation in blood pressure and heart rate and result in CNS stimulation. Use with caution in patients with diabetes, glaucoma, hyperthyroidism, hypokalemia, renal impairment, pheochromocytoma, seizure disorder, or unusual responsiveness to other sympathomimetic amines.

Monitoring. Assess for improvement in symptoms and PFTs. Monitor for adverse effects, changes in vital signs, and alterations in blood chemistries. Monitor patients with hepatic impairment since salmeterol is metabolized in the liver.

Anticholinergic/Antimuscarinic Medications

Anticholinergics are also called muscarinic antagonists. They are available as a short-acting muscarinic antagonist (SAMA) or long-acting muscarinic antagonist (LAMA). Anticholinergics have a slower onset of action than beta2-agonists, and because of this, they are not intended as rescue inhalers.

Short-Acting Muscarinic Antagonists (SAMAs)
Ipratropium
Pharmacokinetics. Use of an MDI may result in less medication reaching the lungs and more reaching the gastrointestinal (GI) tract. Ipratropium is not readily absorbed into systemic circulation. The initial onset of action after inhalation is within 3 to 30 minutes, with a half-life of 2 hours. Maximum bronchodilation occurs within 90 to 180 minutes. Excretion occurs via the urine.

Indications. Ipratropium is indicated for maintenance therapy of cholinergic-mediated bronchospasm (Table 7.2). Ipratropium decreases smooth muscle contractility, resulting in bronchodilation and relief of bronchospasms. For patients with mild, stable COPD, inhaled or nebulized ipratropium may be used as a first-line monotherapy, but combination therapy with SABAs is more helpful for COPD exacerbations (GOLD, 2020).

Adverse Effects. Adverse effects related to MDI use include potentially life-threatening paradoxical bronchospasm. In this event, stop ipratropium and use an alternate therapy. Adverse effects reported with nebulizer use include bronchospasm and urticaria. Adverse effects common to both delivery methods include bronchitis, exacerbation of COPD, sinusitis, headache, dyspepsia, urinary tract infection (UTI), dyspnea, and flu-like symptoms. Ipratropium is a derivative of atropine, with a similar chemical structure, which may result in dizziness and blurred vision.

Contraindications. Ipratropium is contraindicated in patients with a previous history of paradoxical bronchospasms, and in patients who have hypersensitivity to atropine or its derivatives. Prescribe with caution in patients with closed-angle glaucoma, bladder or urinary obstructions, cardiac arrhythmias, or older patients, due to the anticholinergic effects. Advise patients to be aware of dizziness or blurred vision, and to take caution while driving or operating machinery.

Monitoring. Routinely monitor for the development of adverse effects. Monitor for vision changes, urinary retention, and cardiac arrhythmias. Monitor PFTs and movement of symptoms.

Long-Acting Muscarinic Receptors (LAMAs)
Tiotropium
Pharmacokinetics. Tiotropium is available as a soft-mist inhaled solution or a DPI. The pharmacokinetics of each formulation are relatively similar, except for the level of bioavailability:
- Soft-mist inhalation solution (Spiriva Respimat): Following inhalation, about 33% of the medication is available.
- DPI (Spiriva HandiHaler): Following inhalation, about 20% of the medication is available.

For both delivery methods, the maximum plasma concentrations are reached in 5 to 7 minutes. The half-life elimination is about 25 hours. Hepatic metabolism occurs via CYP 2D6 and CYP 3A4 and metabolism is via the urine. Important considerations are impaired renal function in the

TABLE 7.2   Anticholinergics/Antimuscarinics

Category/Medication	Indication	Dosage	Considerations and Monitoring
Short-Acting Muscarinic Antagonist (SAMA)			
Ipratropium bromide	Bronchospasm due to COPD	**Inhalation aerosol: 17 mcg/actuation:** *Adults:* 2 oral actuations three to four times daily at least 4 hr apart. Maximum dosage: 12 actuations/day.	Titrate dose depending on patient response or the development of adverse effects.
		Nebulizer solution: *Adults:* 500 mcg (1 vial) by nebulized inhalation three or four times daily at least 6–8 hr apart. Maximum dosage: 2000 mcg/day via nebulizer.	
Long-Acting Muscarinic Antagonists (LAMAs)			
Aclidinium bromide	Maintenance treatment of COPD	**Inhalation powder: 400 mcg/actuation:** *Adults:* 1 oral actuation twice daily every 12 hr at the same time. Maximum dosage: 2 actuations per day.	Do not use LAMAs with another LAMA. LAMAs may be monotherapy or combined with LABA or ICS.
Tiotropium	Maintenance treatment of COPD Reduce exacerbations of COPD	**Inhalation powder: 18 mcg/capsule:** *Adults:* 2 oral inhalations of 1 capsule (18 mcg) once daily. Maximum dosage: 1 capsule (18 mcg) in 24 hr.	
		Inhalation spray: 2.5 mcg/actuation: *Adults:* 2 oral actuations once daily. Maximum dosage: 1 dose daily.	
Umeclidinium	Maintenance treatment of COPD	**Inhalation powder: 62.5 mcg/actuation:** *Adults:* 1 oral actuation once daily. Maximum dosage: 1 dose every 24 hr.	
Revefenacin	COPD	**Nebulizer solution:** *Adults:* 175 mcg unit-dose vial once daily by oral inhalation using mouthpiece. Maximum dosage: 1 vial per day.	Avoid use with hepatic impairment.

older population, in which the medication clearance may be reduced, resulting in increased plasma concentrations.

Indications. Tiotropium (as Spiriva HandiHaler or Spiriva Respimat) is a long-acting antimuscarinic medication approved for once-daily maintenance therapy and to reduce exacerbations of COPD (see Table 7.2). Tiotropium is not used to treat acute symptoms or bronchospasms. LAMAs are more effective than LABAs at relieving COPD exacerbations (GOLD, 2020).

Adverse Effects. In patients with COPD, the most common adverse effects were upper respiratory tract infections, pharyngitis, cough, dry mouth, and sinusitis. Less common adverse effects resulting from the anticholinergic properties were constipation, dizziness, and cognitive problems.

Serious adverse effects include paradoxical bronchospasms and hypersensitivity reactions.

Contraindications. Avoid in patients with hypersensitivity to tiotropium, ipratropium, or any component of the product. This medication should be used with caution in patients with narrow-angle glaucoma, urinary retention, severe renal impairment, and the concomitant use of other anticholinergic medications.

Monitoring. Primary care providers and patients should be alert for signs and symptoms of acute narrow-angle glaucoma. Renal status should be monitored, but no dose adjustment is needed in renal insufficiency. Screen patients for anticholinergic effects. Monitor for improvement in PFTs, symptoms, and pulmonary status.

Methylxanthines

Theophylline is the most well-known methylxanthine. In COPD, the use of theophylline has become limited as guidelines favor the use of beta2-agonists and anticholinergics. Theophylline is a bronchodilator, which suppresses the response of the airway to stimuli. It has significant and serious adverse effects that require careful monitoring of health status and therapeutic blood levels.

Theophylline

Pharmacokinetics. Pharmacokinetic principles of theophylline will center on the oral extended-release 12-hour tablet, the oral extended-release 24-hour tablet, and the oral elixir (solution). Absorption varies between 8 and 12 hours, with food intake delaying the rate of absorption of the extended-release tablets only. Food does not affect the amount of absorption. Peak concentration occurs in 1 to 2 hours. Hepatic metabolism via the liver uses CYP 450, CYP 1A2, CYP 2E1, and CYP 3A3; excretion is in the urine. Elimination half-life ranges from 1 to 10 hours and is affected by age, disease process, other drugs, smoking tobacco or marijuana, and pregnancy. Smoking marijuana may increase the metabolic clearance of theophylline, therefore decreasing its effect.

Indications. Theophylline is a bronchodilator approved for the management of COPD (Table 7.3). Theophylline is rarely indicated as initial therapy but may be considered if other treatments are not adequately controlling symptoms (GOLD, 2020). The recommended therapeutic serum concentration is 10 to 15 mcg/mL per the U.S. Food and Drug Administration (FDA), and the dose is adjusted to maintain therapeutic response.

Adverse Effects. Adverse effects are possible when the medication is within therapeutic range. These include tachycardia, headache, nausea, vomiting, insomnia, restlessness, tremors, and seizures. Theophylline may cause arrhythmia, seizures, or worsening gastroesophageal reflux or GI ulcers. Serious adverse effects include atrial fibrillation, tachyarrhythmias, Stevens-Johnson syndrome, and intracranial hemorrhage.

Contraindications. Use theophylline with caution in patients with cystic fibrosis, cardiovascular disease, thyroid disease, peptic ulcer disease, or moderate to severe hepatic impairment. Theophylline may increase glucose, uric acid, lipids, and urine-free cortisol excretion. Theophylline may decrease triiodothyronine (T3) levels. Older adults may require cautious titration due to decreased hepatic function with aging. Numerous drug–drug interactions may occur (Table 7.4). Erythromycin can delay theophylline's metabolism and increase serum plasma levels. Some dosage forms may contain propylene glycol, which has been known to cause hyperosmolality, lactic acidosis, seizures, and respiratory depression.

Monitoring. Monitor serum concentration of theophylline after initiation of therapy, when status or treatment regimens change, and yearly. Patients who smoke will need a higher dose of theophylline due to polycyclic hydrocarbons in tobacco

TABLE 7.3 Methylxanthines

Medication	Indication	Dosage	Considerations and Monitoring
Theophylline	Maintenance treatment of COPD COPD exacerbations	**Extended-release tablet or 24 hr extended release: 100, 200, 300, 400, 450, and 600 mg:** *Adults:* 300 mg/day orally in divided doses every 8-12 hr. If tolerated, after 3 days, increase to 400 mg/day orally in divided doses every 8-12 hr; if tolerated, after 3 days, increase to 600 mg/day orally in divided doses every 8-12 hr. Maximum dosage: 400–1600 mg/day. *Adults ≥60 yr:* 300 mg/day orally in divided doses every 8–12 hr. If tolerated, after 3 days, increase dose to 400 mg orally every 8–12 hr. Maximum dosage: 400 mg/day. **Elixir/solution: 80 mg/15 mL:** *Initial:* 300 mg/day orally in divided doses every 8–12 hr. If tolerated, after 3 days, increase to 400 mg/day orally in divided doses every 8–12 hr; if tolerated, after 3 days, increase to 600 mg/day orally in divided doses every 8–12 hr.	In general, not a first-line treatment for maintenance therapy or treatment of exacerbations due to narrow therapeutic window and risk of toxicity and side effects. Calculate dose based on body weight. Adjust dosage based on serum theophylline concentrations to prevent theophylline toxicity. Use caution and adjust dosing with hepatic impairment.

TABLE 7.4   Potential Interactions[a]

Medication	Interactions
Systemic steroids	Rotavirus vaccine: Increased risk of infection by the live vaccine
	Desmopressin: Increased risk of severe hyponatremia
	Select fluoroquinolones: Increased risk of tendon rupture
	Digoxin: False increases in digoxin levels due to digoxin assay interference
Roflumilast	Inhibitors of CYP 3A4 or dual inhibitors of CYP 3A4 and CYP 1A2: Increased risk of adverse reactions
	Oral contraceptives containing gestodene and ethinyl estradiol: Increased risk of adverse reactions
	CYP P450 inducers: Decreased therapeutic effectiveness of roflumilast
Fluticasone/ umeclidinium/ vilanterol	Strong CYP 3A4 inhibitors: Increased systemic corticosteroid and cardiovascular effects
Formoterol/ budesonide	Strong CYP 3A4 inhibitors: Increased systemic exposure to budesonide
Theophylline	Alcohol, caffeine, cimetidine, fluoroquinolones: Increased serum theophylline levels
	Phenobarbital, phenytoin, and rifampin, tobacco, marijuana: Decreased serum theophylline levels

[a]There are many other drug–drug interactions. The primary care provider should check all drug interactions among the patient's medications before prescribing any new medications.

smoke affecting CYP 1A2. Monitor and reduce the dose of theophylline if the patient stops smoking; smoking cessation increases serum theophylline concentration, which increases the risk of severe and potentially fatal theophylline toxicity. Monitor PFTs, vital signs, signs of adverse reactions, and toxicity.

Corticosteroids

Corticosteroids reduce inflammation in the airways when administered on a fixed schedule. Corticosteroids may be administered in oral form or by inhalation (MDI, DPI, or nebulizer). Prior to initiating therapy, establish baseline assessment of symptoms and PFTs.

Oral Corticosteroids

Prednisone

Pharmacokinetics. Pharmacokinetics provided in this section are based on oral regular-release tablets. Peak concentration is reached in 2 hours and the half-life is 2 to 3 hours. Extensive liver metabolism of prednisone by 11-β-HSD liver enzymes produces prednisolone, which is eliminated by the kidneys. No dosing adjustments are required for older patients or those with renal or kidney impairment.

Indications. Corticosteroids are useful for the treatment of acute COPD exacerbations (Table 7.5). Oral corticosteroids are not recommended for maintenance therapy of COPD. Titration or dose packs are the more common method of delivery in the treatment of exacerbations. Refer to GOLD for specific information.

Adverse Effects. The frequency and seriousness of adverse effects depend on dose and duration of therapy. Adverse effects impact multiple body systems, including the cardiovascular, endocrine, ophthalmic, GI, hematologic, immunologic, musculoskeletal, and neurological systems. Some serious adverse effects include steroid psychosis, steroid myopathy, adrenal insufficiency, seizures, and hyperglycemia.

Contraindications. Use is contraindicated in patients with hypersensitivity to corticosteroids or any component

TABLE 7.5   Systemic Corticosteroids

Medication	Indication	Dosage	Considerations and Monitoring
Prednisone	Management of COPD exacerbation in outpatient setting	*Adults:* 40 mg orally once daily for 5–7 days.	Systemic corticosteroids are not FDA approved, but GOLD recommends use for exacerbations. Taper dosing based on clinical response and patient history. BEERS Criteria alert for delirium.
Methylprednisolone	Management of COPD exacerbation in outpatient setting	**Tablet 2, 4, 8, 16, 32 mg:** *Adults:* 4–48 mg orally in 4 divided doses.	
Prednisolone	Management of COPD exacerbation in outpatient setting	*Adults:* 40 mg daily for 5 days.	

of the product. Common interactions include nonsteroidal antiinflammatory drugs (NSAIDs), antiinfectives, immunosuppressants, diuretics, and anticoagulants. Avoid the administration of live vaccines during or for 1 month after immunosuppressive therapy. As with other corticosteroids, observe for increased adverse effects in patients with immune and adrenocortical dysfunction, recent myocardial infarction or cardiovascular disease, endocrine disorders, thyroid disease, and ocular disease. Corticosteroids can mask or increase the severity of fungal, viral, or bacterial infections.

Monitoring. Monitor for adverse effects, particularly in patients receiving long-term therapy. Monitor for improvement in symptoms, frequency of SABA use, and PFTs. Monitor for cardiac tachyarrhythmias, hypertension, vasculitis, thrombosis, electrolyte imbalances, lipid changes, and elevated liver enzymes. In patients concomitantly on digoxin therapy, monitor for false increases in digoxin levels. Frequently monitor glucose levels in diabetic patients and adjust therapies as needed. Also monitor intraocular pressure in patients who are glaucoma suspects. Bone mineral density should be assessed prior to initiation of therapy and periodically.

Inhaled Corticosteroids (ICS)

Inhaled corticosteroids are not FDA approved as monotherapy in the treatment of COPD. Combining low-dose ICS with bronchodilators decreases the frequency of exacerbations and slows the progressive decline in lung function (FEV1) but does not reduce overall mortality (Calverley et al., 2018; Izquierdo & Cosio, 2018). Inhaled corticosteroids will be included with the discussion of combination medications.

Combination Medications

Short-Acting Muscarinic Antagonist/Short-Acting Beta2-Agonist (SAMA/SABA)

Ipratropium/Albuterol
Pharmacokinetics. Bronchodilation begins 15 minutes following MDI and nebulized treatments. However, MDI inhalation has a peak response time of 1 hour and a duration of 4 to 5 hours. Nebulized treatments peak at 90 minutes with a slightly shorter duration of 3 to 5 hours. Metabolism of both medications is via the liver and excretion is via the kidneys. Half-life of ipratropium is 2 hours, and half-life of albuterol is 4 hours via MDI and 6.7 hours when nebulized.

Indications. This is a combination therapy containing ipratropium (a SAMA) and albuterol (a SABA) for maintenance and exacerbations of COPD (Table 7.6). Together, these medications increase bronchodilation of the airways to a greater extent than if used alone. Available delivery methods are inhaler and nebulizer.

Adverse Effects. The respiratory and neurological systems are targets of adverse effects. These include bronchitis, upper respiratory infections, dyspnea, cough, pharyngitis, and sinusitis. Serious adverse effects are noted in the cardiovascular, immunologic, and ophthalmic systems. Hypersensitivity reactions may also occur. Primary care providers should consider adverse reactions specific to the individual medication in the combination of ipratropium and albuterol.

Contraindications. Avoid ipratropium and albuterol combination use in patients with hypersensitivity to albuterol, ipratropium, atropine or its derivatives, or any other component of the product. Due to the combined LABA and LAMA adverse effects, avoid use in patients with a history of cardiovascular disease, seizures, thyrotoxicosis, narrow-angle glaucoma, prostatic hyperplasia, or bladder-neck obstruction. Evaluate risk versus benefit in patients on MAOIs or tricyclics (wait 14 days before starting LABA). Use with caution in patients taking beta blockers, non–potassium-sparing diuretics, or QTc interval-prolonging medications.

Monitoring. Older patients require monitoring as they are more susceptible to adverse effects, especially cardiovascular monitoring. Observe for improved symptoms, lung function, and PFTs. Laboratory monitoring includes blood chemistry for glucose, potassium, and renal function.

Long-Acting Beta2-Agonist/Long-Acting Muscarinic Antagonist (LABA/LAMA)

Umeclidinium Bromide/Vilanterol Trifenatate
Pharmacokinetics. Onset of action occurs within 27 minutes following inhalation. Peak concentrations are reached within 5 to 15 minutes, and peak effects (measured by FEV1) occur within 6 hours. Half-life of the combination medication is 11 hours. Umeclidinium (metabolized by CYP 2D6) and vilanterol (metabolized by CYP 3A4) are excreted in the urine and feces.

Indications. This combination medication contains umeclidinium (a LAMA) and vilanterol (a LABA). Combination LAMA/LABA therapy is more effective at reducing exacerbations, improving lung function, and decreasing dyspnea than monotherapy (GOLD, 2020). Umeclidinium/vilanterol is approved for long-term maintenance therapy in adult patients with COPD. Umeclidinium/vilanterol is a once-daily (every 24 hours) DPI (see Table 7.6). This combination is not for use as a rescue inhaler during acute bronchospasms. No dose adjustments are necessary in older patients, renal insufficiency, or mild to moderate hepatic impairment (severe hepatic impairment is not well studied). Patients prescribed umeclidinium/vilanterol should also be prescribed a short-acting beta2-agonist (inhaled) for relief of acute symptoms.

Adverse Effects. The most common adverse reactions are pharyngitis, diarrhea, and extremity pain. Less common effects included upper respiratory and sinus infections, constipation, musculoskeletal pain, and general chest pain. Serious postmarketing reports include palpitations,

TABLE 7.6   Combination Medications

Category/ Medication	Indication	Dosage	Considerations and Monitoring
Short-Acting Muscarinic Antagonist/Short-Acting Beta2-Agonist (SAMA/SABA)			
Ipratropium/albuterol	Treatment of COPD patients requiring addition of second bronchodilator	**Inhalation aerosol: 20 mcg ipratropium bromide/100 mg albuterol per 3 mL:** *Adult:* 1 vial by oral inhalation every 4–6 hr. Maximum dosage: 6 vials/day. **Inhalation nebulizer: 0.5 mg ipratropium bromide/2.5 mg albuterol per 3 mL vial:** *Adult:* One vial by oral inhalation every 4–6 hr. Maximum dosage: 6 vials/day.	Titrate to symptoms and adverse effects.
Long-Acting Beta2-Agonist/Long-Acting Muscarinic Antagonist (LABA/LAMA)			
Glycopyrrolate/formoterol fumarate	Treatment of COPD	**Inhalation aerosol: 9 mcg glycopyrrolate/4.8 mcg formoterol fumarate per 1 actuation:** *Adults:* 2 oral actuations twice daily. Maximum dosage: 2 actuations twice daily.	Do not use in combination with another LABA or LAMA.
Umeclidinium/vilanterol	Treatment of COPD	**Inhalation powder: 62.5 mcg umeclidinium bromide/25 mcg vilanterol trifenatate per actuation:** *Adult:* 1 oral actuation once daily, taken at the same time every day. Maximum dosage: 1 actuation every 24 hr.	
Tiotropium/olodaterol	Treatment of COPD	**Inhalation aerosol: 2.5 mcg tiotropium/2.5 mcg olodaterol per actuation:** *Adult:* 2 oral actuations once daily at the same time each day. Maximum dosage: 2 actuations in 24 hr.	
Long-Acting Beta2-Adrenergic/Inhaled Corticosteroids (LABA/ICS)			
Budesonide/formoterol	Treatment of COPD	**Inhalation aerosol: 160 mcg budesonide/4.5 mcg formoterol per actuation:** *Adults:* 2 oral actuations every 12 hr. Maximum dosage: 2 actuations per day.	Do not use in combination with another LABA or LAMA.
Fluticasone/salmeterol	Maintenance of COPD	**Inhalation powder diskus: 250 mcg Fluticasone/50 mcg salmeterol per actuation:** *Adults:* 1 oral actuation every 12 hr. Maximum dosage: 2 actuations per day.	
Fluticasone furoate/ vilanterol	Maintenance of COPD Reduction of exacerbations of COPD	**Inhalation powder: 100 mcg fluticasone furoate/25 mcg vilanterol per actuation:** *Adults:* 1 inhalation once daily. Maximum dosage: 1 actuation per day.	
Inhaled Corticosteroids, Long-Acting Muscarinic Antagonists, and Long-Acting Beta2-Adrenergic Combinations (ICS/LAMA/LABA)			
Fluticasone furoate/ umeclidinium/ vilanterol	Maintenance of COPD	**Inhalation powder: 100 mcg fluticasone/62.5 mcg umeclidinium/25 mcg vilanterol per inhalation:** *Adults:* 1 oral inhalation once daily at the same time every day. Maximum dosage: 1 inhalation per 24 hr.	Do not use in combination with another LABA or LAMA.

TABLE 7.6	Combination Medications—cont'd		
Category/ Medication	Indication	Dosage	Considerations and Monitoring
Budesonide/glycopyrrolate/formoterol fumarate	Maintenance of COPD	**Inhalation aerosol: 160 mcg budesonide/9 mcg glycopyrrolate/4.8 mcg formoterol per actuation:** *Adults:* 2 oral actuations twice daily in the morning and evening. Maximum dosage: 2 actuations twice daily.	

eye disorders, hypersensitivity reactions, tremor, anxiety, dysuria, urinary retention, and paradoxical bronchospasm.

Contraindications. The use of umeclidinium/vilanterol is contraindicated in patients with severe hypersensitivity to milk proteins or any components of umeclidinium or vilanterol. Avoid umeclidinium/vilanterol use in patients with a history of cardiovascular disease, seizures, thyrotoxicosis, narrow-angle glaucoma, prostatic hyperplasia, or bladder-neck obstruction. Evaluate risk versus benefit in patients on MAOIs or tricyclics (wait 14 days before starting LABA). Use with caution in patients taking beta blockers, non–potassium-sparing diuretics, or QTc interval-prolonging medications. Vilanterol may result in adverse effects common to other LABAs (altered vital signs, significant ECG changes). The use of umeclidinium/vilanterol at higher doses, or in conjunction with other LABA therapy, may result in cardiovascular effects, overdose, or death. Significant drug–drug interactions occur with concomitant use with CYP 3A4 inhibitors (see Table 7.4).

Monitoring. Monitor for improvement in symptoms, PFTs, overuse of SABA inhalers, and adverse effects. No specific laboratory monitoring is recommended by the manufacturer; however, hypokalemia and hyperglycemia have been reported with this medication. As with other LABA medications, vital signs should be monitored.

Long-Acting Beta2-Adrenergic/Inhaled Corticosteroids (LABA/ICS)

Formoterol/Budesonide

Pharmacokinetics

Formoterol. Following inhalation, rapid absorption occurs. Peak plasma concentrations are reached within 5 to 10 minutes. Hepatic metabolism is via CYP 2D6, CYP 2C19, CYP 2C9, and CYP 2A6 pathways. Single-dose half-life is about 8 hours. Renal excretion surpasses fecal excretion.

Budesonide. Peak plasma concentrations are reached in 20 minutes, with a half-life of 2 to 3 hours. Hepatic metabolism is extensive, with metabolites formed via CYP 450 and CYP 3A4. Metabolite excretion occurs in the urine and feces.

Indications. The combination inhaler contains formoterol (a LABA) and budesonide (an ICS). This medication

is approved as a maintenance therapy for COPD (see Table 7.6). It also reduces COPD exacerbations and may be used as the initial therapeutic agent for patients at high risk for exacerbations or in patients with blood eosinophil counts greater than 200 cells/microliter. This medication is not recommended for acute bronchospasm. No dosage adjustments are recommended for the older patient or patients with renal or hepatic impairments.

Adverse Effects. The most common adverse reactions resulting from the combination of formoterol/budesonide were headaches, nasopharyngitis, oral candidiasis, bronchitis, sinusitis, and viral upper respiratory infections. Adverse effects resulting from formoterol include all those commonly noted with all corticosteroids. Hypersensitivity reactions may be immediate or delayed.

Contraindications. Contraindications to formoterol/budesonide result from the individual medication classifications. Consider each medication classification prior to prescribing. Evaluate risk versus benefit in patients on MAOIs or tricyclics (wait 14 days before starting LABA). Use with caution in patients taking beta blockers, non–potassium-sparing diuretics, or QTc interval-prolonging medications. Use with caution in patients with narrow-angle glaucoma, urinary retention, prostatic hyperplasia, bladder-neck obstruction, seizure disorders, thyrotoxicosis, or those who are unusually responsive to sympathomimetic amines. No drug–drug interactions have been studied with the combination of formoterol/budesonide. In patients with asthma and COPD overlap syndrome, the use of long-acting beta2-adrenergic agonists increases the risk of asthma-related death.

Monitoring. Monitor for improvement in symptoms, PFTs, frequency and severity of exacerbations, overuse of SABA inhalers, and adverse effects. Observe for systemic corticosteroid adverse effects.

Inhaled Corticosteroids, Long-Acting Muscarinic Antagonists, and Long-Acting Beta2-Adrenergic Combinations (ICS/LAMA/LABA)

This combination is referred to in the guidelines as LABA, LAMA and ICS, but medication resources place the corticosteroid in the first position. For the purposes of this section, the combination order will be referred to as ICS, LAMA, and LABA.

Fluticasone/Umeclidinium/Vilanterol

Pharmacokinetics. No pharmacokinetic studies have been conducted with the three-drug combination. Pharmacokinetic information is included for each drug.

- Fluticasone furoate: Peak concentration levels are reached in 30 to 60 minutes with a half-life of 24 hours. Extensive hepatic metabolism occurs via CYP 3A4. Excretion is primarily in the feces.
- Umeclidinium: Peak concentration levels are reached within 15 minutes with a half-life of 11 hours. Extensive hepatic metabolism occurs via CYP 450 and CYP 2D6. Excretion is primarily in the feces.
- Vilanterol: Peak concentration levels are reached in 5 to 15 minutes with a half-life of 11 hours. Extensive hepatic metabolism occurs via CYP 3A4 and is a substrate for the P-gp transporter. Excretion is primarily in the feces.

No drug–drug interaction studies have been conducted with the combination of fluticasone, umeclidinium, and vilanterol.

Indications. This medication is a combination of fluticasone (an ICS), umeclidinium (a LAMA), and vilanterol (a LABA). This combination medication is approved as a step-up therapy for patients already using a LABA/LAMA combination who continue to have COPD exacerbations (see Table 7.6). It is not intended as a rescue inhaler or for use in patients with acute, life-threatening, or deteriorating COPD.

Adverse Effects. The most common adverse effects are headache, back pain, bad taste in the mouth, diarrhea, cough, oropharyngeal pain, and gastroenteritis. Lesser reported adverse effects include oropharyngeal candidiasis, upper and lower respiratory tract infections, dysphonia, and UTIs. Potential serious reactions are rare but may include paradoxical bronchospasms, hypersensitivity reactions, and cardiovascular effects.

Contraindications. This medication is contraindicated in patients with severe hypersensitivity to milk proteins or fluticasone furoate, umeclidinium, vilanterol, or any of its components. Primary care providers should consider each medication within the combination when prescribing and assess the patient history for contraindication to each medication. Evaluate risk versus benefit in patients on MAOIs or tricyclics (wait 14 days before starting LABA).

Use with caution in patients taking beta blockers, non–potassium-sparing diuretics, or QTc interval-prolonging medications. Use with caution in patients with narrow-angle glaucoma, urinary retention, prostatic hyperplasia, bladder-neck obstruction, convulsive disorders, thyrotoxicosis, or those who are unusually responsive to sympathomimetic amines.

Monitoring. Monitoring parameters include those from each medication within the combination.

Phosphodiesterase-4 Inhibitor (PDE-4)

Roflumilast

Pharmacokinetics. Extensive liver metabolism occurs via CYP 450, CYP 3A4, and CYP 1A2. Steady-state concentration is reached in 4 days, the half-life is 17 hours, and the active metabolite lasts for 30 hours. Roflumilast is excreted in the urine.

Indications. Roflumilast is approved to treat adults with severe to very severe COPD with frequent exacerbations not controlled by a LABA (Table 7.7). Roflumilast increases cellular levels of cyclic adenosine monophosphate (cAMP), which reduces inflammation, cough, and excessive mucus production in the lung. The use of roflumilast may decrease the risk for exacerbations in patients with severe, chronic COPD. Roflumilast is not intended for the treatment of acute bronchospasm.

Adverse Effects. Adverse effects include weight loss, diarrhea, nausea, reduced appetite, headache, back pain, and dizziness. Psychiatric effects include insomnia, anxiety, depression, and suicidal ideations. Adverse effects in postmarketing literature include hypersensitivity reactions including angioedema, urticaria, and rash, though no frequency or causality is reported.

Contraindications. Roflumilast should not be used in combination with tiotropium, a LABA, or an inhaled glucocorticoid. Roflumilast is contraindicated in patients with moderate to severe hepatic impairment (Child-Pugh B or C). No dosage adjustment is necessary for older patients or patients with renal insufficiency. Safety in pregnancy has not been established.

Monitoring. Prior to prescribing roflumilast, evaluate patients for a history of psychiatric disorders. Monitor for depression, behavior changes, and suicidality. Monitor for weight loss at each follow-up and evaluate the need to discontinue medication. Monitor PFTs, symptom severity, and the frequency of exacerbations.

TABLE 7.7	Phosphodiesterase-4 Inhibitors (PDE-4)		
Medication	**Indication**	**Dosage**	**Considerations and Monitoring**
Roflumilast	Prevention of severe COPD exacerbations in patients with severe COPD with frequent exacerbations not controlled by LABA	**Tablet:** *Adults:* 250-mcg tablet orally once daily for 4 weeks, then 500-mcg tablet orally once daily. Maximum dosage: 500 mcg daily.	Use in combination with at least one long-acting bronchodilator. Caution with hepatic impairment.

Mucolytic Agents

GOLD (2020) offers limited data on the use of mucolytic agents in COPD. The guidelines include three medications: erdosteine, carbocysteine, and N-acetylcysteine. In patients not on ICS, mucolytics may offer improvements in COPD exacerbations. Erdosteine is currently undergoing studies in the United States. In the RESTORE study, researchers noted a decrease in the rate and severity of COPD exacerbations in patients with moderate to severe disease (Calverley et al., 2019). Carbocysteine is not FDA approved, though off-label use is indicated for acute bronchitis.

Acetylcysteine (N-acetylcysteine)

Pharmacokinetics. The peak mucolytic response occurs 45 minutes after inhalation and lasts almost 2 hours. Metabolism is via the liver and intestinal wall. Half-life varies by formula. Half-life data are not available for inhaled acetylcysteine.

Indications. Acetylcysteine is used in nebulizer form as an adjunct therapy in patients with chronic pulmonary disorders and is effective at reducing COPD exacerbations (Table 7.8). The mucolytic effects decrease mucus viscosity, resulting in thinner secretions.

Adverse Effects. The most common adverse effects are vomiting and hypersensitivity reactions. Pruritus, rash, urticaria, diarrhea, and nausea are considered less frequent common reactions. Serious adverse effects include bronchospasm and respiratory distress, cardiovascular changes, and status epilepticus.

Contraindications. Use is contraindicated in patients with hypersensitivity to acetylcysteine. Use is also contraindicated in pregnancy or breastfeeding. Weigh benefits against potential risk.

Monitoring. Monitor for the risk of airway obstruction due to increase in liquified secretions. Assess the patient's ability to effectively produce secretions with cough. Monitor for bronchospasm.

Prescriber Considerations for COPD Therapy

Clinical Practice Guidelines

GOLD (2020) recommendations provide an international standard of practice in the pharmacologic management of COPD. These comprehensive guidelines are a beneficial resource in developing a maintenance plan or in treating exacerbations. Providers using the standards established in GOLD decreased overtreatment with inhaled corticosteroids and undertreatment with inhaled bronchodilators (Grewe et al., 2020).

Clinical Reasoning for COPD Therapy

Consider the individual patient's health problem requiring therapy. The goals of COPD management are to reduce respiratory symptoms of exacerbations including dyspnea, wheezing, and increased cough. It is important to improve immediate lung function, slow long-term decline, and improve physical activity and quality of life. Bronchodilators, corticosteroids, and antibiotics are used to manage more than 80% of COPD exacerbations in an outpatient setting (GOLD, 2020). In symptomatic patients with hypoxemia at rest, supplemental oxygen is helpful to improve quality of life and survival.

Determine the desired therapeutic outcome based on the degree of pulmonary impairment. The overall therapeutic outcome is symptom relief. Symptoms and PFTs are used to classify the stage of disease progression. There are four stages of severity: Stage 1 (mild COPD); Stage II (moderate COPD); Stage III (severe COPD); and Stage IV (very severe COPD) (Fig. 7.1).

Assess the medication selected for its appropriateness for an individual patient by considering the medication's side effects

---

BOOKMARK THIS!

Clinical Guidelines

- Global Initiative for Chronic Obstructive Lung Disease. Global Strategy for the Diagnosis, Management, and Prevention of Chronic Obstructive Pulmonary Disease. 2020 Report. https://goldcopd.org/
- Global Initiative for Chronic Obstructive Lung Disease. Pocket Guide to COPD Diagnosis, Management, and Prevention. A Guide for Health Care Professionals. https://goldcopd.org/gold-reports/
- Prevention of Acute Exacerbations of COPD. American College of Chest Physicians and Canadian Thoracic Society Guideline (Criner et at., 2014).

TABLE 7.8	**Mucolytic Medications**		
Medication	Indication	Dosage	Considerations and Monitoring
Acetylcysteine	Adjunctive treatment of COPD	**20% solution:** *Adults:* 3–5 mL inhaled by nebulizer three or four times daily. Maximum dosage: 10 mL daily.	
		10% solution: *Adults:* 6–10 mL inhaled by nebulizer three or four times daily. Maximum dosage: 20 mL/day.	

and the patient's age, race/ethnicity, comorbidities, and genetic factors. Once the disease is staged appropriately, begin step-wise therapy based on GOLD. Evaluate the patient's ability to manipulate the medication device (MDI, DPI, nebulizer). If the patient is unable to use the selected device, switch to an alternate delivery system. Assess for comorbid conditions that may impact the efficacy of the selected medication or increase the risk of adverse effects.

Initiate the treatment plan with the selected medication by first providing adequate patient education to ensure the patient's understanding and promote full participation in medication management therapy. For each medication, review the name of the medication, dosage, route, and potential adverse effects. A short-acting beta2-agonist should be prescribed for all patients as a rescue inhaler. Provide information on how to recognize exacerbations, emergency use of rescue inhalers, and when to seek care for shortness of breath. Instruct the patient on how to use and properly care for the inhaler and/or nebulizer devices at initiation and subsequent visits.

Ensure complete patient and family understanding about the medication prescribed for management of COPD using a variety of education strategies. Provide written material covering details of each office visit, including adjustment of medications, the use of supplemental oxygen therapy, follow-up appointments, and referrals to other providers. Online educational resources are readily available and include organizations such as the American Lung Association, the COPD Foundation, and the CDC.

Conduct follow-up and monitoring of patient responses to medication therapy and overall COPD management. Establish an office procedure for immediate response to patient messaging through electronic portals or phone calls. At each visit, ask the patient and their caregiver about symptom exacerbations or improvement using the CAT questionnaire and the mMRC scale to assess symptom severity and the impact of COPD on their daily activities. Assess the frequency of using rescue medications. Assess for medication adherence and adverse effects. Monitor therapeutic responses to medications and adjust accordingly. Determine a plan to seek emergency treatment of exacerbations.

Teaching Points for COPD Therapy

Health Promotion Strategies

- Assess lifestyle risk factors such as smoking and continually reinforce the need to eliminate (or reduce) smoking to slow the progression of COPD.
- Offer smoking cessation medications (Chapter 52).
- Provide routine health maintenance such as immunizations (especially the influenza, coronavirus [COVID-19], pneumococcal, and pertussis vaccines).
- The use of antibiotics in preventing and treating exacerbations is a major objective in COPD management. Prophylactic, continuous, or intermittent antibiotic therapy may be used as maintenance therapy to prevent exacerbations (Miravitlles & Anzueto, 2017).

- Maintaining a healthy diet and taking antioxidants, especially vitamin C, protects against impaired lung function (Shaheen et al., 2010).
- Staying active at an exercise level that does not induce significant dyspnea improves lung health and decreases overall shortness of breath.
- Consider referral to a pulmonary rehabilitation program, which can provide exercise, education, and support for people with pulmonary lung diseases.

Patient Education for Medication Safety

- Tell your primary care provider about all the medicines you take, including prescription and over-the-counter (OTC) medicines, vitamins, and herbal supplements.
- If you smoke, try to stop smoking or decrease the amount you smoke each day. Talk to your primary care provider about smoking cessation therapy.
- Use all medications as instructed. Do not use more or less of the medication.
- Rinse your mouth with water or mouthwash after inhalation to prevent corticosteroid accumulation on the oropharyngeal mucosa.
- Keep all medication devices clean, following manufacturers' recommendations.

Application Questions for Discussion

1. What resources are available to primary care providers to guide the care of COPD patients?
2. Describe the four stages of COPD severity and each PFT criterion.
3. What are the recommendations for prescribing inhaled corticosteroids in COPD patients?
4. What medication should all COPD patients have prescribed for emergency use, and what medications are used for maintenance therapy?

Selected Bibliography

Calverley, P. M. A., Page, C., Dal Negro, R. W., Fontana, G., Cazzola, M., Cicero, A. F., Pozzi, E., & Wedzicha, J. A. (2019). Effect of erdosteine on COPD exacerbations in COPD patients with moderate airflow limitations. *International Journal of Chronic Obstructive Pulmonary Disease, 14,* 2733–2744. http://doi.org/10.2147/COPD.S221852.

Calverley, P. M. A., Anderson, J. A., Brook, R. D., Crim, C., Gallot, N., Kilbride, S., Martinez, F. J., Yates, J., Newby, D. E., Vestbo., Wise, R., Celli, & B., R. SUMMIT Investigators. (2018). Fluticasone furoate, vilanterol, and lung function decline in patients with moderate chronic obstructive pulmonary disease and heightened cardiovascular risk. *American Journal of Respiratory and Critical Care Medicine, 197*(1), 47–55. http://doi.org/10.1164/rccm.201610-2086OC.

Centers for Disease Control and Prevention. (2019). *Basics about COPD.* Available at https://www.cdc.gov/copd/basics-about.html.

Criner, G. J., Bourbeau, J., Diekemper, R. L., Ouellette, D. R., Goodridge, D., Herandez, P., Curren, K., Balter, M. S., Bhutani,

M., Camp, P. G., Celli, B. R., Dechman, G., Dransfield, M. T., Fiel, S. B., Foreman, M. G., Hanania, N. A., Ireland, B. K., Marchetti, N., Marchiniuk, D. D., Mularski, R. A., & Stickland, M. K. (2014). Prevention of acute exacerbations of COPD. American College of Chest Physicians and Canadian Thoracic Society guidelines. *Chest, 147*(4), P894–P942. https://doi.org/10.1378/chest.14-1676.

GlaxoSmithKline. (n.d.). *The COPD assessment test (CAT) for healthcare professionals & researchers.* Available at https://www.catestonline.org/hcp-homepage/clinical-practice.html.

Global Initiative for Chronic Obstructive Lung Disease. (2020). *Global strategy for the diagnosis, management, and prevention of chronic obstructive pulmonary disease. 2020 Report.* Available at https://goldcopd.org/.

Grewe, F. A., Sievi, N. A., Bradicich, M., Roeder, M., Brack, T., Brutsche, M. H., & Clarenbach, C. F. (2020). Compliance of pharmacotherapy with GOLD guidelines: A longitudinal study in patients with COPD. *International Journal of Chronic Obstructive Pulmonary Disease, 15*, 627. https://doi.org/10.2147/COPD.S240444.

Izquierdo, J. L., & Cosio, B. G. (2018). The dose of inhaled corticosteroids in patients with COPD: When less is better. *International Journal of Chronic Obstructive Pulmonary Disease, 13*, 3539–3547. http://doi.org/10.2147/COPD.S175047.

MD+Calc. (n.d.). *mMRC (modified medical research council) dyspnea scale.* Available at https://www.mdcalc.com/mmrc-modified-medical-research-council-dyspnea-scale.

Miravitlles, M., & Anzueto, A. (2017). Chronic respiratory infection in patients with chronic obstructive pulmonary disease: What is the role of antibiotics? *International Journal of Molecular Sciences, 18*(7), 1344. http://doi.org/10.3390/ijms18071344.

Shaheen, S. O., Jameson, K. A., Syddall, H. E., Sayer, A. A., Dennison, E. M., & Cooper, C. Hertfordshire Cohort Study Group. (2010). The relationship of dietary patterns with adult lung function and COPD. *European Respiratory Journal, 36*(2), 277–284. http://doi.org/10.1183/09031936.00114709.

Sim, Y. S., Lee, J. H., Lee, W. Y., Suh, D. I., Oh, Y. M., Yoon, J. S., & Chang, J. H. (2017). Spirometry and bronchodilator test. *Tuberculosis and Respiratory Diseases, 80*(2), 105–112. http://doi.org/10.4046/trd.2017.80.2.105.

8

Antihyperlipidemic Medications

CHERYL H. ZAMBROSKI

Overview

Atherosclerotic cardiovascular disease (ASCVD) remains the leading cause of death in the United States and around the world (Benjamin Emelia et al., 2019). In the United States, cardiovascular diseases account for nearly one out of every three deaths. According to the Centers for Disease Control and Prevention, National Center for Health Statistics (2021), approximately 27% of males and 23% of females meet the criteria for hypercholesterolemia (serum total cholesterol of at least 240 mg/dL or are taking cholesterol-lowering medications). Unfortunately, of those adults who meet the criteria for hypercholesterolemia, only slightly more than half are taking medications that could reduce their cholesterol (CDC, 2019). As adults age, their risk for hypercholesterolemia increases. This chapter focuses primarily on antihyperlipidemic medications as they relate to patients with hypercholesterolemia, and ASCVD prevention and treatment.

Antihyperlipidemic medications are generally divided into four categories based on the mechanisms they implement to reduce lipid levels (Table 8.1) and on which subtype of lipids they influence the most. The most effective medications for patients with primary hyperlipidemia are the *hydroxymethylglutaryl Coenzyme-A (HMG-CoA) reductase inhibitors*, also known as *statins*. The other three categories are used far less often and may be used as adjuncts to dietary interventions, in combination with statins, or if the patient is unable to tolerate statins. For example, *selective cholesterol absorption inhibitors* may be used as monotherapy or in combination with statins to reduce elevated total cholesterol (TC) or low-density lipoprotein cholesterol (LDL-C), and in patients with primary hypercholesterolemia. *Fibric acid derivatives* are typically used as an adjunct to diet to treat adults with severe hypertriglyceridemia or to elevate high-density lipoprotein cholesterol (HDL-C). *Bile acid sequestrants* may be used to reduce an elevated LDL-C. Of note, niacin, once used to increase HDL-C or used as adjunctive therapy to diet to reduce elevated TC, LDL-C, apolipoprotein B (Apo B), and triglyceride (TG) concentrations, is no longer recommended due to questionable effectiveness and an undesirable side-effect profile.

Relevant Physiology

Cholesterol and triglycerides are classified as lipids, and both are normal and vital constituents of plasma. *Cholesterol* is a major component of cell membranes and provides structural stability of the cell. In addition, cholesterol is a basic component of steroid hormones, vitamin D, and bile acids. The vast majority of cholesterol (approximately 80%) is produced by the liver. The remainder is provided from dietary sources. *Triglycerides* are large lipid molecules that are primarily derived from dietary sources (including carbohydrates) and ultimately stored as fat tissue.

Because cholesterol and triglycerides are hydrophobic and insoluble, they are transported in the plasma via lipoproteins. Lipoproteins have a central hydrophobic core surrounded by a hydrophilic membrane that consists of phospholipids, free cholesterol, and apolipoproteins (proteins that bind lipids). These lipoproteins are then subdivided into classes according to their size, lipid composition, and apolipoproteins. Major classes of lipoproteins include chylomicrons, very low-density lipoproteins (VLDLs), intermediate low-density lipoproteins (ILDLs), low-density lipoproteins (LDLs), and high-density lipoproteins (HDLs). Chylomicrons are the largest and least dense of the lipoproteins, followed in order of increasing density and decreasing size by VLDLs (or pre-β), ILDLs (or broad β), LDLs (or β), and HDLs (or α). Chylomicrons and VLDLs are considered triglyceride-rich lipoproteins, whereas IDLs, LDLs, and HDLs are considered cholesterol-rich lipoproteins.

Production of various types of cholesterol and other lipids is an important liver function for maintenance of homeostasis and good health. Lipids, including cholesterol, have life-sustaining essential functions in many body systems. Liver lipid production occurs through several multistep pathways. The major pathway is called the mevalonate pathway, with the HMG-CoA reductase enzyme as the commitment step in first converting a precursor substance (HMG-CoA) into mevalonate. If mevalonate is not formed, cholesterol is not synthesized. So, the presence and activity of HMG-CoA reductase determine whether and how much liver cholesterol is synthesized.

TABLE 8.1 **Antihyperlipidemic Medications**

Drug Category/ Medication	Indication	Dosage	Considerations and Monitoring
HMG-CoA Reductase Inhibitors			
Atorvastatin[a]	Primary/secondary prevention of cardiovascular events by reducing TC, LDL-C, and TG	10–20 mg orally initially, then titrate to 10–80 mg once daily guided by need for LDL-C reduction.	After initiation or increasing dose, check fasting lipid levels after 4–12 weeks to determine effect.
Rosuvastatin	Primary/secondary prevention of cardiovascular events by reducing elevated TC, LDL-C, Apo B, and TGs and to increase HDL-C	For primary prevention, the usual starting dose is 10–20 mg orally once daily. Usual dosage range is 5–40 mg. For Asian patients, start dosing at 5 mg orally once daily.	Dosage adjustments should be made every 2–4 weeks to achieve LDL reduction goal. Monitor symptoms carefully to determine patient tolerance. Assess effectiveness through serum cholesterol panel 4–12 weeks after initiating therapy and after dosage change. A dosage of 40 mg/day is associated with a higher risk of myopathy and should be reserved for patients who require further LDL reduction after receiving 20 mg/day.
Simvastatin[a]	Used for treatment of hypercholesterolemia and for cardiovascular risk reduction by decreasing TC, LDL-C, and TG and by increasing HDL-C	Initially, 10–20 mg orally once daily in the evening. Patients with coronary heart disease or risk factors should start at a dose of 40 mg orally once daily in the evening. Usual dosage range is 5–40 mg orally.	Monitor patient's response to dose after 4–12 weeks and adjust dose to desired response. Maximum dosage is 80 mg/day orally if no evidence of myopathy. Contraindicated in patients with liver disease or heavy alcohol use.
Lovastatin	Treatment of hypercholesterolemia, including hyperlipidemia, hyperlipoproteinemia, or hypertriglyceridemia, as an adjunct to dietary management	Initially, 10–20 mg orally once daily with the evening meal. Patients requiring LDL reductions of ≥20% to achieve their goal may begin with 20 mg orally. Recommended dosage range is 10–80 mg orally once daily in 1 or 2 divided doses. *Extended-release tablets:* Initially, 20–60 mg orally once daily given in the evening at bedtime.	Food reduces absorption of the extended-release tablets so should be avoided. Not recommended for patients with hepatic disease. Dosage adjustments should be made at intervals of 4 weeks or more to reach desired cholesterol reduction.
	For primary prevention of MI	Begin with 20–40 mg orally once daily with the evening meal. Recommended dose is 10–80 mg/day orally in 1 or 2 divided doses *Extended release:* Begin with 20–60 mg once daily at bedtime. For older adults with multiple comorbidities, begin with 20 mg once daily at bedtime.	
	For slowing progression of coronary atherosclerosis	Begin with 20 mg orally once daily with the evening meal. The recommended dosing range is 10–80 mg/day in 1 or 2 divided doses. *Extended-release tablets:* Begin with 20–60 mg orally once daily given at bedtime. For older adults with multiple comorbidities, begin with 20 mg orally at bedtime.	

Continued

TABLE 8.1   Antihyperlipidemic Medications—cont'd

Drug Category/ Medication	Indication	Dosage	Considerations and Monitoring
Pravastatin	Treatment of hypercholesterolemia, including reducing TC, LDL-C, apolipoprotein B and increasing HDL-C as an adjunct to dietary control For MI prophylaxis or stroke prophylaxis	The recommended starting dose is 40 mg once daily. Dosage range is 10–80 mg/day orally. *Adolescents with hyperlipidemia, 14–18 yr:* Begin with 40 mg orally once daily May begin with 10 mg orally once daily, then titrate up in 10-mg increments every 2 months to maximum dosage of 60 mg/day. *Children and adolescents with hyperlipidemia 8–13 yr:* Begin with 20 mg orally once daily. May also begin with 10 mg once daily and titrate up 10 mg every 2 months to maximum dosage of 60 mg/day.	Monitor patient's response to dose after 4–12 weeks and adjust dose to desired response. May be given without regard to meals. Monitor LFTs if patient exhibits signs or symptoms of liver dysfunction. CPKs should be assessed for persistent muscle pain, weakness, or tenderness.
Fluvastatin[a]	For treatment of hypercholesterolemia and for reducing cardiovascular risk. Reduces TC, LDL-C, TG and raises HDL-C	20–40 mg orally once daily titrated up to 40 mg orally twice daily. *Extended-release tablets:* For patients requiring more than 25% LDL-C reduction, may use 80 mg orally once daily. *Children and adolescents 10–17 yr (females should be at least 1 year postmenarche):* Begin with 20 mg orally once daily; may titrate up to 40 mg twice daily. May transition to extended-release tablets 80 mg/day orally.	Maximum dosage is 80 mg/day. May be administered without regard to meals. Monitor patient's response to dose after 4 weeks and adjust dose to desired response. For children and adolescents, monitor response after 6 weeks and adjust dose as needed.
Pitavastatin	For treatment of hypercholesterolemia, hyperlipoproteinemia, and/or hypertriglyceridemia as an adjunct to dietary management	Usual dose is 2 mg orally once daily. Monitor response 4 weeks after beginning therapy or after dose adjustment. Maximum dosage is 4 mg/day.	Patients with diabetes may need increased monitoring of blood glucose. May be taken with or without food.
Selective Cholesterol Absorption Inhibitors			
Ezetimibe	Considered as second-line therapy in addition to maximally tolerated statin therapy in patients with clinical ASCVD and comorbidities that require <25% additional LDL-C reduction Adjunct to diet and exercise to decrease TC, LDL-C, Apo B, and non-HDL-C	As monotherapy or for use in combination with an HMG-CoA inhibitor, 10 mg orally once daily. May be used in adolescents and children ≥10 yr, 10 mg orally once daily	Coadministration with statin is more effective in improving serum TC, LDL-C, Apo-B, TG, and HDL-C. If given with statins, make sure to monitor for myopathy, drug interactions, and elevated liver as with statins.
Fibric Acid Derivatives			
Gemfibrozil	Treatment of hyperlipoproteinemia and hypertriglyceridemia as adjunct to diet Second-line therapy for patients with elevated cholesterol, triglycerides, and VLDL who have low HDL (<35 mg/dL) and no evidence of coronary artery disease	600 mg orally twice daily, given 30 minutes before the morning and evening meals.	Should be discontinued if no changes in lipoprotein concentration after 3 months. Periodic liver function studies are recommended. Monitor patient complaints of abdominal pain as there is an increased risk of cholelithiasis. More likely to cause leg pain than fenofibrate.

TABLE 8.1	Antihyperlipidemic Medications—cont'd		
Drug Category/ Medication	**Indication**	**Dosage**	**Considerations and Monitoring**
Fenofibrate	Used for treatment of severe hypertriglyceridemia as an adjunct to dietary management	50–150 mg orally once daily with a meal. Maximum dosage is 150 mg.	Evaluate lipid serum concentrations at 4–8-week intervals. Multiple formulations and brand names of fenofibrate. Use caution in prescribing. Due to increased risk of renal injury, use caution in prescribing to patients with CrCl 30–80 mL/min. Contraindicated in patients with CrCl <30 mL/min.
Bile Acid Sequestrants			
Cholestyramine	Treatment of hypercholesterolemia, especially elevated LDL-C	Initially, 4 Gm orally once or twice daily before meals. Maintenance dosage range is 4–16 Gm/day given in 2 divided doses. Maximum antihyperlipidemic dosage is 24 Gm/day.	Maximum dosage is 24 Gm/day. Give other medications at least 1 hr before or at least 4–6 hr after each dose. Liquid forms may be mixed with water, milk, fruit juice, or other noncarbonated liquid to be more palatable. Powder can be mixed with applesauce or crushed pineapple.
Colestipol	For treatment of primary hypercholesterolemia (elevated LDL-C)	Initially, 5 Gm orally once or twice daily. Usual dosage range is 5–20 Gm/day orally.	May increase by 5 Gm/day at 1–2-month intervals, up to 30 Gm/day orally given in 2–4 divided doses. Monitor LFTs. TGs increase with colestipol therapy.
Colesevelam	For the treatment of primary hypercholesterolemia or as adjunct to diet and exercise in the reduction of LDL-C in combination with statins	Initially, 3 tablets orally twice daily or 6 tablets orally once daily; administer with liquid and a meal. Doses of 4–6 tablets daily have been shown to be safe and effective in combination with an HMG-CoA reductase inhibitor.	Contraindicated in patients with triglycerides >500 mg/dL and in patients with a history of hypertriglyceridemia-induced pancreatitis. Evaluate serum lipids 4–6 weeks after initiating therapy and with dosage change.

^aSimvastatin, atorvastatin, and fluvastatin are most likely to cause leg pain.

Apo B, Apolipoprotein B; *ASCVD*, atherosclerotic cardiovascular disease; *CPKs*, creatine phosphokinases; *HDL-C*, high-density lipoprotein cholesterol; *HMG CoA*, hydroxymethylglutaryl Coenzyme-A reductase; *LDL*, low-density lipoprotein; *LDL-C*, low-density lipoprotein cholesterol; *LFTs*, liver function tests; *MI*, myocardial infarction; *TC*, total cholesterol; *TG*, triglyceride; *VLDL*, very low-density lipoprotein.

The rate of this enzyme's production is well regulated through several different complex negative feedback mechanisms. When these mechanisms are functioning normally, a person's levels of various blood cholesterol lipoproteins remain within the normal range. Much like how negative feedback regulates blood glucose homeostasis, liver receptors are able to "monitor" blood lipid levels and adjust cholesterol production based on need. Higher blood lipid levels, even those ingested in excess, suppress production of HMG-CoA reductase, which results in less production of lipids and more removal of lipids from the blood. All of the proteins and other substances involved in monitoring and relaying blood lipid information back to the liver are themselves products of many different genes. Variations or mutations in any of these genes can alter the gene product and reduce the effectiveness of the feedback mechanisms, resulting in higher-than-needed blood lipid levels that increase the risk for ASCVD. Some medications used to manage hyperlipidemia focus on external regulation of HMG-CoA reductase.

Of the lipoproteins, evaluation of LDL and HDL levels is of primary importance. These two lipoproteins differ in several respects, including their cholesterol transport activities. Simply stated, LDL transports cholesterol from the liver to peripheral tissues; conversely, HDL removes cholesterol from the periphery and transports it to the liver.

TABLE 8.2   Familial Dyslipidemia and Associated Abnormalities

Dyslipidemia	Primary Abnormality	Frequency[a]
Familial hypercholesterolemia	Defective or absent LDL receptors (increased LDL)	0.2%
Familial defective Apo B	LDL receptor binding decreased because of abnormal Apo B (increased LDL)	0.2%
Familial combined hyperlipidemia	Apo B and VLDL overproduction	0.5%
Familial hypertriglyceridemia	Decreased lipoprotein lipase activity, high VLDL production	1%
Familial hypoalphalipoproteinemia	Decreased Apo-A-1 production, increased HDL catabolism	1%

[a]Percent of general population.

Apo B, Apolipoprotein B; *HDL*, high-density lipoprotein; *LDL*, low-density lipoprotein; *VLDL*, very low-density lipoprotein.

Pathophysiology: Hyperlipidemia

Hyperlipidemia can result from a variety of causes, including genetic disorders, concomitant disease states, and lifestyle factors. Familial *dyslipidemias* (faulty lipid metabolism resulting in higher-than-normal blood lipid levels) such as familial hypercholesterolemia (Table 8.2) are genetic disorders associated with overproduction or impaired removal of lipoproteins. These disorders are associated with mutations of the *LDLR*, *APOB*, or *PCSK9* gene and have an autosomal dominant pattern. Although these disorders are relatively rare, they can significantly increase the risk of premature cardiovascular disease. In fact, males with familial hypercholesterolemia, if untreated, may have their first myocardial infarction before they reach the age of 55 (some even as early as age 20). Females may have signs of coronary heart disease by the age of 60 (Nordestgaard et al., 2013). Screening for children with a family history of early onset of cardiovascular disease or with a family history of elevated cholesterol should begin at the age of 2. To compare, screening of asymptomatic children and adolescents, without a history of lipid disorders, before the age of 20 is not considered necessary or beneficial (United States Preventive Services Task Force, 2016).

PRACTICE PEARLS

Familial Hypercholesterolemia

Pediatrics

- Screening for increased cholesterol is recommended beginning at the age of 2 for children with a family history of elevated cholesterol or early onset cardiovascular disease.
- Familial hypercholesterolemia should be considered in children younger than 20 years of age with an LDL-C of at least160 mg/dL.
- Assess for the presence of secondary causes of elevated lipid levels.
- Evaluate the effectiveness of dietary interventions prior to initiating medication therapy.

Far more common is *polygenic hypercholesterolemia*. Polygenic hypercholesterolemia is a result of genetic mutations that are influenced by dietary intake of unhealthy fats (such as saturated fats and trans fats), obesity, and sedentary

lifestyle. It is associated with increased risk of ASCVD. Elevated LDL-C may be the result of either increased LDL-C production or diminished LDL-C uptake by the liver. Increased LDL then transports cholesterol to the tissues, where it may be deposited within the artery walls.

Diets that are high in saturated fat, trans fat, and cholesterol can decrease the number of LDL-C receptors in the liver, resulting in decreased breakdown of LDL-C in the liver. Saturated fats are usually found in animal fats (such as in meats). They can also be found in eggs, butter, cheeses, and other dairy products.

An important point to remember is that chronic hyperlipidemia reflects a problem in one or more steps in the complex liver regulation of cholesterol biosynthesis, most likely from a gene variation. Just as a person who has perfect glucose regulation can ingest a very large amount of sugars and other carbohydrates without becoming hyperglycemic, a perfectly functioning feedback system for lipids prevents hyperlipidemia.

Loss or reduced proper feedback regulation results in excess liver production of LDL-C. These excess and unnecessary molecules move through the intimal lining of arteries and form irregularly shaped atheromatous plaques that narrow these vessels and initiate inflammatory responses. In addition, less HDL is synthesized. HDL is a beneficial scavenger that removes lipids from existing plaques and transports them to the liver for processing and elimination. With less HDL present, the risk for ASCVD is increased, even when LDLs are within the normal range.

TABLE 8.3   Examples of Secondary Conditions or Medications That Can Cause Hyperlipidemia

Secondary Condition	Medications
Obesity	Select beta-blockers
Diabetes	Thiazide diuretics
Cirrhosis of the liver	Loop diuretics
Heavy alcohol use or alcoholism	First- and second-generation antipsychotics
Chronic kidney disease	Corticosteroids
Cushing's syndrome	Anabolic steroids
Hypothyroidism	Protease inhibitors
	Sodium-glucose co-transporter 2 inhibitors

In addition to dietary and genetic factors, hyperlipidemia can be related to a secondary condition or medication (Table 8.3). If this is the case, correction or modification of this condition should be addressed before or in conjunction with pharmacologic intervention for hyperlipidemia alone.

Antihyperlipidemic Therapy

HMG-CoA Reductase Inhibitors

HMG-CoA reductase inhibitors (statins) competitively inhibit HMG-CoA reductase. Recall that this enzyme is essential in the first step of the conversion of HMG-CoA to mevalonate, a precursor of cholesterol. By inhibiting HMG-CoA reductase, statins work exogenously to reduce production of cholesterol in the liver. Lower intracellular cholesterol stimulates the synthesis of LDL receptors, resulting in increased LDL clearance from the blood. In addition to their LDL-C lowering effects, HMG-CoA reductase inhibitors increase HDL and decrease triglycerides modestly. These medications can decrease levels of C-reactive protein, decreasing inflammatory processes that may be associated with atherosclerosis.

HMG-CoA reductase inhibitors are currently the most effective medications for reducing cardiovascular risk and improving cardiovascular health outcomes. Beyond their effect on lipoproteins, therapeutic benefits include plaque stabilization by decreasing the lipid content of the plaque, as well as reduction of inflammation and apoptosis within the plaque. Statins have been shown to reduce mortality and morbidity in patients with known atherosclerotic heart disease and are recommended in many at-risk patients for primary prevention. Box 8.1 provides descriptions of those patients most benefitting from the use of statins for their hyperlipidemia.

Statins are typically classified by impact on cardiovascular risk as high intensity, moderate intensity, or low intensity (Table 8.4). Specific medications are designated to the category by dose and by average ability to reduce LDL-C. For example, a

high-intensity statin may reduce LDL-C by more than 50%, whereas a low-intensity statin would reduce it by less than 30%. Therefore, it is important for the primary care provider to clearly understand the patient's cardiovascular risk and their LDL-C reduction goals. In patients with clinical atherosclerotic heart disease, the more LDL-C that is reduced while on statin therapy, the greater the benefit to the overall cardiovascular risk.

Statins have a characteristic side-effect profile or *statin-associated side effects* (SASE) (Table 8.5) that can occur in as many as 10% of the population. The most common SASE is myalgia (also called statin-associated m symptoms or SAMS) associated with a normal serum creatine phosphokinase (CPK) level. SASE are important to share with patients as they can reduce adherence to the statin. In most cases, switching to another type of statin or adjusting the dosage of statin can be effective in relieving the symptom and enhancing adherence.

PRACTICE PEARLS

Statin Therapy

The American College of Cardiology (ACC) and American Heart Association (AHA) updated the cholesterol management guidelines in 2018. The new guidelines provide a more detailed cardiovascular risk assessment and new cholesterol-lowering medication options for those with the greatest risk for cardiovascular disease. The assessments for 10-year and lifetime risk can be used to guide the provider in selecting the most personalized approach for cholesterol management. The following link can be used for determining risk assessment: https://tools.acc.org/ASCVD-Risk-Estimator-Plus/#!/calculate/estimate.

Rosuvastatin

Pharmacokinetics. Rosuvastatin is administered orally and may be given in the morning or evening without significant difference in therapeutic effects. Food reduces the absorption rate slightly but does not affect overall bioavailability, so this medication may be given without regard to meals. It is about 88% bound to plasma proteins. Peak rosuvastatin plasma concentrations are reached 3 to 5 hours after oral dosing, with a plasma half-life of about 20 hours. It is eliminated primarily unchanged via the fecal route with only about 10% of the dose eliminated by the kidneys.

Caution must be taken when prescribing rosuvastatin to patients of Asian descent. Pharmacokinetic studies have shown that patients of Japanese and Chinese ancestry may have an increased blood level of the medication from the same dosage as Caucasians. This may require reduction in initial dosing, because although the medication may be more effective, it also will have more intense side effects.

PRACTICE PEARLS

Prescribing Statins to Asian Patients

Asian patients, including those of Japanese, Chinese, or Malay descent and Asian Indians, may be more sensitive to dosing levels of select statins. Providers must use care in initiating dosing in Asian patients as lower doses of statins in this patient population can achieve similar responses as higher doses in White patients.

• Box 8.1 Four Major Statin Benefit Groups

1. Patients with any form of clinical ASCVD such as a history of stable or unstable angina, myocardial infarction, coronary or other arterial vascularization, stroke, transient ischemic attack, or peripheral arterial disease
2. Patients with primary LDL-C levels of 190 mg/dL or greater
3. Patients with diabetes mellitus, 40 to 75 years of age, with LDL-C levels of 70 to 189 mg/dL
4. Patients without diabetes, 40 to 75 years of age, with an estimated 10-year ASCVD risk of at least 7.5% according to the ASCVD Risk Calculator (https://tools.acc.org/ldl/ascvd_risk_estimator/index.html#!/calulate/estimator/patient)

From Grundy, S. M., Stone, N. J., Bailey, A. L., Beam, C., Birtcher, K. K., Blumenthal, R. S., . . . Yeboah, J. (2019). 2018 AHA/ACC/AACVPR/AAPA/ABC/ACPM/ADA/AGS/APhA/ASPC/NLA/PCNA guideline on the management of blood cholesterol. A Report of the American College of Cardiology/American Heart Association Task Force on Clinical Practice Guidelines. *Journal of the American College of Cardiology, 73*(24), e285–e350. http://doi.org/10.1016/j.jacc.2018.11.003.

TABLE 8.4 High-, Moderate-, and Low-Intensity Statin Therapy

	High Intensity	Moderate Intensity	Low Intensity
LDL-C lipid lowering potential	>50%	30% to 49%	<30%
Statins	Atorvastatin 40–80 mg Rosuvastatin 20–40 mg	Atorvastatin 10–20 mg Rosuvastatin 5–10 mg Simvastatin 20–40 mg Pravastatin 40–80 mg Lovastatin 40–80 mg Fluvastatin XL 80 mg Fluvastatin 40 mg twice daily Pitavastatin 1–4 mg	Simvastatin 10 mg Pravastatin 10–20 mg Lovastatin 20 mg Fluvastatin 20–40 mg

From Grundy, S. M., Stone, N. J., Bailey, A. L., Beam, C., Birtcher, K. K., Blumenthal, R. S., . . . Yeboah, J. (2019). 2018 AHA/ACC/AACVPR/AAPA/ABC/ACPM/ADA/AGS/APhA/ASPC/NLA/PCNA guideline on the management of blood cholesterol. A Report of the American College of Cardiology/American Heart Association Task Force on Clinical Practice Guidelines. *Journal of the American College of Cardiology, 73*(24), e285–e350. http://doi.org/10.1016/j.jacc.2018.11.003

TABLE 8.5 Common Statin-Associated Side Effects

Statin-Associated Muscle Symptoms	Frequency	Predisposing Factors
Myalgia (CK normal)	<10%	Older age Female Low BMI Asian descent Increased alcohol intake High levels of physical activity Medications that inhibit CYP 3A4 or OATP1B1 Comorbidities including HIV, renal, liver, thyroid, or preexisting myopathy
Myositis/myopathy (CK > normal limits)	Rare	
Rhabdomyolysis (CK >10 x normal limits)	Rare	
New onset diabetes mellitus	More frequent if risk factors for diabetes such as BMI >30, FBS >100 mg/dL; metabolic syndrome or HbA1c >6%	Diabetes risk factors factors/metabolic syndrome High-intensity statin therapy
Liver Transaminase elevation 3 x normal limits	Infrequent	
CNS Memory/cognition	Rare/no increase in three large RCTs	

HbA1c, Hemoglobin A1C; *BMI*, Body mass index; *CK*, creatine kinase; *CNS*, central nervous system; *CYP*, cytochrome; *FBS*, fasting blood sugar; *HIV*, human immunodeficiency virus; *RCTs*, randomized controlled trials.
Adapted from Grundy, S. M., Stone, N. J., Bailey, A. L., Beam, C., Birtcher, K. K., Blumenthal, R. S., . . . Yeboah, J. (2019). 2018 AHA/ACC/AACVPR/AAPA/ABC/ACPM/ADA/AGS/APhA/ASPC/NLA/PCNA guideline on the management of blood cholesterol. A Report of the American College of Cardiology/American Heart Association Task Force on Clinical Practice Guidelines. *Journal of the American College of Cardiology, 73*(24), e285–e350. http://doi.org/10.1016/j.jacc.2018.11.003.

Indications. Depending on dose, rosuvastatin is considered a high-intensity or medium-intensity statin to reduce total cholesterol, LDL-C, Apo B, and TG, and increase HDL-C to treat patients with primary hypercholesterolemia. It is used for primary prevention of cardiovascular disease including myocardial infarction and stroke, as well as to reduce the progression of atherosclerosis in coronary heart disease and carotid disease.

Adverse Effects. Common reactions include mild arthralgia and myalgia. Risk of myalgia is higher if the statin is given with other medications that cause myopathy or in doses of 40 mg/day or greater. *Rhabdomyolysis* (skeletal muscle breakdown) is a rare but life-threatening adverse effect. Other adverse effects include diarrhea or constipation, headache, diabetes mellitus, and elevated liver enzymes. Although rare, severe hepatotoxicity may occur during HMG-CoA reductase inhibitor therapy. In addition, some patients may experience memory loss, forgetfulness, confusion, or depression.

Contraindications. Rosuvastatin is contraindicated in patients with active liver disease or who are pregnant or breastfeeding. Patients 65 years of age or older, those with renal disease or renal insufficiency, females, and those who have recently had surgery or trauma are at greater risk for myopathy and/or rhabdomyolysis with acute renal failure secondary to myoglobinuria.

Monitoring. Liver function studies should be obtained prior to initiating statins and then as needed for symptoms suggesting liver injury. Assess for medication adherence, adverse effects, and patient response to therapy (fasting lipid level) within 4 to 12 weeks after beginning therapy or after a change in dose. Because of the risk of diabetes mellitus in patients taking statins, blood glucose should be monitored, particularly in patients with prediabetes.

Atorvastatin

Pharmacokinetics. Atorvastatin is administered orally and is 98% plasma protein bound. Peak plasma levels are typically achieved within 1 to 2 hours. Food reduces absorption of atorvastatin; however, this does not affect overall LDL-C reduction. It may be given regardless of time of day. Renal disease does not affect plasma concentration or LDL-C reduction, so dosage adjustments are not needed for patients with renal insufficiency.

Coadministration of medications that are strong cytochrome (CYP) 3A4 inhibitors with atorvastatin can markedly increase the statin serum concentration and increase the patient's risk of myopathy, rhabdomyolysis, and acute renal failure.

PHARMACOGENETICS

Statins

Coadministration of medications that are strong CYP 3A4 inhibitors with select statins (atorvastatin, lovastatin, and simvastatin) can markedly increase the statin serum concentration and increase the patient's risk of myopathy, rhabdomyolysis, and acute renal failure. Examples include clarithromycin, ketoconazole, erythromycin, amiodarone, and diltiazem.

Indications. Atorvastatin is used for treatment of hypercholesterolemia, including hyperlipidemia, lipoproteinemia, and hypertriglyceridemia, and can be used for prevention of myocardial infarction and stroke. It is considered a high-intensity or moderate-intensity statin.

Adverse Effects. Atorvastatin is generally well tolerated, with fewer than 2% of patients discontinuing the medication because of adverse effects. Most common adverse effects include gastrointestinal (GI) symptoms such as mild flatulence, dyspepsia, nausea, and diarrhea. Fewer than 10% of patients experience mild arthralgia, myalgia, or musculoskeletal pain. The most frequent central nervous system (CNS) adverse reaction was insomnia in 1.1% to 5.3% of patients. Diabetes mellitus and hyperglycemia have been reported in 6.1% of patients.

Contraindications. Patients who are pregnant or breastfeeding, have cholestasis, or have active liver disease should not take atorvastatin. It should be used with caution in older adults, females, children, and individuals who have received an organ transplant.

Monitoring. In addition to monitoring adherence to lifestyle changes, atorvastatin's impact on LDL-C should be assessed by measurement of fasting serum lipid levels within 4 to 12 weeks after initiating the medication and after dosage adjustment. After reaching satisfactory reduction in LDL-C, guidelines recommend monitoring every 3 to 12 months. Liver function tests (LFTs) and creatine kinase (CK) levels should be assessed if the patient experiences any symptoms associated with liver failure or significant musculoskeletal symptoms.

Lovastatin

Pharmacokinetics. Lovastatin is given orally and undergoes significant first-pass metabolism in the liver. It is highly bound to plasma proteins (greater than 95%). Peak concentrations occur within 2 to 4 hours after oral administration of immediate-release lovastatin. Food enhances oral absorption. Grapefruit juice can increase absorption of lovastatin by at least 30%. Enhanced absorption increases depending on the amount of juice taken. Immediate- or extended-release forms of lovastatin are most effective when given in the evening due to diurnal patterns of cholesterol synthesis.

PRACTICE PEARLS

Grapefruit Juice and Statins

It has long been recommended that grapefruit juice be avoided in patients taking statins. Recent evidence suggests, however, that typical amounts of grapefruit juice may increase the benefit of statins without increasing the risks (Lee et al., 2016). In addition, grapefruit juice affects certain statins more than other. Be sure to discuss with patients their dietary intake of grapefruit juice so that you can prescribe the best medication.

Indications. Lovastatin is considered a moderate- or low-intensity statin therapy for the reduction of LDL-C and is used to slow progression of coronary atherosclerosis, prevention of stroke, and prevention of myocardial infarction. Although the primary effect is reduction of LDL-C, lovastatin may have a minor impact in raising HDL-C and reducing triglycerides.

Adverse Effects. The most common adverse effect from the use of lovastatin is infection, with incidence ranging from 11% in patients taking extended-release to 16% in patients taking immediate-release tablets. Other, less common side effects include headache, constipation, arthralgia, sinusitis, and influenza. Progression of cataracts may occur in some patients. Unexplained muscle pain, tenderness, or weakness may indicate myopathy, particularly if accompanied by malaise or fever, suggesting rhabdomyolysis. Severe hepatotoxicity may occur in fewer than 1% of patients.

Contraindications. Lovastatin is contraindicated in patients with a history of liver disease or who are pregnant or breastfeeding. Use of lovastatin in patients requiring antiretroviral protease inhibitors is contraindicated due to the increased risk of development of acute renal failure, myopathy, or rhabdomyolysis. It should be used very cautiously in patients with a history of renal or liver impairment. Patients should reduce alcohol intake while taking lovastatin to prevent liver impairment. If there is a concern about alcoholism, lovastatin should not be prescribed.

Monitoring. The primary care provider should determine baseline serum cholesterol panel and LFTs prior to initiation of lovastatin therapy. LFTs should be checked 4 to 12 weeks after starting therapy and then at 6- to 12-month intervals or more often if dosage adjustments are required. Carefully monitor older adults who are receiving lovastatin as they may respond to lower dosages.

PRACTICE PEARLS

Lovastatin

Geriatrics

Older adults who are receiving immediate-release lovastatin have been reported to have 45% higher mean plasma levels of HMG-CoA reductase inhibition than do younger patients, so may respond to lower total dosages.

Pravastatin

Pharmacokinetics. Pravastatin is administered orally. Efficacy of pravastatin is slightly higher (but not significantly different) with evening dosing compared to morning dosing. Pravastatin is rapidly absorbed from the GI tract. Peak plasma concentrations are achieved in 1 to 1.5 hours. Pravastatin undergoes extensive first-pass extraction and metabolism by the liver. Approximately 20% of a dose is eliminated in the urine and 70% in the feces.

Indications. Pravastatin is used for reduction of elevated TC, LDL-C, Apo B, and triglyceride concentrations, and to increase HDL-C. It can be used for prevention of myocardial infarction and stroke and has been shown to reduce cardiovascular mortality. Depending on the dose, pravastatin can be considered a low-intensity or moderate-intensity statin.

Adverse Effects. The most common adverse effect of pravastatin is abdominal pain, experienced by between 1.4% and 6% of patients. Others include dyspepsia, nausea, constipation, and flatulence. Although rhabdomyolysis has been reported, this is extremely rare, occurring in fewer than 0.1% of patients.

Contraindications. Pravastatin is contradicted in females who are pregnant or breastfeeding and for patients with active hepatic disease. It should be avoided in patients with alcoholism or those who are heavy users of alcohol. Caution should be used in older adults as they may be more likely to experience myopathy. Pravastatin should generally be avoided in children with hyperlipidemia before the ages of 8 to 10 years.

PRACTICE PEARLS

Statin Use in Pregnancy and Lactation

Statins are contraindicated in patients who are pregnant or may become pregnant due to the impact on cholesterol pathways that are essential for fetal or infant development, especially brain development. Statins are also contraindicated in patients who are breastfeeding as they can be excreted in the liver. If medication therapy is indicated, bile acid sequestrants such as cholestyramine may be considered.

Monitoring. Liver function studies should be obtained prior to initiating statins and then as needed for symptoms suggesting liver injury. Assess medication adherence, adverse effects, and patient response to therapy (fasting lipid levels within 4 to 12 weeks after beginning therapy or after a change in dose). Due to the risk of diabetes mellitus, blood glucose should be monitored, particularly in patients with prediabetes.

Fibric Acid Derivatives

Fibric acid derivatives (also called fibrates) are typically used to decrease TG and raise HDL-C levels. In general, they reduce TG concentrations by 20% to 50% and increase HDL-C concentrations by 10% to 35% within 6 weeks of their initiation, with greater changes occurring in individuals with severe hypertriglyceridemia. Fibric acid derivatives do not have a significant impact on LDL-C, reducing it by only 5% to 10%. The ability of gemfibrozil to lower TG is attributed to an increase in lipoprotein lipase activity, which results in increased catabolism of VLDL. Gemfibrozil also may suppress lipolysis in adipose tissue, decrease free fatty acid flux, and lower the rate of TG synthesis. The increase in HDL observed with gemfibrozil may result from increased synthesis of Apo A-1, or it may be indirectly related to the medication's ability to lower VLDL.

Gemfibrozil

Pharmacokinetics. Gemfibrozil is administered orally and then is rapidly and completely absorbed from the GI tract. It is highly protein bound (approximately 95%). Gemfibrozil is metabolized by the liver and excreted by the kidney.

Indications. Gemfibrozil can be used in patients with hyperlipidemia and hypertriglyceridemia. It is considered most effective in reducing TG and minimally effective in reducing LDLs or increasing HDLs.

Adverse Effects. The most common adverse effect of gemfibrozil is dyspepsia, experienced by nearly 20% of patients. Other adverse effects include abdominal pain, diarrhea, and nausea. Approximately 8% of patients may experience cholelithiasis (gallstone disease). Mild hemoglobin, hematocrit, and white blood cell decreases have occasionally been observed in patients after gemfibrozil initiation; however, these stabilize with long-term administration. If given in addition to statins, the risk of myopathy and rhabdomyolysis increases significantly.

Contraindications. Gemfibrozil is contraindicated in patients with renal failure, liver disease, gallbladder disease, and primary biliary cirrhosis. It should be used cautiously in patients with a history of cholelithiasis, those who are pregnant or breastfeeding, and children younger than 18 years of age.

Monitoring. Lipid panels, including triglycerides, should be monitored to determine effectiveness within 4 to 12 weeks after initiating gemfibrozil. Complete blood count (CBC), LFTs, and serum bilirubin (direct and indirect) may be measured if the patient experiences signs or symptoms of liver disease, bile duct obstruction, or anemia.

Fenofibrate

Pharmacokinetics. Fenofibrate is more than 99% protein bound, primarily to albumin. Approximately 60% of a dose is excreted in the urine and 25% in the feces.

Indications. Gemfibrozil can be used as an adjunct to diet for the treatment of adult patients with severe hypertriglyceridemia. In addition, it can reduce TC, LDL-C, and Apo B as well as increase HDL in adult patients with primary hypercholesterolemia or mixed dyslipidemia.

Adverse Effects. Approximately 8% of patients experienced elevated LFTs while taking fenofibrate. LFTs returned to normal following medication cessation. Other adverse effects include headache, abdominal pain, backache, and constipation.

Contraindications. Fenofibrate is contraindicated in patients with renal disease, hepatic disease, gallbladder disease, or biliary stenosis. It is also contraindicated in breastfeeding patients as it can disrupt lipid metabolism in the developing infant. It should be used cautiously in patients with known cardiac disease. Patients with a history of thromboembolic disease may be at risk for thromboembolism while taking fenofibrate.

Monitoring. Establish baseline serum lipids, including TGs as well as baseline LFTs. After beginning therapy, monitor follow-up fasting serum lipid panels to determine response within 4 to 12 weeks. Monitor LFTs as needed should the patient experience any signs or symptoms of liver disease.

Bile Acid Sequestrants

Bile acid sequestrants were one of the first antihyperlipidemic agents used to reduce LDL-C by binding with bile acids in the intestine: they are not absorbed systemically. Although individual medications in this category differ in their chemical structure, all are large copolymers that function as anion-exchange resins in the lumen of the intestine. They then bind to bile acids, forming an insoluble complex and producing a significant increase in excretion of bile acids in the feces. The pathways involved in cholesterol and bile acid metabolism are closely related. Although the medications are sequestering bile acids and are interrupting their enterohepatic recirculation, they also result in the diversion of cholesterol into bile acid synthesis. Intracellular cholesterol concentrations decrease and lead to two compensatory changes: acceleration of HMG-CoA reductase activity and upregulation of LDL cell surface receptors. These two homeostatic changes increase intracellular cholesterol concentrations for conversion to bile acids, either by increased cholesterol synthesis or by increased uptake and removal of LDL from plasma. Therefore, bile acid sequestrants increase the diversion of cholesterol to bile acid synthesis, lower intracellular stores of cholesterol, and result in increased catabolism of LDL by the liver.

Because bile acid sequestrants are not absorbed systemically, they may be considered as an alternative to statins in patients requiring antihyperlipidemic therapy during pregnancy or breastfeeding. These medications also may reduce absorption of fat-soluble vitamins A, D, E, and K. Risks and benefits to the mother and infant must be carefully considered.

Cholestyramine

Pharmacokinetics. Cholestyramine is not systemically absorbed, so it doesn't affect serum concentrations. Cholestyramine binds intestinal bile acids, increasing bile acid fecal elimination and preventing reabsorption. Plasma cholesterol levels typically are reduced within 1 month of therapy and then return to pretreatment levels approximately 1 month following drug cessation.

Indications. Cholestyramine is used for treatment of hypercholesterolemia, especially elevated LDL cholesterol (types IIa and IIb hyperlipoproteinemia). It can also be used for pruritus associated with biliary stasis.

Adverse Effects. Adverse effects are predominantly related to the GI tract. The most common is constipation in more than 10% of patients (moderate to severe in rare cases). Other, less frequent adverse effects include abdominal pain, diarrhea, eructation, nausea, and changes in taste. Chronic use of cholestyramine can result in vitamin deficiencies, especially vitamins K and D. Vitamin K deficiency can increase the risk for bleeding and vitamin D deficiency can result in osteoporosis. Rarely, patients may experience cholelithiasis, GI obstruction, or night blindness.

Contraindications. Cholestyramine is contraindicated in patients with biliary obstruction. In addition, because it can increase serum triglycerides, cholestyramine is contraindicated in patients with serum triglyceride concentrations greater than 400 mg/dL and is relatively contraindicated in patients with serum triglyceride concentrations greater than 200 mg/dL. It should be used cautiously in patients with a history of constipation, because of increased risk for fecal impaction. Cholestyramine may interfere with absorption of fat-soluble vitamins and should be avoided in patients who have a history of coagulopathy or who are pregnant or breastfeeding.

Monitoring. Assess the patient carefully to determine GI side effects. Serum lipid levels should be monitored approximately 4 weeks after initiation of therapy.

Colestipol

Pharmacokinetics. Colestipol is administered orally. Since colestipol is not absorbed orally, serum concentrations and half-life parameters do not apply. It is not affected by digestive enzymes and is eliminated in the stool. Reduction of the plasma cholesterol concentration usually is seen within 24 to 48 hours of starting therapy, and maximum effects are achieved within 1 month of starting therapy.

Indications. Colestipol is used in the treatment of primary hypercholesterolemia (elevated LDL cholesterol hyperlipoproteinemia) in conjunction with dietary control in patients with hypertriglyceridemia. In addition, it can be used for the treatment of diarrhea due to increased bile acids after surgery as well as for the treatment of pruritus associated with partial biliary obstruction.

Adverse Effects. By far, the most common side effects are GI related. More than 10% of patients can experience constipation. Constipation is typically mild and short lived but can be severe in rare cases. Other GI side effects include abdominal discomfort, eructation, bloating, flatulence, and nausea. Because colestipol can bind with and impair the absorption of dietary vitamin K, hypoprothrombinemia can occur.

Contraindications. Bile acid resins such as colestipol are absolutely contraindicated in patients with a serum triglyceride concentration greater than 400 mg/dL as it may increase serum triglycerides. Colestipol should be used cautiously in patients with cholelithiasis or complete biliary obstruction. Additionally, use colestipol with caution in patients with primary biliary cirrhosis since it can further raise serum cholesterol. It should be used with caution in patients with preexisting constipation, dysphagia, or GI motility disorders.

Monitoring. Check lipid levels after 1 month of therapy to determine effectiveness of colestipol. Encourage patients to drink plenty of fluids and include additional fiber in the diet to prevent constipation. Because bile acid sequestrants impair the absorption and reduce the bioavailability of folate, it may lead to folate deficiency. Therefore, monitor patients for folate deficiency and supplement when indicated.

Selective Cholesterol Synthesis Inhibitors

Selective cholesterol absorption inhibitors are also known as sterol transporter inhibitors because they selectively inhibit the absorption of cholesterol and related phytosterols (plant sterols) by the small intestine. They do not affect cholesterol synthesis or increase bile acid secretion. When absorption of cholesterol is reduced, decreased cholesterol is delivered to the liver, cholesterol stores are reduced, and increased

cholesterol is cleared from the blood. At this time, ezetimibe is the only agent in this class. Current guidelines recommend use of these medications in addition to statins to reduce cardiovascular risk when unable to obtain sufficient reduction in LDLs with statins alone.

Ezetimibe

Pharmacokinetics. Ezetimibe is administered orally. After oral administration of a single 10-mg dose to fasting adults, mean ezetimibe peak plasma concentrations are attained within 4 to 12 hours. Although administration with food (high-fat vs. nonfat meals) has no effect on the extent of absorption of ezetimibe, administration with a high-fat meal can increase the peak serum concentration of ezetimibe by 38%. No specific dosage adjustments are required in patients with mild hepatic impairment, but ezetimibe should not be given to patients with moderate to severe liver impairment.

Indications. Ezetimibe can be used as an adjunct to diet and exercise therapy to reduce elevated total cholesterol, LDLs, Apo B, and non-HDL-C in patients with primary hyperlipidemia. It is used in combination for reduction of elevated total cholesterol and LDLs in patients with homozygous familial hypercholesterolemia.

Adverse Effects. Ezetimibe is infrequently associated with side effects such as mild diarrhea, abdominal pain, or arthralgia. Risk of myalgia and/or rhabdomyolysis/myoglobinuria increases when this medication is given in combination therapy with a statin.

Contraindications. Ezetimibe should be used with caution in patients with moderate to severe hepatic disease. It should be avoided in patients who are pregnant or breastfeeding.

Monitoring. Patients receiving ezetimibe should be monitored for signs and symptoms of myopathy and/or rhabdomyolysis/myoglobinuria (myalgia, muscle cramps, musculoskeletal pain, lethargy, fatigue, fever, and/or myasthenia). Risk for these problems increases if given with statins.

Prescriber Considerations for Antihyperlipidemic Therapy

Clinical Practice Guidelines

In 2018, the ACC and AHA released a full revision of the 2013 ACC/AHA Cholesterol Guidelines (Grundy et al., 2019). Highlights include emphasis on the use of the ASCVD Risk Calculator (https://tools.acc.org/ASCVD-Risk-Estimator-Plus/#!/calculate/estimate) for all patients between the ages of 40 and 75. If risk is still uncertain, providers can recommend a coronary artery calcium test to further evaluate the need for statin therapy. The guidelines include the principle that "lower is better" for LDL-C and that optimal total cholesterol level is about 150 mg/dL, with LDL-C at or below 100 mg/dL to reduce risk of heart disease and stroke. The guidelines further include a series of risk-enhancing factors as well as emphasizing the need for identifying and managing high LDL-C in children, adolescents, and young adults to reduce their lifetime exposure to the health effects of high cholesterol.

BOOKMARK THIS!

Clinical Guidelines for Hyperlipidemia

- Updated 2018 AHA/ACC/AACVPR/AAPA/ABC/ACPM/ADA/AGS/APhA/ASPC/NLA/PCNA Guideline on the Management of Blood Cholesterol is found at https://www.ahajournals.org/doi/10.1161/CIR.0000000000000625.
- In addition, the primary care provider can find a simplified version of the guidelines at https://www.acc.org/~/media/Non-Clinical/Files-PDFs-Excel-MS-Word-etc/Guidelines/2018/Guidelines-Made-Simple-Tool-2018-Cholesterol.pdf.

Clinical Reasoning for Antihyperlipidemic Therapy

Consider the individual patient's health problem requiring antihyperlipidemic therapy. Start by determining the patient's overall risk factors for cardiovascular disease. What is their blood pressure? Do they smoke? What is their average weekly amount of physical activity? Then, carefully assess the patient's baseline cholesterol to determine the specific lipoprotein phenotype. For primary prevention, use the data to aid determination of the patient's 10-year risk for cardiovascular events using the pooled cohort equation ASCVD Risk Calculator. The results will assist the primary care provider in determining whether the patient is at low risk (less than 5%), borderline risk (5% to 7.4%), intermediate risk (7.5% to 19.9%), or high risk (greater than 20%). If the patient's LDL-C is 190 mg/dL, consider familial hypercholesterolemia. For patients with known ASCVD, identify the major statin benefit category and begin high-intensity statin therapy as indicated.

Determine the desired therapeutic outcome based on the degree of antihyperlipidemic therapy needed for the patient's health problem. Reduction of hyperlipidemia is part of an overall goal of reducing cardiovascular risk. What is the goal based on the patient's cardiovascular risk profile? While there is no ideal target blood level for LDL-C, the new guidelines suggest that it should be less than 100 mg/dL, with total cholesterol at approximately 150 mg/dL. Then the guidelines should be used to determine whether the patient requires high-intensity, medium-intensity, or low-intensity statins. Choose the statin based on the patient's overall risk for primary or secondary prevention. If the patient has cholesterol levels consistent with familial hypercholesterolemia, consider referral to a specialist.

Assess the antihyperlipidemic selected for its appropriateness for an individual patient by considering the medication's side effects and the patient's race/ethnicity, comorbidities, and genetic factors. Use the risk calculator and the clinical practice guidelines to determine the patient's cardiovascular

risk. Carefully evaluate the patient's current medications to avoid drug–food interactions (Table 8.6). Remember that statins are contraindicated in patients who are pregnant or breastfeeding, so for patients of childbearing age, discuss the use of adequate contraception to prevent pregnancy or determine alternative meds to statins. Once the appropriate medication is determined, patients with hepatic disease will require dosage adjustment. For patients with renal disorders, only atorvastatin will not require dosage adjustment. Statin doses should be adjusted for patients of Asian descent. Assess factors that predispose patients to SASE. If side effects of statins are intolerable, use practice guidelines to determine next steps.

Initiate the treatment plan with the selected medication by first providing adequate patient education to ensure the patient's understanding and promote full participation in the antihyperlipidemic therapy. Antihyperlipidemic therapy is not a substitute for nonpharmacologic interventions to ensure reduction of cardiovascular risk. All patients should receive dietary guidance to avoid dietary saturated and trans fats and to increase intake of fruits and vegetables (Fig. 8.1). Provide patients with guidance for follow-up appointments to judge effectiveness of the therapy as well as determine the patient's ability to adhere to dietary and exercise recommendations. Statins may interact with a variety of other medications, so remind the patient to check with their primary care provider prior to adding any over-the-counter (OTC) medications, or herbal or dietary supplements.

Ensure complete patient and family understanding about the medication prescribed for antihyperlipidemic therapy using a variety of education strategies. Provide the patient with written and verbal instructions at each visit. Refer to a dietitian as needed for patients with complex dietary needs. Some patients may benefit by websites and/or smartphone apps that provide dietary information, such as My Fitness Pal (www.myfitnesspal.com) or MyPlate (www.choosemyplate.gov). Both can provide information regarding calories as well as types of fats available in a wide variety of foods.

Conduct follow-up and monitoring of patient responses to antihyperlipidemic therapy. Discuss the patient's ability to follow a low-cholesterol diet, reviewing facilitators and barriers to adherence as well as recommending resources that may be helpful. Monitor the patient's response to antihyperlipidemic therapy using clinical practice guidelines to determine overall goals. If indicated by patient symptoms, assess the patient's liver function, renal status, and creatine phosphokinase. Cholesterol levels should be assessed 4 to 12 weeks after therapy is initiated and after dosage changes.

Teaching Points for Antihyperlipidemic Therapy

Health Promotion Strategies

Hyperlipidemia is one of the major risk factors for cardiovascular disease, and as such, management is part of overall health promotion. The following strategies should be

TABLE 8.6	Examples of Medication–Food Interactions with Statins[a]
Substance	**Interaction**
Amiodarone	May decrease metabolism of statin, increase risk for myopathy
Amlodipine	May increase concentration of statin, increase risk for muscle-related toxicity such as myopathy and rhabdomyolysis
Antacids	May decrease plasma concentrations if given within 2 hours of taking select statins
Colchicine	Increased risk for muscle-related toxicity such as myopathy or rhabdomyolysis; increased statin or colchicine exposure
Cyclosporin	May increase concentration of statin, increase risk for muscle-related toxicity such as myopathy and rhabdomyolysis
Diltiazem	May increase concentration of statin, increase risk of muscle-related toxicity such as myopathy or rhabdomyolysis
Fenofibrate/fenofibric acid	May increase risk of muscle-related toxicity such as myopathy or rhabdomyolysis
Gemfibrozil	May increase risk of muscle-related toxicity such as myopathy or rhabdomyolysis; contraindicated in select statins
Grapefruit and grapefruit juice	Large quantities may increase risk for muscle-related toxicity in select statins
Ranolazine	May increase concentration of statin, increase risk for muscle-related toxicity
Red yeast rice	Contraindicated in patients taking statins; similar compounds in red yeast rice have HMG-CoA reductase inhibitor actions; may increase risk of drug-related toxicity.
Ticagrelor	May increase concentration of statin; may increase risk of muscle-related toxicity such as myopathy or rhabdomyolysis
Verapamil	May increase concentration of statin; may increase risk of muscle-related toxicity such as myopathy or rhabdomyolysis
Warfarin	Increases INR; increases risk for bleeding

[a]There are many other medication–medication and medication–food interactions with statins. The primary care provider should check all medication interactions among the patient's medications before prescribing statins. In some cases, doses may be adjusted to reduce risk of adverse effects.

Data from Clinical Pharmacology powered by Clinical Key. (2019). from Elsevier Clinical Solutions; and Wiggins, B. S., Saseen, J. J., Page, R. L., Reed, B. N., Sneed, K., Kostis, J. B., . . . Morris, P. B. (2016). Recommendations for management of clinically significant drug-drug interactions with statins and select agents used in patients with cardiovascular disease: A scientific statement from the American Heart Association. *Circulation, 134*(21), e468-e495. doi:10.1161/CIR.0000000000000456.

recommended to patients to help them become full partners in their care:

- Choosing unsaturated fats rather than saturated fats is a great way to reduce dietary cholesterol.
- Cooking with unsaturated oils such as olive, corn, sunflower, soybean, or peanut oil is preferred to oils such as coconut or palm oil that are high in saturated fats.
- Substitute low-fat, plain yogurt for sour cream or heavy cream in cooking.
- Switch from whole (4%) or reduced-fat (2%) to low-fat (1%) or skim milk (fat-free).
- Reduce intake of fatty meats and replace with lean cuts of meat.
- Limit intake of sweets and sugar-sweetened beverages.
- Regularly include whole grains, fruits, and vegetables in the diet.
- Consider the DASH Eating Plan (https://www.nhlbi.nih.gov/health-topics/dash-eating-plan) as an option for dietary guidance.
- To reduce LDL-C and overall cardiovascular risk, regularly engage in physical activity in consultation with

your primary care provider. If permitted, perform at least 40 minutes of moderate- to vigorous-intensity activity three or four times each week.
- Emphasize that all patients, even those over 65 years of age, can benefit from diet, exercise, and statin use.
- If the patient smokes or uses other tobacco products, recommend resources such as the National Cancer Institute Helpline (877.448.7848 or www.smokefree.gov).

Patient Education for Medication Safety

- Depending on the statin you are prescribed, you may be asked to avoid grapefruit juice due to the possibility of food–drug interaction.
- If you become pregnant while taking a statin, notify your primary care provider immediately.
- Avoid alcohol while taking statins. If you do drink alcohol, limit to no more than 2 drinks daily for males and 1 drink daily for females. Drink equivalencies are 12 oz of beer equals 5 oz of wine equals 1.5 oz of hard liquor.
- Report increased muscle aches, muscle weakness, fever, or dark urine to your primary care provider for evaluation

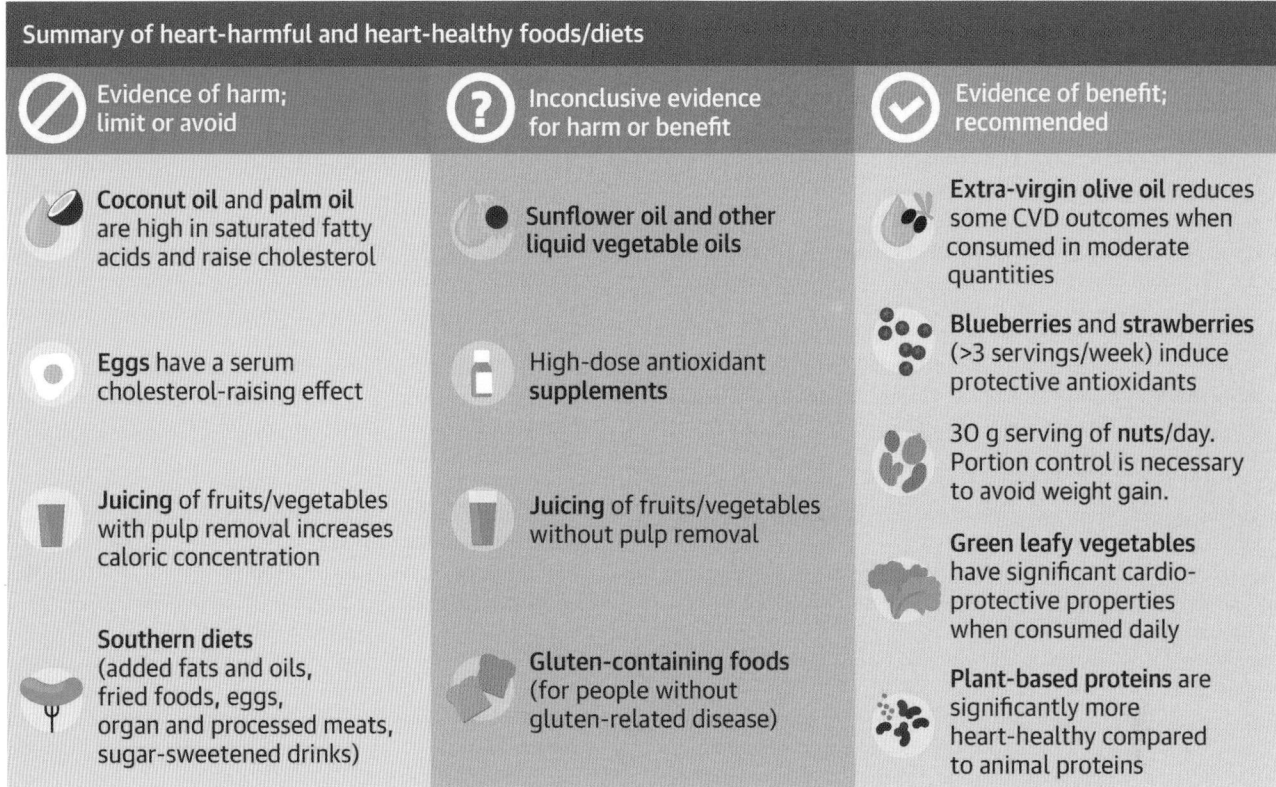

Summary of heart-harmful and heart-healthy foods/diets

⊘ Evidence of harm; limit or avoid

- **Coconut oil** and **palm oil** are high in saturated fatty acids and raise cholesterol

- **Eggs** have a serum cholesterol-raising effect

- **Juicing** of fruits/vegetables with pulp removal increases caloric concentration

- **Southern diets** (added fats and oils, fried foods, eggs, organ and processed meats, sugar-sweetened drinks)

❓ Inconclusive evidence for harm or benefit

- **Sunflower oil** and other **liquid vegetable oils**

- **High-dose antioxidant supplements**

- **Juicing** of fruits/vegetables without pulp removal

- **Gluten-containing foods** (for people without gluten-related disease)

✓ Evidence of benefit; recommended

- **Extra-virgin olive oil** reduces some CVD outcomes when consumed in moderate quantities

- **Blueberries** and **strawberries** (>3 servings/week) induce protective antioxidants

- 30 g serving of **nuts**/day. Portion control is necessary to avoid weight gain.

- **Green leafy vegetables** have significant cardio-protective properties when consumed daily

- **Plant-based proteins** are significantly more heart-healthy compared to animal proteins

• **Fig. 8.1** Evidence-based dietary guidelines to reduce cardiovascular risk and cholesterol (From Freeman, A. M., Morris, P. B., Barnard, N., Esselstyn, C. B., Ros, E., Agatston, A., . . . Kris-Etherton, P. [2017]. Trending cardiovascular nutrition controversies. *Journal of the American College of Cardiology, 69*[9]), 1172–1187.)

as these may be signs of severe muscle damage affecting the kidneys.

- Take statins as directed. If you miss a dose, take it as soon as possible on the same day but skip the dose if less than 8 hours before the next dose.
- Patients with prediabetes or diabetes should monitor their blood sugar as diabetes is an infrequent but possible adverse effect of statins.
- Contact your primary care provider prior to taking any OTC medications, herbals, or dietary supplements to prevent drug–drug interactions.

Application Questions for Discussion

1. What are the implications for prescribing hyperlipidemia treatment to a patient who has a history of AS-CVD and diabetes?
2. Discuss teaching implications for a 40-year-old patient with no history of cardiovascular disease who is newly diagnosed with hyperlipidemia.
3. What data should be included in adjusting doses and intensity of statin in patients with hyperlipidemia?##

SELECTED BIBLIOGRAPHY

Benjamin Emelia, J., Muntner, P., Alonso, A., Bittencourt Marcio, S., Callaway Clifton, W., & Carson April, P. (2019). Heart disease and stroke statistics—2019 update: A report from the American Heart Association. *Circulation, 139*(10), e56–e528. http://doi.org/10.1161/CIR.0000000000000659.

Buck, H. G., Mcghee, S., Polo, R. L., & Zambroski, C. (2019). Hypercholesterolemia management in older adults: A scoping review of recent evidence. *Journal of Gerontological Nursing, 45*(3), 31–42. http://doi.org/10.3928/00989134-20190211-04.

Centers for Disease Control and Prevention, National Center for Health Statistics: (2021). Health, United States, Table 23 Hyattsville, MD. https://www.cdc.gov/nchs/hus/contents2019.htm.

Centers for Disease Control and Prevention (CDC). (February 6, 2019). *High cholesterol facts*. Retrieved from https://www.cdc.gov/cholesterol/facts.htm.

Clark, D., & Virani, S. S. (2019). 2018 Cholesterol guidelines: Key topics in primary prevention. *Current Atherosclerosis Reports, 21*(5), 17. http://doi.org/10.1007/s11883-019-0776-8.

Clinical Pharmacology powered by Clinical Key. (2019). Elsevier Clinical Solutions.

Elagizi, A., Lavie, C. J., Marshall, K., DiNicolantonio, J. J., O'Keefe, J. H., & Milani, R. V. (2018). Omega-3 polyunsaturated fatty acids and cardiovascular health: A comprehensive review. *Progress in Cardiovascular Diseases, 61*(1), 76–85. https://doi.org/10.1016/j.pcad.2018.03.006.

Freeman, A. M., Morris, P. B., Aspry, K., Gordon, N. F., Barnard, N. D., Esselstyn, C. B., & Kris-Etherton, P. (2018). A clinician's guide for trending cardiovascular nutrition controversies: Part II. *Journal of the American College of Cardiology, 72*(5), 553–568. https://doi.org/10.1016/j.jacc.2018.05.030.

Grundy, S. M., Stone, N. J., Bailey, A. L., Beam, C., Birtcher, K. K., Blumenthal, R. S., & Yeboah, J. (2019). 2018 AHA/ACC/AACVPR/AAPA/ABC/ACPM/ADA/AGS/APhA/ASPC/NLA/PCNA guideline on the management of blood cholesterol. A Report of the American College of Cardiology/American Heart Association Task Force on Clinical Practice Guidelines. *Journal of the American College of Cardiology, 73*(24), e285–e350. http://doi.org/10.1016/j.jacc.2018.11.003.

Lee, J. W., Morris, J. K., & Wald, N. J. (2016). Grapefruit juice and statins. *American Journal of Medicine, 129*(1), 26–29. http://doi.org/10.1016/j.amjmed.2015.07.036.

Liao, J. K. (2007). Safety and efficacy of statins in Asians. *The American Journal of Cardiology, 99*(3), 410–414. http://doi.org/10.1016/j.amjcard.2006.08.051.

Lloyd-Jones, D. M., Braun, L. T., Ndumele, C. E., Smith, S. C., Sperling, L. S., Virani, S. S., & Blumenthal, R. S. (2019). Use of risk assessment tools to guide decision-making in the primary prevention of atherosclerotic cardiovascular disease: A special report from the American Heart Association and American College of Cardiology. *Circulation, 139*(25), e1162–e1177. http://doi.org/10.1161/CIR.0000000000000638.

Nordestgaard, B. G., Chapman, M. J., Humphries, S. E., Ginsberg, H. N., Masana, L., & Descamps, O. S. (2013). Familial hypercholesterolaemia is underdiagnosed and undertreated in the general population: Guidance for clinicians to prevent coronary heart disease: Consensus statement of the European Atherosclerosis Society. *European Heart Journal, 34*(45), 3478–3490a. http://doi.org/10.1093/eurheartj/eht273.

Okopien, B., Buldak, L., & Boldys, A. (2018). Benefits and risks of the treatment with fibrates—A comprehensive summary. *Expert Review of Clinical Pharmacology, 11*(11), 1099–1112. http://doi.org/10.1080/17512433.2018.1537780.

Palma, L., Welding, M., & O'Shea, J (2016). Diagnosis and treatment of familial hypercholesterolemia: The impact of recent guidelines. *The Nurse Practitioner, 41*(8), 36–43. http://doi.org/10.1097/01.NPR.0000488711.52197.bd.

Sanin, V., Pfetsch, V., & Koenig, W. (2017). Dyslipidemias and cardiovascular prevention: Tailoring treatment according to lipid phenotype. *Current Cardiology Reports, 19*(7), 61. http://doi.org/10.1007/s11886-017-0869-3.

U.S. Preventive Services Task Force. (2016). Screening for lipid disorders in children and adolescents: U.S. Preventive Services Task Force recommendation statement. *JAMA, 316*(6), 625–633. http://doi.org/10.1001/jama.2016.9852.

Wiggins Barbara, S., Saseen Joseph, J., Page Robert, L., Reed Brent, N., Sneed, K., Kostis John, B., & Morris Pamela, B. (2016). Recommendations for management of clinically significant drug–drug interactions with statins and select agents used in patients with cardiovascular disease: A scientific statement from the American Heart Association. *Circulation, 134*(21), e468–e495. http://doi.org/10.1161/CIR.0000000000000456.

Yu, E., Malik, V. S., & Hu, F. B. (2018). Cardiovascular disease prevention by diet modification: JACC Health Promotion Series. *Journal of the American College of Cardiology, 72*(8), 914–926. https://doi.org/10.1016/j.jacc.2018.02.085.

9

Antihypertensive Medications

CHERYL H. ZAMBROSKI

Overview

Newly developed practice guidelines have caused a major shift in thinking about the prevention, evaluation, and treatment of high blood pressure. An analysis of evidence from a wide range of individual studies and meta-analyses has revealed that cardiovascular risk increases progressively as blood pressure rises above the normal level of 120/80 mm Hg. The new guidelines, from the American College of Cardiology (ACC) and the American Heart Association (AHA) (Whelton et al., 2018), address cardiovascular risk by revising the definition of hypertension to improve health outcomes.

Hypertension is now defined as a systolic blood pressure greater than 130 mm Hg or a diastolic blood pressure greater than 80 mm Hg based on two separate readings obtained on two separate occasions (Table 9.1). In addition, the use of the term *elevated* is now preferred over *prehypertension*. This designation signals to the provider and the patient the importance of addressing the problem earlier rather than waiting until the blood pressure reaches Stage 1. The new guidelines clearly emphasize the need for rigorous treatment of hypertension to improve long-term health outcomes by reducing cardiovascular risk.

The new definition of hypertension has significantly affected prevalence estimates of hypertension in males and females. Based on the new cut point of 130/80 mm Hg or greater, roughly 46% of the adult population has hypertension versus the 32% identified by using the previous cut point of 140/90 mm Hg or greater. Using these data, the prevalence of hypertension is highest in non-Hispanic Black males (approximately 59%), non-Hispanic Black females (56%), and non-Hispanic White males (47%) (Whelton et al., 2018). An important factor in promoting blood pressure health is to fully consider hypertension *awareness*, *treatment*, and *control* among adults who are diagnosed with high blood pressure. Previous data suggest that hypertension control is better in females than in males, in Whites than in Blacks and Hispanics, and in older adults than in younger adults. In addition, adults with higher socioeconomic status tend to have a higher rate of blood pressure control.

Relevant Physiology

Optimal blood pressure is essential to maintain tissue perfusion throughout a range of physiologic conditions. The primary determinants of blood pressure are represented in Fig. 9.1. In summary, arterial pressure is the product of cardiac output and peripheral resistance. *Cardiac output* (the volume of blood pumped from the heart in 1 minute) is further determined by heart rate, myocardial contractility, blood volume, and venous return. *Peripheral resistance* (resistance of the arteries to blood flow) is determined by the diameter of the arterioles; constriction of the arterioles increases blood pressure and dilation results in a decrease in blood pressure. If there are changes in cardiac output without sufficient adjustment in peripheral resistance, there can be insufficient capillary blood flow to maintain tissue perfusion (Table 9.2).

As indicated earlier, recent clinical practice guidelines have refined the desired blood pressures for optimal cardiovascular health. Ideally, normal systolic pressure should be less than 120 mm Hg and normal diastolic pressure should be less than 80 mm Hg. *Systolic pressure* is the highest blood pressure following ventricular contraction (systole). *Diastolic pressure* is the lowest arterial pressure following ventricular filling (diastole). *Mean arterial pressure* (MAP) is the average pressure in the arteries throughout the cardiac cycle. Elasticity of the arterial walls and mean blood volume in the arterial system influence arterial pressure. A normal MAP ranges between 70 and 110 mm Hg. In a healthy adult, MAP remains relatively consistent through a variety of physiologic conditions (e.g., changes in body position, increased physical activity, and during rest) to maintain adequate tissue perfusion. If MAP drops below the normal ranges for an extended period, tissue damage from poor perfusion and hypoxia can occur. The body has a variety of compensatory mechanisms to help maintain MAP and ensure adequate blood flow and tissue perfusion.

The major influencers of blood pressure control include baroreceptors/chemoreceptors, the autonomic nervous system (primarily via the sympathetic nervous system), the renin-angiotensin-aldosterone system (RAAS), and the antidiuretic

Blood Pressure Category	Systolic Blood Pressure		Diastolic Blood Pressure
Normal	<120 mm Hg	And	<80 mm Hg
Elevated[b]	120–129 mm Hg	And	<80 mm Hg
Hypertension			
Stage 1	130–139 mm Hg	Or	80–89 mm Hg
Stage 2	≥140	Or	≥90

TABLE 9.1 Categories of Blood Pressure in Adults[a]

[a]Individuals with systolic blood pressure and diastolic blood pressure in two categories should be considered to be in the higher blood pressure category.

[b]The term *elevated* has replaced the term *prehypertension*.

From Whelton, P. K., Carey, R. M., Aronow, W. S., et al. (2018). 2017 ACC/AHA/AAPA/ABC/ACPM/AGS/APhA/ASH/ASPC/NMA/PCNA guideline for the prevention, detection, evaluation, and management of high blood pressure in adults: A report of the American College of Cardiology/American Heart Association Task Force on Clinical Practice Guidelines. *Hypertension, 71*(6) 1269–1324. https://doi.org/10.1161/hyp.0000000000000065.

hormone (ADH). These work together to ensure adequate tissue perfusion throughout constantly varying conditions.

Baroreceptors respond to local changes in blood pressure by increasing or decreasing heart rate and constricting or relaxing local smooth muscle to change blood flow. The baroreceptors are located in the carotid sinuses and aortic arch and respond through the autonomic nervous system. Stimulation of the parasympathetic nervous system leads to a decrease in heart rate, whereas stimulation of the sympathetic nervous system leads to an increase in heart rate and stroke volume and/or constriction or dilation of blood vessels.

Chemoreceptors, which are sensory nerve cells located in the medulla oblongata and the carotid and aortic bodies, detect changes in pH, carbon dioxide (CO_2), and oxygen. In response to these changes, either the vasomotor center or the cardioregulatory center in the brain leads to compensatory changes in heart rate, stroke volume, and blood pressure.

The RAAS responds to changes in blood pressure through a series of actions that help regulate systemic vascular resistance and blood volume. The three major components of RAAS are *renin* (a peptide produced by the juxtaglomerular cells in the kidneys), *angiotensin* (a peptide hormone), and *aldosterone* (a steroid hormone). Renin is released into the general circulation under three conditions: 1) stimulation of β_1 receptors in the sympathetic nervous system; 2) decreased blood pressure to the kidneys; or 3) decreased sodium to the distal tubules. The renin then acts on angiotensinogen produced in the liver to form angiotensin I. Angiotensin I is converted into angiotensin II by the angiotensin-converting enzyme (ACE), which is found in vascular endothelium, particularly in the lungs. Angiotensin II is a potent vasoconstrictor, primarily of the arterioles. In addition, angiotensin II acts on the adrenal cortex to release aldosterone, which increases reabsorption of sodium in the kidneys, leading to water retention, increased blood volume, and increased

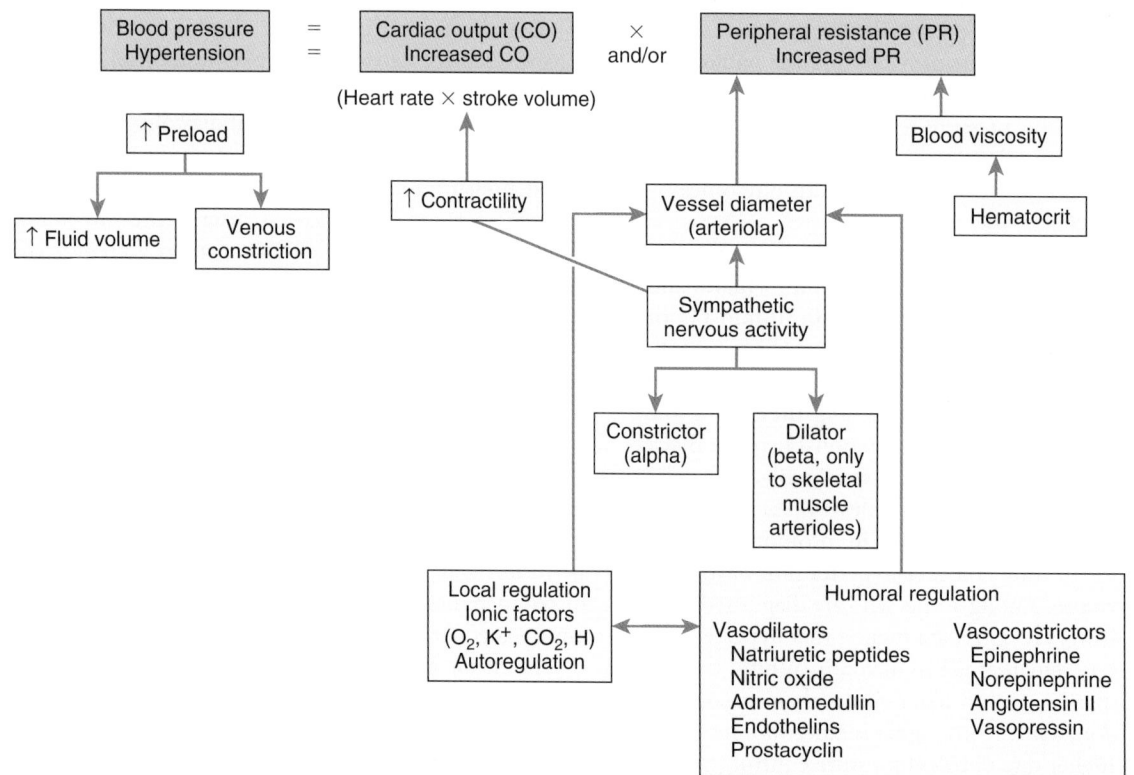

• **Fig. 9.1** Primary determinants of blood pressure. (From McCance, K., & Huether, S. [2019]. *Pathophysiology* [8th ed.]. St. Louis: Elsevier.)

		Mean Arterial Flow	Capillary Flow
Peripheral Resistance[a]	Increased	Increased	Decreased
	Decreased	Decreased	Increased
Heart Rate[b]	Increased	Increased	Increased
	Decreased	Decreased	Decreased
Stroke Volume[c] (determined by myocardial contractility, blood volume, venous return)	Increased	Increased	Increased
	Decreased	Decreased	Decreased

TABLE 9.2 Factors That Affect Mean Arterial Pressure and Capillary Flow

[a]Cardiac output maintained constant
[b]Peripheral resistance and stroke volume maintained constant
[c]Peripheral resistance and heart rate maintained constant
Modified from Little, R. C., & Little, W. C. [1985]. *Physiology of the heart and circulation* [3rd ed.]. St. Louis: Year Book Medical Pub. In McCance, K., & Huether, S. [2019]. *Pathophysiology* [8th ed.]. St. Louis: Elsevier.

blood pressure. Aldosterone increases the excretion of potassium and hydrogen from the distal tubules of the nephron.

The ADH is synthesized in the hypothalamus and released by the posterior pituitary. When it is released, it causes further reabsorption of sodium and water in the kidneys. This increases blood volume and subsequently increases blood pressure.

Pathophysiology: Hypertension

Hypertension is the most common diagnosis in the United States, with nearly 50% of patients meeting criteria for the diagnosis. The vast majority of patients (more than 90%) are diagnosed with *primary hypertension*. Primary hypertension differs from *secondary hypertension* in that in primary hypertension, there is no specifically identifiable cause (i.e., it is idiopathic). Secondary hypertension, on the other hand, is a result of an underlying condition or medication that, when identified and treated sufficiently, allows blood pressure to return to normal levels (Box 9.1). Secondary hypertension is commonly suspected if the patient has a sudden onset of high blood pressure, if the onset of hypertension is in a patient younger than 30 years of age with no obvious risk factors, or if the onset is associated with initiation of certain medications.

Primary hypertension is a result of a set of complex interactions between genetics and the environment (Fig. 9.2). Varying genetic phenotypes in combination with environmental risks ultimately contribute to chronically increased peripheral resistance and increased blood volume. In primary hypertension, one or more normal compensatory mechanisms for controlling blood pressure are no longer effective. Problems leading to primary hypertension include increased or inappropriate sympathetic nervous system activation, dysfunction of the RAAS, and inadequate amounts of natriuretic hormones that normally balance extracellular fluid and electrolytes. In addition, inflammation and insulin resistance can further contribute to vasoconstriction and sodium and water retention in the kidneys. As a result, chronic imbalance of peripheral resistance and increased

• Box 9.1 **Possible Causes of Secondary Hypertension**

- Obstructive sleep apnea
- Chronic kidney disease
- Primary aldosteronism
- Hyperthyroidism
- Heavy alcohol use
- Use of amphetamines
- Use of serotonin norepinephrine reuptake inhibitors
- Use of tricyclic antidepressants
- Use of oral contraceptives
- Use of nonsteroidal antiinflammatory drugs (NSAIDs)
- Use of recreational drugs
- Use of decongestants
- Coarctation of the aorta
- Use of atypical antipsychotics
- Use of Ma Huang (ephedra) herbal supplement
- Use of certain immunosuppressants

blood volume lead to vascular remodeling with damage to end organs including the heart, brain, kidneys, and retina.

A variety of risk factors have been identified for primary hypertension (Box 9.2). Although only some may be modified through lifestyle education, knowledge of less modifiable risk factors can help guide education and screening. It is important to fully screen patients for other risk factors for cardiovascular disease to provide comprehensive and patient-centered care.

PRACTICE PEARLS

Antihypertensive Therapy

Use the AHA/ACC's ASCVD CV Risk Calculator (http://static.heart.org/riskcalc/app/index.html#!/baseline-risk), which estimates a patient's 10-year and lifetime risk for atherosclerotic cardiovascular disease (ASCVD), to guide selection of the most personalized approach to hypertension management.

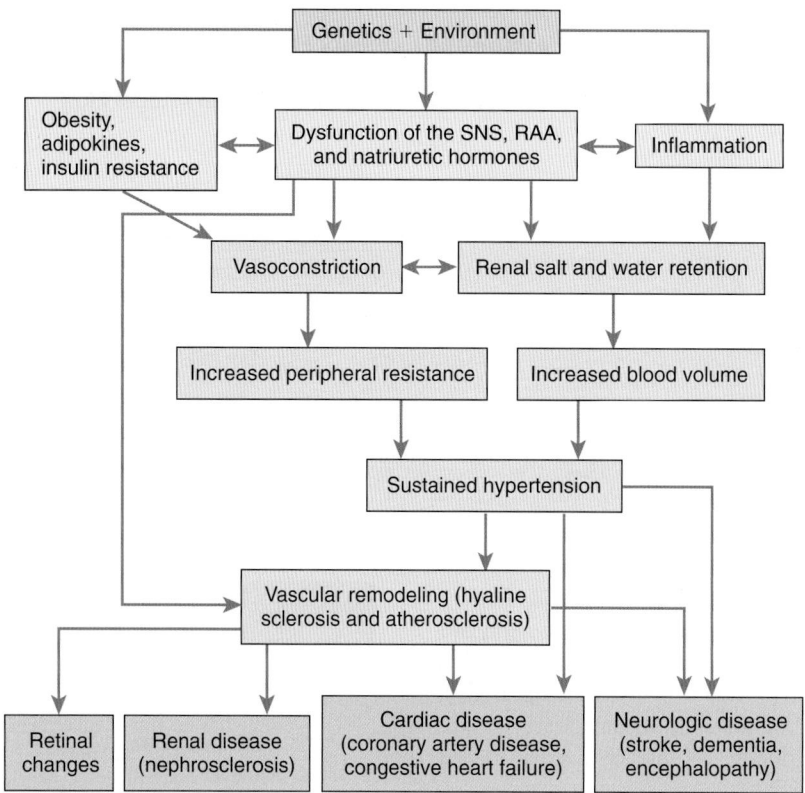

• **Fig. 9.2** Pathophysiology of hypertension. (From McCance, K., & Huether, S. [2019]. *Pathophysiology* [8th ed.]. St. Louis: Elsevier.)

An additional strategy to evaluate blood pressure control in patients is the use of out-of-office and self-monitoring tactics. Self-monitoring provides important data that can be used to enhance the diagnosis of hypertension and help differentiate conditions such as *white coat hypertension* and *masked hypertension*. White coat hypertension is defined as systolic/diastolic pressures that are 20/10 mm Hg higher when blood pressure is obtained while the patient is in the provider's office than when the patient is at home. This phenomenon is more common in older adults, females, and nonsmokers who are screened in an office setting by primary care providers. Masked hypertension is defined as in-office blood pressure readings that are *lower* than out-of-office blood pressure readings. Patients with masked hypertension have a greater cardiovascular risk than patients with white coat hypertension or normal blood pressure. In addition, self-monitoring can help the primary care provider evaluate the patient's response to medications and the need for titration of doses. Box 9.3 provides recommended procedures for use of home blood pressure monitoring by patients. In general, automated devices are recommended for most patients because of their ease of use compared to manual devices. Automated devices are commercially available and can be found at a variety of major retailers in communities and online. Note that adults with some chronic dysrhythmias may be unable to obtain accurate blood pressure measurements with an automatic device and should be assessed using a standard sphygmomanometer by a trained health care provider.

Antihypertensive Therapy

Current clinical practice guidelines in combination with the patient's stage of hypertension, comorbidities, and ability to participate in self-care will influence the primary care provider's decisions regarding the best choices for medication therapy. All antihypertensive therapy should be combined

Teach patients to include blood pressure self-monitoring using the following steps:
1. Use the same validated instrument with each measurement for best comparison.
2. Make sure to place the blood pressure cuff above the bend in the elbow as directed on the device.
3. Take at least two readings 1 minute apart in the morning before taking blood pressure medication and before dinner in the evening. Do this weekly for at least 2 weeks after each treatment change and the week before a clinic visit.
4. Record readings for easy access. This can be done using paper and pencil, a blood pressure self-monitoring unit with built-in memory, or one of a variety of apps available for smartphones.

• Box 9.4   Nonpharmacologic Recommendations for Hypertension

- Weight loss to ideal body weight if possible; each kg of weight lost can reduce blood pressure by 1 mm Hg
- Follow a heart-healthy diet (e.g., the DASH diet, https://www.nhlbi.nih.gov/health-topics/dash-eating-plan)
- Reduce dietary sodium intake to goal of 1500 mg/day or at least decrease intake by 1000 mg/day
- Eat a diet high in potassium (unless contraindicated) with a target of 3500–5000 mg/day
- Regular physical activity with 90–150 min/week aerobic exercise as well as inclusion of dynamic resistance and isometric resistance activities
- Moderate alcohol intake: for females, no more than one drink daily; for males, no more than two drinks daily

Adapted from Whelton et al. [2018]. 2017 ACC/AHA/AAPA/ABC/ACPM/AGS/APhA/ASH/ASPC/NMA/PCNA guideline for the prevention, detection, evaluation, and management of high blood pressure in adults—Executive summary: A report of the American College of Cardiology/American Heart Association Task Force on Clinical Practice Guidelines. *Hypertension, 71*[6], 1269–1324. http://doi.org/10.1161/HYP0000000000000066.

with patient-centered recommendations for nonpharmacologic lifestyle changes to further enhance blood pressure control (Box 9.4). Follow-up and monitoring of interventions is outlined in Fig. 9.3.

First-line therapies for Stage 1 hypertension include *thiazide diuretics*, *ACE inhibitors (ACE-Is)* or *angiotensin receptor blockers (ARBs)*, and *calcium channel blockers (CCBs)* (Table 9.3). For patients with Stage 2 hypertension, a combination of two different pharmacologic classes is recommended. Second-line therapies include *direct renin inhibitors, alpha-1 blockers, centrally acting alpha-2 agonists,* and *direct vasodilators* (Table 9.4). Loop diuretics and beta-blockers are also considered second-line therapies but will be discussed in Chapter 10, Coronary Artery Disease Medications, and Chapter 11, Heart Failure Medications. Basic actions of selected medications are illustrated in Fig. 9.4.

Thiazide Diuretics

Thiazide diuretics are considered a first-line medication for patients with hypertension. They act by inhibiting the reabsorption of sodium and chloride at the distal renal tubule in the nephron. There are two subtypes of thiazide diuretics: *thiazide-type diuretics* and *thiazide-like diuretics.* Thiazide-like diuretics are very similar pharmacologically and structurally to thiazide diuretics with similar diuretic effects.

Initially, thiazide diuretics lower blood pressure by reducing plasma and extracellular fluid volume, thereby decreasing cardiac output. Over time, cardiac output returns to normal, as do plasma and extracellular fluid levels. Nevertheless, peripheral resistance is reduced, ultimately lowering blood pressure. The reason peripheral resistance is reduced is not fully understood. While the major effect is a decrease in blood pressure, a secondary effect is a loss of potassium, chloride, and bicarbonate, which reduces the excretion of calcium and uric acid. Recent evidence suggests that thiazide-like diuretics may reduce the incidence of hypokalemia and hyponatremia. In addition, thiazide-like diuretics such as chlorthalidone may have less impact on cholesterol and blood glucose levels. Because chlorthalidone has a longer half-life than thiazide-type diuretics, it also may lead to better 24-hour blood pressure reduction (Rik et al., 2015).

Chlorothiazide

Pharmacokinetics. Chlorothiazide can be administered either intravenously or orally. The half-life is typically 45 to 120 minutes. Chlorothiazide crosses the placenta and is excreted in breast milk. If it is given orally, diuresis begins within 2 hours, peak response occurs in 4 hours, and duration of action is 6 to 12 hours. Absorption of chlorothiazide is increased if it is taken with food.

Indications. Chlorothiazide is used for the treatment of hypertension. It can also be used in patients with edema secondary to heart failure, ascites, or corticosteroid or estrogen therapy, and in patients with renal dysfunction.

Adverse Effects. The most common adverse effect is hypokalemia, affecting more than 10% of patients. Potassium supplementation is recommended for patients at risk for hypokalemia. Patients who are taking cardiac glycosides in addition to chlorothiazide are at increased risk for dysrhythmias. Chlorothiazide can cause hyperglycemia in patients with diabetes. While hypercholesterolemia and/or hypertriglyceridemia have been associated with thiazide diuretic therapy, data suggest these cholesterol changes are not clinically significant and do not contribute to long-term coronary heart disease risk. Rare adverse effects that have been associated with chlorothiazide diuretics include agranulocytosis, aplastic anemia, Stevens-Johnson syndrome, and toxic epidermal necrolysis.

Contraindications. Absolute contraindications for use of chlorothiazide include thiazide diuretic and/or sulfonamide hypersensitivity and anuria. Chlorothiazide should be used cautiously in patients with hyperkalemia, hypokalemia, hypochloremia metabolic alkalosis, hypomagnesemia, or hypercalcemia;

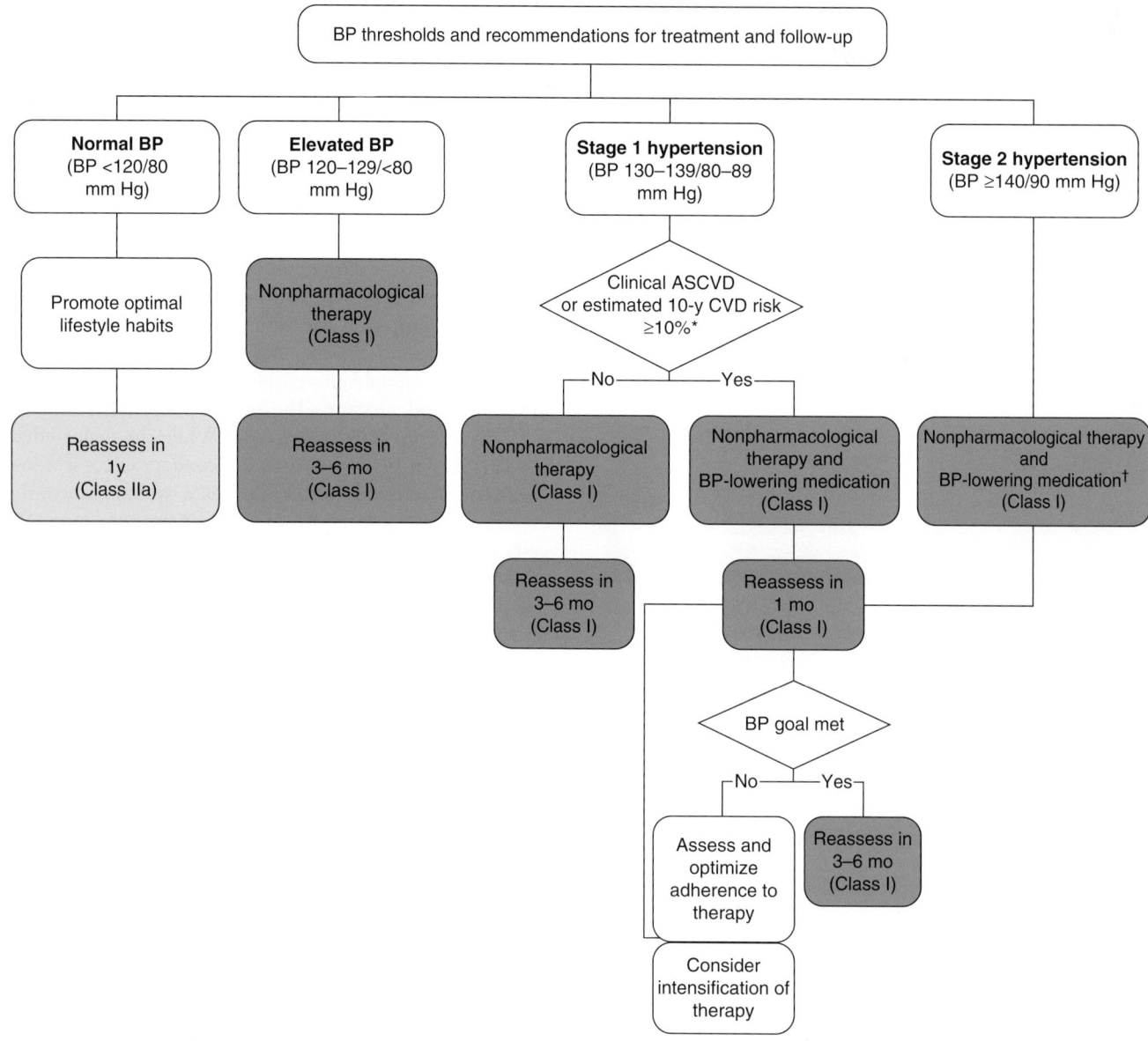

• **Fig. 9.3** Blood pressure thresholds and recommendations for treatment and follow-up (From Whelton, P. K., Carey, R. M., Aronow, W. S., et al. [2018]. 2017 ACC/AHA/AAPA/ABC/ACPM/AGS/APhA/ASH/ ASPC/NMA/PCNA guideline for the prevention, detection, evaluation, and management of high blood pressure in adults: A report of the American College of Cardiology/American Heart Association Task Force on Clinical Practice Guidelines. *Hypertension, 71*[6]: 1269–1324. https://doi.org/10.1161/ hyp.0000000000000065)

these electrolyte imbalances must be corrected prior to use. Older adults are at greater risk for dilutional hyponatremia. Chlorothiazide should be used cautiously in patients with gout due to increased risk for hyperuricemia.

Monitoring. Blood sugar should be monitored frequently in diabetic patients because chlorothiazide can increase hyperglycemia. Extravasation can cause tissue necrosis, so chlorothiazide should never be given subcutaneously or intramuscularly; if given intravenously, assess site frequently. Monitor electrolytes, particularly for those who are at high risk for electrolyte imbalances.

Hydrochlorothiazide

Pharmacokinetics. Hydrochlorothiazide is given orally and absorbed from the gastrointestinal (GI) tract. Absorption depends on the formulation and dose and is reduced in patients with cardiac, renal, or hepatic disease. Onset of action is approximately 2 hours after administration, with peak effects at about 4 hours. Duration of action is 6 to 12 hours. Hydrochlorothiazide is excreted unchanged in the urine. Half-life increases in patients with renal insufficiency and renal failure.

TABLE 9.3	First-Line Antihypertension Medications			
Category/ Medication	Indication[a]	Dosage[b]		Considerations and Monitoring

Thiazide Diuretics

Chlorothiazide	Treatment of hypertension	Usual dose is 500–1000 mg/day orally, given in 1–2 divided doses. *Adolescents:* Dose is the same as for adults. *Children 2–12 yr:* Recommended dose is 10–20 mg/kg/day orally in 1–2 divided doses, not to exceed 1000 mg/day.	Use cautiously in patients with a history of gout related to the risk of hyperuricemia. Chlorthalidone is the preferred choice because studies have shown that use reduces overall risk of cardiovascular disease. Monitor patient for hyponatremia, hypokalemia, hyperglycemia, hyperuricemia, and hypercalcemia.
Hydrochlorothiazide	Treatment of hypertension	Begin with 12.5–25 mg orally once daily. Patients may be given up to 50 mg/day in 1–2 divided doses. Usual dose is 25–50 mg/day. *Adolescents >12 yr:* 1 mg/kg/day orally once daily, titrated as needed up to 3 mg/kg/day based on clinical response. Maximum dosage: 50 mg/day. *Children 2–12 yr:* 1 mg/kg/day orally once daily, titrated as needed up to 3 mg/kg/day. Maximum dosage: 50 mg/day.	
Metolazone	Treatment of hypertension	Usual dose is 2.5–5 mg orally once daily. *Children:* 0.2–0.4 mg/kg/day orally in divided doses every 12–24 hr.	
Chlorthalidone	Treatment of hypertension	Begin with 12.5–25 mg orally once daily. Patients may be given up to 100 mg daily. Usual dose is 12.5–25 mg/day.	
Indapamide[c]	Treatment of hypertension	Begin with 1.25 mg orally once daily. May be increased to 2.5 mg once daily after 1 month if needed. Usual dose is 1.25–2.5 mg/day. Maximum dosage: 5 mg once daily	

Angiotensin-Converting Enzyme Inhibitors

Quinapril	Treatment of hypertension	Begin with 10–20 mg orally once daily in patients who are not receiving diuretics. Doses can be adjusted at 2-week intervals to achieve blood pressure goals. Usual dose is 20–80 mg/day, given in 1–2 divided doses. For older adults, begin at low end of usual adult dose. If given in combination with a diuretic, reduce the initial dose to 5 mg orally once daily. In general, twice-daily dosing may have great end effect at higher doses of 40–80 mg. Maximum dosage: 80 mg/day	Do not use in combination with ARBs or direct renin inhibitors. Increased risk of hyperkalemia, particularly in patients with renal disease. Do not use in patients who are pregnant or may become pregnant. Educate patients to avoid salt substitutes.
Ramipril		Begin with 2.5 mg orally once daily. If given with a diuretic, reduce the initial dose to 1.25 mg once daily. Usual dose is 2.5–20 mg/day in 1–2 divided doses. In some patients, using divided dosing may increase antihypertensive effects.	

Continued

**TABLE
9.3   First-Line Antihypertension Medications—cont'd**

Category/ Medication	Indication[a]	Dosage[b]	Considerations and Monitoring
Benazepril	Treatment of hypertension	Begin with 10 mg orally once daily. If receiving diuretics, begin with 5 mg. Usual dose is 20–40 mg/day, with a maximum dosage of 80 mg/day. May be given in 1–2 divided doses. Older adults should be given lowest dose at beginning of therapy. If blood pressure goals are not met, a thiazide diuretic may be added. *Adolescents and children 6–17 yr:* Use weight-based dosing of 0.2 mg/kg/day up to 10 mg initially. Titrate as needed up to a maximum dosage of 40 mg/day.	
Lisinopril	Treatment of hypertension	Begin with 10 mg orally once daily. Usual dose is 20–40 mg/day. Maximum dosage: 80 mg/day Lower dose may be necessary in patients with impaired renal function, older adults, and in those receiving diuretics. In patients with a creatinine clearance <30 mL/min, begin therapy with 5 mg once daily. *Children 6–17 yr:* 0.07 mg/kg (maximum of 5 mg) orally once daily initially; adjust dosage according to clinical response. Maximum dosage: 0.6 mg/kg/day or 40 mg/day orally, whichever is less	
Fosinopril	Treatment of hypertension	Initial dose is 10 mg orally once daily. Adjust dosage according to response. Usual dose is 20–40 mg/day in 1–2 divided doses, with maximum dosage of 80 mg/day. Older adults may be more sensitive to antihypertensive effects. *Adolescents and children 6 to 17 yr and ≥50 kg:* Begin with 5 mg once daily, then titrate to patient response. Maximum dosage: 40 mg/day	
Trandolapril	Treatment of hypertension	For patients not receiving diuretics, begin with 1 mg orally once daily (for Black patients, use 2 mg as initial dose once daily). Adjust dosage according to the blood pressure response at intervals of at least 1 week. Usual dose is 2–4 mg once daily, with maximum dosage of 8 mg/day. If patient is on a diuretic, it is recommended to discontinue use 2–3 days prior to beginning trandolapril to reduce symptomatic hypotension. If blood pressure is not controlled with trandolapril alone, may add the diuretic. If the diuretic cannot be discontinued, initial dose is 0.5 mg given with careful medical supervision. Usual dose range in patients receiving diuretics is 1–8 mg by mouth once daily.	
Captopril	Treatment of hypertension	Begin with 12.5–25 mg orally two or three times daily; if already on a diuretic, begin with lower doses. May increase to 50 mg three times daily after 1–2 weeks if needed. May add a diuretic after 1–2 weeks if needed. Maximum dosage is considered to be 150 mg/day in divided doses.	

TABLE 9.3 **First-Line Antihypertension Medications—cont'd**

Category/ Medication	Indication[a]	Dosage[b]	Considerations and Monitoring
Angiotensin II Receptor Blockers			
Candesartan	Treatment of hypertension	Begin with 16 mg orally once daily. Usual dose is 8–32 mg/day given in 1–2 divided doses. Maximal blood pressure effect usually occurs within 4–6 weeks. *Adolescents and children >6 yr:* If weight >50 kg, begin with 8–16 mg orally once daily or divided into 2 equal doses. Usual dose is 4–32 mg/day orally given in 1–2 doses/day. Maximum blood pressure reduction is generally obtained within 4 weeks. If weight <50 kg, can begin with 4–8 mg orally once daily or divided into 2 equal doses. Usual dose is 2–16 mg/day given in 1–2 doses/day. *Children ≥1–6 yr:* Can begin with 0.2 mg/kg/day orally as a suspension, given once daily or divided into 2 doses daily. Usual dosage range is 0.05–0.4 mg/kg/day orally, given in 1–2 doses/day. Maximal effect typically achieved in about 4 weeks.	Do not use in combination with ACE inhibitors or direct renin inhibitors. Do not use in patients who are pregnant or may become pregnant. May cause hyperkalemia in patients with chronic kidney disease or in patients taking potassium supplements or potassium-sparing medications. Avoid use in patients with a history of angioedema from ARBs. Adjust dosage according to blood pressure response. If patient is volume depleted, begin therapy with a lower dose under close supervision. Monitor patient for symptomatic hypotension. If needed to manage blood pressure further, a diuretic such as hydrochlorothiazide can be added. Patients with a history of renal artery stenosis are at higher risk of acute renal failure.
Irbesartan	Treatment of hypertension	Begin with 150 mg orally once daily unless patient is volume depleted, then begin with 75 mg once daily.	
Losartan	Treatment of hypertension	*Adults and adolescents:* Begin with 50 mg orally once daily. Maintenance dosage range is 25–100 mg/day given in 1–2 divided doses. Maximum effect typically occurs 3–6 weeks after starting on losartan. *Children ≥6 yr:* Begin with 0.7 mg/kg orally once daily (maximum dosage is 50 mg/day).	
Valsartan		*Adults and adolescents ≥17 yr:* If given as tablet, begin with 80–160 mg when used as monotherapy. Usual dose is 80–320 mg once daily. *Children and adolescents 1–16 yr:* Begin with 1 mg/kg orally once daily (maximum dosage is 40 mg/day). Titrate to patient response (to maximum of 4 mg/kg/day or 160 mg/day). *Adults and adolescents ≥17:* If given as oral solution, 40–80 mg orally twice daily. Maximum dosage: 320 mg/day *Children and adolescents 6–16 yr:* 0.65 mg/kg orally twice daily. Maximum dosage: 40 mg daily initially, then titrate to maximum 1.35 mg/kg twice daily or 160 mg/day.	

Continued

TABLE 9.3 **First-Line Antihypertension Medications—cont'd**

Category/ Medication	Indication[a]	Dosage[b]	Considerations and Monitoring
Olmesartan		*Adults and adolescents ≥17 yr:* Begin with 20 mg once daily, then increase to 40 mg if needed after 2 weeks of therapy. Usual dose is 20–40 mg once daily. If needed, add diuretic such as hydrochlorothiazide. Maximum dosage: 40 mg/day.	
		Children and adolescents 6–16 yr and weight ≥35 kg: Begin with 20 mg once daily, then increase to 40 mg once daily after 2 weeks of therapy, if needed. Maximum dosage: 40 mg/day	
		Children and adolescents 6–16 yr and weight 20–34 kg: Begin with 10 mg orally once daily, then increase to maximum dosage of 20 mg/day after 2 weeks of therapy, if needed.	
Telmisartan	Treatment of hypertension	Begin with 40 mg once daily. If volume depleted, begin with 20 mg once daily. Usual dose is 20–80 mg once daily. Maximum reduction of blood pressure typically occurs after 4 weeks. If not controlled with telmisartan alone, may add diuretic.	

Calcium Channel Blockers: Dihydropyridines

Amlodipine		Begin with 5 mg once daily, with a maximum of 10 mg/day. Full clinical response typically takes 7–14 days.	Dihydropyridines are associated with increased pedal edema, which occurs more commonly in females than in males.
		Older adults or patients who are more debilitated should begin with 2.5 mg.	Avoid use in patients with reduced ejection fraction heart failure. If essential, may use amlodipine or felodipine.
		Usual dose is 2.5–10 mg once daily.	
		Children and adolescents 6–17 yr: Begin with 2.5 mg to maximum of 5 mg daily.	
Felodipine		Begin with 5 mg orally once daily. May take up to 2 weeks for full patient response for titration. Usual dose is 2.5–10 mg once daily. Maximum dosage: 10 mg/day	When using amlodipine for children, may adjust dose every 5–7 days; it may require several weeks for the maximum hypotensive effect.
		For older adults, begin with 2.5 mg once daily and adjust to maximum of 10 mg. Dosage adjustment interval should be at least 2 weeks.	
Nicardipine		*Immediate-release capsules:* Begin with 20 mg orally three times daily. Usual dose 20–40 mg three times daily.	
		Extended-release capsules: Begin with 30 mg orally twice daily. Can be increased to 60 mg orally twice daily if necessary.	
Isradipine		*Regular-release forms:* Begin with 2.5 mg orally twice daily, alone or in combination with a thiazide diuretic. Adjust dosage by 5-mg increments at 2- to 4-week intervals based on clinical response. Usual dose is 5–10 mg twice daily. Maximum dosage: 10 mg orally twice daily.	
		Extended-release forms: Begin with 5 mg orally once daily as monotherapy or in combination with a diuretic. If needed, increase by 5-mg increments at 2- to 4-week intervals to a maximum of 20 mg once daily.	
		NOTE: Adverse effects are increased with doses greater than 10 mg daily.	

TABLE 9.3 First-Line Antihypertension Medications—cont'd

Category/ Medication	Indication[a]	Dosage[b]	Considerations and Monitoring
Nisoldipine		*Extended-release tablets:* Begin with 17 mg once daily. Titrate daily dose based on clinical response. May increase dose by 8.5 mg at 1-week intervals up to maximum of 34 mg/day. For older adults, begin with 8.5 mg orally once daily. Usual dose is 17–34 mg daily.	
Nifedipine		*Extended-release forms:* Begin with 30–60 mg orally once daily. For older adults, begin with lower end of adult dosage range. Maximum dosage: 90 mg for most formulations; maximum dosage for Procardia XL is 120 mg/day.	
Calcium Channel Blockers: Non-Dihydropyridines			
Diltiazem	Treatment of hypertension	*Extended-release forms:* Begin with 180–240 mg orally once daily and titrate to patient response to 360 mg/day. Maximum effect is typically observed within 2 weeks. For older adults, begin with the lower end of dosage range. *Sustained-release capsules:* Begin with 60–120 mg orally twice daily. Increase dose if necessary. Usual dosage range is from 120–180 mg orally twice daily. Maximum dosage is 360 mg/day. For older adults, begin therapy at the lower end of the dosage range.	Non-dihydropyridines should not be used in patients with reduced ejection fraction heart failure. Should be avoided in patients taking beta-blockers due to risk for bradycardia and heart block. Drug interactions are common (CYP 3A4 major substrate and moderate inhibitor).
Verapamil		*Regular-release forms:* Begin with 80 mg orally three times daily. May increase at weekly intervals up to 360 mg/day in divided doses for full effect. For patients of small stature, patients with hepatic disease, or older adults, begin with 40 mg orally three times daily. *Calan SR caplets or Isoptin SR extended-release 12-hour tablets:* Begin with 180 mg orally once daily in the morning. Dosage may be increased to 240 mg twice daily. For patients of small stature, patients with hepatic disease, or older adults, begin with 120 mg orally once daily in the morning. *Verelan extended-release 24-hour capsules:* Begin with 240 mg orally once daily in the morning. May increase, stepwise, to 360 mg and then 480 mg once daily, if needed. Usual daily dose is 240 mg. Antihypertensive effect is typically evident within the first week of therapy. For patients of small stature, patients with hepatic disease, or older adults, begin with 120 mg once daily in the morning. Usual daily dose is 240 mg. *Verelan PM extended-release capsules, controlled onset:* Begin with 200 mg orally once daily at bedtime. Dosage may be increased by 100 mg/day up to 400 mg/day. For patients with hepatic disease or short stature or with older adults, begin with 100 mg once daily at bedtime.	

[a]The table addresses medications as they are specifically indicated for hypertension.
[b]Dosages are for adults unless otherwise noted.
[c]Indapamide is a sulfonamide-type diuretic similar to the thiazides. Adapted from Whelton et al. (2018). 2017ACC/AHA/AAPA/ABC/ACPM/AGS/APhA/ASH/ASPC/NMA/PCNA guideline for the prevention, detection, evaluation, and management of high blood pressure in adults—Executive summary: A report of the American College of Cardiology/American Heart Association Task Force on Clinical Practice Guidelines. *Hypertension, 71*[6], 1269–1324. http://doi.org/10.1161/HYP0000000000000066; Elsevier. [n.d.]. *Clinical pharmacology powered by ClinicalKey®.* Retrieved from http://www.clinicalkey.com.

Second-Line Medications for Antihypertensive Therapy[a]

Drug Category/ Medication	Indications	Dosage[b]	Considerations and Monitoring
Direct Renin Inhibitors			
Aliskirin	Treatment of hypertension	Begin with 150 mg orally once daily, then may be increased to 300 mg/day. *Children and adolescents 6–17 yr and weight ≥50 kg:* 150 mg/day initially; can be increased to 300 mg if needed. In patients weighing 20–50 kg, begin at 75 mg orally once daily, up to 150 mg/day.	Blood pressure response is typically at 85% to 90%, with maximum effect at 2 weeks. Do not combine with ACE inhibitors or ARBs. Avoid use during pregnancy. Increased risk of hyperkalemia for patients with chronic kidney disease or who are taking potassium supplements. May cause renal failure in patients with renal artery stenosis or severe heart failure.
Alpha-1 Receptor Blockers (Antagonists)			
Prazosin	Treatment of hypertension	1 mg orally two or three times daily. Average dose is 6–15 mg/day in divided doses. Maximum dosage is 20 mg/day orally in divided doses.	The first dose can be given at bedtime to minimize orthostatic hypotension. Provide patient with recommendations to reduce fall risk secondary to orthostatic hypotension. Older adults may be more sensitive to risk of hypotension and other adverse effects. May also be used by patients with benign prostatic hypertrophy.
Doxazosin	Treatment of hypertension	Begin with 1 mg orally once daily; may increase up to 16 mg/day. Dosage may be increased every several days as needed to titrate response.	
Terazosin	Treatment of hypertension	Begin with 1 mg orally once daily at bedtime. Average dose is 1–5 mg once daily. May give up to 20 mg/day in divided doses every 12 hours.	

TABLE 9.4   Second-Line Medications for Antihypertensive Therapy[a]—cont'd

Drug Category/ Medication	Indications	Dosage[b]	Considerations and Monitoring
Centrally Acting Alpha-2 Agonists			
Clonidine	Treatment of hypertension	*For oral immediate-release forms:* Begin with 0.1 mg orally twice daily. Then increase by 0.1 mg/day at 1-week intervals until desired effect is achieved. Usual range is 0.2–0.6 mg/day. Older adults may require lower initial dose. *For patch:* Initially apply 1 Catapres TTS-1 (delivers 0.1 mg/24 hr) patch. Adjust dose every 1–2 weeks by changing or combining dosage systems. Doses above two Catapres TTS-3 patches are usually not associated with increased efficacy.	Considered a last-line drug for older adults because of risk of adverse effects, particularly those affecting the CNS. Clonidine must be tapered to avoid rebound hypertension and hypertensive crisis. If using the patch, it is recommended that previous hypertensive medications be continued and gradually reduced, as the transdermal system effects may take several days to be evident. Rotate site of patch to an intact area of hairless skin on the upper arm or torso once every 7 days. Avoid abrupt discontinuation of guanfacine.
Methyldopa	Treatment of hypertension	*Adults and adolescents:* Begin with 250 mg orally two or three times daily. Adjust dose every 2 days as needed. Usual dosage is 500–2000 mg/day orally given in 2–4 divided doses. Lower doses typically required in older adults. *Children:* Begin with 10 mg/kg/day orally or 300 mg/m²/day orally in 2–4 divided doses, followed by an increase in dose at intervals of at least 2 days until blood pressure control is achieved. Maximum daily dose is 65 mg/kg/day orally or 3 g/day, whichever is less.	
Guanfacine	Treatment of hypertension	Begin with 1 mg orally once daily at bedtime. May increase dose if patient does not achieve blood pressure goals after 3–4 weeks to up to 2 mg orally once daily.	
Direct Vasodilators			
Hydralazine	Treatment of hypertension	Begin with 10 mg orally up to four times daily for the first 2–4 days, then may increase to 25 mg four times daily. For the second and subsequent weeks, increase dose to 50 mg orally up to four times daily. Maximum recommended dose is 300 mg/day orally.	Direct vasodilators are associated with sodium and water retention as well as reflex tachycardia. As a result, they should be given with a diuretic and a beta-blocker to reduce these effects. Hydralazine doses >300 mg daily are associated with increased incidence of systemic lupus erythematosus.

Continued

TABLE 9.4	Second-Line Medications for Antihypertensive Therapy[a]—cont'd			
Drug Category/ Medication	**Indications**	**Dosage[b]**		**Considerations and Monitoring**
Minoxidil	Recommended only for treatment of symptomatic hypertension or hypertension associated with target organ damage and not manageable with other maximum therapeutic doses of diuretic plus two other antihypertensive agents	Begin with 5 mg orally once daily. May be increased in intervals of at least 3 days to 10 mg, 20 mg, and then 40 mg in single or divided doses.		Minoxidil should be given with a diuretic and the patient should maintain dietary sodium restriction. In patients taking minoxidil, if supine diastolic pressure has been reduced by less than 30 mm Hg, administer total daily dose once daily; if supine diastolic pressure has been reduced by 30 mm Hg or more, divide the daily dosage into 2 equal doses.

[a]Second-line agents including loop diuretics, potassium sparing diuretics, and aldosterone antagonists are covered in Chapter 11, Heart Failure Medications. Beta-blockers are discussed in greater detail in Chapter 10, Coronary Artery Disease; Chapter 11, Heart Failure Medications; and Chapter 12, Antiarrhythmic Medications.
[b]Dosages are for adults unless otherwise noted.
Adapted from Whelton et al. [2018]. 2017 ACC/AHA/AAPA/ABC/ACPM/AGS/APhA/ASH/ASPC/NMA/PCNA guideline for the prevention, detection, evaluation, and management of high blood pressure in adults—Executive summary: A report of the American College of Cardiology/American Heart Association Task Force on Clinical Practice Guidelines. *Hypertension, 71*[6], 1269–1324. http://doi.org/10.1161/HYP0000000000000066; Elsevier. [n.d.]. *Clinical pharmacology powered by ClinicalKey®.* Retrieved from http://www.clinicalkey.com.

Indications. Hydrochlorothiazide is used for the treatment of hypertension. In addition, it can be used to treat peripheral edema associated with heart failure, ascites, and renal dysfunction. It can also be used to treat peripheral edema associated with corticosteroid or estrogen therapy.

Adverse effects. The most common adverse effects experienced by patients taking hydrochlorothiazide are hypokalemia (30%–50%) and hyperuricemia (fewer than 40%). Hypokalemia is particularly dangerous in patients taking cardiac glycosides as it can increase the risk of cardiac dysrhythmias. Hyperuricemia is more common in males than in females. Other adverse effects include dehydration, dizziness, and hypotension. Older adults are more likely to have hypoglycemia and are at increased risk for falls. Patients with diabetes or prediabetes may experience hyperglycemia. Dermatologic reactions such as photosensitivity, alopecia, purpura, urticaria, and Stevens-Johnson syndrome have occurred with hydrochlorothiazide use. As a sulfonamide, hydrochlorothiazide can cause an idiosyncratic reaction leading to temporary myopia and acute angle-closure glaucoma, which, if left untreated, can lead to blindness.

Contraindications. Hydrochlorothiazide is contraindicated in patients with anuria or hypersensitivity to sulfonamide or thiazide diuretics. It should be used cautiously in patients with electrolyte imbalances such as hypokalemia, hyponatremia, and hypochloremia; these imbalances should be corrected prior to initiating therapy. Photosensitivity has been reported, so patients should avoid extensive exposure to sunlight. Hydrochlorothiazide is generally considered pregnancy category B; however, it is only recommended for use during pregnancy in patients with cardiac disease or hypertension because thiazide diuretics have been reported to cross the placenta. The risk increases to pregnancy category D if the patient is at risk for reduced uteroplacental perfusion. Hydrochlorothiazide is considered safe during breastfeeding with doses less than 50 mg daily. Higher doses may impact milk production. Older adults may be more sensitive to the effects of hydrochlorothiazide and therefore may be started at a lower dose.

Monitoring. Patients should be monitored for signs and symptoms of electrolyte imbalance, particularly hypokalemia. Serum electrolytes should be monitored and, if present, should be corrected prior to or during hydrochlorothiazide therapy. Patients with prediabetes should be monitored at follow-up appointments for elevated blood sugar levels. Evaluate the patient's blood pressure to determine the need to add a second antihypertensive for optimal health outcomes.

Metolazone

Pharmacokinetics. Metolazone is given orally, with complete absorption through the GI tract. A small portion of the drug is metabolized in the liver, but the majority is excreted unchanged in the urine. The half-life is approximately 14 hours. Metolazone crosses the placenta and is distributed in breast milk.

Indications. Metolazone is a thiazide-like diuretic used for the treatment of hypertension. In addition, it can be used for treatment of edema associated with heart failure or renal diseases such as nephrotic syndrome.

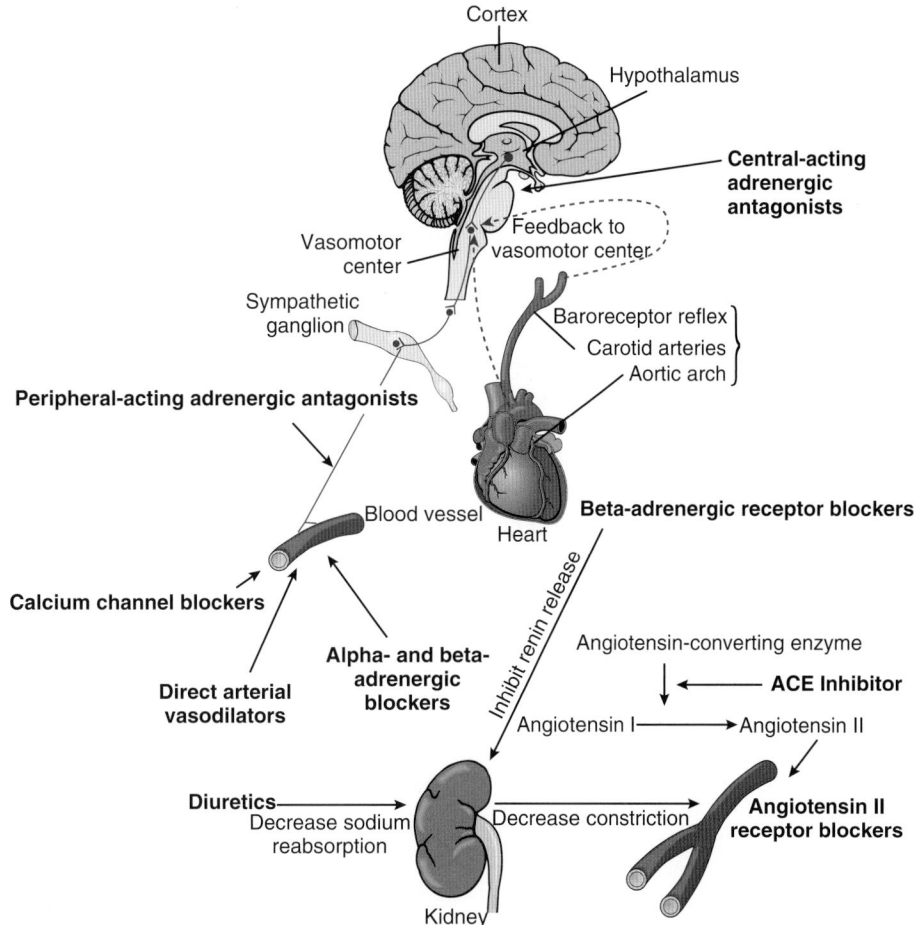

• **Fig. 9.4** Common sites of action of antihypertensive medications (Modified from Lewis, S. L., Dirksen, S. R., Heitkemper, M. M., & Bucher, L. [2013]. *Medical-surgical nursing: Assessment and management of clinical problems* [9th ed.]. St. Louis: Mosby. In Lilley, L., Collins, S., & Snyder, J. [2020]. *Pharmacology and the nursing process* [8th ed.]. St. Louis: Elsevier.)

Adverse effects. Metolazone is generally well tolerated. The most common side effect is hyperuricemia (more than 10% of patients). Gout, a condition caused by hyperuricemia, has been known to occur in people without a history of gout. Electrolyte imbalances including hyponatremia, hypokalemia, hypochloremia, hypomagnesemia, hypercalcemia, and hypophosphatemia may occur. Other side effects include orthostatic hypotension, arthralgia, myalgia, and muscle cramps. Central nervous system (CNS) effects include dizziness, headache, and weakness. Photosensitivity may occur. Erectile dysfunction has been reported to occur in patients taking metolazone. Serious adverse effects are rare (fewer than 1% of patients) and include agranulocytosis, aplastic anemia, Stevens-Johnson syndrome, and toxic epidermal necrolysis. Metolazone can precipitate rapid fluctuations in electrolytes, which can precipitate hepatic coma in susceptible patients.

Contraindications. Metolazone is contraindicated in patients with hepatic encephalopathy or hepatic coma. This medication may cause pancreatitis in patients with a history of pancreatitis. Use cautiously in patients with renal impairments or renal failure. Metolazone is pregnancy category B; however,

experts suggest that diuretic use may decrease placental perfusion. Metolazone is excreted in breast milk. Older adults may be at greater risk for orthostatic hypotension.

Monitoring. Teach patients signs and symptoms of dehydration and electrolyte imbalance. Monitor serum electrolytes, magnesium, blood urea nitrogen (BUN) and creatinine, and uric acid. Risk factors for electrolyte imbalance include severe diarrhea, decreased intake of sodium and potassium, hot weather, and high levels of physical activity. Patients with diabetes are at increased risk for hyperglycemia, so monitor blood sugar carefully. If there is insufficient response to diuretic therapy, follow current guidelines to include a CCB, ACE-I, or ARB to achieve blood pressure goals.

Chlorthalidone

Pharmacokinetics. Chlorthalidone is given orally and is best administered with food. Onset of action is about 2 hours and peak effect is between 2 and 6 hours. Chlorthalidone has a half-life of 40 to 60 hours and a typical duration of action of 48 to 72 hours. The majority of the drug is excreted in the urine, with some biliary excretion.

Indications. Chlorthalidone is a thiazide-like diuretic that may be used to treat hypertension. It is also used to treat edema associated with heart failure, cirrhosis of the liver, and chronic renal failure, and it can be used to treat edema associated with corticosteroid or estrogen therapy.

Adverse Effects. Patients taking chlorthalidone have similar adverse effects as those taking thiazide-type diuretics, including hypotension, dizziness, and GI distress. Patients may also experience hypokalemia, hyperglycemia (particularly diabetic patients), or hyponatremia.

Contraindications. Chlorthalidone is contraindicated in patients with a history of thiazide diuretic hypersensitivity, sulfonamide hypersensitivity, and anuria. Of note, while chlorthalidone is a derivative of sulfonamides, cross-sensitivity has been rarely documented. While chlorthalidone is classified as pregnancy category B, diuretics can reduce placental perfusion, and therefore, chlorthalidone should be used cautiously. In addition, chlortalidone may be passed in breast milk; however, once breastfeeding is established, the American Academy of Pediatrics considers it compatible with breastfeeding due to lack of adverse effects in the infant. Older adults are more sensitive to the effects of the drugs, so they should be started at lower doses than younger adults.

Monitoring. Patients taking chlortalidone should be assessed for hypokalemia, hyponatremia, hyperglycemia, and hypercalcemia. Monitor the medication's effect on blood pressure to ensure that blood pressure targets are achieved. If they are not, consider adding an additional antihypertensive of a different class. In addition, as with other thiazide diuretics, monitor the impact on lipids.

Angiotensin-Converting Enzyme Inhibitors

ACE-Is are recommended as a first-line treatment for patients with hypertension. They can be used especially in patients who are diagnosed with complex illnesses including heart failure, diabetes, chronic kidney disease, or post-myocardial infarction. ACE-Is reduce blood pressure by blocking the conversion of angiotensin I to angiotensin II through competitive inhibition of the ACE. Decreases in plasma angiotensin II reduce aldosterone secretion, leading to a decrease in retention of sodium and water. ACE-Is also inhibit the breakdown of bradykinin, a potent vasodilator that may increase levels of nitric oxide. Of note, reduction of blood pressure is similar for all the ACE-Is, with no specific difference in treatment of hypertension.

PRACTICE PEARLS

Ethnicity and ACE-Is

- ACE-Is are less effective in reducing blood pressure in Black patients (including African Americans) than in non-Black patients.
- Angioedema is more common in Black patients (including African Americans) than in non-Black patients.

Quinapril

Pharmacokinetics. Quinapril is administered orally. As a prodrug, quinapril is converted by the liver to the active metabolite quinaprilat. Peak levels are achieved in 1 to 2 hours. Active drug is primarily excreted unchanged through the kidneys.

Indications. Quinapril is used for the treatment of hypertension alone or may be used in combination with diuretics. For treatment of heart failure, it may be used in combination with a beta-blocker and aldosterone antagonist.

Adverse Effects. Mild dizziness is the most common adverse effect (approximately 8% of patients). Other adverse effects occurring in fewer than 6% of patients include chest pain, headache, fatigue, and cough. Hyperkalemia is infrequent but more likely in patients with heart failure or renal insufficiency.

Contraindications. Quinapril is contraindicated in patients with a history of ACE-I–induced angioedema or ACE-I hypersensitivity. As with all ACE-Is, quinapril is contraindicated in pregnancy, as it can cause injury and even death to the developing fetus if taken during the second and third trimesters.

BLACK BOX WARNING!

ACE-Is

- ACE-Is used during the second and third trimesters can cause injury and even death to the developing fetus.
- ACE-Is should be discontinued as soon as pregnancy is detected.
- Patients of child-bearing ages should be made aware of the risks of taking ACE-Is, and all risks and benefits must be considered prior to prescribing.

Monitoring. While the patient is taking quinapril, the primary care provider should monitor serum BUN, creatinine, and electrolytes. Follow-up blood pressure readings are essential to determine the effectiveness of the medication.

Ramipril

Pharmacokinetics. Ramipril is administered orally, with maximum effect in 3 to 6 hours. The half-life is dependent on renal function; however, in normal patients, half-life can range between 3 and 17 hours. Dosing is once daily. Ramipril is excreted in the urine and feces. It may be given without regard to meals.

Indications. Ramipril is used for treatment of hypertension and often in combination with a diuretic. It is also used for reduction of cardiovascular mortality, myocardial infarction, and stroke in adults 55 years of age or older who are at risk for experiencing major cardiovascular events.

Adverse Effects. The most common side effects are a mild cough in 8% to 12% of patients and moderate hypotension in 0.5% to 11% of patients. Symptomatic hypotension is rare in patients with uncomplicated hypertension but more likely in patients who are volume or salt depleted. Hypotension may occur after the initial dose or after a dosage increase, but this can be transient. Rarely, patients experience hearing loss, angioedema, hepatic failure, anxiety, or depression. Patients who receive other drugs that increase serum potassium or those with decreased renal function are at increased risk for hyperkalemia.

Contraindications. Ramipril is contraindicated in patients with a history of ACE-I–induced angioedema or sensitivity to ACE-Is. Angioedema is more likely in Black patients than in non-Black patients using ACE-Is. This drug should be used with caution in patients who are at risk for hyperkalemia, such as those who have renal insufficiency or who currently use potassium-sparing diuretics.

Monitoring. Carefully monitor patients' blood pressure and renal function while they are taking ramipril. Serum electrolytes should also be monitored, particularly potassium and sodium.

Benazepril

Pharmacokinetics. Benazepril is administered orally and is rapidly absorbed from the GI tract. It is a prodrug that is metabolized by the liver into the active metabolite benazeprilat. Peak plasma levels are typically achieved within 1 to 2 hours if fasting and 2 to 4 hours if taken with meals. The hypotensive effect lasts approximately 24 hours; therefore, dosing is once daily.

Indications. Benazepril is used for the treatment of hypertension.

Adverse Effects. Adverse effects are relatively infrequent, occurring in fewer than 10% of patients. The most common side effects are dizziness, headache, nausea, and fatigue. Dyspnea, cough, and bronchitis have occurred. Patients with heart failure and those with renal insufficiency are at risk for developing hyperkalemia.

Contraindications. ACE-Is should be used cautiously in Black patients due to increased risk of angioedema. They are also less effective in lowering blood pressure in Black patients, including African Americans.

Monitoring. Monitor the patient's fluid balance, as symptomatic hypotension is more likely to occur in those who are volume or sodium depleted. Serum electrolytes and renal function should be monitored closely after therapy is initiated.

Lisinopril

Pharmacokinetics. Lisinopril is administered orally and is widely distributed throughout the body. Onset of action is typically within 1 hour, with peak action within 6 hours. Half-life depends on renal function. Decreased renal function with a glomerular filtration rate less than 30 mL/min increases the half-life. It is eliminated unchanged in the urine.

Indications. Lisinopril is used for the treatment of hypertension. It can also be used for the treatment of heart failure in combination with diuretics or in combination with a beta-blocker and aldosterone antagonist.

Adverse Effects. The most common side effects are moderate hypotension (up to 11% of patients) and mild dizziness (up to 19% of patients); dosage adjustment or discontinuation of the medication may be required in some cases. Cough has been reported in fewer than 3% of patients, although rarely has this required discontinuation of the therapy. Hyperkalemia has been reported in approximately 2% of patients with hypertension and nearly 5% of patients with heart failure. Other infrequent adverse effects include photophobia, headache, fatigue, changes in taste, and chest pain.

Contraindications. Lisinopril is contraindicated in patients with a history of ACE-I angioedema or ACE-I hypersensitivity, and in patients with hereditary angioedema. ACE-Is are contraindicated in pregnancy; there are no data on the safety of lisinopril use while breastfeeding, so alternate medication for blood pressure control should be initiated.

Monitoring. Carefully follow patients' responses to lisinopril to ensure achievement of blood pressure goals. Serum electrolytes, including potassium and chloride, and serum BUN and creatinine should be monitored, particularly in patients with a history of renal insufficiency.

Angiotensin II Receptor Blockers

Angiotensin II receptor blockers (ARBs) lower blood pressure in ways quite similar to ACE-Is. The major difference is that, while ACE-Is block the formation of angiotensin II, ARBs selectively block angiotensin II at the AT_1 receptors in smooth muscle and the adrenal glands, thereby reducing systemic vascular resistance (and thus reducing blood pressure). By blocking angiotensin II at the AT_1 receptors, ARBs reduce the secretion of aldosterone (decreasing the reabsorption of sodium and water from the renal tubules) and reduce angiotensin-mediated vasoconstriction. In addition, because of the effect that ARBs have on the AT_1 receptors, there is an increase of circulating angiotensin II. Increased circulating angiotensin II results in stimulation of AT_2. This leads to vasodilation and production of nitric oxide and bradykinin.

Candesartan

Pharmacokinetics. Candesartan is administered orally and may be given with or without food. It is highly protein bound. Most of the hypertensive effects occur within the first 2 weeks of therapy, with full effects typically achieved at 4 weeks after initial dosing. The blood pressure–lowering effect is additive with hydrochlorothiazide or the CCB amlodipine.

Indications. Candesartan is used for the treatment of hypertension. It also may be used in combination with a thiazide diuretic for enhanced blood pressure control. In addition, it is used for the treatment of heart failure when given with a beta-blocker and aldosterone antagonist.

Adverse Effects. Side effects are infrequent with candesartan and include dizziness (approximately 4% of patients), elevated liver enzymes (fewer than 10%), and hyperbilirubinemia (approximately 6%). Upper respiratory infection may occur in approximately 6% of patients. As with patients taking ACE-Is, ARBs have been rarely associated with angioedema. Other rare adverse effects include arthralgia, cough, fatigue, and peripheral edema.

Contraindications. Candesartan should be discontinued in patients once pregnancy is detected due to increased risk to the developing fetus. While no specific studies show that candesartan is excreted into breast milk, it is recommended that it not be used while breastfeeding and that alternatives to blood pressure control be considered. Candesartan should be used cautiously in older patients who may be experiencing age-related decline in renal function as it may increase the risk for hypotension.

Monitoring. Monitor patients taking candesartan carefully for symptomatic hypotension. In addition, it is essential to prevent or correct volume depletion and/or sodium depletion.

PRACTICE PEARLS

ARB Use in Black Patients

While ARBs are effective at reducing blood pressure in Black patients, the response is typically smaller than in other ethnic groups. Better blood pressure control is achieved when ARBs are combined with a diuretic.

Irbesartan

Pharmacokinetics. Irbesartan is administered orally and may be given without regard to meals. It is about 90% protein bound. Peak effects occur within 3 to 6 hours of administration. It is excreted via both the renal and biliary routes. Pharmacokinetics are not altered based on the patient's age, sex, or renal impairment.

Indications. Irbesartan is used for the treatment of hypertension and may be used in combination with a thiazide diuretic. It may also be used for the treatment of diabetic nephropathy or proteinuria.

Adverse Effects. The most common side effect of irbesartan is dizziness, which can occur in slightly more than 10% of patients. Other side effects include orthostatic hypotension (approximately 5% of patients), fatigue (4%), mild cough (3%), and mild diarrhea (3%). Rarely, patients may experience cardiac symptoms including exacerbation of dysrhythmias, angina, myocardial infarction, heart failure, and cardiac arrest.

Contraindications. As with ACE-Is, ARBs generally and irbesartan specifically has a black box warning for pregnant patients, as it can cause fetal death or injury. It should be discontinued during breastfeeding due to increased risk to the nursing infant. Angioedema can occur in patients with a previous history of ACE-I angioedema. Older adults may have greater sensitivity to hypotensive adverse effects due to age-related decline in renal function.

Monitoring. Monitor patient response to irbesartan. Because AT_1 receptors are nearly saturated at the starting doses of irbesartan (and most ARBs), proportionally small decreases in blood pressure are associated with increased dosing. As a result, improved blood pressure control may be achieved by adding a thiazide diuretic rather than increasing the dose of irbesartan.

Losartan

Pharmacokinetics. Losartan is administered orally and may be administered without regard to food. Losartan and its metabolites are highly protein bound. It is excreted in the urine and feces. Maximal effects typically occur within 1 week; however, they may require as long as 3 to 6 weeks to achieve in some patients. Patients with liver impairment may require dosage adjustments due to decreased plasma clearance.

Indications. Losartan is used to treat essential hypertension alone or in combination with thiazide diuretics for optimal blood pressure control. It may also be used in combination with beta-blockers and aldosterone antagonists in patients with heart failure. Losartan has been shown to be renoprotective in patients with diabetic nephropathy or proteinuria.

Adverse Effects. Losartan is generally well tolerated in adult and pediatric patients. The most common adverse effects are mild respiratory concerns with upper respiratory infections (7%–8% of patients) and nasal congestion (approximately 2%). Mild back pain, headache, or dizziness can occur in fewer than 1% to 3% of patients. Rarely, patients may experience exacerbation of cardiac dysrhythmias.

Contraindications. Losartan should be used cautiously in patients with liver and/or renal dysfunction as well as in patients with hyperkalemia or a history of hyperkalemia. It is not recommended for patients who are pregnant or breastfeeding.

Monitoring. Patient response to losartan varies, but maximum effects are typically achieved within 1 week. Elevated liver enzymes and hyperbilirubinemia have been reported in patients taking losartan. Patients with renal insufficiency should be carefully monitored for hyperkalemia.

Valsartan

Pharmacokinetics. Valsartan is administered orally and may be given without regard to food. It is highly protein bound. Peak antihypertensive activity occurs within about 6 hours. The duration is approximately 24 hours. Maximum blood pressure reduction is typically achieved within about 4 weeks after initiation of therapy.

Indications. Valsartan can be used for patients with hypertension and may be combined with a thiazide diuretic. It can also be used to reduce cardiovascular mortality in stable patients with left ventricular failure or in patients with left ventricular dysfunction after myocardial infarction. Valsartan is effective in Class II through Class IV heart failure and may be given in combination with a beta-blocker and an aldosterone antagonist.

Adverse Effects. Up to 17% of patients may experience mild dizziness. Dizziness and headache are the most common reasons for discontinuation of valsartan. Infrequent adverse effects include cough, fatigue, back pain, and orthostatic hypotension. Hyperkalemia is more likely in patients with renal impairment.

Contraindications. Valsartan is contraindicated in patients who are pregnant, due to the risk of harm to the developing fetus. While no specific data are available on the effects of valsartan in patients who are breastfeeding, it is not recommended due to potential risks. Older adults may be more sensitive to the hypotensive side effects of valsartan. It should be used cautiously in patients with a history of hyperkalemia.

Monitoring. Therapeutic effects of valsartan on blood pressure are typically seen within 1 week of beginning therapy. Monitor adverse effects, as they may reduce patients' likelihood of adhering to valsartan therapy.

Calcium Channel Blockers

Calcium channel blockers (CCBs) are used primarily for the management of hypertension and angina. In general, these drugs inhibit voltage-gated L-type calcium channels on vascular smooth muscle, cardiac myocytes, and cells within the sinoatrial (SA) and atrioventricular (AV) nodes, preventing influx of extracellular calcium. A decrease in intracellular calcium results in inhibition of the contractile process of the myocardial and vascular smooth muscle cells, resulting in dilation of the coronary and peripheral arterial vasculature. Peripheral resistance is decreased, leading to a decrease in systemic blood pressure. In addition, CCBs can improve oxygen delivery to myocardial tissue. CCBs that affect myocardial cells can decrease heart rate and slow AV conduction.

There are two classes of CCBs: dihydropyridines (DHPs) and non-dihydropyridines (non-DHPs). Because DHPs have greater selectivity for vascular smooth muscle, they are the focus for this discussion. Non-DHPs have greater selectivity for cardiac muscle cells and serve as negative inotropes and positive chronotropic drug. Therefore, they will be discussed in greater detail in Chapter 10, Coronary Artery Disease Medications, and Chapter 12, Antiarrhythmic Medications.

Dihydropyridines

Amlodipine

Pharmacokinetics. Amlodipine is administered orally and is highly protein bound. Food does not affect absorption, so it can be given without regard to meals. Amlodipine is extensively metabolized in the liver and excreted in the urine. Peak plasma levels occur in 6 to 12 hours. The half-life is prolonged in older adults, so these patients may require a lower dose. Steady-state plasma concentrations typically occur in 7 to 8 days of consecutive dosing. Clearance is decreased in adults with hepatic illnesses. Pharmacokinetics are similar in children older than 6 years of age, adolescents, and adults.

Indications. Amlodipine is primarily used for the treatment of hypertension. It can also be used to reduce the risk of rehospitalization and of coronary revascularization in patients with coronary artery disease without heart failure or a reduced ejection fraction less than 40%. Amlodipine can be used to treat variant angina.

Adverse Effects. The most common adverse effect is moderate peripheral edema, occurring in approximately 14% to 32% of patients. This appears to be dose related and more common in females than in males. Other side effects include mild flushing, mild fatigue, and palpitations that can occur in up to 4.5% of patients. Sexual dysfunction has been recorded in fewer than 2% of males and fewer than 1% of females. Mild dizziness, nausea, pruritus, and rash may occur. Severe side effects are rare and include angioedema, arrhythmia exacerbation, and pancreatitis.

Contraindications. Amlodipine should be used cautiously in patients with hepatic disease. It should be started at a lower dose in older adults. Data regarding use of amlodipine during pregnancy are not sufficient to inform drug-associated risk. No adverse effects on infants have been shown as a result of breastfeeding. Amlodipine is not indicated for patients with reduced ejection fraction.

Monitoring. Patients taking amlodipine may not experience the full benefit of the drug until at least 1 week after initiating therapy. Since amlodipine has a prolonged half-life in older adults, a lower dose may be required initially.

Felodipine

Pharmacokinetics. Felodipine is administered orally and should be given without food or with a light meal, as giving felodipine with high-fat or high-carbohydrate meals can increase bioavailability. It is highly protein bound, metabolized by the liver and excreted in the urine and feces. Half-life is approximately 11 to 16 hours. Felodipine is a substrate of CYP 3A4, so administration with CYP 3A4 inhibitors can increase plasma concentrations. It should not be taken with grapefruit juice.

Indications. Felodipine is used for the treatment of hypertension. It has been shown to be effective in adults and older adults. Safety and efficacy have not been established in children or adolescents.

Adverse Effects. The most common adverse effect associated with felodipine is headache, occurring in as many as 14.7% of patients. Other adverse effects are associated with peripheral vasodilation and include dizziness, flushing, and hypotension. Peripheral edema has been reported in slightly more than 17% of patients. Of note, the peripheral edema is more likely related to the peripheral vasodilation than left ventricular dysfunction. Nevertheless, worsened heart failure has been reported in some patients taking CCBs.

Contraindications. Felodipine is contraindicated in patients with known hypersensitivity to dihydropyridines. It is classified as pregnancy category C. It is not known whether felodipine is excreted in breast milk, so it is not recommended for use during breastfeeding unless it is essential to the health of the mother. If felodipine is given, the infant must be carefully monitored for effects. Felodipine should not be used in patients with a systolic blood pressure that is less than 90 mm Hg as it can cause severe hypotension. Felodipine can cause reflex tachycardia in patients with severe coronary artery disease. As a result, it could worsen angina pectoris or ischemic heart disease. Avoid use in patients with a history of aortic stenosis or hypertrophic cardiomyopathy. Hepatic dysfunction can decrease clearance of felodipine, so it should be avoided or used cautiously in patients with hepatic disease. Dosages should be started at the low range in older adults and gradually increased to reduce the risk of adverse effects.

Monitoring. Determine the patient's response to felodipine by evaluating blood pressure and heart rate. For patients with coronary heart disease, make sure to assess for increasing angina. Other symptoms that may indicate more serious reactions include fainting spells, irregular heartbeat, and palpitations.

Non-Dihydropyridines

Diltiazem

Pharmacokinetics. Diltiazem can be administered orally and intravenously. Bioavailability is reduced due to extensive first-pass metabolism. It is widely distributed throughout the body, with approximately 75% protein bound. Onset of action for oral immediate-release diltiazem is 1 hour, with the peak effect occurring at 2 to 3 hours. For the sustained-release forms, the onset is 2 to 3 hours, with peak effect at 6 to 11 hours. Release of extended-release tablets is dependent on GI transit times. Patients with hepatic disease have an increased half-life and increased bioavailability. Older adults have an increased half-life and decreased clearance of diltiazem. Diltiazem is an inhibitor and a substrate of CYP 3A. While grapefruit juice does not affect bioavailability, it does increase the half-life slightly.

Indications. Diltiazem can be used in regular-release, sustained-release, or extended-release form to treat hypertension in adults by reducing systemic blood pressure through dilation of peripheral arteries. At this time, only regular release is recommended for children and adolescents. Diltiazem can also be used for patients with chronic stable angina or variant angina to dilate coronary arteries and improve myocardial oxygen supply. It is an effective agent for treatment of paroxysmal supraventricular tachycardia or control of the ventricular rate in atrial fibrillation and atrial flutter (see Chapter 12, Antiarrhythmic Medications).

Adverse Effects. The most common adverse effect for patients taking diltiazem is moderate peripheral edema (approximately 15% of patients) due to peripheral vasodilation. Infrequently, patients experience dizziness, fatigue, or lack of energy. Upper respiratory symptoms including pharyngitis and rhinitis occur in fewer than 6% to 10% of patients. Approximately 4% of patients experience constipation with diltiazem. Skin reactions are typically mild and resolve with cessation of therapy; however, there have been cases that progressed to erythema multiforme, exfoliative dermatitis, toxic epidermal necrolysis, or Stevens-Johnson syndrome.

Contraindications. Diltiazem can precipitate or exacerbate heart failure in a variety of conditions, including acute myocardial infarction, cardiogenic shock, conduction disturbances associated with ventricular dysfunction, or in patients taking beta-blockers. It is contraindicated in patients with select dysrhythmias including bradycardia, second- or third-degree atrioventricular block, sick sinus syndrome, Wolff-Parkinson-White syndrome, or Lown-Ganong-Levine syndrome.

Fewer than 1% of patients taking diltiazem experience moderate to marked elevations in liver function tests. These typically occur within 1 to 8 weeks after starting therapy and are transient. Liver enzymes usually return to normal levels following discontinuation of the drug.

Diltiazem should be used cautiously in patients with gastroesophageal reflux disease (GERD) as it can reduce the tone of the lower esophageal sphincter. There are no well-controlled studies to determine use during pregnancy, so diltiazem should only be used if the benefits justify the risk. It is considered by the American Academy of Pediatrics to be safe to use during breastfeeding.

Monitoring. Follow up to determine the patient's response to antihypertensive therapy. Teach the patient to report any dizziness, palpitations, or shortness of breath that may warrant further diagnostic testing, including an electrocardiogram (ECG). Assess for adverse effects that may impact the patient's adherence to antihypertensive therapy. Remind patients that sustained-release and extended-release forms of the medication must not be chewed or crushed.

Verapamil

Pharmacokinetics. Oral verapamil undergoes significant first-pass metabolism, leading to bioavailability of 20% to 35%. Immediate-release and 24-hour sustained-release forms can be given without regard to food; the 12-hour sustained-release form should be taken with food to decrease the differences between peak and trough levels. Grapefruit juice increases the availability and concentration of verapamil. Onset of action is approximately 1 to 2 hours after oral administration, with peak effect in 1 to 2 hours for immediate-release and 5 hours for sustained-release forms.

Verapamil is extensively metabolized in the liver to more than 12 metabolites. Elimination is primarily through the kidneys. Verapamil interacts with inducers or inhibitors of CYP 3A4.

Indications. Verapamil is used in regular-release or extended-release form to treat hypertension. In addition, verapamil is used to manage symptoms associated with chronic stable angina and variant angina. Verapamil is also used in intravenous (IV) or oral forms to treat a variety of supraventricular dysrhythmias, including chronic atrial fibrillation and atrial flutter.

Adverse Effects. The two most common complications of verapamil are mild headache and moderate constipation in up to 12.1% and 11.7% of patients, respectively. Slightly fewer than 4% of patients may experience peripheral edema. Other adverse effects include fatigue, hypotension, and dizziness. Fewer than 2% of patients experience GI symptoms such as abdominal pain, nausea, and dyspepsia. Patients taking verapamil may experience cardiac disturbances including chest pain, palpitations, bradycardia, or AV block. Reflex tachycardia is possible, however not as common with verapamil as with other CCBs.

Contraindications. Verapamil is contraindicated in patients with left ventricular dysfunction, heart failure, and select dysrhythmias including AV block, sick sinus syndrome, and Wolff-Parkinson-White syndrome. It should not be administered to patients with systolic pressures less than 90 mm Hg. It should be avoided in patients taking beta-blockers, as verapamil can precipitate heart failure in these patients. Patients with renal or hepatic disease are at increased risk for adverse effects of verapamil. Because of the risk of constipation, it should be used cautiously in patients with a history of constipation or fecal impaction. Verapamil should be used cautiously in patients with neuromuscular illnesses. While no well-controlled studies have been conducted in pregnant patients, verapamil has been shown to cross the placenta, so it is recommended that it only be used if it is essential for the health of the mother. Verapamil has been shown to pass into breast milk; however, the American Academy of Pediatrics suggests that it is compatible with breastfeeding as there is a lack of adverse effects in infants. Older adults may have decreased clearance and increased half-life, so use of a lower dose is recommended at onset.

Monitoring. Determine patient response to ensure that therapeutic goals are reached without significant adverse effects. Obtain an ECG if the patient is experiencing symptoms indicating dysrhythmia.

Direct Renin Inhibitors

Direct renin inhibitors are considered secondary agents for the management of hypertension. They reduce blood pressure through inhibition of renin, the proteolytic enzyme released by the kidneys as a response to reduction in blood pressure. By inhibiting renin, direct renin inhibitors ultimately decrease the production of angiotensin II. A decrease in angiotensin II results in arterial and venous vasodilation and decreased blood volume.

Aliskiren

Pharmacokinetics. Aliskiren is administered orally. While it may be given without regard to meals, it is recommended that patients be consistent with their choice. High-fat meals can decrease absorption and may alter efficacy. The major enzyme responsible for metabolism is CYP 3A4. Approximately 90% is eliminated unchanged in the feces. Aliskiren does not inhibit or induce any CYP 450 isozymes, including CYP 3A4. Of note, Black patients experience slightly smaller reductions in blood pressure compared to other patient subgroups.

Indications. Aliskiren is used for the treatment of hypertension. It can be used as monotherapy or in combination with other antihypertensives including valsartan, hydrochlorothiazide, and/or amlodipine.

Adverse Effects. Aliskiren is generally well tolerated with usual doses. The most common adverse effects were mild diarrhea (2.3% of patients) and mild cough (2.3%). Other rare effects include headache, fatigue, rash, and back pain. Hyperkalemia is rare, occurring in fewer than 1% of patients, but may be severe. Angioedema is very rare but has been reported in patients taking aliskiren. Severe cutaneous adverse reactions including Stevens-Johnson syndrome and toxic epidermal necrolysis may occur, but the incidence is unknown.

Contraindications. Aliskiren is absolutely contraindicated in neonates, infants, and children younger than 6 years of age. A black box warning notes that aliskiren should be stopped as soon as possible if pregnancy is detected. Females of child-bearing age should understand potential fetal risks associated with aliskiren. Patients with electrolyte imbalances, including hyper- or hypokalemia, should have these corrected before beginning aliskiren. It is not known how aliskiren affects patients with renal failure, so caution should be used in these cases.

Monitoring. Evaluate blood pressure response to aliskiren. Serum electrolytes, BUN, and creatinine should be evaluated.

Alpha-1 Receptor Blockers (Antagonists)

Alpha-1 receptor blockers selectively block the alpha-1 receptors located in vascular smooth muscles. When the receptors are blocked, these drugs reduce vasoconstriction and, to a lesser extent, reduce venous return. As a result, blood pressure decreases. While alpha-1 receptor blockers can be effective, they commonly cause orthostatic hypotension, particularly after the first few doses and especially in older adults. Other common side effects include nasal congestion related to dilation of arterioles in the nasal mucosa and reflex tachycardia. Some patients experience peripheral edema that may be addressed by combining the alpha-1 receptor blocker with a diuretic. Alpha-1 receptor blockers also relax smooth muscles in the bladder neck and prostate, reducing bladder outlet obstruction without affecting bladder contractility. These medications are considered second-line therapies for hypertension and may be particularly useful for patients with concomitant benign prostatic hypertrophy.

Prazosin

Pharmacokinetics. Prazosin is administered orally and may be given with food. While food may delay absorption slightly, it does not interfere with the overall effect of prazosin. Prazosin is highly protein bound and distributed throughout the body tissues. Prazosin is metabolized by the liver, with the majority of the dose excreted in the feces. Antihypertensive effects peak in 2 to 4 hours after administration, with the duration of effect less than 24 hours. Full antihypertensive effects may not occur until 4 to 6 weeks after initiation of therapy.

Indications. Prazosin is used as a second-line agent for patients with hypertension. Of note, recent evidence suggests that it may be effective in treating posttraumatic stress disorder (PTSD) and related nightmares in combat veterans.

Adverse Effects. Prazosin is associated with orthostatic hypotension and syncope, particularly in older adults. This may be sudden and unrelated to plasma prazosin. The risk of first-dose hypotension may be decreased by beginning therapy at a low dose and taking the medication with food. Syncope is also associated with increases in dosage and with the addition of antihypertensive medications. Additional adverse effects include dizziness, headache, fatigue, and weakness. Cardiovascular effects include palpitations, peripheral edema, and sinus tachycardia. Rarely, patients may experience adverse effects such as angina, bradycardia, elevated liver enzymes, and pancreatitis. Urinary incontinence, erectile dysfunction, and priapism are rare.

Contraindications. Prazosin should be used cautiously in patients with angina due to the possibility of severe hypotension. Patients should be notified of the possibility of first-dose hypotension, which can result in syncope. As a result, prazosin should be given at bedtime for the first few doses and titrated for best effect. Older adults may be more likely to experience hypotension and syncope, so prazosin should be used with caution and only if there are no better alternatives. Prazosin is pregnancy category C and should be used only if the benefits to the mother are greater than the risks to the fetus. Prazosin distributes into breast milk.

Monitoring. Monitor the patient's blood pressure and heart rate to determine outcome. Teach patients to report significant adverse effects and to avoid discontinuing the medication without discussion with the primary care provider.

Doxazosin

Pharmacokinetics. Doxazosin is administered orally and may be given without regard to food. It is highly protein bound (98%). It is metabolized by the liver and excreted mainly via the feces, with approximately 9% excreted in the urine. Onset of action is about 2 hours, with peak effect in 5 to 6 hours. Duration is approximately 24 hours.

Indications. Doxazosin is used for the treatment of hypertension. Of note, it can also be used for the treatment of benign prostatic hypertrophy alone or in combination with finasteride.

Adverse effects. The most common adverse effects are dizziness (5.3%–19% of patients) and fatigue (8%–12%). Infrequently, patients experience asthenia, headache, drowsiness, hypotension, or vertigo.

Contraindications. Doxazocin is contraindicated in patients with hypersensitivity to doxazocin or other quinazolines (e.g., prazosin, terazosin). Doxazocin should be used cautiously in patients with hepatic disease as it is primarily metabolized in the liver. Avoid use in pregnant and breastfeeding patients.

Monitoring. Doxazosin may cause first-dose hypotension. If feasible, blood pressure should be monitored for the first 2 to 6 hours after the first dose is administered and after each dose adjustment. Administering at bedtime may reduce this effect.

Terazosin

Pharmacokinetics. Terazosin is administered orally. While food may delay the time to peak concentrations by about 1 hour, the presence of food does not affect overall bioavailability. Terazosin is highly protein bound and is metabolized by the liver. It is excreted in the feces (60%) and kidneys (40%). Onset of action is typically within 15 minutes, with peak plasma levels about 1 hour after administration. Half-life of terazosin is approximately 12 hours.

Indications. Terazosin is used for the treatment of hypertension. It can also be used to treat benign prostatic hypertrophy.

Adverse effects. The most common adverse effects are typically mild and include dizziness (up to 19.3% of patients), headache (approximately 16%), and asthenia (up to 11.3%). Infrequently, patients experience orthostatic hypotension, drowsiness, nasal congestion, peripheral edema, or palpitations.

Contraindications. Terazosin meets the Beers Criteria as being potentially inappropriate for older adults unless it is essential when compared to other antihypertensives. It should be used cautiously in patients with a history of angina as severe hypotension may increase risk of ischemia. There are no significant studies that support the use of terazosin in pregnant and breastfeeding patients. Rarely, as with other alpha-1 adrenergic blockers, priapism is possible and should be recognized as a medical emergency.

Monitoring. Avoid prescribing priapism for older adults who are at greater risk for adverse effects; if prescribed, monitor the patient's blood pressure on a regular basis to ensure that they are achieving the best response with the lowest possible dose. Recommend that the patient take the first doses at bedtime to avoid first-dose hypotension.

Centrally Acting Alpha-2 Agonists

Centrally acting alpha-2 agonists stimulate presynaptic alpha-2 receptors in the medulla. Stimulation of these receptors inhibits sympathetic outflow and vascular tone. As a result, there is decreased peripheral resistance and decreased vascular tone. These medications are considered last-line therapy because of significant CNS effects, particularly in older adults.

Clonidine
Pharmacokinetics. Clonidine can be prescribed orally or via a transdermal patch. About half of the dose is metabolized in the liver to inactive compounds. Unchanged drug and metabolites are excreted in the urine and feces.

Food does not affect the absorption of oral forms of clonidine. The oral dose has a half-life of 12 to 16 hours. Onset of action for immediate-release forms is typically between 30 and 60 minutes, with maximum effects within 2 to 4 hours. Peak clonidine concentrations after oral administration of extended-release forms were approximately 50% of those achieved with the immediate-release forms and occurred approximately 5 hours later.

The transdermal patch is released and absorbed through the skin at a constant rate over 24 hours. Steady-state concentrations are reached within 3 days after application to the upper arm or chest. The steady state remains consistent after removal of one patch and application of the next. Half-life after removal of the patch is approximately 20 hours. Half-life is up to 41 hours in patients with renal impairment.

Indications. Clonidine is considered a last-line drug for the treatment of hypertension. It can be used in adults as well as children and adolescents older than 12 years of age. It is not recommended for use in children younger than 12 years of age. Clonidine has been shown to be an effective immediate-release tablet for the treatment of hypertensive urgency or emergency.

Adverse Effects. Clonidine meets the Beers Criteria for older adults due to a high risk of adverse CNS effects including bradycardia and orthostatic hypotension. Other adverse effects include weakness, fatigue, headache, nervousness, and insomnia. Transdermal forms of clonidine typically result in less severe adverse systemic effects and include drowsiness, fatigue, headache, lethargy, and dizziness. Rarely, ileus, GI obstruction, angioedema, depression, thrombocytopenia, and liver dysfunction/hepatitis are seen.

Contraindications. Clonidine is contraindicated in patients who are on anticoagulant therapy or who have any coagulopathy. The hypotensive effects of clonidine may worsen ischemia in patients with severe heart failure, cerebrovascular disease, or recent myocardial infarction.

Clonidine is not recommended during pregnancy unless it is clearly required for the health of the mother, as it crosses the placenta easily. Clonidine is excreted in breast milk and may affect prolactin and oxytocin levels in the mother.

Abrupt discontinuation of clonidine can lead to a withdrawal syndrome with a sudden increase in catecholamines. This can lead to rebound hypertension as well as symptoms of headache, anxiety, agitation, and tremor. In rare cases, abrupt discontinuation can lead to cerebrovascular accident, hypertensive encephalopathy, and even death.

Monitoring. Monitor blood pressure while initiating therapy to determine patient response. If discontinuation is required, doses should be slowly tapered every 3 days for patients who are taking oral forms to avoid withdrawal syndrome. Extended-release forms should be reduced every 3 to 7 days. Monitor heart rate and blood pressure while tapering.

Methyldopa
Pharmacokinetics. Oral methyldopa is approximately 50% absorbed through the GI tract. Maximum hypotensive effects typically occur within 4 to 6 hours and last 12 to 24 hours. Half-life is typically about 2 hours, although in patients with renal impairment, half-life increases to 4 to 6 hours.

Indications. Methyldopa is used for patients with hypertension. It can also be used in an IV form for hypertensive urgency or emergency. It should be used cautiously in older adults due to increased risk of adverse effects.

Adverse Effects. The most common adverse effect is drowsiness, which usually occurs within 48 to 72 hours after initiation of therapy. This typically diminishes with continued therapy. Larger doses can result in increased sedation, memory lapses, or inability to concentrate. In addition, patients can experience headache, depression, weakness, or even neurological symptoms of parkinsonism, Bell's palsy, or paresthesia. If sodium and fluid retention occur, thiazide diuretics can be used to reduce the symptoms. GI symptoms include nausea, vomiting, diarrhea, dry mouth, increased flatulence, and constipation. Methyldopa has been associated with thrombocytopenia, leukopenia, and agranulocytosis.

Methyldopa has been linked with the onset of a drug-induced fever within 3 weeks of initiation of therapy. This can be associated with elevated liver enzymes. Cirrhosis, hepatitis, and cholestasis have been reported. These usually return to normal function after methyldopa is discontinued.

Contraindications. Methyldopa is contraindicated in patients with hepatic disease and hepatitis. It is also contraindicated in patients receiving monoamine oxidase inhibitor (MAOI) therapy due to the risk of headache, severe hypertension, and hallucinations.

Monitoring. Patient blood pressure and heart rate should be monitored regularly. Patients should have their hemoglobin, hematocrit, and red blood cell count checked before initiating therapy, as well as during therapy because of the risk of hemolytic adverse reactions. Approximately 15% of patients will have a positive Coombs test. This usually reverses within weeks to months after therapy has been discontinued; however, if there is evidence of anemia or a positive Coombs test, it is important to rule out hemolysis.

Direct Vasodilators

Direct vasodilators primarily act on arteriolar smooth muscle, resulting in decreased peripheral resistance and decreased blood pressure. As a result of the decreased blood pressure, the baroreceptor reflex is triggered and there is a release of norepinephrine and epinephrine. The major medication in this category, hydralazine, increases renin release as a response to the sympathetic nervous system stimulation. The release of renin triggers the production of angiotensin II, resulting in aldosterone secretion and eventually fluid retention secondary to sodium reabsorption. Ultimately, there is an increased heart rate, increased venous return, and increased cardiac output. These compensatory responses can diminish the antihypertensive effect. The compensatory sympathetic response observed with direct vasodilators such as hydralazine may be reduced if the drug is combined with a beta-blocker.

Hydralazine

Pharmacokinetics. Hydralazine is administered orally and may be given parenterally if needed in cases of urgent/emergent hypertension. While hydralazine is approximately 90% absorbed after oral administration, it goes through extensive first-pass metabolism. Hydralazine is distributed approximately 87% protein bound. It is metabolized by the liver and excreted in the urine and feces. Onset of action is approximately 20 to 30 minutes after administration, with peak plasma concentration at 1 to 2 hours and duration of 2 to 4 hours. Half-life for the oral form is typically 3 to 7 hours. Taking hydralazine with meals can increase absorption of the medication but also can reduce plasma levels and ultimately antihypertensive effects. It is recommended that patients take hydralazine on a fixed schedule related to mealtimes for consistent results.

Indications. Hydralazine is used for the treatment of hypertension and in hypertension urgency/emergency situations. It can also be used to treat severe preeclampsia and eclampsia in pregnant patients. In addition, it can be used to treat patients with heart failure in combination with an ACE-I, ARB, or angiotensin receptor-neprilysin inhibitor for Black patients with a reduced ejection fraction.

Adverse Effects. The most common adverse effects of hydralazine are mild headache and mild nausea. In addition, because hydralazine is a potent vasodilator, patients can experience reflex tachycardia, dizziness, palpitations, and orthostatic hypotension. Hydralazine may cause peripheral edema, fluid retention, and weight gain. This can be reduced through the addition of a thiazide diuretic. While rare, hydralazine is the most frequent drug associated with lupus-like symptoms.

Contraindications. Hydralazine is contraindicated in patients with coronary heart disease and in patients with mitral valve rheumatic heart disease. Patients with coronary heart disease are at risk for reflex tachycardia and subsequent increased myocardial oxygen demand. Patients with mitral valve rheumatic heart disease are at risk for increased pulmonary artery pressure. Hydralazine should be used cautiously in patients with acute myocardial infarction or acute stroke, and in patients with increased intracranial pressure.

Hydralazine is considered pregnancy category C. While it has been used in patients with preeclampsia, other drugs such as labetalol and/or CCBs have been used with improved maternal and fetal outcomes. It should be used cautiously in breastfeeding patients.

Monitoring. Patient response to hydralazine should be monitored carefully due to risk of orthostatic hypotension and reflex tachycardia. Monitor BUN/creatinine levels as renal failure can increase half-life.

Prescriber Considerations for Antihypertensive Therapy

In 2017, the ACC and AHA Task Force released clinical practice guidelines for antihypertensive therapy (Whelton et al., 2018). Highlights include a new definition of hypertension, the recommendation for more aggressive treatment for Stage 2 hypertension, and the need to calculate overall cardiovascular risk using the ASCVD Risk Calculator. The guidelines also include a focus on self-monitoring to improve diagnosis, treatment, and management.

> ### BOOKMARK THIS!
>
> **Clinical Guidelines for Antihypertensive Therapy**
>
> Updated AHA/ACC Clinical Practice Guidelines for Prevention, Detection, Evaluation and Management of High Blood Pressure in Adults: https://www.acc.org/latest-in-cardiology/ten-points-to-remember/2017/11/09/11/41/2017-guideline-for-high-blood-pressure-in-adults

Clinical Reasoning for Antihypertension Therapy

Consider the individual patient's health problem requiring antihypertensive therapy. One of the most important strategies for determining the need for antihypertensive therapy is accurate determination of blood pressure. Ensure that guideline recommendations for accurate blood pressure management are followed. This can be accomplished with thorough training of providers and staff. In addition, partnering with patients is important as out-of-office and self-monitoring of blood pressure can contribute to the diagnostic process (Box 9.3). Carefully review the patient's medical history, ASCVD risk factors, current medications, lab work, and general health status. While secondary causes of hypertension are far less common, it is critical to rule them out. If the patient is diagnosed with primary hypertension, determine their overall cardiovascular risk and review their current lifestyle and the potential lifestyle changes they can make to reduce cardiovascular risk.

Determine the desired therapeutic outcome based on the degree of blood pressure management needed for the patient's health problem. Use current clinical practice guidelines to determine blood pressure thresholds and goals (Table 9.5) for pharmacologic therapy according to the patient's clinical conditions. Recent guidelines recommend a blood pressure less than 130/80 for best clinical outcomes. Carefully follow up with patients to determine the effectiveness of blood pressure medications and the need to adjust the dose or change to a different medication.

Assess the medication therapy selected for its appropriateness for an individual patient by considering the medication's side effects and the patient's age, race/ethnicity, comorbidities, and genetic factors. Choose medications based on patient age, race, and comorbidities, stage of hypertension, estimated ASCVD risk, and factors that can affect medication adherence. The majority of first-line medications can be given once daily, improving the likelihood of adherence. In addition, most medications can be started at lower doses and increased gradually for best patient response.

Black patients with hypertension but without heart failure or chronic kidney disease should begin with a thiazide-type diuretic or CCB to achieve blood pressure goals. Most patients will require at least two medications to achieve blood pressure goals. Patients of childbearing age who plan to become pregnant should not be treated with ACE-Is, ARBs, or direct renin inhibitors because of risks to the fetus.

For children and adolescents, ensure that lifestyle changes are thoroughly addressed. Carefully choose medications that have been shown to be effective for children and adolescents. Older adults may be more sensitive to antihypertensive medications with greater risk of hypotension, so begin at lower doses and monitor their effects.

Initiate the treatment plan with the selected medication by first providing adequate patient education to ensure the patient's understanding and promote full participation in the antihypertensive therapy. Provide the patient with information including the name of the medication, expected benefits, possible adverse effects, and when to call their primary care provider. Ensure adequate follow-up appointments after initiating therapy and with dosage adjustments. Drug adherence is a major factor in achieving optimal blood pressure control. Table 9.6 provides a list of evidence-based interventions to enhance patient adherence. Patient teaching and ambulatory monitoring can contribute to improved outcomes.

Ensure complete patient and family understanding about the medication prescribed for antihypertensive therapy using a variety of education strategies. Provide the patient and their family with oral and written instructions, and use teach-back strategies to assess patient understanding. Resources such as the AHA provide excellent patient information regarding a variety of cardiovascular topics, including hypertension.

TABLE 9.5 Blood Pressure Thresholds for and Goals of Pharmacologic Therapy in Patients with Hypertension According to Clinical Conditions

Clinical Condition(s)	BP Threshold (mm Hg)	BP Goal (mm Hg)
General		
Clinical CVD or 10-year ASCVD risk ≥10%	≥130/80	<130/80
No clinical CVD and 10-year ASCVD risk <10%	≥140/90	<130/80
Older persons (≥65 yr; noninstitutionalized, ambulatory, community-living adults)	≥130 (SBP)	<130 (SBP)
Specific Comorbidities		
Diabetes mellitus	≥130/80	<130/80
Chronic kidney disease	≥130/80	<130/80
Chronic kidney disease after renal transplantation	≥130/80	<130/80
Heart failure	≥130/80	<130/80
Stable ischemic heart disease	≥130/80	<130/80
Secondary stroke prevention	≥140/90	<130/80
Secondary stroke prevention (lacunar)	≥130/80	<130/80
Peripheral arterial disease	≥130/80	<130/80

ASCVD: Atherosclerotic cardiovascular disease; *BP:* blood pressure; *CVD:* cardiovascular disease; and *SBP:* systolic blood pressure.
(Adapted from Whelton et al. [2018]. 2017 ACC/AHA/AAPA/ABC/ACPM/AGS/APhA/ASH/ASPC/NMA/PCNA guideline for the prevention, detection, evaluation, and management of high blood pressure in adults—Executive summary: A report of the American College of Cardiology/American Heart Association Task Force on Clinical Practice Guidelines. *Hypertension, 71*[6], 1269–1324. http://doi.org/10.1161/HYP0000000000000066)

TABLE 9.6	Interventions That Can Improve Drug Adherence in Hypertension
Level of Intervention	**Examples of Interventions**
Primary care providers	• Provide information on risks and benefits of treatment. • Partner with patients to determine strategies to achieve lifestyle goals. • Use single-pill treatment strategies. • Prescribe medications that can be taken once daily. • Give positive feedback on behavioral and clinical improvements. • Use an interdisciplinary approach to care (include pharmacy, dietitian, nursing, medicine, and social services as needed). • Help patient determine solutions to barriers that affect adherence.
Patients	• Self-monitor blood pressure using ambulatory monitoring strategies. • Use reminders such as personal organizers or reminder apps for smartphones. • Determine partners in care such as family, friends, or health care supporters. • Participate in health-related activities available in your community. • Use one pharmacy to refill all medications to help prevent harmful drug interactions. • Work with your pharmacist to determine a schedule for refilling medications to avoid making multiple trips to the pharmacy for different medications.

Adapted from Burnier, M., & Egan, B. M. (2019). Adherence in hypertension. *Circulation Research, 124*(7), 1124–1140. http://doi.org/10.1161/CIRCRESAHA.118.313220

Conduct follow-up and monitoring of patient responses to antihypertensive therapy. Careful follow-up for patients with hypertension is essential. Patients who present with Stage 1 hypertension and an estimated 10-year ASCVD risk of less than 10% should begin with nonpharmacologic interventions and repeat blood pressure evaluation in 3 to 6 months. If the ASCVD risk is greater than 10%, teach the patient about nonpharmacologic interventions and begin first-line medication therapy. Then repeat in 1 month to determine response. For patients with Stage 2 hypertension, initiate nonpharmacologic therapy and combination therapy of drugs from two different classes, and reevaluate in 1 month. Again, partnering with the patient to include home monitoring can be very useful in contributing to patient care.

Teaching Points for Antihypertensive Therapy

Health Promotion Strategies

Hypertension is a major risk factor for cardiovascular disease and requires ongoing health promotion. The following evidence-based strategies should be incorporated into the plan of care. Care must be patient centered to help achieve the best patient outcomes.

- Include ambulatory or home self-monitoring of blood pressure to inform diagnosis, treatment, and management of hypertension. Have patients record their blood pressure using paper and pencil or an app on their smartphone.
- Prescribe a heart-healthy diet, such as the DASH diet. More information can be found at https://www.nhlbi.nih.gov/health-topics/dash-eating-plan.
- Maintaining a healthy body weight can help manage blood pressure. Every kg (2.2 lb) of body weight reduction toward a healthy body weight can reduce blood pressure.
- Promote participation in regular physical activity, including aerobic and resistance exercises.

- Advise patients to reduce their sodium intake by avoiding processed foods and reading labels; set a target of 1500 mg daily or a reduction in intake of 1000 mg daily.
- Advise patients to reduce alcohol intake to no more than one drink daily for females and no more than two drinks daily for males.
- Advise patients to increase their potassium intake, with the goal of eating 3500 to 5000 mg daily (unless the patient has a health condition that prohibits this).
- Advise patients to avoid taking diuretics in the evening as they can impact sleep.
- Advise patients to contact their primary care provider before taking herbal or over-the-counter (OTC) medications that may interact with blood pressure medications.

Patient Education for Medication Safety

- The American Heart Association website provides current and easily accessible information on high blood pressure at https://www.heart.org/en/health-topics/high-blood-pressure.
- Make sure to take your medications at the same time every day for best effects.
- Avoid smoking as it increases the risk for high blood pressure.
- Talk to your primary care provider about strategies to help manage weight and increase levels of physical activity.
- Talk to your primary care provider or pharmacist about the best time of the day to take your blood pressure medications.
- Do not take over-the-counter or herbal medications without discussing with your primary care provider or your pharmacist to avoid harmful drug interactions.
- If you take ACE-Is, notify your primary care provider if you have a dry cough or any swelling of your face or lips, as these may be adverse effects associated with the medication. If you have any severe swelling, call 911.

- If you are pregnant or plan to become pregnant, make sure to notify your primary care provider as some antihypertensives can affect the fetus.
- Make sure to sit or stand up slowly as you may have some temporary dizziness (called orthostatic hypotension). This should decrease after a few seconds. If your dizziness persists, make sure to tell your primary care provider as the medication doses may need to be adjusted.
- Do not stop taking your blood pressure medication without discussing with your primary provider. Stopping your medication suddenly may lead to adverse effects.

Application Questions for Discussion

1. One of the major concerns regarding blood pressure medications is the lack of symptoms, which may be one of the factors that can affect patients' adherence to their prescribed therapy. What strategies would be most effective in improving adherence?
2. What are some strategies to differentiate between primary and secondary hypertension and how should they affect treatment decisions?
3. What data should be included in determining whether to use single or combination medications when initiating or changing therapies for patients with Stage 1 hypertension?

Selected Bibliography

Arnett, D. K., Blumenthal, R. S., Albert, M. A., Buroker, A. B., Goldberger, Z. D., Hahn, E. J., & Ziaeian, B. (2019). ACC/AHA guideline on the primary prevention of cardiovascular disease. *Circulation, 140*(11), e596–e646. CIR.0000000000000678. http://doi.org/10.1161/CIR.0000000000000678.

Benjamin, E. J., Muntner, P., Alonso, A., Bittencourt, M. S., Callaway, C. W., Carson, A. P., et al. (2019). Heart disease and stroke statistics—2019 update: A report from the American Heart Association. *Circulation, 139*(10), e56–e528. http://doi.org/10.1161/CIR.0000000000000659.

Booth, J. N., Li, J., Zhang, L., Chen, L., Muntner, P., & Egan, B. (2017). Trends in prehypertension and hypertension risk factors in US adults: 1999–2012. *Hypertension, 70*(2), 275–284. http://doi.org/10.1161/HYPERTENSIONAHA.116.09004.

Burnier, M., & Egan, B. M. (2019). Adherence in hypertension. *Circulation Research, 124*(7), 1124–1140. http://doi.org/10.1161/CIRCRESAHA.118.313220.

Dorans, K. S., Mills, K. T., Liu, Y., & He, J. (2018). Trends in prevalence and control of hypertension according to the 2017 American College of Cardiology/American Heart Association (ACC/AHA) guideline. *Journal of the American Heart Association, 7*(11), e008888. http://doi.org/10.1161/JAHA.118.008888.

Elsevier. (n.d.). *Clinical pharmacology powered by ClinicalKey®*. Retrieved from http://www.clinicalkey.com.

Engberink, R. H. G. O., Frenkel, W. J., Bogaard, B. v. d., Brewster, L. M., Vogt, L., & Born, B.-J. H. v. d. (2015).Effects of thiazide-type and thiazide-like diuretics on cardiovascular events and mortality. *Hypertension, 65*(5), 1033–1040. http://doi.org/10.1161/HYPERTENSIONAHA.114.05122.

Kario, K., Thijs, L., & Staessen, J. A. (2019). Blood pressure measurement and treatment decisions. *Circulation Research, 124*(7), 990–1008. http://doi.org/10.1161/CIRCRESAHA.118.313219.

Liang, W., Ma, H., Cao, L., Yan, W., & Yang, J. (2017). Comparison of thiazide-like diuretics versus thiazide-type diuretics: A meta-analysis. *Journal of Cellular and Molecular Medicine, 21*(11), 2634–2642. http://doi.org/10.1111/jcmm.13205.

Lloyd-Jones, D. M., Braun, L. T., Ndumele, C. E., Smith, S. C., Sperling, L. S., Virani, S. S., & Blumenthal, R. S. (2019). Use of risk assessment tools to guide decision-making in the primary prevention of atherosclerotic cardiovascular disease: A special report from the American Heart Association and American College of Cardiology. *Circulation, 139*(25), e1162–e1177. http://doi.org/10.1161/CIR.0000000000000638.

McCance, K. L., & Huether, S. E. (Eds.) (2019). *Pathophysiology: The biologic basis for disease in adults and children* (8th ed.). St. Louis: Elsevier.

Nerenberg, K. A., Zarnke, K. B., Leung, A. A., Dasgupta, K., Butalia, S., McBrien, K., & Daskalopoulou, S. (2018). Hypertension Canada's 2018 guidelines for diagnosis, risk assessment, prevention, and treatment of hypertension in adults and children. *Canadian Journal of Cardiology, 34*(5), 506–525. http://doi.org/10.1016/j.cjca.2018.02.022.

Qato, D. M., Ozenberger, K., & Olfson, M. (2018). Prevalence of prescription medications with depression as a potential adverse effect among adults in the United States. *JAMA, 319*(22), 2289–2298. http://doi.org/10.1001/jama.2018.6741.

Reboussin, D. M., Allen, N. B., Griswold, M. E., Guallar, E., Hong, Y., Lackland, D. T., & Vupputuri, S. (2018). Systematic review for the 2017 ACC/AHA/AAPA/ABC/ACPM/AGS/APhA/ASH/ASPC/NMA/PCNA guideline for the prevention, detection, evaluation, and management of high blood pressure in adults. *Journal of the American College of Cardiology, 71*(19), 2176–2198. http://doi.org/10.1016/j.jacc.2017.11.004.

Tamargo, J., Segura, J., & Ruilope, L. M. (2014). Diuretics in the treatment of hypertension. Part 1: Thiazide and thiazide-like diuretics. *Expert Opinion on Pharmacotherapy, 15*(4), 527–547. http://doi.org/10.1517/14656566.2014.879118.

Whelton, P. K., Carey, R. M., Aronow, W. S., Casey, D. E., Collins, K. J., Himmelfarb, C. D., & Wright, J. T. (2018). 2017 ACC/AHA/AAPA/ABC/ACPM/AGS/APhA/ASH/ASPC/NMA/PCNA guideline for the prevention, detection, evaluation, and management of high blood pressure in adults—Executive summary: A report of the American College of Cardiology/American Heart Association Task Force on Clinical Practice Guidelines. *Hypertension, 71*(6), 1269–1324. http://doi.org/10.1161/HYP0000000000000066.

Yu, E., Malik, V. S., & Hu, F. B. (2018). Cardiovascular disease prevention by diet modification: JACC Health Promotion Series. *Journal of the American College of Cardiology, 72*(8), 914–926. https://doi.org/10.1016/j.jacc.2018.02.085.

10

Coronary Artery Disease Medications

ELIZABETH REMO, ANDREA EFRE, AND CHERYL H. ZAMBROSKI

Overview

Coronary artery disease (CAD) is a narrowing of the coronary arteries most commonly caused by atherosclerotic plaque buildup and inflammation, which affect the elasticity and strength of the vessels. The coronary arteries supply oxygenated blood to the heart muscles, heart valves, and conductivity pathways. Limited blood flow and reduced oxygen supply can result in myocardial ischemia or, if extensive and prolonged, myocardial infarction.

The impacts of CAD on overall heart health can be widespread, from decreased exercise tolerance to sudden death. Prevention is key, and reducing risk factors through lifestyle modifications and pharmacologic management limits advancement of the disease process. The American College of Cardiology (ACC) and the American Heart Association (AHA) provide clinical guidelines on the pharmacologic management of CAD, which is the focus of this chapter. Although a variety of medications are used to prevent and manage CAD, the focus here is antianginal medications—specifically, statin therapy, anticoagulants, beta-blockers, calcium channel blockers (CCBs), a partial fatty-acid oxidation inhibitor known as ranolazine, and nitrates.

Relevant Physiology

The normal coronary blood supply consists of the right and left coronary arteries, pulmonary artery, and aorta. From the right and left coronary arteries, which lie on the surface of the heart, smaller arteries branch off from the surface into the cardiac muscle. The left coronary artery supplies the anterior and lateral areas of the left ventricle, and the right coronary artery supplies the blood supply to the right ventricle, as well as the posterior part of the left ventricle in about 90% of individuals.

Seventy-five percent of the total coronary venous blood flow from the left ventricle returns to the right atrium through the coronary sinus, whereas venous blood flow from the right ventricle is returned through small anterior cardiac veins directly into the right atrium. Resting coronary blood flow averages 70 mL/min/100 Gm of heart weight, which averages to 225 mL/min. Blood flow through the coronary arteries is regulated by arterial vasodilation in response to the nutrient needs of the cardiac muscle. During exercise, cardiac output and coronary blood flow both increase to supply the additional oxygen and nutrients needed. Approximately 70% of the oxygen in the coronary arterial blood is removed as blood flows throughout the heart and cardiac muscle. It is thought that in response to a decrease in oxygen concentration in the heart, vasodilators such as adenosine, potassium and hydrogen ions, carbon dioxide, prostaglandins, and nitric acid are released from the muscle cells to dilate the coronary arterioles. Coronary blood flow is also affected by the autonomic nervous system. Stimulation of the sympathetic nervous system results in the release of epinephrine and norepinephrine, leading to increased heart rate and myocardial contractility as well as increased cardiac metabolism with increased coronary artery blood flow. On the other hand, stimulation of the parasympathetic nervous system via the vagus nerve leads to the release of acetylcholine with decreased heart rate, decreased myocardial contractility, decreased cardiac oxygen consumption, and constriction of coronary arteries with decreased blood flow.

During systole (contraction), the coronary capillary blood flow of the left ventricle falls due to the strong compression of the left ventricle around the vessels. In diastole, the cardiac muscle relaxes and blood flows through the left ventricular muscle capillaries at a rapid rate during diastole. Although blood flow in the right ventricle also changes in systole and diastole, the right-sided contraction force is less than that of the left ventricle, so the inverse changes in blood flow are only partial.

Pathophysiology: Coronary Artery Disease

Coronary artery circulation starts at the aortic root and feeds the myocardium with oxygenated blood through the right and left coronary arteries during diastole. In CAD, blood flow is hindered when an atheroma or atherosclerosis alters the vessel size and limits perfusion of the cardiac muscle. An *atheroma* is an accumulation of lipids, connective tissue, macrophages, and calcium that generates plaque in the vessels. The formation of plaque creates an inflammatory response as neutrophils are attracted to the area and proinflammatory cytokines are released.

Atherosclerosis refers to a narrowing of the coronary arteries that occurs with plaque formation inside the vessel walls.

The exact pathogenesis of atherosclerosis is not completely understood. The coronary artery walls have three layers. The innermost layer, the *tunica intima*, is where the plaque begins to form (Fig. 10.1). The atherosclerosis process begins when the endothelium lining the tunica intima becomes damaged due to glycation (from diabetes) or oxidation (from

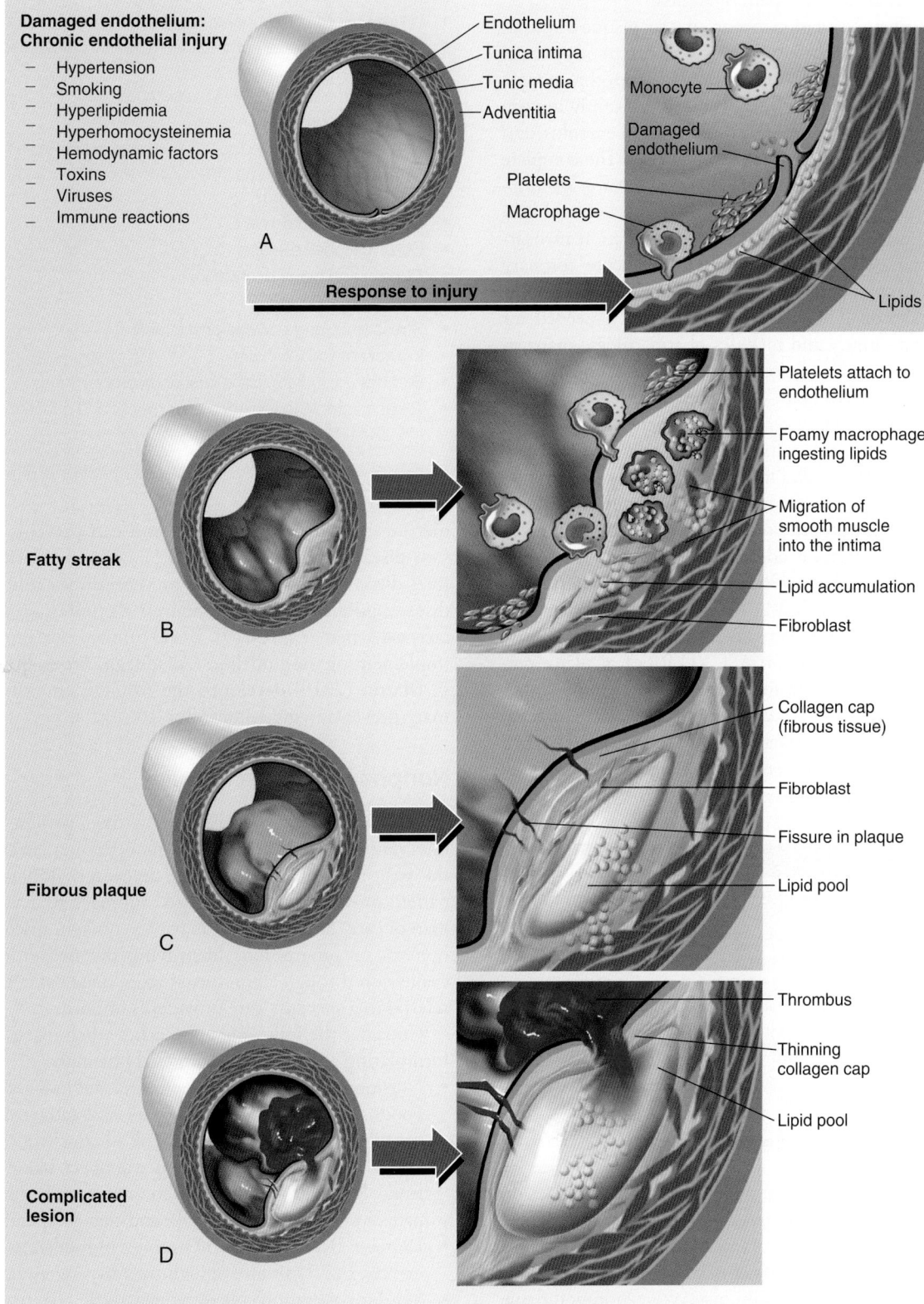

• **Fig. 10.1** Progression of atherosclerosis. (A) Damaged endothelium. (B) Diagram of fatty streak and lipid core formation (C) Diagram of fibrous plaque. Raised plaques are visible: some are yellow, others are white. (D) Diagram of complicated lesion: thrombus is red, collagen is blue. Plaque is complicated by red thrombus deposition. (From Huether, S., & McCance, K. [2020]. *Understanding pathophysiology* [7th ed.]. St. Louis: Elsevier.)

smoking and hyperlipidemia). This triggers the formation of plaque. As the plaque grows within the layers of the vessel wall, coronary blood flow is impeded. Deprivation of oxygen to the cardiac muscle leads to symptoms of coronary ischemia, such as the chest pain of angina.

A more urgent situation occurs if the plaque ruptures and the injured endothelial cells excrete thrombotic factors (such as von Willebrand factor), leading to atherothrombosis. The resultant *thrombus* (blood clot) can significantly impede blood flow, or it may break away, becoming an embolus, and travel downstream to occlude the distal vessel. The complete restriction of the blood supply leads to *ischemia of the myocardium* (acute myocardial infarction). Complete blood flow obstruction often triggers an ST-segment elevation myocardial infarction (STEMI). Symptoms of an acute coronary event include chest pain, dyspnea, diaphoresis, nausea, vomiting, and syncope. Emergency intervention is needed for acute coronary injury and includes pharmacologic management, interventional cardiology procedures, and potentially a coronary artery bypass graft. Time is extremely important in managing acute coronary events. The patient should receive intervention as soon as possible.

Limiting risk factors and introducing preventive therapies early in the disease process can make a significant impact in reducing disease progression. For example, lifestyle modifications and medication adjustments may be initiated to reduce the risk of coronary ischemia. In addition, a prevention tool such as the ASCVD Risk Calculator can be used to evaluate the risk of atherosclerotic cardiovascular disease (ASCVD). The pooled cohort ASCVD Risk Calculator predicts patients' 10-year risk for a first atherosclerotic cardiovascular event (Goff et al., 2014) and is regularly updated with the most currently available guidelines. Based on the results of the calculation, nonpharmacologic and pharmacologic treatment plans can be developed.

PRACTICE PEARLS

ASCVD Risk Estimator Plus

The ASCVD Risk Estimator Plus is a free mobile app version of the ASCVD Risk Calculator that is available in the iTunes and Google Play app stores and on the American College of Cardiology website. More information is available at https://www.acc.org/tools-and-practice-support/mobile-resources/features/2013-prevention-guidelines-ascvd-risk-estimator.

Coronary Artery Disease Therapy

Living a healthy lifestyle can make a significant impact on CAD prevention and progression. There are modifiable and nonmodifiable risk factors to consider when developing a plan of care for patients at risk for or diagnosed with CAD. Age, gender, and family history are nonmodifiable risk factors that contribute to disease progression. Smoking, elevated blood pressure, elevated cholesterol levels, diabetes, obesity, physical inactivity, high stress, and an unhealthy

---

• Box 10.1 Factors Associated With Increased Risk for Atherosclerotic Cardiovascular Disease

- Advanced age
- Males or post-menopausal females
- History of premature menopause
- Family history of premature atherosclerotic cardiovascular disease
- Diabetes mellitus and insulin resistance
- Ethnicity (South Asia ancestry)
- Chronic inflammatory disease such as rheumatoid arthritis, lupus, or HIV/AIDS
- Metabolic syndrome
- Primary hyperlipidemia
- Chronic kidney disease
- Obesity and being overweight
- Sedentary lifestyle
- Stress (including occupational stress)
- Increased alcohol intake
- Diet high in sodium, trans fats, and carbohydrates
- Tobacco smoking (includes prior history and exposure to secondhand smoke)

---

diet are modifiable risk factors and can prevent CAD or slow disease progression (Box 10.1). Clinical practice guidelines directed toward primary prevention of cardiovascular disease, published in 2019, address a number of these risk factors (Arnett et al., 2019). To aid primary care providers in implementing the guidelines, Alfaddagh, Arpes, Blumenthal & Martin (2019) developed the ABCDE checklist of primary prevention guidelines (Box 10.2).

Nonpharmacologic Therapy

A collaborative approach highlighting patient-centered interventions, such as behavior modification, is critical in the treatment of CAD. Shared decision-making with the patient provides an individualized approach to developing a plan of care. Several factors may play a role in disease development or progression. Identifying the need for further evaluation through laboratory studies, diagnostic testing, or referral to a specialty care provider is important.

Consider the following approaches when discussing and formulating a plan of care with CAD patients:

- Nutrition: Consider a low-cholesterol and low-sodium diet. Foods that are high in cholesterol and saturated fat will contribute to the development of atherosclerotic plaques. Foods that are high in sodium will affect blood pressure levels. Adequate hydration is also important. Encourage the patient to balance caloric intake and energy expenditure.
- Exercise: Recommend 150 minutes of moderate-intensity exercise or 75 minutes of high-intensity exercise per week.
- Smoking cessation: Nicotine negatively affects the coronary blood vessels, increasing the risk of heart disease (Fig. 10.1). Smoking cessation should be encouraged at every visit.

Adapted from Alfaddagh, A., Arps, K., Blumenthal, R. S., & Martin, S. S. (2019, March 21). *The ABCs of primary cardiovascular prevention: 2019 update.* American College of Cardiology. https://www.acc.org/latest-in-cardiology/articles/2019/03/21/14/39/abcs-of-primary-cv-prevention-2019-update-gl-prevention.

• Box 10.2   ABCDE Checklist of Primary Prevention Guidelines

Assess Risk and Use of **A**ntiplatelet Therapy

- Estimate ASCVD risk using the Pooled Cohort Equation for adults 40–75 years of age
- Refine risk assessment using coronary artery calcium scoring
- Reserve use of aspirin (antiplatelet therapy) for high-risk individuals (consider other risk factors)

Blood Pressure Control

- Lifestyle interventions (heart-healthy, low-sodium diet and physical activity)
- Goal blood pressure of <130/80 mm Hg for those on antihypertensive medications

Cholesterol Management and **C**igarette Smoking

- Statin use for adults 40–75 years of age with:
- 10-year ASCVD risk of ≥7.5%
- Diabetes
- LDL-C ≥190 mg/dL
- Tobacco use cessation:
  - Behavioral intervention plus pharmacotherapy recommended for tobacco users to assist in quitting
  - Dedicated trained staff for tobacco treatment

Diabetes Screening/Management and **D**iet/Weight Gain

- A diet rich in vegetables, fruits, legumes, nuts, whole grains, and fish is recommended
- Avoid intake of trans and saturated fats
- Overweight or obese adults: reduce caloric intake by >500 kCal daily and increase physical activity to >150 minutes weekly

Exercise and **E**conomic/Social Risk Factors

- Recommend 150 minutes of moderate-intensity exercise or 75 minutes of vigorous-intensity exercise weekly
- Avoid sedentary behavior
- Assess for socioeconomic barriers to patient's ability to follow treatment recommendations
- Patient-centered approach

- Mental health: Stress impacts CAD and contributes to disease progression. Therefore, stress reduction methods should be discussed.

Pharmacologic Therapy

A multistep approach is often needed to treat CAD and prevent further cardiac damage. Pharmacologic management involves the treatment of associated medical conditions, risk factors, and underlying CAD. Patients with a CAD diagnosis may have other comorbid conditions that impact their disease process. Therefore, a variety of drugs may be needed to manage CAD (Table 10.1).

- Aspirin: Aspirin reduces the risk of blood clots, which can help prevent obstruction of the coronary arteries (see Chapter 14, Anticlotting Medications). Aspirin and clopidogrel (Plavix) are no longer recommended for primary prevention of CAD but are used following percutaneous coronary interventions or in high-risk cases. For this reason, clopidogrel is most often initiated by cardiology. For more information, refer to ACC/AHA guidelines for the primary prevention of cardiovascular disease (Arnett et al., 2019).
- Cholesterol-modifying medications: Cholesterol reduction plays an important role in CAD prevention and management. Medications to reduce cholesterol levels include statins, fibrates, bile acid sequestrants, and selective cholesterol inhibitors (see Chapter 8, Antihyperlipidemic Medications, for more information).
- Beta-blockers: Beta-blockers (beta-adrenergic antagonists) reduce the sympathomimetic effects of epinephrine and norepinephrine on beta-adrenergic receptors. As a result, beta-blockers can decrease heart rate, myocardial contractility, and blood pressure. Cardioselective beta1-blockers are preferred in patients as they primarily affect the receptors in the heart. Nonselective beta-blockers are used with greater caution due to their impact on beta2 receptors in the lungs. Beta-blockers approved for use in

---

TABLE 10.1   List of Drug Classifications for Management of CAD

Drug Classification/ Medications	Indications	Dosage	Comments
Aspirin			
Acetylsalicylic acid	For primary prevention in patients with low to moderate risk for coronary event if not taking warfarin	75–162 mg orally once daily.	Moderate risk of a coronary event is based on age and 10-year cardiac risk greater than 10%.
	For secondary prevention and a reduction of cardiovascular mortality in patients with stable coronary artery disease, including angina or previous myocardial infarction or acute coronary syndrome	75–162 mg orally once daily indefinitely.	Lower doses of 100 mg/day or less are recommended for patients with a history of aspirin-induced bleeding or with risk factors for bleeding. In patients with a high likelihood of a myocardial infarction, administer aspirin in combination with clopidogrel.

Continued

TABLE 10.1   List of Drug Classifications for Management of CAD—cont'd

Drug Classification/ Medications	Indications	Dosage	Comments
Cholesterol-Modifying Medications			
Statins			
Atorvastatin (Lipitor)	Treatment of hypercholesterolemia as an adjunct to dietary control to reduce the risk of cardiovascular events, including myocardial infarction and stroke	Begin with 10–20 mg orally once daily. May start at 40 mg once daily if patients require greater than 45% LDL reduction. Dose range is 10–80 mg orally. May adjust dose every 2–4 weeks. *Children and adolescents ≥10 yr:* Begin with 10 mg orally once daily. May be increased to 20 mg/day after a minimum of 4 weeks if needed.	Older adults may have an increased cholesterol-lowering response to statins. Atorvastatin may be given at any time of day and without regard to meals. Adolescent females should be at least 1 yr postmenarche.
Fluvastatin	Treatment of hypercholesterolemia as an adjunct to dietary control to reduce the risk of cardiovascular events	**Regular release:** *Adults:* 20–40 mg orally once daily (22%–25% LDL reduction), titrated up to 40 mg twice daily (or switch to extended-release fluvastatin 80 mg once daily) to achieve 35%–36% LDL reduction. *Children and adolescents 10–17 yr:* 20 mg orally once daily; may titrate up to 40 mg twice daily. Adjust dosage at intervals of 6 weeks as needed. **ER tablet:** *Adults:* 20–80 mg orally once daily. *Children and adolescents 10–17 yr:* Patients who have been titrated up to 40 mg of regular release twice daily may be transitioned to 80 mg once daily of the extended-release formulation.	Adolescent females should be at least 1 yr postmenarche.
Lovastatin (Mevacor, Altoprev)	Treatment of hypercholesterolemia as an adjunct to dietary control	**IR forms:** *Adults:* 10–20 mg orally once daily with the evening meal. Dose range 10–80 mg in 1 or 2 divided doses. *Adolescents and children ≥10 yr, including girls who are at least 1 yr postmenarche:* Begin with 10–20 mg orally once daily with the evening meal. Maximum dosage: 40 mg/day. **ER:** *Adults:* Begin with 20–60 mg orally at bedtime. *Older adults or patients with complicated medical conditions:* May give 20 mg once daily.	For patients with renal impairment, use caution if CrCl <30. Food decreases absorption of extended-release forms. Dosage adjustments should be made at intervals of 4 weeks or more to achieve desired outcomes. Patients requiring less than a mean LDL reduction range of 30%–41% should not receive extended-release forms.

TABLE 10.1   List of Drug Classifications for Management of CAD—cont'd

Drug Classification/ Medications	Indications	Dosage	Comments
	Slowing of the progression of coronary atherosclerosis	**IR tablets:** Begin with 20 mg orally daily. Dose ranges between 10–80 mg with evening meal. **ER:** Initially, 20–60 mg orally once daily (mean LDL reduction range: 30%–41%).	
Pitavastatin	Treatment of hypercholesterolemia, hyperlipoproteinemia, and/ or hypertriglyceridemia as an adjunct to dietary control	*Adults, adolescents, and children 8–17 yr:* Begin with 2 mg orally once daily. Maximum dosage: 4 mg/day.	May be given without regard to meals. For patients with eGFR less than 60 mL/min/1.73 m², begin with 1 mg orally once daily; maximum dosage: 2 mg/day.
	For regression of ASCVD in patients with acute coronary syndrome (ACS)	4 mg orally once daily.	
Pravastatin (Pravachol)	For prevention of myocardial infarction or stroke	Begin with 40 mg orally daily; may adjust dose every 4 weeks. Maximum dosage: 80 mg/day. *Patients with severe renal impairment:* Start at 10 mg orally daily.	May be given without regard to meals.
Rosuvasatin (Crestor)	For primary prevention of ASCVD and to reduce the risk of arterial revascularization procedures in patients who have risk factors for cardiovascular disease	Usual beginning dosage is 10–20 mg orally daily. Dosage range is 5–40 mg orally daily. *Asian patients:* Start at 5 mg orally daily (increased risk of drug levels).	For patients with CrCl <30, start at 5 mg daily, with maximum dosage of 10 mg/day.
Simvastatin (Zocor)	Treatment of hypercholesterolemia as an adjunct to dietary control, and for reduction in cardiovascular mortality, including myocardial infarction prophylaxis and stroke prophylaxis	Begin with 10–20 mg orally once daily in the evening Usual dose is 5–40 mg daily in the evening. May adjust dose every 4 weeks.	For patients with severe renal impairment, dose should begin with 5 mg orally in the evening.
Beta-Blockers			
Atenolol	Chronic stable angina	Begin with 50 mg orally once daily. May increase to 100 mg/ day if needed after 7 days. Maximum dosage: 200 mg/ day orally.	In older adults, use lower starting doses. For patients with renal impairment, CrCl 15–35: maximum dosage of 50 mg/day. For patients with renal impairment, CrCl <15: maximum dosage of 25 mg/day.
Metoprolol	Chronic stable angina	**Regular-release tablets:** Begin with 25–50 mg orally twice daily; dose may be titrated at weekly intervals to clinical response. Usual effective dose range is 100–400 mg/day given in 2 divided doses. **ER tablets:** Sprinkle capsules 100–400 mg orally daily; start at 100 mg orally daily; may increase dose every week, with a maximum dosage of 400 mg/day; tablet may be cut in half but do not crush or chew.	Taper dosing over 1–2 weeks to discontinue. Regular-release tablets should be taken with food or right after meals to enhance absorption. Extended release may be given without regard to meals.

Continued

TABLE 10.1 **List of Drug Classifications for Management of CAD—cont'd**

Drug Classification/ Medications	Indications	Dosage	Comments
Nadolol (Corgard)	Chronic stable angina	Begin with 40 mg orally daily; may increase by 40–80 mg/day every 3–7 days, with maximum dosage of 240 mg/day.	
Propranolol hydrochloride	Chronic stable angina	**IR forms:** Begin with 10–20 mg orally two to four times per day. May increase at 3- to 7-day intervals up to 160–320 mg/day given in 2 to 4 divided doses. Begin with lower doses in older adults. **ER capsules:** Begin with 80 mg orally once daily, then increase at 3- to 7-day intervals up to 160–320 mg once daily.	Similar clinical efficacy (e.g., exercise tolerance, chest pain, blood pressure, heart rate control) are seen with equivalent daily doses of sustained-release propranolol (Inderal LA) compared with regular-release propranolol tablets (given in divided doses). Use caution in older adults.
Calcium Channel Blockers			
Amlodipine	Chronic stable angina, vasospastic angina, and CAD documented by angiography and without heart failure or ejection fraction less than 40%	Begin with 5–10 mg orally daily; for older adults, start at 5 mg orally daily.	For patients with hepatic impairment, begin with 5 mg daily.
Diltiazem	Chronic stable angina	**IR dosing:** 30–90 mg orally four times daily; start at 30 mg orally four times daily and increase every 1–2 days, with a maximum dosage of 480 mg/day given in 3–4 divided doses. **ER dosing:** 120–480 mg orally daily; start at 120–240 mg orally daily and titrate over 7–14 days; maximum dosage of 480 mg/day; do not open, crush, chew, or dissolve contents.	NOTE: Confirm extended-release doses with manufacturer, as diltiazem extended-release forms are provided under multiple varying trade names. Differing trade names also have varying administration instructions.
Nicardipine	Chronic stable angina	20–40 mg orally three times daily; start at 20 mg orally three times daily and may increase dose every 3 days, with a maximum dosage of 120 mg/day.	
Nifedipine	Chronic stable angina and vasospastic angina	**IR dosing:** 10–20 mg orally three times daily; start with 10 mg orally three times daily and may increase dose every 7–14 days, with a maximum dosage of 180 mg/day in divided doses; dosages greater than 120 mg/day are rarely needed. **ER dosing:** 30–90 mg orally daily; start at 30–60 mg orally daily and may increase dose every 7–14 days, with a maximum dosage of 90 mg/day; do not cut, crush, or chew ER tablet.	For IR dosing, single dose maximum is 30 mg.

TABLE 10.1 **List of Drug Classifications for Management of CAD—cont'd**

Drug Classification/ Medications	Indications	Dosage	Comments
Verapamil	Unstable angina, chronic stable angina, and vasospastic angina in adults	**Regular-release tablets:** 80–120 mg orally every 8 hr, then up to 480 mg/day in divided doses. For older adults, those with hepatic disease, or those of small stature, begin with 40 mg every 8 hr and increase based on clinical response to 480 mg/day in divided doses. **ER capsule:** *Adults:* Start at 180 mg daily at bedtime; may be titrated to 240, 360, and 480 mg as tolerated, with all doses administered at bedtime. For older adults, begin at lower dose and titrate as tolerated.	
Antianginal Medications			
Ranolazine	Chronic stable angina	500–1000 mg orally twice daily; start at 500 mg orally twice daily, with a maximum dosage of 2000 mg/day. Older adults should begin with lower dose. For any adult patients taking diltiazem, verapamil, aprepitant, erythromycin, or fluconazole, limit dosage to 500 mg daily.	Improves symptom of chest pain. Use of ranolazine with CYP3A inducers or strong CYP3A inhibitors is contraindicated. Effects of ranolazine on angina frequency and exercise tolerance are considerably smaller in women than in men.
Nitrates			
Isosorbide dinitrate	For long-term angina protection	**Angina Prophylaxis** **IR dosing:** 10–40 mg orally two or three times daily; start at 5–20 mg orally two or three times daily, with a maximum dosage of 480 mg/day. **SR dosing:** 40–80 mg orally once or twice daily; start at 40 mg orally daily, with maximum dosage of 160 mg/day.	Nitrate-free interval of 14 hours is recommended to prevent nitrate tolerance for both immediate-release and sustained-release forms.
Isosorbide mononitrate	Treatment of chronic stable angina pectoris	**IR dosing:** 20 mg orally twice daily, with maximum dosage of 40 mg/day; spaced 7 hr apart; in small-stature or older patients, consider starting dose of 5 mg orally twice daily and may increase to 10 mg twice daily by day 2 or 3 of therapy. **ER dosing:** 30–120 mg orally daily in the morning; start at 30–60 mg orally daily in the morning and may increase dose over several days, with maximum dosage of 240 mg/day.	Older adults and patients of small stature may be more sensitive to effects.

Continued

List of Drug Classifications for Management of CAD—cont'd

Drug Classification/ Medications	Indications	Dosage	Comments
Nitroglycerin	Acute angina pectoris or acute angina prophylaxis	**Angina Prophylaxis** **Sublingual dosing:** 0.3–0.6 mg × 1 tablet; start 5–10 min before strenuous activity. **Translingual spray dosing:** 1–2 actuations × 1; start 5–10 min before strenuous activity. **Acute Angina** **Sublingual dosing:** 0.3–0.6 mg/5 min, with a maximum of 3 doses within 15 minutes. **Translingual spray dosing:** 1–2 actuations/5 min as needed, with maximum dosage of 3 actuations within 15 min.	
	Chronic stable angina	**Transdermal patch:** Apply 1 patch (0.1–0.8 mg/ hour) to intact skin once daily. Begin with the smallest dose and increase as tolerated to manage symptoms. To prevent nitrate tolerance, leave the patch on 12–14 hours, then remove for 10–12 hours before applying the next patch. **Topical 2% ointment:** 15–30 mg (2.5–5 cm as squeezed from the tube, about 1–2 inches) applied to the skin every 8 hr while awake and at bedtime; frequency of application may be increased to every 6 hr if needed. Alternatively, a regimen providing a 12-hour nitrate-free interval may be used; apply dosage once each morning, then reapply 6 hr later. Maximum daily dosage is 75 mg (12.5 cm as squeezed from the tube).	2% ointment is applied in a thin layer covering approximately 2–3 inches of skin but *should not be massaged into the skin*.

ASCVD, Atherosclerotic cardiovascular disease; *CrCl,* creatinine clearance; *EF,* ejection fraction; *eGFR,* estimated glomerular filtration rate; *ER,* extended release; *HD,* hemodialysis; *MI,* myocardial infarction; *HTN,* hypertension; *IR,* immediate release; *NYHA,* New York Heart Association; *SR,* sustained release.

treating angina pectoris include atenolol, metoprolol, nadolol, and propranolol. Carvedilol can be used in patients with left ventricular dysfunction (ejection fraction of 40% or higher) following acute myocardial infarction. Atenolol, metoprolol, carvedilol, propranolol, and timolol have been shown to reduce cardiovascular mortality. For more discussion of beta-blockers, see Chapter 11, Heart Failure Medications, and Chapter 12, Antiarrhythmic Medications.

- CCBs: CCBs are most commonly used in the treatment of hypertension and angina pectoris. In addition, select CCBs may also be used in the treatment of arrhythmias. There are two subclasses of CCBs: dihydropyridines (DHPs) and nondihydropyridines (non-DHPs). DHPs have greater selectivity for vascular smooth muscle cells whereas non-DHPs have greater selectivity for cardiac muscle cells. The DHPs amlodipine and nicardipine as well as non-DHPs such as diltiazem are approved for the treatment of chronic stable angina. Verapamil can be used for the treatment of stable and unstable angina. Finally, medications from both subclasses, including amlodipine, nifedipine, diltiazem, and verapamil, can be used to treat variant angina. See Chapter 9, Antihypertensive Medications, and Chapter 12, Antiarrhythmic Medications, for more discussion on the use of CCBs in treating hypertension and arrhythmias, respectively.

- Angiotensin-converting enzyme inhibitors (ACE-Is): ACE-Is are considered first-line treatment for patients with hypertension, particularly those with heart failure, post-myocardial infarction, diabetes, and chronic kidney disease, and for secondary stroke prevention. Two ACE-Is have been shown to reduce cardiovascular mortality: ramipril and perindopril. For more in-depth discussion of the use of ACE-Is in patients with hypertension and heart failure, see Chapter 9, Antihypertensive Medications, and Chapter 11, Heart Failure Medications, respectively.
- Angiotensin receptor blockers (ARBs): Two ARBs have been shown to reduce cardiovascular mortality. Telmisartan can be used to prevent stroke and myocardial infarction as well as reduce cardiovascular mortality in adults 55 years of age or older who are at high risk for major cardiovascular events and are unable to take ACE-Is. Valsartan can be used to reduce cardiovascular mortality in stable patients with left ventricular failure or left ventricular dysfunction after acute myocardial infarction. For more discussion of ARBs, see Chapter 9, Antihypertensive Medications, and Chapter 11, Heart Failure Medications.

Additional Antianginal Medications

Along with the medications mentioned previously, additional antianginal medications include ranolazine and nitrates. Ranolazine may be prescribed with or instead of a beta-blocker to reduce chest pain. Nitroglycerin temporarily dilates the coronary arteries and reduces coronary demand for oxygenated blood. Long-acting nitrate preparations such as isosorbide mononitrate and isosorbide dinitrate are useful in long-term management of CAD with angina.

Ranolazine (Ranexa)

Used for its antianginal effects, ranolazine belongs to a group of drugs known as partial fatty-acid oxidation inhibitors. While its exact mechanism of action is not fully understood, it may work by inhibiting the late sodium current, leading to a reduction of intracellular sodium and calcium overload in ischemic cardiac myocytes. Ranolazine can reduce myocardial oxygen demand, decrease the production of lactic acid, and improve cardiac function. It does not affect heart rate or blood pressure.

Pharmacokinetics. Ranolazine is metabolized in the liver by the cytochrome (CYP) 3A4 and CYP 2D6 enzymes. Plasma concentration peaks in 2 to 5 hours and half-life is 7 hours. Steady state is achieved in 3 days.

Indications. Ranolazine is used for the treatment of chronic angina. Of note, the effects of ranolazine on exercise tolerance and frequency of anginal attacks are lower in females than in males.

Adverse Effects. The most common adverse effects associated with ranolazine are dizziness and headache (in about 6% of patients). Other adverse effects are relatively infrequent (occurring in about 4% of patients) and include mild gastrointestinal (GI) issues such as anorexia, nausea, vomiting, dyspepsia, and constipation. Possible cardiovascular effects include orthostatic hypotension, palpitations, sinus bradycardia, and peripheral edema. Patients with renal impairment may experience increased levels of potassium, blood urea nitrogen (BUN), and creatinine.

Contraindications. Ranolazine is contraindicated in patients with cirrhosis of the liver and those who are on dialysis treatment. Dose adjustment is required when taken with CYP 3A4 inhibitors such as verapamil, diltiazem, fluconazole, and erythromycin, as these can increase ranolazine levels. P-glycoprotein inhibitors such as cyclosporine may also increase ranolazine levels. Patients taking CYP 3A4 and P-glycoprotein inhibitors should not exceed a ranolazine dosage of 500 mg twice daily. Concomitant use with CYP 3A4 inducers such as rifampin, carbamazepine, phenytoin, and St. John's wort can decrease ranolazine levels and is not recommended. Patients with a family history of long QT syndrome and with a known history of prolonged QT interval should be closely monitored. There are limited data on the use of this medication in patients who are pregnant, during lactation, or in the pediatric population.

Monitoring. Electrocardiogram (ECG) monitoring, specifically the evaluation of QT measurements, is required. The use of ranolazine in combination with metformin may increase metformin levels in patients with a creatinine clearance (CrCl) less than 60 mL/minute. Monitor serum creatinine closely and discontinue therapy if renal failure occurs. It is important not to use this medication in patients with a CrCL that is less than 30 mL/minute. Monitor BUN and urine output, as well as for the presence of neurologic side effects. Close monitoring is recommended in patients 75 years of age or older.

PRACTICE PEARLS

Ranolazine

- Because grapefruit juice is a moderate CYP 3A inhibitor, remind patients to avoid it while taking ranolazine as this could result in increased drug levels.
- Remind patients that ranolazine does not relieve an acute angina episode but is used on a regularly scheduled basis to reduce the symptoms of chronic stable angina.
- High doses can cause dose-dependent increases in dizziness, tremor, dysphagia, hallucinations, unsteady gait, nausea, and vomiting.

Nitroglycerin

Nitroglycerin converts nitric oxide (NO) in the body and activates the enzyme guanylyl cyclase. It then converts guanosine triphosphate (GTP) to guanosine 3′,5′-monophosphate (cGMP) in the vascular smooth muscles and tissues. Additionally, cGMP activates protein kinase-dependent phosphorylation, resulting in smooth muscle relaxation within the blood vessels. Venodilation occurs primarily, causing pooling of blood within the venous system; it also reduces preload to the heart, lessens the cardiac workload, and decreases anginal symptoms secondary to demand

1. At the first sign of an angina attack (chest pain or tightness), place 1 tablet under your tongue.
2. Let the tablet dissolve under the tongue.
3. Do not swallow whole.
4. Replace the dose if you accidentally swallow it. It will help if your mouth is not dry. Saliva around the tablet will help it dissolve more quickly. Do not eat or drink, or smoke or chew tobacco, while a tablet is dissolving.
5. If you are not better within 5 minutes after taking ONE dose of nitroglycerin, call 9-1-1 immediately to seek emergency medical care.
6. Do not take more than 3 nitroglycerin tablets over 15 minutes.

If you take this medicine often to relieve symptoms of angina, your doctor or health care professional may provide you with different instructions to manage your symptoms. If symptoms do not go away after following these instructions, it is important to call 9-1-1 immediately.

Adapted from Elsevier. (n.d.). *Clinical pharmacology powered by ClinicalKey®*. http://www.clinicalkey.com.

TABLE 10.2   Route-Specific Onset and Duration of Nitroglycerin

Route	Onset	Duration of Action
Sublingual	1–3 minutes	30 minutes
Translingual (spray)	2–4 minutes	30–60 minutes
Extended-release capsules and tablets	2–3 minutes	8–12 hours
Transdermal ointment	20–60 minutes	4–8 hours[a]
Transdermal patch	40–60 minutes	18–24 hours[a]

[a]Prescription of transdermal ointment or transdermal patch should include a 10–12-hour drug-free period to avoid nitrate tolerance and help preserve antianginal effect.

TABLE 10.3   Common Drug Interactions with Nitrate Products

Precipitant Drug	Adverse Interaction
Alcohol	Severe hypotension, cardiovascular collapse
Aspirin	May increase nitrate serum concentrations or actions
Calcium channel blockers	Marked orthostatic hypotension may occur
Dihydroergotamine	Bioavailability of the ergot may increase, causing an increase in mean standing systolic blood pressure or a functional antagonism between the two agents and a decrease in antianginal effects
Heparin	May decrease heparin pharmacologic effects
Sildenafil (Viagra)	May precipitate severe hypotension, syncope, myocardial infarction, or death

ischemia. Arterial vasodilation also occurs, increasing blood flow and perfusion to the heart.

Pharmacokinetics. Nitroglycerin can be given via a number of routes, including oral, lingual (spray), sublingual, and transdermal (Table 10.2). Of note, organic nitrates are nearly completely metabolized by the enzyme glutathione-organic nitrate reductase. This is important, as biotransformation is the overall determinant of bioavailability. When nitroglycerine is given orally, most of the dose is destroyed through first-pass metabolism. Nitroglycerin distributes widely, with approximately 60% protein bound. Metabolites of nitroglycerin are predominantly excreted by the kidneys.

Indications. Nitroglycerin is used as an antianginal medication. It is a vasodilatory drug that provides acute relief during a coronary event (Box 10.3). It is also used for acute prophylaxis of angina pectoris secondary to CAD.

Adverse Effects. Adverse effects of nitroglycerin are typically related to its vasodilatory and hypotensive effects, which include dizziness, weakness, palpitations, vertigo, headaches, nausea, vomiting, diaphoresis, pallor, and syncope. Headaches may be severe, throbbing, and persistent and usually occur right after taking the medication. Orthostatic hypotension may also occur, with associated symptoms of dizziness, weakness, palpitations, and vertigo. Additional symptoms include flushing, exfoliative dermatitis, and drug rash.

Contraindications. Allergic reactions to the medication can occur. Nitroglycerin is contraindicated in patients with a history of increased intracranial pressure, severe anemia, right-sided myocardial infarction, and hypersensitivity to nitroglycerin. Concurrent use with phosphodiesterase type 5 (PDE 5) inhibitors, such as sildenafil citrate, vardenafil hydroxide, and tadalafil, is contraindicated. Additional drug interactions are listed in Table 10.3.

Monitoring. Patients' vital signs should be monitored for hemodynamic effects. This includes monitoring of blood pressure, heart rate, respiratory rate, and oxygen saturation. Interactions are common when nitroglycerin is used with tricyclic antidepressants and anticholinergic drugs. Patients are instructed to limit alcohol intake. The medication is classified under pregnancy category C; use with caution in patients who are breastfeeding.

Isosorbide Mononitrate

Pharmacokinetics. Isosorbide mononitrate can be given orally. It is rapidly absorbed from the GI tract and does not undergo first-pass metabolism, allowing bioavailability at nearly 100%. Isosorbide mononitrate is metabolized in the liver to mononitrate glucuronide and other inactive metabolites. At least 99% of the drug is metabolized prior to excretion in the urine. Half-life is approximately 5 hours. Peak effect is typically within 1 to 4 hours.

Indications. Isosorbide mononitrate is used for the chronic treatment of angina pectoris due to CAD. It should not be used to treat acute anginal attacks.

Adverse Effects. The most common adverse effects associated with isosorbide mononitrate are headaches (in as many as 57% of patients) and dizziness (up to 11%). While less frequent, serious exacerbation of arrhythmias including atrial arrythmias, sinus bradycardia or tachycardia, and ventricular tachycardia have occurred. Other serious reactions include severe hypotension, heart failure, myocardial infarction, and methemoglobinemia.

Contraindications. Use of isosorbide mononitrate is contraindicated in patients who are hypersensitive to nitrates or who have severe anemia. It should be used cautiously in patients with volume depletion, recent myocardial infarction, hypertrophic cardiomyopathy, and closed-angle glaucoma. It should not be discontinued abruptly due to the risk of rebound angina.

Monitoring. Monitor blood pressure closely. Laboratory monitoring is not necessary.

Isosorbide Dinitrate

Pharmacokinetics. Isosorbide dinitrate is rapidly absorbed from the GI tract and, like other nitrates, undergoes extensive first-pass metabolism, resulting in approximately 25% bioavailability. Capsules and tablets have an onset of about 8 to 45 minutes with a duration of 2 to 6 hours; extended-release capsules and tablets have an onset of 60 to 90 minutes and a duration of 10 to 14 hours. Isosorbide dinitrate is metabolized in the liver and excreted in the urine.

Indications. Isosorbide dinitrate is used for the prevention or treatment of angina pectoris in patients with CAD. Of note, a dosing interval of more than 14 hours may be necessary to avoid nitrate tolerance.

Adverse Effects. The most common adverse effects are headache (40% of patients), dizziness (30%), and hypotension (10%). Others include nausea (about 4%), and vomiting and xerostomia (both at less than 1%). In extremely rare situations, isosorbide dinitrate can cause methemoglobinemia.

Contraindications. Isosorbide dinitrate is contraindicated in patients with hypersensitivity to nitrates, severe anemia, and closed-angle glaucoma due to the risk of drug-induced intraocular pressure. Use with caution in patients with hypotension, volume depletion, acute myocardial infarction, or hypertrophic cardiomyopathy. Isosorbide dinitrate may cause increased intracranial pressure in patients with head trauma. Safety in pregnancy and breastfeeding has not be established.

Monitoring. Monitor blood pressure closely. Laboratory monitoring is not necessary.

Alternative Pharmacologic Therapy

There are several alternative supplements that may be recommended to patients with CAD. Due to the impact of inflammatory changes on the heart, supplements that help reduce inflammation, such as fish oil, flaxseed oil, and other sources of omega-3 fatty acids, have been recommended. These supplements are available over the counter (OTC) and in prescription form. Supplements that can reduce blood pressure and lower cholesterol have also been recommended, including alpha-linolenic acid, barley, cocoa, coenzyme Q10, fiber, garlic, and plant stanols/sterols. These alternative medications may have some benefits in preventing or reducing risk factors for heart disease; however, additional research is needed to determine evidence-based benefits and dosage recommendations. Drug interactions with the use of OTC medications may be detrimental. Therefore, health care providers should be aware of their side effects prior to advising their use.

> **BOOKMARK THIS!**
>
> **National Center for Complementary and Integrative Health**
>
> The National Center for Complementary and Integrative Health (NCCIH) provides links to clinical practice guidelines that may guide practice related to the use of alternative substances in cardiovascular care; see https://www.nccih.nih.gov/health/providers/clinicalpractice. The NCCIH also provides resources on a variety of additional health topics, consumer information, facts about herbal and botanical drugs, and information regarding access to clinical trials.

Prescriber Considerations for Coronary Artery Disease Therapy

Clinical Reasoning for Coronary Artery Disease Therapy

The ACC and AHA have published practice guidelines recommending strategies for preventing cardiovascular disease, including atherosclerotic vascular disease, heart failure, and atrial fibrillation. Both organizations emphasize the critical need for a team-based approach to cardiovascular care, shared decision-making, and considerations of the social determinants of health to inform practice recommendations.

> **BOOKMARK THIS!**
>
> **Clinical Guidelines**
>
> ACC/AHA ASCVD Risk Estimator: https://tools.acc.org/ldl/ascvd_risk_estimator/index.html#!/calulate/estimator/
> ACC/AHA Guidelines for Primary Prevention of Cardiovascular Disease (2019): https://www.ahajournals.org/doi/full/10.1161/CIR.0000000000000678

Consider the individual patient's health problem requiring CAD therapy. Initial assessment and evaluation of the patient's medical condition, including the use of diagnostic tests for screening purposes, is necessary to detect the presence of cardiovascular disease. Risk factors must be considered, including familial coronary history, smoking, hyperlipidemia, diabetes mellitus, and hypertension. Additionally, prevention is the key to CAD management (Box 10.2).

Determine the desired therapeutic outcome based on the degree of CAD management needed for the patient's health problem. A patient-centered approach to care is critical in developing a focused plan specific to the patient's needs. Communicating the health problem of concern to the patient and presenting evidence-based recommendations for management allows a collaborative opportunity to achieve the desired health outcome. CAD management consists of both nonpharmacologic and pharmacologic approaches addressing primary, secondary, and tertiary prevention of the disease process. It is important to consider associated health problems and risk factors when determining an individualized plan of care.

Assess the medication therapy selected for its appropriateness for an individual patient by considering the medication's side effects and the patient's age, race/ethnicity, comorbidities, and genetic factors. Prevention and management of CAD includes the use of prescribed medications and OTC supplements. Patients with CAD may have additional medical conditions requiring adjunct medication therapy. It is important to assess and review the patient's medications to ensure their appropriateness. The polypharmacy required to manage the multiple disease processes surrounding CAD may impede or affect the patient's quality of life. Additionally, some medication classes may be less effective in certain patient populations; therefore, patient sex and race should be considered.

Initiate the treatment plan with the selected medication by first providing adequate patient education to ensure the patient's understanding and promote full participation in the CAD therapy. A collaborative approach between the patient and the health care provider in developing an individualized plan of care sets the foundation for success in achieving desired health outcomes. The patient's awareness of their medical condition and management plan allows for understanding and acceptance of the health care provider's treatment recommendations. Focused education on risk factors and associated comorbid conditions can prevent worsening of the disease process. Clear communication of the purpose of the medication, dosage, use, side effects, and other associated information provides clarity on its necessity and what to expect.

Ensure complete patient and family understanding about the medication prescribed for CAD therapy using a variety of education strategies. For most patients, preventive and maintenance medications are taken long term. Patients must understand that committing to daily nonpharmacologic and pharmacologic treatments is the only way to prevent further development of the disease. Taking prescriptions as they are recommended and following lifestyle modifications are essential in preventing CAD.

Conduct follow-up and monitoring of patient responses to CAD therapy and overall CAD management. Routine follow-up with primary and specialty health care providers is part of the medical management of CAD. Regular symptom assessment, electrocardiograms, laboratory studies, and other pertinent diagnostic testing will be integrated to ensure the appropriate level of therapy. Unresolved chest pain or angina after use of nitroglycerine requires emergency care.

Teaching Points for Coronary Artery Disease Therapy

Health Promotion Strategies

- Lifestyle and risk factors should be assessed on a continued basis, with a focus on discussing preventive measures, such as smoking cessation, at each visit. Offer smoking cessation medications as appropriate (see Chapter 52, Smoking Cessation Medications).
- Discuss weight loss, diet, and exercise at every visit. Encourage patients to increase physical activity to 150 minutes per week, or more if possible. Include teaching about signs of overexertion and the possible need for emergency nitroglycerin.
- Discuss food choices and recommend a diet rich in vegetables, fruits, legumes, nuts, whole grains, and fish. Advise the patient to avoid foods high in trans and saturated fats and to limit their intake of fast food.
- Cholesterol management should be a priority in the preventive plan, and statin therapy is recommended in moderate or high-intensity dosages based on the ASCVD Risk Calculator.
- Diabetic patients have a greater risk for CAD. Screening for diabetes and careful management helps in the prevention of CAD.
- Blood pressure must be managed, with a goal of systolic pressure less than 130 mmHg and diastolic pressure less than 80 mmHg.
- The primary care provider should discuss the risks and benefits of each medication used in the treatment of CAD prior to initiating therapy as part of the shared decision-making process.

Patient Education for Medication Safety

- Be alert for signs of coronary ischemia and contact emergency services if you experience pain in the chest, back, neck, or arms that lasts more than a few minutes. Additional symptoms include shortness of breath, sweating, nausea, or vomiting. These are all signs of a myocardial infarction and need emergency evaluation and treatment.
- Tell your health care provider if your symptoms change or increase; adaptations in your medical plan may be necessary.
- Follow the ABCDE checklist of primary prevention guidelines (Box 10.2).
- If you smoke, try to stop smoking or decrease the amount you smoke each day. Talk to your health care provider about smoking cessation therapy.

- Tell your health care provider about all the medicines you take, including prescription and OTC medicines, vitamins, and herbal supplements.
- Use all medications as instructed. Do not use more or less of the medication.
- Keep nitroglycerin with you at all times for emergency use.

Application Questions for Discussion

1. What resources are available to primary care providers to guide the care of CAD patients?
2. Discuss the medications included in the ABCDE checklist of primary prevention guidelines.
3. What medication should all CAD patients have prescribed for emergency use? What medications are used for maintenance therapy?

Selected Bibliography

Alfaddagh, A., Arps, K., Blumenthal, R. S., & Martin, S. S. (2019). The ABCs of primary cardiovascular prevention: 2019 update. *American College of Cardiology.* https://www.acc.org/latest-in-cardiology/articles/2019/03/21/14/39/abcs-of-primary-cv-prevention-2019-update-gl-prevention.

American College of Cardiology and American Heart Association. (n.d.). *ASCVD risk estimator.* https://tools.acc.org/ldl/ascvd_risk_estimator/index.html#!/calulate/estimator/.

American Heart Association (2020). *American Heart Association recommendations for physical activity in adults and kids.* https://www.heart.org/en/healthy-living/fitness/fitness-basics/aha-recs-for-physical-activity-in-adults.

Arnett, D. K., Blumenthal, R. S., Albert, M. A., Buroker, A. B., Glodberger, Z. D., & Ziaeian, B. (2019). 2019 ACC/AHA guideline on the primary prevention of cardiovascular disease: A report of the American College of Cardiology/American Heart Association task force on clinical practice guidelines. *Circulation, 140*(11), e596–e646. https://www.ahajournals.org/doi/10.1161/CIR.0000000000000678.

Buttaro, T. M., Polgar-Bailey, P., Sandberg-Cook, J., & Trybulski, J. (2021). *Primary care: Interprofessional collaborative practice* (6th ed.). St. Louis: Elsevier.

Elsevier. (n.d.). *Clinical pharmacology powered by ClinicalKey®.* http://www.clinicalkey.com.

Goff, D. C., Jr., Lloyd-Jones, D. M., Bennett, G., et al. (2014). 2013 ACC/AHA guideline on the assessment of cardiovascular risk: A report of the American College of Cardiology/American Heart Association task force on practice guidelines. *Journal of the American College of Cardiology, 63*(25 Pt B), 2935–2959. http://doi.org/10.1016/j.jacc.2013.11.005.

Hall, J. E. (2011). *Guyton and Hall textbook of medical physiology* (12th ed.). Philadelphia: Elsevier.

Mayo Clinic. (2020). *Coronary artery disease.* https://www.mayoclinic.org/diseases-conditions/coronary-artery-disease/symptoms-causes/syc-20350613.

McCance, K. L., & Huether, S. E. (2019). *Pathophysiology: The biologic basis for disease in adults and children* (8th ed.). St. Louis: Elsevier.

Pflieger, M., Winslow, B. T., Mills, K., & Dauber, I. M. (2011). Medical management of stable coronary artery disease. *American Family Physician, 83*(7), 819–826. https://www.aafp.org/afp/2011/0401/afp20110401p819.pdf.

Virani, S. S., Alonso, A., Benjamin, E. J., Bittencourt, M. S., Callaway, C. W., Carson, A. P., & Tsao, C. W. (2020). Heart disease and stroke statistics—2020 update: A report from the American Heart Association. *Circulation, 141*(9), e139–e596. http://doi.org/10.1161/CIR.0000000000000757.

11

Heart Failure Medications

JANET ROMAN

Overview

Heart failure (HF) medications are prescribed most often using guideline-directed medical therapy (GDMT). HF disease is the heart's inability to pump and/or fill effectively to supply adequate cardiac output and tissue perfusion. This chapter focuses on the HF medications used most often in the primary care setting. These include beta-blockers, inhibitors of angiotensin-converting enzymes, angiotensin II receptors, aldosterone, renin, diuretics, nitrates, digoxin, and some newer medications proven effective in HF treatment. It is very important for the advanced practice nurse (APN) to understand which medications are appropriate for the various types of HF, how to titrate to targeted dosages, appropriate monitoring, and lifestyle modifications necessary to facilitate medication effectiveness.

Relevant Physiology

Heart and Vascular Structures

The heart contains three layers: the epicardium, myocardium, and endocardium. The *pericardium* forms a protective sac around the heart and has two layers, parietal and visceral, that are separated by pericardial fluid which provides a cushion for the heart. The heart has four chambers: the right and left atria and the right and left ventricles. The right side of the heart, consisting of the right atrium and ventricle, is a low-pressure system that pumps blood into the lungs. The left side of the heart, consisting of the left atrium and ventricle, is a high-pressure system that pumps blood throughout the body.

Blood moves passively from the atria to the ventricles. The ventricles must overcome resistance and pump the blood through the pulmonary or systemic vessels. Normal blood flow through the heart begins with deoxygenated blood entering the right atrium from the system through the superior and inferior vena cava. The blood is pumped from the right ventricle into the pulmonary arteries and then into the right and left lungs. The oxygenated blood exits the lungs through the pulmonary veins to the left atrium and left ventricle. The blood then exits the heart through the aorta to the systemic vessels.

The *cardiac cycle* consists of one ventricular contraction (*systole*) and the relaxation period (*diastole*) before the next contraction. During systole, the ventricle contracts and the blood is ejected into the pulmonary and systemic circulation. The heart muscle relaxes during diastole and the ventricles fill with blood from the atria, completing one cardiac cycle. The sympathetic and parasympathetic nerves innervate all parts of the atria and ventricles and affect the speed of the cardiac cycle or heart rate as well as the force of the contraction. The sympathetic nervous system (SNS) increases the heart rate, while norepinephrine is released by the nervous system and the circulating catecholamines interact with the β-adrenergic receptors. This cascade results in an influx of calcium ions, which increase the strength and speed of the contraction. The parasympathetic nervous system decreases the heart rate through the release of acetylcholine, which reduces the strength of the contraction.

Sympathetic stimulation is contingent on several factors: whether the α- or β-adrenergic receptors are plentiful on the effector tissue cells; whether the neurotransmitter is epinephrine or norepinephrine; and the extent of receptor responsiveness based on its structure. There are nine types of adrenergic receptors. The cardiovascular structures contain more β- receptors than α- receptors. *Chronotropy* increases the heart rate by stimulating the β_1 and β_2 receptors, and *inotropy* increases the force of the contraction. *Vasodilation* occurs when β_2 receptors located on the smooth muscle are stimulated. *Vasoconstriction* occurs when norepinephrine binds with α_1 receptors. The *pathogenesis of HF* occurs when there is dysfunction of the α- or β- adrenergic receptors.

Cardiac output is the amount of blood the heart pumps through the circulatory system in one minute. *Stroke volume* is the amount of blood pumped out by the left ventricle in one contraction. The stroke volume (SV) and the heart rate (HR) determine the *cardiac output* (CO). The *ejection fraction* (EF) is the amount of blood pumped out of the ventricles with each heartbeat.

$$EF\left(\%\right) = SV\,/\,EDVx100$$

The EF is calculated by dividing the stroke volume by the volume of blood remaining in the ventricle at the end of diastole (the end diastolic volume [EDV]). The normal

EF is approximately 65% for females and 60% for males +/- 8% for either gender. The EF can be increased by factors that increase contractility. A decreased EF indicates ventricular failure.

Factors that have a direct effect on cardiac output include heart rate, contractility, preload, and afterload. *Preload* is the amount of blood in the ventricle at the end of diastole. HF can develop because of an increase in the preload, which causes a decreased stroke volume and increased ventricular pressure. This cascade causes blood volume to back up into pulmonary and/or systemic circulation. *Afterload* is described as the resistance the ventricle must overcome during systole. The amount of blood ejected from the heart is directly related to the heart's stretching and filling ability, or the *Frank-Starling Law of the Heart*: that is, the length to tension relationship of the heart muscle or the sarcomere length and the volume of blood in the heart at the end of diastole to the tension generated or ventricular pressure. The *Law of Laplace* is calculated using the amount of tension in the ventricle wall and is contingent upon ventricular wall thickness and radius to produce intraventricular pressure.

Stroke volume is the amount of blood ejected per heartbeat and is dependent on myocardial contractility. There are three contributing factors to myocardial contractility: preload, inotropic stimulation of the ventricles, and myocardial oxygen supply. Stroke volume is decreased when there is excessive preload. Inotropic agents affect contractility. Positive inotropes include the SNS neurotransmitters epinephrine and norepinephrine. Acetylcholine is released by the vagus nerve and is a negative inotrope. Myocardial contractility is decreased when there is low oxygen saturation (less than 50%). Preload, afterload, and contractility are interdependent and determine stroke volume and cardiac output.

The Circulatory System

The circulatory system is made up of the *arterial system*, which takes oxygenated blood from the left side of the heart and distributes it throughout the body; and the *venous system*, which returns the deoxygenated blood to the heart through the right side. There are two types of arteries: elastic and muscular. The *elastic arteries* include the aorta and the pulmonary trunk, which contain thick walls of elastic and smooth muscle fibers. The *muscular arteries* contain more muscle than elastic, and they control blood flow via smooth muscle contraction and dilation. *Vasoconstriction* is reduced blood flow due to narrowing of the vessel. Conversely, *vasodilation* occurs when the smooth muscles relax, allowing increased blood flow through the lumen.

Veins are composed of fibrinous tissue and thin walls with a large diameter. There are more veins than arteries, and veins are larger than arteries within the surrounding tissue. Some veins contain valves that facilitate one-way flow of blood toward the heart, as in the legs; compression of leg veins helps facilitate the return of blood to the heart. Blood flow is influenced by the pressure, resistance, velocity, and

compliance of the vasculature. Organ perfusion depends on the pressure difference in the arteries and veins supplying that organ. Arteries have a higher pressure gradient than veins do, and fluid moves from the higher-pressure arteries to the lower-pressure veins. *Resistance* is the opposition of blood flow (Fig. 11.1).

Arterial pressure is calculated by multiplying cardiac output by peripheral resistance. The highest arterial blood pressure following ventricular contraction (systole) is the systolic blood pressure. The diastolic blood pressure in the lowest arterial blood pressure that occurs during ventricular filling (diastole). The difference between systolic and diastolic blood pressures is the pulse pressure, which averages 40 to 50 mm Hg.

Cardiac output is controlled by the sympathetic and parasympathetic nervous systems. The arterial baroreceptors and chemoreceptors send signals to the brain to regulate sympathetic and vagal output to modify heart rate, contractility, and vascular diameter. Hormones affect blood pressure regulation through their effects on vascular smooth muscle and blood volume. The vasoconstrictor hormones are angiotensin II, vasopressin, epinephrine, and norepinephrine. The vasodilator hormones are atrial natriuretic peptide (ANP), B-type natriuretic peptide (BNP), C-type natriuretic peptide, and urodilatin. In addition to vasodilation, these hormones regulate sodium and water excretion (natriuresis and diuresis).

Pathophysiology: Heart Failure

HF is a chronic, debilitating disease for which there is no cure. The heart's main function is to propel blood forward, in a one-way motion. HF is the inability of the heart to supply adequate blood flow to peripheral tissues and organs. Inadequate perfusion of organs leads to reduced exercise capacity, fatigue, and shortness of breath due to resultant hypoxemia.

There are more than 7 million HF cases in the United States, and approximately 700,000 new cases are diagnosed annually. There are more than 1 million HF hospitalizations annually, of which 25% are rehospitalizations that occur within 30 days of discharge. Morbidity and mortality rates are high, with a five-year mortality in 50% of HF patients. HF-associated costs exceed $40 billion annually. These staggering numbers make HF management paramount.

Heart Failure With Reduced Ejection Fraction

Heart failure with reduced ejection fraction (HFrEF), or systolic HF, is characterized by the heart's inability to generate adequate cardiac output to perfuse the tissues due to an ejection fraction of less than 40%. The renin angiotensin aldosterone system (RAAS) is activated when cardiac output is diminished and renal perfusion is decreased. RAAS activation increases preload and afterload by increasing peripheral resistance and blood volume. Baroreceptors sense the decreased cardiac output and change in pressure, and

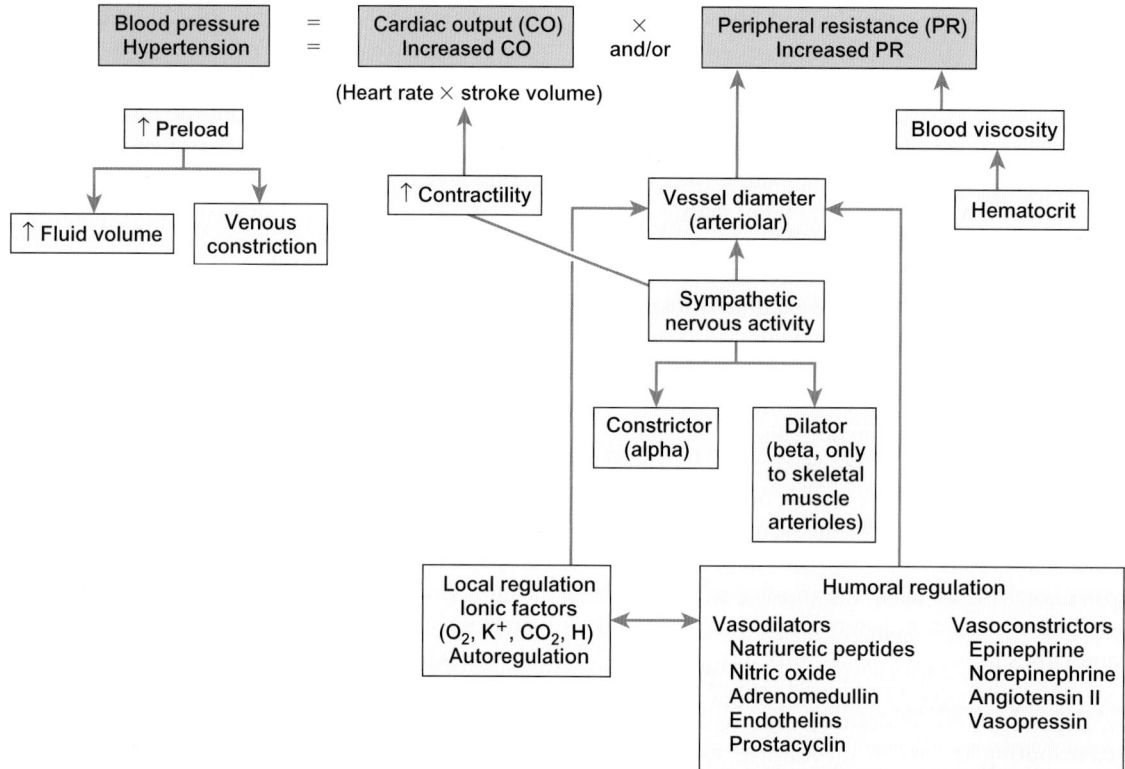

• **Fig. 11.1** Factors regulating blood pressure. (From McCance, K. L., & Huether, S. E. [Eds.]. [2019]. *Pathophysiology: The biological basis for disease in adults and children* [8th ed.]. St. Louis: Elsevier.)

then the circulating catecholamines stimulate the SNS. This excitement causes vasoconstriction and attempts to compensate for the decrease in cardiac output by increasing the heart rate.

This cascade of decreased contractility with increased preload and afterload perpetuates myriad neurohormonal, inflammatory, and metabolic processes. Aldosterone causes sodium and fluid retention and contributes to dysrhythmias. The antidiuretic hormone is released in response to low cardiac output and causes peripheral vasoconstriction and renal fluid retention, which exacerbates hyponatremia and edema. Symptoms of congestion seen with HFrEF include dyspnea, dependent edema, orthopnea, ascites, and paroxysmal nocturnal dyspnea. Symptoms that result from decreased perfusion seen in HFrEF are fatigue, hypoxia, lethargy, cool extremities, and daytime sleepiness.

The goal of medication management in HFrEF is to stop the cyclical decrease in contractility, decrease preload and afterload, and block neurohormonal responses. It takes a combination of medications to block these responses: beta-blockers inhibit SNS activations; angiotensin-converting enzyme (ACE) inhibitors interrupt the RAAS and reduce preload and afterload; and diuretics reduce preload. Angiotensin II receptor blockers (ARBs) have been proven to be as effective as ACE inhibitors in treating HFrEF in patients who cannot tolerate ACE inhibitors. ACE inhibitors, ARBs, and beta-blockers have all been determined to reduce morbidity and mortality in HFrEF patients. A new

class of medications, neprilysin inhibitors, has been combined with ARBs and is proven to reduce morbidity, mortality, and hospitalizations in HFrEF patients.

Heart Failure With Preserved Ejection Fraction

Heart failure with preserved ejection fraction (HFpEF), also called diastolic HF, is characterized by an EF greater than 50%. The pathophysiologic changes in the ventricle include decreased compliance and lusitropy (the rate of myocardial relaxation), which results in abnormal diastolic relaxation. This occurs when the myocytes have been damaged and their intracellular proteins are disrupted, which inhibits their ability to pump calcium. Due to noncompliance within the ventricle walls, the ventricle cannot fill properly. The ventricular walls must overcome the noncompliance and lusitropy with increased resistance and increased wall tension. This increased resistance and wall tension causes a high-pressure state within the left ventricle and left atrium, which then increases pulmonary circulation, causing pulmonary edema. The diagnosis of HFpEF is more challenging than the diagnosis of HFrEF and is based on signs and symptoms of HF along with diastolic dysfunction with a normal EF. Management of HFpEF targets prolongation of diastolic filling times and improved ventricular relaxation. The same medications used in HFrEF are used in HFpEF: beta-blockers, ACE inhibitors, ARBs, and aldosterone antagonists, with varying degrees of success.

Right Heart Failure

Right heart failure is the inability of the right ventricle to provide adequate blood flow to pulmonary circulation. Right heart failure can result from left ventricle dysfunction or *cor pulmonale* (right heart failure due to pulmonary disease). The increased pressure in pulmonary circulation causes increased resistance to the right ventricle during systole. The right ventricle suffers damage due to the high pressure and then hypertrophies, eventually dilating and failing over time. The right ventricle failure causes increased systemic venous circulation, distended jugular veins, hepatosplenomegaly, and peripheral edema. Management involves treatment of the underlying cause.

Heart Failure Therapy

Medication management and treatment therapies for HF are based on classifications developed by the American College of Cardiology (ACC) and the American Heart Association (AHA). There are four stages that emphasize the progression of the disease:

- Stage A identifies the patient who is at high risk for developing HF but has no structural disorder of the heart.
- Stage B refers to a patient with a structural disorder of the heart, but who has never developed symptoms of HF.
- Stage C denotes the patient with past or current symptoms of HF associated with underlying structural heart disease.
- Stage D designates the patient with end-stage disease.

Structural disorders of the heart include left ventricular hypertrophy, fibrosis, dilation or hypercontractility, valvular heart disease, or previous myocardial infarction. Only Stages C and D qualify for the traditional clinical diagnosis of HF for diagnostic or coding purposes. These stages are meant to be used in conjunction with the New York Heart Association (NYHA) functional classifications (Table 11.1), which focus on exercise capacity and the symptomatic status of the disease and primarily gauge the severity of symptoms in patients who are in Stage C or D. Treatments for Stage A

HF patients focus on prevention of structural heart damage by modifying and treating risk factors, Stage B on treating structural heart disease, and Stages C and D on reducing morbidity and mortality.

ACE Inhibitors

ACE inhibitors improve HF by decreasing preload and afterload; they also reduce cardiac myocyte hypertrophy. Angiotensin II causes direct vasoconstriction of precapillary arterioles and postcapillary venules; inhibits the reuptake of norepinephrine; stimulates the release of catecholamines from the adrenal medulla; reduces urinary excretion of sodium and water; stimulates synthesis and release of aldosterone; and stimulates hypertrophy of both vascular smooth muscle cells and cardiac myocytes. ACE inhibitors block angiotensin-converting enzymes that convert angiotensin I to angiotensin II. Decreased production of angiotensin II enhances natriuresis, lowers blood pressure, and prevents remodeling of smooth muscle and cardiac myocytes. Lowered arterial and venous pressure reduces preload and afterload.

ACE inhibitors are recommended for use in HF patients in Stage B, C, or D, and in Stage A as needed. GDMT for HF indicates that patients with HFrEF should be on ACE inhibitors, as the risks of death and hospitalization are reduced. ACE inhibitors should be used with caution in patients with very low systolic blood pressure (systolic BP <80 mmHg), increased serum creatinine (>3 mg/dL), or elevated serum potassium (>5 mEq/L).

Within the ACE inhibitors class of drugs, all medications have the same impact on symptom management and long-term survival. Treatment with an ACE inhibitor should begin with low doses and gradually increase by doubling the dose every 1 to 2 weeks until target dosage is achieved. Increase in dosage should only occur after lower doses have been tolerated. These target doses have been determined through clinical trials to evaluate survival. If the target dose cannot be achieved, titrate to the highest dose tolerable. Lab values for serum potassium and renal function should be monitored

TABLE 11.1 NYHA Classes/ACC/AHA Stages

Functional Capacity	Objective Assessment
Class I. Patients with cardiac disease but without resulting limitations of physical activity. Ordinary physical activity does not cause undue fatigue, palpitation, dyspnea, or anginal pain.	**A.** No objective evidence of cardiovascular disease.
Class II. Patients with cardiac disease resulting in slight limitation of physical activity. They are comfortable at rest. Ordinary physical activity results in fatigue, palpitation, dyspnea, or anginal pain.	**B.** Objective evidence of minimal cardiovascular disease.
Class III. Patients with cardiac disease resulting in marked limitation of physical activity. They are comfortable at rest. Less-than-ordinary physical activity causes fatigue, palpitation, dyspnea, or anginal pain.	**C.** Objective evidence of moderately severe cardiovascular disease.
Class IV. Patients with cardiac disease resulting in inability to carry on any physical activity without discomfort. Symptoms of heart failure or the anginal syndrome may be present even at rest. If any physical activity is undertaken, discomfort is increased.	**D.** Objective evidence of severe cardiovascular disease.

Data from Shah, A., Gandhi, D., Srivastava, S., Shah, K. J., & Mansukhani, R. (2017). Heart failure: A class review of pharmacotherapy. *Pharmacy and Therapeutics*, 42(7), 464–472. https://www.ncbi.nlm.nih.gov/pmc/articles/PMC5481297/.

within 1 to 2 weeks of initiation and periodically thereafter. A serum creatinine increase of up to 30% is tolerable and does not warrant stopping ACE inhibitor therapy. Adverse effects of ACE inhibitors include dry, nonproductive paroxysmal cough; angioedema; hyperkalemia; increases in serum creatinine (SCr); and symptomatic hypotension (Table 11.2).

Lisinopril

Pharmacokinetics. Lisinopril is administered orally and is not metabolized. The drug is distributed throughout the body and is excreted unchanged in the urine. The half-life is contingent upon renal function.

Indications. Lisinopril is indicated in HFrEF NYHA Class I to IV to reduce morbidity and mortality.

Adverse Effects. Lisinopril is generally well tolerated, with mild, transient adverse effects. Hypotension can occur in 3% to 11% of patients and is most often associated with higher dosages (more than 32 mg/day). Dizziness (3.5% to 19% of patients) and headache (3.8%) are among the most commonly reported adverse reactions and occasionally require discontinuation of therapy. Orthostatic hypotension and fatigue were reported in more than 1% of patients with HF. A persistent, nonproductive cough has been reported in 2.5% of patients and was a reason for discontinuation of therapy in 0.5% of patients. If lisinopril is used with concomitant diuretic therapy, consider lowering the dose to minimize hypovolemia. Hypotension after the initial dose does not preclude further titration.

Contraindications. Lisinopril is contraindicated in patients with a history of ACE inhibitor–induced angioedema. Therapy should be discontinued if angioedema occurs. The incidence of ACE inhibitor–induced angioedema is higher in Black patients than non-Black patients, and ACE inhibitors are less effective in lowering blood pressure in Black patients. Concomitant use with or within 36 hours of switching to or from a neprilisyn inhibitor should be avoided.

Monitoring. The following parameters should be monitored with use of an ACE inhibitor: blood pressure, serum creatinine/blood urea nitrogen (BUN), potassium, and sodium.

Ramipril

Pharmacokinetics. Ramipril is administered orally. It is mostly plasma protein bound, and is excreted in the urine and the feces, primarily as ramiprilat. Ramipril is converted to ramiprilat, which delays maximum effects to 3 to 6 hours post dose. It is 50% to 60% absorbed from the gastrointestinal (GI) tract. Hepatic esterases convert the oral formulation to ramiprilat, and noticeable cardiovascular effects begin within 1 to 2 hours.

Indications. Ramipril is indicated for the treatment of stable patients with clinical signs of HF and in HFrEF patients in NYHA Class I to IV to reduce morbidity and mortality.

Adverse Effects. Adverse reactions associated with the use of ramipril are usually mild and transient. Dizziness, headache, and fatigue were the most common adverse effects

reported. Ramipril can cause symptomatic hypotension after the initial dose or after a dosage increase. A persistent, nonproductive cough has been reported in 8% to 12% of patients and was a reason for discontinuation of therapy in 1% to 7% of patients.

Contraindications. Ramipril should be used with caution in patients with risk factors for hyperkalemia. It is contraindicated in patients with a history of ACE inhibitor–induced angioedema. Therapy should be discontinued if angioedema occurs. The incidence of ACE inhibitor–induced angioedema is higher in Black patients than non-Black patients, and ACE inhibitors are less effective in lowering blood pressure in Black patients.

Monitoring. The following parameters should be monitored with use of ramipril: blood pressure, serum creatinine/BUN, potassium, and sodium.

Fosinopril

Pharmacokinetics. Fosinopril is administered orally. Hepatic metabolism is required to generate the active metabolite fosinoprilat. Fosinoprilat is approximately 99.4% bound to plasma proteins. It is excreted in the urine and feces and is eliminated equally by the liver and kidney. The half-life is about 14 hours in patients with HF.

Indications. Fosinopril is indicated in HFrEF patients in NYHA Class I to IV to reduce morbidity and mortality.

Adverse Effects. In HF patients, significant hypotension after the first dose of fosinopril occurred in 2.4% of patients; 0.8% of patients discontinued therapy due to first-dose hypotension. Symptomatic hypotension is most likely to occur in patients who have been volume and/or salt depleted as a result of prolonged diuretic therapy, dietary salt restriction, dialysis, or dehydration. The most commonly seen hypotensive symptoms include orthostatic hypotension (1.4% to 1.9% of patients), sinus tachycardia (0.4% to 1%), dizziness (1.6% to 11.9%), and syncope (0.2% to 1%). These symptoms occasionally require discontinuance of therapy.

Contraindications. Fosinopril should be used with caution in patients with risk factors for hyperkalemia. It is contraindicated in patients with a history of ACE inhibitor–induced angioedema. Therapy should be discontinued if angioedema occurs. The incidence of ACE inhibitor–induced angioedema is higher in Black patients than non-Black patients, and ACE inhibitors are less effective in lowering blood pressure in Black patients.

Monitoring. The following parameters should be monitored with use of fosinopril: blood pressure, serum creatinine/BUN, potassium, and sodium.

Angiotensin Receptor Blockers

Angiotensin receptor blockers (ARBs) inhibit the RAAS by blocking the binding of angiotensin II to its receptor, causing the vessels to vasoconstrict and preventing the release of aldosterone. ARBs do not cause an inhibition of kininase, which reduces the incidence of cough in comparison with

TABLE 11.2 Indication: Goal-Directed Medication Therapy for Stage C HFrEF

Medication	Initial Daily Dose	Target Daily Dosage	Adverse Effects	Considerations and Monitoring
ACE Inhibitors				
Captopril	6.25 mg three times	50 mg three times	Hypotension	Monitor serum potassium, serum Cr, and BUN.
Enalapril	2.5 mg twice	10–20 mg twice	Serum Cr and BUN increase	Do not use if previous angioedema due to any ACE-inhibitor hypersensitivity.
Fosinopril	5–10 mg once	40 mg once	Hyperkalemia	
Lisinopril	2.5–5 mg once	20–40 mg once	Cough	
Perindopril	2 mg once	8–16 mg once		
Quinapril	5 mg twice	20 mg twice		
Ramipril	1.25–2.5 mg once	10 mg once		
Trandolapril	1 mg once	4 mg once		
Angiotensin-Receptor Blockers				
Candesartan	4–8 mg once	32 mg once	Hypotension	Monitor serum potassium, Cr, and BUN.
Losartan	25–50 mg once	50–150 mg once	Serum Cr and BUN increase	Do not use: hypersensitivity or concomitant use with aliskiren.
Valsartan	20–40 mg twice	160 mg twice	Hyperkalemia	
Angiotensin Receptor–Neprilysin Inhibitor				
Sacubitril/valsartan	49/51 mg twice (therapy may be initiated at 24/26 mg twice)	97/103 mg twice	Hypotension Serum Cr and BUN increase Hyperkalemia Cough Dizziness	Do not use within 36 hr of taking ACE or ARB or concomitantly if previous angioedema due to any ACE inhibitor.
Beta-Blockers				
Bisoprolol	1.25 mg four times	10 mg four times	Hypotension	Monitor blood glucose as may increase risk for hyperglycemia in previously nondiabetic patients.
Carvedilol	3.125 mg twice	50 mg twice	Dizziness	
Carvedilol CR	10 mg four times	80 mg four times	Bradycardia	
Metoprolol succinate extended release (metoprolol CR/XL)	12.5–25 mg four times	200 mg four times	Headache Fatigue	
Aldosterone Antagonists				
Spironolactone	12.5–25 mg four times	25 mg twice or four times	Dizziness Hypotension	Monitor for hyperkalemia.
Eplerenone	25 mg four times	50 mg four times	Hyperkalemia	
I_f Channel Inhibitors				
Ivabradine	5 mg twice	7.5 mg twice	Bradycardia Atrial fibrillation Hypotension	Contraindicated in patients with pacemaker dependence. Contraindicated in patients with severe hepatic disease. Monitor ECG, heart rate.

Continued

TABLE 11.2   Indication: Goal-Directed Medication Therapy for Stage C HFrEF—cont'd

Medication	Initial Daily Dose	Target Daily Dosage	Adverse Effects	Considerations and Monitoring
Isosorbide dinitrate and hydralazine (African Americans only)				
Fixed-dose combination	20 mg isosorbide dinitrate/37.5 mg hydralazine three times	40 mg isosorbide dinitrate/75 mg hydralazine three times	Hypotension Dizziness Drowsiness, particularly during initiation of therapy	Avoid in patients with dehydration or hypotension.
Isosorbide dinitrate and hydralazine	20–30 mg isosorbide dinitrate/25–50 mg hydralazine three or four times	40 mg isosorbide dinitrate 3 times with 100 mg hydralazine three times		
Loop Diuretics				
Use in any stage HFrEF or HFpEF when congestion is present.				
Bumetanide	0.5–1.0 mg once or twice daily	10 mg daily	Hypotension Dizziness Hypokalemia Hypocalcemia Hypomagnesemia	Monitor all electrolytes. Do not use: hypersensitivity anuria.
Furosemide	20–40 mg daily or twice daily	600 mg daily		
Torsemide	10–20 mg daily	200 mg daily		
Ethacrynic acid	25–50 mg daily	100 mg twice daily		
Thiazide Diuretics Used in Combination With Loop Diuretics				
Metolazone	2.5–10 mg daily + loop diuretic	N/A	Hypotension Hypokalemia Gout attacks Dizziness	Monitor all electrolytes. Do not use: hypersensitivity anuria.
Hydrochlorothiazide	25–100 mg once or twice daily plus loop diuretic	N/A		
Cardiac Glycosides				
Digoxin	0.125–0.25 mg daily	0.25 mg daily	Arrythmias Heart block Nausea/vomiting Diarrhea Anorexia Visual changes Headache Gynecomastia Confusion	Target serum concentration in HF 0.5–0.9 ng/mL. Contraindicated in patients with ventricular fibrillation or carotid sinus hypersensitivity.

ACE inhibitors. ARBs are recommended in patients who cannot tolerate ACE inhibitors because of cough or angioedema, and are used to reduce hospitalizations, morbidity, and mortality.

ARBs are initiated at lower doses and are titrated by doubling the dose every 1 to 2 weeks until target dosage is achieved, similar to ACE inhibitors. The side effects of ARBs include potential elevation of serum potassium and alterations in renal function. For that reason, baseline renal function and serum potassium should be established prior to initiating ARBs and should be monitored regularly throughout therapy. There have been trials to ascertain whether ARBs are as efficacious as ACE inhibitors. The CHARM trial results revealed that ARBs are just as effective as ACE inhibitors in HF patients who could not tolerate an ACE inhibitor, and that they reduce morbidity and mortality rates. Inhibition of kinase II decreases bradykinin breakdown and is thought to be the primary mechanism for ACE inhibitor–induced cough.

Candesartan

Pharmacokinetics. Candesartan is administered orally. Protein binding is greater than 99%, and about 26% of an oral dose is excreted unchanged in the urine. Blood pressure response is dose related over the range of 2 to 16 mg every 12 hours. Most of the antihypertensive effect is seen within 2 weeks of initial dosing; however, the full effect may not be observed for up to 4 weeks.

Indications. Candesartan is indicated in HF. HF guidelines recommend an ARB in combination with an evidence-based beta-blocker and aldosterone antagonist in patients with HFrEF NYHA Class I to IV to reduce morbidity and mortality. Use of an ARB is recommended in patients who are intolerant of ACE inhibitors because of cough or angioedema. ARB use is recommended for patients with HFpEF to decrease hospitalizations and control blood pressure.

Adverse Effects. The following adverse reactions occurred in at least 1% of candesartan-treated patients: back pain (3%), upper respiratory tract infection (6%), pharyngitis (2%), rhinitis (2%), and dizziness (4%). Dizziness was also one of the most common (0.3%) reasons for discontinuation of therapy with candesartan.

Contraindications. Candesartan should be used with caution in patients with hypovolemia, including patients receiving high doses of diuretics. Intravascular volume depletion may increase the risk of symptomatic hypotension. Candesartan should be used with great care in patients who exhibit signs of hypotension, and it should be used with caution in patients whose renal function is critically dependent on RAAS activity. Patients with HF who are given candesartan commonly have some reduction in blood pressure, including symptomatic hypotension. Increases in serum creatinine may also occur. In HF patients with symptomatic hypotension and/or an increase in serum creatinine, these complications may require temporarily holding or reducing the dose or the adjunctive diuretic. Candesartan should be used with caution in patients with hyperkalemia.

Anaphylactic reactions and angioedema have been reported with angiotensin II receptor antagonists. Candesartan should be discontinued in pregnancy. Use of drugs that affect RAAS during pregnancy can cause fetal death or injury such as hypotension, neonatal skull hypoplasia, or reversible or irreversible renal failure. It is unknown whether candesartan is excreted in breast milk. To avoid injury to the breastfeeding infant, discontinue breastfeeding or discontinue candesartan therapy.

Monitoring. Monitoring of blood pressure, serum electrolytes, BUN, and creatinine is recommended during dose titration and periodically during follow-up in treating patients with HF.

Valsartan

Pharmacokinetics. Valsartan is administered orally. Approximately 95% is bound to serum proteins, primarily serum albumin. Valsartan is primarily recovered in the feces (83%) and urine (13%). Following oral administration in HF patients, the apparent clearance of valsartan is approximately 4.5 L/hour. The elimination half-life averages 6 hours.

Indications. Valsartan is indicated in the treatment of HF (Class II to IV). It is also indicated in the treatment of HF in patients intolerant to ACE inhibitors but is not recommended for combined use with ACE inhibitors due to unfavorable outcomes. HF guidelines recommend an ARB in combination with an evidence-based beta-blocker and aldosterone antagonist in patients with HFrEF NYHA Class I to IV to reduce morbidity and mortality. Use of an ARB is recommended in patients who are intolerant of ACE inhibitors because of cough or angioedema. ARB use is recommended for patients with HFpEF to decrease hospitalizations and control blood pressure.

Adverse Effects. Valsartan is generally well tolerated. The most common reasons for discontinuation are headache (1% of patients) and dizziness (8%). Hypotension occurs in approximately 7% of patients. Orthostatic hypotension (2% or less) and syncope (more than 1%) are infrequent but have occurred with valsartan therapy. Azotemia and renal impairment may occur during therapy; these reactions are most often mild and transient and are most likely to occur in patients with preexisting renal impairment. Hyperkalemia was reported in 10% of patients with HF. Patients receiving valsartan also reported viral infection (3%), back pain (3%), fatigue (2% to 3%), and abdominal pain (2%). The incidence of cough is lower with valsartan than with ACE inhibitors. Valsartan does not inhibit ACE (kinase II). Anaphylactic reactions and angioedema have been reported rarely with valsartan use. Breastfeeding is not recommended during treatment with valsartan.

Contraindications. Valsartan is a teratogenic and should not be used during the second or third trimester of pregnancy. Use valsartan with caution in patients with hypovolemia, including patients receiving high doses of diuretics. Intravascular volume depletion increases the risk of symptomatic hypotension. Valsartan is contraindicated in patients with a known hypersensitivity to valsartan or any of its components. Use valsartan with caution in patients whose renal function is critically dependent on RAAS activity. Increases in serum potassium have been reported in patients with HF and are more likely to occur in patients with preexisting renal impairment. Although these effects are usually minor and transient, dose reduction or discontinuation of valsartan may be required. To minimize hypotensive effects in patients with HF or left ventricular dysfunction post myocardial infarction, initial doses are lower than those used in the treatment of hypertension. Use valsartan with caution in patients with severe hepatic disease and in patients with hyperkalemia. Although hyperkalemia is infrequent with valsartan, angiotensin II blockade can elevate serum potassium concentrations by blocking aldosterone secretion and could worsen preexisting hyperkalemia.

Monitoring. The following parameters should be monitored: blood pressure, liver function tests (LFTs), renal function, serum electrolytes, and serum bilirubin (total and direct).

Angiotensin Receptor–Neprilysin Inhibitors

Angiotensin receptor–neprilysin inhibitors (ARNIs) are a new class of drug that inhibits the RAAS and are proven to reduce morbidity, mortality, and hospitalizations in HFrEF patients.

Sacubitril-Valsartan

This drug consists of the neprilysin inhibitor sacubitril and the ARB valsartan. Neprilysin is a neutral endopeptidase that metabolizes endogenous vasoactive peptides, including natriuretic peptides, bradykinin, and substance P, into their inactive metabolites. When neprilysin is inhibited, the levels of these substances rise and reduce vasoconstriction, sodium retention, abnormal growth, and remodeling. Angiotensin II is a substrate of neprilysin. Therefore, an ARB is added to the neprilysin inhibitor to prevent RAAS activation.

In HFrEF patients who are tolerating an ACE inhibitor or ARB but remain symptomatic, replacement with an ARNI is recommended. ARNIs cannot be given with ACE inhibitors or other ARBs. Additionally, initiation of an ARNI cannot occur within 36 hours of the last dose of an ACE inhibitor. The adverse effects are similar to those of ACE inhibitors and ARBs and include hypotension, hyperkalemia, increased serum creatinine, angioedema, cough, and renal failure. Labs (serum potassium and renal function) are monitored 1 to 2 weeks after initiation, with dosage changes, and periodically. The initial dose of sacubitril-valsartan is based upon whether the patient is already taking an ACE inhibitor or ARB and at what dose (Table 11.2).

Pharmacokinetics. Sacubitril-valsartan is administered orally. Sacubitril and valsartan are highly bound to plasma proteins (more than 94%). After oral administration, 52% to 68% of sacubitril (primarily as metabolite) and approximately 13% of valsartan and its metabolites are excreted in the urine. The remaining drug and metabolites are excreted in the feces. In patients with HF and reduced ejection fraction, sacubitril-valsartan administration resulted in significantly increased urine atrial natriuretic peptide (ANP), cyclic guanosine monophosphate (cGMP), and plasma cGMP, and decreased plasma N-terminal pro b-type natriuretic peptide (NT-proBNP), aldosterone, and endothelin-1. Sacubitril-valsartan blocked the AT1-receptor, resulting in increased plasma renin activity and plasma renin concentrations. Oral absolute bioavailability of sacubitril is estimated to be 60% or more. Valsartan, when combined in the sacubitril-valsartan combination product, is more bioavailable than valsartan tablets alone. In the sacubitril-valsartan combination tablet, the valsartan is more bioavailable than in the valsartan tablet alone; 26, 51, and 103 mg of valsartan in the combination tablet is equivalent to 40, 80, and 160 mg of the valsartan tablet alone, respectively.

Indications. Sacubitril-valsartan is indicated in HF. HF guidelines recommend sacubitril-valsartan in combination with an evidence-based beta-blocker and aldosterone antagonist in patients with HFrEF NYHA Class II to III to reduce morbidity and mortality. In patients with chronic symptomatic HFrEF Class II or III who tolerate an ACE inhibitor or ARB, replacement with ARNI therapy is recommended.

Adverse Effects. Angioedema has been reported with the use of sacubitril-valsartan. Due to the potential for teratogenesis, every effort should be made to discontinue sacubitril-valsartan and consider alternative therapy during pregnancy. Hypotension and a decrease in renal function have been reported with the use of sacubitril-valsartan. Hyperkalemia was reported in 12% of patients and cough was reported in 9% of patients receiving sacubitril-valsartan.

Contraindications. Sacubitril-valsartan is contraindicated with concomitant use of ACE inhibitors or ARBs. Allow a 36-hour washout period if switching from an ACE inhibitor to sacubitril-valsartan. Sacubitril-valsartan is contraindicated in patients with hypersensitivity to any component of the product. It is also contraindicated in patients with a history of ACE inhibitor–induced angioedema and in those with ARB therapy–induced angioedema. Sacubitril-valsartan lowers blood pressure and may cause symptomatic hypotension, and it may decrease renal function in patients whose renal function depends on RAAS activity. Sacubitril-valsartan therapy may also result in hyperkalemia and should be used cautiously in patients with risk factors for hyperkalemia. Administration of sacubitril-valsartan is not recommended in patients with severe hepatic disease. Breastfeeding is not recommended during treatment with sacubitril-valsartan.

Monitoring. The following parameters should be monitored: serum creatinine/BUN and serum potassium.

Beta-Blockers

The use of beta-blockade in HFrEF patients has been proven to reduce symptom burden and improve symptom-related quality of life. Research data have shown that the use of carvedilol, or sustained-release metoprolol succinate, reduces morbidity and mortality in HFrEF patients. These are the only beta-blockers tested in large clinical trials to show a mortality benefit. They all block the β_1-adrenergic receptor located on the heart. HFrEF stimulates the RAAS and sympathetic system to compensate for the reduced EF. When the β_1 receptors are inhibited, ventricular remodeling, which refers to changes in the size, shape, structure, and function of the heart, is prevented by the stimulated RAAS and sympathetic system. While metoprolol is selective for the β_1 receptor, carvedilol also blocks the β_2 and α_1 receptors, leading to vasodilation. Due to the effects on multiple receptors, carvedilol should be initiated cautiously, with frequent monitoring of orthostatic blood pressure readings. The impact of carvedilol on the β_2 receptor can exacerbate chronic obstructive pulmonary disease (COPD) and asthma as it alters the bronchial tone, alveolar reabsorption, and gas diffusion.

Beta-blockers should be initiated when HFrEF is diagnosed at low doses and titrated slowly to target doses if tolerable. Beta-blockers should be prescribed to all patients with stable HFrEF to reduce risks of disease progression and clinical deterioration.

Adverse events include fluid retention and worsening HFrEF, fatigue, bradycardia or heart block, and hypotension. Beta-blocker–induced bradycardia is generally asymptomatic and requires no treatment unless the patient becomes symptomatic. The dose of the beta-blocker should be decreased if symptoms of dizziness, lightheadedness, or second- or third-degree heart block develop. In patients with fluid retention, beta-blockers should not be prescribed without diuretics. The diuretics are used to maintain sodium and fluid balance. The risks of hypotension can be reduced by administering beta-blockers and ACE inhibitors at different times of the day. Beta-blocker therapy is generally introduced soon after initiation of an angiotensin system blocker with an ARNI, ACE inhibitor, or ARB. Beta-blockers can be introduced prior to reaching the target dose of angiotensin system blocker.

Metoprolol Succinate

Pharmacokinetics. Metoprolol is administered orally and intravenously and is widely distributed throughout the body, with a reported volume of distribution of 3.2 to 5.6 L/kg. The drug is approximately 10% to 12% bound to serum albumin. Metoprolol is moderately lipid soluble. Metoprolol crosses the blood–brain barrier, with 78% of plasma concentration distributing to cerebrospinal fluid. It also crosses the placenta and is concentrated in breast milk. Metoprolol is quickly absorbed from the GI tract; however, estimated oral bioavailability is only about 50% due to a significant first-pass effect. Significant beta-blockade effect occurs within 60 minutes of administration. Duration is variable and dose related; a 50% reduction of maximum heart rate after single doses of 20, 50, and 100 mg occurs at 3.3, 5, and 6.4 hours, respectively.

Indications. Metoprolol is indicated for the treatment of HF, including idiopathic dilated cardiomyopathy in adults with stable, symptomatic (NYHA Class II or III) HF of ischemic, hypertensive, or cardiomyopathic origin.

Adverse Effects. The adverse effects of metoprolol are generally mild and temporary; they usually occur at the onset of therapy and diminish over time. Shortness of breath and bradycardia were each reported in about 3% of patients receiving metoprolol. Some of the adverse reactions reported during the trial included hypotension (27.4%), bradycardia (15.9%), atrioventricular block (4.7% to 5.3%), and HF (27.5%). CNS effects can occur with beta-blockers, resulting in mental depression, dizziness, fatigue, and in some cases vivid dreams, nightmares, or hallucinations. Bronchospasm, wheezing, and dyspnea were each reported in about 1% of patients receiving metoprolol. Patients with preexisting bronchospastic disease are at greater risk. Metoprolol can also mask signs of hypoglycemia, especially tachycardia, palpitations, and tremors; in contrast, diaphoresis and the hypertensive response to hypoglycemia are not suppressed with beta-blockade. Sexual dysfunction, such as impotence (erectile dysfunction), is a less frequent adverse effect of metoprolol. Exacerbation of peripheral vasoconstriction can occur with metoprolol administration. Withdrawal symptoms, including headache, diaphoresis, palpitations, sinus tachycardia, tremor, and hypertension, have been associated with abrupt discontinuation of metoprolol.

Contraindications. Abrupt discontinuation of metoprolol can result in the development of myocardial ischemia, myocardial infarction, ventricular arrhythmias, or severe hypertension, particularly in patients with preexisting cardiac disease. Metoprolol should be used with caution in patients with hyperthyroidism or thyrotoxicosis because the drug can mask tachycardia. Metoprolol is contraindicated in patients with severe bradycardia, sick sinus syndrome, or advanced atrioventricular block (second- or third-degree block) unless a functioning pacemaker is present. Metoprolol should be used with caution in patients with cerebrovascular insufficiency or stroke. Beta-1-selective beta-blockers such as metoprolol are preferred over nonselective agents in patients with asthma or other pulmonary disease. Beta-blockers may be associated with dizziness or drowsiness in some patients. Metoprolol should be used with caution in severe hepatic disease. Metoprolol crosses the placenta. Available data for published studies have not demonstrated an association of adverse developmental outcomes with the maternal use of metoprolol during pregnancy. Limited data from published reports indicate that metoprolol is present in breast milk.

Monitoring. The following parameters should be monitored: blood pressure and heart rate.

Carvedilol

Pharmacokinetics. Carvedilol is administered orally. It is a lipophilic beta-blocker and is distributed extensively to all body tissues, including breast milk. Plasma protein binding is approximately 98%. The elimination half-life ranges from 5 to 11 hours, and it is excreted in the feces and urine. Carvedilol is rapidly and extensively absorbed after oral administration; however, the absolute bioavailability is relatively low (less than 40%) due to extensive first-pass metabolism.

Indications. Carvedilol is indicated for the treatment of mild, moderate, or severe HF in adult patients as a single agent or in conjunction with digoxin, diuretics, hydralazine, or ACE inhibitor therapy.

Adverse Effects. Most adverse reactions to carvedilol are associated with its pharmacologic effects. When beginning treatment with carvedilol, patients may experience worsening HF or fluid retention/edema (4% to 6% of patients) during the initial up-titration period. The dosage of carvedilol may need to be reduced or temporarily discontinued; subsequent increases in carvedilol dosage are not precluded in these patients. Orthostatic hypotension affects a significant percentage of carvedilol recipients; however, this adverse reaction is an infrequent cause of discontinuation of carvedilol therapy. Adverse reactions reported with carvedilol use include vertigo (2% to 3%), headache (5% to 8%), and fatigue (24%).

Nonselective beta-blockers such as carvedilol are more likely than selective agents to precipitate pulmonary disorders. Adverse pulmonary events reported during carvedilol clinical trials included cough (5% to 8%), dyspnea (11%), and rales (4%). Patients with preexisting bronchospastic disease are at greater risk. Male patients have also experienced impotence (erectile dysfunction) (2% to 3%) and a decrease in libido (0.1% to 1%) after receiving carvedilol. Withdrawal symptoms, including headache, diaphoresis, palpitations, sinus tachycardia, tremor, and hypertension, have been associated with abrupt discontinuation of carvedilol.

Contraindications. Carvedilol is contraindicated in patients who have demonstrated a serious hypersensitivity reaction. Do not use carvedilol in patients with known beta-blocker hypersensitivity. Carvedilol should be used with caution in patients with hyperthyroidism or thyrotoxicosis because the drug can mask tachycardia.

Beta-blockers depress conduction through the atrioventricular node, so these drugs are contraindicated in patients with severe bradycardia, sick sinus syndrome, or second- or third-degree atrioventricular block unless a functioning pacemaker is present. Although carvedilol is indicated for the treatment of patients with mild to severe chronic HF, it should not be used in patients with acute decompensated HF, particularly in those requiring intravenous (IV) inotropic therapy. Hypotension and orthostatic hypotension are commonly encountered during the initial dosing period. Because of potential effects of beta-blockade on blood pressure and pulse, carvedilol should be used with caution in patients with cerebrovascular insufficiency or stroke. Carvedilol is a nonselective beta-blocker and, as such, should be avoided in patients with bronchial asthma and generally avoided in patients with other pulmonary disease.

Monitoring. The following parameters should be monitored: blood pressure and heart rate.

Aldosterone Receptor Antagonists

Aldosterone receptor antagonists (ARAs) are recommended for HFrEF <35% in patients with NYHA Class II to IV. Morbidity, mortality, and hospitalizations are reduced with the use of ARAs. Careful consideration must be taken with initiation of an ARA, as use of an ARA in patients who have a glomerular filtration rate <30 mL/min/1.73 m^2 and a potassium level >5.0 mEq/dL is potentially harmful because of hyperkalemia or renal insufficiency. Potassium and renal function should be checked prior to initiation; 2 to 3 days after and again at 7 days after initiation; monthly for 3 months; and then every 3 months thereafter. Spironolactone is a nonselective aldosterone antagonist, while eplerenone is selective to the aldosterone receptor. Aldosterone is an endogenous steroid hormone that increases sodium retention and facilitates magnesium and potassium loss. While ACE inhibitors and aldosterone antagonists are often used concomitantly for patients with HFrEF, concurrent use of these agents can increase risks for development of hyperkalemia. Due to the risk of elevated potassium levels, potassium supplements should be discontinued (or reduced and carefully monitored) in those with a history of hypokalemia.

Spironolactone

Pharmacokinetics. Spironolactone is administered orally. It is metabolized by the liver and excreted unchanged in the urine and feces. The half-life of spironolactone after a single dose is 1 to 2 hours.

Indications. Spironolactone is indicated in HFrEF. It is recommended in patients with HFrEF NYHA Class II to IV with a GFR >30 mL/minute and serum potassium <5mEq/L. Spironolactone may be considered in patients with HFpEF with EF >45%, elevated B-type natriuretic peptide, or HF admission within 1 year, and GFR >30mL/minute, SCr <2.5mg/dL, and serum potassium <5mEq/L.

Adverse Effects. Spironolactone causes hyperkalemia and can cause life-threatening cardiac arrhythmias. Spironolactone can cause hyponatremia, hypomagnesemia, hypocalcemia, hypochloremic metabolic alkalosis, hyperglycemia, and asymptomatic hyperuricemia. Adverse GI effects reported include nausea, vomiting, cramping, diarrhea, gastritis, abdominal pain, gastric bleeding, and ulceration. Adverse nervous system effects that have been reported in patients receiving spironolactone therapy include headache, dizziness, drowsiness, lethargy, ataxia, and mental confusion. Muscular weakness may be a sign of drug-induced hyperkalemia. Excessive diuresis may cause symptomatic dehydration, hypovolemia, hypotension, gynecomastia, and worsening renal function, including renal failure.

Contraindications. Spironolactone is contraindicated in patients with hyperkalemia, Addison's disease, or other conditions associated with hyperkalemia and should not be administered to those who are receiving other potassium-sparing agents. Spironolactone tablets are contraindicated in patients with anuria or any renal disease associated with severe renal impairment (CrCl <10 mL/minute) or acute renal failure. Avoid spironolactone use in pregnancy or advise pregnant patients of the potential risk to a male fetus.

Monitoring. Monitor serum potassium and renal function 3 days and 1 week after initiation of therapy or dose increase, monthly for 3 months, quarterly for 1 year, and every 6 months thereafter. Also, monitor the following parameters: blood pressure, serum creatinine/BUN, and serum electrolytes.

I_f Channel Inhibitors

Ivabradine

Ivabradine can reduce hospitalizations in patients with HFrEF lower than 35%. These HF patients should be on GDMT, in sinus rhythm with a resting HR greater than 70 beats per minute. Ivabradine is a heart-rate–reducing agent in patients with symptomatic HFrEF. It is also an inhibitor of the I_f *channel.* The I_f channel controls HR through modulation of autonomic neurotransmitters, such as epinephrine. Specific blockade of these channels removes the contribution I_f has on pacemaker depolarization and thus slows HR.

Ivabradine is typically initiated at 5 mg orally twice daily, and is titrated every 2 weeks to a target HR of 50 bpm to 60 bpm. At that time, if HR is greater than 60 bpm, the dose of ivabradine should be increased by 2.5 mg per dose. The maximum dosage is 7.5 mg orally twice daily. In comparison, if HR is less than 50 bpm, or if the patient presents with symptomatic bradycardia, the dose should be decreased by 2.5 mg per dose and discontinued if necessary. Ivabradine should be avoided in patients with a resting HR that is less than 60 bpm, low blood pressure, decompensated HFrEF, and conduction abnormalities, including sick sinus syndrome, sinoatrial block, or third-degree heart block. Due to its hepatic metabolism, ivabradine should be avoided in patients with severe hepatic impairment.

Pharmacokinetics. Ivabradine is administered orally and is approximately 70% plasma protein binding. Metabolites are excreted to a similar extent in the feces and urine.

Indications. Ivabradine is indicated to reduce hospitalization in patients with symptomatic HFrEF and an EF less than 35%, NYHA Class II or III who are receiving a beta-blocker at the maximum tolerated dose or have contraindication to beta-blocker use, and who are in sinus rhythm with a resting HR of 70 bpm or more.

Adverse Effects. Ivabradine increases the risk of atrial fibrillation. Bradycardia, sinus arrest, and heart block have occurred with ivabradine. Ivabradine can cause visual impairment presenting as luminous phenomena. Angioedema, erythema, rash, pruritus, and urticaria have been reported during use of ivabradine in adults. Vertigo has been reported during use of ivabradine in adults. There are no adequate and well-controlled studies of ivabradine use during pregnancy to inform any drug-associated risks. There is no information about the presence of ivabradine in breast milk or the effects of ivabradine on the breast-fed infant or milk production.

Contraindications. Ivabradine is contraindicated in adults with pacemaker dependence. Ivabradine is also contraindicated in patients with severe hepatic disease as well as those with decompensated acute HF, clinically significant hypotension, sick sinus syndrome, sinoatrial block, or third-degree AV block unless a functioning pacemaker is present; and clinically significant bradycardia.

Monitoring. The following parameters should be monitored: ECG, blood pressure, and HR.

Isosorbide Dinitrate and Hydralazine

The combination of hydralazine and isosorbide dinitrate vasodilators has been shown to reduce morbidity and mortality in patients self-described as African Americans with NYHA Class III to –IV HFrEF. The combination of hydralazine and isosorbide dinitrate is recommended in African Americans who remain symptomatic despite concomitant use of GDMT with an ACE-I, ARB, or ARNI; a beta-blocker; and aldosterone antagonist. Isosorbide dinitrate causes a release of nitric oxide that relaxes vascular smooth muscle, affecting both arteries and veins. Hydralazine works to selectively relax arterial smooth muscle.

A starting dose of hydralazine 37.5 mg/isosorbide dinitrate 20 mg (available as a combination tablet) three times daily is recommended. When administering hydralazine and isosorbide dinitrate separately, the recommendation is to start with hydralazine 25 mg to 50 mg three or four times daily and isosorbide dinitrate 20 mg to 30 mg three or four times daily. The medication dosages should be doubled after 2 weeks if tolerated. The maximum recommended dose is hydralazine 75 mg/isosorbide dinitrate 40 mg three times daily or hydralazine 300 mg daily in divided doses with isosorbide dinitrate 120 mg daily in divided doses. Continue doubling the dosage until maximum dosing is reached. Adverse effects of hydralazine and isosorbide dinitrate include nausea, fatigue, palpitations, joint pain, and rash. The use of phosphodiesterase-5 inhibitors is contraindicated with nitrates due to the increased risk of adverse events such as symptomatic hypotension. Adherence to this combination is challenging due to the frequency of administration and quantity of pills.

Pharmacokinetics. Hydralazine/isosorbide dinitrate is administered orally. When given in combination, the half-life is 4 hours and 2 hours for the hydralazine and isosorbide dinitrate components, respectively. Following oral administration of hydralazine/isosorbide dinitrate, peak plasma concentrations are reached in 1 hour. No information is available regarding the effects of food on the bioavailability of hydralazine and isosorbide dinitrate. Hydralazine is excreted in the urine and feces, and the half-life of the drug in a normal patient is 3 to 7 hours. Isosorbide is excreted renally in urine.

Indications. Hydralazine/isosorbide dinitrate is indicated in the adjunctive treatment of HF in patients self-identified as Black taking standard HF therapy. HF guidelines recommend hydralazine and isosorbide dinitrate in combination with an ACE-I, ARB, or ARNI for Black patients with

HFrEF NYHA Classes III and IV to reduce morbidity and mortality.

Adverse Effects. The two most commonly reported adverse events were headache (50% of patients) and dizziness (32%). Impotence (erectile dysfunction) has also been reported. Hypotension and ventricular tachycardia were observed in 8% and 4%, respectively, of patients treated with hydralazine/isosorbide dinitrate. Some patients may experience symptomatic hypotension, even with small doses. Orthostatic hypotension, syncope, and lightheadedness may develop in some individuals. Other cardiovascular adverse events associated with the use of hydralazine/isosorbide dinitrate include flushing, palpitations, weakness, peripheral edema, fluid retention, and weight gain. Hydralazine has been associated with the development of lupus-like symptoms. Tinnitus and vertigo have been reported during use of hydralazine/isosorbide dinitrate.

Contraindications. Hydralazine/isosorbide dinitrate is absolutely contraindicated in patients who have known nitrate hypersensitivity. Specific precautions should be taken appropriate to each component of this product. Hydralazine/isosorbide dinitrate should be used with caution in patients with preexisting hypotension, orthostatic hypotension, or hypovolemia because the drug can worsen hypotension, cause syncope and/or reflex tachycardia, and/or produce chest pain. This medication can also induce significant drowsiness, impaired cognition, or asthenia, particularly during the initiation of treatment. Hydralazine/isosorbide dinitrate should not be used in patients with increased intracranial pressure, closed-angle glaucoma, severe anemia, or hyperthyroidism. In addition, this medication should not be used in patients taking phosphodiesterase-5 inhibitors. There are no studies on the use of hydralazine/isosorbide dinitrate during pregnancy, or on its presence in breast milk, effects on the breast-fed infant, or effects on milk production.

Monitoring. The following parameters should be monitored: antinuclear antibody (ANA) titer, blood pressure, HR, and serum creatinine/BUN.

Diuretics

Diuretics are indicated in patients with HFrEF and HFpEF if there are signs of volume overload. Diuretics do not improve morbidity or mortality; however, they are the only class of drugs that adequately control fluid retention. Diuretics inhibit sodium and chloride reabsorption in the kidney nephron. Loop diuretics inhibit approximately 80% of sodium and chloride reabsorption at the Loop of Henle, while thiazide and aldosterone receptor antagonists (also called potassium sparing diuretics) inhibit 15% and 5%, respectively, of sodium and chloride reabsorption at the distal tubule. Loop diuretics include furosemide, torsemide, and bumetanide, and are the preferred diuretic class in HFrEF and HFpEF treatment. Metolazone is a thiazide-like diuretic that is less potent than loop diuretics but has a synergistic effect when given with a loop diuretic.

Diuretic therapy is initiated at low doses and is titrated up as needed and as tolerated. Diuretic dosing is based on signs and symptoms of fluid retention. Adequate treatment is not determined by reaching a set target dose. Daily weights are used to judge efficacy of diuretics, with reduction in weight of 1 lb to 2 lb daily being ideal. Adverse effects of diuretics include fluid depletion, hypotension, azotemia, and depletion of sodium, potassium, magnesium, chloride, and calcium. Typical monitoring parameters for these agents include daily weight and blood pressure measurements, and periodic monitoring of renal function and electrolytes.

Furosemide

Pharmacokinetics. Furosemide is a loop diuretic administered orally and intravenously. It is 95% plasma protein bound, crosses the placenta, and appears in breast milk. Furosemide undergoes minimal metabolism in the liver, with 50% to 80% of a dose excreted in the urine within 24 hours. The half-life of furosemide is approximately 30 minutes to 1 hour. Furosemide is absorbed erratically when taken orally. Diuresis generally begins 30 to 60 minutes after oral administration. Diuresis generally begins about 5 minutes after IV administration of furosemide.

Indications. Furosemide is indicated for the treatment of edema in HF patients.

Adverse Effects. Polyuria during furosemide therapy can cause excessive fluid loss and dehydration. This results in hypovolemia and electrolyte imbalance. Hypovolemia can lead to orthostatic hypotension, syncope, and hemoconcentration, and can be potentially more serious in chronic cardiac or older patients. Adverse CNS effects associated with furosemide therapy include dizziness, lightheadedness, vertigo, headache, blurred vision, xanthopsia, restlessness, and paresthesia.

Contraindications. Hyponatremia, hypokalemia, hypocalcemia, hypochloremia, or hypomagnesemia should be corrected before initiating furosemide therapy. Furosemide is contraindicated in patients with anuria and should be used cautiously in renal impairment. Since furosemide can reduce the clearance of uric acid, patients with gout or hyperuricemia can have exacerbations of their disease. High doses and accumulation of furosemide may cause ototoxicity. Sulfonylurea hypersensitivity is a contraindication in furosemide administration. Do not use furosemide during pregnancy unless the potential benefit justifies the potential risk to the fetus. Furosemide is excreted in breast milk.

Monitoring. The following parameters should be monitored: audiometry, blood glucose, blood pressure, serum creatinine/BUN, serum electrolytes, and serum uric acid. Close monitoring is necessary to check for hyponatremia, hypokalemia, hypocalcemia, hypochloremia, and hypomagnesemia.

Bumetanide

Pharmacokinetics. Bumetanide is a loop diuretic administered orally, intramuscularly, or intravenously. Bumetanide is 96% plasma protein bound. It is not clear whether the drug crosses the placenta, enters the cerebrospinal fluid (CSF), or appears in breast milk. Bumetanide is metabolized in the liver; the half-life of bumetanide is 1 to 1.5 hours.

Indications. Bumetanide is indicated for the treatment and prevention of edema in HF patients.

Adverse Effects. Muscle cramps (1.1% of patients), dizziness (1.1%), low blood pressure (0.8%), and headache (0.6%) are the most frequent adverse effects reported with bumetanide use. Electrolyte abnormalities reported during therapy have included hypochloremia (14.9%), hypokalemia (14.7%), and hyponatremia (9.2%). Bumetanide may also increase urinary calcium and phosphate excretion with resultant hypocalcemia and/or hypophosphatemia. Hypotension has been reported in 0.8% of bumetanide-treated patients. Hypovolemia and dehydration can occur during therapy due to polyuria and excessive electrolyte losses.

Contraindications. Bumetanide is contraindicated in patients with severe electrolyte imbalance, anuria, and hepatic encephalopathy. Sulfonylurea hypersensitivity is a contraindication in bumetanide administration. High doses and accumulation of bumetanide may cause ototoxicity.

Monitoring. The following parameters should be monitored: blood glucose, serum creatinine/BUN, serum electrolytes, and serum uric acid. Patients receiving bumetanide should be taught the signs and symptoms of electrolyte imbalances (e.g., lethargy, mental confusion, fatigue, faintness, dizziness, muscle cramps, headache, paresthesia, thirst, anorexia, nausea, or vomiting) and report these signs immediately.

Torsemide

Pharmacokinetics. Torsemide is a loop diuretic administered orally and intravenously. Torsemide is cleared through hepatic metabolism (80%); the remaining 20% is cleared in the urine as unchanged drug. The elimination half-life is about 3.5 hours. Torsemide taken orally is rapidly absorbed, with about 80% bioavailability.

Indications. Torsemide is indicated for the treatment and prevention of edema in HF patients.

Adverse Effects. Electrolyte imbalance and hypovolemia are common adverse reactions; excessive urination was reported in 6.7% of torsemide-treated patients. Hypovolemia may precipitate orthostatic hypotension or hemoconcentration, which may lead to syncope or thrombosis, especially in older or chronic cardiac patients. Symptomatic gout has been reported during therapy with torsemide.

Contraindications. Torsemide is contraindicated in patients with known hypersensitivity to this drug. Sulfonylurea hypersensitivity is also a contraindication in torsemide administration; however, sulfonamide cross-sensitivity has been rarely documented with torsemide. Torsemide is contraindicated in patients with anuria. High doses and accumulation of torsemide may cause ototoxicity.

Monitoring. The following parameters should be monitored with torsemide use: audiometry, blood glucose, serum creatinine/BUN, serum electrolytes, and weight.

Monitoring of serum electrolytes is recommended during torsemide therapy. Patients with ventricular arrhythmias should be monitored closely since torsemide-induced hypokalemia can exacerbate these conditions.

Metolazone

Pharmacokinetics. Metolazone is a thiazide-like diuretic administered orally. The drug crosses the placenta and is distributed into breast milk. A small portion of an oral dose is metabolized, while the majority of the drug (70%) is excreted unchanged in the urine. The half-life of metolazone is approximately 14 hours.

Indications. Metolazone is indicated in the treatment of edema associated with HF. Metolazone used in combination with a loop diuretic is indicated for HFrEF patients experiencing diuretic resistance.

Adverse Effects. Metolazone is generally well tolerated. Adverse effects are rare and are usually attributable to the expected pharmacologic effects of the drug. Electrolyte imbalance may occur at any time with metolazone therapy and can result in hyponatremia, hypokalemia, hypochloremia, hypomagnesemia, hypercalcemia, or hypophosphatemia. Metolazone may induce metabolic alkalosis associated with hypokalemia and hypochloremia. Metolazone can cause hyperuricemia and can occasionally precipitate gout, even in patients without a prior history of gout.

In diabetic patients, metolazone can produce impaired glucose tolerance, glycosuria, and hyperglycemia. Hypercholesterolemia and/or hypertriglyceridemia have been reported with metolazone. Orthostatic hypotension can occur with metolazone therapy and can be exacerbated by concomitant therapy with other antihypertensive agents. Hypotension may result in syncope in some patients. Complications of aggressive diuretic therapy may include intravascular hypovolemia, with potential for development of prerenal azotemia. Palpitations, chest pain, and venous thrombosis have also been reported with metolazone. GI adverse reactions reported in patients receiving metolazone include nausea, vomiting, diarrhea, abdominal pain, abdominal bloating, epigastric pain, xerostomia, dyspepsia, and constipation. CNS adverse reactions include dizziness, lightheadedness, paresthesias, drowsiness, restlessness, insomnia, and vertigo.

Contraindications. Metolazone is contraindicated in patients with metolazone hypersensitivity. Metolazone is a sulfonamide derivative; however, sulfonamide cross-sensitivity is rare.

Monitoring. The following parameters should be monitored with torsemide use: blood glucose, serum calcium, serum cholesterol profile, serum creatinine/BUN, serum electrolytes, serum magnesium, and serum uric acid. Patients receiving metolazone should be monitored closely for signs of electrolyte imbalance including hyponatremia, hypokalemia, hypomagnesemia, and hypochloremia. Patients may require potassium supplementation to counteract excessive potassium loss; monitor serum potassium at regular intervals. Patients should be educated on the symptoms of these disturbances, (e.g., lassitude, mental confusion, fatigue, faintness, dizziness, muscle cramps, headache, paresthesia, thirst, anorexia, nausea, or vomiting).

Cardiac Glycosides

Digoxin

Digoxin has been proven to decrease hospitalizations and improve exercise tolerance but has not been shown to improve mortality. Digoxin is recommended in HFrEF patients who have persistent symptoms while on GDMT. Digoxin has a positive inotropic effect by increasing the force of contractions and deactivating neurohormonal effects by decreasing sympathetic and RAAS responses. The initial dose of digoxin is 0.125 mg to 0.250 mg daily, with higher doses rarely used in HF management. There is no need for a loading dose, and plasma concentration should range between 0.5 ng/mL and 0.9 ng/mL.

There are many adverse effects of digoxin and they are generally dose dependent. Digoxin toxicity typically occurs with serum levels greater than 2 ng/mL, and presents with the combination of cardiac arrhythmias, neurologic effects (visual changes, anxiety, dizziness, etc.), or GI effects (anorexia, nausea, vomiting, and abdominal pain). The concomitant use of digoxin with many drugs, including amiodarone, dronedarone, verapamil, erythromycin, clarithromycin, and cyclosporine, can increase the likelihood of digoxin toxicity. Consult a drug interactions database for more detailed information.

Pharmacokinetics. Digoxin is administered orally, intravenously, or intramuscularly. Approximately 20% to 30% of the drug is plasma protein bound. Digoxin crosses the placenta, and maternal and fetal plasma concentrations of the drug are equal. A small amount of digoxin is metabolized in the liver to inactive metabolites. From 30% to 50% is excreted unchanged in the urine. The elimination half-life in adults is normally 30 to 40 hours, but HF or renal impairment can prolong digoxin elimination.

Indications. Digoxin is indicated for the treatment of HF. Digoxin has a narrow therapeutic index. In all populations, the dosage is individualized based on patient weight, renal function, clinical goals, patient response, and when needed, serum digoxin concentrations.

Adverse Effects. Digoxin can induce almost any type of cardiac arrhythmia. Common cardiac effects associated with digitalis toxicity include variable degrees of AV block, including complete heart block, PR prolongation, unifocal or multifocal premature ventricular contractions, supraventricular tachycardia, atrial tachycardia with or without block, sinus bradycardia with junctional escape, AV dissociation, and an accelerated junctional rhythm. Other rhythm disturbances have included bigeminal or trigeminal rhythms, premature atrial contractions, atrial fibrillation, sinus tachycardia, ventricular fibrillation, and ventricular tachycardia. Mental disturbances were reported as anxiety, depression, delirium, and hallucinations. Other CNS effects that have been reported include weakness,

apathy, and confusion. Digoxin therapy can produce visual disturbances.

Contraindications. Digoxin is not recommended in patients with acute myocardial infarction; use of digoxin in these patients may result in undesirable increases in myocardial oxygen demand and ischemia. Digoxin should be avoided in patients with myocarditis because it can precipitate vasoconstriction and may promote production of pro-inflammatory cytokines. Digoxin should be used with great caution in patients with severe bradycardia or significant AV block. Digoxin can exacerbate bradycardia or SA block, and it should be used with caution in patients with sick sinus syndrome.

Digoxin should also be used with caution in patients with severe pulmonary disease, acute cor pulmonale, hypoxemia, hypothyroidism or myxedema, severe HF, amyloid cardiomyopathy, restrictive cardiomyopathy, or an otherwise damaged myocardium. Digoxin should not be used in patients with left ventricular failure associated with predominant diastolic dysfunction, since increased cytosolic calcium levels could worsen diastolic dysfunction and digoxin is less effective for this type of HF. Digoxin can lower HR and paradoxically worsen low CO states of patients with valvular stenosis, chronic pericarditis, or chronic cor pulmonale.

Digoxin use is relatively contraindicated in patients with ventricular arrhythmias including premature ventricular contractions or ventricular tachycardia, and in patients with carotid sinus hypersensitivity. Digoxin is absolutely contraindicated in patients with ventricular fibrillation. Digoxin should be used with caution in patients with hepatic disease. There are no data on the effects of digoxin on the breast-fed infant or the effects on milk production.

Monitoring. The following parameters should be monitored: periodic electrocardiograms (ECGs), serum calcium, serum creatinine/BUN, serum magnesium, and serum potassium. Most importantly, serum digoxin concentrations should be monitored. This should be done at least 6 to 8 hours after the last dose.

Sodium-Glucose Cotransporter 2 (see Chapter 38)

Dapagliflozin

Dapagliflozin is a sodium-glucose cotransporter 2 (SGLT2) initially designed to aid in the treatment of diabetes. Dapagliflozin reduces the reabsorption of filtered glucose by inhibiting the SGLT2 in the renal tubules. This results in increased urinary excretion of glucose and reduced plasma glucose concentrations. Dapagliflozin reduces sodium reabsorption and increases sodium delivery to the distal tubule for excretion. This results in decreased cardiac preload/afterload and reduced sympathetic activity. Recent clinical trials have studied the use of dapagliflozin in HF patients related to its effects on sodium reabsorption. The results of multiple trials reveal that dapagliflozin is effective in reducing hospitalizations, mortality, and emergent visits in HFrEF patients with or without a diabetes diagnosis. Dapagliflozin was approved for use by the U.S. Food and Drug Administration (FDA) in HF patients in May 2020, and is recommended in HFrEF patients with NYHA Class II to IV as an additive to treatment therapy. The adverse effects include hypotension due to intravascular depletion or concomitant use of antihypertensives and renal impairment.

Pharmacokinetics. Dapagliflozin is administered orally and is approximately 91% protein bound. Elimination of dapagliflozin and its metabolites occurs primarily via the renal pathway. Following oral administration, 75% and 21% of the dose is excreted in the urine and feces, respectively. Following a single oral dose of dapagliflozin 10 mg, the mean plasma terminal half-life is approximately 12.9 hours.

Indications. Dapagliflozin is indicated for the reduction of HF hospitalizations in adults with type 2 diabetes mellitus and established cardiovascular (CV) disease or multiple CV risk factors. Dapagliflozin is also indicated for the treatment of HF with reduced EF (NYHA Class II to IV) to reduce the risk of cardiovascular death and hospitalization for HF.

Adverse Effects. Dapagliflozin can increase the risk of hypoglycemia when combined with insulin. Dapagliflozin results in an osmotic diuresis, which may lead to reductions in intravascular volume. Adverse reactions related to volume depletion include hypotension, orthostatic hypotension, dehydration, and hypovolemia. Acute kidney injury, in some cases requiring hospitalization and dialysis, has been reported, as has increased urinary frequency, including polyuria and increased urine output. Use dapagliflozin cautiously in patients with a history of UTI or genital fungal infection, including vaginitis or balanitis, and in uncircumcised males. Hyperlipidemia can occur with dapagliflozin.

Constipation was reported in 2.2% of patients and nausea was reported in 2.8% of patients receiving dapagliflozin. Naso-pharyngitis was reported in 6.3% of patients. Dapagliflozin can cause increases in serum phosphorus and hematocrit, and it has been associated with Fournier's gangrene (also called necrotizing fasciitis of the perineum), a serious, rare, and life-threatening infection. Use of dapagliflozin may increase the risk for ketoacidosis or diabetic ketoacidosis.

Contraindications. Dapagliflozin is contraindicated in patients with a known serious hypersensitivity reaction to dapagliflozin, including a history of angioedema. Additional hypersensitivity reactions, including serious anaphylactic reactions, severe cutaneous adverse reactions, and angioedema, were reported in 0.3% of dapagliflozin-treated patients. Dapagliflozin causes intravascular volume contraction. Symptomatic hypotension can occur after initiating dapagliflozin.

Monitoring. The following parameters should be monitored: blood glucose, BP, HbA1c, serum cholesterol profile, and serum creatinine/BUN.

Treatments by Stage

Stage A Recommendations

- Control of hypertension and lipid disorders in accordance with contemporary guidelines to lower the risk of HF
- Control or avoidance of other conditions that may lead to or contribute to HF, such as obesity, diabetes mellitus, tobacco use, and known cardiotoxic agents
- ACE inhibition in patients with a history of atherosclerotic vascular disease, diabetes mellitus, or hypertension and associated cardiovascular risk factors
- Treatment of thyroid disorders
- Periodic evaluation for signs and symptoms of HF
- Noninvasive evaluation of left ventricular function in patients with a strong family history of cardiomyopathy or in those receiving cardiotoxic interventions
- Exercise to prevent the development of HF
- Reduction of dietary salt beyond that which is prudent for healthy individuals in patients without hypertension or fluid retention
- Routine testing to detect left ventricular dysfunction in patients without signs or symptoms of HF or evidence of structural heart disease
- Routine use of nutritional supplements to prevent the development of structural heart disease

Stage B Recommendations

Stage B refers to patients without symptoms but who have had a myocardial infarction and patients without symptoms who have evidence of left ventricular dysfunction and are at considerable risk for developing HF.

- Measures listed as recommendations for patients in stage A
- ACE inhibition in patients with a recent or remote history of myocardial infarction regardless of EF
- ACE inhibition in patients with a reduced EF whether or not they have experienced a myocardial infarction
- Beta-blockade in patients with a recent myocardial infarction regardless of EF
- Beta-blockade in patients with a reduced EF whether or not they have experienced a myocardial infarction
- Regular evaluation for signs and symptoms of HF
- Treatment with digoxin in patients with left ventricular dysfunction who are in sinus rhythm
- Reduction of dietary salt beyond that which is prudent for healthy individuals in patients without hypertension or fluid retention
- Exercise to prevent the development of HF
- Routine use of nutritional supplements to treat structural heart disease or to prevent the development of symptoms of HF

Stage C and Stage D Recommendations

Patients with Stage C or D HF should be treated by or in conjunction with cardiology or advanced HF cardiology clinics.

Referrals should be considered before the patient starts to exhibit end-organ damage from the systematic impact of HF syndrome in order to optimize the benefit of advanced therapies. Rehospitalization within 12 months for decompensated HF is an early trigger for referral to an advanced HF clinic. For patients with new-onset systolic HF who are ambulatory and have not yet had an attempt at GDMT, it is certainly reasonable to deliver care in their current clinical environment as long as GDMT can be optimized in that location.

Stage C Recommendations

Stage C refers to patients with structural heart disease and prior or current symptoms of HF.

- Measures listed as recommendations for patients in Stage A and Stage B are also recommended for Stage C.
- GDMT with a beta-blocker and an ACEI/ARB/ARNI should be started in any order for patients with reduced EF.
- GDMT agents should be up-titrated to maximally tolerated or target dose.
- Diuretics are recommended in patients with HFrEF who have evidence of fluid retention.
- Addition of an aldosterone antagonist should be considered after initiation of a beta-blocker and an angiotensin antagonist.
- Sodium-glucose cotransporter-2 (SGLT-2) inhibitors should also be considered for patients with HFrEF who are NYHA Class II to IV.
- Hydralazine and isosorbide dinitrate should be considered for Black patients who are persistently symptomatic despite the above therapies.

Stage D Recommendations

Stage D refers to refractory HF requiring specialized interventions.

- Referral to a HF specialist should be considered in patients needing inotropes and in patients with NYHA Class IIIB/IV symptoms or persistently elevated natriuretic peptides, end-organ dysfunction, EF 35% or less, ICD shocks, recurrent hospitalizations, congestion despite escalating diuretics, low blood pressure and/or high heart rate, and progressive intolerance to GDMT needing down-titration.
- Goals of care should be addressed during the course of illness with HF, and expectations should be calibrated to guide timely decisions.
- End-of-life care in HF involves meticulous management of HF therapies, and palliative care consultation may help with other noncardiac symptoms such as pain.

Considerations for Heart Failure Medication Therapy

Clinical Practice Guidelines

In 2013 the American College of Cardiology Fellows and the American Heart Association created guidelines for the management of HF patients. Highlights from the 2013 update are:

- A thorough history and physical examination should be obtained/performed in patients presenting with HF to identify cardiac and noncardiac disorders or behaviors that might cause or accelerate the development or progression of HF.
- Volume status and vital signs should be assessed at each patient encounter. This includes serial assessment of weight, estimates of jugular venous pressure, and assessment for the presence of peripheral edema or orthopnea.
- Treatment recommendations for Stage A: Hypertension and lipid disorders should be controlled in accordance with contemporary guidelines to lower the risk of HF.
- Treatment recommendations for Stage B: ACE inhibitors should be used in all patients with a reduced EF to prevent symptomatic HF, even if they do not have a history of MI.
- Treatment recommendations for Stage C: GDMT is the mainstay for HFrEF.
- Treatment recommendations for Stage D: Consider referral to an advanced heart failure cardiologist to confirm diagnosis and develop an advanced treatment plan.
- Beta-blockers should be used in all patients with a reduced EF to prevent symptomatic HF, even if they do not have a history of MI.
- Patients with HF should receive specific education to facilitate HF self-care.
- Calcium channel–blocking drugs are not recommended as routine treatment for patients with HFrEF.
- Diuretics should be used for relief of symptoms due to volume overload in patients with HFpEF.
- Implantable cardioverter-defibrillator (ICD) therapy is recommended for primary prevention of sudden cardiac death (SCD) to reduce total mortality in selected patients with left ventricular ejection fraction (LVEF) of 30% or less and NYHA Class I symptoms while receiving GDMT and who have a reasonable expectation of meaningful survival for more than 1 year.
- Goals of care should be addressed during the course of illness with HF, and expectations should be calibrated to guide timely decisions.

BOOKMARK THIS!

Clinical Guidelines for Management of Heart Failure

Guidelines for the management of heart failure from the American College of Cardiology Foundation and the American Heart Association can be found at: https://www.ahajournals.org/doi/10.1161/cir.0b013e31829e8776.

Clinical Reasoning and Heart Failure Medication Therapy

Adjustment of therapies should be considered every 2 weeks to achieve guideline-directed medical therapy (GDMT) in the outpatient setting. An echocardiogram should be repeated

3 to 6 months after achieving target doses of therapy for consideration of an implantable cardioverter-defibrillator (ICD)/cardiac resynchronization therapy (CRT).

Medication adherence should be assessed regularly. Interventions that help with adherence include patient education, medication management, pharmacist comanagement, cognitive behavioral therapies, medication reminders, and incentives to improve adherence.

Advanced practice nurses should risk-stratify patients routinely, and many validated tools are available for use. The Seattle HF model provides robust information about the risk of mortality in ambulatory patients with HF.

To optimize the benefit of advanced therapies, referrals to cardiology should be considered before the patient starts to exhibit end-organ damage from the systematic impact of HF syndrome. Collaboration between the advanced practice nurse and cardiology is key to promote optimal patient health. Rehospitalization within 12 months for decompensated HF is an early trigger to referral to an advanced HF clinic.

Determine the desired therapeutic outcome based on the stage of HF. For patients at risk for HF, the desired therapeutic outcome is prevention through BP control, reduction of elevated cholesterol, and maintenance of optimal glycemic control and ideal body weight. Other preventive measures include smoking cessation and stress reduction.

Assess the selected HF treatment for its appropriateness for an individual patient by considering the patient's age, race/ethnicity, comorbidities, side effects of medications, and genetic factors. Initial treatment for HF is based on the stage and classification of the disease. Race is a consideration when GDMT is not effective, especially in Black patients. Referrals to cardiology should be considered before the patient starts to exhibit end-organ damage.

Initiate the treatment plan with the selected medication by first providing adequate patient education to ensure patient's understanding to promote full participation in the HF therapy. Patient education is paramount in the HF treatment process. Several medications are used in addition to diet, fluid intake, and exercise recommendations. Patients and their families need a good understanding of how the medications, foods, and fluids consumed affect their HF status. Daily maintenance of HF with measurements of weight and blood pressure should be explained and include how to properly obtain measurements.

Ensure complete patient and family understanding about the medication prescribed for HF therapy using a variety of education strategies. Important medication information to provide includes expected therapeutic effects, side effects, adverse effects, any monitoring or follow-up needed, and the importance of checking with the primary care provider for potential drug and food interactions before starting any new medications and supplements. Instruct the patient on symptoms of heart failure exacerbation, what to report to the primary care provider, and when to seek emergency care.

Follow-up and monitoring of patient responses to HF therapy is required to ensure patient safety. Electrolyte disturbance occurs with HF medication therapy. Monitoring of electrolytes should occur with initiation and dose adjustments in diuretics, ARBs, and aldosterone antagonists. Patients should be educated on the signs and symptoms of depleted and excessive electrolytes, especially potassium and magnesium.

Initial laboratory evaluation of patients presenting with HF should include complete blood count, urinalysis, serum electrolytes (including calcium and magnesium), blood urea nitrogen, serum creatinine, glucose, fasting lipid profile, liver function tests, and thyroid-stimulating hormone.

In ambulatory patients with dyspnea, measurement of BNP or N-terminal pro-B-type natriuretic peptide (NT-proBNP) is useful to support clinical decision making regarding the diagnosis of HF, especially in the setting of clinical uncertainty. Measurement of BNP or NT-proBNP is useful for establishing prognosis or disease severity in chronic HF.

A chest X-ray to assess heart size and pulmonary congestion should be obtained in patients with suspected or new-onset HF or in patients who present with acute decompensated HF. A 2-dimensional echocardiogram with Doppler should be performed during the initial evaluation of patients presenting with HF to assess ventricular function, ventricle size, wall thickness, wall motion, and valve function. Repeat measurement of EF and measurement of the severity of structural remodeling are useful in providing information in patients with HF who have had a significant change in clinical status.

Effective systems of care coordination with special attention to care transitions should be deployed for every patient with chronic HF. Every patient with HF should have a clear, detailed, and evidence-based plan of care that ensures the achievement of GDMT goals, effective management of comorbid conditions, timely follow-up with the health care team, appropriate dietary and physical activities, and compliance with secondary prevention guidelines for cardiovascular disease. This plan of care should be updated regularly and made readily available to all members of the patient's health care team. Palliative and supportive care is effective in improving quality of life for patients with symptomatic advanced HF.

In addition to evaluating the effectiveness of the treatment plan, personal points to discuss at follow-up include the acceptability of the treatment to the patient and whether changes to the plan may be needed. Medication adherence must be determined and patient knowledge about the medication and treatment plan reassessed to determine any need for education reinforcement. Ensure that the patient has an adequate supply of medication until the next follow-up appointment.

Teaching Points for HF Medication Therapy

Disease management through a self-care regimen will assist medication therapy. Patients need to understand how to monitor their symptoms and weight fluctuations, restrict their sodium intake, take their medications as prescribed, and stay physically active.

Daily weights and blood pressures should be taken prior to taking medications. Primary care providers should set parameters for when patients should hold their medications if their weight and/or blood pressure is outside the established parameters.

Health Promotion Strategies

Hypertension and lipid disorders should be controlled in accordance with contemporary guidelines to lower the risk of HF. Other conditions that may lead to or contribute to HF, such as obesity, diabetes mellitus, tobacco use, and known cardiotoxic agents, should be controlled or avoided. The following strategies and practices should be presented to patients to help them become full partners in their health care:

- Reduce your risk for cardiac disease by engaging in routine physical activity in consultation with your primary care provider. If other conditions permit, perform at least 150 minutes a week of moderate-intensity aerobic physical activity or 75 minutes a week of vigorous-intensity aerobic physical activity.
- Reduce your intake of sodium to lower blood pressure or to maintain a healthy blood pressure.
- If you are overweight (body mass index [BMI] = 25 to 29 kg/m^2) or obese (BMI >30 kg/m^2), lose weight with guidance from your primary care provider to reduce your risk for stroke.
- If you are a smoker, work with your primary care provider to quit smoking with drug therapy using nicotine replacement, bupropion, or varenicline in combination with counseling.

Patient Education for Medication Safety

HF medication treatment therapy generally involves one or more medications, some resulting in similar adverse outcomes. Specific attention should be placed on blood pressure monitoring and daily weights. Primary care providers need to stress the following points and actions to patients for safe medication management:

- Take your HF medications as directed. If you miss a dose, take the missed dose as soon as possible on the same day, but skip if it is less than 6 hours before the next scheduled dose.
- Take daily weight and blood pressure measurements prior to taking diuretics and other medications that can lower your blood pressure.
- Never double up a dose to make up for a missed dose.
- Get emergency medical help if you have signs of an allergic reaction, such as hives, difficulty breathing, or swelling of your face, lips, tongue, or throat.
- Keep all clinic and laboratory appointments for blood tests related to your HF management. If you need to miss an appointment, notify your primary care provider and reschedule as soon as possible.

Application Questions for Discussion

1. As a primary care provider, when should you consider referral of HF patients to cardiology or an advanced HF specialist?
2. What should be included in the education plan for a patient and/or caregiver who has been diagnosed with HF?
3. What resources are available in your community to assist with the management of HF patients?

Selected Bibliography

McCance, K. L., & Huether, S. E. (2019). *Pathophysiology: The Biological Basis for Disease in Adults and Children.* St. Louis: Elsevier.

Petrie, M. C., Verma, S., Docherty, K. F., Inzucchi, S. E., Anand, I., Belohlavek, J., Bohn, M., Chiang, C-E., Chopra, V. K., DeBoer, R. A., Desai, A. S., Diez, M., Drozdz, J., Dukat, A., Ge, J., Howlett, J., Katova, T., Kitakaze, M., & McMurray, J. V. (2020). Effect of dapagliflozin on worsening heart failure and cardiovascular death in patients with heart failure with and without diabetes. *Journal of the American Medical Association, 323*(14), 1353–1368. http://doi.org/10.1001/jama.2020.1906.

Ponikowski, P. (2020). Dapagliflozin in patients with heart failure and reduced ejection fraction DAPA-HF. *American College of Cardiology.* https://www.acc.org/latest-incardiology/clinical-trials/2019/08/30/21/33/dapa-hf.

Shah, A., Gandhi, D., Srivastava, S., Shah, K. J., & Mansukhani, R. (2017). Heart failure: A class review of pharmacotherapy. *Pharmacy and Therapeutics, 42*(7), 464–472. https://www.ncbi.nlm.nih.gov/pmc/articles/PMC5481297/.

Yancey, C. W., Jessup, M., Butler, J., Draaner, M. H., Geraci, S. A., Januzzi, J. L., Kasper, E. K., Masoudi, F. A., McMurray, J. J. V., Petereson, P. N., Sam, F., Tang, W. H. W., & Wilkoff, B. L. (2013). 2013 ACCF/AHA guideline for the management of heart failure. *Journal of the American College of Cardiology, 62*(16), 47–213. http://dx.doi.org/10.1016/j.jacc.2013.05.020.

Yancey, C. W., Jessup, M., Bozkurt, B., Butler, J., Casey, D. E., Colvin, M. M., Drazner, M. H., Filippatos, G., Fonarow, G. C., Givertz, M. M., Hollenberg, S. M., Lindenfeld, S. M., Masoudi, F. A., McBride, P. E., Peterson, P. N., Stevenson, L. W., & Westlake, C. (2016). 2016 ACC/AHA/HFSA focused update on new pharmacological therapy for heart failure: An update of the 2013 ACCF/AHA guideline for the management of heart failure. *Journal of the American College of Cardiology, 68*(13), 1476–1488. http://doi.org/10.1016/j.jacc.2016.05.011.

Yancey, C. W., Jessup, M., Bozkurt, B., Butler, J., Casey, D. E., Colvin, M. M., Drazner, M. H., Filippatos, G., Fonarow, G. C., Givertz, M. M., Hollenberg, S. M., Lindenfeld, S. M., Masoudi, F. A., McBride, P. E., Peterson, P. N., Stevenson, L. W., & Westlake, C. (2017). 2017 ACC/AHA/HFSA focused update of the 2013 ACCF/AHA guideline for the management of heart failure. *Journal of the American College of Cardiology, 70*(6), 776–797. http://dx.doi.org/10.1016/j.jacc.2017.04.025.

12

Antiarrhythmic Medications

ELIZABETH REMO AND CHERYL H. ZAMBROSKI

Overview

A disruption in the pathway of electrical impulses in the heart creates irregularities in the heart rhythm. Changes in calcium, sodium, and potassium ions generate an electrical activity that flows through the heart—an impulse that originates in the sinoatrial (SA) node. These electrical activities reflect how quickly or slowly a heart beats, as well as the regularities and consistencies of the rhythm.

Arrhythmias occur when there are irregularities in the heart rhythm. The type of arrhythmia may vary depending on the origin of the electrical disruption. Indications for antiarrhythmic medications include the management of various atrial and ventricular arrhythmias. Common disease-related etiology may be hypertension, chronic heart failure (HF), valvular heart disease, myocardial ischemia, thyroid abnormalities, electrolyte abnormalities, and hypoxemia. Prescribed or over-the-counter (OTC) medications, drug toxicity, food/nutritional supplements (such as caffeine-containing products), and alcohol may also lead to arrhythmias. In some clinical settings, anxiety and exercise may provoke arrhythmias, especially in patients with underlying disease and/or known consumption of certain types of medication or food.

In general, pharmacologic management of complex arrhythmias should be accomplished through collaboration with specialty practices. The cardiology specialist typically determines the appropriate medication and initiates treatment. The patient, once stable, may be turned over to the primary care provider for long-term monitoring. The primary care provider will also regularly assess the patient for adverse effects of prescribed medications, monitor lab work, and reinforce healthy lifestyle habits.

Relevant Physiology

The heart is composed of specialized myocardial muscle cells that have the capacity to generate an electrical potential (*automaticity*) and spread the electrical current from cell to cell (*conductivity*) (Fig. 12.1). These bundles of cells within the myocardium serve as a pacemaker for the heart. The primary pacemaker is the SA node. Electrical waves of depolarization spread through the atrium, the atria-ventricular

(AV) junction, and the bundle of His, and then move down the left- and right-bundle branches, producing synchronized atrial and ventricular muscular contractions. When the dominant pacemaker slows or does not fire, other cells take over and continue the heartbeat, although at a slower rate. Sometimes aberrant cells take over the pacemaker role, creating irregular rhythms and/or tachyarrhythmias.

Changes in the electrical pathways create a cellular response that triggers electrical impulses. Differences in electrical charge across the myocardial cell membrane, known as *action potential*, may occur, resulting in polarization and depolarization (Fig. 12.2). *Polarization* can be further described by its action—that is, whether it sets a charge before or after muscle contraction. *Depolarization* is the electrical impulse that precedes the mechanical contraction of cardiac tissue. It is caused by the movement of sodium, potassium, calcium, and chloride across cardiac cell membranes. *Repolarization* is the recovery stage after muscle contraction.

Pathophysiology

The effectiveness of antiarrhythmic medications depends on three factors: whether the clinician has accurately addressed the mechanism of the arrhythmia, whether the clinician knows the origin of the disruption in electrical impulses, and the impact the disruption has had on the heart's electrical response. Two basic arrhythmic mechanisms within the heart are increased automaticity that results in an ectopic focus, and reentry through abnormal conduction pathways. It is often clinically impossible to determine the mechanism without an electrophysiology mapping study. Arrhythmias that are caused by irritability or increased automaticity are treated with drugs that prolong the action potential, thus decreasing the rate at which impulses can be generated (Fig. 12.3). Sustained ventricular tachycardia usually occurs as a reentry type of tachycardia, and it is treated with a drug that prolongs the effective refractory period.

Types of Arrhythmias

The origin or location of the arrhythmias may vary, but in general, they can be categorized as either atrial or ventricular. Understanding the etiology of the disruption in

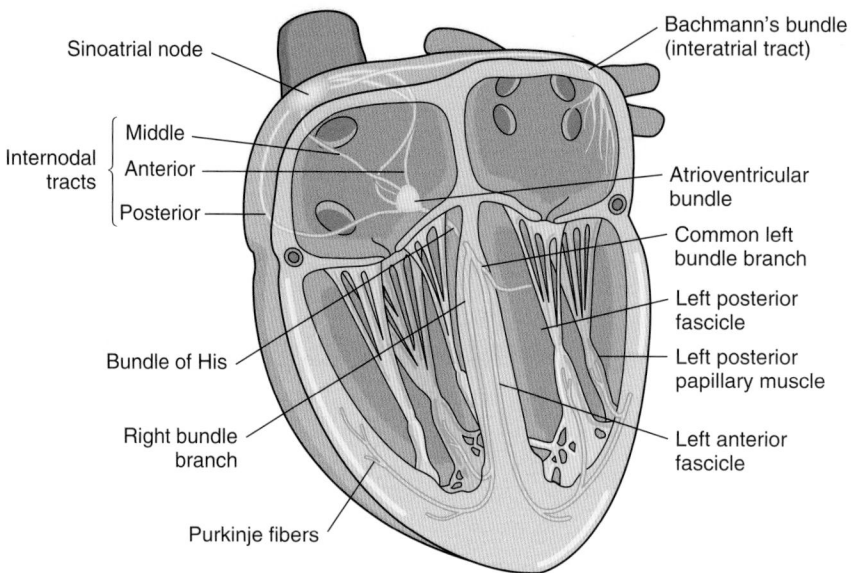

• **Fig. 12.1** Conduction system of the heart. (From Monahan, F., Sands, J. K., , Neighbors, M., Marek, J. F., & Green, C. J. [2006]. *Phipps' medical-surgical nursing: Health and illness perspectives* [8th ed.]. St. Louis: Mosby.)

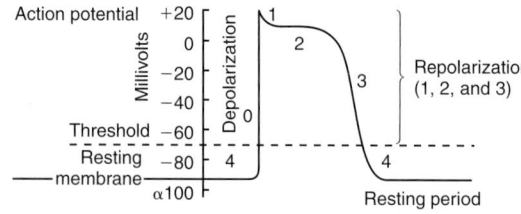

Depolarization
Phase 0—membrane becomes permeable to Na⁺, which rapidly flows into the cell

Repolarization
Phase 1—membrane potential becomes slightly positive because of the rapid influx of Na⁺
Phase 2—slow inward flow of Ca⁺⁺ and outward flow of K⁺
Phase 3—rapid outward flow of K⁺

Resting period
Phase 4—cell membrane actively transports Na⁺ outside and K⁺ inside, returning cell membrane to state of polarization

A

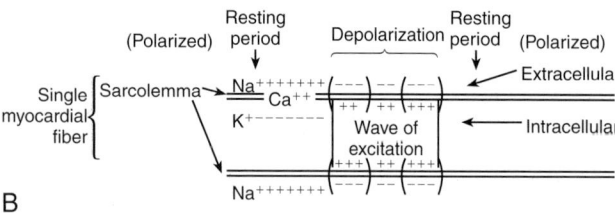

B

• **Fig. 12.2** (A) Action potential of a single myocardial fiber (cell). (B) Ionic exchanges that occur across the cell membrane of a single myocardial fiber during an action potential. (From McKenry, L. M., & Salerno, E. [2006]. *Mosby's pharmacology in nursing* [22nd ed.]. St. Louis: Mosby.)

the electrical pathway can help the clinician determine an appropriate treatment plan. Management of arrhythmias is influenced by the type of arrhythmia and how it impacts the patient's heart rate and cardiac structure. Classification

of the antiarrhythmic medications will be discussed later in this chapter.

Atrial Arrhythmias

Atrial Fibrillation

Atrial fibrillation (AF) is a relatively common type of arrhythmia that shows a lack of organized electrical activity in the atria. AF can be further classified according to the duration of the arrhythmia—either *paroxysmal* or *persistent*—and whether the timing or duration of symptoms is *new onset* or *chronic*. Risk factors include male gender, underlying cardiovascular disease, surgery, emotional stress, increasing age, and use of painkillers such as nonsteroidal antiinflammatory drugs (NSAIDs) and cyclooxygenase-2 (COX-2) inhibitors.

Paroxysmal AF refers to episodes that self-terminate and may last fewer than 7 days or even fewer than 24 hours. This type of AF can be terminated by electrical cardioversion after the absence of clots in the left atrium has been confirmed by transesophageal echocardiogram (TEE). If clots are found during a TEE screening, treatment with anticoagulation therapy is initiated. *Permanent AF* lasts longer than 1 year and may be due to failure to attempt termination of the arrhythmia or an unsuccessful termination attempt.

Treatment of patients with AF focuses on rate and/or rhythm control and the use of anticoagulation therapy to prevent systemic clot embolization. The presence of AF puts a patient at higher risk for developing a clot that can embolize and cause ischemic stroke. Rate control can be achieved with the use of beta-blockers, calcium channel blockers (CCBs), or digoxin. Rhythm control is attained through electrical cardioversion, radiofrequency ablation, or medications. Antiarrhythmics, such as amiodarone, are used for

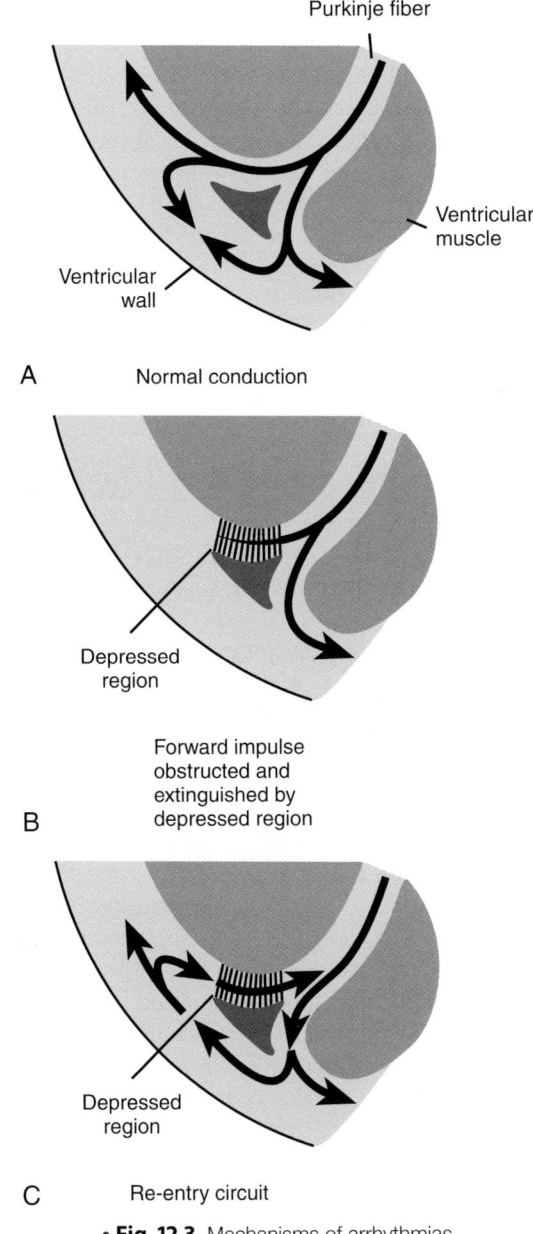

A Normal conduction

Depressed region

Forward impulse obstructed and extinguished by depressed region

B

Depressed region

C Re-entry circuit

• **Fig. 12.3** Mechanisms of arrhythmias.

clots are released into the systemic circulation, causing arterial occlusion and stroke.

If appropriate, nonpharmacologic therapy is initiated prior to drug therapy. Radiofrequency ablation of foci around the pulmonary veins, the root of the left/right atrium, and the isthmus of the mitral valve may be an appropriate intervention for those with symptomatic AF who are unresponsive to pharmacologic therapy. In patients with chronic AF, treatment is threefold: control of rate, rhythm, and thromboembolic events.

Control of rapid ventricular response is accomplished with the use of a beta-blocker or a nondihydropyridine calcium channel antagonist for patients with persistent or permanent AF. In the absence of preexcitation, intravenous (IV) administration of beta-blockers (e.g., esmolol, metoprolol, and propranolol) or nondihydropyridine calcium channel antagonists (e.g., verapamil and diltiazem) is recommended to slow the ventricular response to AF in the acute setting. Caution is exercised in patients with hypotension or HF. IV administration of digoxin or amiodarone is recommended to control the heart rate in patients with AF and HF who do not have an accessory pathway. Prevention of thromboembolic events is accomplished by anticoagulation.

Amiodarone may be used for pharmacologic cardioversion or suppression of AF and maintenance of normal sinus rhythm. Dronedarone may be an option for the treatment of nonpermanent AF in those whose condition cannot be controlled through first-line therapy (usually including beta-blockers). A single oral bolus dose of propafenone or flecainide can be administered to terminate persistent AF outside the hospital once treatment has proved to be safe in the hospital. This treatment option is for select patients without sinus or AV node dysfunction, bundle-branch block, QT interval prolongation, Brugada syndrome, or structural heart disease. Before antiarrhythmic medication is initiated, a beta-blocker or a nondihydropyridine calcium channel antagonist should be given to prevent rapid AV conduction in the event that atrial flutter occurs.

Atrial Flutter

Regular, rapid atrial contractions are referred to as *atrial flutter*. This type of arrhythmia differs from AF because the atrial contractions are organized. That is, although the heart rate may be rapid, the rhythm remains consistent, and the flutter waves in between the QRS in an electrocardiogram (ECG) remain regular and continuous. Atrial flutter can be either typical or atypical and paroxysmal or persistent.

Typical atrial flutter is commonly seen in the clinical setting. In this type of atrial flutter, a large reentrant electrical circuit is activated in the right atrium with passive conduction from the left atrium. This reentry commonly occurs in a clockwise direction. This type of flutter rhythm is often seen in male patients, in older adults, and in those with medical conditions such as hypertension, diabetes, and chronic obstructive pulmonary disease (COPD). Excessive alcohol intake and high-endurance sports or activities may

either medical conversion to normal sinus rhythm or maintenance of a normal rhythm after electrical cardioversion. Anticoagulation therapy, such as the use of direct oral anticoagulation (DOAC) or warfarin, is considered first-line therapy for stroke prevention.

Long-term maintenance of normal sinus rhythm is usually unsuccessful if the patient has a history of valvular disease or chronic hypertension. Unmanaged AF can lead to rapid ventricular response and/or thromboembolism. *Rapid ventricular response* usually occurs at a rate of 150 to 220 beats per minute (bpm). This accelerated rate may be poorly tolerated and may precipitate structural heart abnormalities if the patient cannot tolerate the loss of atrial kick. Subsequently, clots may form in the atria as a result of blood stasis that occurs with chaotic electrical impulses and a lack of contractility. *Thromboembolism* may result when these also contribute to this type of arrhythmia. About half of the patients with this type of flutter may also develop AF.

Management depends on the clinical presentation. Typically, a fast ventricular rate is present (around 120 to 150 bpm), and the ECG may show a 2:1 or 1:1 AV conduction. Patients with 1:1 AV conduction, an extremely fast ventricular rate, and symptoms such as low blood pressure, chest pain, palpitations, and dizziness will require immediate attention. Atrial flutter can also result in a syncopal episode and may cause HF. Although the likelihood of thromboembolism is low compared to AF, left atrial appendage thrombi have been detected.

The treatment plan should follow a stepwise approach, focusing on rate control first, then rhythm control. AV nodal-blocking medications such as digoxin, beta-blockers, and calcium antagonist are first-line therapy. If the patient remains unstable, cardioversion to sinus rhythm is the next step. Class III antiarrhythmics, such as dofetilide and ibutilide, may be effective; however, there is a small risk of QT prolongation and torsades de pointes. Anticoagulation may be considered prior to and after cardioversion.

Ventricular Arrhythmias

Supraventricular Arrhythmias

Supraventricular arrhythmias originate above the ventricles and may include the atria, SA node, and AV node. As a result, these types of arrhythmias may affect the rate and regularity of the heart's rhythm. AV nodal arrhythmias originate from the AV node and are likely caused by delayed or absent conduction from the SA node to the AV node. These types of arrhythmias may reduce ventricular filling, leading to reduced cardiac output.

Paroxysmal supraventricular tachycardia (*PSVT*) is a term that applies to all supraventricular tachycardias except for AF and atrial flutter. Approximately 60% of cases of PSVT are due to reentry within or close to the AV node, known as *atrioventricular nodal reentrant tachycardia* (*AVNRT*). This condition results from atrioventricular reentrant tachycardia (AVRT) in 30% of cases. *AVRT* refers to the accessory pathways that connect the atrium with the ventricle, and it is characterized by a heart rate of 130 to 250 bpm, 1:1 conduction, and a narrow QRS complex. PSVTs are often seen in patients with no underlying heart disease. Treatment depends on the patient's ability to tolerate the tachycardia, the mechanism of the arrhythmia, and how frequently the arrhythmia presents.

Prophylaxis of PSVT usually involves digoxin or beta-blockers, with verapamil as a second choice. These medications may also be used in combination. Note that verapamil increases digoxin serum levels. If the patient has significant heart disease, they may require Class IA, IC, or III drugs. Radiofrequency ablation is frequently used to eliminate the accessory pathway, which avoids the potential safety concerns of antiarrhythmic drugs. Digoxin and CCBs should never be used if an accessory pathway is diagnosed or suspected.

Ventricular Arrhythmias

Ventricular arrhythmias typically originate in the ventricle or the bundle of His. Patients may present clinically with a fast heart rate (ventricular tachycardia). These types of arrhythmias are generally life threatening as they can lead to loss of consciousness and sudden cardiac death.

Premature ventricular complexes (PVCs) are caused by increased automaticity and are classified according to prevalence as well as morphologic characteristics. The most important QT factor in determining whether to treat PVCs is the presence of underlying heart disease. Underlying heart disease (especially myocardial ischemia or recent myocardial infarction) in the presence of PVCs can be a marker for the development of malignant ventricular arrhythmias. Additional factors that place the patient at increased risk are the presence of cardiac scarring, hypertrophy, and/or left ventricular dysfunction. PVCs that are frequent, paired, or sustained are particularly dangerous. PVCs that occur during the QT interval present a risk for initiating ventricular fibrillation.

In general, PVCs that are complex, that occur less than 1 year after a myocardial infarction, or that present with underlying heart disease and symptoms (such as angina) should be treated. Asymptomatic/simple PVCs in patients without a cardiac history and those that disappear during an exercise test should be closely monitored. Because of the risks inherent in antiarrhythmic therapy, patients should not be treated unless clearly indicated.

Torsades de pointes is a life-threatening ventricular tachycardia that is associated with prolongation of the QT interval. Long QT syndrome (LQTS) can also arise separately, usually from a genetic defect. In many cases, antiarrhythmic medications may precipitate sudden acute cardiac arrest in individuals who have a genetic tendency toward LQTS. Using certain medications to protect these individuals and avoiding medications that may precipitate the event is lifesaving for patients diagnosed with this genetic mutation.

Long-term treatment to suppress ventricular arrhythmias is usually selected after provocative testing in an acute care setting. Drugs that may be effective include Class IA drugs and amiodarone. Although these drugs may be effective, caution and close monitoring are recommended as they may also cause the arrhythmia that is being treated.

Long QT Syndrome

As mentioned in the preceding section, LQTS is a unique physiologic condition in which medications are often the cause of the problem and not the treatment for it. LQTS is a channelopathy characterized by prolongation of the QT interval on an ECG. Time is measured from the beginning of the QRS complex to the end of the T wave, and intervals longer than 0.44 seconds are generally considered abnormal; the problem is usually best seen in the right precordial leads. The QT interval represents the duration of activation and recovery of ventricular myocardial activity. Prolonged recovery from electrical excitation increases the likelihood of dispersing the recovery refractoriness, leaving some parts of the myocardium refractory to subsequent depolarization.

The clinical consequence of delayed repolarization may be polymorphic ventricular tachycardia, or torsades de pointes, which may lead to ventricular fibrillation and sudden cardiac death. This arrhythmia may result from physiologic changes that cause reactivation of calcium channels, reactivation of a delayed sodium current, or a decreased outward potassium current that results in early afterdepolarization. The LQT cardiac repolarization defect is often caused by a variety of genetic mutations that may be present congenitally or acquired. The LQT interval may be lengthened by different factors in different people, such as exercise, drugs, or a startle reflex. It may be that all individuals with this problem have an underlying genetic defect and that medications only reveal the syndrome. Current research is examining whether many cases of sudden infant death syndrome (SIDS) or sudden acute cardiac deaths in young athletes are related to LQTS.

A number of medications have been associated with prolonged QT interval. For example, cardiac drugs identified with prolonging the QT include certain Class IA antiarrhythmic agents (e.g., disopyramide, quinidine, and procainamide) and Class III antiarrhythmic agents (e.g., sotalol and amiodarone). Other examples include select antimicrobial agents (e.g., macrolides and fluoroquinolones), antipsychotics (e.g., haloperidol, risperidone, and quetiapine), and tricyclic antidepressants (e.g., imipramine and amitriptyline). It is important to consider the impact of medications on conduction. When a medication is found to be the causative agent in LQTS, the drug should be discontinued.

In some high-risk patients, an implantable cardioverter-defibrillator (ICD) is highly effective in preventing sudden cardiac death. Patients with aborted cardiac arrest or recurrent cardiac events (e.g., syncope or torsades de pointes), despite their treatment with more conventional therapy (i.e., beta-blocker alone), and those with a very prolonged QT interval (>500 ms) are viewed as high-risk patients and good candidates for ICD. Beta-blockade in combination with a pacemaker and/or stellectomy may be used in selected patients. Patients who are not sensitive to beta-blockers would also be good candidates for ICD.

Arrhythmia Therapy

Management of cardiac arrhythmias may be prioritized based on the patient's hemodynamic stability and heart rate. The treatment plan may be developed and altered based on the clinical presentation and acuity of symptoms. Although medications are available for the treatment of many arrhythmias, it is important to understand that synchronized cardioversion may be the initial intervention in many cases. If this therapy fails or is determined to be inappropriate for a patient, then antiarrhythmic therapy should be initiated.

An antiarrhythmic drug's mechanism of action is to reduce the electrical irregularity of the heart by altering the action potential of cardiac cells (Fig. 12.4). All antiarrhythmics may directly or indirectly affect heart rate and electrical pathways and have the potential to cause an arrhythmia (Table 12.1). These disruptions in the electrical pathway may be captured by an ECG, an echocardiogram, portable event recorders, a Holter monitor, or implantable loop recorders. They can also be diagnosed through a stress test, a tilt table test, or if needed, an electrophysiological study.

Classification of Antiarrhythmic Agents (Vaughn-Williams Classification System)

The Vaughn-Williams classification system has been used to guide providers in carefully selecting appropriate antiarrhythmics as clinically indicated. This system categorizes the antiarrhythmic agents into four classes based on the mechanism of action and the targeted cell. Table 12.2, Table 12.3, and Table 12.4 provide information on pharmacokinetics of common antiarrhythmic medications, dosage and administration recommendations, and common adverse effects, respectively.

Class I: Sodium Channel Blockers

Sodium channel blockers (SCBs) block sodium pathways affecting the cell's ability to respond to depolarization. This raises the action potential firing and slows the rate of depolarization. As a result, the heart rate is decreased. Additionally,

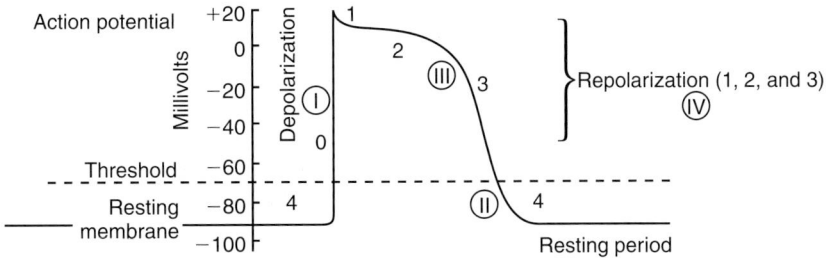

• **Fig. 12.4** Phases of the action potential and locations of action of the classes of antiarrhythmics. Circled roman numerals indicate the major site of action of that category of antiarrhythmic.

| TABLE 12.1 | **Mechanism of Action of Antiarrhythmic Medications** | | | | | | | | | |

Category/ Medication	Heart Rate	Automaticity of Foci	CONDUCTION VELOCITY		REFRACTORY PERIOD		Accessory Pathway	ECG CHANGES		QT Interval
			AV Node	Ventricle	Atrium	Ventricle		PR Interval	QRS	
Class IA										
Quinidine	±	↓	±	↓	↓↓	↑	↑	±	↑	↑
Procainamide	±	↓	±	↓	↑	↑	↑↑	±	↑	↑
Class IB										
Mexiletine	0	↓	0	0	0	↑	↑	0	0	0
Tocainide	0	↓	0	0	↓	↓	↑	0	0	↓
Class IC										
Flecainide	0	↓	↓	↓↓	0	↑	↑↑	↑	↑↑	↑
Propafenone	0	↓	↓	↓	0	↑	↑	↑	↑	↑
Class II (Beta-Adrenergic Blockers)										
Propranolol	↓	↓	↓	↓	±	0	↑	↑	0	↓
Metoprolol	↓	↓	↓	0	±	0	↑	↑	0	↓
Class III										
Amiodarone	↓	↓	↓	↓	↑	↑	↑	↑	↑	↑↑
Class IV (Calcium Channel Blockers)										
Verapamil	↓	↓	↓	0	0	0	0	↑	0	0
Other										
Digoxin	↓	↑	↓	↓	±	↓	↑↓	↑	0	↓

SCBs affect the ventricle by decreasing upstroke conduction velocity and precipitate dysthymia.

Class IA: Antiarrhythmics

Class IA drugs (quinidine, disopyramide, and procainamide) depress rapid depolarization, or phase 0, of the action potential. These drugs slow conduction by lengthening the effective refractory period of the atrial and ventricular myocardium, depressing the inward sodium current, and decreasing the automaticity and excitability of cardiac muscle. These agents may also block potassium channels, slowing the conduction speed by reducing membrane repolarization and increasing the effective refractory period. Procainamide is only available for IV or intramuscular doses in the United States. Oral forms are no longer available, so they will not be discussed here.

Quinidine

Pharmacokinetics. Oral quinidine is readily absorbed from the gastrointestinal (GI) tract and is unaffected by food. Bioavailability, distribution, and elimination vary widely among individuals, with absolute bioavailability varying between 45% and 100%. Quinidine is 80% to 90% plasma protein bound, and it is metabolized by the liver and excreted in the urine. Approximately 10% is excreted unchanged in the urine. Grapefruit juice delays the absorption of quinidine and inhibits cytochrome (CYP) 3A4 metabolism of quinidine to 3-hydroxyquinidine in the liver.

Indications. Quinidine can be used for conversion to and/or maintenance of sinus rhythm in patients with AF, atrial flutter, or ventricular tachycardia. It can also be used to treat PSVT, and to prevent PSVT in patients with reentrant tachycardias (including Wolff-Parkinson-White [WPW] syndrome). Quinidine is rarely used due to its adverse effect profile and has been replaced by Class III agents.

Adverse Effects. The most common adverse effects associated with quinidine are GI-related and include diarrhea (24% to 35% of patients), esophagitis (22%), and pyrosis (22%). Less commonly, patients may experience headache, fatigue, and palpitations. Potential ECG changes associated with quinidine therapy include PR prolongation, widening of the QRS, and prolongations of the QT interval. There is an increased risk for torsades de pointes and ventricular tachycardia with elevated serum levels in patients treated with quinidine.

TABLE 12.2 Pharmacokinetics of Common Antiarrhythmic Medications

Drug	Absorption	Drug Availability (After First Pass)	Onset of Action	Time to Peak Concentration	Half-Life	Duration of Action	Protein Bound	Metabolism	Excretion	Therapeutic Serum Level
Class IA										
Quinidine (as sulfate)	—	80%	—	1–3 hr	6–8 hr	6–8 hr	80%–88%	Hepatic	Urine	2–6 mcg/mL
Procainamide	85%	—	30 min	—	3 hr	3 + hr	20%	Hepatic	Renal	Procainamide 4–10 mcg/mL; N-acetylprocainamide (NAPA) 10–20 mcg/mL
Class IB										
Mexiletine	90%	—	—	2–3 hr	10–12 hr	24 hr	50%–60%	Hepatic	Renal	0.5–2 mcg/mL
Tocainide	100%	100%	—	0.5–2.5 hr	11–14 hr	5 hr	10%	Hepatic	Renal	5–12 mcg/mL
Class IC										
Flecainide	100%	100%	—	1.5–3 hr	12–27 hr	—	40%	Hepatic	Renal	0.2–1 mcg/mL
Propafenone	100%	3%–10%	—	2–3 hr	2–8 hr	—	97%	Hepatic	Hepatic	—
Class II										
Propranolol	100%	30%–40%	1–2 hr	—	4–6 hr	6 hr	90%–95%	Hepatic	Renal	50–100 ng/mL
Acebutolol	90%	40%	1–2 hr	2–4 hr	3–4 hr	12–24 hr	5%–15%	Hepatic	Renal	—
Class III										
Amiodarone	35%–65%	50%	2–3 months unless loading dose is used	3–7 hr	40–55 days	Weeks–months	96%	Hepatic	Hepatic	0.5–2.5 mcg/mL
Class IV										
Verapamil	—	20%–35%	1–2 hr	1–2 hr	5–12 hr	6–8 hr	88%–92%	Hepatic	Renal	50–200 ng/mL
Other										
Digoxin	—	70%–80%	0.5–2 hr	1 hr	30–40 hr	24 hr	20%–25%	Nonhepatic	Renal	0.5–2 ng/mL

TABLE 12.3	Antidysrhythmic Medications[a]		
Category/ Medication	**Indication**	**Dosage**	**Considerations and Monitoring**
Class I: Sodium Channel Blockers			
Class IA			
Quinidine	Conversion to and/or maintenance of sinus rhythm in patients with atrial fibrillation, atrial flutter, or ventricular tachycardia Treatment of paroxysmal supraventricular tachycardia (PSVT); or for PSVT prophylaxis in patients with reentrant tachycardias, including patients with Wolff-Parkinson-White (WPW) syndrome	**Immediate-release tablets:** *Adults:* Begin with 200–300 mg orally every 6–8 hr. May be increased to 600 mg orally every 6 hr if needed, based on serum quinidine concentrations. **Extended-release tablets:** *Adults:* 300–600 mg orally every 8–12 hr.	Give with a full glass of water 1 hour before or 2 hours after meals for better absorption. Avoid grapefruit juice while taking quinidine. Monitor serum quinidine concentrations due to narrow therapeutic index. Normal range 2–6 mcg/mL Use reduced dosing in patients with CrCl ≤10 mL/min.
Class IB			
Mexiletine	Treatment of life-threatening ventricular arrhythmias, such as ventricular tachycardia	Begin with 200 mg orally every 8 hr (may load with 400 mg if needed). Dosage may be increased by 50–100 mg at intervals every 2–3 days if needed. Usual dosage is 200–300 mg orally every 8 hr. Maximum dosage: 1200 mg/day.	Typically prescribed by specialty practitioners. ECG and LFTs should be monitored. May be administered with food or antacids to decrease GI distress.
Tocainide	Treatment of patients with sustained ventricular tachycardia that is considered to be life-threatening	Begin with 400 mg orally every 8 hr. Usual dosage range of 1200–1800 mg/day in divided doses. Maximum dosage: Up to 2400 mg/day in divided doses.	Typically prescribed by specialty practitioners. Dose adjustment required in patients with renal impairment. Electrophysiological testing should be done prior to and during therapy to assess whether continued treatment is warranted.
Class IC			
Propafenone	Treatment of patients with sustained ventricular tachycardia deemed to be life-threatening	**Immediate-release tablets:** Begin with 150 mg orally every 8 hr. May be increased if needed after 3–4 days to 225 mg orally every 8 hr. Maximum dosage: 300 mg every 8 hr.	Dosage should be initiated in a hospital setting. Avoid use in patients with heart failure and/or left ventricular dysfunction. May be taken with or without food.
	Maintenance of sinus rhythm in patients with paroxysmal atrial fibrillation or atrial flutter associated with disabling symptoms	**Immediate-release tablets:** Begin with 150 mg orally every 8 hr. May be increased if needed after 3–4 days to 225 mg orally every 8 hr. Maximum dosage: 300 mg every 8 hr. **Extended-release tablets:** Begin with 225 mg orally every 12 hr. Increase dosage at intervals of 5 days or more to 325 mg every 12 hr and, if necessary, to 425 mg every 12 hr.	

TABLE 12.3 Antidysrhythmic Medications[a]—cont'd

Category/ Medication	Indication	Dosage	Considerations and Monitoring
Class II Beta-Blockers			
Propranolol	For heart rate control in patients with atrial fibrillation and/or atrial flutter Treatment of paroxysmal supraventricular tachycardia or prevention of paroxysmal supraventricular tachycardia	**Immediate-release tablets:** Begin with 10–30 mg orally three or four times daily. Dosage may be increased up to 160–320 mg/day in 3–4 divided doses.	In older adults, start with lower doses and increase slowly as tolerated. Should be given with meals and at bedtime.
Acebutolol	Treatment of premature ventricular contractions	Begin with 200 mg orally twice daily. Usual dosage range is 600–1200 mg/day.	Taper over at least 2 weeks if discontinuing.
Class III-Potassium Channel Blockers			
Amiodarone	Treatment and prevention of frequently recurring ventricular fibrillation in patients who are refractory to other therapy.	Begin with 800–1600 mg/day orally in single or divided doses for a minimum of 1 to 3 weeks. followed by 600–800 mg/day in one or divided doses for about 1 month. Reduce to lowest effective dose. Usual dose is 400 mg/day in one or divided doses.	Treatment should be initiated in a monitored setting until therapeutic response is achieved. Requires baseline and periodic pulmonary function tests, laboratory tests, and ophthalmologic examination. Monitor ECG closely for prolonged QT interval with initiation or increase in therapy.
Dronedarone	Used for reduction in the risk of hospitalization for atrial fibrillation in patients in sinus rhythm with a history of paroxysmal or persistent atrial fibrillation	400 mg orally twice daily with meals.	Contraindicated in patients with permanent atrial fibrillation who cannot be converted to NSR. Class I or Class III antiarrhythmics or drugs that are strong CYP3A4 inhibitors must be discontinued prior to dronedarone being initiated. Not used in patients with NYHA Class III or IV heart failure or recent episode of decompensated heart failure.
Sotalol	Maintenance of NSR in patients with symptomatic atrial fibrillation or atrial flutter who are currently in sinus rhythm Treatment of life-threatening ventricular arrythmias	80 mg orally twice daily. May be increased to 120 mg twice daily. Maximum dosage 320 mg/day orally for atrial fibrillation/atrial flutter, 640 mg/day orally for life-threatening ventricular arrhythmias.	Treatment should be initiated in a monitored setting until therapeutic response is achieved. Monitor serum potassium and serum magnesium. Reduced dosage for impaired creatinine clearance.
Class IV			
Verapamil	For paroxysmal supraventricular tachycardia (PSVT) prophylaxis due to reentry For ventricular rate control in patients with chronic atrial fibrillation and/ or atrial flutter in combination with digoxin	**Regular release tablets:** 240–480 mg/day orally in 3–4 divided doses.	Avoid grapefruit juice. May be given without regard to food.
Other			
Digoxin	May be used to control ventricular rate in patients with chronic atrial fibrillation and/or atrial flutter or for the prevention and treatment of narrow-complex paroxysmal supraventricular tachycardia	0.125 mg orally once daily. Maximum dosage: 0.5 mg once daily.	Meets Beers Criteria as potentially inappropriate medication in older adults and not recommended as first-line drug. Narrow therapeutic index.

[a]Antidysrhythmic medications are typically prescribed by specialty practitioners in acute care settings rather than in primary care.

TABLE 12.4   Examples of Adverse Effects of Antiarrhythmic Agents

Drug	Common Adverse Effects	Serious Adverse Effects
Class IA		
Quinidine	Light-headedness, diarrhea, nausea, vomiting, heartburn, esophagitis, fatigue, palpitations, weakness, rash, visual problems, and tremor	Hepatotoxicity, bronchospasm, lupus erythematosus–like syndrome, seizures, ventricular tachycardia, ventricular fibrillation, and torsades de pointes
Procainamide	Myalgias, anorexia, nausea, vomiting, diarrhea, and rash	Lupus erythematosus–like syndrome, blood dyscrasia, agranulocytosis, neutropenia, hypoplastic anemia, thrombocytopenia, HF, asystole, ventricular fibrillation, hypotension, and hepatic dysfunction
Class IB		
Mexiletine	Palpitations, increased PVCs, nausea, vomiting, diarrhea, heartburn, constipation, dizziness, tremor, fatigue, weakness, blurred vision, and paresthesias	Hepatic dysfunction, blood dyscrasias, ventricular tachycardia, ventricular fibrillation, angina, hypotension, bradycardia, second- or third-degree heart block, supraventricular arrhythmias, and cardiogenic shock
Tocainide	Fatigue, palpitations, chest pain, nausea, vomiting, anorexia, diarrhea, dizziness, paresthesias, tremor, headache, anxiety, blurred vision, diaphoresis, and increased PVCs	Blood dyscrasias, agranulocytosis, leukopenia, neutropenia, aplastic/hypoplastic anemia, thrombocytopenia, pulmonary fibrosis/edema, interstitial pneumonitis, HF, hypotension, bradycardia, ventricular tachycardia, and ventricular fibrillation
Class IC		
Flecainide	Dizziness, visual disturbances, dyspnea, headache, nausea, fatigue, palpitations, chest pain, asthenia, tremor, constipation, and edema	HF, bradycardia, second- or third-degree heart block, ventricular tachycardia, ventricular fibrillation, supraventricular arrhythmias, hepatic dysfunction, blood dyscrasias, and death
Propafenone	Unusual taste, nausea, vomiting, headache, fatigue, weakness, palpitations, diarrhea, anorexia, anxiety, and blurred vision	HF, bradycardia, second- or third-degree heart block, ventricular tachycardia, ventricular fibrillation, torsades de pointes, and bronchospasm
Class II		
Propranolol	Fatigue, light-headedness, depression, short-term memory loss, nausea, vomiting, and diarrhea	Bronchospasm, bradycardia, HF, hypotension, and second- or third-degree heart block
Acebutolol	Fatigue, dizziness, depression, headache, nightmares, insomnia, peripheral edema, nausea, diarrhea, pruritus, and rash	Bronchospasm, bradycardia, HF, hypotension, and second- or third-degree heart block
Class III		
Amiodarone	Photosensitivity, hyperthyroidism, hypothyroidism, malaise, fatigue, tremor, poor coordination, nausea, vomiting, constipation, and anorexia	Pulmonary toxicity, hepatic failure, second- or third-degree heart block, blue-gray skin discoloration, bradycardia, ventricular tachycardia, ventricular fibrillation, torsades de pointes, optic neuropathy/neuritis, vision loss, peripheral neuropathy, and HF
Dronedarone	Diarrhea, nausea, vomiting, abdominal pain, dyspepsia, increased creatinine, rash, photosensitivity, and electrolyte abnormalities	Bradycardia, QT prolongation, cardiovascular death (largely arrhythmic), HF, liver failure, interstitial pneumonitis, and pulmonary fibrosis
Class IV		
Verapamil	Constipation, headache, rash, bleeding, visual problems, upper respiratory infection, dizziness, fatigue, edema, nausea, and flushing	Second- or third-degree heart block, bradycardia, HF, and hypotension
Other		
Digoxin	Palpitations, ventricular extrasystoles, tachycardia, anorexia, nausea, vomiting, diarrhea, headache, dizziness, mental disturbances, and rash	Cardiac arrest, second- or third-degree heart block, ventricular tachycardia, and ventricular fibrillation

PVCs, Premature ventricular complexes; *HF,* heart failure.

Contraindications. Quinidine is contraindicated in patients with AV block, left bundle-branch block, digitalis-induced AV conduction disorders, and myasthenia gravis. It should be used cautiously in patients with liver disease, renal impairment, or HF. Avoid in patients with QT prolongation. There are insufficient data to recommend the use of quinidine during pregnancy. It should not be used in patients who are breastfeeding.

Monitoring. Monitor digoxin levels as quinidine can increase plasma levels. Monitor potassium levels as patients may experience decreased efficacy, exacerbation of QT prolongation, and torsades de pointes. Perform periodic complete blood count (CBC) and hepatic and renal function tests. The therapeutic plasma level is 2 to 5 mcg/mL in most laboratories, although a patient-dependent therapeutic response has been shown to occur at levels of 3 to 6 mcg/mL.

Disopyramide

Disopyramide is only used in patients with life-threatening ventricular arrhythmias. Of note, an active metabolite of disopyramide has significant anticholinergic effects that contribute to the medication's overall adverse effects. Treatment should be initiated in a hospital setting due to the medication's proarrhythmic potential.

Pharmacokinetics. Disopyramide is well absorbed following oral administration, with bioavailability ranging between 87% and 95%. It is more than 90% protein bound and well distributed throughout the body. Disopyramide is metabolized by the liver and excreted primarily in the urine. Onset of action is approximately 30 minutes, with peak within 3 hours and duration between 1.5 and 8.5 hours.

Indications. Disopyramide is used for the treatment of life-threatening arrhythmias including sustained ventricular tachycardia.

Adverse Effects. The most common adverse effects are associated with disopyramide's anticholinergic side effects, including xerostomia (32% of patients), urinary retention (15%), and constipation (11%). Patients may also experience urinary frequency, urgency, and hesitation. Infrequent side effects include headache, fatigue, nausea, and vomiting. Rarely, patients may experience AV blockade, prolonged QT, torsades de points, ventricular tachycardia, or other arrhythmia exacerbations. Patients may also experience increased risk for hypoglycemic reactions if they are taking medications that impact blood glucose metabolism.

Contraindications. Disopyramide is contraindicated in patients with AV block and decompensated HF. It should not be used in patients with myasthenia gravis due to its anticholinergic effects. Avoid using in patients taking anticholinergic medications or in patients with glaucoma and urinary retention. Dosage adjustments may be required in patients with renal impairment.

Monitoring. Patients who are taking medications that regulate glucose metabolism should have their blood glucose monitored regularly. Also regularly monitor serum potassium, blood urea nitrogen (BUN) and creatinine, and ECG.

Class IB: Antiarrhythmics

Class IB drugs (mexiletine and lidocaine) exert less effect on sodium channels at rest but are more prominent during depolarization, so their effect on phase 0 is only slight. They bind to both open and closed sodium channels and shorten the repolarization effect. Mexiletine is available in oral form for patients with life-threatening ventricular arrhythmias. Lidocaine is available in an IV form and is indicated for use in ventricular arrythmias in an acute care setting.

Mexiletine

Mexiletine is an analog of lidocaine with efficacy like quinidine. However, it does not prolong the QT interval or precipitate vagal stimulus effects.

Pharmacokinetics. Mexiletine is well absorbed following oral administration. It is distributed approximately 50% to 60% protein bound. Mexiletine is metabolized in the liver; elimination occurs primarily via the biliary tract, with only about 10% excreted unchanged in the urine. Plasma half-life is generally 10 to 12 hours but can be significantly increased in patients with HF, myocardial infarction, or hepatic failure (25 hours). While mexiletine is not primarily excreted by the kidneys, its half-life can be increased to 15.6 hours in patients with renal failure.

Indications. Mexiletine is primarily used in patients with life-threatening ventricular arrhythmias. It is also used in combination with quinidine to increase antiarrhythmic efficacy while reducing adverse effects. Additionally, it is used in conjunction with amiodarone in patients with implantable cardioverter defibrillators and those with recurrent ventricular tachycardia.

Adverse Effects. The most common adverse effects associated with mexiletine are nausea, vomiting, and pyrosis, occurring in nearly 40% of all patients. Neurologic adverse effects include tremors (12.6%), dizziness (10.5%), ataxia (10.2), and headache (7.5%). Mexiletine can worsen arrhythmias, including ventricular tachycardia, AV block, and bradycardia.

Contraindications. Mexiletine is contraindicated in patients who have AV block or are in cardiogenic shock. Use with caution in patients with a history of myocardial infarction, HF, hepatic or renal impairment, and seizure disorder. Mexiletine increases the risk for hypotension.

Monitoring. Obtain baseline creatinine and electrolyte levels and then monitor as needed. Obtain baseline ECG and monitor routinely for changes in rhythm. GI adverse effects may be reduced by administering mexiletine with food. Tobacco smoking can significantly increase the elimination of mexiletine. As a result, it is important to assess the patient's smoking behaviors.

Class IC: Antiarrhythmics

Class IC drugs (flecainide and propafenone) depress phase 0 markedly and slow conduction profoundly. The medications in this class are the most powerful of all the SCBs. They block the sodium channels during the upstroke of the ventricular cells and result in suppression of premature ventricular contractions, PSVT, and AF. They have a marked effect on cardiac function and are usually reserved for patients with severe ventricular tachycardia.

Flecainide

Pharmacokinetics. Flecainide is well absorbed orally, with about 40% to 50% distributed bound to plasma proteins. It is primarily metabolized in the liver by CYP 2D6. Half-life ranges from 12 to 30 hours, with duration of approximately 1 to 2 days. Flecainide has a narrow therapeutic range and must be monitored carefully. Approximately 30% is excreted in the urine and 5% is excreted in the feces.

Indications. Flecainide is clinically indicated in patients with life-threatening ventricular arrhythmias that are unresponsive to other measures. However, it can also be used at certain dosages to prevent paroxysmal AF and/or atrial flutter, and to prevent PSVT in patients who experience disabling symptoms and have no structural heart disease.

Adverse Effects. Serious reactions may include ventricular arrhythmias, congestive heart failure (CHF), heart block, QT prolongation, torsades de pointes, cardiac arrest, cholestasis, hepatic failure, blood dyscrasias, leukopenia, granulocytopenia, thrombocytopenia, and exfoliative dermatitis. Pneumonitis may occur with long-term use.

Contraindications. Use is contraindicated in patients with second- or third-degree AV block without a pacemaker, bifascicular block without a pacemaker, cardiogenic shock, and recent myocardial infarction. Use with caution in patients with structural heart disease, myocardial dysfunction, CHF, QT prolongation, sick sinus syndrome, pacemaker, electrolyte abnormalities, creatinine clearance less than 36, and hepatic impairment.

Monitoring. Obtain baseline electrolytes, including magnesium levels, and monitor creatine levels and serum drug levels. Obtain baseline ECG and routinely monitor for rhythm changes. A black box warning has been issued with this medication because of the increase in mortality in patients with non–life-threatening ventricular arrhythmias. Patients should be made aware of the importance of reporting new or worsening symptoms.

Propafenone

Pharmacokinetics. Propafenone is administered orally and undergoes extensive first-pass metabolism. Distribution is about 85% to 97% protein bound. Metabolism of the drug is primarily dependent on CYP 2D6 isoenzyme activity and generates active metabolites. Dosage and patient response should be carefully monitored due to large intersubject variability in propafenone and metabolite concentrations. Half-life of propafenone extensive metabolizers is typically between 2 and 10 hours, while half-life in poor metabolizers is between 10 and 32 hours. About 38% of metabolites are excreted in the urine, while about 58% are excreted in the feces. Severe hepatic dysfunction increases bioavailability significantly.

Indications. Propafenone is indicated for treatment in patients with life-threatening sustained ventricular tachycardia. It is important to note that propafenone therapy should be initiated in the hospital setting.

Adverse Effects. The most common adverse effects include dysgeusia, nausea, and vomiting (more than 10% of patients). Other adverse effects include dizziness, dyspnea, fatigue, anxiety, constipation, upper respiratory infections, edema, headache, bradycardia, first-degree heart block, palpitations, chest pain, blurred vision, ecchymosis, and weakness.

Serious reactions include ventricular arrhythmias, QT prolongation, torsades de pointes, CHF, AV block, unmasking of Brugada syndrome, asystole, agranulocytosis, myasthenia gravis exacerbation, and hepatotoxicity.

Contraindications. Propafenone is contraindicated in bronchospastic disorders, CHF, cardiogenic shock, severe hypotension, sick sinus syndrome without a pacemaker, AV block without a pacemaker, bradycardia, congenital long QT syndrome, Brugada syndrome, and uncorrected electrolyte abnormalities. Use caution in prescribing propafenone in patients with QT prolongation, family history of QT prolongation, history of torsades de pointes, ventricular arrhythmias, myocardial infarction within 2 years, hepatic and renal impairment, myasthenia gravis, pacemaker, and poor CYP 2D6 metabolizers.

Monitoring. Obtain baseline electrolytes, including magnesium level. Obtain ECG at baseline, after starting the medication and periodically thereafter.

Class II: Beta-Blockers/Beta-Adrenergic Antagonists

Beta-blockers are Class II antiarrhythmics that work by inhibiting sympathetic stimulation. They increase threshold potential and prolong the effective refractory period, resulting in slow HR and conduction velocity. In addition, they antagonize the effects of catecholamines released from the adrenergic nerve endings and the adrenal medulla. Blocking sympathetic activity reduces the rate of discharge of the sinus and other foci that act as pacemakers, and increases the effective refractory period of the AV node.

Beta-blockers are most frequently used in the treatment of ventricular arrhythmias, including supraventricular tachycardias, precipitated by sympathetic stimulation. They are effective in reducing mortality after myocardial infarction, even in patients with relative contraindications such as severe diabetes or asthma. Beta-blockers can be categorized as selective or nonselective. *Selective beta-blockers* act predominantly on the cardiac muscle, while *nonselective beta-blockers* can alter noncardiac tissues.

Propranolol

Pharmacokinetics. Propranolol is a first-generation agent with nonselective-blocking beta-1 and beta-2 receptors. Oral doses of propranolol are almost completely absorbed. This drug undergoes extensive first-past metabolism, with bioavailability at about 25%. Food can increase bioavailability of immediate-release forms up to 50% but does not affect the time of peak concentrations. Peak concentrations for immediate-release forms range between 1 and 4 hours while peak concentration for long-acting capsules is about 6 hours. Propranolol is highly protein bound and crosses the blood–brain barrier. It can cross the placenta and is distributed into breast milk. Propranolol undergoes extensive metabolism in the liver, with half-life prolonged in patients with liver impairment. Excretion is primarily in the urine.

Indications. Propranolol is used in catecholamine-stimulated tachyarrhythmias, which are usually experienced during exercise and emotional stress. It may also be used in patients experiencing AF and/or flutter for the purposes of HR control.

Adverse Effects. A side effect of this medication is smooth muscle spasm, which is typically related to nonselectivity and results in bronchospasm, cold extremities, and impotence.

Contraindications. Propranolol is contraindicated in patients with cardiogenic shock, sinus bradycardia without a pacemaker, sick sinus syndrome without a pacemaker, second- or third-degree AV block without a pacemaker, decompensated HF, and bronchial asthma. Use with caution in older adults, patients in the second or third trimester of pregnancy, patients who have recently undergone or will soon have major surgery, and patients with renal impairment, hepatic impairment, peripheral vascular disease, bronchospastic disease, diabetes mellitus, thyroid disorder, Wolff-Parkinson-White syndrome, pheochromocytoma, myasthenia gravis, history of severe anaphylactic reaction, and musculoskeletal disease.

Monitoring. Routine monitoring of blood pressure and heart rate is recommended. Avoid abrupt withdrawal of this medication due to risk of adverse effects, including chest pain, myocardial infarctions, sudden increase in blood pressure, or arrhythmias.

Acebutolol

Pharmacokinetics. Acebutolol is selective to β1 receptors with little effect on peripheral β2 receptors. Acebutolol is well absorbed from the GI tract following oral administration. It undergoes extensive first-pass metabolism, producing the major active metabolite diacetolol. Half-life is 3 to 4 hours for the parent compound and 8 to 13 hours for diacetolol. Elimination of the parent drug and the metabolite is about 30% to 40% in the urine. In addition, it is eliminated via the bile and through the intestinal wall. Older adults have an increased acebutolol bioavailability and may require a lower dose at initiation.

Indications. Acebutolol is indicated for the treatment of premature ventricular contractions. It can also be used in patients to treat hypertension.

Adverse Effects. The most common adverse effect associated with acebutolol is fatigue, occurring in more than 10% of patients. Patients can also experience dizziness, headache, abnormal dreams, insomnia, and nausea. Other common effects are related to the cardiovascular effects of acebutolol

and include sinus bradycardia, hypotension, angina, and HF. Like other beta-blockers, acebutolol can cause and/or mask symptoms of hypoglycemia.

Contraindications. Acebutolol is contraindicated in patients with AV block, bradycardia, HF, and cardiogenic shock. It should not be used in patients with hyperthyroidism or thyrotoxicosis. Acebutolol should be used cautiously in patients with asthma, COPD, diabetes mellitus, or hepatic or renal disease. It should not be abruptly discontinued due to the risk of myocardial ischemia, myocardial infarction, severe hypertension, and ventricular dysrhythmias.

Monitoring. Regularly monitor heart rate and blood pressure. Advise patients to avoid abruptly stopping their medication due to the risk of adverse cardiac effects. Monitor serum BUN/creatinine.

Class III: Potassium Channel Blockers

Class III drugs (amiodarone, dronedarone, and sotalol) prolong phase 3 repolarization by blocking potassium channels. The QT interval is thus prolonged on the ECG, which can also increase the risk of torsades de pointes, a ventricular tachycardia.

However, amiodarone does not appear to have this effect. This medication is considered a mixed-class agent—that is, it is mainly a Class III agent but also has Class I, II, and IV antiarrhythmic effects. As a Class I agent, it decreases the firing rate in pacemaker cells; as a Class II agent, it noncompetitively antagonizes alpha and beta receptors; and as a Class IV agent, it blocks calcium channels, which results in significant AV node block and bradycardia. Amiodarone's vasodilatory action decreases cardiac workload and therefore decreases myocardial oxygen consumption. Dronedarone is a benzofuran derivative of amiodarone that was recently approved by the U.S. Food and Drug Administration (FDA). There is some indication that it prolongs the QT interval. As a nonselective beta-blocker, sotalol exhibits both Class II and Class III antiarrhythmic effects.

Amiodarone

Pharmacokinetics. Oral amiodarone is absorbed incompletely and slowly from the GI tract, with average absolute bioavailability at 50%. Variable systemic availability of oral amiodarone may be attributed to large interindividual variability in CYP 3A4 activity. Once in the systemic circulation, amiodarone distributes widely throughout the body. Amiodarone and its metabolites are extensively bound to plasma proteins. Because of its wide distribution, including to adipose tissue, elimination of amiodarone is prolonged, with a mean half-life of approximately 53 days. This can lead to persistent adverse effects even after discontinuation. Onset of action can be as long as 2 to 3 months unless loading doses are used. Amiodarone and its metabolite are extensively metabolized and eliminated by the liver.

Indications. Amiodarone is used for the treatment and prevention of frequently recurring ventricular fibrillation and unstable ventricular tachycardia in patients who are refractory to other therapy. It is most effective in low doses and in patients experiencing HF or recent myocardial infarction.

Adverse Effects. Nausea and vomiting, constipation, loss of appetite, dysgeusia, and mild abdominal pain are common with oral amiodarone therapy. GI adverse effects may be reduced by dosage reduction or division or by giving the medication with food and/or fluids. Major adverse effects typically occur with long-term therapy and/or higher doses. These include pulmonary toxicity, cardiac arrhythmias, liver failure, blood dyscrasias, and renal impairment.

Photosensitivity can occur in about 10% of those on amiodarone. Blue-gray skin discoloration can occur with sun exposure over long-term use. This typically dissipates with discontinuation of the drug.

BLACK BOX WARNING!

Amiodarone

- Amiodarone is intended only for patients with life-threatening arrhythmias due to the risk of severe adverse effects.
- Pulmonary toxicity can occur in patients with long-term use and can be fatal. Obtain baseline CXR and pulmonary function tests when initiating amiodarone.
- Amiodarone can cause fatal hepatoxicity. Risk is increased in patients with preexisting liver disease.
- Amiodarone can exacerbate arrhythmias including ventricular fibrillation, increased resistance to cardioversion, ventricular tachycardia and QT prolongation, torsade de pointes, sinus bradycardia, and sinus arrest.

Contraindications. Hypersensitivity to amiodarone or its components may occur. This medication is contraindicated in patients with severe sinus node dysfunction, marked sinus bradycardia, second- and third-degree AV block, syncope caused by bradycardia, or cardiogenic shock.

QUALITY AND SAFETY

Beers Criteria and Amiodarone

Amiodarone is considered a potentially inappropriate medication for use in older adults. It should be avoided in patients with AF unless the patient has HF or significant left ventricular hypertrophy. It has greater toxicities than other antiarrhythmics used in AF.

Monitoring. Closely monitor CBC, thyroid function, HR, and blood pressure with each visit. Advise patients that they may take amiodarone with or without food but that they should be consistent to avoid variation in absorption between doses. Plasma concentrations may be helpful in evaluating nonresponsiveness or unexpectedly severe toxicity. Advise patients to use sunscreen and protective clothing.

Perform baseline chest radiographs and pulmonary function tests, including diffusion capacity, before initiation of therapy. Patient history, physical examination, and chest radiograph should be performed every 3 to 6 months. Thyroid function is needed at baseline and periodically during therapy. Assess liver enzymes at baseline and at least twice yearly. Additionally, obtain annual ophthalmic examination, including funduscopic and slit-lamp examinations, to detect optic neuritis.

Dronedarone

Dronedarone is a new agent, structurally similar to amiodarone in that it has the antiarrhythmic effects of amiodarone but without the adverse effects. It does not include iodine in its structure and has a short half-life; therefore it has a lower risk of thyroid toxicity. In addition, dronedarone has decreased lipophilicity compared to amiodarone, which also contributes to its shorter half-life, and lower tissue accumulation compared with amiodarone.

Pharmacokinetics. Dronedarone is administered orally. It is highly bound to plasma proteins and metabolized in the liver, primarily by the CPY 3A isoenzyme. Steady-state concentration is reached within 4 to 8 days at the usual dose. Half-life is 13 to 18 hours, with excretion primarily as metabolites in the feces (approximately 84%). Exposure to dronedarone is approximately 23% higher in older adults, 30% higher in females, and twofold higher in Japanese males than White males.

PHARMACOGENETICS

Dronedarone

- Dronedarone is a substrate of the CYP 3A isoenzyme, a moderate inhibitor of CYP 3A and CYP 2D6, and an inhibitor of P-glycoprotein transport.
- Plasma concentration of dronedarone may be affected by inhibitors and inducers of CYP 3A.
- Dronedarone may interact with drugs that are substrates of CYP 3A and CYP 2D6.
- All drugs that are CPY 3A4 inhibitors should be discontinued prior to beginning dronedarone therapy.

BLACK BOX WARNING!

Dronedarone

- Dronedarone is contraindicated in patients with New York Heart Association (NYHA) Class IV HF or who have symptomatic HF with recent decompensation that required hospitalization due to the increased risk of mortality.
- Dronedarone is contraindicated in patients with permanent AF due to the increased risk for stroke, HF, and death.

Indications. Dronedarone is used for patients who are in sinus rhythm and have a history of paroxysmal AF or persistent AF in order to reduce the risk of hospitalization for AF. It is contraindicated for patients who cannot be cardioverted to normal sinus rhythm.

Adverse Effects. The most common adverse effect associated with dronedarone is QT prolongation, which can occur in up to 28% of patients. GI effects are common and include diarrhea, nausea, vomiting, and dyspepsia. HF, bradycardia, and stroke are infrequent but may be severe. Hepatic and renal failure have been reported in patients receiving dronedarone. Electrolyte abnormalities (hypokalemia, hypomagnesemia) have occurred if dronedarone was administered with potassium-depleting diuretics.

Contraindications. Absolute contraindications include sick sinus syndrome, QT prolongation, bradycardia, and AV block. In addition, dronedarone is contraindicated in patients with HF, patients who are pregnant or breastfeeding, and those with amiodarone-induced lung or liver toxicity. There are black box warnings specifically addressing patients with NYHA Class IV HF or patients with permanent AF. Dronedarone should be used cautiously in females, older adults, and those with sickle cell anemia or systemic inflammatory or autoimmune disorders due to risk of QT prolongation. Use with caution in patients of Asian descent.

Monitoring. Obtain ECG and serum creatinine, magnesium, and potassium levels prior to administration. Monitor liver enzymes closely. ECG should be monitored every 3 months. Because of a high mortality rate from cardiovascular events such as stroke and CHF in patients taking this drug, the FDA required relabeling of the product and it is unclear whether it will remain on the market. It is intended for short-term use only in those with nonpermanent AF.

Sotalol

Sotalol is a mixed-class antiarrhythmic: it is a nonselective beta-blocker (Class II characteristic), and it can increase the action potential by blocking potassium channels (Class III characteristics).

Pharmacokinetics. Sotalol is well absorbed following oral administration. Food reduces bioavailability by about 20%, but this medication may be taken with or without food. Peak plasma concentrations are reached within 2.5 to 4 hours, with steady-state plasma concentrations reached within 2 to 3 days. Sotalol is not metabolized and is primarily excreted unchanged in the urine.

Indications. Sotalol is indicated in severe ventricular arrhythmias and in patients who do not tolerate the side effects of amiodarone. It is also used to prevent atrial flutter and AF.

Adverse Effects. The most common adverse effect of sotalol is fatigue, occurring in up to 26% of patients. Other common adverse effects include asthenia, headache, dyspnea, and dizziness. Symptomatic bradycardia can occur in as many as 13% of patients taking sotalol. Infrequently, sotalol can cause palpitations and torsades de pointes. Nausea, vomiting, and diarrhea can also occur.

Contraindications. Sotalol is contraindicated in patients with sinus bradycardia, sick sinus syndrome without a pacemaker, second- or third-degree AV block without a pacemaker, congenital or acquired QT prolongation, baseline QTc greater than 450 msec, uncorrected electrolyte abnormalities, cardiogenic shock, decompensated HF, and bronchospastic disorders. Sotalol is also contraindicated in patients with a creatinine clearance less than 40 mL/min, AF, atrial flutter, or in IV use. Use with caution in patients with ventricular arrhythmias, history of torsades de pointes, family history of QT prolongation, recent myocardial infarction, coronary artery disease (CAD), hypotension, creatinine clearance less than 60 mL/min, diabetes mellitus, thyroid disorder, peripheral vascular disease (PVD), pheochromocytoma, myasthenia gravis, history of severe anaphylactic reaction, or before, during, and/or after major surgery.

Monitoring. Obtain creatinine level and electrolytes, including magnesium, at baseline and before dose increase. Obtain blood pressure at baseline, then periodically. Obtain ECG and monitor QT interval after dose initiation and dose increase. Avoid abrupt withdrawal of the medication.

Class IV: Calcium Channel Blockers

CCBs are used to slow conduction in order to prevent reentry. Their antiarrhythmic properties are still controversial. In patients with CAD, there is a decrease in calcium inflow to the myocytes, resulting in the alteration of cardiac muscle contraction. CCBs also cause vasodilation, decreased cardiac muscle contractions, decreased heart rate, and slowed conduction through the AV node, which in turn limits reentry. There are two different receptor types and their differences are seen in the blocking action of the agents. Both types, however, reduce afterload with little effect on preload. They also differ in selectivity of cardiac calcium channels versus vascular calcium channels. Type 1 CCBs (nondihydropyroidines), which impact both myocardial cells and vascular smooth muscle cells, will be discussed here. Type II CCBs (dihydropyridines) have the strongest affinity to the vascular calcium channel and are most often used in the treatment of hypertension and angina. They are discussed in Chapters 9 and 10.

Type I Calcium Channel Blockers or Nondihydropyridines

The nondihydropyridine CCBs (verapamil and diltiazem) inhibit calcium ion influx through slow channels into conductive and contractile myocardial cells and vascular smooth muscle cells. They also slow AV conduction and prolong the effective refractory period within the AV node. These agents do not play a role in ventricular arrhythmias. They are useful in select SVTs because of the slowing of AV node conduction. Additionally, they have the propensity to worsen ventricular arrhythmias, so assessment for the presence of ventricular arrhythmias before starting a patient on this type of medication is vital.

Verapamil

Pharmacokinetics. Oral verapamil undergoes an extensive first-pass effect. It is approximately 90% protein bound and is widely distributed throughout the body, including the central nervous system (CNS). It is distributed in the placenta and in breast milk. Verapamil is extensively metabolized in the liver into more than 12 metabolites, with one of the metabolites, norverapamil, possessing about 20% activity of the parent compound. In addition, in older adults the bioavailability of verapamil and norverapamil is increased 87% and 77%, respectively. Duration of action generally ranges from 8 to 10 hours for standard-release forms and 24 hours for extended-release forms. Verapamil is excreted, primarily as its metabolites, in the urine.

PHARMACOGENETICS

Verapamil

Verapamil inhibits CYP 3A4 isoenzymes. Inducers or inhibitors of CYP 3A4 may cause significant interactions with verapamil. All patients who receive verapamil should be monitored carefully for drug interactions.

QUALITY AND SAFETY

Verapamil

- Verapamil is marketed in several oral dosage forms that are not completely interchangeable. Always carefully review the administration instructions regarding timing and the impact of taking the medication with food.
- Avoid drinking grapefruit juice before or after administration to avoid increases in verapamil bioavailability.

Indications. In addition to its antihypertensive properties, verapamil is indicated in the conversion and prevention of paroxysmal SVT and AF/atrial flutter. It is also used in patients with angina and as prophylaxis for migraine headaches.

Adverse Effects. Serious reactions include CHF, severe hypotension, AV block, severe bradycardia, hepatotoxicity, and paralytic ileus. Common reactions include constipation, dizziness, nausea, hypotension, headache, edema, and fatigue.

Contraindications. Verapamil is contraindicated in severe left ventricular dysfunction, sick sinus syndrome without a pacemaker, second- or third-degree AV block without a pacemaker, AF/atrial flutter with accessory bypass tract, systolic blood pressure less than 90 mmHg, and cardiogenic shock. Use with caution in patients with CHF, bradycardia, hepatic impairment, renal impairment, muscular dystrophy, myasthenia gravis, or gastroesophageal reflux disease (GERD), and in older adults.

Monitoring. Obtain baseline ECG. Monitor liver function tests, blood pressure, and heart rate.

Diltiazem

Pharmacokinetics. This agent has selectivity toward vascular calcium channels and intermediate properties of type I and type II CCBs. It holds both cardiac depressant and vasodilation properties, so it can reduce arterial pressure without generating a similar effect on the heart that is observed in type II CCBs.

Indications. In addition to its antihypertensive properties, diltiazem is indicated in conversion of PSVT and in AF/atrial flutter. It is also used in patients with angina.

Adverse Effects. Serious reactions include bradycardia, AV block, arrhythmias, severe hypotension, syncope, cardiac failure, CHF, acute hepatic injury, hypersensitivity reactions, erythema multiforme, exfoliative dermatitis, and acute generalized exanthematous pustulosis. Common reactions include peripheral edema, headache, nausea, dizziness, asthenia, orthostatic hypotension, constipation, rash, bradycardia, first-degree AV block, and elevated alanine transaminase (ALT) and aspartate aminotransferase (AST) levels.

Contraindications. Diltiazem is contraindicated in sick sinus syndrome without a pacemaker, second- or third-degree AV block without a pacemaker, systolic blood pressure less than 90 mmHg, acute myocardial infarction with pulmonary congestion, AF/atrial flutter with accessory bypass tract (with IV use), and ventricular tachycardia (with IV use). Use with caution in patients with renal and hepatic impairment, CHF, cardiac conduction defects, and left ventricular dysfunction.

Monitoring. Obtain baseline ECG. Monitor BUN and creatinine levels, liver function tests, blood pressure, and HR.

Other

Digoxin

Although digoxin was once commonly used to treat HF and AF, it has largely been replaced by other, more effective and less toxic medications. Digoxin is a cardiac glycoside that has a substantial effect on the electrical activity of the heart. It acts to increase the slope of phase 4 depolarization, shortens the duration of the action potential, and decreases maximal diastolic potential. Digoxin also slows the ventricular rate in patients with AF by decreasing atrial depolarizations that reach the ventricle.

Pharmacokinetics. Oral digoxin is rapidly absorbed from the GI tract. Approximately 20% to 30% is plasma protein bound and is distributed throughout body tissues. Digoxin crosses the placenta and can be found in breast milk. Onset of effect usually occurs within 30 minutes to 2 hours after dosing, with peak effect between 2 and 6 hours. A small amount of digoxin is metabolized to inactive metabolites in the liver. Between 30% and 50% is excreted unchanged in the urine. Half-life is normally between 30 and 40 hours. Renal impairment can increase half-life to up to 4 to 6 days.

Indications. Labeled use of digoxin is for ventricular rate control in patients with chronic AF or in patients with HF. It also has unlabeled use in patients with atrial flutter, for treatment of narrow-complex PSVT, and for prevention of PSVT in patients without a delta wave on an ECG during sinus rhythm.

Adverse Effects. Patients taking digoxin may experience mild nausea, headache, and dizziness or diarrhea. Digoxin has caused visual disturbances, including blurred or yellow vision, in about 3% of patients. This is more likely in toxic doses but may continue after other signs of toxicity have resolved. Cardiac arrhythmias including palpitations, PVCs, and cardiac arrest are uncommon (fewer than 1% of patients). Rarely, digoxin has also been associated with abdominal pain, bowel ischemia, and hemorrhagic bowel necrosis of the intestines. Of note, loss of appetite, nausea, vomiting, and diarrhea may also be signs of digoxin toxicity, so patients should be monitored carefully (Table 12.5).

Contraindications. Digoxin is contraindicated in patients with ventricular fibrillation. It should be used cautiously in patients with sick sinus syndrome, any AV block, or any ventricular arrythmias; patients with electrolyte imbalances, including hypokalemia, hypercalcemia, and hypomagnesemia; patients with COPD, as acute hypoxemia can increase cardiac sensitivity to digoxin; and patients who are pregnant or breastfeeding.

Monitoring. Monitor patients for development of toxicities. Report any occurrence of patients seeing a yellow halo around objects, as well as symptoms of nausea, decreased appetite, or episodes of extreme fatigue, as these may indicate early toxicity. See Table 12.5 for digoxin levels associated with therapeutic and toxic concentrations.

Prescriber Considerations for Antiarrhythmic Therapy

In 2017, the American Heart Association (AHA), the American College of Cardiology (ACC), and the Heart Rhythm Society (HRS) released guidelines for management of patients with ventricular arrhythmias and prevention of sudden cardiac death (Al-Khatib et al., 2018). More recently, they updated their guidelines for management of patients with AF (January et al., 2019). Another source of practice guidelines is the American Academy of Family Physicians (AAFP), which updated the pharmacologic management of newly diagnosed AF. Both guidelines recommend the use of CCBs over digoxin, although the AAFP recommends a more lenient rate control than the AHA/ACC/HRS guidelines (Savoy, 2017).

> ### BOOKMARK THIS!
>
> **Clinical Guidelines for Antiarrhythmic Therapy**
>
> - Updated clinical guidelines for various arrhythmias and other clinical topics can be found at the American College of Cardiology website, https://www.acc.org/Education-and-Meetings/Products-and-Resources/Guideline-Education. These include guidelines for AF, bradycardia and cardiac conduction delays, ventricular arrhythmias, and sudden cardiac death.
> - The American Academy of Family Physicians provides clinical recommendations on a variety of acute and chronic conditions, including management of AF. Visit https://www.aafp.org/family-physician/patient-care/clinical-recommendations.A.html#adl-az-list.
> - The American Heart Association has an extensive database of guidelines and statements at https://professional.heart.org/en/guidelines-and-statements/guidelines-and-statements-search.

Clinical Reasoning for Antiarrhythmic Therapy

Consider the individual patient's health problem requiring antiarrhythmic therapy. Carefully evaluate the patient's risk factors that may contribute to the arrhythmia, including electrolyte or acid/base imbalances, thyroid disorders, heavy use of alcohol or caffeine, substance use disorders, and medications. The AHA published a scientific statement regarding drugs that may cause or exacerbate cardiac arrhythmias including bradyarrhythmias, supraventricular tachyarrhythmias, and ventricular arrhythmias (Tisdale et al., 2020).

Determine the desired therapeutic outcome based on the degree of antiarrhythmic therapy needed for the patient's health problem. Consult clinical practice guidelines to help determine appropriate goals for each patient. For example, what is the most appropriate degree of rate control for patients with AF? In addition to rate control, what anticoagulant medications will be used to prevent stroke in these patients? Maintain strong communication with specialty practices to ensure shared goals.

TABLE 12.5 Digoxin (Serum, Plasma) Levels

Type of Level	Traditional Units	Scientific International Units	Comments
Therapeutic concentration (Congestive heart failure)	0.5–1 ng/mL	0.6–1.3 nmol/L	
Therapeutic concentration (Arrhythmias)	0.8–2 ng/mL	1–2.6 nmol/L	Titrate dose to goal heart rate
Toxic concentration	>2.5 ng/mL	>3.2 nmol/L	
Toxic concentration (Child)	>3 ng/mL	>3.8 nmol/L	

From Elsevier. (2019). *Clinical pharmacology powered by ClinicalKey®.* Retrieved from http://www.clinicalkey.com.

Assess the antiarrhythmic selected for its appropriateness for an individual patient by considering the medication's side effects and the patient's age, race/ethnicity, comorbidities, and genetic factors. A normal change as a result of aging is the loss of conduction fibers in the heart, which can predispose patients to benign arrhythmias; therefore, older patients should be evaluated carefully. Older adults are also at increased risk for adverse effects of antiarrhythmics and may require adjusted dosages to avoid possible impaired renal or hepatic function. The safety and efficacy of many of these drugs have not been established in pediatric patients. It is essential to maintain strong communication with specialty providers. Exposure to dronedarone is higher in older adults and females and has a twofold higher exposure in Japanese males compared to White males. As a result, it is imperative to monitor patients carefully if dronedarone is prescribed by specialists for these populations.

Initiate the treatment plan with the selected medication by first providing adequate patient education to ensure the patient's understanding and promote full participation in the antiarrhythmic therapy. Ensure complete patient and family understanding about the medication prescribed for antiarrhythmic therapy using a variety of education strategies. Important medication information to reinforce includes expected therapeutic effects, potential adverse effects, any monitoring or follow-up needed, and the importance of checking with the primary care provider before starting any new medications and supplements in order to prevent any potential drug and food interactions. Instruct the patient on adverse effects to report to the health care provider and when to seek emergency care.

Conduct follow-up and monitoring of patient responses to antiarrhythmic therapy to note any adverse effects and to ensure strong communication with the patient's specialty practitioners. Obtain baseline laboratory values such as CBC, electrolytes, thyroid panel, and renal and hepatic function tests and then follow-up labs as indicated. While total elimination of all arrythmia medications may not be realistic, prevention of potentially fatal ventricular arrhythmias as well as prevention of complications of arrhythmias (e.g., stroke in patients with AF) is critical. Discuss with the patient their ability to adhere to the medication and whether changes are required. Ensure that the patient has an adequate supply of medication to last until the next follow-up appointment with either the primary care provider or the specialty practitioner.

Teaching Points for Antiarrhythmic Therapy

Health Promotion Strategies

- Advise the patient to wear a medical alert bracelet and to carry medical information specifying that they are taking an antiarrhythmic drug.

- Teach the patient to report any new or uncomfortable symptoms to their primary care provider.
- Carefully review the patient's caffeine, tobacco, and alcohol intake as use of these substances may increase the possibility for arrhythmias.
- Examine carefully all cardiovascular risk factors, including hypertension, hyperlipidemia, tobacco use, and lack of physical activity, to advise the patient of their cardiovascular health status.
- Encourage regular physical activity to improve overall cardiovascular outcomes.

Patient Education for Medication Safety

- Be sure to take all medications as prescribed by your health care provider.
- Before you add any medication, including OTC or herbal medications, speak to your provider or pharmacist to avoid drug interactions.
- The American Heart Association at www.heart.org is a great source for information on overall cardiovascular health.
- Avoid products that contain nicotine or tobacco or any stimulant drugs that may increase your risk of arrhythmias.
- Discuss alcohol use with your health care provider. If alcohol triggers your arrhythmia, eliminate it from your diet. If it does not, limit alcohol use according to current guidelines.
- Contact your health care provider if your symptoms worsen, if you have new symptoms, or if you feel depressed.
- If you are interested in increasing your physical activity, contact your health care provider to discuss what exercises are best for you.
- If you have AF or atrial flutter, it is likely that you will also be taking anticoagulant medications. These are critical to your overall well-being and to reducing complications. Work closely with your health care provider to ensure that you are receiving all the benefits of these medications while decreasing the risk of adverse effects.

Application Questions for Discussion

1. As a primary care provider, what are the patient and safety factors that should be considered in managing the care of a patient requiring an antiarrhythmic?
2. What should be included in the education plan for a patient and/or caregiver who has been prescribed a Class II antiarrhythmic? Class III?
3. What role may genetics play in the treatment response to some antiarrhythmics?

Selected Bibliography

Al-Khatib, S. M., Stevenson, W. G., Ackerman, M. J., Bryant, W. J., Callans, D. J., Curtis, A. B., & Page, R. L. (2018). 2017 AHA/ACC/HRS Guideline for Management of Patients with Ventricular Arrhythmias and the Prevention of Sudden Cardiac Death: Executive Summary. *Journal of the American College of Cardiology, 72*(14), 1677–1749. http://doi.org/10.1016/j.jacc.2017.10.053.

Chalmers, S. W., & Champion, C. R. (2019). Pharmacotherapeutics in cardiovascular dysrhythmias. *The Journal for Nurse Practitioners, (15)*, 1132–1138.

Cosio, F. G. (2017). Atrial flutter, typical and atypical: A review. *Arrhythmia and Electrophysiology Review, 6*(2), 55–62. Retrieved from https://www.ncbi.nlm.nih.gov/pmc/articles/PMC5522718/pdf/aer-06-55.pdf.

Elsevier. Clinical pharmacology powered by ClinicalKey®. (2019). Retrieved from http://www.clinicalkey.com.

Farzam, K., & Tivakaran, V. S. (2020). QT Prolonging Drugs. [Updated 2020 Nov. 27]. In: *StatPearls [Internet]*. Treasure Island (FL): StatPearls Publishing; 2020 Jan-Available from. https://www.ncbi.nlm.nih.gov/books/NBK534864/.

Hauk, L. (2017). Newly detected atrial fibrillation: AAFP updates guideline on pharmacologic management. *American Family Physician, 96*(5), 332–333.

January, C. T., Wann, L. S., Calkins, H., Chen, L. Y., Cigarroa, J. E., Cleveland, J. C., & Yancy, C. W. (2019). 2019 AHA/ACC/HRS Focused Update of the 2014 AHA/ACC/HRS Guideline for the Management of Patients with Atrial Fibrillation. *Journal of the American College of Cardiology, 74*(1), 104–132. http://doi.org/10.1016/j.jacc.2019.01.011.

Katzung, B. G., Kruidering-Hall, M., & Trevor, A. J. (2019). *Katzung & Trevor's Pharmacology: Examination & Board Review* (12th ed.). New York: McGraw-Hill. https://accesspharmacy-mhmedical-com.ezproxy.hsc.usf.edu/content.aspx?bookid=2465&sectionid=197943453.

McCance, K. L., & Huether, S. E. (2019). *Pathophysiology: The Biologic Basis for Disease in Adults and Children* (8th ed.). St. Louis: Elsevier.

Savoy, M. L. (2017). Differences Between the AAFP Atrial Fibrillation Guideline and the AHA/ACC/HRS Guideline. *American Family Physician, 96*(5), 284–285.

Tilton, J. J., Sanoski, C., & Bauman, J. L (2020). The arrhythmias. In J. T. DiPiro, G. C. Yee, L. Posey, S. T. Haines, T. D. Nolin, & V. Ellingrod (Eds.), *Pharmacotherapy: A Pathophysiologic Approach* (11th ed.). New York: McGraw-Hill https://accesspharmacy-mhmedical-com.ezproxy.hsc.usf.edu/content.aspx?bookid=2577&sectionid=233592457.

Tisdale, J. E., Chung, M. K., Campbell, K. B., Hammadah, M., Joglar, J. A., Leclerc, J., & Rajagopalan, B. (2020). Drug-Induced Arrhythmias: A Scientific Statement from the American Heart Association. *Circulation, 142*(15), e214–e233. http://doi.org/10.1161/CIR.0000000000000905.

Additional Resources

Medscape: https://reference.medscape.com/
Prescribers Digital Reference: https://www.pdr.net/
Epocrates: https://online.epocrates.com/

13

Anemia Medications

CONSTANCE G. VISOVSKY

Overview

Anemia is considered the most common blood disorder in the United States, affecting about 5.6% of the population. Primary care visits for anemia account for 5.5 million visits annually (Shappert & Rechtsteiner, 2008). *Anemia* is defined as having a hemoglobin (Hb) less than 13 Gm/dL in males and less than 12 Gm/dL in females. Children 6 months to 6 years of age are considered anemic at Hb levels less than 11 Gm/dL, and children 6 to 14 years of age are considered anemic at Hb levels less than 12 Gm/dL (World Health Organization, 2011). A diagnosis of iron deficiency anemia (IDA) requires laboratory evidence of low iron stores (*serum ferritin*) and an abnormal (high or low) reticulocyte count. Anemia itself is not considered a specific disease state. Rather, it can result from acute blood loss, chronic disease, or hereditary conditions that cause decreased or faulty red blood cell (RBC) production or increased destruction of RBCs.

The production of RBCs is affected by genetic factors that interfere with the proper structure of RBC components and by a deficiency of any one of the elements/components that are required for proper RBC production or function. Some conditions associated with these causes of anemia include sickle cell anemia, IDA, vitamin B_{12} deficiency, and bone marrow or stem cell disease. IDA is the most common type of anemia, accounting for 50% of all cases of anemia worldwide. According to Hempel & Bollard (2016), IDA affects approximately 1% to 2% of the U.S. population.

The destruction of RBCs can be triggered by inherited conditions, such as sickle cell anemia and thalassemia, or as a consequence of snake or spider venom. Acute blood loss resulting in anemia can be caused by trauma, gastrointestinal (GI) bleeding, gastric acid-suppressing medications, and chronic conditions such as renal failure, heart failure, human immunodeficiency virus (HIV) infection, cancer, inflammatory bowel disease, and malabsorption syndromes.

Relevant Physiology

Erythropoietin is a hormone that is made in the kidney and secreted by renal cortical interstitial cells in response to tissue hypoxia. Erythropoietin is the main regulator of the production of RBCs and also stimulates the synthesis of Hb. *Erythropoiesis* is the process by which new RBCs are formed. RBCs are produced in the bone marrow in response to the presence of erythropoietin. The process from stem cell to mature RBC takes 7 days. Under normal conditions, RBCs survive in the bloodstream 120 days before being degraded and cleared from the circulation by phagocytic cells in the liver and spleen. The juxtaglomerular cells in the kidney respond to decreased oxygen delivery to tissues by producing erythropoietin. Erythropoietin works to stimulate the proliferation and differentiation of red cell precursors found in the bone marrow and protects these precursor cells from *apoptosis* (cell death). Erythropoietin also works with other growth factors such as IL-3, IL-6, and glucocorticoids in the development of erythroid cells. Erythropoietin binds to the erythropoietin receptor on red blood progenitor cell surfaces to activate signaling cascades involved in cell survival, differentiation, and communication, resulting in the proliferation of erythroid cells.

Iron, folate, vitamin B_{12}, and several other elements are also needed for RBC production. Iron is a key component of Hb in RBCs. Typically, adults have at least 3 to 4 Gm of stored iron that is balanced between physiologic iron loss and dietary intake. About 25 mg of iron is needed daily for heme synthesis. Most iron is incorporated into Hb, with the remainder stored as ferritin or myoglobin. As iron is not excreted and can accumulate to toxic levels, the intake of iron is tightly regulated. *Hepcidin*, a peptide hormone produced primarily in the liver, regulates systemic iron homeostasis. When systemic iron levels are low, hepcidin decreases, and more iron is released into the plasma.

To maintain adequate numbers of RBCs, immature RBCs known as *reticulocytes* are continually released into the circulation in small amounts by the bone marrow. A feedback loop involving erythropoietin helps regulate erythropoiesis so that the rate of RBC production equals the rate of removal of older, defective RBCs from the body to ensure adequate tissue oxygenation (Nandakumar, Ulirsch, & Sankaran, 2016) (Fig. 13.1).

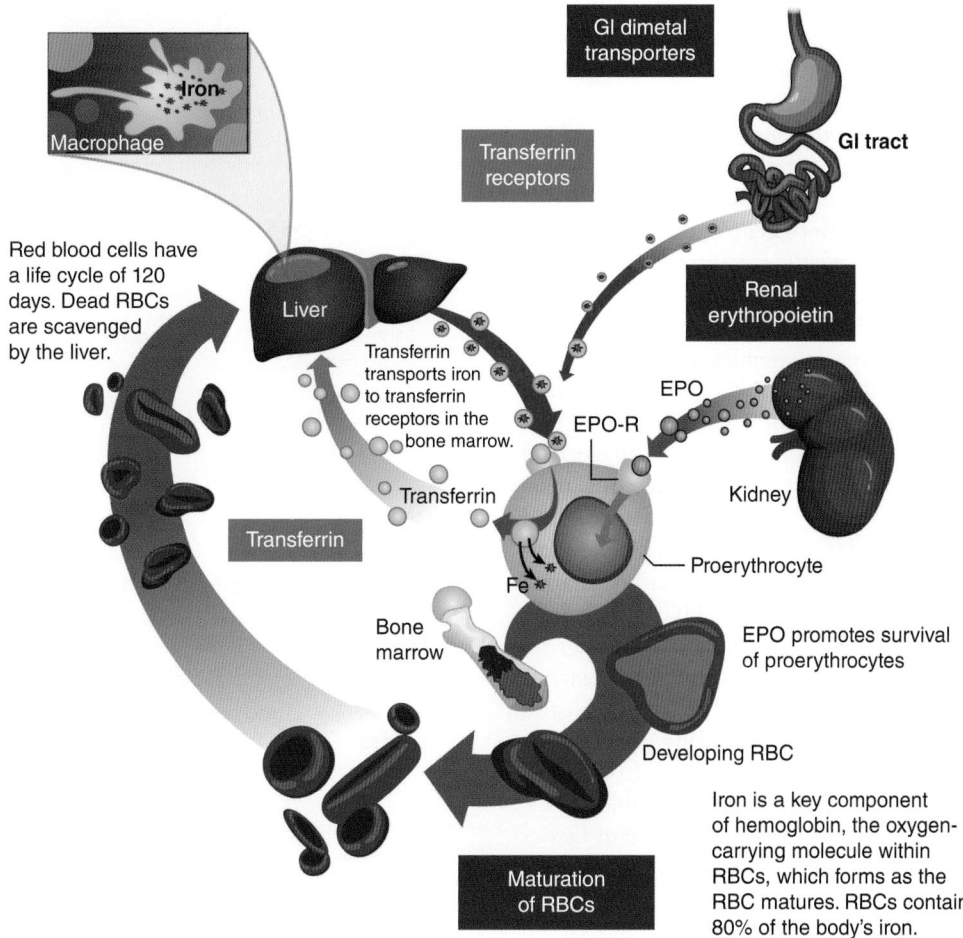

• **Fig. 13.1** Erythrocyte production and life cycle. (From Provenzano, R, Lerma, E. V., & Szczech, L. [Eds.]. [2017]. *Management of anemia: A comprehensive guide for clinicians.* New York: Springer.

Pathophysiology: Anemia

All types of anemia ultimately result in the decreased ability of the blood to carry and transport oxygen to the target tissues and organs. With decreased oxygen available to the tissues, cellular mitochondria are adversely affected, which in turn results in a decrease in adenosine triphosphate (ATP) production. ATP can still be produced through glycolysis. In addition to being a less-efficient energy production pathway, the glycolic pathway increases the renin-angiotensin-aldosterone response, which causes fluid and electrolyte shifts and results in the formation of lactic acid, adversely affecting the body's acid–base balance.

The reduced number of circulating RBCs and decreased Hb results in hypoxia and tissue ischemia, causing fatigue, weakness, pale skin and mucosa, exertional dyspnea, and dizziness. To compensate for the decrease in circulating RBCs available to oxygenate tissues, the rate and depth of respirations increase. Hypoxia also affects the cardiovascular system, forcing it to compensate by increasing stroke volume, heart rate, and myocardial oxygen demand, which increases the risk for heart failure.

This chapter focuses on IDA caused by impairment in RBC production and includes pernicious anemia, as this condition is commonly treated in the primary care setting. Pernicious anemia is characterized by impairment in erythrocyte production and absorption of vitamin B_{12} resulting from a lack of *intrinsic factor*. Intrinsic factor is normally produced by the parietal cells of the stomach. When intrinsic factor is not produced or vitamin B_{12} is not absorbed, pernicious anemia results. The deficiency in vitamin B_{12} is thought to be the result of an autoimmune response against intrinsic factor. Without intrinsic factor, deoxyribonucleic acid (DNA) synthesis is impaired, negatively affecting RBC production (Chaparro & Suchdev, 2019).

Anemia Classification and Grading

Anemias are classified by erythrocyte size and amount of Hb. Size is classified as *normocytic* (normal size), *microcytic* (smaller than normal), or *macrocytic* (larger than normal). Size is related to the amount of various products and fluid within each cell. The amount of Hb is evaluated by degree or depth of color because Hb is a pigmented compound. *Normochromic* cells have normal depth of color and *hypochromic* cells have less depth of color (and less Hb), making them appear pale.

In patients with anemia, the *mean corpuscular volume* (MCV)—a measure of the average volume of an RBC—is used to classify the anemia as normocytic, microcytic, or macrocytic. The amount of Hb present in the RBC is measured by the *mean cell hemoglobin concentration* (MCHC), which represents the average concentration of Hb in erythrocytes in a given volume of blood.

Normocytic, normochromic anemias are characterized by normal MCV and normal MCHC and include anemias of chronic disease, hemolytic anemias (destruction of RBCs), anemia resulting from acute hemorrhage, and aplastic anemias (lack of RBC precursors in bone marrow). Microcytic, hypochromic anemias are characterized by low MCV and low MCHC and include IDA and thalassemia. Macrocytic, normochromic anemias are characterized by high MCV and normal MCHC and include vitamin B_{12} deficiencies and folate deficiencies. Table 13.1 lists the MCV/MCHC values and differential diagnoses for each anemia characterization. The World Health Organization (2011) developed a grading schema for classifying the severity of anemia that ranges from grade 0 (normal) to grade 4 (life threatening) (Table 13.2). Characterization and grading of anemia are useful tactics in primary care to help determine the origin and severity of a patient's anemia.

Anemia Therapy

Once the origin of the anemia has been determined, the primary care provider's next task is the selection of appropriate therapy. It is important to understand that the anemia's etiology drives therapy selection. Before patients begin treatment, they should discontinue all medications that can adversely impact the development of erythroid precursors, and any underlying illnesses known to be associated with anemia should be appropriately treated. Another important consideration is the grade or severity of the anemia. Maintaining hemodynamic stability is crucial, especially in acute hemorrhage, so if anemia is severe, transfusion may be required in lieu of oral or parenteral therapy.

Iron Preparations

Iron products are used to provide additional iron required for Hb synthesis to replenish body stores of iron. Iron may be administered prophylactically during pregnancy due to fetal requirements, dilution of maternal Hb from hormone-induced increased fluid volume, or anticipated loss of iron that can occur during delivery. Oral iron supplementation is the most common treatment for IDA because of an established safety profile, ease of administration, and low cost of therapy. Parenteral iron is

PRACTICE PEARLS

Understanding Pharmacogenomics and Anemia

- The *transmembrane protease, serine 6 (TMPRSS6) gene* signals the production of a protein called matriptase, which in turn controls hepcidin levels.
- When blood iron levels are low, this signaling pathway decreases hepcidin production, allowing more iron from the diet to be absorbed through the intestines and transported out of the liver and spleen and into the bloodstream.
- Mutations in the TMPRSS6 gene cause a rare iron-refractory IDA.
- Patients with a mutated TMPRSS6 gene fail to absorb dietary iron despite systemic iron deficiency and may also fail to respond to parenteral iron.

TABLE 13.1   Anemia Type and Differential Diagnosis

Anemia Classification	MCV Value	Differential Diagnosis
Normocytic anemia	Normal MCV of 80–100 fL	Anemia of chronic disease
		Hemolytic anemia
		Aplastic anemia
Microcytic anemia	Small MCV of <80 fL	Iron deficiency anemia
		Thalassemia
Macrocytic anemia	Large MCV of >100 fL	Vitamin B_{12} deficiency
		Folate deficiency

MVC, Mean corpuscular volume.

TABLE 13.2   World Health Organization Anemia Grading Scale

Anemia Grade	Hemoglobin Level	Anemia Severity
0	11–14 Gm/dL	Normal
1	9.5–10.9 Gm/dL	Mild
2	8.0–9.4 Gm/dL	Moderate
3	6.5–7.9 Gm/dL	Severe
4	<6.5 Gm/dL	Life threatening

typically given to patients who have a demonstrated intolerance, had an inadequate response to oral iron preparations in the past, or require a rapid increase in iron stores (replenishment).

Ferrous Sulfate

Pharmacokinetics. Ferrous sulfate is an oral iron salt most commonly prescribed for the prophylaxis or treatment of IDA. Absorption of ferrous sulfate is variable and incomplete, with a bioavailability of 5% to 10% that increases to 20% to 30% during iron deficiency states. For maximum absorption, ferrous sulfate should be taken on an empty stomach, but it may be taken with or after meals to minimize GI irritation. Vitamin C tablets or foods rich in vitamin C (orange juice, peppers, tomatoes) may enhance absorption of ferrous sulfate. Dairy products, whole grains, and legumes decrease absorption of ferrous sulfate.

Ferrous sulfate is protein bound to transferrin. *Reticulocytosis*, which is an increase in the level of circulating immature RBCs and indicates an improvement in RBC production, occurs within 3 to 10 days, with increased Hb values notable within 2 to 4 weeks of therapy. Ferrous sulfate is eliminated in the urine and is excreted into breast milk.

Indications. Ferrous sulfate is indicated for the treatment of IDA. Ferrous sulfate may also be administered for prophylaxis in pregnancy, and in childhood anemia when nutritional sources of iron are insufficient.

Adverse Effects. The most common adverse effects are constipation (39% of patients), dark stools (80%), GI irritation and stomach pain (70%), and nausea (63%) (Tolkien, 2015). Oral solutions can cause superficial tooth discoloration.

Contraindications. Hypersensitivity reactions to iron salts have been reported. Ferrous sulfate is contraindicated in conditions of high iron storage, such as hemochromatosis, or in hemolytic anemia. Ferrous sulfate should be avoided in active peptic ulcer disease, ulcerative colitis, and regional enteritis as iron preparations can worsen ulcerative conditions. Ferrous sulfate should also be avoided in premature infants until vitamin E stores are replenished to avoid hemolytic anemia. Unintentional iron overdose is the leading cause of fatal poisoning in children younger than 6 years of age; keep ferrous sulfate out of the reach of children. Avoid administering ferrous sulfate for more than 6 months, except in patients with continuous bleeding or menorrhagia.

Monitoring. A rise in Hb can be expected within 3 weeks of therapy. Monitor Hb levels as an increase in Hb by 1 Gm/dL after 1 month is considered an adequate response. Three months of therapy is recommended to replenish iron stores. Serum iron, total iron binding capacity (TIBC), and reticulocyte count should also be monitored.

Ferrous Gluconate

Ferrous gluconate is an iron salt that works to replace iron found in Hb, myoglobin, and enzymes in the prevention and treatment of IDA. This medication permits the transport of oxygen to cells and tissues via Hb.

Pharmacokinetics. Under normal conditions, iron is absorbed in the duodenum and upper jejunum. With iron supplementation, 10% of an oral dose is absorbed, and this increases to 20% to 30% in patients with inadequate iron stores. Ferrous gluconate is excreted in the urine,

PRACTICE PEARLS

Iron Preparations

- Care must be taken in ordering and administering oral or parenteral iron preparations as multiple concentrations of the oral liquid exist, and incorrect selection may result in serious over- or underdosing.
- Accidental overdose of iron-containing products is a leading cause of fatal poisoning in children younger than 6 years of age. Advise parents to keep ferrous sulfate out of the reach of children.
- Ferrous sulfate interacts with some antibiotics, antacids, and other supplements that contain calcium, phosphorous, or zinc.

PRACTICE PEARLS

Ferrous Sulfate Use in Pregnancy and Lactation

- The use of iron supplementation is acceptable during pregnancy.
- Maternal anemia increases the risk of having a low-birthweight, premature infant and may affect the infant's cognitive development. Iron supplementation can prevent IDA and related adverse consequences to the infant.

through perspiration, and during menses. The onset of reticulocytosis occurs in 5 to 10 days, with an increase in Hb within 2 to 4 weeks of therapy. Ferrous gluconate is protein bound to transferrin.

Indications. Ferrous gluconate is indicated for the treatment of IDA. Ferrous sulfate may also be administered for prophylaxis in pregnancy, and in childhood anemia when nutritional sources of iron are insufficient.

Adverse Effects. Constipation, darkening of stools, nausea, stomach cramps, and vomiting have been reported. Oral solutions can cause superficial tooth discoloration.

Contraindications. Ferrous gluconate is contraindicated for any type of hypersensitivity to iron salts. It is also contraindicated in hemochromatosis and in hemolytic anemia states. Ferrous gluconate should be avoided in active peptic ulcer disease, ulcerative colitis, and regional enteritis as iron preparations can worsen ulcerative conditions. Avoid using ferrous gluconate in premature infants until birth-related vitamin E deficiency is replenished.

Monitoring. Monitoring of Hb levels, serum iron, TIBC, and reticulocyte count should be performed after 3 to 4 weeks of therapy. Monthly testing can be performed after that for at least 3 months.

Iron Dextran

Iron dextran is an injectable form of iron salt. When the parenteral iron is released from the plasma, it replenishes the depleted iron stores in the bone marrow where it is then incorporated into Hb.

BOOKMARK THIS!

Iron Deficiency Anemia in Pregnancy

- National Center for Biotechnology Information, U.S. National Library of Medicine: Iron supplementation and screening for iron deficiency anemia in pregnant women: A systemic review to update the U.S. Preventive Services Task Force recommendation: https://www.ncbi.nlm.nih.gov/books/NBK285987/
- Obstetrics & Gynecology FIGO Committee Report: Good clinical practice advice: Iron deficiency anemia in pregnancy: https://obgyn.onlinelibrary.wiley.com/doi/10.1002/ijgo.12740

Pharmacokinetics. When iron dextran is administered intramuscularly, 60% of the medication is absorbed after 3 days and 90% is absorbed after 1 to 3 weeks, with the remainder being slowly absorbed over months. Intravenously administered iron dextran is taken up by the reticuloendothelial system in a constant manner at approximately 10 to 20 mg/hour. Similar to the response to oral iron preparations, reticulocytosis occurs in 5 to 10 days, with an increase in Hb values within 2 to 4 weeks. Serum ferritin levels peak in 7 to 9 days after an intravenous (IV) dose is administered. The half-life of iron dextran is 48 hours; it is excreted in the urine and feces.

Indications. Parenteral iron dextran is used in the treatment of iron deficiency in patients who have failed to respond to oral iron salts. It can also be used when the oral route is not feasible, or when a more rapid response is needed to increase Hb levels.

Adverse Effects. The most severe adverse effect is the risk for anaphylaxis. Life-threatening hypersensitivity infusion reactions, while infrequent, remain a concern with high molecular-weight dextran preparations. Patients can experience cardiac arrhythmias, chest pain, diaphoresis, urticaria, flushing, seizures, loss of consciousness, and shock. A 25-mg test dose should be administered prior to starting iron dextran therapy, and patients should be observed for at least 1 hour prior to administering the prescribed therapeutic dose. Dermatologic adverse effects include pruritus and urticaria. Abdominal pain, diarrhea, nausea, and vomiting have also been reported, as well as hematuria and other types of urine discoloration. Reactions including pain, swelling, and inflammation at the injection site, injection site phlebitis, and discoloration at the site of intramuscular (IM) injection can be problematic for patients receiving iron dextran.

Contraindications. Use iron dextran with caution in patients with preexisting cardiovascular disease as it may exacerbate cardiovascular complications. This drug is contraindicated for any type of hypersensitivity to iron products.

Monitoring. Monitoring of Hb levels, serum iron, TIBC, and reticulocyte count should be performed after 3 to 4 weeks of therapy. Testing can continue monthly after that for at least 3 months.

Iron Sucrose

Iron sucrose is an iron salt administered by parenteral infusion that becomes separated into iron and sucrose by the reticuloendothelial system when administered. When the iron is released into the system, it works to increase serum iron concentrations that are then incorporated into Hb.

Pharmacokinetics. The onset of action to either oral or parenteral iron salts is essentially the same, with peak reticulocytosis occurring within 5 to 10 days and Hb values increasing within 2 to 4 weeks. In healthy adults, the half-life of iron sucrose is 6 hours, and it is excreted in the urine.

Indications. Intravenous iron sucrose is indicated in the treatment of IDA in chronic kidney disease.

Adverse Effects. Hypersensitivity reactions, including some fatal anaphylactic reactions, have been reported. Significant hypotension can occur in hemodialysis-dependent and peritoneal dialysis–dependent patients.

Contraindications. Iron sucrose is contraindicated in patients with known hypersensitivity to iron sucrose or any component of the formulation. Because of similarities in chemical structure and pharmacologic actions, there remains a possibility of cross-sensitivity to iron that cannot be discounted.

Monitoring. Due to the risk for hypersensitivity reactions, monitor patients during and for at least 30 minutes following administration. Discontinue the infusion immediately if signs/symptoms of a hypersensitivity reaction (shock, hypotension, loss of consciousness) or signs of intolerance occur. Equipment for resuscitation should always be immediately available.

BLACK BOX WARNING!

Parenteral Iron Preparations

- Anaphylactic-type reactions, including fatal events, have been associated with parenteral iron dextran. Patients with other known allergies are at increased risk for anaphylactic-type reactions.
- The administration of parenteral iron dextran should occur in settings with resuscitation equipment and trained personnel available.
- A test dose is administered prior to the first dose.
- The full therapeutic dose can be continued if there are no signs or symptoms of anaphylaxis.
- Observe patient for signs and symptoms of anaphylactic-type reactions during all treatment as fatal reactions have occurred following a tolerated first-dose test.
- Iron dextran is used only in patients with laboratory-confirmed iron-deficient state not amenable to oral iron.

Monitor Hb, ferritin, serum iron, serum phosphate, and transferrin levels before and during treatment. Serum iron levels greater than 300 mcg/dL, elevated ferritin levels, and transferrin oversaturation may indicate iron overload. Iron therapy should be withheld in patients with evidence of iron overload. Transferrin saturation values will increase rapidly after IV administration of iron sucrose. For reliable values, obtain serum iron values 48 hours after IV dosing.

PRACTICE PEARLS

Calculation of Iron Deficit

- To calculate iron deficit: Total replacement dose (mg of iron) = 0.6 × weight (kg) × [100 − (actual Hb /12 × 100)].
- For this equation, the target Hb concentration is 12 mg. However, in some patients, a different target may be desired.

Ferric Carboxymaltose

Ferric carboxymaltose is a stable, nondextran iron formulation that permits uptake of iron by the reticuloendothelial system without the release of free iron. It is administered via slow IV infusion and is used in the treatment of IDA and in anemia of chronic disease.

Pharmacokinetics. A rapid, dose-dependent increase in total serum iron concentration has been observed following a single IV dose of 0.1 to 1 Gm of ferric carboxymaltose, with a peak iron concentration noted within 1 hour following infusion. Ferric carboxymaltose is rapidly distributed to the bone marrow, liver, and spleen. The half-life of ferric carboxymaltose is 7 to 12 hours. A small amount of the medication is excreted in the urine.

Indications. This medication is used in the treatment of IDA in adults who are intolerant of or have had an unsatisfactory response to oral iron preparations.

Adverse Effects. Life-threatening hypersensitivity reactions, while rare, have been reported. Extravasation of the medication can cause brown discoloration at the site and may be long lasting. Hypertension has been reported in 3.8% of patients receiving ferric carboxymaltose. Short-term elevations in systolic blood pressure, with facial flushing, dizziness, or nausea, have been reported in 6% of patients immediately after administration, but have resolved within 30 minutes (Onken et al., 2014).

Contraindications. Ferric carboxymaltose is contraindicated in patients with known hypersensitivity to ferric carboxymaltose. Caution should be used when administering this medication to patients who may be at risk for hypersensitivity reactions.

Monitoring. Monitor for extravasation during administration; if extravasation occurs, discontinue administration at the affected site. Monitor for signs and symptoms of hypersensitivity reactions for at least 30 minutes after administration. Monitor for signs and symptoms of hypertension following each dose of ferric carboxymaltose. Monitor Hb, ferritin, serum iron, and transferrin levels before and during treatment.

PRACTICE PEARLS

Ferric Carboxymaltose Use in Pregnancy and Lactation

- Use IV ferric carboxymaltose with caution in lactating patients.
- In breastfeeding patients with postpartum IDA, mean breast-milk iron concentrations were higher in those receiving IV ferric carboxymaltose than in those receiving oral ferrous sulfate.

Ferumoxytol

Ferumoxytol is a pharmacologic iron salt coated with a low-molecular-weight carbohydrate. It forms an iron-containing complex that can enter the reticuloendothelial system macrophages of the liver, spleen, and bone marrow. After entering, iron is released from the complex. The iron is then transported via plasma transferrin for incorporation into Hb. Ferumoxytol is administered via IV infusion and is used in the treatment of IDA and in anemia of chronic disease.

Pharmacokinetics. Ferumoxytol is administered intravenously and is eliminated in a dose-dependent manner from plasma, with a half-life of approximately 15 hours. In normal adults, 90% of metabolized iron is preserved for repeated use, with very little iron being eliminated. In patients with renal impairment, ferumoxytol is not removed by hemodialysis.

Indications. Ferumoxytol is used in the treatment of IDA in adults who have either an intolerance or an unsatisfactory response to oral iron. It is also used in patients with anemia from chronic kidney disease.

Adverse Effects. Fatal and serious hypersensitivity reactions including anaphylaxis have occurred. Intravenous ferumoxytol can cause hypotension, so use caution when administering ferumoxytol to patients with preexisting hypotension or in those receiving hemodialysis.

Contraindications. Ferumoxytol is contraindicated in patients with known hypersensitivity to ferumoxytol or other iron products. Do not administer ferumoxytol to patients with evidence of iron overload (e.g., patients with hemochromatosis).

Monitoring. Observe for signs or symptoms of hypersensitivity reactions during and for at least 30 minutes following ferumoxytol infusion. Monitor blood pressure and pulse during and after administration. Monitor Hb, serum ferritin, serum iron, and transferrin saturation 1 month following the second IV dose, and then periodically.

Erythropoietin-Stimulating Agents

Recombinant erythropoietin medications are known as *erythropoietin-stimulating agents* (ESAs). ESAs are given by injection and work in the bone marrow to stimulate the production of RBCs for release into the bloodstream. Prior to the development of ESAs, blood transfusions were the mainstay of treatment for anemia from kidney disease. Although blood transfusions increase Hb levels and provide relief of anemia symptoms, transfusions were also associated with hospitalization, iron overload, and transfusion-related viral hepatitis. Early studies showed that ESAs reduced the need for RBC transfusions; however, increases in mortality, cardiovascular events, and cancer progression were also observed. Therefore, guidelines for the use of ESAs in the treatment of anemia from all causes have become increasingly conservative. It is important to understand that all ESAs have the potential to cause high blood pressure; thus, use extreme caution when prescribing ESAs to patients with hypertension or to those at high risk for cardiovascular events.

The first therapeutic agent to be used for the stimulation of erythropoiesis was recombinant human erythropoietin (epoetin). Darbepoetin alfa and methoxy polyethylene glycol-epoetin beta (a continuous erythropoietin-receptor activator [CERA]) are newer synthetic forms of naturally occurring erythropoietin that have a longer duration of action (Macdougall, 2008; Lopez, Cacoub, Macdougall, & Peyrin-Biroulet, 2016). The choice of which ESA to use in the treatment of anemia in primary care is dependent on several factors, including patient and provider preference, cost, and frequency of administration (Table 13.3).

Erythropoietin Alfa

Erythropoietin alfa is a recombinant form of the hormone erythropoietin alfa and belongs to the drug class known as ESAs or colony-stimulating factors. Erythropoietin alfa works in the bone marrow to induce erythropoiesis by stimulating the division and differentiation of erythroid progenitor cells and facilitates the release of reticulocytes from the bone marrow into the bloodstream, where they mature to erythrocytes. These actions result in an increase in the reticulocyte count and a rise in hematocrit and Hb levels. Assess the iron status in all patients before and during treatment with erythropoietin alfa. Causes of anemia such as vitamin deficiency, metabolic or chronic inflammatory conditions, and bleeding should be corrected before initiating epoetin alfa.

Pharmacokinetics. Reticulocyte counts increase within 10 days, with a peak effect noted within 2 to 6 weeks. The half-life of erythropoietin alfa in adults is dependent on dose and route (IV or subcutaneous) and is approximately 4 to 7 hours. In infants and in pediatric populations with chronic kidney disease, the half-life of an IV dose is between 4 and 13 hours.

Indications. Erythropoietin alfa is indicated in the treatment of anemia from chronic kidney disease, and for anemia secondary to HIV treatment. Erythropoietin alfa is also used in selected patients with nonmyeloid malignancies when anemia is due to concomitant myelosuppressive chemotherapy.

Adverse Effects. The most common adverse effect of erythropoietin alfa is an increase in blood pressure (33% of patients), which occurs in the first few months of therapy. Embolism and thrombosis (15%), nausea (56%), vomiting (28%), diarrhea (up to 30%), and fever (up to 42%) are also common. Local effects such as injection site reaction (up to 18%) and injection site pain (up to 13%) have been reported.

Contraindications. Erythropoietin alfa is contraindicated in patients with allergic reactions to epoetin alfa products and in those with uncontrolled hypertension. The multidose vials contain benzyl alcohol and are contraindicated in neonates, infants, pregnant women, and breastfeeding women.

Monitoring. Assess Hb weekly until stable to minimize the need for RBC transfusions, and then monthly. Transferrin saturation and serum ferritin should be assessed prior to and during treatment. Monitor blood pressure throughout treatment. Monitor for signs and symptoms of pulmonary embolism or deep vein thrombosis. The development of a sudden loss of response to epoetin, accompanied by severe anemia and low reticulocyte count, requires the primary care provider to assess the patient for the presence of binding and neutralizing antibodies to erythropoietin. If antierythropoietin antibody-associated anemia is suspected, withhold epoetin and other erythropoietic proteins.

PRACTICE PEARLS

ESA Therapy

- Evaluate iron status in all patients before and during treatment.
- Correct or exclude deficiencies of iron, vitamin B_{12}, and/or folate, as well as other factors that may impair erythropoiesis (inflammatory conditions, infections, bleeding).
- Reduce or withhold ESAs if blood pressure becomes difficult to control. Advise patients about the importance of compliance with antihypertensive therapy.
- If the Hb does *not* increase by more than 1 Gm/dL after 4 weeks, increase the dose by 25%. Do not increase the dose more frequently than once every 4 weeks.
- If the desired response is not met over a 12-week dose-escalation period, discontinue therapy.
- For patients who do not respond to therapy, potential factors impairing erythropoiesis, acute bleeding, possible malignant processes, and/or hematologic disease (e.g., thalassemia, refractory anemia, myelodysplastic disorder) should be investigated.
- If the Hb increases by more than 1 Gm/dL in any 2-week period, reduce the dose by at least 25%.

TABLE 13.3   Anemia Medications

Category/ Medication	Indication	Dosage	Considerations and Monitoring
Iron Salts			
Ferrous sulfate	IDA	*Regular-release:* 325 mg orally three times daily. *ER:* 160 mg orally once or twice daily.	Maintain therapy for minimum of 3 months Monitor Hb after 3–4 weeks of therapy, and then monthly for 3 months
	Anemia in pregnancy/ lactation	325 mg orally once daily.	
	IDA in children	*0–5 yr:* 15–30 mg/kg/day. *5–12 yr:* 300 mg/day. *Males 12–18 yr:* 2 300-mg tablets orally daily. *Females 12–18 yr:* 300–600 mg/day.	
Ferrous gluconate	IDA	*Oral:* 100–200 mg daily in 2–3 divided doses.	Monitor Hb after 3–4 weeks of therapy, and then monthly for 3 months
Iron dextran	IDA not responsive to oral iron salts	The formula for dosing is based on Hb Gm/dL and LBW in kg or ABW in kg if <LBW, or for children ≤15 kg.	Monitor Hb, serum iron TIBC, and reticulocyte count after 3–4 weeks of therapy, and then monthly for 3 months
Iron sucrose	IDA in chronic kidney disease	*Initial dose:* IV: 5–7 mg/kg/dose; maximum initial dose: 100 mg/dose. *Maintenance dose:* IV: 5–7 mg/kg/dose every 1–7 days until total replacement dose achieved; maximum single dose: 300 mg/dose.	Monitor Hb, ferritin, serum iron, serum phosphate, and transferrin levels
Ferric carboxymaltose	IDA unresponsive to total preparations	*Adult IV dose (weight ≥50 kg):* 750-mg dose separated by at least 7 days; do not exceed 1500 mg of iron/course. *Adult IV dose (weight <50 kg):* 15 mg/kg dose for 2 doses separated by at least 7 days.	Monitor Hb, ferritin, serum iron, and transferrin levels.
Ferumoxytol	IDA in chronic kidney disease	*Adult IV dose:* 510 mg IV followed by a second dose 3–8 days later.	Monitor Hb, ferritin, serum iron, and transferrin levels after 1 month.
Erythropoietin-Stimulating Agents			
Erythropoietin alfa	Anemia of chronic disease and HIV treatment	*Adults:* 50–100 units/kg/dose IV or subcutaneously three times weekly initially when Hg <10 Gm/dL. *Infants, children, and adolescents:* Dosage varies depending on indication, frequency of administration, and individual response. *Neonates:* Optimal dosing regimen and indications are not defined; doses ranging from 300 to 2500 units/kg/dose IV daily or every other day for a short duration after birth.	Monitor Hb weekly until stable, then monthly; monitor transferrin saturation and serum ferritin before and during treatment; monitor BP throughout treatment

Continued

TABLE 13.3   Anemia Medications—cont'd

Category/ Medication	Indication	Dosage	Considerations and Monitoring
Darbepoetin alpha	Anemia of chronic disease and HIV treatment	*Adults (no hemodialysis):* 0.45 mcg/kg IV or subcutaneously once every 4 weeks when Hg <10 Gm/dL; if Hg increases >1 Gm/dL in 2 weeks, reduce dose by ≥25%. *Adults (on hemodialysis):* 0.45 mcg/kg subcutaneously or IV once weekly or 0.75 mcg/kg IV once every 2 weeks as appropriate; if Hg increases >1 Gm/dL in 2 weeks, reduce dose by ≥25%. *Infants and children:* Dosage may vary depending on indication, frequency of administration, and individual response; safety not established in neonates.	Evaluate iron status in all patients before and during treatment; monitor ferritin, iron, transferrin, and Hb/hematocrit levels throughout treatment.
Methoxy polyethylene glycol-epoetin beta	Treatment of anemia from chronic renal failure	*Adults:* 0.6 mcg/kg IV subcutaneously once every 2 weeks.	Evaluate iron status in all patients before and during treatment; monitor ferritin, iron, transferrin, and Hb/hematocrit levels throughout treatment. Supplemental iron can be added if serum ferritin <100 mcg/L or serum transferrin saturation <20%.
Peginesatide	Treatment of anemia from chronic renal failure in patients on dialysis	*Adults:* 0.04 mg/kg IV or subcutaneously once/month if not currently treated with an ESA; initiate treatment when Hg <10 Gm/dL. Safety not established in neonates, infants, children, or adolescents.	Monitor BP and for neurologic symptoms; monitor ferritin, iron, transferrin, and Hb/hematocrit levels throughout treatment. Supplemental iron can be added if serum ferritin <100 mcg/L or serum transferrin saturation <20%.
Nandrolone decanoate	Treatment of anemia from chronic renal failure	*Adult and adolescent males >14 yr:* 50–200 mg IM every 1–4 weeks. *Adult and adolescent females >14 yr:* 50–100 mg IM every 1–4 weeks. *Children and adolescents 2–13 years:* 25–50 mg IM every 3–4 weeks.	Monitor liver function tests, glucose, and lipid levels at baseline and throughout treatment.
Anabolic Steroids			
Oxymetholone	Treatment of anemia from aplastic anemia, myelofibrosis, and hypoplastic anemia from myelotoxic agents	*Adults, children, and adolescents:* 1–2 mg/kg/day orally; can be given up to 5 mg/kg/day orally; therapy length is a minimum of 3–6 months.	Monitor growth rate, liver function tests, hepatic enzymes, serum iron and iron binding capacity, and Hb/hematocrit levels.
Vitamin B₁₂			
Cyanocobalamin	Treatment and prevention of vitamin B₁₂ deficiency	*Adults, pregnant and lactating females:* 2.4–2.8 mcg orally daily. *Children:* 0.9–1.8 mcg orally daily. *Infants:* 0.4–0.5 mcg orally daily. Recommended daily allowance not established.	Monitor hematocrit, platelet and reticulocyte count, vitamin B₁₂, folate, iron concentrations, and serum potassium levels.

ABW, Actual body weight; *BP,* blood pressure; *ER,* extended release; *ESA,* erythropoietin-stimulating agent; *Hb,* hemoglobin; *HIV,* human immunodeficiency virus; *IDA,* iron deficiency anemia; *IM,* intramuscular; *IV,* intravenous; *LBW,* lean body weight; *TIBC,* total iron binding capacity.

Darbepoetin Alfa

Darbepoetin alfa has two additional carbohydrate chains compared to erythropoietin alfa, resulting in different dosing regimens. Darbepoetin alfa does induce erythropoiesis in the same fashion as erythropoietin alfa—by stimulating the division and differentiation of erythroid progenitor cells—and facilitates the release of reticulocytes from the bone marrow into the bloodstream, where they mature to erythrocytes. These actions result in an increase in reticulocyte count, hematocrit, and Hb levels. However, the half-life of darbepoetin alfa is three times that of erythropoietin alfa concentrations, making it a longer-lasting preparation.

Pharmacokinetics. Darbepoetin alfa is administered intravenously or subcutaneously with a dose-dependent response. It remains unknown whether darbepoetin alfa crosses the placenta or is distributed into breast milk. Metabolism and elimination of darbepoetin alfa are not fully known. Approximately 10% of the administered dose appears to be excreted in the urine. Increased Hb levels are not generally observed until 2 to 6 weeks after initiating treatment.

Indications. Darbepoetin alfa is indicated in the treatment of anemia due to chronic kidney disease, for anemia secondary to HIV or hepatitis C treatment, and in selected patients with nonmyeloid malignancies when anemia is due to concomitant myelosuppressive chemotherapy.

Adverse Effects. Like erythropoietin alfa, darbepoetin alfa may increase the risk of death, serious adverse cardiovascular reactions, and stroke in patients with chronic kidney disease who achieve Hb concentrations greater than 11 Gm/dL. Darbepoetin alfa may shorten the overall survival time and increase the risk of tumor progression or recurrence in patients with cancer. A rare but serious adverse effect of this drug is PRCA, in which bone marrow production and maturation of erythrocytes is greatly reduced or stopped. PRCA with darbepoetin is associated with neutralizing antibodies to erythropoietin that result in the loss of erythropoiesis, mostly in patients with chronic kidney failure receiving subcutaneous injections. Another serious adverse effect of darbepoetin alfa is the increased risk of seizures in patients with chronic kidney disease, possibly as a result of lowering the seizure threshold. Patients who have existing seizure disorders must be carefully observed and may require dosage adjustment of prescribed antiepilepsy agents.

Contraindications. Darbepoetin alfa is contraindicated for use by patients with uncontrolled hypertension. During the early phase of darbepoetin therapy in patients with chronic kidney disease, patients will often require either initiation of or intensification of antihypertensive therapy.

Monitoring. Evaluate the iron status in all patients before and during treatment and maintain iron repletion. During therapy, monitor ferritin, iron, transferrin, and Hb/hematocrit levels. Correct or exclude other causes of anemia, such as vitamin deficiency, metabolic or chronic inflammatory conditions, and bleeding, before initiating

BLACK BOX WARNING!

ESAs

- ESAs increase the risk of death, myocardial infarction, stroke, and venous thromboembolism.
- Potentially serious allergic reactions, although rare, have been reported and include anaphylactic reactions, angioedema, bronchospasm, rash, and urticaria. Discontinue immediately (and permanently) in patients who experience serious allergic/anaphylactic reactions.
- ESAs have shortened overall survival and/or increased the risk of tumor progression or recurrence in clinical studies of patients with breast, non-small-cell lung, head and neck, lymphoid, and cervical cancers.
- Use ESAs only for anemia from myelosuppressive chemotherapy. Discontinue following the completion of a chemotherapy course.
- Erythema multiforme and Stevens-Johnson syndrome/toxic epidermal necrolysis have been reported with ESAs (including epoetin alfa products). *Discontinue immediately if a severe cutaneous reaction develops.*
- Pure red cell aplasia (PRCA), a condition that affects RBC precursors, can develop during treatment with ESAs due to antibodies to erythropoietin that can form.

darbepoetin alfa. During the first several months after darbepoetin initiation, closely monitor patients for neurologic symptoms, especially new onset of seizures or increased seizure activity.

Methoxy Polyethylene Glycol-Epoetin Beta

Methoxy polyethylene glycol-epoetin beta (MPG-epoetin beta) is a synthetic, continuous erythropoietin-receptor activator. MPG-epoetin beta contains a methoxy polyethylene-glycol polymer attached to recombinant human erythropoietin. As a result, MPG-epoetin beta degrades at a slower rate and remains in the circulation much longer than endogenous erythropoietin (approximately 134 hours versus 8 hours). This longer biologic activity allows for dosing intervals of every 2 to 4 weeks.

Pharmacokinetics. MPG-epoetin beta can be administered either intravenously or subcutaneously. Metabolism and elimination of any form of erythropoietin is poorly understood. Steady-state concentrations increased by 12% after repeat dosing every 2 weeks, but no accumulation is observed when dosing is repeated every 4 weeks. A change in Hb may not be observed for 2 to 6 weeks after the dose of MPG-epoetin beta is modified. The pharmacokinetics of MPG-epoetin beta are not affected by liver or renal impairment or hemodialysis.

Indications. MPG-epoetin beta can be administered for the treatment of anemia associated with chronic renal failure. It is an appropriate treatment in both dialysis-dependent and non–dialysis-dependent patients.

Adverse Effects. PRCA associated with neutralizing antibodies to erythropoietin have been reported in patients with chronic kidney failure receiving subcutaneous injections.

Serious fatal and nonfatal cardiovascular and thromboembolic events have occurred with all ESAs. MPG-epoetin beta caused hypertension in 13% of adult patients and 19% of pediatric patients in clinical trials. Thrombocytopenia was observed in 6% of pediatric patients who received MPG-epoetin beta injection. Serious hypersensitivity reactions that include anaphylaxis, angioedema, bronchospasm, and Stevens-Johnson syndrome have been reported with the use of MPG-epoetin beta.

Contraindications. MPG-epoetin beta is contraindicated in patients whose PRCA begins after treatment. Cases of PRCA with MGP-epoetin beta also have been associated with neutralizing antibodies to erythropoietin. This drug is contraindicated for use by patients with uncontrolled hypertension because hypertensive encephalopathy and seizures have been reported.

Monitoring. Blood pressure and neurologic symptoms should be monitored closely during therapy, with special attention in the first several months of treatment. During therapy, monitor ferritin, iron, transferrin, and Hb/hematocrit levels.

Peginesatide

Peginesatide is a synthetic peptide that binds to the erythropoietin receptor and stimulates erythropoiesis in RBC precursors. Peginesatide increases the reticulocyte count and Hb in a dose-dependent fashion; however, the dose response can vary among patients.

Pharmacokinetics. Peginesatide can be administered by the IV or subcutaneous route. Peginesatide is not metabolized and is eliminated through urinary excretion. In healthy individuals, the mean half-life of peginesatide is 25 ± 7.6 hours after IV administration and 53 ± 17.7 hours after subcutaneous administration.

Indications. Peginesatide is primarily indicated for the treatment of anemia due to chronic kidney disease. It is used specifically for patients who are receiving dialysis.

Adverse Effects. Patients receiving peginesatide may develop hypertension. All ESAs increase the risk of death, myocardial infarction, stroke, and venous thromboembolism. Infusion-related reactions including anaphylaxis, hypotension, bronchospasm, and angioedema have been reported in patients receiving peginesatide. There is a risk of provoking an immune response to erythropoietin with antibody formation, leading to development of PRCA. Any patient experiencing a lack or loss of Hb response to peginesatide should be evaluated to determine the potential cause. Seizures have also been reported with peginesatide therapy. GI adverse effects including diarrhea, nausea, and vomiting have been reported. Musculoskeletal reactions such as arthralgia, back pain, and muscle cramps or spasms have been reported. ESAs have been shown to increase the risk of tumor progression or recurrence in patients with breast, non–small-cell lung, head and neck, lymphoid, and cervical cancers.

Contraindications. Peginesatide is contraindicated for use by patients who have known serious allergic reactions (anaphylaxis) to the medication. Peginesatide is contraindicated in patients with *uncontrolled* hypertension; hypertension should be controlled prior to beginning peginesatide

therapy in all patients. Peginesatide is classified as pregnancy category C. There are currently no well-controlled studies of peginesatide in pregnant women.

Monitoring. During the first few months of therapy, monitor blood pressure and the presence of neurologic symptoms closely. Patients should contact their primary care provider immediately if they experience new-onset seizures or changes in seizure frequency.

Anabolic Steroids

Nandrolone Decanoate

Nandrolone decanoate is a parenteral (IM-only) anabolic steroid used to manage the anemia of chronic renal failure. This agent increases Hb levels and red cell mass and promotes erythrocyte production. Increased erythrocyte production is due to enhanced production of erythropoietic stimulating factors. While anabolic steroids also promote body building and reverse catabolic processes, drug misuse and abuse also occur, with adverse effects such as changes in libido, hepatotoxicity, increased risk of cardiovascular disease, and antisocial behavior reported.

PRACTICE PEARLS

Nandrolone Decanoate Use in Pregnancy and Lactation

- Androgens can cause teratogenesis and are absolutely contraindicated during pregnancy because of adverse effects on the fetus.
- Nandrolone decanoate is known to cause embryotoxicity, fetotoxicity, and masculinization of female animal offspring.
- Nandrolone decanoate is also contraindicated in females who are or may become pregnant.

Pharmacokinetics. Once nandrolone decanoate is administered via IM injection, plasma enzymes hydrolyze the drug into free nandrolone that rapidly diffuses into cells. Nandrolone is then metabolized in the liver. Data on the excretion of the nandrolone and its metabolites are lacking. The elimination half-life of nandrolone decanoate is 6 to 8 days.

Indications. Nandrolone decanoate is used in the treatment of anemia resulting from chronic renal failure.

Adverse Effects. Since nandrolone decanoate acts as an endogenous androgen, disturbances of growth and sexual development can occur if given to young children. Reversible increases in low-density lipoprotein (LDL) and decreases in high-density lipoprotein (HDL) have also occurred. Menstrual irregularity can occur with nandrolone decanoate therapy in females because of gonadotropin suppression. Masculinization of females can occur and may be irreversible, especially with prolonged treatment.

Contraindications. Nandrolone decanoate is absolutely contraindicated during pregnancy because of probable adverse effects on the fetus (pregnancy category X). Androgens such as nandrolone decanoate must be used cautiously in patients with diabetes mellitus. Extreme caution should be taken when using nandrolone decanoate in children as androgens may accelerate bone maturation ahead of linear growth. This medication can stimulate the growth of cancer and should not be used in male patients with prostate or breast cancer. Nandrolone decanoate is contraindicated for use in patients with preexisting hepatic or renal disease. The drug also should be used cautiously in patients with hypercholesterolemia or a history of cardiac disease, especially heart failure, as androgen therapy can result in edema secondary to sodium retention.

Monitoring. Loss of diabetic control with nandrolone decanoate can occur, so close monitoring of blood glucose is recommended during therapy. Because of the potential for hepatoxicity, baseline liver function tests are recommended prior to nandrolone decanoate initiation, with periodic liver function test assessments performed during therapy. Alterations in the serum lipid profile consisting of decreased HDL and increased LDL occur with anabolic steroids including nandrolone, so the monitoring of lipoprotein concentrations is recommended.

PRACTICE PEARLS

Nandrolone Decanoate

- Nandrolone decanoate therapy may be administered for up to 12 weeks at 3- to 4-week intervals.
- If needed, a second course may be administered after a 3- to 4-week rest period.
- Therapy should be discontinued if no hematologic improvement is seen within the first 6 months.
- Adequate iron intake is required for a maximal response.

Oxymetholone

Oxymetholone is an anabolic steroid that stimulates the production of erythropoietin. This medication is used in the treatment of anemia due to bone marrow failure and deficient RBC production.

Pharmacokinetics. Limited information is available on the pharmacokinetic profile of oral oxymetholone. Oxymetholone undergoes both phase I and phase II metabolism. While oxymetholone interacts with the cytochrome (CYP) P450 system in vitro, it is not metabolized by these enzymes. Approximately 5% of oxymetholone is present in the urine when eliminated. Oxymetholone therapy has resulted in a fivefold increase in erythropoietin levels.

Indications. Oxymetholone is used for the treatment of anemia caused by conditions that are characterized by reduced RBC production. These conditions include aplastic anemia, myelofibrosis, and hypoplastic anemia due to myelotoxic drugs.

Adverse Effects. Cholestatic hepatitis and jaundice may occur with oxymetholone use, with more severe effects resulting in hepatic necrosis, coma, and/or death. Adverse effects on the central nervous system (CNS), such as excitability and insomnia, have been reported in patients receiving oxymetholone. IDA has been reported in patients receiving oxymetholone. The development of leukemia has also been reported in patients with aplastic anemia who received oxymetholone. Musculoskeletal adverse effects including premature closure of epiphyses in children have occurred. Changes in serum lipids, including decreased HDL and increased LDL concentrations, may occur with oxymetholone therapy. Edema has been reported in patients receiving oxymetholone. Anabolic steroids, such as oxymetholone, may suppress clotting factors II, V, VII, and X and increase prothrombin time.

Contraindications. Use is contraindicated in patients with severe hepatic or renal disease. Oxymetholone can cause loss of diabetic control and should be used with caution in patients with diabetes mellitus. As with other androgens, females are at risk for masculinization from oxymetholone. Oxymetholone is contraindicated in male and female patients with breast cancer and in male patients with prostate cancer, as oxymetholone can stimulate the growth of cancer. Male geriatric patients who receive androgenic anabolic steroids may be at increased risk for developing prostate hypertrophy and prostate cancer. Oxymetholone is classified as pregnancy category X. Fetal harm can occur and use is contraindicated in patients who are pregnant or may become pregnant while on therapy.

Monitoring. Reversible changes in liver function tests have been reported, including elevated hepatic enzymes. Periodic monitoring of liver function tests is recommended. Prepubertal patients receiving oxymetholone should have X-rays every 6 months to evaluate the rate of bone maturation and epiphyseal center changes that can result from oxymetholone. Monitor serum iron and iron binding capacity periodically, and start supplemental iron therapy if iron deficiency is detected. Also monitor Hb and hematocrit levels periodically (for polycythemia) in patients receiving high doses of oxymetholone.

Cyanocobalamin (Vitamin B$_{12}$)

The terms *cyanocobalamin* and *vitamin B$_{12}$* are used interchangeably. However, vitamin B$_{12}$ is also available as hydroxocobalamin, a less commonly prescribed medication. Cyanocobalamin is available orally, intranasally, and parenterally. Cyanocobalamin is used to diagnose (via the Schilling test) and treat pernicious anemia or other types of vitamin B$_{12}$ deficiency.

Pharmacokinetics. Cyanocobalamin is administered intranasally, orally, and parenterally, while hydroxocobalamin is administered only parenterally. The intranasal formulation is not approved to treat acute B$_{12}$ deficiency. Once cyanocobalamin is absorbed, vitamin B_{12} is distributed and stored primarily in the liver as coenzyme B_{12}. The bone marrow also stores a significant amount of the absorbed vitamin B_{12}. Vitamin B_{12} crosses the placenta and is distributed into breast milk. Elimination of cyanocobalamin occurs primarily through the liver, with excess cyanocobalamin excreted unchanged in the urine.

Indications. Vitamin B_{12} is used for the treatment and prevention of vitamin B_{12} deficiency. It is also used for the treatment of vitamin B_{12} deficiency in megaloblastic anemia or macrocytic anemia.

Adverse Effects. Pulmonary edema and heart failure developing shortly after the start of treatment have been reported with parenteral cyanocobalamin. Long-term cyanocobalamin therapy can result in hypokalemia and thrombocytosis when severe megaloblastic anemia converts to normal erythropoiesis. Hypersensitivity reactions to the medication preservative benzyl alcohol can also occur.

Contraindications. Cyanocobalamin is contraindicated in patients with known hypersensitivity reactions to vitamin B_{12}, and in those with hypersensitivity to cobalt (cyanocobalamin contains cobalt). If hypersensitivity is suspected, an intradermal test dose should be administered. Cyanocobalamin should not be used in patients with early hereditary optic nerve atrophy (Leber's disease) as optic nerve atrophy can worsen.

Monitoring. Hematocrit, reticulocyte count, vitamin B_{12}, folate, and iron concentrations should be obtained prior to treatment. If folate concentrations are also low, folic acid should be administered in combination with B_{12}. Platelet counts and serum potassium should also be monitored during treatment. Vitamin blood concentrations and peripheral blood counts should be monitored at 1 month of treatment and then at intervals of 3 to 6 months.

PRACTICE PEARLS

Cyanocobalamin Injection Toxicity

- Cyanocobalamin injection contains aluminum, and aluminum toxicity may occur with prolonged administration in high-risk patients, including those with renal impairment and premature neonates.

- Premature neonates are at particular risk for aluminum toxicity because of immature renal function and because they require large amounts of calcium and phosphate solutions, which contain aluminum.

- Cyanocobalamin preparations containing benzyl alcohol should be avoided in premature neonates because benzyl alcohol has been associated with gasping syndrome, a potentially fatal condition characterized by metabolic acidosis and CNS, respiratory, circulatory, and renal dysfunction.

- Research indicates that patients with renal impairment who receive parenteral aluminum at more than 4 to 5 mcg/kg/day may develop aluminum-related CNS (dizziness, incoordination, paresthesia, abnormal gait) and bone (back pain, arthritis) toxicities.

Prescriber Considerations for Anemia Therapy

Anemia is a common finding in patients with chronic disease, including people affected by acute blood loss, malignancy, HIV, heart failure, chronic kidney disease, chronic inflammatory bowel disease, pregnancy, hemolytic or acquired anemias, malabsorption syndromes, and nutritional deficiencies in folate and vitamin B_{12}. Symptoms caused by anemia are consistent with deficient oxygen delivery to tissues and include fatigue, shortness of breath, weakness, light-headedness, and tachycardia (Palmer et al., 2014; Cascio & DeLoughery, 2016). Paleness of the skin, conjunctivae, and nail beds are other common findings (Lopez et al., 2016). The symptoms of anemia are dependent on the severity of the anemia, the patient's age, the patient's underlying comorbidities, and the cause of the anemia.

Because anemia has many etiologies, uncovering its cause is the first critical step before determining a pharmacologic therapy. A thorough review of systems (ROS) for underlying chronic conditions predisposing a patient to anemia, plus the history of present illness, will assist in formulating a plan for any diagnostic or laboratory testing needed. In cases of acute blood loss accompanied by severe anemia (Table 13.2), blood transfusion may be necessary. Once the etiology of anemia is established, if pharmacologic treatment is planned, the primary care provider needs to establish the treatment and follow-up plan. There are currently no gold-standard indices for follow-up laboratory testing, but some experts recommend assessment of a complete blood count (CBC) to examine RBC size, hematocrit/Hb levels, ferritin, iron, and transferrin 1 month after treatment begins, and every 3 months thereafter for 1 year.

Clinical Reasoning for Anemia Therapy

Consider the individual patient's health problem requiring anemia therapy. The first step in the initiation of a treatment plan is to determine the underlying cause of the patient's anemia. Anemia has many different potential sources, including acute bleeding, pregnancy/lactation, malnutrition, folic acid deficiency, hemolysis, inherited conditions, and chronic disease. Once the cause of anemia is established, determine whether the therapy required will be short or long term. Acute GI bleeding may require short-term therapy to correct the cause of the blood loss and reverse the anemia. However, a patient with chronic kidney disease receiving dialysis will require long-term therapy because of decreased erythropoietin production. When designing therapy, it is helpful to understand the patient's risk factors for anemia. A thorough history of present and past conditions and genetic and dietary factors will help to identify the risk factors for future episodes of anemia, and the necessary follow-up.

Determine the desired therapeutic outcome based on the degree of anemia therapy needed for the patient's health problem. The overall purpose of anemia therapy is to reverse the anemia to adequately oxygenate the tissues of the body, reduce the patient's symptoms, and reduce the risk for morbidity and mortality. First, ensure that other causes of anemia such as vitamin deficiency, metabolic or chronic inflammatory conditions, and bleeding have been addressed. As a general guideline when using IV iron therapy, the desired therapeutic outcome is to prescribe the lowest dose sufficient to reduce the patient's need for RBC transfusions.

Assess the anemia therapy selected for its appropriateness for an individual patient by considering the medication's side effects and the patient's age, race/ethnicity, comorbidities, and genetic factors. Oral iron therapy is used in the treatment of mild to moderate IDA. In the absence of severe anemia, oral iron is a preferred treatment because it is low cost, is noninvasive, and has an established safety profile. Oral iron at 325 mg three times daily with meals provides 60 mg of elemental iron with each dose. Iron bioavailability is increased in an acidic environment, so combining vitamin C with oral iron can optimize the treatment.

Oral iron can cause several unpleasant GI side effects, such as constipation/diarrhea, dark-colored stools, epigastric pain, and nausea. Taking oral iron with meals may reduce these side effects. Slower-acting formulations are more expensive but may reduce GI effects and require only once-daily dosing. While the percentage of severe or fatal anaphylactic reactions is low (<2%), reduction of severe adverse effects could be achieved by premedication with diphenhydramine and acetaminophen before IV iron infusions (see Table 13.3).

Initiate the treatment plan with the selected medication by first providing adequate patient education to ensure the patient's understanding and promote full participation in the anemia therapy. Discuss the planned anemia therapy with the patient and family. Explain the goal of the selected therapy, the anticipated duration of treatment, any instructions for increasing dietary iron intake, and the importance of treatment adherence to the anemia therapy prescribed.

Ensure complete patient and family understanding about the medication prescribed for anemia using a variety of education strategies. The most important information to provide concerning anemia therapy is the name of the medication, the expected therapeutic effects and side effects, adverse effects to be reported, and the laboratory testing and follow-up needed. Both verbal and written instruction methods should be included. Instruct the patient about an iron-rich diet, and provide a list of foods to be incorporated into the diet. If ESAs are prescribed, the patient and family should be advised to monitor the patient's blood pressure at home and should know when to alert the primary care provider about elevated findings. Patients prescribed subcutaneous ESAs will need to be taught to draw up and inject the medication. Kinesthetic skills such as injection administration are best taught using verbal, written, and demonstration techniques. Also, most pharmaceutical manufacturers have demonstration videos accessible on the internet that patients and families can use to reinforce correct injection techniques.

Conduct follow-up and monitoring of patient responses to anemia therapy. Prior to and during therapy, monitor the patient's iron status, including transferrin saturation and serum ferritin. The therapeutic response to iron begins after approximately 5 to 10 days of treatment with a rise in the reticulocyte count. Monitor Hb at least every 2 weeks, and at least monthly thereafter. Once stable, the Hb can be checked every 3 months and then annually. Monitor trends in Hb and consider the rate of Hb variability in response to the prescribed therapy, especially prior to adjusting the prescribed dose. A single Hb concentration outside of the therapeutic range may not necessitate a dosage change. Several weeks are needed to observe Hb levels as they normalize, and therapy is typically needed for months to reach the necessary iron stores.

Administer additional oral iron when transferrin saturation is less than 20% or ferritin is less than 100 mcg/L. If the desired response to oral iron therapy is not achieved after 4 weeks, consider IV iron therapy. IV iron appears to be better tolerated by some patients who could not tolerate oral iron, or who have a hemoglobin (Hb) increase of less than 2 Gm/dL within 4 weeks. A referral to a hematologist is usually required.

Patients with preexisting hypertension may require an increase in antihypertensive therapy. Take special care to closely monitor and control the patient's blood pressure. Advise patients regarding the importance of compliance with antihypertensive therapy and any dietary sodium restrictions to reduce hypertensive episodes. The patient should be asked to report new-onset neurologic symptoms, seizure activity, or an increase in seizure activity related to anemia therapy.

The primary care provider should suspect the development of pure red cell aplasia if a sudden loss of response to ESA therapy accompanied by severe anemia and low reticulocyte count is noted. The presence of binding and neutralizing antibodies to erythropoietin should be assessed. If antierythropoietin antibody-associated anemia is suspected, withhold epoetin and other erythropoietic proteins. Again, a referral to a hematologist is in order if red cell aplasia is suspected.

Teaching Points for Anemia Therapy

Worldwide, IDA is a common problem across the life span. Patients can reduce their risk for IDA by adopting a healthy lifestyle. The following health promotion strategies and practices should be presented to patients to help them become full partners in their health care.

Health Promotion Strategies

- Advise patients to increase their dietary intake of iron. Heme iron, which is found only in meat, poultry, and fish, is two to three times more absorbable than non-heme iron, which is found in plant-based foods and iron-fortified foods.
- Vitamin C improves the absorption of non-heme iron from plant sources. Advise patients to include sources of vitamin C in their regular diet. Dietary sources of vitamin C include oranges, lemons, grapefruit, cranberries, bananas, and kiwi.
- Polyphenols (in certain vegetables), tannins (in tea), phytates (in bran), and calcium (in dairy products) can

inhibit the absorption of iron. Advise patients to include in their diet foods that are high in folate, such as citrus fruits, leafy greens, nuts, seeds, and legumes.

- Vegetarian diets are low in heme iron. However, iron bio-availability in a vegetarian diet can be increased by careful planning of meals to include other sources of iron and enhancers of iron absorption.
- Advise patients to limit alcohol consumption. Alcohol can aggravate the symptoms of IDA.
- If the patient is taking iron supplements, advise them not to consume tea or coffee for several hours before and after taking them.
- For lactating patients, encourage *exclusive* breastfeeding of infants for 6 months after birth. When exclusive breastfeeding is stopped, encourage use of an additional source of iron from supplementary foods or iron-fortified infant formula.

Patient Education for Medication Safety

All medications used in the treatment of anemia must be taken as prescribed to have the optimum therapeutic effect. Primary care providers need to stress the following to patients for safe medication management:

- Ferrous sulfate or ferrous gluconate can cause you to have dark, tarry stools and constipation. Prevent constipation by eating a high-fiber diet, by ensuring that you are adequately hydrated (based on medical history), and by taking a stool softener daily.
- Iron dextran may discolor your urine.
- Get emergency medical help if you have signs of an allergic reaction at home, such as hives, difficulty breathing, or swelling of your face, lips, tongue, or throat.
- Tell your primary care provider about any medication allergies you may have as you may be at higher risk of hypersensitivity reactions to iron.
- Oral iron preparations can cause fatal poisoning in children. Keep these medications safely out of reach.
- Tell your primary care provider about all the medications you are taking to avoid medication interactions with iron preparations.
- If you are taking an ESA, report any new or worsening seizure activity to your primary care provider.
- Monitor your blood pressure at home and report unusual or higher-than-normal values to your primary care provider.
- Take your medication for hypertension as prescribed, and avoid missing doses as anemia treatments can cause hypertension.
- Keep all clinic and laboratory appointments for blood tests related to your anemia. If you need to miss an appointment, reschedule it as soon as possible.

Application Questions for Discussion

1. What are the clinical considerations for laboratory testing and iron supplementation for pregnant patients?

2. What are the primary and secondary prevention strategies for patients at high risk for or who are newly diagnosed with IDA?

3. What data should be included in a decision for increasing or changing iron therapy in patients with anemia?

Selected Bibliography

Blanchette, N. L., Manz, D. H., Torti, F. M., & Torti, S. V. (2016). Modulation of hepcidin to treat iron deregulation: Potential clinical applications. *Expert Review of Hematology, 9*(2), 169–186.

Cascio, M. J., & DeLoughery, T. G. (2017). Anemia: Evaluation and diagnostic tests. *Medical Clinics of North America, 101*(2), 263–284. http://doi.org/10.1016/j.mcna.2016.09.003.

Chaparro, C. M., & Suchdev, P. S. (2019). Anemia epidemiology, pathophysiology, and etiology in low- and middle-income countries. *Annals of the New York Academy of Sciences, 1450*(1), 15–31. http://doi.org/10.1111/nyas.14092.

Hempel, E. V., & Bollard, E. R. (2016). The evidence-based evaluation of iron deficiency anemia. *Medical Clinics of North America, 100*(5), 1065–1075. http://doi.org/10.1016/j.mcna.2016.04.015.

Lopez, A., Cacoub, P., Macdougall, I. C., & Peyrin-Biroulet, L. (2016). Iron deficiency anaemia. *Lancet, 387*(10021), 907–916. http://doi.org/10.1016/S0140-6736(15)60865-0.

McDonagh, M., Cantor, A., Bougatsos, C., et al. (2015). Routine iron supplementation and screening for iron deficiency anemia in pregnant women: A systematic review to update the U.S. Preventive Services Task Force Recommendation. https://www.ncbi.nlm.nih.gov/books/NBK285987/.

Nandakumar, S. K., Ulirsch, J. C., & Sankaran, V. G. (2016). Advances in understanding erythropoiesis: Evolving perspectives. *British Journal of Haematology, 173*(2), 206–218. http://doi.org/10.1111/bjh.13938.

Onken, J. E., Bregman, D. B., Harrington, R. A., et al. (2014). A multicenter, randomized, active controlled study to investigate the safety and efficacy of intravenous ferric carboxymaltose in patients with iron deficiency anemia. *Transfusion, 54,* 306–315.

Palmer, S. C., Saglimbene, V., Mavridis, D., Salanti, G., Craig, J. C., Tonelli, M., Wiebe, N., & Strippoli, G. F. (2014). Erythropoiesis stimulating agents for anaemia in adults with chronic kidney disease: A network meta-analysis. *The Cochrane Database of Systemic Reviews*(12), Article CD010590. http://doi.org/10.1002/14651858.CD010590.pub2.

Shappert, S. M., & Rechtsteiner, E. A. (2008). *Ambulatory care utilization estimates for 2006.* National Health Statistics Report, National Center for Health Statistics. https://pubmed.ncbi.nlm.nih.gov/18958997/.

Tolkien, Z., Stecher, L., Mander, A. P., Pereira, D. I., & Powell, J. J. Ferrous sulfate supplementation causes significant gastrointestinal side-effects in adults: A systematic review and meta-analysis. *PLoS One, 10*(2): e0117383. http://doi.org/10.1371/journal.pone.0117383.

WHO. (2011). *Haemoglobin concentrations for the diagnosis of anaemia and assessment of severity.* Geneva: World Health Organization. Vitamin and Mineral Nutrition Information System (WHO/NMH/NHD/MNM/11.1) Accessed April 15, 2019. http://www.who.int/vmnis/indicators/haemoglobin.pdf.

14

Anticlotting Medications

CONSTANCE G. VISOVSKY

Overview

Medications that interfere with blood clotting are divided into two broad categories: anticoagulants and fibrinolytic (thrombolytic) agents. *Anticoagulants* reduce a patient's blood-clotting potential. *Fibrinolytics* help dissolve formed clots and are used in critical care settings. This chapter focuses on the anticoagulant medications used most often in the primary care setting. These include platelet activation/aggregation inhibitors, indirect thrombin inhibitors, direct thrombin inhibitors, and vitamin K antagonists. Some categories of anticoagulants have subcategories that differ by mechanism of action. Understanding the implications in primary care for patients who received or are receiving anticoagulants (often initiated in the acute care setting) is very important for the primary care provider in terms of evaluating the need for continued anticoagulation and for appropriate follow-up care. A thorough understanding of the mechanisms of action for the various types of anticoagulants ensures more precise prescribing, taking into consideration the exact cause of the clotting problem, interactions with other medications, and individual patient factors. Too much anticoagulation increases the risk for bleeding, while too little increases the risk for thrombotic events.

Relevant Physiology

Extrinsic and Intrinsic Coagulation Pathways

Coagulation is necessary in normal physiology to maintain adequate whole-body perfusion. Our understanding of the complex molecular mechanisms involved in the initiation of coagulation pathways is still evolving and continues to shed light on the delicate balance between homeostasis and pathologic thrombotic events. Blood normally circulates through the vasculature of the body as a liquid, which is the form needed for organ and tissue perfusion. In the event of an injury involving the blood vessels in which blood leaves the vasculature, the blood-clotting cascade must quickly start coagulation, limited to the area of injury, to minimize blood loss while maintaining circulation and perfusion to all other areas.

Normal blood clotting has two distinct pathways: the *extrinsic pathway* (outside the blood vessels) and the *intrinsic pathway*, which begins with changes in the blood rather than with trauma. These pathways compose the multistep processes of the blood-clotting cascade reaction, which leads to a rapid response to maintain circulation and homeostasis (Fig. 14.1). Both pathways are similar and eventually merge later in the cascade, forming a common path to result in the formation of a stable fibrin clot capable of hemostasis. Essentially the extrinsic pathway is a "shortcut" to the final result of the cascade: the formation of a stable fibrin clot. The required substances common to both pathways are activated platelets, appropriate amounts of *all* clotting factors, and calcium. Platelets (*thrombocytes*) are small, disk-shaped bodies formed as fragments from *megakaryocytes* in the bone marrow. These cell-like disks circulate freely as independent single entities in the blood until they are activated and then adhere to each other and to blood vessel walls. Platelet activation and aggregation is the critical step in initiating both the intrinsic and extrinsic pathways of the blood-clotting cascade, starting the formation of a *platelet plug*. The plug is *not* a clot, but ultimately clot formation is very dependent on this aggregation.

As shown in Fig. 14.1, the steps of both pathways rely on the presence of blood-clotting factors. Many of the "factors" are actually inactive enzymes synthesized in the liver. Once a factor is activated, it can act as a functional enzyme and activate the next factor in the cascade. (Although the factors are numbered, the numbering system only indicates the order in which the factors were discovered and not the order in which they function in the cascade.) With injury to blood vessels, blood clotting begins with aggregation of platelets at the beginning of the extrinsic pathway when a substance known as *tissue factor* (also called *tissue thromboplastin*) is released from injured cells. This factor becomes a *prothrombin activator*, which then acts as an enzyme to convert inactive prothrombin (Factor X) into the active enzyme *thrombin* (Factor Xa). It is at this juncture of Xa production that the extrinsic pathway and the intrinsic pathway converge as a final common pathway in which thrombin converts inactive *fibrinogen* (Factor I) into active *fibrin* molecules that assemble into long threads, forming a mesh to trap platelets,

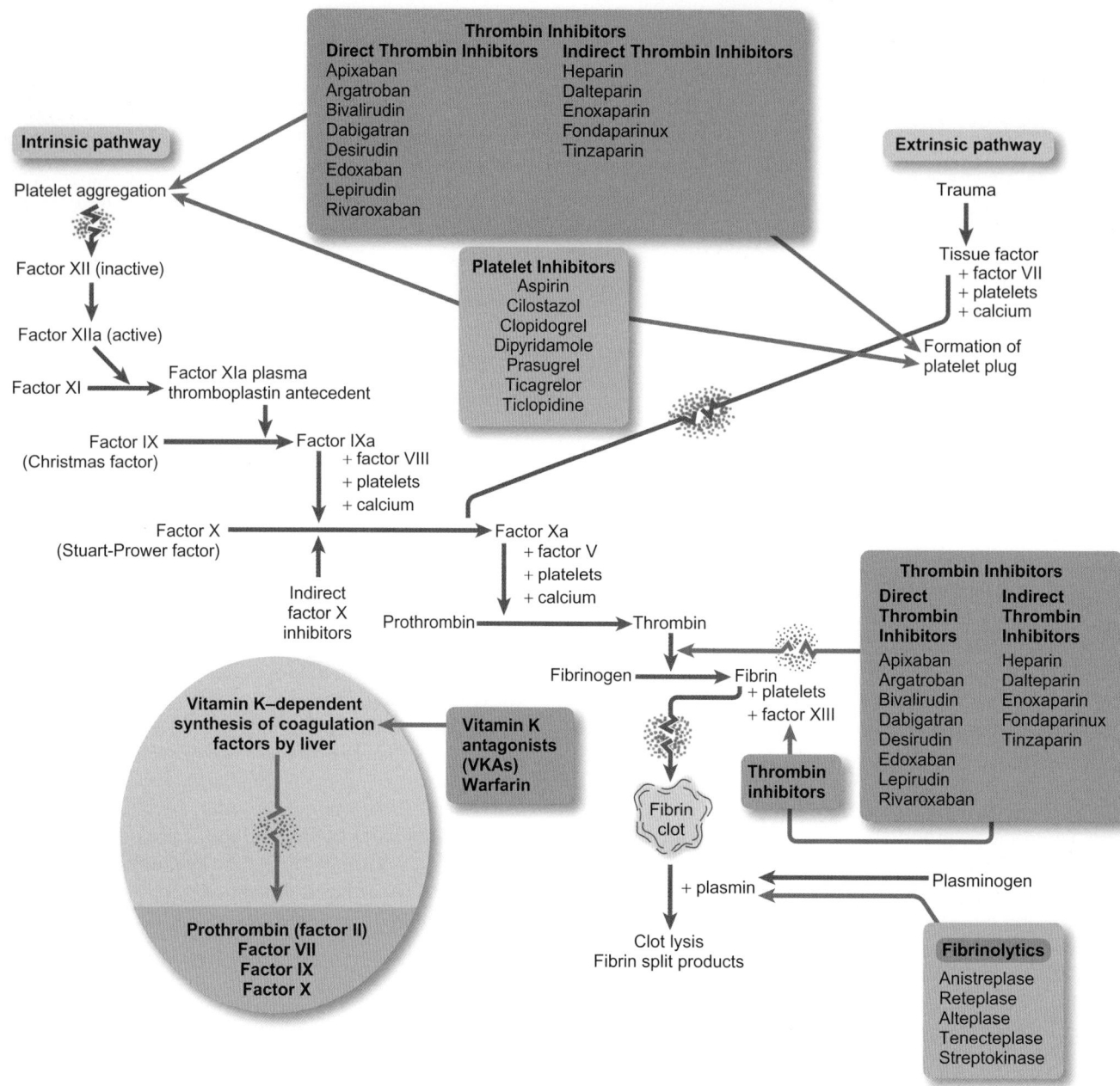

• **Fig. 14.1** Summary of the blood-clotting cascade. RBC: red blood cell. (From Ignatavicius, D. D., Workman, M. L., Rebar, C., & Heimgartner, N. [2021]. *Medical surgical nursing: Concepts for interprofessional collaborative care* [10th ed.]. St. Louis: Elsevier.)

red blood cells (RBCs), and plasma proteins to form a fibrin clot. (This step also activates more platelets.) This clot is stabilized to its final structure by fibrin-stabilizing factor (*Factor XIII*). The extrinsic (tissue factor) pathway functions in normal homeostasis. The intrinsic pathway is initiated by abnormal conditions inside the blood vessel, and it is this pathway that has been implicated in thrombotic diseases. Although all factors and steps are needed for blood to clot, the ones that are important at critical control points and are most affected by anticoagulation therapy are discussed here in more detail.

Platelet Activation/Aggregation

Platelets are not truly cells, because they have no nuclei and cannot reproduce. However, they do have intracellular organelles filled with chemical mediators that allow them to not only respond to certain conditions and substances by becoming activated, but also reinforce this activation among themselves and induce activity or secretion of proclotting substances by other cells. Each platelet is surrounded by a glycoprotein coating (known as GBIIb/IIIa complex) that normally does not adhere to other platelets, blood cells, or vascular linings unless activated. Embedded within this complex are receptors for fibrinogen and thromboxane A2 (TXA2). In response to tissue or vascular injury, platelets become activated by thrombin, adenosine diphosphate (ADP), serotonin, and epinephrine when these substances bind to their specific receptors in or on platelets. These activators change the shape of the glycoprotein coat and expose more receptors, especially for fibrinogen and TXA2, causing the activated platelets to adhere to the damaged endothelium or collagen as well as to each other and form a platelet plug at the site of vessel injury. In addition, the presence of activated platelets signals the formation and release of clotting Factors VII and X, thus enhancing other steps in clot formation. This action then stimulates (by positive feedback) the activation of additional platelets and increased release of TXA2, serotonin, and ADP to enhance platelet aggregation and reinforce the formed clot. Additionally, the binding of ADP to G-protein receptors P2Y12 and P2Y1 initiates more platelet aggregation and increases the response of platelets to TXA2 and thrombin in the process of clot formation.

Coagulation is dependent on the activation and function of platelets to begin and maintain the blood-clotting cascade. Thus, platelet activation/aggregation is a logical point for pharmacologic intervention of coagulation and is a common site of action for some categories of anticoagulants.

Activation of Fibrinogen to Fibrin

Without thrombin activation of fibrinogen to fibrin, a clot cannot form, even when platelet plugs are plentiful. Platelet plugs alone cannot prevent widespread bleeding caused by vascular injury. Thus, conversion of fibrinogen to fibrin, which can only be performed by thrombin, remains another key control point and site of action for anticoagulation therapy.

Antithrombin III

A key point for homeostasis is to maintain circulation to the body with appropriate blood clotting where needed by limiting the cascade to areas of injury. One factor helping to control the extension of clotting beyond its area of utility is the presence of the factor *antithrombin III*. This factor binds to excess loose fibrin molecules and prevents them from assembling into the long fibrin threads and the meshwork that form the scaffold of fibrin clots. It also binds to and removes activated clotting Factors IX, X, XI, and XII, thus slowing the cascade reaction. With these actions, manipulation of antithrombin III is another key control point and site of action for anticoagulation therapy.

Pathophysiology: Thromboembolic Risks and Events

Virchow's triad is an explanation for thrombus formation that results from the interaction of impaired blood flow, hypercoagulability of the blood, and damage to the vascular endothelium. One or more of Virchow's triad of

pathophysiologic actions is typically a part of any risk associated with the development of thromboembolic events and *thrombophilia* (hypercoagulation).

Several risk factors are known to be involved in the development of thromboembolic events (Box 14.1). In general, the events leading to thrombosis involve conditions or disease states associated with decreased circulation, obstruction to blood flow, reduced mobility, poor lifestyle choices (smoking, obesity), or genetically inherited risk factors.

Research evidence has demonstrated that the role of platelets extends beyond that of clot formation, as platelets are key mediators of inflammation, atherosclerosis, and thrombosis. Platelets gather at the site of vascular injury to form platelet plugs to minimize excessive bleeding risk. Platelets also aggregate intravascularly following blood vessel wall injury or rupture of existing atherosclerotic plaques, exposing blood cells to collagen. For example, in patients with atherosclerosis, an intracoronary thrombus can form, narrowing the coronary artery and restricting blood flow to the myocardium. An atherosclerotic plaque in the coronary artery can become disrupted, leading to partial or complete coronary artery occlusion, and ultimately, a myocardial infarction. These same processes can occur in the internal carotid artery or atria of the heart (secondary to atrial fibrillation) and can result in stroke. The main causes of coronary thrombosis are elevated low-density lipoprotein (LDL) cholesterol, smoking, sedentary lifestyle, and hypertension.

Patients with underlying conditions prone to venous stasis or inherited clotting disorders are at risk for deep vein thrombosis (DVT). Dislodgement of a DVT can result in a pulmonary embolus (PE). Atherosclerosis can lead to chronic peripheral arterial occlusive disease in the

---

• BOX 14.1 Risk Factors for Thromboembolic Events

- Major surgery (trauma, coronary artery bypass, abdominal or neurosurgery)
- Major orthopedic surgery (hip, pelvis, femur)
- History of cancer
- Age (>40 years)
- History of venous thromboembolism
- Varicose veins
- Pregnancy
- Oral contraceptives of estrogen-based hormone replacement therapy
- Acquired hematologic conditions
- Heart failure
- Immobility/bedrest
- Spinal cord injury
- Obesity (BMI >30 kg/m^2)
- History of ischemic stroke
- Inflammatory bowel disease

femoropopliteal, tibioperoneal, aortoiliac, carotid, vertebral, splanchnic, renal, or brachiocephalic arteries.

Patients with elevated homocysteine levels are at threefold risk for thromboembolic events (Spence, 2016). Homocysteine binds with a variety of plasma proteins, including fibrinogen, and can activate them. When fibrinogen is activated excessively to fibrin when there is no need for coagulation, pathologic thrombi and emboli can form.

Inherited Coagulopathies

In the case of inherited coagulopathies, protein C and protein S are vitamin K–dependent glycoproteins that act as natural anticoagulants, with additional actions that include antiapoptotic, antiinflammatory gene expression regulation and endothelial barrier protection. Protein C deficiency is found in 6% of families with inherited thrombophilia and in 3% of patients with a first-time DVT (Wypasek & Undas, 2013). Protein S deficiency is less common, with an estimated prevalence of less than 0.5% in the general European population and presence in about 2% to 12% of patients with known coagulopathy (Wypasek & Undas, 2013). Protein C and Protein S deficiencies arise from genetic mutations. Patients with either deficiency have a 2- to 11-fold increased risk for developing DVT or PE compared to those without a deficiency (McCance et al., 2019).

Inherited antithrombin III deficiency is a rare genetic disorder that greatly increases the risk for thromboembolic disease. In antithrombin III deficiency, antithrombin antigen and heparin cofactor levels are both reduced to about 50% of normal. Patients are often diagnosed after experiencing multiple thromboembolic events such as venous thrombosis or PE, often at ages much younger than expected (McCance et al., 2019).

Coagulation risk increases in anyone who has a higher-than-normal level of any clotting factor. Several genetic disorders result in an increased circulating level of specific clotting factors. Factor V Leiden mutation is a thrombophilia associated with a mutation in the gene for clotting Factor V. The mutated Factor V functions normally but is degraded much more slowly than normal Factor V, and clotting activity continues beyond the time that it is needed, which greatly increases the risk for DVT and, to a lesser extent, PE (van Langevelde et al., 2012).

Prothrombin G20210A mutations arise when guanine is changed for adenine at position 20210 of the prothrombin (Factor X) gene. Prothrombin G20210A is the second most frequently acquired polymorphism in females and presents an overall 5% risk in venous thrombotic events (Dziadosz & Baxi, 2016). This mutation increases plasma prothrombin levels and allows more thrombin (Factor Xa) to be present, which then increases fibrin levels and contributes to hypercoagulability.

Factor VIII is an important blood-clotting protein known as antihemophilic factor. Elevations in Factor VIII increase the risk for recurrent thrombosis by as much as

37% (Jenkins et al., 2012). Lifetime anticoagulation may be warranted for the genetic mutation that results in chronically increased circulating levels of Factor VIII.

Anticoagulant Therapy

Anticoagulant medications interfere with one or more steps in the blood-clotting processes, preventing new clots from forming and existing clots from extending. Remember that anticoagulants cannot dissolve formed clots. The goal of anticoagulant therapy is to achieve the desired effect while minimizing bleeding risk. Anticoagulants are classified as platelet inhibitors, indirect thrombin inhibitors, direct thrombin inhibitors, and vitamin K antagonists. Although some medications have more than one mechanism of action, the anticoagulants described in this chapter are categorized by primary mechanism of action and are the drugs most commonly prescribed in or used in primary care following an acute thromboembolic event or percutaneous coronary intervention (PCI).

Platelet Inhibitors

All platelet inhibitors function to inhibit platelet activation and aggregation. As described earlier, activation of platelets is accomplished by several interacting substances and reactions. In addition, activated platelets use positive feedback mechanisms to ensure continued activation of more platelets and are also key elements in enhancing other proclotting areas of the blood coagulation cascade. The three major mechanisms by which platelet inhibitors prevent or suppress platelet activation and aggregation are by inhibiting TXA2, interfering with ADP induction of platelet activation, and inhibiting the enzyme phosphodiesterase III (PDE3).

The major role of platelet inhibitors in clinical practice is to prevent consequences of thrombosis in atherosclerotic arteries to the heart (atrial fibrillation, cardiac devices), brain (ischemic stroke), and peripheral vascular system (intermittent claudication and pain). Determining the needed onset of action, duration of therapy of choice, indication for therapy, and patient characteristics drives selection of a specific platelet inhibitor. In recent years, bleeding has been identified as an important risk factor for adverse outcomes and has led to a renewed emphasis on individual bleeding risk when choosing appropriate therapy.

All platelet inhibitors can cause easy bruising and bleeding and carry black box warnings for potential, significant, or sometimes fatal bleeding risk. While the risk of excessive bleeding is relatively low, the advanced practice nurse (APN) must monitor for signs and symptoms related to bleeding and teach patients and families to report ecchymosis; petechiae; lightheadedness; dizziness; tachycardia; abnormal bleeding from any source; dark, tarry stools; coffee-ground vomitus; and shortness of breath. All antiplatelet medications have numerous drug–drug interactions, and a thorough medication reconciliation is vital before beginning

TABLE 14.1	Platelet Inhibitor Medications		
Category/ Medication	**Indication**	**Dosage**	**Considerations and Monitoring**
Thromboxane Inhibitors			
Aspirin	Primary/secondary prevention of thrombotic stroke, MI, ACS, PVD, thromboembolism	Loading dose: 160–325 mg Maintenance dosage: 80 or 81 mg daily	Monitor for bleeding, abdominal pain, and angioedema; stop aspirin 7 days before surgery.
Dipyridamole	Thromboembolism prophylaxis post-cardiac valve replacement	75–100 mg orally every 6 hr as an adjunct to warfarin	Monitor for bronchospasm, chest pain, and liver dysfunction.
ADP-Induction Inhibitors			
Clopidogrel	Secondary prevention of thrombotic stroke MI, ACS, PVD, or after PCI; often prescribed in addition to aspirin	Loading dose of 600 mg or 300 mg before stent placement depending on condition and patient demographics. Maintenance dosage: 75 mg daily	Usually taken for up to 12 months; many drug–drug interactions.
Prasugrel	Prevention of cardiac thrombotic stroke in acute coronary syndromes (with confirmed MI) who underwent PCI and/or have unstable angina	10 mg daily for 1 year; given with aspirin for prevention of thrombosis in stent placement	Monitor for bleeding, hypersensitivity reactions, and TTP.
Ticlopidine	Prevention of thrombotic stroke in patients who fail aspirin therapy, prevention of stent thrombosis	250 mg every 12 hr; given with aspirin for prevention of thrombosis in stent placement	Monitor CBC and LFTs before starting, and then every 2 weeks for first 3 months. Monitor serum cholesterol and triglycerides. Discontinue 10–14 days before major surgery in patients with bleeding diathesis.
Ticagrelor	For the reduction in risk of first myocardial infarction (myocardial infarction prophylaxis) or stroke in patients with coronary artery disease (CAD) at high risk for these events	Maintenance dosage: 90 mg orally twice daily (for 1 year) Maintenance dosage (after 1 year with history of MI): 60 mg orally twice daily	Aspirin maintenance dose >100 mg reduces the effectiveness of ticagrelor and should be avoided.
PDE3 Inhibitors			
Cilostozol	Intermittent claudication	100 mg orally every 12 hr either 30 minutes before or 2 hr after meals	Monitor for signs and symptoms of angina or MI; monitor CBC for adverse hematologic effects.
Anagrelide	Essential myeloproliferative disorders, polycythemia vera	0.5 mg orally every 6 hr, or 1 mg orally every 12 hr Dose escalation: increase dose no more frequently than 0.5 mg/day/week Not to exceed 10 mg/day or 2.5 mg/dose	Platelet count responds typically in 7–14 days; time to complete response is 4–12 weeks. Monitor platelet counts.

ACS, acute coronary syndrome; *ADP,* adenosine diphosphate; *CBC,* complete blood count; *LFTs,* liver function tests; *MI,* myocardial infarction; *PCI,* percutaneous coronary intervention; *PDE3,* phosphodiesterase III; *PVD,* peripheral vascular disease; *TTP,* thrombotic thrombocytopenia purpura.

treatment with these agents. Table 14.1 provides a summary of platelet inhibitors.

TXA2 Inhibitors

TXA2 inhibitors have the same essential mechanism of action, although some are more efficient than others. As described earlier, TXA2 promotes coagulation by activating platelets, making their membranes sticky for better adhesion to each other. It also enhances the binding of fibrinogen to platelet membrane surfaces. TXA2 is produced in many cells, including platelets, by the cyclooxygenase-1 (COX-1) pathway of the arachidonic acid cascade that also synthesizes many other inflammatory mediators and prostaglandins.

TXA2 inhibitors bind to the enzyme responsible for converting an intermediate substance in the arachidonic acid pathway into TXA2, thereby blocking its production within platelets. Some inhibitor medications bind to this enzyme so tightly and irreversibly that the platelet exposed to the drug is unable to produce any TXA2 for the rest of its life span. For other medications, the binding is reversible and the exposed platelet begins TXA2 synthesis within 24 hours after the medication has been cleared.

Aspirin

Aspirin, the most commonly prescribed platelet inhibitor, prevents platelet aggregation by *irreversibly* inhibiting COX-1, blocking the formation of TXA2. As a result, platelets are unable to regenerate cyclooxygenase, and the immediate antithrombotic effect of aspirin remains for the life span of the platelet (8 to 10 days).

Pharmacokinetics. Aspirin is rapidly absorbed from the gastrointestinal (GI) tract and reaches peak effect in 1 to 3 hours. The half-life of aspirin is dose dependent, with 2 to 3 hours for an 81-mg tablet and up to 15 to 30 hours for large doses. Aspirin at moderate dosage (160 to 325 mg) produces rapid and immediate antiplatelet effects. Return to full platelet activity after even one 325-mg dose requires 5 to 10 days for the affected platelets to be destroyed and replaced by new platelets unexposed to aspirin.

PHARMACOGENETICS

Aspirin Therapy

- While aspirin is widely prescribed as an antiplatelet agent to reduce the risk of thrombus and recurrent cardiovascular events, a considerable number of patients have a less-than-optimal response to aspirin.
- Approximately 15% of the suboptimal aspirin response is influenced by age, gender, and smoking status, as well as by comorbidities (obesity, diabetes, hyperlipidemia), with 14% to 39% explained by genetic factors that influence COX-1 platelet activation pathways.
- Aspirin can cause hemolysis in patients with glucose-6-phosphate dehydrogenase (G6PD) deficiency.

Indications. Despite evidence of the effectiveness of aspirin therapy, patients with established thromboembolic disease were found to be undertreated. A global study of 67,888 patients with three or more risk factors for thrombosis found that only 76.2% were prescribed aspirin (Bhatt et al., 2006).

Subgroups of patients present with aspirin resistance and continue to experience ischemic events on aspirin therapy. Aspirin resistance may be indicative of therapeutic variability and incomplete suppression of TXA2 synthesis among some patient populations.

Adverse Effects. The major adverse effect of aspirin therapy is uncontrolled bleeding. Caution must be taken in using aspirin with patients who are at risk for bleeding or

---

PRACTICE PEARLS

Aspirin Therapy

In 2021 the U.S. Preventive Services Task Force (USPSTF) modified the recommendations for the use of aspirin in the primary prevention of cardiovascular disease.

- Initiation of low-dose aspirin for the primary prevention of cardiovascular disease in adults 40 to 59 years of age with a 10% or greater 10-year risk should be individualized as the evidence of aspirin use in this group is small.
- The USPSTF recommends against initiating low-dose aspirin use for the primary prevention of cardiovascular disease in adults 60 years of age or older.
- No current data exist to support prescribing daily low-dose aspirin to patients younger than 50 or older than 70 years of age.
- Counsel patients to avoid taking aspirin on a long-term basis without consulting their health care provider.

U.S. Preventive Services Task Force. (2021). *Aspirin use to prevent cardiovascular disease: Preventive medication.* https://www.uspreventiveservicestaskforce.org/uspstf/draft-recommendation/aspirin-use-to-prevent-cardiovascular-disease-preventive-medication.

---

are using concomitant nonsteroidal antiinflammatory drugs (NSAIDs), corticosteroids, or other drugs that interfere with platelet activity to avoid hemorrhage.

Aspirin also suppresses the production of many helpful prostaglandins, including those that produce the thick, gel-like mucous that protects the stomach lining from the action of hydrochloric acid. Combined with aspirin-induced reduced blood flow to the stomach lining, the reduced stomach mucus increases the risk for peptic ulcer disease.

Contraindications. Aspirin is contraindicated for patients with sensitivity or allergy to salicylates, those with a history of GI bleeding, those who have a coagulation disorder, and anyone with G6PD deficiency. Aspirin should be used cautiously in patients with renal impairment, thrombocytopenia, recent surgery, or trauma. Do not use in children and teenagers with varicella or influenza because of the risk of Reye's syndrome.

Monitoring. Patients should be monitored for signs and symptoms of abnormal bleeding, abdominal pain indicative of peptic ulcer formation, and hypersensitivity reactions, such as angioedema.

Dipyridamole

The primary mechanism of action for dipyridamole is not yet clearly known. One effect is similar to aspirin as a TXA2 inhibitor. It appears to block the release of arachidonic acid, which in turn prevents synthesis of TXA2. In addition, dipyridamole appears to inhibit the phosphodiesterase enzymes that break down cyclic adenosine monophosphate (cAMP), which in turn increases intracellular cAMP concentrations and blocks the platelet aggregation response to ADP. Dipyridamole also inhibits RBC uptake of adenosine and TXA2, thereby inhibiting

BLACK BOX WARNING!

Aspirin

- Do not use in patients who have active bleeding or a history of transient ischemic attack (TIA) or stroke.
- Do not start in patients planning to undergo urgent coronary artery bypass graft (CABG) surgery; when possible, discontinue at least 5 days prior to any surgery (ticagrelor).
- Aspirin is not recommended for people older than 75 years of age due to increased risk of fatal and intracranial bleeding.
- Discontinue aspirin at least 7 days before any surgical procedure.
- If possible, manage bleeding without discontinuing aspirin due to risk of subsequent cardiovascular events.
- Do not prescribe to patients weighing less than 60 kg due to increased bleeding risk.
- Avoid use with increased bleeding risk due to recent trauma, surgery, recent or recurrent GI bleeding, active peptic ulcer disease, severe hepatic impairment, or moderate to severe renal impairment.
- Avoid concomitant use of other drugs that are known to increase bleeding risk.

platelet activation. Even with all these antiplatelet actions, dipyridamole alone does not sufficiently inhibit platelet activation to therapeutic levels and is often used in conjunction with other platelet inhibitors or other types of anticoagulants in patients at higher risk for inappropriate clot formation.

Pharmacokinetics. Following oral administration of standard preparations, peak plasma concentrations of dipyridamole are attained in 1 to 2.5 hours with a duration of action of about 3 hours. The half-life of dipyridamole is 10 to 12 hours. With extended-release tablets containing dipyridamole and aspirin, peak plasma dipyridamole concentrations are attained in about 2 hours with twice-daily dosing. Dipyridamole is metabolized by the liver and eliminated through the feces.

Indications. Patients with a history of ischemic stroke may benefit from aspirin plus dipyridamole therapy initially, with a subsequent switch to clopidogrel therapy after 1 year. A recently published meta-analysis found the combination of aspirin plus dipyridamole to be more effective as compared to aspirin alone (Niu et al., 2016). Aspirin plus dipyridamole was also associated with better short-term outcomes in patients with ischemic stroke than aspirin alone. Extended-release dipyridamole with aspirin is not interchangeable with the individual components of aspirin and conventional dipyridamole tablets.

Adverse Effects. Adverse effects of dipyridamole include chest pain, angina, abnormal electrocardiogram (ECG), headache, and dizziness. Fewer than 10% of patients experience ST changes, abdominal discomfort, and abnormal heart rhythm. Patients with a history of asthma may be at greater risk for bronchospasm when

taking this medication. Elevated liver function tests (LFTs) have been reported.

Contraindications. Dipyridamole is contraindicated in patients with thrombocytopenia. Use during pregnancy and breastfeeding is contraindicated as small amounts cross the placenta and can be found in breast milk, placing the fetus and infant at risk for excess bleeding.

Monitoring. Patients should be monitored for difficulty breathing or for wheezing related to bronchospasm. Patients with coronary artery disease (CAD) should be monitored for chest pain that can develop with dipyridamole. Monitor LFTs for signs of liver dysfunction.

ADP-Induction Inhibitors

All current ADP-induction inhibitors work at the glycoprotein coating (GBIIb/IIIa complex) of platelets. These medications act as antagonists by binding tightly and irreversibly to the ADP receptors at the P2Y12 site on the membrane complex without activating the receptors. This action prevents the agonist ADP from binding to its membrane receptors. As a result, the receptors for fibrinogen and TXA2 remain embedded in the complex and the positive feedback enhancement of platelet activation/aggregation is disrupted to varying degrees. With the irreversible binding of these medications to the ADP receptors, platelet function does not return to normal until at least 72 hours after the medication has been discontinued and fresh platelets repopulate the blood.

Clopidogrel

Pharmacokinetics. Clopidogrel is ingested as an inactive parent compound. After being metabolized in the liver by hepatic cytochrome (CYP) 450 enzymes, the active metabolite exerts its effect on circulating platelets and is excreted in urine and feces. The half-life of clopidogrel is approximately 6 hours following a single 75-mg dose.

PHARMACOGENETICS

Clopidogrel Therapy

- Clopidogrel's antiplatelet activity is dependent on conversion to an active metabolite by the CYP 450 system, principally CYP 2C19. The efficiency of this enzyme in drug metabolism varies by genetic inheritance of one or more small mutations known as *polymorphisms*.
- More than 50% of Asians have CYP 2C19 genetic variants that inhibit clopidogrel metabolism. Such individuals are known as *poor metabolizers* or *slow metabolizers*. If clopidogrel is used in poor metabolizers or in patients taking other medications that inhibit the CYP 2C19 enzyme, such as proton pump inhibitors, more drug is excreted as an inactive compound and the antiplatelet effect is reduced.
- Patients who may be CYP 2C19 poor metabolizers should be tested for this polymorphism, and if present, use of another platelet P2Y12 inhibitor should be considered.

Indications. Clopidogrel is used to prevent myocardial infarction and ischemic stroke in patients with known cardiovascular disease, those who have had a recent stroke, and those who have been diagnosed with peripheral vascular disease. Clopidogrel is also used along with aspirin therapy following cardiac stent placement. Clopidogrel use is associated with improved mortality outcomes when compared with aspirin alone.

Adverse Effects. Thrombotic thrombocytopenia purpura (TTP) is the most commonly reported adverse effect of clopidogrel. Neutropenia, acquired hemophilia, thrombocytopenia or idiopathic thrombocytopenia, and TTP with hemolytic uremic syndrome occur rarely in patients taking clopidogrel. Patients treated with clopidogrel should be carefully monitored for hematologic adverse effects, especially in the first 2 to 3 months after initiation of therapy. Early recognition and prompt initiation of treatment can be lifesaving in patients who have hematologic adverse effects to clopidogrel.

Contraindications. Like aspirin, clopidogrel can cause easy bruising, poses a risk for excessive bleeding, and must be used with extreme caution in patients with bleeding or platelet disorders. A significant increase in excessive bleeding has been reported in patients receiving clopidogrel plus aspirin compared with those receiving aspirin alone. Although rare, patients can develop TTP at any time after starting this medication.

PRACTICE PEARLS

Clopidogrel Use in Pregnancy and Lactation

- Pregnancy: Well-controlled studies of clopidogrel use during pregnancy are lacking and fetal risk is unknown. Thus, clopidogrel should be used during pregnancy only if absolutely needed.
- Lactation: The presence of clopidogrel in breast milk is unknown; but due to the potential for serious adverse reactions in the breastfeeding infant, a determination should be made whether to discontinue breastfeeding or discontinue the clopidogrel, with consideration of the health of the mother.

Monitoring. Clopidogrel should be used with caution in patients with a history of hepatic or renal disorders. Patients treated with clopidogrel should be carefully monitored for hematologic adverse effects, especially in the first 2 to 3 months after initiation of therapy.

Prasugrel

Pharmacokinetics. Prasugrel is rapidly absorbed following oral administration as an inactive parent compound. The medication is rapidly broken down in the intestine to form an active metabolite. The half-life of prasugrel's active metabolite is approximately 7 hours, with a range of 2 to 15 hours. Prasugrel reaches peak plasma time in 30 minutes and is eliminated in the urine and feces. This medication

has a greater antiplatelet effect compared with clopidogrel. Following discontinuance, platelet aggregation gradually returns to baseline values in about 5 to 9 days.

PHARMACOGENETICS

Prasugrel Therapy

The genetic polymorphism of CYP 2C19 does not appear to affect pharmacodynamic or clinical response to prasugrel. Thus, this medication may be used in patients identified as poor metabolizers of clopidogrel.

Indications. Prasugrel is used primarily for the prevention of cardiac thrombotic events in patients who have acute coronary syndromes (with confirmed myocardial infarction) who underwent PCI and/or have unstable angina. Medication therapy is continued for at least 12 months following placement of a coronary artery stent.

Adverse Effects. Anemia, bradycardia, dizziness, and atrial fibrillation have been reported in 1% to 10% of patients taking this medication. As with any other platelet inhibitor, there is a risk for severe, potentially fatal bleeding. TTP, hypersensitivity reactions with accompanying angioedema, hepatic dysfunction hemolysis, and hemorrhage have been reported in fewer than 1% of patients.

Contraindications. Prasugrel is contraindicated for use in patients with active bleeding, prior TIA, or stroke. Prasugrel is not recommended in patients older than 75 years of age due to increased risk of severe bleeding and intracranial bleeding.

Monitoring. Patients should be monitored for signs and symptoms of abnormal bleeding, such as bleeding gums, blood in the urine or stool, tachycardia, and shortness of breath. Patients should also be monitored for signs of TIA or stroke that may arise from bleeding. Swelling of the lips, face, or tongue may indicate angioedema. Patients should be monitored for TTP, especially within the first 2 weeks of therapy, by checking the platelet count.

BLACK BOX WARNING!

Prasugrel

- Prasugrel can cause significant bleeding. Do not use prasugrel in patients with active bleeding or a history of TIA or stroke.
- To avoid severe bleeding, discontinue prasugrel at least 7 days prior to any surgery.

Ticagrelor

Pharmacokinetics. Ticagrelor is rapidly absorbed as an inactive parent compound and then metabolized by the liver via CYP 3A4/5 to the active metabolite. It is excreted in the feces and urine. Peak plasma levels are achieved in approximately 1 hour, with a half-life of 7 to 9 hours.

Indications. Ticagrelor is indicated for patients with acute coronary syndrome (ACS) (unstable angina, non-ST elevation myocardial infarction, or ST elevation myocardial infarction) or a history of myocardial infarction to reduce the rate of thrombotic cardiovascular events. Ticagrelor also reduces the rate of stent thrombosis. Ticagrelor is prescribed for at least the first 12 months following ACS and is thought to be superior to clopidogrel in its action and in the fact that activation is not dependent on the CYP 2C19 enzyme.

Adverse Effects. Common adverse effects of ticagrelor include dyspnea (6.5% of patients), bleeding (8%), and higher incidences of severe post–CABG-related bleeding that can be fatal (Bonaca et al., 2016). Ticagrelor should be stopped 5 days before any surgery. Mild to moderate dyspnea has been reported in patients treated with ticagrelor, and resolves with discontinuance. Ticagrelor has been associated with the occurrence of bradyarrhythmias in 2.2% of patients, including some incidences of ventricular pauses and atrioventricular (AV) block (Sciraca et al., 2011).

Contraindications. Ticagrelor is contraindicated in patients with active intracranial or GI bleeding and in those who developed angioedema while taking it. There are no well-conducted clinical trials in patients during pregnancy, but fetal abnormalities have been observed with ticagrelor use in animal studies. Ticagrelor is contraindicated in patients with severe hepatic impairment as the risk of bleeding is increased due to reduced synthesis of coagulation proteins. This medication is used with caution in patients with a history of hyperuricemia. Renal uptake and transport of uric acid are inhibited by ticagrelor and the risk of hyperuricemia and gout may be increased.

Monitoring. Monitor patients for signs of bleeding; check hemoglobin and hematocrit at routine intervals. Check renal function and uric acid levels in patients with gout or at risk of hyperuricemia.

Ticlopidine

Pharmacokinetics. Ticlopidine is metabolized by the liver and excreted in the urine and feces. The medication is rapidly absorbed following oral administration, with peak action seen in 2 hours and a reported half-life of 12 hours. Breastfeeding is not recommended while using ticlopidine, because it is not known whether the medication enters breast milk.

Indications. Ticlopidine is used for the prevention of thromboembolic events, including in patients with a history of stroke, TIA, myocardial infarction, or stent placement. It is also used prophylactically in some patients with sickle cell disease and for patients with diabetic retinopathy at risk for clot formation in retinal vessels.

Adverse Effects. Ticlopidine has caused elevations in alkaline phosphatase and AST in approximately 3% to 10% of patients. Life-threatening TTP (1%), aplastic anemia (2.4%), and agranulocytosis (2.4%) have been reported related to the development of auto-antibodies (Jacob et al., 2012). The incidence of neutropenia, TTP, or aplastic anemia peaks between 3 and 8 weeks following initiation of

therapy and declines thereafter. Adverse hematologic effects occur 3 months after initiation of therapy. Long-term use with concurrent aspirin is not recommended due to elevated bleeding risk.

Contraindications. Ticlopidine is contraindicated for patients with preexisting hematologic disorders, such as neutropenia, thrombocytopenia, or active bleeding; with a history of either TTP or aplastic anemia; and who are currently prescribed other anticoagulants. It is also contraindicated in patients who have active bleeding or have a high risk for bleeding (i.e., peptic ulcer), and those with severe hepatic impairment. It is reserved for patients who have hypersensitivity to aspirin or who failed to respond therapeutically to aspirin, because of the potentially life-threatening adverse effects.

Monitoring. Close clinical monitoring is needed, especially during the first 3 months of ticlopidine therapy. Complete blood counts (CBCs), including platelet count and leukocyte differentials, should be performed prior to initiation of therapy and every 2 weeks to the end of the third month of therapy. LFTs and serum cholesterol and triglycerides should be monitored as these can become elevated with ticlopidine. Therapy should be discontinued immediately if laboratory testing confirms neutropenia, TTP, aplastic anemia, or thrombocytopenia.

PDE3 Inhibitors

As discussed earlier, ADP is a potent activator of platelets. Inside cells, adenosine triphosphate (ATP) is split to produce ADP, which is then broken down into cAMP. This substance is important in regulating many cellular actions and reactions. The trigger for splitting ATP into ADP is a low intracellular level of cAMP. When intracellular concentrations of cAMP are high, ATP is not induced to split and form ADP. The PDE3 enzyme acts to open cAMP, thus reducing the intracellular levels of cAMP and triggering ATP to form more ADP. When PDE3 is not present, cAMP levels remain high and inhibit ATP from making more ADP. Thus, inhibiting PDE3 prevents platelet activation and aggregation by indirectly reducing the amount of ADP available but does not interact with the ADP receptors. The PDE3 inhibitors reversibly inhibit the enzyme.

Cilostazol

Pharmacokinetics. Cilostazol is an active parent compound and its metabolites are also active in preventing platelet activation. It is metabolized in the liver by CYP 3A4 and CYP 2C19 enzymes and excreted in the urine (74%) and feces. The half-life of cilostazol is approximately 11 to 13 hours for both the drug and active metabolite. Cilostazol has been found in the breast milk of rats. There is a lack of human studies of cilostazol in breast milk, but due to the potential risk for serious adverse effects, breastfeeding should be discontinued while taking cilostazol.

Indications. The major indication for use of cilostazol is the treatment of intermittent claudication because of its femoral artery vasodilating action. It is also used after percutaneous cardiac intervention to prevent clot formation.

Adverse Effects. Dizziness, tachycardia, edema, and abnormal bleeding can occur in 1% to 10% of patients receiving cilostazol. The most common adverse effects include headache (27% to 34%), diarrhea (12% to 19%), and infection (10% to 14%) (Farkas et al., 2017). Patients with a history of ischemic heart disease may be at risk for angina or myocardial infarction. Thrombocytopenia or leukopenia progressing to agranulocytosis have been reported. Agranulocytosis is reversible upon discontinuation of therapy.

Contraindications. Cilostazol has been shown to decrease the survival of patients with heart failure, and thus is contraindicated in patients with heart failure of any severity.

Monitoring. Patients with ischemic heart disease should be monitored for chest pain; pain in the shoulder, back, or jaw; and shortness of breath that may indicate angina or myocardial infarction. CBCs should also be monitored for any adverse hematologic effects of cilostazol.

Anagrelide

Pharmacokinetics. Anagrelide is well absorbed following oral administration and is metabolized in the liver into active metabolites. The peak plasma time is 1 hour, with a duration of action of 6 to 24 hours and a half-life of 1.3 hours. Platelet counts typically begin to decline in 7 to 14 days. Anagrelide is excreted in the urine as metabolites (more than 70%) and unchanged drug (less than 1%). Approximately 10% is excreted in feces through bile.

Indications. Anagrelide is prescribed in the treatment of chronic (essential) myeloproliferative disorders that result in thrombocythemia to decrease risk for thrombosis, and thrombohemorrhagic events. Essential thrombocythemia is associated with an increase in platelet precursors in the bone marrow. Complications of myeloproliferative disorders include blood clotting and/or bleeding. Anagrelide has been designated as an orphan drug by the U.S. Food and Drug Administration (FDA) for the treatment of *polycythemia vera*, a slow-growing cancer of the bone marrow that produces excessive RBCs, thickening the blood and increasing the risk for thrombotic events.

Adverse Effects. The most common adverse effects include headaches (11% of patients), palpitations (19%), diarrhea (26%), weakness/loss of energy (23%), edema (21%), dizziness (15%), and dyspnea (12%) (Rey et al., 2014). Adverse cardiovascular effects (e.g., tachycardia, edema, heart failure) have been reported with anagrelide, including rare cases of sudden death.

Contraindications. Anagrelide is contraindicated for use in patients with severe hepatic dysfunction. Its use is avoided in patients with known or suspected cardiovascular disease. Anagrelide crosses the placenta, and thus could pose harm to the developing fetus. Although presence of anagrelide in breast milk is unknown, recommendations are to discontinue breastfeeding due to the potential risk in nursing infants.

Monitoring. Platelet counts should be monitored every 2 days for 1 week following initiation of therapy, then at least weekly thereafter until maintenance dosage is established individually. CBCs, LFTs, and renal function tests should be monitored while platelet counts are being decreased during the first 2 weeks of therapy. Cardiac status should be monitored prior to and during therapy.

Indirect Thrombin Inhibitors

Indirect thrombin inhibitors are a type of anticoagulant that does not have inhibition of platelet activation as its main mechanism of action. Table 14.2 summarizes the types of non–platelet inhibitor anticoagulants. These medications reduce clot formation through the action of antithrombin III. Recall from the Relevant Physiology section that antithrombin III actually removes activated Factor Xa and also binds loose fibrin molecules. These two actions prevent the assembly of fibrin into the meshwork needed for clot formation. The indirect thrombin inhibitors enhance the activity of antithrombin III.

Unfractionated Heparin

Heparin, also known as unfractionated heparin (UFH), is made up of a mixture of polysaccharides (sugar molecules) with varying molecular weights but with similar biologic activity. The larger polysaccharides in heparin exert their anticoagulant effect by interacting with antithrombin III, changing its shape to make it more active. The modified antithrombin III then inactivates thrombin and inhibits the activity of activated Factor X in the coagulation process. Only about one-third of a dose of UFH binds to antithrombin III, and it is this fraction that results in anticoagulant activity. Heparin itself has no direct action on the clotting factors. However, at high doses, heparin can inhibit platelet activation to some degree.

Pharmacokinetics. The bioavailability of subcutaneous UFH is dose dependent, ranging from 30% (lower doses) to 70% (higher doses). Following subcutaneous injection, the anticoagulation effect is seen in 1 to 2 hours. When there is a need for rapid anticoagulation, heparin is given intravenously. Following direct intravenous (IV) injection, the onset of anticoagulation activity is immediate. Subcutaneous administration is not recommended for rapid anticoagulation. The half-life of UFH is 30 to 90 minutes but may be shorter in patients with thromboembolic disorders.

PHARMACOGENETICS

Heparin Therapy

- Heparin resistance may be observed in patients with hereditary antithrombin III deficiency. However, the anticoagulant effect of heparin is enhanced when patients are treated with antithrombin III.
- To reduce risk of bleeding, reduce the heparin dose during concomitant treatment with human antithrombin III.

TABLE 14.2 Non–Platelet Inhibitor Anticoagulants

Category/ Medication	Indication	Dosage	Considerations and Monitoring
Indirect Thrombin Inhibitors			
Heparin	DVT and PE prophylaxis and treatment, acute coronary syndrome,[a] maintain patency of venous and arterial catheters[a]	*DVT or PE prophylaxis:* 5000–7500 units subcutaneously every 8–12 hr *Treatment of DVT or PE:* 5000 units IV bolus, then continuous infusion of 1300 units/hr	Several different concentrations available, so use caution in prescribing to avoid error. Monitor therapy with aPTT, anti-Xa; monitor platelet count and hematocrit in all patients receiving heparin. Consider DEXA scan in patients on therapy >6 months.
Low molecular weight heparin	DVT and PE prophylaxis	30 mg subcutaneously every 12 hr for 10–35 days postoperatively	No routine monitoring of coagulation factors required.
Vitamin K Antagonists			
Warfarin	DVT and PE prophylaxis and treatment Prevent thrombosis from atrial fibrillation or MI, thromboembolic stroke, heart valve replacement	Dosage and administration must be individualized according to the patient's INR and condition being treated *Typical dosages for prevention of thromboembolism:* Initial dosage: 2–5 mg orally once daily Maintenance dosage: 2–10 mg orally once daily	Baseline INR prior to initiation of warfarin, then monitor INR every 4 weeks. Target INR: 2–3
Direct Thrombin Inhibitors			
Dabigatran	Prevention and treatment of DVT and PE, or thrombosis prevention in atrial fibrillation or following hip surgery	*DVT prophylaxis:* 150 mg orally twice daily *Thrombosis prevention following hip surgery:* 220 mg orally once daily	Anticoagulation not typically measured, but if necessary, use aPTT, not INR, to assess anticoagulant activity. Assess renal function prior to initiation of treatment and periodically as needed; adjust therapy accordingly.
Rivaroxaban	Prevention and treatment of DVT and PE, or thrombosis prevention in atrial fibrillation or following hip surgery	*Typical dosage for atrial fibrillation:* 20 mg orally once daily *Typical dosage for DVT or PE:* Initial dosage: 15 mg orally twice daily for first 21 days of therapy Maintenance dosage: 20 mg orally once daily for the duration of treatment *Typical dosage for prevention of DVT after hip replacement surgery:* 10 mg orally once daily starting 6–10 hr after surgery; continue treatment for approximately 35 days	Monitor for bleeding, hypersensitivity reactions, and neurologic deficits.
Apixaban	Prevention and treatment of DVT and PE, or thrombosis prevention in atrial fibrillation or following hip surgery	*Typical dosage:* 2.5 mg daily *Stroke prevention in atrial fibrillation:* 5 mg orally twice daily *DVT or PE prophylaxis following hip surgery:* 2.5 mg orally twice daily beginning 12–24 hr after surgery	Monitor for hypersensitivity reactions, bleeding, and signs and symptoms of intercranial or intraocular bleeding.
Edoxaban	Reduction of stroke risk in patients with nonvalvular atrial fibrillation, and treatment of DVT and PE	60 mg once daily	Monitor for abnormal bleeding or neurologic deficit; monitor CBC.

[a]Treatment is administered in the hospital and not in a primary care setting.

aPTT, Activated partial thromboplastin time; *CBC,* complete blood count; *DVT,* deep vein thrombosis; *INR,* international normalized ratio; *PE,* pulmonary embolism.

Indications. Heparin is used primarily for DVT and PE prophylaxis and treatment, for acute coronary syndrome, and to maintain patency of venous and arterial catheters. The route of heparin is determined by the treatment indication. Heparin is administered subcutaneously when the goal of therapy is prevention of venous thromboembolism. A patient requiring immediate anticoagulation should be given a weight-based IV bolus, followed by continuous infusion. When transitioning from IV heparin to warfarin, heparin administration is co-administered with warfarin for 4 to 5 days until the international normalized ratio (INR) is between 2 and 3 times the control, because warfarin's onset of initial action requires 48 to 72 hours since circulating vitamin K-dependent clotting Factors II, VII, IX, and X must first be cleared.

Adverse Effects. Heparin administration can result in a serious adverse effect known as *heparin-induced thrombocytopenia (HIT)*, an immunologic effect that results in the degradation of platelets and thrombocytopenia. HIT typically begins 5 to 14 days after the start of therapy and can result in venous thromboembolism, PE, or even myocardial infarction. HIT is not generally characterized by bleeding, and the disorder is sometimes termed *heparin-induced thrombocytopenia and thrombosis (HITT)*. HIT is suspected when a patient's platelet count drops by about 50%. Patients who have had cardiac or orthopedic surgery and received UFH have a higher risk of developing HIT (1% to 5%) as opposed to medical or obstetric patients (0.1% to 1%). Heparin may suppress aldosterone and cause hyperkalemia in some patients. Osteoporosis may occur with prolonged (more than 6 months) therapy due to a reduction in mineral bone density.

Contraindications. Heparin is contraindicated for patients with known HIT or who have had HIT in the past. Active bleeding is also a contraindication to heparin use.

Monitoring. Heparin therapy is monitored using activated partial thromboplastin time (aPTT). The prothrombin time (PT) often is monitored as well, as heparin can prolong PT. Platelet count and hematocrit should be

---

PRACTICE PEARLS

Bleeding Risk Factors for Heparin Therapy

Patients older than 65 years of age who have a history of the following may have increased risk for severe bleeding or hemorrhage from heparin therapy:

- Concurrent NSAID use
- History of peptic ulcer
- Renal failure
- Cirrhosis
- Recent surgery or trauma

PRACTICE PEARLS

Heparin Use During Pregnancy and Lactation

UFH does not cross the placenta and is not distributed into breast milk. For this reason, it is the anticoagulant of choice when severe clotting problems occur during pregnancy. It is not used when active vaginal bleeding is present.

---

monitored in all patients receiving heparin to detect complications of therapy. If the anticoagulant effect of heparin needs to be neutralized, protamine sulfate is given, and works to neutralize heparin by binding to it and preventing its interaction with antithrombin III.

Low Molecular Weight Heparin

Low molecular weight heparin (LMWH) is given subcutaneously for the prevention of DVT in patients at high risk for PE and for thrombosis prevention following knee or hip replacement surgery. LMWH was developed based upon observations that heparin fractions lose their ability over time to prolong the aPTT while still able to inhibit activated Factor X (Xa). So, LMWH preparations consist of polysaccharide fragments that act by inhibiting the activity of activated Factor X. LMWH has a longer half-life and increased bioavailability compared with UFH. Plasma levels of LMWH are predictable, permitting fixed-schedule dosing of once or twice daily subcutaneously, and as a result, routine monitoring of aPTT is not necessary.

While all anticoagulants, including UFH, pose a risk for bleeding, LMWH preparations result in less risk of severe bleeding. Another potential advantage of LMWH is a lower risk for the development of HIT. A recent meta-analysis of 15 randomized control trials showed an absolute risk for HIT was 0.2% with LMWH compared with 2.6% in those receiving UFH.

The use of LMWH is contraindicated for patients with a known heparin allergy, allergies to sulfites or benzyl alcohol, active bleeding, or HIT. The half-life of LMWH may be prolonged in patients with renal failure, and LMWH should be avoided in patients with a creatinine clearance rate (CrCl) less than 30 mL/minute as their excretion is renal dependent.

Direct Thrombin Inhibitors

Medications categorized as direct thrombin inhibitors prevent thrombin, activated Factor X (Xa), from catalyzing the conversion of fibrinogen into fibrin molecules. The exact mechanisms of action differ slightly among each medication and are listed in the following sections accordingly. Direct thrombin inhibitors do not prevent the synthesis or activation of thrombin.

TABLE 14.3	Dabigatran Dosing Adjustment Based on Creatinine Clearance	
Creatinine Clearance	**Recommended Dose**
>30 mL/min	150 mg orally twice daily
15–30 mL/min	75 mg orally twice daily
<15 mL/min	Not recommended

Dabigatran

Dabigatran is a competitive, reversible direct thrombin inhibitor that inhibits free and fibrin-bound thrombin (Factor Xa). This medication also has inhibitory effects on clotting Factors V, VIII, and XIII. Chemically, dabigatran closely resembles activated thrombin. When large amounts of dabigatran are present, the medication competes with activated thrombin in the conversion reaction. Although dabigatran closely resembles activated thrombin, it cannot catalyze the reaction. As long as more dabigatran is present than activated thrombin, it greatly reduces the amount of fibrin formed from fibrinogen.

Pharmacokinetics. Once dabigatran is absorbed, it undergoes hydrolyzation by microsomal liver enzymes to its active compound, producing immediate anticoagulation. Peak plasma concentrations occur within 2 hours of oral administration; food intake can delay this process. The half-life of dabigatran is between 12 and 17 hours. Thirty-five percent of dabigatran is bound to plasma proteins and is not metabolized. Dabigatran is excreted by the kidneys, and dosing is renal–function dependent. Table 14.3 lists dosing adjustments needed based on creatinine clearance in patients with reduced kidney function.

PHARMACOGENETICS

Dabigatran Therapy

Individual variability in serum concentrations of dabigatran have been reported, and variants in two genes (*ABCB1* and *CES1*) that encode for hepatic proteins may be responsible for variations in dabigatran absorption and metabolism. Future decisions for anticoagulation therapy with this medication may be based on genetic variants.

Indications. Dabigatran is indicated for the reduction of stroke risk and PE in patients with atrial fibrillation. It is also indicated for risk reduction or treatment of DVT and for PE inpatients who have undergone hip surgery.

Adverse Effects. The most common adverse effect of dabigatran is severe bleeding. The risk for bleeding increases with co-administration of other anticoagulants. GI disturbances are common, including dyspepsia, abdominal pain and discomfort, gastroesophageal reflux, esophagitis, peptic ulcer, and gastritis. There is a risk of epidural or spinal hematomas and neurologic injury, including paralysis, in patients taking dabigatran who undergo neuraxial (spinal/epidural) anesthesia or spinal puncture.

Contraindications. Dabigatran is contraindicated in patients with any form of active bleeding, with a history of sensitivity to the drug, or with mechanical prosthetic heart valves. Information regarding the use of dabigatran during pregnancy and lactation is lacking, but studies of rats show an increase in fetal and maternal death due to hemorrhage.

Monitoring. Patients should be monitored for signs and symptoms of abnormal bleeding and educated about what to report to the health care provider (heavy menstrual flow, bleeding gums, petechiae, bloody urine or stools). While there is no need for routine laboratory monitoring of coagulation parameters, dosing depends on creatinine clearance, so creatinine levels should be taken at baseline and before dose adjustments. Patients receiving neuraxial (spinal/epidural) anesthesia or spinal puncture should be monitored for neurologic impairment such as midline back pain; numbness, tingling, or weakness in lower limbs; or bowel or bladder dysfunction. Patients should be referred for urgent treatment if neurologic compromise is noted.

Rivaroxaban

Rivaroxaban is an anticoagulant that selectively and reversibly inhibits Factor Xa in both the intrinsic and extrinsic coagulation pathways to prevent fibrin clot formation. This medication binds to activated thrombin and covers its active site, rendering it unable to convert fibrinogen into fibrin.

Pharmacokinetics. Rivaroxaban is rapidly absorbed, reaching peak plasma levels in 2 to 4 hours, with a half-life of 6 to 9 hours. It is metabolized in the liver via CYP 3A4/5 and CYP 2J2. Approximately 60% of rivaroxaban is excreted in the urine, with 30% as unchanged drug and 30% as inactive metabolites. The remainder of the drug is excreted as an inactive metabolite in the feces. In patients with renal or hepatic impairment, drug levels can reach higher thresholds, with subsequent increased effects.

Indications. Rivaroxaban is used to treat DVT or PE as initial therapy or to reduce the risk of DVT and PE recurrence in patients at high risk who have completed 6 months of initial full therapeutic anticoagulant treatment for DVT and/or PE. Rivaroxaban is an option for prophylaxis of postoperative DVT in patients undergoing total hip arthroplasty or total knee arthroplasty. This medication is also indicated for prevention of stroke and systemic embolism in patients with nonvalvular atrial fibrillation.

Adverse Effects. Rivaroxaban increases risk of hemorrhage and can cause serious bleeding that may be fatal. Administration of other antiplatelet medications can increase bleeding risk. Patients who have undergone spinal surgery or spinal procedures are more likely to suffer bleeding around the spine that can result in paralysis. Hypersensitivity reactions, including anaphylaxis, have been reported. Rivaroxaban should be stopped at least 24 hours prior to surgery to prevent excessive bleeding. Rivaroxaban should be used very cautiously during pregnancy because of the lack of adequate safety data and the risk of pregnancy-related hemorrhage and/or emergent delivery.

Contraindications. Rivaroxaban is contraindicated in patients with active bleeding and hypersensitivity reactions. Rivaroxaban should be avoided in patients with moderate to severe liver disease or impairment associated with coagulopathy.

Monitoring. Patients should be monitored frequently for signs and symptoms of bleeding, and the risks and benefits of treatment continuation must be considered. Patients receiving neuraxial (spinal/epidural) anesthesia or spinal puncture should be monitored for neurologic impairment such as midline back pain; numbness, tingling, or weakness in lower limbs; or bowel or bladder dysfunction. Patients should be referred for urgent treatment if neurologic compromise is noted.

Apixaban

Apixaban is an oral anticoagulant that directly and reversibly acts as an activated Factor Xa inhibitor. This medication binds selectively to activated thrombin and covers its active site, rendering it unable to convert fibrinogen into fibrin.

Pharmacokinetics. Apixaban is absorbed throughout the GI tract, with 55% of the administered dose absorbed in the distal small intestine. The absolute bioavailability of apixaban is 50%, with peak plasma levels occurring 3 to 4 hours after administration. This drug is metabolized principally by CYP 3A4/5, with a half-life of about 6 hours. Apixaban is eliminated through hepatic metabolism, intestinal, biliary, and renal routes.

PHARMACOGENETICS

Apixaban Therapy

- Recent studies indicate that polymorphisms in the ABCG2 421A/A and CYP 3A5*3 genotypes can affect apixaban pharmacokinetics.
- These polymorphisms influence time to the peak but not the trough of apixaban plasma concentrations.

Indications. Apixaban is indicated for the prevention of strokes in patients with nonvalvular atrial fibrillation and may be useful in patients with moderate stroke risk who

BLACK BOX WARNING!

Direct Thrombin Inhibitors

- In patients with atrial fibrillation, direct thrombin inhibitors should not be abruptly discontinued unless another rapidly acting anticoagulant is started to avoid the risk for stroke.
- The risk for spinal or epidural hematoma increases in patients taking direct thrombin inhibitors who undergo neuraxial anesthesia or lumbar puncture.

cannot comply with coagulation monitoring required with warfarin therapy. It is also used for the prevention of DVT after hip or knee replacement surgery, and for both prevention and treatment of DVT and PE resulting from any cause.

Adverse Effects. Apixaban can result in severe hypersensitivity reactions in fewer than 1% of patients. Severe bleeding, including GI bleeding, intracranial bleeding, and intraocular bleeding, has also occurred.

Contraindications. Apixaban is contraindicated in active bleeding and in patients who have a known hypersensitivity reaction (skin rash, anaphylaxis) to the medication.

Monitoring. Patients should be monitored for signs and symptoms of bleeding and for symptoms of hypersensitivity reactions. Patients receiving neuraxial (spinal/epidural) anesthesia or spinal puncture should be monitored for neurologic impairment such as midline back pain; numbness, tingling, or weakness in lower limbs; or bowel or bladder dysfunction. Patients should be referred for urgent treatment if neurologic compromise is noted.

PRACTICE PEARLS

Direct Thrombin Inhibitor Use During Pregnancy and Lactation

- Complete data are lacking for direct thrombin inhibitor use during pregnancy; however, increased maternal bleeding has been noted in animal studies.
- Due to the risk of bleeding during pregnancy and delivery, use direct thrombin inhibitors only when the benefits outweigh the potential risks.
- The presence of direct thrombin inhibitors in breast milk is unknown. Breastfeeding should be discontinued when using direct thrombin inhibitors.

Edoxaban

Edoxaban is an elective Factor Xa inhibitor that inhibits free Factor Xa and prothrombinase activity and inhibits thrombin-induced platelet aggregation. Inhibition of Factor Xa in the coagulation cascade reduces thrombin generation and thrombus formation.

Pharmacokinetics. Edoxaban is metabolized by the liver via CYP 3A4 and is excreted unchanged through the urine. Plasma concentrations of edoxaban become increased in patients with renal impairment. Edoxaban reaches a peak plasma level in 1 to 2 hours, with a half-life of 10 to 14 hours.

Indications. Edoxaban is used to reduce the risk of stroke in patients with nonvalvular atrial fibrillation, and for the treatment of DVT and PE after parenteral anticoagulant therapy of 5 to 10 days.

Adverse Effects. Edoxaban confers a risk of serious, sometimes fatal bleeding, and this risk is increased in patients with renal failure. Edoxaban should be discontinued at least 24 hours prior to surgery or other invasive procedures. If surgery cannot be delayed, weigh the potential increased risk of bleeding against the urgency of intervention. Epidural or spinal hematoma may occur with concurrent use of edoxaban in patients undergoing neuraxial (spinal/epidural) anesthesia or spinal puncture procedures. Such injuries are serious and can result in paralysis. An increase in LFTs can also occur.

Contraindications. Edoxaban is contraindicated in patients with active bleeding and should not be used in patients with a CrCl of more than 95 mL/minute due to reduced efficacy in patients with renal insufficiency. Edoxaban is not recommended for patients with mechanical heart valves or moderate to severe mitral stenosis due to the lack of safety and efficacy data.

Monitoring. Routine coagulation monitoring is not recommended due to the inconsistent results of coagulation studies. Frequently monitor for signs of neurologic impairment (numbness or weakness in the lower extremities, bowel or bladder dysfunction). If neurologic symptoms are present, transfer to a hospital should be arranged for immediate treatment. Patients should also be monitored for signs of hypersensitivity.

PRACTICE PEARLS

Anticoagulant Therapy

- Premature discontinuance of any oral anticoagulant can increase the risk of thromboembolic events.
- When transitioning patients from one anticoagulant medication to another, continuous anticoagulation must be maintained, while minimizing the risk of bleeding.
- When switching patients from a Factor Xa inhibitor to warfarin therapy, a longer transition may be needed due to warfarin's comparatively slower onset of action.
- In general, anticoagulant therapy for venous thromboembolism should be continued for at least 3 months, and possibly longer in patients with a high risk of recurrence and low risk of bleeding.

Vitamin K Antagonists: Warfarin

As discussed earlier, all clotting factors are needed at various points in the blood-clotting cascade for coagulation to occur. Many of these factors are synthesized in the liver, and the synthesis/activation of Factors II, VII, IX, and X

are dependent on adequate amounts of vitamin K (phytonadione). The only medication currently in this class is warfarin, which is a derivative of the chemical coumarin. Warfarin inhibits at least one of the two enzymes responsible for synthesizing and activating vitamin K, vitamin K epoxide reductase (VKORC1), and possibly the enzyme vitamin K reductase. Thus, the presence of warfarin prevents the activation of vitamin K, which in turn prevents the synthesis/activation of clotting Factors II, VII, IX, and X (recall that Factor X is prothrombin, an extremely important clotting factor). The actions of warfarin have no effect on the clotting factors that have already been formed and are circulating.

Pharmacokinetics. Warfarin is completely absorbed after oral administration, with peak plasma concentration reached within 4 hours and a duration of 2 to 5 days following a single dose. Warfarin is metabolized by hepatic cytochrome P-450 (CYP 450) microsomal enzymes. Warfarin metabolites are excreted by the kidneys. Warfarin has a long half-life (20 to 60 hours) and need only be given once daily. The action of warfarin is not seen until it has been taken for several days, because the already existing clotting factors must be depleted before the lack of newly synthesized Factors II, VII, IX, and X can affect clotting.

PHARMACOGENETICS

Warfarin Therapy

- Polymorphisms in the genes for CYP P450 2C9 (CYP 2C9), P450 2C19 (CYP 2C19), and vitamin K epoxide reductase (VKORC1) influence warfarin response.
- Not all patients with mutations or polymorphisms in these genes respond to warfarin therapy in the same way, because some polymorphisms confer resistance to warfarin therapy and other polymorphisms increase the patient's sensitivity to the medication.
- Patients who have a variation that confers *resistance* require much higher warfarin doses to achieve coagulation.
- African Americans are relatively resistant to warfarin due to VKORC1 polymorphisms, whereas Asian Americans are generally more sensitive.
- Among Caucasians, CYP 2C9 and CYP 2C19 polymorphisms explain 10% of the dose variation between patients.
- These known polymorphisms are probably not the only ones that influence the effectiveness of the medication, and pharmacogenomic testing for patients prescribed warfarin currently remains controversial.

Indications. Warfarin has been and remains a very commonly prescribed anticoagulant. It is used for the prevention and treatment of venous thrombosis, PE, thromboembolic complications associated with atrial fibrillation, myocardial infarction, thromboembolic stroke, and for patients with heart valve replacement.

Adverse Effects. Warfarin can cause severe, potentially fatal bleeding. Box 14.2 lists risk factors known to potentiate warfarin-induced bleeding. The risk for bleeding is highest within the first month of treatment. Maintenance of INR in the therapeutic range does not eliminate the risk of bleeding. Necrosis of the skin is a serious risk but is relatively uncommon (fewer than 0.1% of patients). Necrosis can be present concurrently with local thrombosis and usually appears within a few days of the start of warfarin sodium therapy. A major drawback of warfarin therapy, particularly when used long term, is its many interactions with other medications, foods, and herbal supplements, some of which can have serious consequences. Box 14.3 lists some specific interactions with commonly prescribed medications. Accurate and complete medication reconciliation is crucial before initiating warfarin therapy, and consultation with a pharmacologist may be needed to avoid serious complications of interactions.

• BOX 14.2	Risk Factors for Bleeding During Warfarin Therapy

- Anticoagulation that achieves INR >4, or highly variable INR levels
- Age >65
- Impaired renal function
- History of GI bleeding, hypertension, cerebrovascular disease, anemia, malignancy, trauma, renal impairment
- Many drugs, herbal supplements, and certain foods/juices can interact with warfarin to increase the risk for bleeding
- Extended duration of warfarin therapy

INR: international normalized ratio; GI: gastrointestinal.

Contraindications. Warfarin is contraindicated for patients with known hematologic disorders associated with bleeding, active bleeding, central nervous system (CNS) hemorrhage, cerebral aneurysms, or aorta dissection. Patients undergoing spinal anesthesia or spinal puncture and those who have a history of malignant hypertension should not take warfarin. Warfarin should not be used as initial therapy in patients with HIT and with heparin-induced thrombocytopenia with thrombosis syndrome (HITTS) due to the risk for limb ischemia, necrosis, or gangrene.

PRACTICE PEARLS

Warfarin Use During Pregnancy and Lactation

- Warfarin is contraindicated in pregnancy, except for patients with mechanical heart valves at high risk for thromboembolism, where the treatment benefit outweighs the risks.
- Warfarin use is associated with many birth defects and fetal loss. Patients must be instructed to use effective contraception methods to prevent pregnancy while taking warfarin and for at least 1 month after the last dose.

• BOX 14.3	Examples of Common Drug Interactions with Warfarin[a]

Medications That Increase Warfarin's Effects	Medications That Decrease Warfarin's Effects
Apixaban	Adalimumab
Aspirin	Cholestyramine
Clopidogrel	Conjugated estrogens
Coumadin	Multivitamins containing vitamin K
Duloxetine	
Enoxaparin	Phytonadione
Heparin	Pravastatin
Nonsteroidal antiinflammatory drugs	Rifampin
	Thyroid medications
Prednisone	Trazadone
Ticlopidine	Vitamin C

[a]There are many other drug–drug and drug–food interactions with warfarin. The primary care provider should check all drug interactions among the patient's medications before prescribing warfarin.

Monitoring. Warfarin has a narrow therapeutic range requiring regular blood monitoring of INR. Daily monitoring of INR may be required initially. Regular monthly monitoring of INR is recommended in all patients treated with warfarin. Patients with stable INR and on longer-term treatment can have INR checked every 3 months. More frequent INR monitoring is needed when starting or stopping other drugs, including botanicals, or when changing dosages of other drugs that interact with warfarin.

Prescriber Considerations for Anticoagulation Therapy

In 2016, the American College of Chest Physicians (CHEST) updated the clinical guidelines for antithrombotic therapy for venous thromboembolic disease, which includes DVT and PE (Grant, 2016). Highlights from the 2016 update are:

- The anticoagulants of choice in patients with acute DVT or PE (without cancer) are the direct oral anticoagulants dabigatran, rivaroxaban, or apixaban in place of warfarin. These drugs are equally effective.
- Consider the use of low-dose aspirin in patients who completed anticoagulant therapy for DVT or PE and have a low risk of recurrence.
- Do not use compression stockings routinely to prevent postthrombotic syndrome (PTS). This recommendation is based on a recent multicenter randomized clinical trial that demonstrated compression stockings did not prevent PTS after an acute proximal DVT.
- Assess the personal and family history of clotting, bleeding, or vascular disorders for all patients with suspect-

ed disorders of hypercoagulability or thromboembolic events.

- Assess the personal lifestyle factors for all patients with suspected disorders of hypercoagulability or thromboembolic events.
- Laboratory assessments for all patients with suspected disorders of hypercoagulability or thromboembolic events should include INR, PTT, CBC with platelets, homocysteine level, serum chemistry, and LFTs.

The complete updated set of clinical guidelines can be found at https://www.the-hospitalist.org/hospitalist/article/121399/updated-accp-guideline-antithrombotic-therapy-vte-disease#.

BOOKMARK THIS!

Clinical Guidelines for Anticoagulant Therapy

Updated ACCP Clinical Guidelines for DVT & PE: https://www.the-hospitalist.org/hospitalist/article/121399/updated-accp-guideline-antithrombotic-therapy-vte-disease#

Clinical Reasoning for Anticoagulation Therapy

Consider the individual patient's health problem requiring anticoagulation therapy. Does the problem constitute a temporary risk for thrombotic events for which primary prevention is important or will anticoagulants be required for primary prevention over the long term? Temporary problems include lower limb joint replacement surgery, extensive abdominal surgery (especially involving revisions to major blood vessels), and disorders requiring prolonged immobility. Primary prevention for the longer term includes conditions that increase the risk but for which lifelong anticoagulant therapy may not be needed, such as after stent placement or other percutaneous cardiac interventions. Primary prevention for lifelong increased risk is often needed for patients who have diagnosed coagulopathies.

Secondary prevention using anticoagulation therapy is common in primary care, although initial therapy may begin in an acute care setting. Primary care providers are responsible for all follow-up care, including determining effectiveness, tolerance, and compliance with therapy as well as assessing the need for therapy continuance. Common health problems include having had a previous thromboembolic event (e.g., DVT, PE), atrial fibrillation, and acute coronary syndromes.

Determine the desired therapeutic outcome based on the degree of anticoagulation needed for the patient's health problem. For patients at high risk for thromboembolic events, the desired therapeutic outcome is prevention of DVT, PE, and other thromboembolic events, but the degree of anticoagulation needed may vary with the health problem. Consider the types of anticoagulants available as first-line

or first-choice therapy and choose one based upon efficacy and safety.

Assess the anticoagulant selected for its appropriateness for an individual patient by considering the medication's side effects and the patient's age, race/ethnicity, comorbidities, and genetic factors. Consider first-, second-, and third-line recommended treatments for the patient's specific health problem, referenced and supported by clinical guidelines (as available). Ideally, the choice of an anticoagulant medication should be effective, have good antithrombotic action and sustained response, and pose little risk of excessive bleeding. None of the current medications discussed in this chapter meets *all* the criteria. Thus, the primary care provider must use clinical judgment to determine the best possible choice based upon the desired therapeutic outcome and patient history.

Medications that impact blood clotting have interactions with many other prescribed medications and over-the-counter (OTC) drugs (such as ibuprofen), herbal preparations, and nutritional supplements. The patient must be asked for a complete list of all medications, herbal preparations, and supplements being taken, and a complete medication reconciliation must be done to avoid over- or undertreatment or adverse effects *before* an anticoagulant is selected.

The choice of anticoagulant may change over time depending on patient response. Another consideration is cost and the patient's ability to pay. Even when the patient has insurance, the health care provider may need to reconsider medication selection based on insurance coverage and approval.

Initiate the treatment plan with the selected medication by first providing adequate patient education to ensure the patient's understanding and promote full participation in the anticoagulant therapy. A thorough explanation to the patient and family about the goal of treatment and the importance of anticoagulant medication adherence needs to be emphasized. For example, following hip replacement surgery, anticoagulants such as apixaban may begin within 24 hours of surgery but continue for up to 35 days after hospital discharge.

Ensure complete patient and family understanding about the medication prescribed for anticoagulation therapy using a variety of education strategies. Important medication information to provide includes expected therapeutic effects, side effects, adverse effects, any monitoring or follow-up needed, and the importance of checking with the health care provider before starting any new medications or supplements to prevent potential drug and food interactions. Instruct the patient on symptoms of excessive bleeding to report to the health care provider, and when to seek emergency care.

Conduct follow-up and monitoring of patient responses to anticoagulant therapy. This is required to some degree for therapy effectiveness and individual idiosyncratic issues regardless of the anticoagulant selected. Timing of follow-up depends on the purpose of the treatment, the condition to be treated, and the health and comorbidities of the patient. Schedule the patient for the appropriate follow-up visits for laboratory tests for blood clotting (if needed) and follow-up.

Ensure that there is a standard practice for following up with patients who miss lab or clinic appointments. In addition to evaluating the effectiveness of the treatment plan, personal points to discuss at follow-up include the acceptability of the treatment to the patient and whether changes to the plan may be needed. Medication adherence and patient knowledge of the medication and treatment plan should be reassessed for the need for education reinforcement. Ensure that the patient has an adequate supply of medication to last until the next follow-up appointment.

Teaching Points for Anticoagulation Therapy

Health Promotion Strategies

Whether the need for anticoagulation therapy is temporary or long term, patients can reduce their risks for VTE by adopting a healthy lifestyle. The following strategies and practices should be presented to patients to help them become full partners in their health care:

- Reduce your risk for stroke by engaging in routine physical activity in consultation with your health care provider. Current guidelines recommend at least 150 minutes weekly of moderate-intensity or 75 minutes weekly of vigorous-intensity aerobic physical activity.
- Reduce your intake of sodium to lower blood pressure or maintain a healthy blood pressure.
- Eat a diet that includes daily intake of multiple servings of fruits and vegetables.
- Eat minimal fats from animal sources and include healthy, plant-based fats.
- If you are overweight (body mass index = 25 to 29 kg/m^2) or obese (body mass index is greater than 30 kg/m^2), lose weight with guidance from your health care provider to reduce your risk for stroke.
- If you are a smoker, work with your health care provider to quit smoking with drug therapy using nicotine replacement, bupropion, or varenicline in combination with counseling.
- Avoid missing appointments for your INR tests. If you have difficulty remembering these appointments, request to receive reminders via phone, text message, email, or regular mail. If you routinely miss these appointments, talk with your health care provider to learn why these tests are important.

Patient Education for Medication Safety

Anticoagulants are commonly prescribed medications that have great potential for harm if taken incorrectly. Too little medication greatly increases the risk for thrombotic events. Excessive medication can lead to serious bleeding issues and even fatal hemorrhage. Primary care providers need to stress the following points and actions to patients for safe medication management:

- Swallow medication capsules whole with a full glass of water.
- Take your anticoagulant as directed. If you miss a dose, take the missed dose as soon as possible on the same day, but skip if it is less than 6 hours before the next scheduled dose.
- Never double up a dose to make up for a missed dose.

- Do not stop taking any medication that affects blood clotting without first talking to your health care provider, because stopping suddenly can increase your risk of blood clot or stroke.
- Anticoagulant medications can cause you to bleed more easily. Call your health care provider at once if you have signs of bleeding such as headaches, feeling very weak or dizzy, bleeding gums, nosebleeds, heavy menstrual periods or abnormal vaginal bleeding, blood in your urine, bloody or tarry stools, coughing up blood, or vomit that looks like coffee grounds.
- Get emergency medical help if you have signs of an allergic reaction, such as hives, difficulty breathing, or swelling of your face, lips, tongue, or throat.
- Taking anticoagulants during pregnancy may cause abnormal bleeding for you or your unborn baby. Tell your health care provider if you are pregnant or plan to become pregnant.
- Some anticoagulants may not be safe during lactation. Ask your health care provider about any risks.
- Keep all clinic and laboratory appointments for blood tests related to your anticoagulant. If you need to miss an appointment, notify your health care provider and reschedule as soon as possible.

Application Questions for Discussion

1. As a health care provider, what are the patient and safety factors that should be considered before prescribing an anticoagulant?
2. What should be included in the patient and/or caregiver education plan for a patient who has been prescribed warfarin?
3. What role may genetics play in the treatment response to some anticoagulants?

Selected Bibliography

Bhatt, D. L., Steg, P. G., Ohman, E. M., Hirsch, A. T., Ikeda, Y., Mas, J. L., Goto, S., Liau, C. S., Richard, A. J., Rother, J., & Wilson, P. W. (2006). International prevalence, recognition, and treatment of cardiovascular risk factors in outpatients with atherothrombosis. *JAMA, 295*(2), 180–189.

Bonaca, M. P., Bhatt, D. L., Ophuis, O., Steg, P. G., Cohen, M., Kuder, J., IM, K., Magnsni, G., Budaj, A., Therox, P., Hamm, C., Spinar, J., Kiss, R. G., Dalby, A. J., Medina, F. A., Kontny, F., Alward, P. E., Jensen, E. C., Held, P., Braunwald, E., & Sabatine, M. S. (2016). Long-term tolerability of ticagrelor for the secondary prevention of major adverse cardiovascular events: A secondary analysis of the PEGASUS-TIMI 54 trial. *JAMA Cardiology, 1*(4), 425–432.

Dziadosz, M., & Baxi, L. V. (2016). Global prevalence of prothrombin gene mutation G2021A and implications in women's health: A systematic review. *Blood Coagulation and Fibrinolysis, 27*, 481–489.

Farkas, K., Jarai, Z., & Kolossvary, E. (2017). Cilostazol is effective and safe option for the treatment of intermittent claudication. Results of the NOCLAUD study. *Orvosi Hetilap, 158*(4), 123–128.

Grant, P. J. (2016). Updated ACCP guideline for antithrombotic therapy for VTE disease. *The Hospitalist*(11), 2016. https://www.the-hospitalist.org/hospitalist/article/121399/updated-accp-guideline-antithrombotic-therapy-vte-disease#.

Jacob, S., Dunn, B. L., Qureshi, Z. P., Bandarenko, N., Kwaan, H. C., Pandey, D. K., McKoy, J. M., Barnato, S. E., Winters, J. L., Cursio, J. F., Weiss, I., Raife, T. J., & Bennett, C. L. (2012). Ticlopidine-, clopidogrel-, and prasugrel-associated thrombotic thrombocytopenic purpura: A 20-year review from the Southern Network on Adverse Reactions (SONAR). *Seminars in Thrombosis and Hemostasis, 38*(8), 845–853.

Jenkins, P. V., Rawley, O., Smith, O. P., & O'Donnell, J. S (2012). Elevated factor VIII levels and risk of venous thrombosis. *British Journal of Haematology, 157*(6), 653–663.

McCance, K., Huether, S., Brashers, V., & Rote, N. (2019). *Pathophysiology: The Biologic Basis for Disease in Adults and Children* (8th ed.). St. Louis: Mosby.

Niu, P. P., Guo, Z. N., Xing, Y. Q., & Yang, Y. (2016). Antiplatelet regimens in the long-term secondary prevention of transient ischaemic attack and ischaemic stroke: An updated network meta-analysis. *BMJ Open, 6*(3), Article e009013. http://doi.org/10.1136/bmjopen-2015-009013.

Pagana, K., & Pagana, T. (2018). *Mosby's Manual of Diagnostic and Laboratory Tests* (6th ed.). St. Louis: Mosby.

Rey, J., Viallard, J. F., Keddad, K., Smith, J., Wilde, P., & Kiladjian, J. J. (2014). Characterization of different regimens for initiating anagrelide in patients with essential thrombocythemia who are intolerant or refractory to their current cytoreductive therapy: Results from the multicenter FOX study of 177 patients in France. *European Journal of Haematology, 92*(2), 127–136.

Scirica, B. M., Cannon, C. P., Emmanuelsson, H., Michelson, E. L., Harrington, R. A., Husted, S., James, S., Katus, H., Pais, P., Raevd, D., Spinar, J., Steg, P. G., Storey, R. F., & Wallentin, L. (2011). The incidence of bradyarrhythmias and clinical bradyarrhythmic events in patients with acute coronary syndromes treated with ticagrelor or clopidogrel in the PLATO trial: Results of the continuous electrocardiographic assessment substudy. *Journal of the American College of Cardiology, 57*(19), 1908–1916.

Spence, J. D. (2016). Homocysteine lowering for stroke prevention: Unraveling the complexity of the evidence. *International Journal of Stroke, 11*(7), 744–747.

van Langevelde, K., Flinterman, L. E., van Hylckama Vlieg, A., Rosendaal, F. R., & Cannegieter, S. C (2012). Broadening the factor V Leiden paradox: Pulmonary embolism and deep-vein thrombosis as 2 sides of the spectrum. *Blood, 120*(5), 933–946.

Wypasek, E., & Undas, A. (2013). Protein C and protein S Deficiency-Practical and diagnostic issues. *Advances in Clinical and Experimental Medicine, 22*(4), 459–467.

15

Gastroesophageal Reflux Disease, Gastritis, and Peptic Ulcer Disease Medications

DEBORAH ADELL

Overview

Gastroesophageal reflux disease (GERD) is a common condition treated in the primary care setting. It is estimated that the prevalence of GERD in North America ranges from 18% to 27% of the population (El-Serag et al., 2014). With the availability of over-the-counter (OTC) antacids, histamine-2 receptor antagonists (H2RAs), and proton pump inhibitors (PPIs), annual spending on OTC treatments for heartburn symptoms in 2020 exceeded $2 billion (Consumer Health Care Products Association, 2021).

Medications used to treat pathology in the upper gastrointestinal (GI) system address excess secretion of hydrochloric acid (HCl), decreased protection of the stomach lining, and tone and motility of the upper gastrointestinal tract, which moves stomach contents forward. The classes of medications utilized are antacids, H2RAs, PPIs, prostaglandins, and prokinetic agents. Many of these medications are available over the counter, and patients may attempt self-care prior to seeking care from a health care professional. The primary care provider may more effectively prescribe these medications as part of a comprehensive evaluation and treatment plan for gastritis, GERD, and peptic ulcer disease (PUD).

Relevant Physiology

Although HCl and pepsin, which are necessary for digestion, are caustic chemicals, they are usually problematic only when intrinsic protective measures are overcome. Those measures are the buffering of HCl by bicarbonate, barriers to regurgitation of stomach contents into the esophagus by the lower esophageal sphincter (LES), the negative biofeedback loop regulating HCl production, and a protective mucous barrier in the stomach. Failure of any of these measures can result in gastritis, GERD, or PUD. Treating PUD can be further complicated by the presence of the bacteria *Helicobacter pylori*.

Digestion of food is accomplished through a complex interaction of physical and chemical processes. Physical processes begin with the act of swallowing and the propulsion of food through the LES toward the pyloric valve. Tone of the LES is an intrinsic protective mechanism for preventing reflux of acidic stomach contents into the neutral or base esophagus. Muscular contractions of the stomach during digestion propel the partially digested food (*chyme*) through the pyloric sphincter into the duodenum.

Chemical processes of digestion are regulated by nerves, hormones, and paracrine substances. The process of digestion begins in the mouth through production of the enzyme ptyalin, which is mixed in food during mastication. In the stomach, secretion of HCl by parietal cells is a complex and variably continuous process. HCl is produced by parietal cells in the body and the fundus of the stomach through stimulation by chemical mediators including histamine type 2 (H2).

H2 differs from histamine type 1, which is responsible for respiratory and cutaneous allergic reaction. H2 receptors reside primarily in the stomach. H2 is released from enterochromaffin-like (ECL) cells in the fundus. Once they are released, proton pumps within the parietal cells are stimulated by the H2 attaching to receptors, resulting in secretion of HCl. Parietal cells are also indirectly affected by gastrin and somatostatin (SST). Gastrin is produced by antral G cells, located within the pyloric glands, in response to central nervous system (CNS) activation (vagal nerve stimulation) as well as local factors such as stomach distention from food ingestion. Once released from the antral G cells, gastrin stimulates the ECL cells to produce H2.

SST is produced by antral D cells in the stomach. SST inhibits gastric acid secretion through a negative biofeedback loop. In patients infected with *H. pylori*, the antral D cells are damaged by urease produced by the bacteria, thereby losing the gastric acid inhibitory action that may account for the hyperacidity of PUD.

Propulsion of food through the digestive system is controlled by peristaltic waves toward the antrum and pyloric valve. Gastric motility is controlled by the enteric nervous system, sympathetic and parasympathetic nervous systems, and multiple hormones.

The stomach is protected from autodigestion by a continuous mucosal layer. Mucus is secreted by the goblet cells as a liquid in response to stimulation by prostaglandins E2 and I2. Once the mucus is secreted, it forms a gel-like layer that is impermeable to HCl and pepsin. Additionally, bicarbonate ions are secreted by superficial gastric epithelial cells, raising gastric pH.

Pathophysiology

GERD is caused by decreased lower esophageal tone, increased intrabdominal pressure related to pregnancy or abdominal obesity, hiatal hernia, or delayed gastric emptying. Reflux of the acidic stomach contents into the esophagus results in painful irritation. Over time, untreated GERD can result in erosive esophagitis and cancer of the esophagus (*Barrett's esophagus*). Excessively acidic or spicy foods, alcohol, peppermint, and other foods can increase the irritative quality of reflux. Some medications can cause decreased tone of the LES, allowing reflux to occur. Medications and foods that can cause or contribute to GERD are listed in Box 15.1.

Patients frequently present with *dyspepsia*, described as upper GI symptoms of heartburn, but may also include epigastric fullness, nausea, or vomiting, with heartburn being the predominant complaint. These symptoms can cross several diagnoses, so a careful medical and social history and physical exam are needed. Particular attention must be paid to excluding cardiac or respiratory causes of the symptoms.

A diagnosis of uncomplicated GERD is usually made by patient history and presenting symptoms (Box 15.2). For unclear or complicated cases, upper GI endoscopy,

---

• BOX 15.1   GERD: Contributing Factors

- Anticholinergic medications
- Nitrates
- Calcium channel blockers
- Nicotine (smoking)
- Alcohol
- Chocolate, peppermint, red wine, acidic food
- Estrogens, progesterone
- Caffeine
- High-fat foods

• BOX 15.2   Symptoms of GERD

- Epigastric burning sometimes experienced as chest pain and often worse when lying down or after eating
- Sour or bitter taste
- Feeling of fullness (globus sensation) in the throat
- Cough or worsening asthma
- Hoarseness

---

esophageal manometry, or ambulatory acid probe testing of the esophagus can be performed.

Gastritis and PUD share many characteristic presentations, etiology, and management. Gastritis, which can be chronic or acute, results from a loss of integrity of the mucosal surface of the stomach, allowing HCl and pepsin to contact the stomach epidermis, which results in inflammation and pain. Erosion of the stomach lining may be superficial, or it may be deep fissures that result in bleeding. Loss of integrity can be caused by long-term or high-dose use of nonsteroidal antiinflammatory drugs (NSAIDs). NSAIDs suppress prostaglandins, resulting in decreased mucous production and loss of protective coating. The bacteria *H. pylori* may cause some cases of gastritis. Hypersecretion of HCl or ingestion of irritating food or alcohol can also result in gastritis. *Zollinger-Ellison syndrome* is rare and is the result of a tumor in the pancreas or duodenum. The tumor, a *gastrinoma*, secretes gastrin, which prompts excess acid production.

PUD takes the form of ulceration of the duodenum or the stomach. In addition to the hyperacidity and loss of the protective mucous layer contributing to gastritis, the presence of the bacteria *H. pylori* is a factor in most cases. It is thought that 50% of the worldwide population is infected with *H. pylori* and approximately 70% of those infected are asymptomatic (Hooi et al., 2017). It is also thought that *H. pylori* infection is acquired in childhood. Less commonly, Zollinger-Ellison syndrome and vagal stimulation related to stress can contribute to development of PUD. Patients admitted to intensive care units (ICUs) for any reason are at risk for developing peptic ulceration.

Peptic ulcers can vary in depth, from penetrating only the mucosal layer to extending into the smooth muscle layers of the stomach, resulting in bleeding and perforation. Once the patient is treated, imperfect regeneration of mucosal layers can result in repeated ulceration.

Gastritis and PUD can present with similar symptoms, making diagnosis difficult (Box 15.3). Definitive diagnosis is made by careful history, endoscopy including biopsy, C urea breath test, stool antigen test, and blood tests for serologic titers. The serologic test can indicate whether a person has been infected with *H. pylori* but cannot determine when infection occurred. Joint recommendations from the ACG and CAG are listed in Box 15.4.

BOX 15.3 Symptoms of Gastritis or PUD

- Pain described as burning, gnawing, or cramping in the abdomen.
- Often located in the epigastric radiating below the costal margins or to the back. May occasionally manifest as upper-back pain.
- Pain may occur more at night or when the stomach is empty and may be relieved by food or antacids.
- Loss of appetite, nausea, vomiting.
- Vomit may contain blood.
- Perforation may manifest as sudden, severe abdominal pain, weakness, dizziness, or other signs of circulatory shock.

Hyperacidity Therapy

Control of excess acidity can take two forms: direct neutralization of HCl or interference with HCl production. Direct control through neutralization of acid by antacids is considered a topical measure despite the possibility of small amounts of absorption of antacid ingredients. Interference with parietal cell production of HCl can occur in two ways: decreasing histamine stimulation of parietal cell receptors through the use of H2RAs, and use of PPIs to directly stop HCl production. Each method has clinical application along with risks and benefits.

Antacids

Antacids are available in different single-ingredient or combination products of calcium carbonate, magnesium hydroxide, and aluminum hydroxide. Most are available as liquid or as chewable tablets. The effect of antacids is direct neutralization of HCl in the stomach, and to a lesser extent, decreased pepsin activity.

Antacids are useful for effective, immediate relief of heartburn symptoms caused by reflux of stomach contents through the LES or gastritis, although the effect is not long lasting and repeated dosing is necessary. Antacids are often used in conjunction with other acid control products for a synergistic effect in managing conditions with hyperacidity. Related to the alteration in pH, antacids can cause significant drug–drug interactions, resulting in changes in how other medications are dissolved, absorbed, and eliminated. The most notable interactions are with ferrous sulfate, isoniazid, sulfonylureas, and fluoroquinolones. Other significant drug–drug interactions are listed in Table 15.1. Antacids may destroy the enteric coating on any drug, resulting in earlier absorption than desired. Administration of antacids should be separated from other drugs by 2 hours.

Although generally considered topically acting medications, long-term use or high doses of antacids can result in absorption of the active ingredient in small amounts. This is clinically significant in patients with renal impairment related to inability to excrete the medication. An

BOX 15.4 ACG/CAG Recommendations for Diagnosis and Management of Patients With Dyspepsia or With Suspected *H. pylori*

1. We suggest dyspepsia patients age 60 or over have an endoscopy to exclude upper gastrointestinal neoplasia. *(Conditional recommendation, very low-quality evidence)*
2. We do not suggest endoscopy to investigate alarm features for dyspepsia patients under the age of 60 to exclude upper GI neoplasia. *(Conditional recommendation, moderate-quality evidence)*
3. We recommend dyspepsia patients under the age of 60 should have a noninvasive test for *H. pylori*, and therapy for *H. pylori* infection if positive. *(Strong recommendation, high-quality evidence)*
4. We recommend dyspepsia patients under the age of 60 should have empirical PPI therapy if they are *H. pylori* negative or who remain symptomatic after *H. pylori* eradication therapy. *(Strong recommendation, high-quality evidence)*
5. We suggest dyspepsia patients under the age of 60 not responding to PPI or *H. pylori* eradication therapy should be offered prokinetic therapy. *(Conditional recommendation, very low-quality evidence)*
6. We suggest dyspepsia patients under the age of 60 not responding to PPI or *H. pylori* eradication therapy should be offered TCA therapy. *(Conditional recommendation, low-quality evidence)*
7. We recommend FD patients that are *H. pylori* positive should be prescribed therapy to treat the infection. *(Strong recommendation, high-quality evidence)*
8. We recommend FD patients who are *H. pylori* negative or who remain symptomatic despite eradication of the infection should be treated with PPI therapy. *(Strong recommendation, moderate-quality evidence)*
9. We recommend FD patients not responding to PPI or *H. pylori* eradication therapy (if appropriate) should be offered TCA therapy. *(Conditional recommendation, moderate-quality evidence)*
10. We suggest FD patients not responding to PPI, *H. pylori* eradication therapy, or tricyclic antidepressant therapy should be offered prokinetic therapy. *(Conditional recommendation, very low-quality evidence)*
11. We suggest FD patients not responding to drug therapy should be offered psychological therapies. *(Conditional recommendation, very low-quality evidence)*
12. We do not recommend the routine use of complementary and alternative medicines for FD. *(Conditional recommendation, very low-quality evidence)*
13. We recommend against routine motility studies for patients with FD. *(Conditional recommendation, very low-quality evidence)*
14. We suggest motility studies for selected patients with FD where gastroparesis is strongly suspected. *(Conditional recommendation, very low-quality evidence)*

FD, functional dyspepsia; *H. pylori*, Helicobacter pylori; *PPI*, proton pump inhibitor; *TCA*, tricyclic antidepressant

Modified from Moayyedi, P., Lacy, B., Andrews, C., Enns, R., Howden, C., & Vakil, N. (2017). ACG and CAG Clinical Guideline: Management of dyspepsia. *American Journal of Gastroenterology, 112*(7), 988–1013. http://doi.org/10.1038/ajg.2017.154.

inability to excrete magnesium can result in hypermagnesemia. Magnesium-based products should be used with caution if there is any degree of renal sufficiency and the use of magnesium products in patients with renal failure is contraindicated. Calcium-based products are contraindicated in patients with renal calculi and hypercalcemia. Antacid products may be high in sodium. Patients needing to restrict sodium intake should be advised to seek low-sodium products. Common doses of antacids are listed in Table 15.2.

Magnesium Hydroxide

Pharmacokinetics. For magnesium hydroxide administered orally, onset of action is immediate, with peak action in 30 minutes and a duration of 30 minutes to 1 hour if taken on an empty stomach. Action can be extended to 3 hours if taken after a meal. The half-life of antacids is unknown. From 15% to 30% of magnesium is absorbed and excreted promptly by the kidneys. The remainder is excreted in the feces.

Indications. Magnesium hydroxide is indicated for use in treating occasional GERD; it is not intended for long-term or high-dose use. It is sometimes used in conjunction with other acid control products for gastritis or PUD. High doses of magnesium products are also used for occasional constipation.

Adverse Effects. Magnesium hydroxide may cause diarrhea, nausea, or vomiting. Caution is indicated in patients with renal insufficiency related to the potential for drug accumulation and magnesium toxicity. When used at standard doses for short periods, use during pregnancy and breastfeeding is generally considered safe.

Contraindications. Magnesium hydroxide should be used cautiously in patients with renal disease due to the risk of hypermagnesemia and magnesium toxicity. It should be avoided in patients with chronic diarrhea, fecal impaction, hemorrhoids, or any undiagnosed GI bleeding. It should be

used cautiously in older adults due to age-related changes in renal function.

Monitoring. No routine monitoring for intermittent use is recommended. For continuous use, monitoring of serum magnesium and creatinine/blood urea nitrogen (BUN) in older patients or in those with renal insufficiency should be performed.

Aluminum Hydroxide

Pharmacokinetics. Onset of action of aluminum hydroxide is slightly slower than magnesium hydroxide related to solubility; however, peak action remains at 30 minutes with a duration of 30 minutes to 1 hour if taken on an empty stomach. Peak action can be extended to 3 hours if taken after a meal. The half-life of antacids is unknown. From 17% to 30% of aluminum hydroxide can be absorbed and eliminated via the kidney. The remainder is excreted in the feces.

Indications. Aluminum hydroxide is used to treat GERD, PUD, gastritis, and erosive esophagitis. It may be also used prophylactically for stress-induced gastritis.

Adverse Effects. Aluminum hydroxide may cause constipation or bowel obstruction. Hypophosphatemia and hypercalcemia may occur with high-dose, prolonged use. Aluminum is generally considered safe in pregnancy, although no pregnancy category is assigned. At normal doses and for short-term use, aluminum hydroxide does not appear significantly in breast milk.

Contraindications. Caution in renal impairment is advised due to the potential for drug accumulation in the bones, lungs, and nerve tissue. Caution is indicated in patients with chronic diarrhea, in patients predisposed to constipation, in older adults, and in patients with renal impairment. Aluminum hydroxide is contraindicated in hypophosphatemia and renal failure.

Monitoring. Routine monitoring for short-term use is not recommended. For long-term or high-dose use, monitoring of serum calcium and phosphate is advised.

TABLE 15.1 Medication Interactions With Antacids

Medication	Interacting Medication	Possible Effects
Magnesium hydroxide	Sulfonylurea, quinidine	Increased effect of the interacting drug
	Benzodiazepines, corticosteroids, H2 blockers, hydantoins, iron salts, nitrofurantoin, phenothiazines, tetracyclines, ticlopidine	Decreased effect of the interacting drug
Aluminum hydroxide	Allopurinol, chloroquine, corticosteroids, ethambutol, H2 blockers, iron salts, phenothiazines, tetracyclines, thyroid hormones, ticlopidine	Decreased effect of the interacting drug
	Benzodiazepines	Increased effect of the interacting drug
Calcium antacids	Fluoroquinolones, hydantoins, iron salts, salicylates, tetracyclines	Decreased effect of the interacting drug
All antacids	Enteric coating	Coating may affect absorption

H2, Histamine type 2.

TABLE 15.2   Dosage for Selected Antacids

Medication	Indication	Dosage	Comments
Aluminum hydroxide	Hyperacidity associated with gastritis, peptic ulcer disease (PUD) (including duodenal ulcer and possibly gastric ulcer), reflux esophagitis, and hiatal hernia	**Oral suspension:** *Adults:* 40–60 mL orally every 3–6 hr or 1–3 hr after meals and at bedtime. Over-the-counter (OTC) dosage is 10 mL five or six times daily after meals and bedtime. *Children:* 5–15 mL orally every 3–6 hr or 1–3 hr after meals and at bedtime. *Infants:* Safer and more effective alternatives exist.	The suspension is available in several different concentrations. Always review product information. Avoid concurrent administration with other oral medications. Review drug interactions carefully. Patients with renal impairment or renal failure are at risk for drug accumulation. Drug should be avoided or dosage adjusted based on patient response
Magnesium hydroxide	Temporary relief of pyrosis, dyspepsia, and/or acid indigestion	**Oral dosage (regular suspension 400 mg/5 mL strength):** *Adults, children, and adolescents ≥12 yr:* 5–15 mL as a single dose orally; may repeat up to four times daily. Maximum dosage: 60 mL/day.	Not for long-term use. May be more palatable if refrigerated. Do not give concurrently with other oral medications due to possible interference with absorption. Review drug interactions and advised times of dose separation to limit drug–drug interactions.
Aluminum hydroxide/ magnesium hydroxide combination	Relief of dyspepsia, pyrosis, or conditions associated with hyperacidity	**Oral dosage (regular strength suspension):** *Adults:* Recommended OTC dosage is 10–20 mL orally four times daily. Maximum OTC dosage: 80 mL/day. *Children:* 5–15 mL orally every 3–6 hr, or 1–3 hr after meals and at bedtime. *Infants:* 1–2 mL/kg orally per dose, given after meals and at bedtime. **Oral dosage (therapeutic concentrate [TC] suspension):** *Adults:* Recommended OTC dosage is 5–10 mL orally four times daily, 20 minutes to 1 hr after meals and at bedtime. Maximum OTC dosage: 40 mL/day orally. *Children:* 2.5–7.5 mL orally every 3–6 hr, or 1–3 hr after meals and at bedtime. *Infants:* 0.5–1 mL/kg orally per dose, given after meals and at bedtime. **Oral dosage (chewable tablets):** *Adults:* Recommended OTC dosage is 1–4 tablets orally as needed, up to 16 tablets/day. **Oral dosage (extra-strength chewable tablets):** *Adults:* Recommended OTC dosage is 1–2 tablets orally as needed, up to 8 tablets/day.	Dosage is variable; however, an acid-neutralizing capacity of 80–140 mEq (e.g., 15–25 mL regular suspension) orally may be required in some adults. Avoid in patients with renal impairment or renal failure as patients may be at risk for accumulation of aluminum and magnesium. To avoid drug interactions, do not administer other medications within 2 hr. Doses should be given every 3–4 hr, or 1 and 3 hr after meals and at bedtime.

Calcium Carbonate

Pharmacokinetics. Onset of action of calcium carbonate is comparable to that of aluminum hydroxide, with peak effect in 30 minutes. Duration of action is 30 minutes to 1 hour, which can be extended if taken with food. The half-life of antacids is unknown. From 25% to 30% of calcium is absorbed and about 40% of the absorbed dose is protein bound to albumin. Absorption is influenced by food and the extent of calcium deficiency in the patient. Excretion is by glomerular filtration and renal tubular resorption, with the unabsorbed dose excreted in the feces.

Indications. Calcium carbonate is indicated for use in management of GERD, stress gastritis prophylaxis, hypocalcemia, hyperphosphatemia in chronic renal failure, and for adjunct use in the treatment of gastritis and PUD, although other antacids are preferred due to rebound effect. Calcium carbonate is used in higher doses in osteopenia or to prevent osteoporosis.

Adverse Effects. Patients may experience constipation, flatulence, and gastric distension. At higher doses or in those who are predisposed, renal calculi or hypercalcemia may develop. Milk-alkali syndrome manifested by hypercalcemia and metabolic acidosis may lead to renal failure. Patients taking calcium carbonate may experience a rebound effect with resultant excess hyperacidity.

Contraindications. Caution should be used in patients with a history of renal calculi, preexisting or a history of constipation or GI obstruction, and decreased bowel motility. Calcium carbonate is contraindicated in patients with renal disease or hypercalcemia. Short-term use at normal dosing appears to be safe in pregnancy and breastfeeding.

Monitoring. For short-term use at normal doses, routine monitoring is not recommended. Serum calcium and serum phosphate may be considered in patients experiencing nausea or vomiting, headache, weakness, or change in mental status, or for those predisposed to renal calculi.

QUALITY AND SAFETY

Avoiding Rebound Gastric Acidity

Rebound increases in gastric acidity can occur with PPIs and H2 antagonist medications as well as calcium carbonate antacids. Prolonged use of these medications can justify a gradual taper when discontinuing.

H2 Receptor Antagonists

H2 receptor antagonists (H2RAs) are used to decrease HCl production in GERD, gastritis, and PUD. Three receptor sites reside on the gastric parietal cell surface: H2, acetylcholine, and gastrin. Stimulation of these receptors results in HCl production by the proton pumps within the parietal cells. H2RAs bind reversibly and selectively to the H2 receptors, thereby blocking endogenous stimulation of the receptor by the patient's H2. The selective receptor action of these medications only partially inhibits HCl and decreases production by about 70%. Acetylcholine and gastrin continue stimulating HCl production. For that reason, PPIs that inhibit HCl by up to 95% often replace H2RAs in practice. Additionally, tolerance to the acid suppression effects of H2RAs can occur as soon as 3 days after starting therapy. Such tolerance is resistant to increased doses.

Cimetidine (Tagamet), famotidine (Pepcid), and nizatidine (Axid) are available as prescription and OTC medications. All are available in oral and intravenous (IV) formulations. Efficacy has been found to be similar among the three.

All are rapidly absorbed after oral administration and exhibit minimal protein binding, with nizatidine having the highest amount bound to albumin. Concomitant administration with antacids can decrease absorption; however, food does not alter absorption. Small amounts of H2RAs are metabolized in the liver, although dose adjustment for hepatic impairment is generally reserved for severe disease, especially with cimetidine. Excretion of the unchanged drug and a small amount of metabolite is by renal tubular secretion. Decreased creatinine clearance (CrCl) requires reduced dosing.

This class of medication is generally well tolerated, with the most common adverse effects being diarrhea, headache, drowsiness, fatigue, and constipation. IV administration may result in CNS effects such as confusion, delirium, hallucinations, and slurred speech. Long-term use can result in atrophic gastritis. Some evidence suggests a link between the use of acid suppression medications and pneumonia. Significant medication interactions can occur when altering the pH of the stomach related to changes in absorption of other medications (Table 15.3). Long-term acid suppression with any agent has been implicated in pernicious anemia. For long-term use, the patient's vitamin B_{12} levels should be monitored.

Within this class, cross-sensitivity among drugs has been noted. Hypersensitivity to one drug should preclude the use of other medications in the class. Typical dosing of the class is found in Table 15.4.

Cimetidine

Pharmacokinetics. After oral administration, absorption is rapid and complete. An extensive first-pass effect is noted, with peak serum concentration in 45 to 90 minutes and a half-life of 2 hours. Although metabolism is hepatic, nearly half the dose is excreted in the urine unchanged, with the remainder excreted in the feces.

Indications. Cimetidine is indicated for the treatment of GERD, gastritis, esophagitis, PUD, and disorders of hypersecretion such as Zollinger-Ellison syndrome. It may also be used prophylactically preanesthesia or intubation, and to prevent stress gastritis in critically ill patients.

Adverse Effects. In addition to diarrhea, CNS-related effects including headache, dizziness, confusion, agitation, depression, and anxiety have been reported. Long-term or high-dose use of cimetidine can result in antiandrogenic effects such as impaired libido, gynecomastia, galactorrhea, hyperprolactinemia, and impotence. Cimetidine inhibits the cytochrome (CYP) P4 enzyme system in a nonselective manner. Related to competition for the renal transport system, cimetidine may alter renal elimination of medications, such as metformin, memantine, trospium, procainamide, adefovir, pramipexole, and entecavir. Although a pregnancy category B is assigned, no adequate studies in pregnant patients exist and the risk/benefit to mother and fetus should be considered. Cimetidine is readily excreted in breast milk and should be avoided in nursing mothers.

Contraindications. Caution should be exercised in patients with renal or hepatic impairment as this may cause drug retention. Related to the CYP P450 inhibition, multiple drug interactions are possible.

Monitoring. When cimetidine is administered concurrently with antibiotics, monitor for pseudomembranous colitis, especially since diarrhea is a known adverse effect. If symptoms do not improve in 2 weeks, further evaluation, including for gastric cancer, should be undertaken.

Famotidine

Pharmacokinetics. With oral administration, time to onset of action is about 1 hour, with peak action in 1 to 4 hours. The half-life is 2.5 to 3.5 hours. Famotidine is partially metabolized in the liver, with the remainder excreted unchanged in the urine.

Indications. Famotidine is indicated for the treatment of GERD, gastritis, esophagitis, PUD, and disorders of hypersecretion such as Zollinger-Ellison syndrome as well as preanesthesia and prevention of stress-induced gastritis.

Adverse Effects. Common adverse effects include diarrhea or constipation, headache, and dizziness. As with cimetidine, CNS effects such as agitation, depression, anxiety, confusion, and hallucinations have been reported, although more commonly in older adults and in those with renal impairment. Famotidine has fewer drug–drug interactions than cimetidine.

Contraindications. Famotidine should be used with caution in patients with hepatic impairment, renal insufficiency, and renal failure. A pregnancy category B is assigned; however, no adequate studies in pregnant patients exist and the risk/benefit to mother and fetus should be considered. Although famotidine is secreted in breast milk, the amount is smaller than with other H2RAs, and use in breastfeeding mothers is generally considered acceptable.

Monitoring. When famotidine is administered concurrently with antibiotics, monitor the patient for pseudomembranous colitis, especially since diarrhea is a known adverse effect. If symptoms do not improve in 2 weeks, further evaluation, including for gastric cancer, should be undertaken.

TABLE 15.3 Medication Interactions With Histamine Type 2 Receptor Antagonist Agents

Drug	Interacting Medication	Possible Effects
Famotidine	Ketoconazole	Reduced absorption of interacting drug = reduced action
	Fluorouracil, procainamide, succinylcholine, narcotic analgesics	Increased action of interacting drugs
Nizatidine	Salicylates	Increased serum salicylate level with high-dose salicylates
	Indomethacin, ketoconazole, tetracyclines, digoxin, fluconazole, tocainide	Decreased action of interacting drugs
Cimetidine	Benzodiazepines, calcium channel blockers, carbamazepine, labetalol, metoprolol, metronidazole, propafenone, sulfonylureas, tacrine, theophylline, tricyclic antidepressants, valproic acid, warfarin	Decreased hepatic metabolism of interacting drugs
	Ferrous salts, indomethacin, ketoconazole, tetracyclines	Decreased action of interacting drugs due to decreased absorption
	Digoxin	Decreased serum digoxin
	Narcotic analgesics	May increase potential for respiratory depression and other toxic effects
	Procainamide	Decreased renal tubular secretion of procainamide may result in increased plasma levels and levels of cardioactive metabolites
	Cigarette smoking	Hinders ulcer healing due to smoking's reversal of cimetidine's nocturnal gastric secretion inhibition
All H2 medications	Ethanol	Increased action of interacting drug

H2, Histamine type 2.

TABLE 15.4 Select H2 Agonist Dosing Schedules[a]

Medication	Indications	Dosages	Comments
Cimetidine (Tagamet)	Treatment of gastric or duodenal ulcer	**Acute treatment:** *Adults and adolescents ≥16 yr:* Give 800 mg orally once daily at bedtime, or 400 mg twice daily or 300 mg four times daily with meals and at bedtime for 8–12 weeks. *For children and adolescents 1–15 yr:* 20–40 mg/kg/day orally in divided doses every 6 hr. **For maintenance therapy:** *Adults and adolescents ≥16 yr:* 400 mg orally once daily at bedtime. Duration up to 3 yr if underlying cause cannot be reversed. Shorter courses are recommended for uncomplicated ulcer.	Usually used with less severe GERD as PPIs offer more relief and faster healing. Do not administer concomitantly with antacids. Administer with food, water, or milk to minimize gastric irritation.
	GERD Esophagitis with GERD	*Adults and adolescents ≥16 yr:* 800 mg orally twice daily or 400 mg four times daily for 12 weeks. *Children and adolescents 1–15 yr:* 20–40 mg/kg/day in divided doses. Usual starting dose is 10 mg/kg orally four times daily before meals and at bedtime.	
	Self-medication of simple heartburn/indigestion	*Adults, adolescents, and children ≥12 yr and older:* OTC doses 200 mg orally twice daily. Maximum dosage: 400 mg/day.	
Famotidine (Pepcid)	Treatment of gastric and duodenal ulcer	**Acute treatment:** *Adults:* 40 mg orally once daily at bedtime for 4–8 weeks. *Adolescents and children:* 0.5 mg/kg/day orally at bedtime or 0.25 mg/kg twice daily initially. Maximum dosage: 40 mg/day. **Maintenance therapy after initial treatment phase has been completed:** *Adults:* 20 mg orally once daily at bedtime.	May administer with food, water, or milk to minimize gastric distress. May be effective in less severe GERD. For more severe cases, PPIs offer more symptom relief and more rapid healing.
	GERD	*Adults:* 20-mg tablets orally twice daily for up to 6 weeks. If esophagitis has developed, 20–40 mg twice daily for up to 12 weeks is recommended. *Children and adolescents:* 0.5 mg/kg orally twice daily (maximum dosage: 40 mg twice daily). Treat for 6–12 weeks.	
Calcium carbonate; famotidine; magnesium hydroxide (Pepcid-Complete)	Heartburn, indigestion	**Tablets (containing calcium carbonate 800 mg, famotidine 10 mg, magnesium hydroxide 165 mg):** *Adults:* Give 1 tablet orally as needed. Maximum dosage: 2 tablets/day. *Children and adolescents ≥12 yr:* 1 tablet orally as needed. Maximum dosage: 2 tablets/day.	Chewable tablets. Chew completely; do not swallow whole.

Continued

TABLE 15.4	Select H2 Agonist Dosing Schedules—cont'd		
Medication	**Indications**	**Dosages**	**Comments**
Nizatidine	Duodenal ulcer	**Capsules or 15 mg/mL solution:**	Give with food, water, or milk to minimize GI distress.
		Active ulcer: *Adults:* 300 mg orally at bedtime, or 150 mg every 12 hr, for 8 weeks.	
		Maintenance therapy: *Adults:* 150 mg orally at bedtime.	
	GERD	**Capsules or 15 mg/mL solution:**	
		Adults: 150 mg orally twice daily for up to 12 weeks.	

ªDosing should be individualized to patients and their diagnosis. Manufacturer's literature should always be consulted.
GERD, Gastroesophageal reflux disease; *GI,* gastrointestinal; *PPIs,* proton pump inhibitors.

Nizatidine

Note that the brand name medication, Axid, as well as generic nizatidine solutions have been withdrawn in the United States. Generic tablets may still be available for prescription.

Pharmacokinetics. Nizatidine has an onset of action of 60 minutes, with peak therapeutic levels of .5 to 3 hours. Slightly higher protein-bound than other H2 antagonists at 35%, nizatidine has a half-life of 1 to 2 hours. Approximately 60% of the dose is excreted unchanged in the urine by glomerular filtration and tubular secretion. Although a minority of the dose is metabolized by the liver, nizatidine may cause hepatocellular injury, which is reversible if the medication is discontinued.

Indications. Nizatidine is indicated for the treatment of GERD, gastritis, esophagitis, PUD, and disorders of hypersecretion such as Zollinger-Ellison syndrome as well as preanesthesia and prevention of stress-induced gastritis.

Adverse Effects. The adverse effects are the same as with other H2 antagonists and include diarrhea or constipation, headache, and dizziness. Other reported adverse effects are rash, runny nose, pharyngitis, and liver damage. Nizatidine has fewer drug–drug interactions than cimetidine.

Contraindications. Caution should be used (i.e., reduce the dose) in patients with renal or hepatic impairment. Use in pregnancy is discouraged because of the lack of human studies and several animal studies with unfavorable results. Excretion in breast milk is minimal; however, risk/benefit analysis should be used when deciding whether to prescribe to those who are nursing.

Monitoring. When nizatidine is administered concurrently with antibiotics, monitor for pseudomembranous colitis, especially since diarrhea is a known adverse effect. If symptoms do not improve in 2 weeks, further evaluation, including for gastric cancer, should be undertaken. Liver function studies should be performed if the patient demonstrates signs and symptoms of liver damage such as jaundice or abdominal pain.

Proton Pump Inhibitors

Proton pump inhibitors (PPIs) are the most potent inhibitors of HCl and decrease production by up to 95% in a 24-hour period. Six PPIs, all with equivalent efficacy at comparable doses, are available for clinical use: omeprazole, esomeprazole, lansoprazole, dexlansoprazole, rabeprazole, and pantoprazole. PPIs block the final step in gastric acid production through irreversible inhibition of the proton pump on the secretory surface of the gastric parietal cells. PPIs effectively block production from all types of stimulation including H2, gastrin, food intake, and vagal stimulation. The effect is dose related and lasts for 72 hours after 1 dose. After continuous administration, gastric acid secretion resumes within 3 to 5 days of stopping the medication, returning to pretreatment levels in 2 weeks to 3 months, depending on the product.

PPIs are administered as a prodrug with an enteric coating to prevent absorption until the product reaches the less acidic duodenum. If administered as tablets, they should be administered whole, not cut or crushed. Granules can be mixed with applesauce or juice, but the granules should not be chewed, and the dose should be administered immediately after mixing.

Absorption is rapid but may be delayed by up to 50% in the presence of food. PPIs should be given on an empty stomach, preferably before the first meal of the day. If dosing twice daily, the second dose should be given before the last meal of the day. Between 2 and 7 days may be necessary for full acid suppression. After absorption and distribution, PPIs are highly protein bound. Entering circulation, they are delivered to the parietal cells, where the acid environment converts the prodrug to active form. The half-life of PPIs is 1 to 2 hours, except in the presence of hepatic disease, which can prolong the half-life up to 9 hours. The duration of action, however, is extended related to the drug binding to enzymes within the parietal gland, resulting in prolonged action. All PPIs are heavily metabolized in the liver. Dose reduction of esomeprazole and lansoprazole in patients with hepatic disease due to reduced clearance is recommended. All PPIs are metabolized via the CYP systems. Omeprazole is metabolized by the CYP 450 system, resulting in interaction with other drugs metabolized by this system (Table 15.5). Up to 90% of excretion occurs via the kidney, with the remainder following a biliary excretion route via the feces. After prolonged use, pretreatment levels of gastric secretion return from 1 week to 3 months after discontinuing the medication, with omeprazole taking the shortest time and pantoprazole taking the longest time.

PPIs are generally considered safe in pregnancy if clinically indicated, although well-controlled studies in pregnancy have not been established. Benefits to the mother should outweigh risks to the fetus. PPIs are excreted in breast milk in both animal and human studies. Administration to the nursing mother should consider the importance of the drug to the mother's treatment.

Given the long-term and widespread use of prescription and OTC PPIs, the risk of serious side effects from this class is modest; however, awareness of potential short- and long-term effects is necessary for safe prescribing. Short-term adverse effects of the class include dizziness, drowsiness, abdominal pain, constipation, diarrhea, and flatulence. Potential long-term adverse effects include vitamin B_{12} deficiency, osteoporosis, bone fractures, hypomagnesemia, pneumonia, lupus-like syndromes, and *C. difficile* infection. All PPIs may stimulate excess gastrin secretion (hypergastrinemia), which may precipitate rebound hyperacidity after discontinuing the medication and may promote the growth of gastric tumors. As with H2 medications, altering the stomach pH can impact the absorption, metabolism, or excretion

of other drugs (see Table 15.5). Typical dosing schedules are found in Table 15.6. For long-term use, tapering patients off the medication is preferred to abrupt cessation.

Lansoprazole

Pharmacokinetics. Lansoprazole is readily absorbed in the duodenum. The onset of action is about 1 hour, with a duration of action of greater than 24 hours related to deposition in the parietal cells. Highly protein bound at 97%, lansoprazole has a half-life of 1 to 1.5 hours. Metabolized in the liver, the medication is excreted as metabolites in the urine. Although it is metabolized by the CYP P450 enzymes, there are no clinically significant drug–drug interactions related to this metabolism. Return to pretreatment levels of gastric secretion can take up to 4 weeks after discontinuing the medication.

Indications. Lansoprazole is indicated for the treatment of GERD, PUD, hypersecretory conditions such as Zollinger-Ellison syndrome, and concurrently with antibiotic therapy for the eradication of *H. pylori*. It is also used to prevent gastritis during long-term NSAID use.

Adverse Effects. Adverse effects are noted to be primarily GI in nature, with constipation, nausea, abdominal discomfort, and diarrhea among the most reported. Less commonly reported are myopathies, arthralgias, and rashes. Decreased vitamin B_{12} levels have been noted with long-term use. Prolonged use may lead to hypomagnesemia.

Contraindications. Caution should be used in patients with risk for or known vitamin B_{12} deficiencies, osteopenia or osteoporosis, and hepatic impairment. For severe hepatic impairment, dose reduction is recommended. Rebound

---

TABLE 15.5 Medications That Interact With Proton Pump Inhibitors

Medication	Interacting Medication	Possible Effects
Omeprazole	Clarithromycin	When administered together, plasma levels of both drugs may be elevated
	Sulfonylureas	May increase hypoglycemia potential
	Benzodiazepines, phenytoin	Half-life of diazepam may be doubled, and phenytoin clearance may be reduced 15%
Lansoprazole	Theophylline	Decreased theophylline clearance
Esomeprazole	Clarithromycin	Increased plasma levels of both drugs
	Benzodiazepines	Benzodiazepine metabolism may be decreased, clearance increased, and half-life prolonged
Rabeprazole	Clarithromycin	When administered together, plasma levels of both drugs may be elevated
All PPIs	Sucralfate	Decreased absorption of PPI
	Azole antifungals	Decreased absorption of azoles
	Digoxin	Increase digoxin levels
	Warfarin	Prolonged administration time of warfarin
	Enteric-coated tablets	Enteric coating may be altered, resulting in unpredictable dissolution of medication

PPI, Proton pump inhibitor.

hyperacidity is possible when discontinuing this medication. Although the class in general may be affected by the use of the CYP 450 system for metabolism, lansoprazole does not appear to be clinically affected and has minimal drug–drug interactions related to the system.

Monitoring. For long-term use, monitoring of liver function and magnesium levels is indicated. If the patient fails to achieve clinical goals after 3 months of therapy, further investigation to determine complications or other diagnostic concerns is warranted.

TABLE 15.6	**Selected Proton Inhibitor Dosages and Schedules**[a]		
Medication	**Indication**	**Dosage**	**Considerations and Monitoring**
Omeprazole (Prilosec)	Duodenal ulcer	**Delayed-release capsules or delayed-release suspension:** *Adults and adolescents ≥17 yr:* 20 mg orally once daily for 4–8 weeks.	Give on an empty stomach 60 minutes before first meal of the day. May be taken with antacids. For patients who have difficulty swallowing, delayed-release capsules may be opened and sprinkled on applesauce or yogurt or given with water or fruit juices. For patients with erosive esophagitis: If a patient does not respond to 8 weeks of treatment, an additional 4 weeks of treatment may be given. If there is recurrence of erosive esophagitis, an additional 4 to 8-week courses of omeprazole may be considered. Long-term maintenance may be up to 5 yr. Dosages greater than 80 mg/day should be administered in divided doses.
	Gastric ulcer	**Delayed-release capsules or delayed-release suspension:** *Adults and adolescents ≥17 yr:* 40 mg orally once daily for 4–8 weeks.	
	Erosive esophagitis and GERD	**Delayed-release capsules or delayed-release suspension:** *Adults:* Give 20 mg orally for 4 weeks. Patients with esophagitis may require 4–8 weeks. *Adolescents and children weighing ≥20 kg:* Give 20 mg orally once daily or 0.7–3.3 mg/kg/day. *Children weighing 10–19 kg:* Give 10 mg once daily OR give 0.7–3.3 mg/kg/day.	
	Hypersecretory disorders (Zollinger-Ellison syndrome)	**Delayed-release capsules or delayed-release suspension:** *Adults and adolescents ≥17 yr:* Give 60 mg orally once daily initially, then titrate dosage up to 120 mg orally three times daily.	
Esomeprazole magnesium (Nexium)	Prevention of NSAID-induced ulcer prophylaxis in at-risk patients	**Capsules or suspension:** *Adults:* 20–40 mg orally once daily.	Give on an empty stomach at least 60 minutes before meals. If given once daily, administer before the first meal of the day. For patients who have difficulty swallowing, may sprinkle contents of capsule on applesauce or yogurt or give with water, apple juice, or orange juice.
	GERD	**Capsules or suspension:** *Adults:* 20 mg orally once daily every morning for 4 weeks. May continue an additional 4 weeks if symptoms persist. *Adolescents and children ≥12 yr:* Give 20 mg once daily. May also give a dosage range of 0.7–3.3 mg/kg/day Do not exceed 20–40 mg/day. *Children 1–11 yr:* Give 10 mg orally once daily for up to 8 weeks.	
	Hypersecretion associated with Zollinger-Ellison syndrome	**Capsules or suspension:** *Adults:* Begin with 40 mg orally twice daily. May increase as needed up to 240 mg/day in divided doses. May need up to 1 yr.	

TABLE 15.6 **Selected Proton Inhibitor Dosages and Schedules[a]—cont'd**

Medication	Indication	Dosage	Considerations and Monitoring
Lansoprazole (Prevacid)	Duodenal ulcer	*Adults, adolescents and children ≥12 yr:* 15 mg orally once daily in the morning at least 30 minutes before a meal for up to 4 weeks. For maintenance, may continue 15 mg once daily.	Give on an empty stomach, 30–60 minutes before first meal of the day. Delayed-release capsules may be opened and contents sprinkled on 15 mL of either applesauce, Ensure pudding, yogurt, cottage cheese, or strained pears. May also be mixed into apple juice, orange juice, or tomato juice. Patient should make sure to rinse mouth well to swallow all of the medication.
	Erosive esophagitis, gastric ulcer	*Adults, adolescents, and children ≥12 yr:* Give 30 mg once daily for up to 8 weeks. If healing is incomplete or recurs, consider an additional 8 weeks of treatment. For maintenance of healing, 15 mg once daily 30–60 min. *Children 1–11 yr weighing ≥30 kg:* 30 mg orally once daily in the morning at least 30 minutes before a meal for up to 12 weeks. *Children 1–11 yr weighing <30 kg:* Give 15 mg orally once daily in the morning at least 30 minutes before a meal for up to 12 weeks.	
	Hypersecretory disorders	*Adults:* Begin with 60 mg orally once daily at least 30 minutes before meals. Dosages up to 90 mg twice daily have been used. If dosage is greater than 120 mg/day, give in divided doses.	
	GERD	*Adults, adolescents, and children ≥12 yr:* Give 15 mg orally once daily 30–60 minutes before first meal of the day for up to 8 weeks. *Children 1–11 yr weighing ≥30 kg:* Give 30 mg orally once daily in the morning at least 30 minutes before a meal for up to 12 weeks. May give 1.4–1.5 mg/kg/day orally. *Children 1–11 yr weighing <30 kg:* 15 mg orally once daily in the morning at least 30 minutes before a meal for up to 12 weeks.	
	Prevention of NSAID-induced ulcers in patients with previous gastric ulcer	*Adults:* Give 15 mg orally once daily in the morning at least 30 minutes before a meal.	

Continued

TABLE 15.6	Selected Proton Inhibitor Dosages and Schedules[a]—cont'd		
Medication	**Indication**	**Dosage**	**Considerations and Monitoring**
Rabeprazole (Aciphex)	GERD	**Delayed-release tablets:** *Adults:* Give 20 mg orally once daily in the morning for up to 4 weeks. *Adolescents and children 12–17 yr:* 20 mg once daily for 8 weeks. **Delayed-release sprinkle capsules:** *Children 1–11 yr weighing ≥15 kg:* Give 10 mg orally once daily for 12 weeks. *Children 1–11 yr weighing <15 kg:* Give 5 mg orally once daily for 12 weeks, with the option to increase to 10 mg/day if inadequate response.	Administer 30–60 minutes before meals. Delayed-release capsules and contents sprinkled on a spoonful of soft food or liquid (at or below room temperature). Take the entire dose within 15 minutes of being sprinkled; do not store mixture for future use.
	Erosive esophagitis	**Delayed-release tablets:** *Adults:* 20 mg orally once daily for 4–8 weeks. May give an additional 8-week course.	
	Healing duodenal ulcer	**Delayed-release tablets:** *Adults:* 20 mg orally once in the morning up to 4 weeks.	

[a]Dosing should be individualized to patients and their diagnosis. Manufacturer's literature should always be consulted.
GERD, Gastroesophageal reflux disease; *NSAID,* nonsteroidal antiinflammatory drug.

Omeprazole

Pharmacokinetics. Omeprazole should be taken approximately 60 minutes before breakfast. Omeprazole is rapidly absorbed **after** oral administration and distributes throughout the body tissues, concentrating in the gastric parietal cells. It is highly metabolized in the liver. Onset of action is approximately 1 hour, and duration is approximately 72 hours. Excretion of omeprazole is via the kidney (72% to 80%) and the feces (18% to 23%).

Indications. Omeprazole is indicated for short-term (fewer than 2 weeks) treatment of dyspepsia or heartburn symptoms, esophageal reflux disease, hypersecretory disorders such as Zollinger-Edison syndrome, as part of therapy to eradicate *H. pylori*, PUD, stress-induced gastritis, and for prophylaxis of NSAID-induced gastritis.

Adverse Effects. As is typical for this class, reported adverse effects are drowsiness, constipation, diarrhea, flatulence, and dizziness. Long-term use carries the potential for iron or vitamin B_{12} deficiency, osteoporosis, and atrophic gastritis.

Contraindications. Because of the increased risk of fractures after long-term use of omeprazole, it should be used cautiously in patients who either have or are at risk for osteopenia or osteoporosis. Because of the increased risk of dysrhythmias, avoid use in patients who may have long QT syndrome. Advise patients to seek medical care if they experience watery stool, abdominal pain, and fever as they may be signs of serious infection, including *Clostridium difficile.* Omeprazole should be avoided in pregnant women. Use of omeprazole during breastfeeding may increase the risk of adverse effects in infants, including suppression of gastric acid secretions. PPIs including omeprazole are considered inappropriate for older adults according to the Beers Criteria due to the increased risk of bone fracture and *Clostridium difficile* infection.

Monitoring. For long-term use, monitoring of liver function, vitamin B_{12}, iron, and magnesium levels is indicated. If the patient fails to achieve clinical goals after 3 months of therapy, further investigation to determine complications or other diagnostic concerns is warranted.

Cytoprotective Medications

The protective mechanism of the mucous layer in the stomach can be interrupted by long-term or high-dose NSAID use, high-dose steroids, and iatrogenic situations such as hospitalization in ICUs or burn units. Cytoprotective medications can be used to treat PUD as well as to prevent the formation of ulceration. Increasing protection of the stomach can be encouraged by decreasing use of antiprostaglandin agents such as NSAIDs or steroids, or through the exogenous administration of prostaglandin. Artificial protection can be provided by gel-like agents that adhere to the stomach lining and form a protective coating.

Sucralfate

Pharmacokinetics. The cytoprotective medication sucralfate (Carafate) is a topical agent with neither significant systemic absorption (3% to 5%) nor acid-neutralizing qualities. Administered as a tablet or suspension, sucralfate is activated by the acid environment of the stomach, forming a gel-like substance that adheres to damaged GI mucosa, although it binds to normal tissue to a lesser extent. This shields the ulcerated area from HCl and pepsin, promoting healing. The gel-like layer adheres to ulcers for up to 6 hours. Up to 90% of the administered dose is excreted in the feces within 48 hours. Although absorption is minimal, in renally impaired patients small amounts of aluminum from absorbed doses can accumulate.

Adverse Effects. Adverse effects include constipation or diarrhea, gastric discomfort, nausea, dry mouth, and headache. Rarely, anaphylactoid-type reactions such as angioedema, edema of the mouth and throat, edema, rash, or pruritis are noted. Persons with renal failure or those who are on dialysis may absorb aluminum. Sucralfate can interfere with the absorption of other medications if administered concurrently.

Contraindications. Caution should be used when prescribing sucralfate to patients with renal impairment. It may increase blood glucose in patients with diabetes.

Monitoring. No routine monitoring is indicated; however, blood glucose should be monitored in patients taking oral antidiabetics related to changes in absorption of the medications.

Prostaglandin Analogs

Endogenous prostaglandins that promote protective mechanisms in the stomach are synthesized in the gastric mucosa and prevent gastric epithelial injury through two mechanisms: by binding to receptors on the parietal cells and by decreasing gastric acid production and stimulating mucin and bicarbonate. Through these effects, a protective coating is developed, present gastric acid is buffered, and further production of gastric acid is blunted, although this last effect is dose dependent. Typical dosing schedules are listed in Table 15.7.

Misoprostol

Pharmacokinetics. Synthetic prostaglandins are administered orally as misoprostol, an inactive compound. The active metabolite, misoprostol acid, inhibits acid production promptly, usually within 30 minutes, with a duration of action of approximately 3 hours. The half-life is 20 to 40 minutes. Misoprostol acid is excreted in the urine, with approximately 1% as the unchanged parent drug.

Indications. Misoprostol is used for prophylaxis of gastroduodenal ulcers induced by NSAIDs, debilitating disease, or corticosteroid use.

Adverse Effects. Diarrhea is the most common adverse effect, occurring in up to 40% of patients, but this tends to be self-limiting. Other adverse effects include abdominal

---

> ### BLACK BOX WARNING!
>
> **Misoprostol**
>
> Misoprostol is contraindicated in patients of childbearing potential, unless the patient is at risk for significant complications from gastric ulcers or at high risk for developing gastric ulcers. If essential for the patient, misoprostol may be prescribed if the patient:
>
> - Exhibits a negative serum pregnancy test within 2 weeks of beginning therapy
> - Uses effective and reliable contraception while taking misoprostol
> - Receives both oral and written warnings of the risks of misoprostol
> - Begins therapy only on the second or third day of the next normal menstrual cycle
>
> The patient should discontinue misoprostol and contact the provider if they become pregnant.
>
> Data from Elsevier. Clinical pharmacology powered by ClinicalKey®. C2019-(cited August 2020). Retrieved from http://www.clinicalkey.com.

---

pain, nausea and vomiting, flatulence, constipation, and dyspepsia. A small percentage of patients (2% to 3%) experience headache.

Contraindications. Misoprostol is contraindicated in pregnancy, as synthetic prostaglandin use can result in uterine contractions, endangering a pregnancy. Use of misoprostol in pregnancy is an absolute contraindication indicated by a black box warning. Misoprostol acid is readily excreted in breast milk, making it unsuitable for nursing patients. Use with caution in patients with renal impairment due to the potential for drug accumulation. Taking misoprostol with magnesium can increase the potential for diarrhea (Table 15.8).

Monitoring. Reinforce the need to avoid pregnancy by using adequate contraception as well as to report pregnancy should it occur. With prolonged use or for those with renal dysfunction, monitor electrolytes and BUN.

Promotility Medications

Prokinetic medication is used to stimulate motility and tone of the upper gastric tract without stimulating gastric, biliary, or pancreatic secretion. The purpose is to increase transit time of food and prompt gastric emptying. Metoclopramide is particularly effective in GERD, prompted by the patient lying down and related not only to gastric emptying but also to increased tone of the LES. The antiemetic action of metoclopramide is a result of dopamine receptor antagonist action in the CNS. Several notable drug–drug indications are listed in Table 15.8.

Metoclopramide

Pharmacokinetics. Metoclopramide is available for oral, intramuscular, and IV use, and is promptly absorbed after oral administration with a peak action of 1 hour and a duration of 1 to 2 hours. The half-life of metoclopramide is 4 to 6 hours and it is excreted in the urine.

TABLE 15.7	Prokinetic and Cytoprotective Dosages		
Medication	**Indication**	**Dosage**	**Comments**
Metoclopramide (Reglan)	Symptomatic GERD	*Adults:* 10–15 mg orally up to four times daily, 30 minutes before meals and at bedtime. Older adults may respond to a dose of 5 mg. If patient is a poor metabolizer of CYP2D6, the recommended dosage is 5 mg orally four times daily or 10 mg orally three times daily. Maximum dosage: 30 mg/day.	Not recommended for longer than 12 weeks. Review drug interactions carefully; dosages may need to be adjusted.
Misoprostol (Cytotec)	NSAID-induced gastric ulcer prophylaxis in patients receiving NSAIDs and at high risk for gastric ulceration	*Adults:* Give 200 mcg orally four times daily, with meals and at bedtime. May reduce to 100 mcg orally four times daily in patients who do not tolerate 200-mcg dose. Continue for duration of NSAID therapy.	**Note:** Misoprostol is indicated to prevent NSAID-induced gastric ulcers but has not been shown to prevent duodenal ulcers. Contraindicated during pregnancy due to increased risk of uterine contractions and miscarriage as well as teratogenic effects.
Sucralfate (Carafate)	Treatment of duodenal ulcer not related to NSAID use:		Take on an empty stomach at least 1 hr before a meal and at bedtime. Do not take antacids 30 minutes before or after a sucralfate dose.
	Active disease	**Oral tablets or suspension:** *Adults:* Give 1 Gm four times daily, 1 hour before meals and at bedtime for 4–8 weeks or less if healing has been effectively demonstrated.	
	Maintenance therapy	**Tablets only:** *Adults* 1 Gm orally twice daily on an empty stomach.	

GERD, Gastroesophageal reflux disease; *NSAID,* nonsteroidal antiinflammatory drug.

TABLE 15.8	Medications That Interact With Cytoprotective and Prokinetic Agents	
Medication	**Interacting Medication**	**Possible Effects**
Metoclopramide	Levodopa	Increased availability of levodopa, decreased availability of metoclopramide
	Digoxin	Decreased absorption and plasma levels of digoxin
	Antidepressants, opioids, alcohol, antihistamines, sedative hypnotics	Increases alcohol absorption, additive CNS depression
	Cimetidine	Reduced bioavailability of cimetidine
	Drugs with potential extrapyramidal effects	Increased risk of extrapyramidal effects
	Anticholinergics and opioids	Metoclopramide may have antagonist effect on these medications
Misoprostol	Magnesium-based antacids	Increased risk of diarrhea
Sucralfate	All medications absorbed in the stomach	Sucralfate's action of coating the stomach wall can decrease absorption of other oral medications

CNS, central nervous system.

Indications. Metoclopramide is used to treat GERD, diabetic gastroparesis, and nausea and vomiting, especially related to chemotherapy.

Adverse Effects. Short-term use can result in drowsiness, confusion, disorientation, and restlessness. Related to its action of blocking dopamine receptors, metoclopramide may cause extrapyramidal effects such as tardive dyskinesia, dystonia, tremors, and bradykinesia. Galactorrhea has also been reported. These effects are usually noted after long-term use.

Contraindications. Insufficient data are available regarding the safety of metoclopramide in pregnancy. Alternative medications should be considered with a careful risk/benefit analysis. Limited data are available on safety in breastfeeding, although it is known that metoclopramide is excreted in breast milk. Low-dose, short-term use in nursing patients is generally considered acceptable with appropriate risk/benefit analysis.

A black box warning is applied to metoclopramide for use of the drug in patients currently experiencing tardive dyskinesia. Absolute contraindications are GI bleed, obstruction, or perforation; pheochromocytoma; and seizure disorder. Caution should be used in patients who are breastfeeding, have breast cancer, or have cardiac disease. Caution, including a dose reduction, is advised for patients with renal disease. Typical dosing schedules are listed in Table 15.7.

BLACK BOX WARNING!

Metoclopramide

Metoclopramide is contraindicated in patients with a history of tardive dyskinesia or dystonic reaction. This is due to its blockage of dopamine receptors, particularly D2 receptors. The risk is related to the length of therapy, and the U.S. Food and Drug Administration (FDA) recommends against using metoclopramide for more than 12 weeks.

Prescriber Considerations for Hyperacidity Therapy

Clinical Practice Guidelines

The ACG provides guidance for the diagnosis and management of dyspepsia, GERD, and *H. pylori* infections. Many hyperacidity conditions appear with similar symptoms and require a detailed history and physical exam to arrive at a diagnosis. In some cases, laboratory, radiographic, or interventional studies will be needed. Lifestyle management is a cornerstone of management, and pharmacologic therapy should be individualized to the patient's needs.

BOOKMARK THIS!

Clinical Guidelines for Hyperacidity Therapy

The ACG (https://gi.org/guidelines/) provides current clinical practice guidelines on topics including dyspepsia as well as other topics relevant to the primary care provider. Guidelines are updated regularly as required for the science.

Clinical Reasoning for Hyperacidity Therapy

Many patients will come to primary care having already attempted OTC self-treatment for symptoms of heartburn, indigestion, nausea, chest pain or discomfort, abdominal discomfort, hoarseness, or belching. Of immediate concern is to evaluate for *alarm symptoms*, which indicate the potential for higher morbidity or mortality diseases such as gastric cancer. Alarm symptoms include dysphagia, odynophagia, anorexia, weight loss, upper GI bleed, and new onset of GI symptoms over the age of 60. Such symptoms should be investigated with upper endoscopy. Evaluation for cardiac causes should be considered in patients describing chest pain or discomfort. Typical presentations with no alarm symptoms can generally be treated empirically with consideration of the severity of symptoms. provides recommendations from the ACG (Katz, 2013).

Mild or transient symptoms can be treated with antacids or H2 antagonists. For moderate to severe symptoms, PPIs are preferred for their profound degree of suppression of gastric acid. Choice of PPI is not complex, as PPIs have been found to have similar efficacy across the class. If the patient fails to improve with consistent therapy, additional testing should be performed to evaluate the esophagus and stomach for erosion, ulceration, or tumor; a bacterial component; or other pathology. Testing may include endoscopy, ambulatory esophageal reflux monitoring, or urea breath test for *H. pylori* (Figure 15.1).

Consider the individual patient's health problem requiring hyperacidity therapy. GERD, PUD, and gastritis can present with similar or overlapping symptoms. In addition, some symptoms are subjective and difficult to quantify. Of importance is that severity of symptoms may not correlate with severity of disease state. If the patient has been self-medicating, this may cloud the clinical picture, calling for careful questioning of the patient's medication, symptom history, and lifestyle to create an individualized plan of therapy. Attention to an individual plan will assist with compliance and medication efficacy. Individualization of treatment can also be accomplished by attention to the degree of acid control that is needed. Increasing acid control is demonstrated across the classes, from topical acid neutralization of antacids to intermediate control with H2RAs, with the greatest amount of acid control coming from administration of a proton pump inhibitor.

Determine the desired therapeutic outcome based on the degree of acid reduction needed for the patient's health problem. In most cases, symptom relief of hyperacidity is being sought by the patient related to the impact the symptoms have on quality of life. Patients find that symptoms disrupt productivity at work, disturb sleep, and generally impact quality of life. Nighttime symptoms appear to interfere more with quality of life than daytime symptoms. With self-treatment, patients tend to use intermittent therapy when symptoms become intolerable, creating a waxing and waning course. With prescribed therapy, encouraging the patient to remain on regular, continuous therapy will provide greater

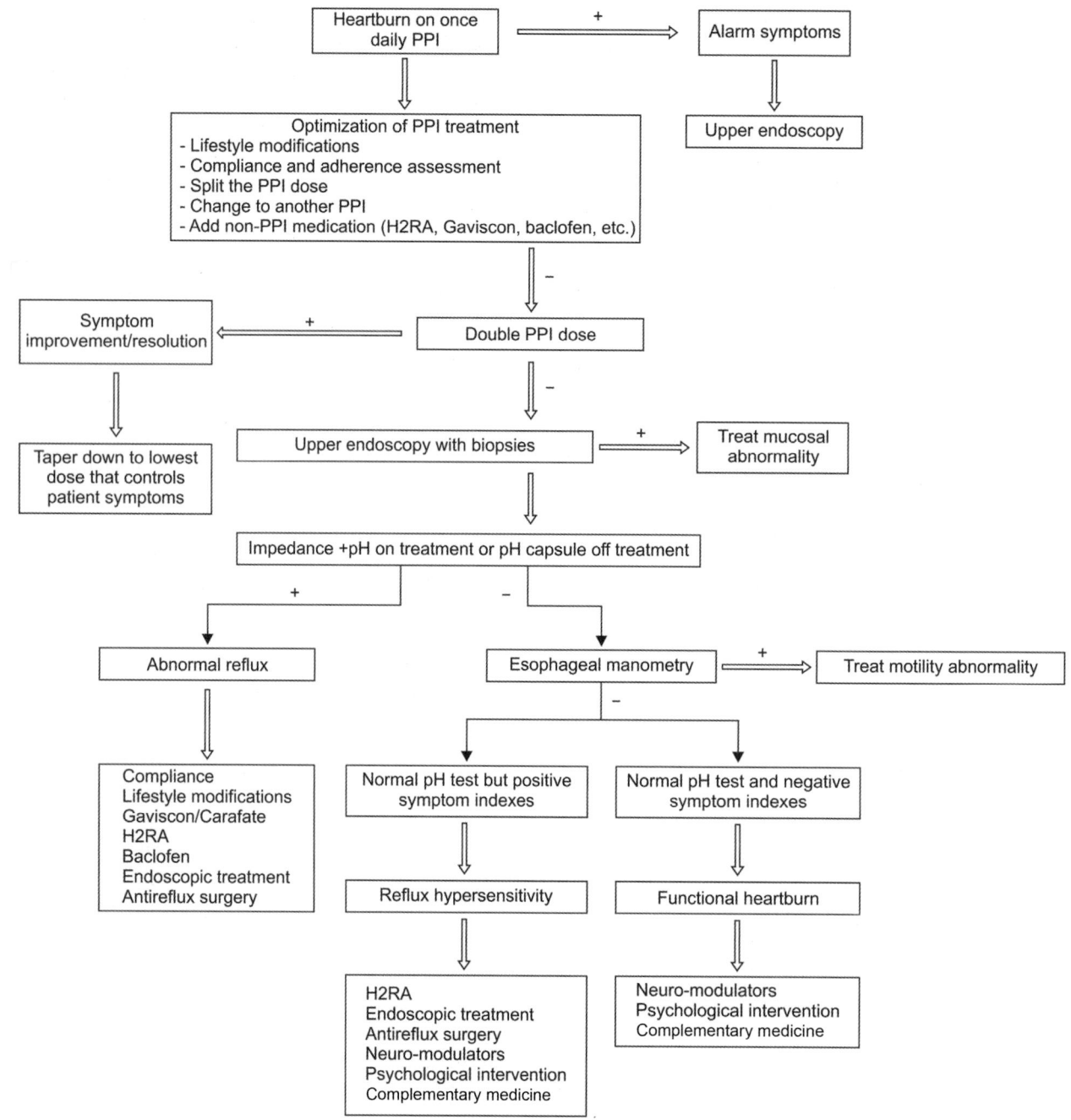

• **Fig. 15.1** Management of the complaint of heartburn uncontrolled on first-line treatment. (From Sandhu, D. S., & Fass, R. [2018]. Current trends in the management of gastroesophageal reflux disease. *Gut and Liver, 12*[1], 7–16. http://doi.org/10.5009/gnl16615.)

symptom control. Additionally, patients should be educated that reduction in symptoms while medicated should not be construed as curative of more severe problems such as PUD or gastritis, and continuing the course of treatment is necessary.

Assess the medication selected for its appropriateness for an individual patient by considering the side effects of the medication and the patient's age, race/ethnicity, comorbidities, and genetic factors. Attention to the risk/benefit profile related to the individual patient's needs and the chosen medication is

important. Across the classes of drugs, there is considerable variability in adverse-effect profile and cost. Choice of medication should provide the highest level of acid suppression necessary with the fewest adverse effects, at a cost that is acceptable to the patient. While the PPI class is considered preferable related to the degree to which it can suppress gastric acid, use of another class of medication may be necessary due to the side-effect profile of the medication or the patient's comorbid conditions. For example, PPIs (except cimetidine) interact with warfarin, which would make the choice of other medications to control acidity necessary. In extreme cases, patients with multiple comorbidities or medications may be treated with topical, minimally absorbed antacids. When cost is of concern, H2 blockers, especially generic ones, are less costly than PPIs. Although they do cost more, PPIs do not need dose adjustments for renal or hepatic impairment. Possibly related to liver enzyme activity, persons of Asian descent may experience higher-than-expected levels of omeprazole at equivalent doses, so dosage reduction is recommended.

Initiate the treatment plan with the selected medication by first providing adequate patient education to ensure the patient's understanding and promote full participation in the hyperacidity therapy. The overall goal of patient education is to ensure adherence to the treatment plan through patient understanding of the pathology being treated, goal of therapy, specifics of the treatment plan, risks of lack of treatment, and importance of adherence to both lifestyle modifications and medications (Box 15.5). The important synergy between lifestyle modifications and medication management should be emphasized.

• BOX 15.5 Patient Education Information

Patient Education Points

Patient education should address the following concepts:
- Cause of hyperacidity and long-term risks if untreated
  - Patients should be advised of the potential for GERD to become chronic in nature. The progression of GERD to erosive esophagitis, premalignancy, or malignancy should be explained.
- Role of lifestyle modifications in management and future prevention
  - It is important that patients understand that medication alone will not resolve the problem and that their lifestyle choices play an important part in management.
- Actions of prescribed medication on both pathology and symptoms
  - Clear expectations of the synergism between medications and lifestyle management should be described.
- When to expect relief of symptoms
  - Setting forth reasonable time frames creates clear expectations.
- Names, doses, and schedule of medications
  - Clear instruction on when and how to take medications should be presented
  - Drug–drug or drug–food interactions and adverse events specific to the medication should be reviewed.
- Importance of adherence
  - Potential barriers to adherence to the treatment plan should be investigated and should include psychosocial as well as financial concerns. The importance of following all medication schedules, including antibiotics to treat PUD, should be stressed.
- When to call the provider with concerns and the importance of maintaining follow-up visits as scheduled or if symptoms do not resolve

Ensure complete patient and family understanding about the medication prescribed for hyperacidity therapy using a variety of education strategies. The education process should be tailored to the needs of the patient considering their education, language spoken, reading ability, previous experience with medical systems, and readiness to learn. Principles of therapeutic communication such as focusing and clarification by having patients restate instructions should be employed. Allowing patients time to express fears or concerns about the diagnosis is important. In addition to oral instruction, providing patients with written materials will assist with remembering instructions when arriving home. While giving oral instruction, simultaneously creating a table for medication administration that can be posted in the home is helpful. The patient's understanding of information should be verified using the teach-back method.

Conduct follow-up and monitoring of patient responses to hyperacidity therapy. Outcome evaluation is dependent upon severity or persistence of symptoms. Mild cases of hyperacidity disorders such as situation or intermittent GERD do not require follow-up unless symptoms do not abate. Patients should be advised of reasonable time frames for expectations of symptom abatement and be encouraged to return to primary care if symptoms do not resolve. For more severe symptoms, initial follow-up of 2 to 4 weeks is recommended for medication adjustment or confirmation of improvement. Patients who do not improve on maximum PPIs in 8 weeks, whose symptoms worsen, or who develop alarm symptoms should be referred to a GI specialist for further evaluation.

Teaching Points for Hyperacidity Therapy

Health Promotion Strategies

The foundation of managing GERD, PUD, and gastritis begins with lifestyle modification. Medication alone has been found to be less effective than when used in combination with healthy changes to diet and habits. Patients should be instructed to avoid spicy, acidic, or greasy foods; chocolate; alcohol; carbonated beverages; and coffee. Noncaffeinated coffee should not be substituted for regular coffee as the acidity may exacerbate symptoms. Several small meals daily are preferable to large quantities at one time. Certain medications should be used cautiously (anticholinergics, corticosteroids, theophylline, meperidine, and calcium channel blockers), and the patient should advise the primary care provider of the use of any newly prescribed medication or OTC products. The patient should be cautioned to discontinue the use of OTC NSAIDs without supervision. Patients should be assisted with smoking cessation.

For GERD that is problematic at night, eating the last meal 3 hours or more before retiring is encouraged. Elevating the head of the bed on blocks is preferable to using pillows to prop the upper body higher. Use of pillows may result in bending at the waist and increased upward pressure on the LES.

Patients should avoid tight clothing at the waist and should avoid exercising for 3 hours after eating. Obesity and intraabdominal fat can create upward pressure on stomach contents. Weight loss and decreased abdominal obesity should be encouraged.

Application Questions for Discussion

1. GERD, PUD, and gastritis can present with similar symptoms. How does the primary care provider determine a suitable pharmacologic treatment plan?
2. Lifestyle modifications are considered synergistic to medications in the treatment of hyperacidity. What important modifiable habits and choices are linked to successful management of hyperacidity conditions, and how might the patient be supported to make necessary changes?
3. Medication to manage hyperacidity can intervene locally, indirectly, or directly on acid-secreting cells or can be used to increase protective mechanisms of the stomach. What patient characteristics would lead the primary care provider to choose from among the various methods?

Selected Bibliography

Badillo, R., & Francis, D. (2014). Diagnosis and treatment of gastroesophageal reflux disease. *World Journal of Gastrointestinal Pharmacology and Therapeutics, 5*(3), 105–112.

Bramhall, S. R., & Mourad, M. M. (2020). Is there still a role for sucralfate in the treatment of gastritis? *World Journal of Meta-Analysis, 8*(1), 1–3.

Brunton, L. L., Hilal-Dandan, R., & Knollmann, B. C. (2017). *Goodman and Gilman's The Pharmacological Basis of Therapeutics* (13th ed.). New York: McGraw Hill Professional.

Chey, W. D., Leontiadis, G. J., Howden, C,W., & Moss, S. F. (2017). ACG Clinical Guideline: Treatment of Helicobacter pylori Infection. *American Journal of Gastroenterology, 112*(2), 212–239. doi:10.1038/ajg.2016.563.

Consumer Health Care Products Association. (2021). *OTC Use Statistics* Retrieved from https://www.chpa.org/about-consumer-healthcare/research-data/otc-use-statistics.

El-Serag, H. B., Sweet, S., Winchester, C. C., & Dent, J. (2014). Update on the epidemiology of gastro-oesophageal reflux disease: a systematic review. *Gut, 63*(6), 871–880. https://doi.org/10.1136/gutjnl-2012-304269.

Elsevier. Clinical pharmacology powered by ClinicalKey®. C2019- (cited August 2020). Retrieved from http://www.clinicalkey.com.

Grossman, S., & Porth, C. (2013). *Porth's Pathophysiology: Concepts of Altered Health States* (9th ed.). New York: Lippincott, Williams & Wilkens.

Heidelbaugh, J. (2013). Proton pump inhibitors and risk of vitamin and mineral deficiency: Evidence and clinical implications. *Therapeutic Advances in Drug Safety, 4*(3), 125–133.

Hooi, J., Lai, Ying, W., Ng, W., K., Suen, M., Underwood, F., Tanyingoh, D., Malfertheiner, P., Graham, D., Wong, V., Wu, J., Chan, F., Sung, J., Kaplan, G., & Ng, S (2017). Global prevalence of *Helicobacter pylori* infection: Systematic review and meta-analysis. *Gastroenterology, 153*(2), 420–429. Retrieved from https://www.gastrojournal.org/article/S0016-5085(17)35531-2/pdf.

International Foundation for Gastrointestinal Disorders. (2019). *Diet & lifestyle changes*. Retrieved from https://www.aboutgerd.org/diet-lifestyle-changes.html.

Katz, P., Gerson, L., & Vela, M. (2013). Guidelines for the diagnosis and management of gastroesophageal reflux disease. *American Journal of Gastroenterology, 108*(3), 308–328. http://doi.org/10.1038/ajg.2012.444.

Khan, A. M., & Howden, C. W. (2018). The role of proton pump inhibitors in the management of upper gastrointestinal disorders. *Gastroenterology & Hepatology, 14*(3), 169–175.

McCance, K. L., & Huether, S. E. (2019). *Pathophysiology: The Biologic Basis for Disease in Adults and Children* (8th ed.): Mosby Elsevier.

Moayyedi, P., Lacy, B., Andrews, C., Enns, R., Howden, C., & Vakil, N. (2017). ACG and CAG Clinical Guideline: Management of dyspepsia. *American Journal of Gastroenterology, 112*(7), 988–1013. http://doi.org/10.1038/ajg.2017.154.

Salisbury, B., & Terrell, J. (2020). Antacids. *StatPearls*. Retrieved from https://www.ncbi.nlm.nih.gov/books/NBK526049/.

Sandhu, D., & Fass, R. (2018). Current trends in the management of gastroesophageal reflux disease. *Gut and Liver, 12*(1), 7–16.

16

Constipation and Diarrhea Medications

STEPHEN McGHEE AND CHERYL H. ZAMBROSKI

Overview

Constipation and diarrhea are two of the most commonly reported gastrointestinal (GI) symptoms resulting in visits to ambulatory care settings. Diarrhea was the third most reported, and constipation was the sixth most reported (Peery et al., 2019). While many cases of constipation and diarrhea are mild and resolve rapidly, both can be very distressing. Diarrhea can be associated with abdominal cramping, fecal incontinence, fluid and electrolyte losses, and even death in at-risk populations. Although constipation rarely is fatal, it can lead to abdominal discomfort or pain, frequent use of over-the-counter (OTC) medications, hemorrhoids, anal fissures, and reduced quality of life.

Antidiarrheals and laxatives are among the most frequently purchased OTC medications in the United States. In 2018, consumers spent more than $1.3 billion on OTC laxatives and $275 million on OTC antidiarrheals (Consumer Healthcare Products Association, 2020). While constipation and diarrhea may be reported to the primary care provider, it is important to recognize that by the time the patient seeks care, they may have already used a variety of OTC medications to treat their symptoms.

Primary care providers must develop excellent assessment and diagnostic skills to determine etiology and follow best practices to treat the distressing symptoms that accompany these diagnoses. Differentiation between acute and chronic constipation and/or diarrhea will determine the best intervention—pharmacologic or nonpharmacologic—and whether referral to a specialty practice is needed.

Relevant Physiology

The large intestine consists of the cecum, appendix, colon, rectum, and anal canal. The colon is divided into four sections: the ascending colon, transverse colon, descending colon, and sigmoid colon. The cecum receives *chyme*, a semifluid mass of partially digested food, water, and digestive juices, from the distal small intestine (ileum). Chyme flows from the cecum through the ascending, transverse, and descending sections of the colon to the sigmoid and into the rectum. The anal canal is surrounded by a thick portion of smooth muscle that forms the *internal anal sphincter*. The *external anal sphincter* (anus) is composed of striated skeletal muscle.

The gastrocolic reflex begins propulsion of chyme through the colon. The movement is segmental in nature as circular muscles move the intestinal contents through the haustra (Fig. 16.1). Epithelial cells and mucus-secreting goblet cells form the mucosa that lines the colon. The epithelial cells absorb fluid and electrolytes while the goblet cells lubricate the mucosa.

The intestinal contents become the fecal mass as water, sodium, potassium, and short-chain free fatty acids are absorbed. By the time the fecal mass reaches the sigmoid colon, it is typically composed of food residue as well as epithelial cells, bacteria, and unabsorbed secretions from the GI tract. The defecation reflex occurs with the movement of feces into the sigmoid colon and rectum. When the stool enters the rectum, the resultant distention typically causes the urge to defecate. Defecation can be delayed by voluntarily contracting the external anal sphincter and the pelvic floor muscles.

The role of microorganisms in the colon is complex and not completely understood. Nevertheless, it is widely considered that gut microbiota act as a barrier from pathogens, have a role in metabolic functions, and can help regulate the inflammatory response. The composition of gut microorganisms depends on a variety of host-specific factors, including genetics, diet, lifestyle, physiological status, and environment. The diversity and number of bacteria vary across the GI tract, with the colon containing the largest microbial load (Schippa & Conte, 2014). In addition, alterations in the gut microbiota secondary to the introduction of pathogens with contaminated food, water, or as adverse effects of certain medications (e.g., antibiotics, chemotherapy agents) can result in diarrhea that may be severe.

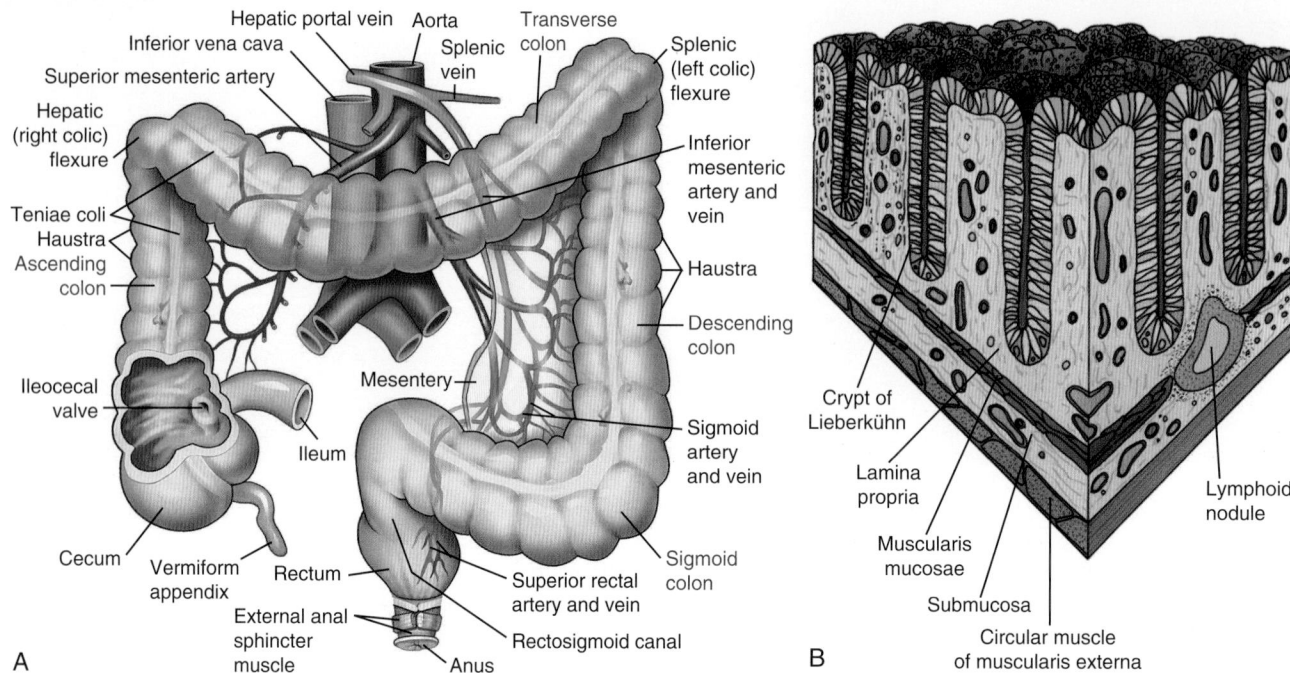

• **Fig. 16.1** (A–B) Structure of the large intestine. (Modified from Patton, K. T., & Thibodeau, G. A. [2018]. *The human body in health & disease* [7th ed.]. St. Louis: Mosby. In Huether, S., & McCance, K. [2021]. *Understanding pathophysiology* [7th ed.]. St. Louis: Elsevier.)

Pathophysiology

Constipation

Constipation is typically defined as difficult or infrequent defecation. Symptoms of constipation include hard stools, straining with stools, a sensation of incomplete evacuation of the bowel, and fewer than normal stools for the patient per week. Because "normal" varies from patient to patient (anywhere from one to three bowel movements each day to a few times per week), determining the patient's normal bowel schedule is important. Risk factors for constipation include depression, lack of physical activity, dehydration, a low-fiber diet, and a variety of medications (Box 16.1). In general, mild constipation can easily be treated with nonpharmacologic interventions such as adequate hydration, a healthy diet that includes fiber, and physical activity. However, if the lack of a bowel movement is associated with significant symptoms or decreased quality of life, pharmacologic intervention may be required. Chronic constipation is characterized by the presence of these symptoms for at least

three out of the previous 12 months. It is more common in adults over 60 and in those who are in long-term care facilities (Mounsey et al., 2015).

Before therapy is initiated, accurate diagnosis is essential to determine whether the etiology of constipation is primary or secondary. *Primary constipation* is typically divided into three subtypes: normal transit, slow transit, and disorders of defecation. *Normal transit constipation* (also called *functional constipation*) is characterized by normal frequency of bowel movements but difficulty with defecation or passage of hard stool (Box 16.2). The most common type of constipation,

• **BOX 16.1   Risk Factors for Constipation**

- Lower socioeconomic status
- Dehydration
- Decreased physical activity
- Depression
- Delay in having a bowel movement
- Older age
- Female
- Pregnancy

• **BOX 16.2   Rome IV Diagnostic Criteria for Functional Constipation**

Patient must have experienced at least two of the following symptoms over the preceding 3 months with symptom onset at least 6 months prior to the diagnosis:

- Straining for more than 25% of defecation attempts
- Lumpy or hard stools for at least 25% of defecation attempts
- Sensation of anorectal obstruction or blockage for at least 25% of defecation attempts
- Sensation of incomplete defecation for at least 25% of defecation attempts
- Manual maneuvering required to defecate for at least 25% of defecation attempts
- Fewer than three spontaneous bowel movements per week

NOTE: Should not meet the criteria for irritable bowel syndrome (IBS) and/or that loose stools are rarely present without the use of laxatives.

From Lacy, B. E., Mearin, F., Chang, L., Chey, W. D., Lembo, A. J., Simren, M., & Spiller, R. (2016). Bowel disorders. *Gastroenterology, 15*(6), 1393–1407.e1395. http://doi.org/10.1053/j.gastro.2016.02.031.

normal transit constipation is associated with decreased physical activity, a diet low in fiber or high in refined foods, or decreased fluid intake. *Slow-transit constipation* is characterized by decreased frequency of bowel movements accompanied by bloating and abdominal discomfort associated with abnormal innervation of the bowel. *Disorders of defecation* are related to a decreased ability to expel stool from the rectum due to dysfunction of the pelvic floor muscles or the anal sphincter. *Secondary constipation* can be attributed to numerous causes, including medications and a variety of medical conditions (Box 16.3). Whether the constipation is primary or secondary, anal fissures, hemorrhoids, and rectal bleeding can occur with passing hard stools. Assessment and diagnosis can guide effective nonpharmacologic and pharmacologic treatments.

Opioid-induced constipation (OIC) is addressed separately here as a type of secondary constipation. Patients with OIC may have been prescribed opioids for the management of cancer- or noncancer-related chronic pain, or may be taking opioids for nonmedical or illicit use (Crockett et al., 2019). Regardless, OIC occurs when exogenous opioids bind to opioid receptors in the GI tract, inhibiting gastric emptying and peristalsis. This leads to increased fluid being absorbed from the stool, which subsequently causes hardening of the stool and more difficult defecation. Opioids also bind to receptors in the submucosa of the GI tract, which decreases sodium and water absorption in the lumen. In addition, opioids decrease the relaxation of the internal anal sphincter with straining and incomplete bowel evacuation. Symptoms of OIC typically occur when starting, changing, or increasing opioid therapy (Box 16.4).

Severe constipation can result in fecal impaction accompanied by abdominal cramping, pain, nausea/vomiting, and rectal bleeding. Fecal impaction is caused by hard, dry stool that becomes lodged in the rectum or sigmoid colon when the patient is unable to evacuate. Risk for fecal impaction increases with age and can be the result of colonic hypomotility, inadequate water intake, and inadequate dietary fiber (Obokhare, 2012). Patients may also experience leaking of stool around the impacted feces (which may be misdiagnosed as diarrhea). Firm feces can be palpated during a digital rectal exam.

Diarrhea

Diarrhea is generally defined as the presence of loose, watery stools occurring three or more times a day. It is important to emphasize that diarrhea should be defined by stool form rather than stool frequency. Diarrhea is not a disease per se, but rather a symptom secondary to a variety of conditions, such as eating certain foods, infection, inflammation, diseases of the intestine (such as ulcerative colitis or Crohn's disease), and adverse effects of medications (Box 16.5).

• BOX 16.4   Rome IV Diagnostic Criteria for Opioid-Induced Constipation

- New or worsening symptoms of constipation that occur when initiating, changing, or increasing opioid therapy. Symptoms must include at least two of the following:
- Straining during more than 25% of defecations
- Lumpy or hard stools more than 25% of defecations
- Sensation of incomplete evacuation more than 25% of defecations
- Sensation of anorectal obstruction/blockage more than 25% of defecations
- Manual maneuvers to facilitate more than 25% of defecations (e.g., digital evacuations, support of pelvic floor)
- Fewer than three spontaneous bowel movements per week
- Loose stools are rarely present without use of laxatives.

From Lacy, B. E., Mearin, F., Chang, L., Chey, W. D., Lembo, A. J., Simren, M., & Spiller, R. (2016). Bowel disorders. *Gastroenterology, 150*(6), 1393–1407.e1395. http://doi.org/10.1053/j.gastro.2016.02.031.

• BOX 16.5   Examples of Causes of Diarrhea

Medications	Broad-spectrum antibiotics Digoxin H2 receptor blockers Proton pump inhibitors ACE inhibitors Magnesium-containing antacids NSAIDs Bisphosphonates
Foods	Foods that contain sugar alcohols including sorbitol, mannitol, and xylitol Increase of foods high in fiber such as whole grains, fruits, and vegetables Foods high in fats or sugar
Bacteria	*Salmonella, Shigella, Campylobacter, Clostridium difficile, Escherichia coli*
Viruses	Norovirus, rotavirus, adenovirus
Parasites	*Giardia lamblia, Entamoeba histolytica*

ACE, Angiotensin-converting enzyme; *NSAIDs,* nonsteroidal antiinflammatory drugs.

• BOX 16.3   Examples of Causes of Secondary Constipation

Medications

- Anticholinergics
- Opiates
- Calcium channel blockers
- Antipsychotics
- Antacids containing calcium carbonate or aluminum hydroxide
- Diuretics
- Anticonvulsants
- Iron supplements
- Antihistamines
- Calcium supplements

Medical Conditions

- Parkinson's disease
- Spinal cord injury
- Hirschsprung's disease
- Diabetes mellitus
- Hypothyroidism
- Stroke
- Colorectal cancer
- Multiple sclerosis
- Bowel obstruction

TABLE 16.1	Definitions and Recommendations for the Treatment of Travelers' Diarrhea	
Type	Definition	Treatment
Mild (acute)	Diarrhea that is tolerable, is not distressing, and does not interfere with planned activities	Antibiotic treatment is not recommended. Loperamide or bismuth subsalicylate may be considered.
Moderate (acute)	Diarrhea that is distressing or interferes with planned activities	Antibiotics may be used, including fluoroquinolones, azithromycin, or rifaximin. Loperamide may be used as adjunctive therapy. Antimotility agents alone are not recommended for patients with bloody diarrhea or those who have diarrhea and fever. Loperamide may be considered for use as monotherapy.
Severe (acute)	Diarrhea that is incapacitating or completely prevents planned activities	Antibiotics should be used. Azithromycin is preferred; however, fluoroquinolones may be used to treat severe, nondysenteric travelers' diarrhea. Rifaximin or rifamycin SV may be used to treat severe, nondysenteric travelers' diarrhea. Single-dose antibiotic regimens.

Adapted from Cooper, B. A. (2019). Travelers' diarrhea. In J. B. Nemhauser & G. W. Brunette (Eds.), *CDC Yellow Book 2020: Health Information for the International Traveler*, Oxford University Press. https://wwwnc.cdc.gov/travel/yellowbook/2020/preparing-international-travelers/travelers-diarrhea.

It can also be associated with functional bowel disorders including irritable bowel syndrome (IBS).

While diarrhea is often mild and may be responsive to common OTC antidiarrheals, it can lead to significant morbidity and mortality secondary to fluid and electrolyte imbalance, dehydration, and malnutrition. Diarrhea can be classified as acute, persistent, or chronic. *Acute diarrhea* is defined as more than three loose stools developing within 24 hours and lasting fewer than 14 days. With *persistent diarrhea*, symptoms last for more than 14 days but fewer than 30 days. *Chronic diarrhea* lasts for more than four weeks.

Diarrhea may be large volume or small volume in nature. *Large-volume diarrhea* results from a large amount of water and/or secretions being absorbed into the intestines, and *small-volume diarrhea* results from excessive motility without a substantial increase in the volume of feces. There are three mechanisms of diarrhea: secretory, osmotic, and motility. *Secretory diarrhea*, a type of large-volume diarrhea, results from increased mucosal secretion of fluid and electrolytes into the lumen of the bowel. It is associated with a variety of causes, including infection, inflammation, malabsorption syndromes, and adverse effects of certain medications. *Osmotic diarrhea*, also considered large-volume diarrhea, is the result of poorly absorbed solutes in the intestine drawing water into the lumen of the intestine leading to increases in stool volume and weight. Examples of causes of osmotic diarrhea include ingestion of magnesium-containing antacids, ingestion of artificial sweeteners such as sorbitol or aspartame, and lactase deficiency. *Motility diarrhea*, a type of small-volume diarrhea, results in rapid transit time through the bowel with decreased opportunity for fluid absorption. Causes include medications such as stimulant laxatives or metoclopramide, as well as a sequela of surgical resections of the small or large bowel.

Travelers' diarrhea is the most common travel-related illness with the greatest incidence. Symptoms range from mild to severe (Table 16.1), and onset of symptoms varies depending on the cause. For example, bacterial and viral cases can cause symptoms lasting from a few hours to three days, while protozoal pathogens may have an incubation period of one to two weeks. Bacterial cases typically last three to seven days without treatment while viral cases may last two to three days (Table 16.2). Infection with protozoal pathogens can persist for weeks or even months if not treated. Rarely, patients may experience persistent GI symptoms without demonstrated infection.

BOOKMARK THIS!

Travelers' Health

The Centers for Disease Control and Prevention (CDC) provides an excellent resource for travelers and providers alike at https://wwwnc.cdc.gov/travel. The site includes specific information regarding destinations from Afghanistan to Zimbabwe. Recommendations are provided regarding current outbreaks, vaccines and medicines recommended, patient counseling, and healthy-travel packing lists. Information about travelers' diarrhea can be found in the *Yellow Book* (2019) at https://wwwnc.cdc.gov/travel/yellowbook/2020/preparing-international-travelers/travelers-diarrhea.

Regardless of the etiology or type of diarrhea, it is essential to evaluate and treat the underlying cause, restore fluid and electrolyte balance, and prevent dehydration. Then it

TABLE 16.2 Antibiotic Recommendations for the Treatment of Acute Diarrhea

Antibiotic[a]	Dose	Duration
Azithromycin[b,c]	1000 mg	Single or divided dose[d]
	500 mg daily	3 days
Levofloxacin	500 mg daily	1–3 days[d]
Ciprofloxacin	750 mg	Single dose[d]
	500 mg twice daily	3 days
Ofloxacin	400 mg twice daily	1–3 days[d]
Rifamycin SV[e]	388 mg twice daily	3 days
Rifaximin[e]	200 mg three times daily	3 days

[a]Antibiotic regimens may be combined with loperamide 4 mg initially followed by 2 mg after each loose stool, not to exceed 16 mg in a 24-hour period.
[b]Use empirically as first-line treatment in Southeast Asia or other areas if fluoroquinolone-resistant bacteria are suspected.
[c]Preferred regimen for dysentery or febrile diarrhea.
[d]If symptoms are not resolved after 24 hours, continue daily dosing for up to 3 days.
[e]Do not use if clinical suspicion for *Campylobacter*, *Salmonella*, *Shigella*, or other causes of invasive diarrhea. Use may be reserved for patients unable to receive fluoroquinolones or azithromycin.
From Cooper, B. A. (2019). Travelers' diarrhea. In J. B. Nemhauser & G. W. Brunette (Eds.), *CDC Yellow Book 2020: Health Information for the International Traveler*, Oxford University Press. https://wwwnc.cdc.gov/travel/yellowbook/2020/preparing-international-travelers/travelers-diarrhea.

• BOX 16.6 Diagnostic Criteria[a] for Irritable Bowel Syndrome

Recurrent abdominal pain, on average, at least 1 day per week in the last 3 months, associated with 2 or more of the following criteria:
- Related to defecation
- Associated with change in frequency of stool
- Associated with change in form (appearance of stool)

[a] Criteria fulfilled for the last 3 months with symptom onset at least 6 months before diagnosis.
From Lacy, B. E., Mearin, F., Chang, L., Chey, W. D., Lembo, A. J., Simren, M., & Spiller, R. (2016). Bowel disorders. *Gastroenterology, 150*(6), 1393–1407.e1395. https://doi.org/10.1053/j.gastro.2016.02.031.

• BOX 16.7 Diagnostic Criteria for Irritable Bowel Syndrome Subtypes

Predominant bowel habits are based on stool form on days with at least one abnormal bowel movement. NOTE: Subtypes can only be established if the patient is not taking any medications that treat bowel habit abnormalities.

- IBS with predominant constipation (IBS-C): more than 25% of bowel movements with BSFS type 1 or 2 and less than 25% of bowel movements with BSFS types 6 or 7
- IBS with predominant diarrhea (IBS-D): more than 25% of bowel movements with BSFS types 6 or 7 and less than 25% of bowel movements with BSFS types 1 or 2
- IBS with mixed bowel habits (IBS-M): more than 25% of bowel movements with BSFS types 1 or 2 and more than 25% of bowel movements with BSFS types 6 or 7
- IBS unclassified (IBS-U): Patients who meet diagnostic criteria for IBS but whose bowel habits cannot be accurately categorized into one of the three groups

BSFS, Bristol Stool Form Scale; *IBS*, irritable bowel syndrome.
Adapted from Lacy, B. E., Mearin, F., Chang, L., Chey, W. D., Lembo, A. J., Simren, M., & Spiller, R. (2016). Bowel disorders. *Gastroenterology, 150*(6), 1393–1407.e1395. https://doi.org/10.1053/j.gastro.2016.02.031.

is important to provide patients with strategies to prevent diarrhea in the future.

Irritable Bowel Syndrome

Irritable bowel syndrome (IBS) is a chronic bowel disorder that is characterized by abdominal pain typically related to defecation in association with changes in frequency or forms of bowel movements (Box 16.6). IBS is divided into four subtypes to better direct therapies: *IBS–predominant diarrhea* (IBS-D); *IBS–predominant constipation* (IBS-C); *IBS–mixed bowel habits* (IBS-M); and *IBS unclassified* (IBS-U). The subtypes are differentiated using the Bristol Stool Form Scale (Fig. 16.2). Each subtype is characterized by the main symptoms the patient experiences (Box 16.7). Of note, diagnosis of the IBS subtype must be determined while the patient is off all medications used to treat the abnormal bowel habits.

Historically, the cause of IBS was attributed primarily to psychological factors with no specific structural or biochemical dysfunction. More recent evidence suggests that a variety of factors contribute to its onset and chronicity. IBS is considered a multisystem disorder that causes a variety of symptoms. The pathophysiology can be conceptualized as a brain–gut disorder as well as a gut–brain disorder (Ford et al., 2017). The brain–gut pathway suggests that environmental

and genetic factors can result in alterations in the central nervous system (CNS) with anxiety, depression, and activation of the stress response. These alterations ultimately result in changes in the gut epithelium and microbiome, with increased intestinal permeability, localized inflammation, and changes in neuromuscular function. These changes lead to symptoms of IBS. The gut–brain pathway suggests that factors such as infection, food antigens, inflammatory processes, and certain medications can trigger the onset of IBS. These can lead to changes in intestinal permeability as well as changes in the gut microbiome with inflammatory response and development of IBS symptoms. Symptoms of IBS, then, can result in the psychological symptoms often associated with IBS.

In addition to the medications discussed in this chapter that can be used to treat IBS, evidence suggests that tricyclic antidepressants may be effective in reducing symptoms. Tricyclic antidepressants are discussed in Chapter 34.

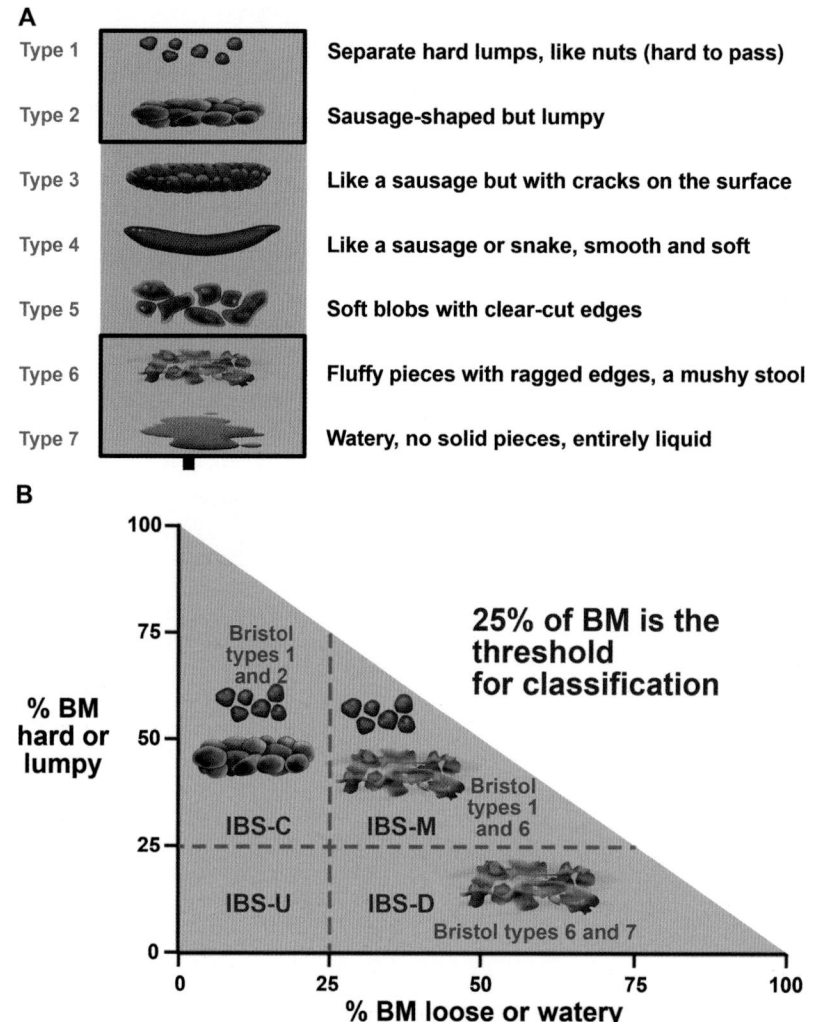

A

Type 1   Separate hard lumps, like nuts (hard to pass)

Type 2   Sausage-shaped but lumpy

Type 3   Like a sausage but with cracks on the surface

Type 4   Like a sausage or snake, smooth and soft

Type 5   Soft blobs with clear-cut edges

Type 6   Fluffy pieces with ragged edges, a mushy stool

Type 7   Watery, no solid pieces, entirely liquid

B

25% of BM is the threshold for classification

% BM hard or lumpy

Bristol types 1 and 2

Bristol types 1 and 6

IBS-C   IBS-M

IBS-U   IBS-D

Bristol types 6 and 7

% BM loose or watery

• **Fig. 16.2** (A) The BSFS is a useful tool to evaluate bowel habit. The BSFS has been shown to be a reliable surrogate marker for colonic transit. (B) IBS subtypes should be established according to stool consistency, using the BSFS. IBS subtyping is more accurate when patients have at least four days of abnormal bowel habits per month. Bowel habit subtypes should be based on BSFS for days with abnormal bowel habits. *BM,* Bowel movement; *BSFS,* Bristol Stool Form Scale; *IBS,* irritable bowel syndrome; *IBS-C,* IBS–predominant constipation; *IBS-D,* IBS–predominant diarrhea; *IBS-M,* IBS–mixed bowel habits; *IBS-U,* IBS unclassified. (From Lacy, B. E., Mearin, F., Chang, L., Chey, W. D., Lembo, A. J., Simren, M., & Spiller, R. [2016]. Bowel disorders. *Gastroenterology, 150*[6], 1393–1407.e1395. https://doi.org/10.1053/j.gastro.2016.02.031.)

Laxative Therapy

Laxatives are used for a variety of purposes, ranging from softening the stool to ease defection to facilitating the rapid evacuation of stool from the bowel. There are four major classes of laxatives: bulk forming, surfactants, stimulants, and osmotics (Table 16.3). In addition, laxatives can be classified by therapeutic response as Group I, Group II, or Group III (Table 16.4). Classes of medications used to treat IBS-C include chloride channel activators, guanylate cyclase-C agonists, and select serotonin receptor agonists.

Bulk-Forming Laxatives

Bulk-forming laxatives are considered safe and effective choices for initial therapy for occasional or idiopathic constipation. They are not absorbed from the GI tract, and they act to increase both the bulk and moisture content of the stool. The increased bulk stimulates peristalsis and the absorbed water softens the stool. Bulk laxatives also may stimulate colonic bacterial growth, which increases the weight of the stool and stretches the intestinal wall, further stimulating peristalsis.

Calcium Polycarbophil

Pharmacokinetics. Polycarbophil is available for oral administration in tablet or chewable tablet form. While polycarbophil is not absorbed from the GI tract and not metabolized, each 625-mg tablet provides about 125 mg of calcium, which can be absorbed systemically. The onset of action is typically between 12 and 72 hours after administration.

Indications. Polycarbophil is used for the prevention and treatment of constipation. It may be used in adults,

TABLE 16.3 Medications for the Treatment of Constipation

Category/Medication	Indication	Dosage	Considerations and Monitoring
Bulk-Forming Agents			
Psyllium	Serves as a dietary fiber supplement and eases occasional constipation	**Granules or powders:** *Adults, children, and adolescents 12–17 yr:* 1 rounded tsp, tbsp, or premeasured packet in 240 mL of fluid orally, one to three times daily. *Children 6–11 yr:* 0.5 rounded tsp, tbsp, or premeasured packet in 240 mL of fluid orally, one to three times daily. **Chewable wafers:** *Adults, children, and adolescents 4–17 yr:* 2 wafers orally one to three times daily with 240 mL of fluid orally. **Oral capsules:** *Adults, children, and adolescents 12–17 yr:* 2-5 capsules orally once daily. May increase to up to four times daily. Administer with 240 mL of water or fluid orally.	Avoid taking other medications within 2 hr before or after bulk-forming laxatives. Take these medications with at least 240 mL (8 ounces) of water with each dose. Granules or powders should be mixed thoroughly with cool liquids for administration.
Calcium polycarbophil	Treatment and prevention of constipation	**Tablets or caplets with 625 mg calcium polycarbophil):** *Adults, children, and adolescents >12 yr:* 2 tablets orally one to four times daily as needed. Maximum dosage: 8 tablets/day. **Chewable tablets with 625 mg calcium polycarbophil:** *Adults, children, and adolescents >12 yr:* 2 tablets orally one to four times daily as needed. Maximum dosage: 8 tablets/day. *Children 6–11 yr:* 1 chewable tablet orally one to four times daily as needed. Maximum dosage: 4 tablets/day. *Children 2–5 yr:* 1 chewable tablet orally once or twice daily as needed. Maximum dosage: 2 tablets/day orally.	Nonchewable tablets usually not recommended for children due to risk of choking. Patients should drink with at least 240 mL of water or other liquid with each dose.

Continued

TABLE 16.3   Medications for the Treatment of Constipation—cont'd

Category/Medication	Indication	Dosage	Considerations and Monitoring
Surfactant Laxatives			
Docusate calcium	Treatment or prevention of constipation	**Oral dosage:** *Adults:* 240 mg/day orally in a single dose. *Children ≥12 yr:* 240 mg/day orally in a single dose.	Should be taken with a full glass of water.
Docusate sodium	Treatment or prevention of constipation	**Oral dosage:** *Adults, adolescents, and children ≥12 yr:* 50–300 mg/day orally in single or divided doses. *Children 2–11 yr:* 50–150 mg/day orally in single or divided doses. **Oral solution containing 10 mg/mL docusate sodium:** *Adults, adolescents, and children ≥12 yr:* 50–200 mg/day orally in single or divided doses. Up to 500 mg/day orally in divided doses recommended for idiopathic childhood constipation. *Children 2–11 yr:* 25–100 mg/day orally in single or divided doses. 12.5–25 mg orally three times daily for patients with idiopathic childhood constipation. **Oral syrup containing 60 mg/15 mL docusate sodium:** *Adults, adolescents, and children ≥12 yr:* 60–360 mg/day (15–90 mL/day) orally in single or divided doses. *Children 2–11 yr:* 60–150 mg/day (15–37.5 mL/day) orally in single or divided doses. **Rectal dosage (283-mg enema):** *Adults, adolescents, and children ≥12 yr:* 1–3 enemas daily as needed. *Children 2–11 yr:* 1 enema (283 mg) daily as needed. **Rectal dosage (100-mg enema):** *Children 2–11 yr:* 1 enema (100 mg) daily as needed. **Oral dosage (50 mg/15 mL docusate sodium):** *Children 2–11 yr:* 50–150 mg/day (15–45 mL/day) orally in single or divided doses.	Multiple formulations/combinations of docusate sodium are available over the counter. Remind patient not to exceed recommended dosage limits for the specific product. Note that OTC products, for example, may specify slightly different recommendations from other products on the product label. Monitor for effectiveness of the medications. Must include adequate nutritional and physical activity counseling to help normalize bowel movements. Tablets or soft-gel capsules should be taken with a full glass of water. Liquid forms should be measured accurately with a calibrated device rather than household measures to ensure adequate dosing. For children and infants, solution should be mixed with 6–8 ounces of milk, fruit juice, or infant formula to mask the bitter taste and prevent throat irritation. Rectal dosage as enema usually produces bowel movement within 2–15 minutes of administration. Do not use enema formulation >1 week.

Medications for the Treatment of Constipation—cont'd

Category/Medication	Indication	Dosage	Considerations and Monitoring
Stimulant Laxatives			
Bisacodyl	Treatment of occasional constipation	**Oral dosage:** *Adults, children, and adolescents 12–17 yr:* 5–15 mg orally once daily or as a single one-time dose. *Children 6–11 yr:* 5 mg orally once daily or as a single one-time dose, no more than three times weekly. **Rectal suppository:** *Adults, children, and adolescents 12–17 yr:* 1 suppository (10 mg) rectally once daily or as a single one-time dose. May be used up to three times weekly. *Children 6–11 yr:* 0.5 suppository (5 mg) rectally once daily or as a one-time single dose no more than three times weekly. **Rectal dosage (enema):** *Adults, children, and adolescents:* 1 retention enema (10 mg/30 mL) rectally once daily or as a single dose.	Oral preparations should be taken the evening before a morning bowel movement is desired. Either a suppository OR oral tablet/capsule(s) may be used up to three times weekly. Taking oral preparations on an empty stomach will produce more rapid results. Swallow enteric-coated preparations whole. Do not crush. Do not take within 1 hr of antacids or milk. Rectal suppositories or enemas may be administered at the time a bowel movement is desired. Instruct patient on proper use of suppository or enema. If suppository is too soft because of storage in a warm place, chill in the refrigerator for 30 minutes or run cold water over it before removing the wrapper. Encourage patient to retain suppository or enema for 15–30 minutes before expelling.
Senna	Treatment of constipation	**Oral dosage (tablets with 8.6 mg sennosides/tablet):** *Adults, children, and adolescents 12–17 yr:* 1–2 tablets orally twice daily. *Children 6–11 yr:* 1 tablet orally at bedtime. *Children 2–5 yr:* 0.5 tablet orally once daily at bedtime. **Oral dosage (soft-gel capsules with 8.6 mg sennosides/capsule):** *Adults, children, and adolescents 12–17 yr:* 2 soft-gel capsules orally at bedtime. *Children 6–11 yr:* 1 soft-gel capsule orally at bedtime. **Oral dosage (solution or syrup containing 8.8 mg sennosides/5 mL):** *Adults, children, and adolescents 12–17 yr:* 10–15 mL orally at bedtime. *Children 6–11 yr:* 5–7.5 mL orally at bedtime. *Children 2–5 yr:* 2.5–3.75 mL orally at bedtime. **Oral dosage (maximum-strength oral solution with 25 mg sennosides/15 mL):** *Adults, children, and adolescents 12–17 yr:* 15–30 mL orally once daily.	Typically recommended to take at bedtime with a full glass of water. The solution or syrup may be given with water or juice to mask the taste.

Continued

TABLE 16.3	Medications for the Treatment of Constipation—cont'd

Category/Medication	Indication	Dosage	Considerations and Monitoring
Osmotic Laxatives			
Polyethylene glycol	Treatment of constipation	**Powder:** *Adults and adolescents ≥17 yr:* 17 Gm of powder mixed in 120–240 mL of fluid given orally once daily. Using for more than 7 days is not recommended.	Powder can be mixed in 4–8 ounces of liquid such as water, juice, soda, coffee, or tea as the patient prefers. Make sure that the powder is fully dissolved before drinking solution. May be taken with food or on an empty stomach. Can be taken at any time of day, but morning is the best time for most people.
Lactulose	Treatment of constipation	**Oral solution or syrup:** *Adults:* Begin with 15–30 mL oral solution or syrup form once daily, increasing to 60 mL once daily if needed. **Powder for oral dilution:** *Adults:* 10–20 Gm daily; may increase up to 40 Gm daily. To administer, dissolve dose (10–20 Gm) in 4 ounces of water.	Response may take 24–48 hr. To improve flavor of oral solution or syrup, mix with a full glass of water, milk, fruit juice, or carbonated citrus beverage. May be administered on an empty stomach for more rapid results. Powder should be dissolved in at least 4 ounces of water.
Magnesium citrate	For intermittent use as a laxative to treat acute constipation	**As an oral solution, 1.745 gm magnesium citrate/30 mL:** *Adults, children, and adolescents 12–17 yr:* 150–300 mL in a single or divided dose. Maximum dosage: 300 mL/24 hr. *Children 6–11 yr:* 90–210 mL in a single or divided dose. Maximum dosage: 210 mL/24 hr. *Children 2–5 yr:* May use 60–90 mL in a single or divided dose. Maximum dosage: 90 mL/24 hr.	Use only intermittent single doses. Routine use is not recommended. 300-mL magnesium citrate solution contains approximately 250 mEq magnesium. Laxative effect typically takes place within 30 minutes to 4 hours. Should not be taken late in the day or at bedtime. Children less than 6 years old should be monitored carefully.

TABLE 16.3 **Medications for the Treatment of Constipation—cont'd**

Category/Medication	Indication	Dosage	Considerations and Monitoring
Magnesium hydroxide	For occasional treatment of constipation	**Oral suspension with magnesium hydroxide 400 mg/5 mL:** *Adults, children, and adolescents 12–17 yr:* 15–60 mL daily as a single dose, preferably at bedtime, or the daily dose may be given in divided doses. *Children 6–11 yr:* 15–30 mL daily as a single dose at bedtime, or the daily dose may be given in divided doses. *Children 2–5 yr:* 5–15 mL daily as a single dose at bedtime, or the daily dose may be given in divided doses. *Children <2 yr:* Available only with prescription 0.5 mL/kg/day as a single dose. **Oral dosage (concentrated suspension with magnesium hydroxide 800 mg/5 mL):** *Adults, children, and adolescents 12–17 yr:* 15–30 mL daily, preferably at bedtime, or the daily dose may be given in divided doses up to four times daily. **Oral dosage (chewable tablets with 400 mg of magnesium hydroxide/tablet):** *Children 6–11 yr:* 3–6 tablets/day in 1 or 2 divided doses. *Children 2–5 yr:* 1–3 tablets/day in 1 or 2 divided doses.	Should not be given concurrently with other oral medications as it may interfere with absorption. Should be taken with full glass of water.
Chloride Channel Activators			
Lubiprostone	Treatment of chronic idiopathic constipation; treatment of IBS-C in females Treatment of opiate agonist-induced constipation in patients with chronic noncancer-related pain, including patients with chronic pain related to prior cancer or its treatment who do not require frequent opioid dose escalation	*For treatment of idiopathic constipation or opioid agonist-induced constipation:* 24 mcg orally twice daily with food and water. *For treatment of IBS-C in females:* 8 mcg orally twice daily with food and water.	Patients should swallow capsules whole. Do not break apart or chew. Administer with food to decrease nausea.

Continued

TABLE 16.3   Medications for the Treatment of Constipation—cont'd

Category/Medication	Indication	Dosage	Considerations and Monitoring
Opioid Antagonist			
Methylnaltrexone	Treatment of OIC in patients with advanced illness or pain caused by active cancer Treatment of OIC in patients taking opioids for chronic noncancer-related pain	**Subcutaneous dosage (weight based):** *Weight >114 kg:* 0.15 mg/kg subcutaneously every other day as needed. *Weight 62–114 kg:* 12 mg subcutaneously every other day as needed. *Weight 38–61 kg:* 8 mg subcutaneously every other day as needed. **Oral dosage:** *Adults:* 450 mg orally once daily in the morning.	Use for >4 months in this population has not been studied. Discontinue all laxative therapy prior to beginning methylnaltrexone. If patient's response is not effective after 3 days, may use laxative(s) as needed. Reassess the continued need for methylnaltrexone if the opioid regimen is changed to decrease the risk of adverse reactions. Oral forms should be taken on an empty stomach at least 30 minutes before the first meal of the day.
Guanylate Cyclase C Agonists			
Linaclotide	Treatment of chronic idiopathic constipation Treatment of IBS-C	**For chronic idiopathic constipation:** *Adults:* 145 mcg orally once daily on an empty stomach, at least 30 minutes before the first meal of the day. If needed, 72 mcg once daily may be used based on patient presentation and tolerability. **For IBS-C:** *Adults:* 290 mcg orally once daily on an empty stomach, at least 30 minutes before the first meal of the day.	Patient should take on an empty stomach, at least 30 minutes prior to the first meal of the day. Do not crush, cut, or chew capsule or capsule contents; swallow whole. For adults with swallowing difficulties, may place 1 tsp of applesauce in a clean container. Open capsule and sprinkle entire contents (beads) over the applesauce. Patient should consume all the beads immediately. DO NOT chew. Do not store the bead-applesauce mixture for later use. **Note:** The drug is coated on the surface of the beads and will dissolve off the beads into the water; the beads will remain intact and not dissolve. Therefore it is not necessary to consume all the beads to deliver the complete dose.
Selective Serotonin (5HT-4) Partial Agonist			
Tegaserod	IBS-C in females <65 yr	*Adult females <65 yr:* 6 mg orally twice daily at least 30 minutes before meals.	Discontinue if the patient has not had adequate relief of symptoms after 4–6 weeks of treatment. Contraindicated in patients with moderate or severe liver impairment. Contraindicated in patients with end stage renal disease or estimated GFR less than 15 mL/min/1.73 m²

GFR, Glomerular filtration rate; *IBS-C,* irritable bowel syndrome with constipation; *OIC,* opioid-induced constipation.

TABLE 16.4	Classification by Therapeutic Response		

Group I: Produce Watery Stool in 2–6 hr	Group II: Produce Semifluid Stool in 6–12 hr	Group III: Produce Soft Stool in 1–3 Days
Osmotic Laxatives (in High Doses)	**Osmotic Laxatives (in Low Doses)**	**Bulk-Forming Laxatives**
Magnesium salts	Magnesium salts	Methylcellulose
Sodium salts	Sodium salts	Psyllium polycarbophil
Polyethylene glycol	Polyethylene glycol	**Surfactant Laxatives**
Others	**Stimulant Laxatives**	Docusate sodium
Castor oil	Bisacodyl, oral[a]	Docusate calcium
Polyethylene glycol-electrolyte solution	Senna	**Others**
		Lubiprostone
		Lactulose

[a]Bisacodyl suppository acts within 15–60 minutes.
From Rosenthal, L. D., & Burchum, J. R. (2018). *Lehne's pharmacotherapeutics for advanced practice providers*. St. Louis: Elsevier.

children, and adolescents. Chewable tablets have been used effectively in children as young as 2 years of age.

Adverse Effects. The most common adverse effects associated with polycarbophil are GI related and include bloating, abdominal cramping, nausea, increased flatulence, and perianal irritation. It should be discontinued if the patient experiences abdominal pain or vomiting. Obstruction of the esophagus is rare and can be avoided if the patient takes adequate amounts of fluid with each dose. Because it contains calcium, hypercalcemia may occur in patients with a risk for hypercalcemia or in patients with renal insufficiency.

Contraindications. Polycarbophil is contraindicated in patients with dysphagia or GI bleeding. It should be used cautiously in patients with a history of hypercalcemia, esophageal stricture, or nephrolithiasis.

Monitoring. The onset of the laxative effect varies from 12 to 72 hours. Patients should take polycarbophil with at least 8 ounces of water to avoid accumulation of the medication in the esophagus, which can lead to obstruction. Laboratory monitoring is typically not indicated for patients taking polycarbophil.

Psyllium

Pharmacokinetics. Psyllium is given orally. It is not absorbed into the general circulation but is distributed locally throughout the intestine. The onset of action varies from 12 hours to 3 days. It is excreted in the feces.

Indications. Psyllium can be used as a dietary fiber supplement and as a laxative for occasional constipation. It may also be used for the treatment of hypercholesterolemia to reduce cholesterol levels when used in doses that provide dietary fiber of approximately 7 Gm daily. Psyllium is considered safe during pregnancy and breastfeeding.

Adverse Effects. The most common adverse effect, occurring in more than 10% of patients, is mild flatulence. Other side effects include bloating, abdominal cramping,

and nausea, although these are relatively rare. Discontinue if the patient experiences abdominal cramps or vomiting. Esophageal obstruction can occur if psyllium is taken with insufficient fluids; therefore, it is important to teach patients to take with psyllium at least 8 ounces of water.

Contraindications. Psyllium is contraindicated in patients with dysphagia. It should not be used in patients with symptoms of acute abdomen, appendicitis, esophageal stricture, or ileus, or any symptoms of GI obstruction. Psyllium products may cause allergic reactions in patients sensitive to inhaled or ingested psyllium. Psyllium should be avoided in infants and children 3 years of age and younger due to a potential choking hazard.

Monitoring. Advise the patient to contact their primary care provider if they experience nausea, vomiting, or rectal bleeding, if they do not produce a bowel movement after 2 to 3 days, or if they experience any increase in symptoms. Monitor the patient to ensure adequate fluid intake.

Surfactant Laxatives

Surfactant laxatives, also known as stool softeners or emollients, typically act by lowering the surface tension at the oil–water interface of the feces. This allows water and lipids to penetrate the stool, resulting in a "softer" stool that is easier for the patient to pass. Surfactants do not typically stimulate defecation, so they are not classic "laxatives"; however, they are often considered within the laxative classification. Onset of action is usually within 1 to 3 days.

Surfactants are usually considered mild acting and are frequently used for long-term treatment and prevention of constipation produced by a delay in rectal emptying. In addition, they can be helpful in reducing straining with bowel movements. They can be beneficial in older patients who are unable to drink adequate fluids for bulk laxatives to be effective, and if their constipation is not opioid or medication induced.

Docusate

Pharmacokinetics. Docusate calcium can be given orally only. Docusate sodium can be administered either orally or rectally. Both forms are minimally absorbed. Onset of action typically begins in 1 to 3 days.

Indications. Docusate is indicated for the prevention and treatment of constipation. It may be given to adults, adolescents, and children. Because docusate is minimally absorbed, it is generally considered safe in those who are pregnant or breastfeeding.

Adverse Effects. In general, adverse effects secondary to stool softeners such as docusate are rare. The patient may experience mild GI cramping. Loose stools or diarrhea may be the result of excessive dosing. Patients using rectal forms of docusate may experience rectal irritation. Discontinue if the patient experiences anal rash from the rectal forms of docusate.

Contraindications. Avoid docusate if the patient has any history of hypersensitivity to docusate salts. Docusate should not be used in patients who are experiencing abdominal pain, nausea, and/or vomiting.

Monitoring. Discontinue docusate if the patient does not experience a bowel movement or has any rectal bleeding. Ensure that patients use proper techniques for rectal administration. Remind patients that results typically take 1 to 3 days.

Stimulant Laxatives

Stimulant laxatives increase the motility of the bowel by directly stimulating peristalsis via irritation of the intestinal mucosa. In addition, stimulant laxatives increase the absorption of water and electrolytes. In general, these laxatives act within 6 to 12 hours and are only recommended for short-term use. Use beyond 4 weeks has not been validated (Hayat et al., 2017).

Bisacodyl

Pharmacokinetics. Oral bisacodyl is minimally absorbed. Any circulating drug undergoes hepatic metabolism and is excreted in the urine. The onset of action is typically 6 to 8 hours. Similarly, the rectal dose is minimally absorbed; however, the onset of action begins approximately 15 to 60 minutes after administration.

Indications. Bisacodyl may be used for occasional constipation. It may also be used as part of a bowel regimen in patients with a spinal cord injury. It may be used during pregnancy when alternatives have not been effective or when absolutely necessary. In addition, it may be used to treat occasional constipation in patients who are breastfeeding.

Adverse Effects. Patients may experience some abdominal cramping, nausea/vomiting, or mild abdominal pain with normal doses. Rectal suppositories may cause mild rectal burning or mild proctitis. If bisacodyl is used on a prolonged/frequent basis, the patient may experience GI irritation, diarrhea, and fluid and electrolyte imbalance.

Prolonged use may result in a physiological dependence, with the cessation of the drug leading to symptoms of constipation.

Contraindications. Bisacodyl is contraindicated in patients with GI bleeding, ileus, or any suspected GI obstruction. It should not be given to patients with an acute abdomen or any condition such as severe ulcerative colitis or diverticulitis. It is not effective for patients with fecal impaction. Older adults may be more susceptible to electrolyte imbalance.

Monitoring. Evaluate patient response to the stimulant laxative. Discourage routine use to manage constipation when other methods such as bulk-forming laxatives may be effective. Remind the patient that rectal suppositories typically act within 15 to 30 minutes. Teach the patient to avoid taking oral forms within 1 hour of any antacids or milk.

Osmotic Laxatives

Osmotic laxatives contain substances that are poorly absorbed from the GI tract and that draw water into the intestine by osmosis. This process softens the stool and helps accelerate intestinal transit. In general, osmotic laxatives work rapidly, so they may serve several purposes. While some may be used for the treatment of constipation, others may be used for rapid bowel evacuation prior to GI procedures such as colonoscopy.

Polyethylene Glycol

Pharmacokinetics. Polyethylene glycol is administered orally and excreted in the feces. Only a very small amount (0.2%) of the dose is absorbed systemically and then excreted in the urine.

Indications. Polyethylene glycol is used for the treatment of constipation. It may be part of bowel prep for patients who require bowel evacuation for colonoscopy. It may be used by pregnant or breastfeeding patients as it is only negligibly absorbed.

Adverse Effects. Diarrhea, flatulence, and nausea are the most common adverse effects, affecting 1% to 10% of patients. These effects are usually temporary and mild (with higher doses more likely to cause diarrhea). Rarely, patients will experience fecal incontinence or allergic reactions.

Contraindications. Polyethylene glycol is contraindicated in patients with GI obstruction. It should be used cautiously in patients with GI bleeding or any symptoms of acute abdomen or ileus. Avoid in patients with dysphagia or impaired cognition.

Monitoring. Instruct the patient on proper measuring or mixing of the prescribed dose. Teach the patient to use the medication exactly as directed and to call if any severe abdominal pain or difficulty in swallowing occurs.

Lactulose

Pharmacokinetics. Lactulose can be administered orally or rectally. It is poorly absorbed and excreted mainly in the feces. At most, only about 3% is absorbed into the blood and is excreted unchanged in the urine within 24 hours.

Indications. Lactulose can be used for the treatment of constipation. Of note, it also may be used in cases of hepatic encephalopathy or barium retention after radiologic procedures.

Adverse Effects. The most common adverse effects are mild abdominal pain, eructation (belching), and flatulence, occurring in approximately 20% of patients. Nausea, vomiting, and diarrhea may occur. A serious fluid, electrolyte, and acid-base imbalance may occur if diarrhea is severe.

Contraindications. Because lactulose contains galactose, a monosaccharide sugar, it is contraindicated in patients who require a galactose-free diet.

Monitoring. While GI adverse reactions are typically mild, dosage reductions may be required in some patients. Acid-base imbalance, hypernatremia, and hypokalemia may occur with severe diarrhea.

Opioid Antagonists

Select opioid antagonists may be used to treat opioid-induced constipation in patients requiring opioids to manage cancer- and noncancer-related chronic pain. They are typically reserved for patients with advanced illness. The opioid antagonists used typically block the peripheral mu-opioid receptors, reducing the effect of opioids on the GI tract.

Methylnaltrexone

Pharmacokinetics. Methylnaltrexone can be administered orally or subcutaneously. Absorption of the oral form is reduced when taken with a meal, so it should be taken at least 30 minutes before the first meal of the day. Methylnaltrexone distributes primarily to the GI tract, binding to peripheral mu receptors. It is metabolized by the liver and excreted in the urine and feces. Half-life is about 45 hours.

Indications. Methylnaltrexone is used for the treatment of opioid-induced constipation. It is typically reserved for patients with advanced cancer- and noncancer-related chronic pain.

Adverse Effects. The most common adverse effects are mild abdominal pain, diarrhea, flatulence, and nausea. Discontinue if severe or persistent abdominal pain or diarrhea occurs. Symptoms of opioid withdrawal have occurred. Dizziness, headache, and vomiting are infrequent.

Contraindications. Methylnaltrexone is contraindicated in patients at risk for GI obstruction. Use cautiously in patients with liver or renal impairment or a history of GI perforation or ulcerative colitis. Data are limited in the use of methylnaltrexone in pregnant and breastfeeding patients.

Monitoring. Dose adjustments are required for patients who have moderate to severe liver or renal impairment and are taking the oral formulation. Dosage adjustments are not required for patients who have mild to moderate liver impairment and are taking the subcutaneous formulation.

Monitor liver function tests (LFTs), blood urea nitrogen (BUN), and creatinine.

Chloride Channel Activators

Chloride channel activators can be used for chronic constipation and IBS-C. These agents increase the secretion of intestinal fluids by activating chloride channels on the apical portion of the GI epithelium. This leads to an increase of chloride and water in the intestinal lumen. The improved intestinal fluid secretion increases motility in the intestine, thereby promoting the passage of stool and alleviating symptoms associated with chronic idiopathic constipation and IBS-C.

Lubiprostone

Pharmacokinetics. Lubiprostone is given orally. It is rapidly metabolized, with the majority excreted in the urine. It has low systemic availability with minimal distribution beyond the GI tract. The dosage should be reduced in patients with severe liver impairment due to the risk of increased incidence and severity of adverse effects. Dosage adjustments are not required in patients with mild liver impairment or renal impairment.

Indications. Lubiprostone is used for the treatment of adults with chronic idiopathic constipation, patients with opiate-agonist–induced constipation resulting from non-cancer-related pain management, and females who have IBS with constipation.

Adverse Effects. The most common adverse effect associated with lubiprostone is nausea, occurring in up to 29% of patients. Headache (2% to 11%) and diarrhea (7% to 12%) may occur but are typically mild. Patients with more severe diarrhea should report to their provider. Fewer than 10% of patients experience abdominal distention, flatulence, mild abdominal pain, dyspepsia, or loose stools.

Contraindications. Lubiprostone is contraindicated in any patient with symptoms of mechanical GI obstruction, such as tumor, inflammatory bowel disease, abdominal adhesions, or fecal impaction. It should not be used in patients with severe diarrhea as it may exacerbate the condition. At this time, there are limited data for recommending lubiprostone to those who are pregnant and no data for recommending it to those who are breastfeeding.

Monitoring. Recommend that the patient take lubiprostone with food or meals to decrease the risk of nausea. In addition, emphasize that the patient should swallow the capsules whole rather than breaking them apart or chewing them. Teach the patient to contact their primary care provider if symptoms do not improve or if they worsen while taking lubiprostone.

Guanylate Cyclase-C Agonists

Guanylate cyclase-C (GC-C) agonists are used for the treatment of chronic idiopathic constipation and IBS-C. Normally, GC-C receptors line the intestines and are involved in a variety of normal physiologic functions, including protection of the mucosal barrier in the intestines, regulation of intestinal pH, and fluid and electrolyte balance. GC-C agonists may have the effect of relieving abdominal pain, decreasing inflammation, and increasing fluid and electrolyte secretion in the intestinal lumen. Additionally, these agents may decrease abdominal bloating and improve stool consistency, leading to an improvement in symptoms.

Linaclotide

Pharmacokinetics. Linaclotide is administered orally on an empty stomach at least 30 minutes before breakfast. It is minimally absorbed with unmeasurable plasma concentrations after the administration of therapeutic doses. Metabolism occurs within the GI tract, with linaclotide and its metabolite degraded within the intestinal lumen. It is excreted in the feces.

Indications. Linaclotide is indicated for the treatment of chronic idiopathic constipation and IBS with constipation.

Adverse Effects. Diarrhea is the most common adverse effect associated with linaclotide, occurring in as many as 22% of patients. Other, less common adverse effects include mild abdominal pain (7%), mild flatulence (6%), and mild headache (4%). Severe diarrhea, rectal bleeding, and fecal incontinence are uncommon.

Contraindications. Linaclotide is contraindicated in infants and children younger than 6 years of age and should be avoided in children 6 to 17 years of age. It is also contraindicated in patients with signs of GI obstruction or who are at risk for GI obstruction, such as patients with inflammatory bowel disease or abdominal adhesions. It should be avoided in those who are pregnant or breastfeeding.

Monitoring. No laboratory monitoring is necessary for patients taking linaclotide. For best results, patients should take the medication on an empty stomach at least 30 minutes before the first meal of the day. Taking linaclotide immediately after a high-fat breakfast resulted in looser stools and a higher stool frequency than when taken as directed.

BLACK BOX WARNING!

Linaclotide

Linaclotide is contraindicated in infants and children up to the age of 6. It should be avoided in children 6 to 17 years of age.

Serotonin Receptor Agonists

Selective serotonin type 4 (5HT-4) agonists stimulate peristalsis in the GI tract. Normally, peristalsis is a result of the release of inhibitory and excitatory neurotransmitters through activation of the intrinsic afferent neurons in the GI mucosa. Tegaserod is the main drug in this category, and it acts as a selective serotonin partial agonist. It has limited approval for use at this time due to previously reported cardiovascular events. Tegaserod is approved only for treatment of females with IBS-C who are younger than 65 years of age.

Tegaserod

Pharmacokinetics. Tegaserod is rapidly absorbed following oral administration, reaching peak plasma levels in about 1 hour. Administration with food decreases bioavailability by 40% to 65%. As a result, the manufacturer recommends that it be given at least 30 minutes before meals. Tegaserod is metabolized by the liver and excreted in the feces and urine.

Indications. Tegaserod is indicated for females younger than 65 years of age who have IBS-C. There is insufficient information to recommend tegaserod for males or for older adults.

Adverse Effects. Diarrhea is the most common adverse effect, typically occurring within the first week and resolving with continued therapy. Fewer than 2% of patients experience adverse effects such as weakness, dizziness, anemia, and increased appetite. Stroke, myocardial infarction, and cardiovascular effects have been reported in patients with cardiovascular risk factors who were taking tegaserod. Suicide, suicidal attempt and ideation, and self-injurious behavior have been reported in fewer than 1% of patients.

Contraindications. Tegaserod is contraindicated in patients with a history of angina, myocardial infarction, transient ischemic attack (TIA), or stroke due to the risk of major cardiovascular events. It should be used cautiously in patients with a risk of cardiovascular disease. Tegaserod should not be used in patients with moderate or severe hepatic or renal impairment. It should also not be used in patients with a history of GI obstruction, symptomatic gallbladder disease, or any form of intestinal ischemia. Avoid using in patients who experience frequent episodes of diarrhea.

Tegaserod should be used cautiously in patients with a history of depression or suicidal ideation, especially during the first few months of treatment. Data are insufficient to recommend its use by those who are pregnant or breastfeeding.

Monitoring. Advise patients and caregivers to monitor changes in mood, particularly worsening of depression or suicidal ideation. If they arise, instruct the patient/caregiver to contact their provider or a crisis line immediately. Laboratory monitoring is not necessary.

Antidiarrheal Therapy

The goal of antidiarrheal therapy is to reduce the symptoms of diarrhea and eliminate the causative agent, particularly if the etiology is infectious. Antibiotics used to treat diarrhea are discussed in Unit 13. The most commonly used types of medication for treating symptoms of diarrhea are opiates, opioid derivatives, and intestinal adsorbents (Table 16.5).

TABLE 16.5 Medications for the Treatment of Diarrhea

Category/Medication	Indication	Dosage	Considerations and Monitoring
Opioid and Opioid Derivatives			
Diphenoxylate with atropine	Adjunct in the treatment of diarrhea in patients with no identifiable infectious agent	**Tablets:** *Adults and adolescents:* Initially, 5 mg (2 tablets) orally four times daily. Do not exceed 20 mg/day orally. **Oral solution:** *Adults and adolescents:* Initially, 5 mg (10 mL) orally four times daily. Do not exceed 20 mg/day orally.	After initial control has been achieved, decrease dose to minimum effective requirements. Acute diarrhea typically resolves within 48 hr. Discontinue as soon as possible with maximum of 10 days if clinical improvement. Not recommended for children 6–12 yr. Do NOT use in children <6 yr. For acute symptoms, if improvement does not occur within 48 hours, it is not likely to be effective. For chronic symptoms, if not improved within 10 days at a maximum daily dose of 20 mg, it is not likely to be effective.
Loperamide	Control of the symptoms of diarrhea, including acute nonspecific diarrhea, travelers' diarrhea, and chronic diarrhea	**For acute and nonspecific or travelers' diarrhea:** *Adults, children, and adolescents ≥12 yr:* If used under prescription, 4 mg orally initially, followed by 2 mg orally after each unformed stool. For self-treatment (OTC use), do not exceed 8 mg/day. *Children 9–11 yr (weight 27.3–43.2 kg):* 2 mg orally after the first unformed stool, followed by 1 mg orally after each subsequent unformed stool. Max: 6 mg/day. *Children 6–8 yr (weight 21.8–26.8 kg):* 2 mg orally after the first unformed stool, followed by 1 mg orally after each subsequent unformed stool. Max: 4 mg/day. *Children 2–5 yr (weight 13–20 kg):* 1 mg orally after the first unformed stool, followed by 0.1 mg/kg orally after each subsequent unformed stool. Max: 3 mg/day. **For chronic diarrhea in adults:** 4 mg orally initially, then 2 mg after each subsequent unformed stool until diarrhea is controlled. Then, reduce total daily dose to meet individual requirements. When the optimal daily dosage is established, may administer as a single dose or in divided doses. Average daily maintenance dosage from clinical trials: 4–8 mg/day.	Instruct patient to seek guidance if fever or mucus in stool or if bloody diarrhea. For patients with chronic diarrhea, if clinical improvement is not observed in 10 days, it is unlikely to be effective and should be discontinued.
Intestinal Adsorbents			
Bismuth subsalicylate	OTC treatment of nonspecific diarrhea	**Oral dosage, tablets or caplets:** *Adults and adolescents:* 524 mg (2 tablets) orally every 30–60 minutes, as needed. Do not exceed 8 doses/day. **Oral dosage, liquids containing 262 mg/15 mL:** *Adults and adolescents:* 524 mg (30 mL) orally/30–60 minutes, as needed. Do not exceed 8 doses/day. **Oral dosage, extra-strength liquids containing 525 mg/15 mL:** *Adults and adolescents:* 1050 mg (30 mL) orally/hr, as needed. Do not exceed 4 doses/day.	Bismuth is not recommended in children due to increased risk of Reye's syndrome after viral illnesses.

Continued

TABLE 16.5	Medications for the Treatment of Diarrhea—cont'd			
Category/ Medication	**Indication**	**Dosage**		**Considerations and Monitoring**
Selective Serotonin 5-HT3 Receptor Antagonists				
Alosetron	Treatment of severe, chronic IBS-D in females for whom conventional therapy has been unsuccessful	*Adult females:* Begin with 0.5 mg orally twice daily for 4 weeks. If tolerated, may increase to 1 mg twice daily for 4 weeks. If does not relieve symptoms after 4 weeks, do not restart. Maximum dosage: 2 mg/day orally.		If constipation develops during the first 4 weeks, stop treatment until constipation resolves, then may restart at 0.5 mg once daily. If constipation continues, discontinue alosetron. Older females, debilitated patients, or patients taking medications that decrease GI motility are more prone to complications. Safety has not been established in males.
Antispasmodic				
Dicyclomine	IBS and other functional disturbances of GI motility	*Adults:* Begin with 20 mg orally four times daily; may increase after 1 week as tolerated to 40 mg four times daily. Maximum oral dosage: 160 mg/day.		Adverse effects are dose related. Discontinue medication if not effective after 2 weeks or if significant adverse effects occur. Older adults are more sensitive to anticholinergic effects.
Opioid Receptor Agonists				
Eluxadoline	Treatment of IBS-D	100 mg orally twice daily with food. For patients unable to tolerate the 100-mg dose or who are taking an OATP1B1 inhibitor, decrease to 75 mg daily.		Discontinue in patients who develop severe constipation.
Other				
Rifaximin	For travelers' diarrhea caused by noninvasive strains of *E. coli*	*Adults, children, and adolescents ≥12 yr:* 200 mg orally three times daily for 3 days. Maximum dosage: 600 mg/day for travelers' diarrhea.		May be taken with or without food.
	For IBS-D	*Adults:* 550 mg orally three times daily for 14 days. May repeat for recurrence up to 2 additional times (maximum 3 treatment cycles). Maximum dosage: 1650 mg/day for IBS-D.		
Rifamycin	For travelers' diarrhea due to noninvasive strains of *E. coli*	*Adults:* 388 mg orally twice daily for 3 days. Maximum dosage: 776 mg/day orally.		Not indicated for patients with diarrhea complicated by fever or bloody stool.

GI, Gastrointestinal; *IBS-D*, irritable bowel syndrome with diarrhea; *OATP*, organic anion transporting polypeptide; *OTC*, over the counter.

PRACTICE PEARLS

Use of *Lactobacillus acidophilus* in Patients With Diarrhea

Probiotics, including *Lactobacillus acidophilus*, can influence the intestinal microbiota and have been recommended to treat pediatric infectious diarrhea, antibiotic-associated diarrhea, and IBS. However, while probiotics have increasing popularity, there is currently insufficient evidence to fully support their use.

Opiate and Opioid Derivatives

Opiate and opioid derivatives act by activating opioid receptors in the GI tract. As a result, these agents decrease GI motility and slow intestinal transit. The slower intestinal transit results in increased time for fluid and electrolytes to be absorbed into the intestine, thus reducing water in the stool. Unlike morphine, these agents do not cause analgesia at the recommended doses. Nevertheless, it is important to determine the effects of higher doses on the patient. For example, higher than recommended doses of diphenoxylate with atropine may cause euphoria and even physical dependence. On the other hand, loperamide does not exhibit opioid-like effects, even at high doses.

Eluxadoline is an opioid agonist/antagonist specifically used for the treatment of IBS-D. It is an agonist of mu and kappa opioid receptors and an antagonist of delta opioid receptors. Eluxadoline decreases secretions from the stomach, pancreas, and biliary tract, leading to delayed digestion and decreases in diarrhea.

Diphenoxylate (With Atropine)

Pharmacokinetics. Diphenoxylate with atropine is administered orally. It is approximately 90% absorbed, with an onset of action typically within 45 minutes to 1 hour and a duration of approximately 3 to 4 hours. Diphenoxylate with atropine is metabolized in the liver and primarily excreted in the feces, with a small amount excreted in the urine. Atropine is not expected to reach therapeutic effects.

Indications. Diphenoxylate with atropine is used as adjunctive therapy in the management of diarrhea with no identifiable infectious agent as the cause. It is available in oral forms combined with low-dose atropine (diphenoxylate HCl 2.5 mg, atropine SO₄ 0.025 mg).

Adverse Effects. Diphenoxylate with atropine may cause mild GI symptoms, including nausea and vomiting (up to 7% of patients) and dry mouth (3%). In addition, patients may experience mild dizziness (5%) or drowsiness (4%).

PRACTICE PEARLS

Life Span Considerations: Diphenoxylate With Atropine

Pediatric patients, especially those with Down syndrome, are at greater risk for atropinism after taking diphenoxylate with atropine, even though the atropine is in subtherapeutic levels. Symptoms of atropinism include dryness of the skin and mucous membranes, tachycardia, urinary retention, and hyperthermia. In addition, pediatric and older adult patients may be at increased risk for respiratory depression caused by diphenoxylate.

Contraindications. Diphenoxylate with atropine is contraindicated in infants and children younger than 6 years of age, patients with jaundice, and patients with pseudomembranous colitis. It has been reported to result in serious GI complications in patients with infectious diarrhea, including sepsis. It should be used cautiously in patients taking any medications with anticholinergic effects. It is not recommended in patients who are pregnant or breastfeeding.

Monitoring. In high doses, diphenoxylate with atropine can cause euphoria and physical dependence, resulting in physical withdrawal symptoms upon discontinuation.

Loperamide

Pharmacokinetics. Loperamide is administered orally, with approximately 40% absorbed from the GI tract.

Approximately 97% is distributed protein bound. Peak plasma concentrations occur 2.5 hours after administration of the oral solution and 5 hours after administration of the capsule form. Loperamide is primarily metabolized by the cytochrome (CYP) 34A and CYP 2C8 isoenzymes. It is also a substrate for P-glycoprotein transport. About 30% of the loperamide dose is eliminated via the feces as an unchanged drug, with less than 2% excreted in the urine.

Indications. Loperamide can be used to treat diarrhea in cases of acute nonspecific diarrhea, travelers' diarrhea, or chronic diarrhea. It may also be used as an adjunct medication for patients with diarrhea-predominant IBS.

Adverse Effects. Loperamide is well tolerated and adverse effects generally are rare. GI effects associated with loperamide include constipation (up to 5.3% of patients), nausea (up to 3.2%), and abdominal effects (up to 3%). Other adverse effects include epigastric or abdominal pain, abdominal distention, flatulence, and xerostomia. High doses may increase the risk for adverse cardiac effects including QT prolongation, torsade de pointes, ventricular dysrhythmias, and cardiac arrest.

PRACTICE PEARLS

Drug Interactions With Loperamide

While loperamide is available over the counter, it is associated with major drug interactions with a variety of commonly prescribed cardiovascular medications, including diltiazem, verapamil, clopidogrel, and amiodarone. Reinforce to patients the importance of checking with their primary care provider or a pharmacist before purchasing any OTC medications.

Contraindications. Loperamide is contraindicated in children younger than 2 years of age. It should be avoided in patients with a history of cardiac dysrhythmias due to the potential for serious cardiac events, particularly with high doses. It is contraindicated in patients with abdominal pain in the absence of diarrhea and in patients with acute ulcerative colitis. Loperamide should not be used in patients with bacterial gastroenteritis or enterocolitis caused by infection with invasive organisms including *Salmonella*, *Shigella*, and *Campylobacter*. It is contraindicated in patients with pseudomembranous colitis. It should be used cautiously in patients with hepatic disease. As there are no adequate studies on the use of loperamide in those who are pregnant, it should only be used if the benefits outweigh the risks. The American Academy of Pediatrics (AAP) has considered loperamide to be safe in breastfeeding for short-term (fewer than 2 days) treatment of acute diarrhea.

BLACK BOX WARNING!

Loperamide

Loperamide is contraindicated for use in infants or children younger than 2 years of age due to an increased risk for respiratory depression and serious cardiac events.

Monitoring. Treatment with loperamide only addresses the symptom of diarrhea, not the cause. If the patient is not responsive within 48 hours, it is important to further investigate the etiology. Moreover, teach the patient to report any rectal bleeding, significant pain, bloating of the abdomen, fever, syncope, or irregular heart rate.

Eluxadoline

Pharmacokinetics. Eluxadoline is given orally and may be administered with food. Following absorption, about 81% is protein bound. Half-life is approximately 4 to 6 hours. Excretion is primarily through the feces.

Indications. Eluxadoline is used for the treatment of IBS-D.

Adverse Effects. The most common adverse effects are GI related. Constipation (7% to 8% of patients) can occur with the use of eluxadoline and may be severe (1%). The majority of these cases occurred within the first 3 months, even as soon as 2 weeks after beginning therapy. In addition, nausea, vomiting, bloating, and flatulence may occur. Rarely, patients experience hypersensitivity reactions to eluxadoline.

Contraindications. Eluxadoline is contraindicated in patients with a risk for pancreatitis, including those with alcoholism or biliary obstruction, patients who have had a cholecystectomy, or those who have a history of pancreatitis. It should not be used in anyone with a history of hypersensitivity reaction to its ingredients. Older adults are more likely to experience adverse effects. Data are limited in the use of eluxadoline by patients who are pregnant or breastfeeding.

Monitoring. Patients taking eluxadoline should be monitored for development of constipation. Discontinue eluxadoline if the constipation is severe. Recommended lab work includes LFTs, BUN/creatinine, and serum lipase.

Intestinal Adsorbents

Intestinal adsorbents act by blocking the effect of toxins produced by enterotoxigenic bacteria. In addition, the absorbents may act by preventing the attachment of microorganisms to the intestinal mucosa. Medications containing salicylates may impact prostaglandin synthesis, ultimately reducing secretions and reducing diarrhea stools.

Bismuth Subsalicylate

Pharmacokinetics. Following oral administration, bismuth subsalicylate is hydrolyzed in the stomach to produce bismuth oxychloride and salicylic acid. Approximately 90% of the salicylic acid is absorbed and distribution is highly protein bound. Absorption of bismuth is negligible, with excretion primarily through the feces. Salicylic acid excretion is primarily renal as free salicylic acid and conjugated metabolites.

Indications. Bismuth subsalicylate may be used for the treatment of nonspecific diarrhea. In addition, it can be used as an OTC treatment for short-term dyspepsia and pyrosis (heartburn).

Adverse Effects. Bismuth subsalicylate is generally well tolerated at recommended doses. A common (harmless) side effect is dark brown or black stools that result from the formation of bismuth sulfide, an insoluble black salt, in the intestine. Bismuth subsalicylate may cause constipation. Excessive doses may cause symptoms associated with salicylate toxicity, including tinnitus, polydipsia, nausea and vomiting, headache, diaphoresis, and hearing loss. The use of bismuth subsalicylate or other salicylate-containing products may lead to Reye's syndrome in children following active varicella infection or other viral illnesses.

Contraindications. Bismuth subsalicylate is contraindicated in patients with hematological diseases, peptic ulcer disease, or GI bleeding due to an increased risk of bleeding. In addition, it is contraindicated in patients with salicylate hypersensitivity or signs of salicylate toxicity including hearing loss and tinnitus. Older adults and patients with renal impairment are at increased risk of salicylate toxicity. Bismuth subsalicylate should be avoided in patients who are pregnant or breastfeeding.

PRACTICE PEARLS

Life Span Considerations: Pediatric Use of Bismuth Subsalicylate

The use of bismuth subsalicylate should be avoided in febrile pediatric patients with varicella, influenza, or other viral infections due to the risk of Reye's syndrome. In addition, it should be avoided for at least 6 weeks after the child receives the varicella vaccine.

Monitoring. Emphasize the importance of using bismuth subsalicylate only at recommended doses. If toxicity is suspected, the patient may require serum salicylate concentrations. Of note, the administration of bismuth subsalicylate within two to four weeks of performing diagnostic tests for the presence of *H. pylori* may result in false-negative results.

Serotonin Receptor Antagonists

Serotonin $5HT_3$ receptors are widely distributed throughout the GI tract as well as other central and peripheral locations. Agents that block these receptors can reduce the hypersensitivity and hyperactivity of the GI tract associated with IBS-D. Alosetron acts as a selective antagonist of $5HT_3$ receptors reducing abdominal pain, bowel urgency, and diarrhea stools.

Alosetron

Pharmacokinetics. Alosetron is rapidly absorbed with oral administration. It is distributed throughout the body approximately 82% bound to plasma proteins. Alosetron is extensively metabolized in the liver and primarily excreted as metabolites in the urine (about 74%) and feces (11%). Plasma concentrations can be elevated up to 40% in older adults, leading to increased risk for adverse effects.

Indications. Alosetron is used for the treatment of severe, chronic IBS-D in females for whom conventional therapy has failed. Safety has not been determined for use in males.

Adverse Effects. The most common adverse effect associated with alosetron is constipation, occurring in nearly 30% of patients. Typically, the constipation is mild or moderate and is self-limited; however, there have been cases of severe constipation requiring hospitalization and surgical intervention. Rarely, patients may experience anxiety, drowsiness, and headache. Elevated LFTs have been reported.

BLACK BOX WARNING!

Alosetron

Serious GI events have occurred in patients taking alosetron, including ischemic colitis and serious complications of constipation. These complications have resulted in hospitalization, surgery, and death. Do not prescribe alosetron to patients with constipation, and advise patients to immediately report symptoms of constipation or ischemic colitis to their provider.

Contraindications. Alosetron should not be used in patients who are constipated or have a history of severe GI disorders including ischemic colitis, inflammatory bowel disease, or GI obstruction or adhesions. It should not be used in patients who have diverticulitis, a history of thrombophlebitis or any hypercoagulable state, or severe liver disease. Use cautiously in patients with mild to moderate liver disease. Avoid in patients with renal impairments. Insufficient data are available to recommend its use in those who are pregnant or breastfeeding.

Monitoring. Advise patients to report constipation or signs of ischemic colitis (e.g., blood in the stool, abdominal pain and cramping, low fever). No specific laboratory monitoring is required. Alosetron may be given with or without food but should be taken with a full glass of water.

Antispasmodic Agents

Dicyclomine

Pharmacokinetics. Dicyclomine can be administered orally or intramuscularly (IM). The oral form is absorbed rapidly from the GI tract and reaches peak plasma concentrations in 1 to 1.5 hours. Half-life is roughly 9 to 10 hours. The oral dose is excreted through the urine (80%) and feces (about 9%). The IM dose is nearly twice as bioavailable as the oral dose.

Indications. Dicyclomine is used in the treatment of IBS-D, predominantly for its antispasmodic effects. While it is an anticholinergic, it typically does not have atropine-like effects on the sweat glands or cardiovascular system.

Adverse Effects. The adverse reactions associated with dicyclomine are generally dose related. The most common adverse effects are dizziness (40% of patients), xerostomia (33%), and blurred vision (27%). Less frequent side effects include nausea, drowsiness, and mild weakness. Dermatologic and allergic responses have also been reported.

Contraindications. Dicyclomine should be used with caution in hot and humid environments due to drug-induced inhibition of sweating (anticholinergic effect). It is contraindicated in patients with esophagitis, ulcerative colitis, myasthenia gravis, GI obstruction, and urinary tract obstruction. It is contraindicated in patients who are breastfeeding, infants, and neonates. It is contraindicated in patients with glaucoma due to the risk of increased intraocular pressure. Use cautiously in patients who may be affected adversely by anticholinergic effects.

Monitoring. Advise patients that dicyclomine may cause drowsiness, so it should not be used while driving or operating heavy machinery until the patient fully evaluates their own response to the medication. If the patient uses contact lenses, they may require lubricating drops to treat dryness of the eyes.

Prescriber Considerations for Laxative and Antidiarrheal Therapy

Clinical Practice Guidelines

Clinical practice guidelines for the treatment of a variety of GI disorders can be found on the American Gastroenterological Association (AGA) website at https://www.gastro.org/guidelines. In addition, the North American Society for Pediatric Gastroenterology, Hepatology & Nutrition (NASPGHAN) provides a series of guidelines for children at https://naspghan.org/professional-resources/clinical-guidelines.

BOOKMARK THIS!

Clinical Practice Guidelines for Constipation

Clinical practice guidelines for infants, children, and adults with functional constipation can be found at https://naspghan.org/professional-resources/clinical-guidelines and https://www.gastro.org/guidelines.

BOOKMARK THIS!

Clinical Practice Guidelines for Irritable Bowel Syndrome

The American College of Gastroenterology (ACG) published its first clinical practice guidelines for the treatment of IBS in 2020 (Lacy et al., 2020). See https://gi.org/guidelines.

Clinical Reasoning for Laxative and Antidiarrheal Therapy

Consider the individual patient's health problem requiring a laxative or antidiarrheal. Carefully evaluate the patient's medication and health history to determine the underlying cause of the change in bowel pattern. Are there medications that could be considered causal? Can medication doses be adjusted, or could the medication be changed to one with a lower side-effect profile? How do the patient's symptoms of constipation or diarrhea compare to the patient's normal bowel habits? Can the onset of symptoms be explained by changes in diet, physical activity, or travel? Does the patient have a history of bowel disorders? Evaluate hydration status in addition to the bowel symptoms. Evaluate the chronicity of the symptoms; are these symptoms evidence of IBS?

Determine the desired therapeutic outcome based on the laxative or antidiarrheal needed for the patient's health problem. The primary goals will be to normalize bowel function and restore hydration or prevent dehydration. The risk of adverse reactions may be reduced by carefully evaluating and educating the patient to prevent overuse of medications. Choose medications that will achieve the best effects based on the onset of action. Patients should be aware of appropriate time frames for use of the medications to prevent further incidences of constipation or diarrhea. Therapeutic outcomes for patients with IBS are typically based on the predominant symptoms.

Assess the laxative or antidiarrheal selected for its appropriateness for an individual patient by considering the medication's side effects and the patient's age, race/ethnicity, comorbidities, and genetic factors. For most patients experiencing acute constipation or diarrhea, the use of nonpharmacologic interventions may be effective in restoring normal bowel function. For older adults with constipation, evaluate swallowing status carefully as bulk-forming laxatives can place the patient at increased risk for obstruction if not taken with adequate amounts of fluid. Stimulant laxatives are the most commonly abused type of laxatives. Patients taking osmotic laxatives should maintain adequate fluid intake to decrease the risk of dehydration. For children with diarrhea, oral rehydration solutions may be necessary to restore normal fluid balance. Do not withhold nutrition from infants or children while treating diarrhea. Certain laxatives such as bulk-forming laxatives and stimulant laxatives may reduce the absorption of medications, so it is important to verify the timing of administration for best effects.

Initiate the treatment plan with the selected medication by first providing adequate patient education to ensure the patient's understanding and promote full participation in the laxative or antidiarrheal therapy. Discuss the patient's normal bowel habits to ensure that the goals for daily bowel movement are realistic for the patient's age and developmental level. Correct any misconceptions that patients and families may have about normal bowel function. Include nonpharmacologic interventions to enhance a return to normal bowel habits.

Ensure complete patient and family understanding about the medication prescribed for laxative or antidiarrheal therapy using a variety of education strategies. Provide patients with information regarding onset of action to reduce any misconceptions about the medication's effectiveness. Discuss lifestyle changes that patients can make to help normalize bowel function. Educate the patient and family regarding signs and symptoms of dehydration. Provide patients with information to prevent infectious diarrhea, particularly travelers' diarrhea.

Conduct follow-up and monitoring of patient responses to the laxative or antidiarrheal therapy. Monitor patients with constipation and/or diarrhea for restoration of normal bowel patterns and for challenges associated with the incorporation of lifestyle changes. Follow up with patients or caregivers to ensure adequate hydration and avoidance of dehydration secondary to diarrhea.

Teaching Points for Laxative and Antidiarrheal Therapy

Health Promotion Strategies

- Ensure that patients fully understand the importance of adequate fluid intake, whether to prevent constipation or to prevent dehydration if experiencing diarrhea.
- Adequate fluids are important for laxatives to be most effective and to prevent constipation, with a 1500-mL daily minimum essential for maintaining normal bowel activity.
- Unless contraindicated, adults should have a daily intake of 20 to 35 Gm of fiber; children should receive 1 Gm per year of age plus 5 Gm per day after 2 years of age. Sources of fiber include fruits, vegetables, and whole grains.
- Encourage regular toileting and avoiding the delay of bowel movements to decrease the risk of constipation.
- Limit foods that are high in fat, low in fiber, or overly processed, which may contribute to constipation.
- Prepare patients for travel by teaching strategies to reduce the incidence of travelers' diarrhea, including choosing foods carefully. Avoid foods that are cooked and served out (buffet style), avoid raw fruits and vegetables unless they have been washed, drink fluids that are in sealed containers, and avoid ice.
- To decrease symptoms of diarrhea, teach patients to avoid foods that are sweetened with high-fructose corn syrup or artificial sweeteners as well as fatty or greasy foods.

Patient Education for Medication Safety

- Contact your primary care provider if you have a fever or increased abdominal pain, blood in your stool, or severe bloating.
- Follow medication directions carefully to ensure best results.
- If using OTC medications for diarrhea, make sure to notify your primary care provider if you experience fever as well as mucus or blood in the stools.
- When traveling, use preventive measures to reduce the risk of travelers' diarrhea, such as avoiding unwashed fruits or vegetables, using bottled drinks, and eating foods that have been cooked thoroughly.
- Drink at least a full glass of water while taking laxatives, particularly bulk-forming medications and stimulants.
- Bismuth subsalicylate should be avoided in children as it may be associated with the occurrence of Reye's syndrome following viral illnesses.

- Do not take loperamide for diarrhea if you have a history of irregular heart rate or another cardiac dysrhythmia.

Application Questions for Discussion

1. A 75-year-old patient is complaining of chronic constipation. How would you approach the patient? What treatment plan would you implement to ensure restoration to normal bowel elimination?
2. You are the nurse practitioner working with a large school system in a region that highly values travel abroad. Trips planned for summer travel experiences include Ireland, Japan, Mexico, Brazil, and Kenya. What measures will you take to ensure the safety of the students and faculty who travel? How will the instructions vary by country? What sources will you use to prepare the students and faculty for travel?
3. You are the primary care provider questioning the patient's symptoms to best differentiate the subtypes of IBS. What strategies will you use to achieve the diagnosis? How will the subtype guide your pharmacologic recommendations? Your nonpharmacologic recommendations?

Selected Bibliography

Andrews, C. N., & Storr, M. (2011). The pathophysiology of chronic constipation. *Canadian Journal of Gastroenterology, 25 Suppl B*, 16b–21b.

Barr, W., & Smith, A. (2014). Acute diarrhea. *American Family Physician, 89*(3), 180–189.

Bharucha, A. E., Wouters, M. M., & Tack, J. (2017). Existing and emerging therapies for managing constipation and diarrhea. *Current Opinion in Pharmacology, 37*, 158–166. http://doi.org/10.1016/j.coph.2017.10.015.

Camilleri, M., & Murray, J. A. (2018). Diarrhea and constipation. In J. L. Jameson, A. S. Fauci, D. L. Kasper, S. L. Hauser, D. L. Longo, & J. Loscalzo (Eds.), *Harrison's principles of internal medicine* (20th ed.). New York: McGraw-Hill Education.

Consumer Healthcare Products Association. (2020). OTC sales by category 2015-2018. Retrieved from https://www.chpa.org/OTCsCategory.aspx.

Cooper, B. A. (2019). Travelers' diarrhea. In J. B. Nemhauser, & G. W. Brunette (Eds.), *CDC yellow book 2020: Health information for the international traveler*: Oxford University Press. https://wwwnc.cdc.gov/travel/yellowbook/2020/preparing-international-travelers/travelers-diarrhea.

Costilla, V. C., & Foxx-Orenstein, A. E. (2014). Constipation: Understanding mechanisms and management. *Clinics in Geriatric Medicine, 30*(1), 107–115. http://doi.org/10.1016/j.cger. 2013.10.001.

Crockett, S. D., Greer, K. B, Heidelbaugh, J. J., Falck-Ytter, Y., Hanson, B. J., Sultan, S (2019). American Gastroenterological Association Institute Guideline on the Medical Management of Opioid-Induced Constipation. *Gastroenterology, 156*(1), 218–226. doi: 10.1053/j.gastro.2018.07.016.

De Giorgio, R., Ruggeri, E., Stanghellini, V., Eusebi, L. H., Bazzoli, F., & Chiarioni, G. (2015). Chronic constipation in the elderly: A primer for the gastroenterologist. *BMC Gastroenterology, 15*, 130. http://doi.org/10.1186/s12876-015-0366-3.

Emmanuel, A., Mattace-Raso, F., Neri, M. C., Petersen, K.-U., Rey, E., & Rogers, J. (2017). Constipation in older people: A consensus statement. *International Journal of Clinical Practice, 71*(1), e12920. http://doi.org/10.1111/ijcp.12920.

Florez, I. D., Niño-Serna, L. F., & Beltrán-Arroyave, C. P. (2020). Acute infectious diarrhea and gastroenteritis in children. *Current Infectious Disease Reports, 22*(2), 4. http://doi.org/10.1007/s11908-020-0713-6.

Ford, A. C., Lacy, B. E., & Talley, N. J. (2017). Irritable bowel syndrome. *The New England Journal of Medicine, 376*(26), 2566–2578.

Hayat, U., Dugum, M., & Garg, S. (2017). Chronic constipation: Update on management. *Cleveland Clinic Journal of Medicine, 84*(5), 397–408. http://doi.org/10.3949/ccjm.84a.15141.

Lacy, B. E., Mearin, F., Chang, L., Chey, W. D., Lembo, A. J., Simren, M., & Spiller, R. (2016). Bowel disorders. *Gastroenterology, 150*(6), 1393–1407. e1395. http://doi.org/10.1053/j.gastro.2016.02.031.

Lacy, B. E., Pimentel, M., Brenner, D. M., Chey, W. D., Keefer, L. A., Long, M. D., & Moshiree, B. (2020). ACG clinical guideline: Management of irritable bowel syndrome. *Official Journal of the American College of Gastroenterology | ACG. Published Ahead of Print.* https://journals.lww.com/ajg/Fulltext/9000/ACG_Clinical_Guideline__Management_of_Irritable.98972.aspx.

Lewis, S. J., & Heaton, K. W. (1997). Stool form scale as a useful guide to intestinal transit time. *Scandinavian Journal of Gastroenterology, 32*, 920–924.

McQuaid, K. R. (2020). Constipation. In M. A. Papadakis, S. J. McPhee, & M. W. Rabow (Eds.), *Current medical diagnosis and treatment 2020*. New York: McGraw-Hill Education.

Mounsey, A., Raleigh, M., & Wilson, A. (2015). Management of constipation in older adults. *American Family Physician, 92*(6), 500–504.

Obokhare, I. (2012). Fecal impaction: a cause for concern? *Clinics in Colon and Rectal Surgery, 25*(1), 53–58. doi:10.1055/s-0032-1301760.

Peery, A. F., Crockett, S. D., Murphy, C. C., Lund, J. L., Dellon, E. S., Williams, J. L., & Sandler, R. S. (2019). Burden and cost of gastrointestinal, liver, and pancreatic diseases in the United States: Update 2018. *Gastroenterology, 156*(1), 254–272. e211. http://doi.org/10.1053/j.gastro.2018.08.063.

Pont, L. G., Fisher, M., & Williams, K. (2019). Appropriate use of laxatives in the older person. *Drugs & Aging, 36*(11), 999–1005. http://doi.org/10.1007/s40266-019-00701-9.

Poulsen, J. L., et al. (2015). Evolving paradigms in the treatment of opioid-induced bowel dysfunction. *Therapeutic Advances in Gastroenterology, 8*(6), 360–372.

Riddle, M. S., Connor, B. A., Beeching, N. J., DuPont, H. L., Hamer, D. H., Kozarsky, P.,. . . & Ericsson, C. D. (2017). Guidelines for the prevention and treatment of travelers' diarrhea: A graded expert panel report. *Journal of Travel Medicine, 24*(suppl_1), S57–S74. http://doi.org/10.1093/jtm/tax026.

Rosenthal, L. D., & Burchum, J. R. (2018). *Lehne's pharmacotherapeutics for advanced practice providers*. St. Louis: Elsevier.

Schippa, S., & Conte, M. P. (2014). Dysbiotic events in gut microbiota: impact on human health. *Nutrients, 6*(12), 5786–5805. doi: 10.3390/nu6125786.

Wald, A. (2015). Constipation: Pathophysiology and management. *Current Opinion in Gastroenterology, 31*(1), 45–49. http://doi.org/10.1097/mog.0000000000000137.

Waldman, S. A., & Camilleri, M. (2018). Guanylate cyclase-C as a therapeutic target in gastrointestinal disorders. *Gut, 67*, 1543–1552.

17

Antiemetic Medications

CHERYL H. ZAMBROSKI

Overview

Nausea and vomiting are common symptoms associated with a wide range of conditions, many of which may bring patients to seek help in primary care. Both are considered defenses of the gastrointestinal (GI) system and can be a sign of other serious conditions. While some symptoms may be transient and respond to nonpharmacologic therapies, persistent and progressive nausea and vomiting require pharmacologic intervention. Left untreated, these symptoms can result in dehydration, electrolyte and acid-base imbalance, and aspiration pneumonia, as well as significant emotional distress.

Common antiemetic classes used in primary care include antihistamine and anticholinergic agents, dopamine antagonists, and serotonin/5-HT$_3$ antagonists. A newer class of substance, P/neurokinin 1 (NK$_1$) antagonists, is used primarily for patients receiving cancer chemotherapy and for postsurgical patients. Other medications include doxylamine/pyridoxine, a combination of an antihistamine and vitamin B$_6$ that is primarily used to treat nausea and vomiting in pregnancy.

Medication therapies directed to the treatment of chemotherapy-induced nausea and vomiting (CINV), postoperative nausea and vomiting (PONV), radiation-induced nausea and vomiting (RINV), and hyperemesis gravidarum (HG) are typically addressed by specialty practices and will be covered here only nominally.

BOOKMARK THIS!

Nausea and Vomiting Related to Cancer Treatment

Primary care providers may work with patients going through cancer treatment within an oncology specialty practice. The National Cancer Institute provides resources for health professionals at https://www.cancer.gov/about-cancer/treatment/side-effects/nausea/nausea-hp-pdq.

Relevant Physiology

Nausea is an unpleasant symptom associated with a variety of causes. Some causes include disorders of the GI tract and central nervous system (CNS), side effects of commonly used medications, and certain metabolic conditions and psychiatric disorders (Box 17.1). Vomiting is described as the forceful emptying of the stomach and intestinal contents through the mouth. This is a complex reflex resulting from activation of the vomiting center in the medulla oblongata. Stimulation of the vomiting center can occur directly or indirectly (Fig. 17.1). Direct stimuli can arise from the cerebral cortex, as in cases of anxiety or fear;

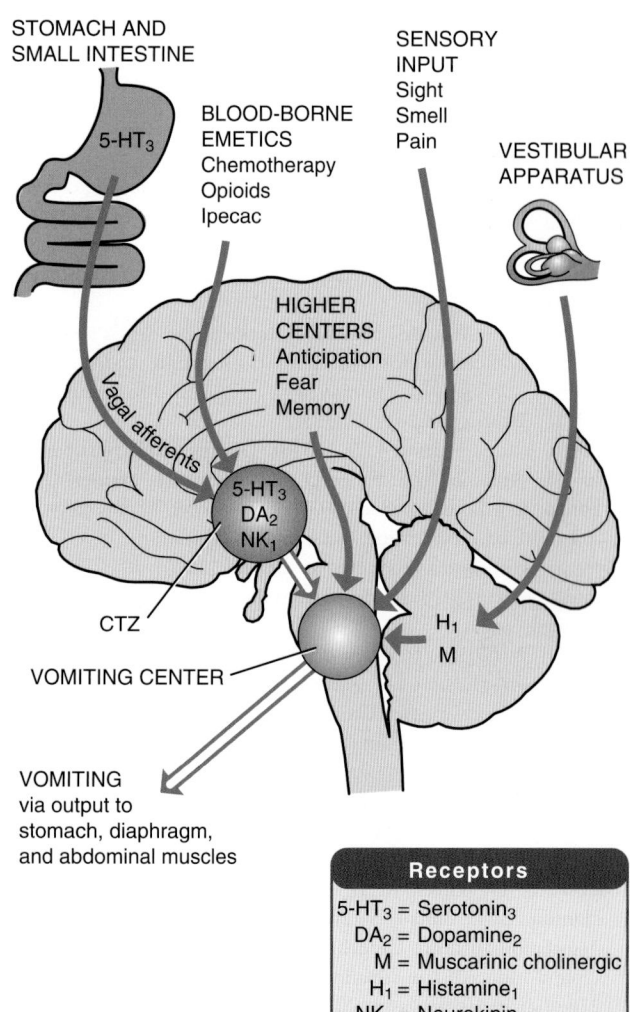

• **Fig. 17.1** The emetic response: stimuli, pathways, and receptors. *CTZ,* Chemoreceptor trigger zone. (From Rosenthal, L. D., & Burchum, J. R. [2018]. *Lehne's pharmacotherapeutics for advanced practice providers.* St. Louis: Elsevier.)

• BOX 17.1   Examples of Etiologies of Nausea and Vomiting

Gastrointestinal

- Acute gastroenteritis
- Irritable bowel syndrome
- Bowel obstruction
- Pancreatitis
- Viral infections
- Bacterial infections
- Biliary colic
- Gastroesophageal reflux

Central Nervous System

- Migraine headache
- Vestibular disorders (e.g., Meniere's disease, motion sickness)
- Pain
- Increased intracranial pressure

Cardiovascular Disorders

- Acute myocardial infarction
- Heart failure

Mental Health Disorders

- Depression
- Anxiety

Medications

- Oral hypoglycemics
- Antibiotics
- Oral contraceptives
- Antidepressants
- Opioids
- Aspirin, NSAIDs
- Cancer chemotherapies
- Radiation therapies
- Anesthesia
- Alcohol overdose

Metabolic

- Pregnancy
- Adrenal disorders
- Uremia
- Thyroid disorders

NSAIDs, Nonsteroidal antiinflammatory drugs.

---

sensory input, such as upsetting sights or odors; and signals from the vestibular apparatus (rich in histamine$_1$ receptors and muscarinic cholinergic receptors) of the inner ear, as in vertigo. Indirect stimuli initially activate the chemoreceptor trigger zone (CTZ), which in turn activates the vomiting center. The CTZ is rich in dopamine$_2$ receptors, serotonin 5-HT$_3$ receptors, and neurokinin$_1$ receptors. It is activated by signals from the stomach and small intestine, and by the direct action of emetogenic agents, such as opioids and cancer chemotherapy agents.

As a result of activation of the vomiting center, signals to the stomach, diaphragm, and abdominal muscles create increased intrathoracic pressure, forcing expulsion of gastric contents. Triggering of the sympathetic nervous system results in associated signs and symptoms including tachycardia, diaphoresis, and tachypnea. Increased parasympathetic stimulation leads to increased salivation, increased gastric motility, and relaxation of the esophageal sphincters.

Pathophysiology

In all cases of nausea and vomiting, the underlying cause should be determined as these are only symptoms of other conditions. As a result, further exploration and workup should be initiated. Most cases are straightforward and have an identifiable cause; however, some are nonspecific in nature and require a thorough history and physical, review of medications, and psychosocial assessment to identify an

underlying cause. For example, nausea and vomiting may arise from excessive stimuli of the senses (e.g., odor or sight), or may be the presenting symptoms of an underlying condition such as a brain tumor, intestinal obstruction, or appendicitis. It is also important to recognize that use of an antiemetic medication may slow the diagnosis. Accurate diagnosis of the cause also determines which class of antiemetic will be most effective in treating symptoms.

Antiemetic Therapy

Most causes of acute nausea and vomiting are self-limiting and require no specific pharmacologic treatment. The general focus of treatment is to treat (or remove) the causative agent and prevent dehydration by replacing fluids and electrolytes. Supportive therapy typically consists of a diet of clear, cool liquids and small quantities of dry/bland foods as tolerated. Complementary or alternative therapies may also be effective and provide some relief (Table 17.1). Nevertheless, if oral intake is disproportionate to fluid loss in addition to signs and symptoms of dehydration, antiemetics should be given.

Antiemetic agents may be given as a comfort measure for patients with severe symptoms without dehydration. In cases of persistent nausea without vomiting, an oral antiemetic should be adequate. Rectal suppositories may be indicated for patients who are unable to tolerate oral medication. These are effective for short-term use of acute nausea

TABLE 17.1   Complementary and Alternative Products Used as Antiemetics

Symptom	Product	Comments
Nausea/ vomiting	Peppermint aromatherapy	There is not enough evidence to recommend peppermint oil for nausea at this time. Peppermint oil applied to skin may cause irritation and skin rash. Peppermint oil should not be applied to the face or chest of infants or young children due to the risk of serious side effects if inhaled.[a]
	Ginger	Ginger may cause mild to moderate interactions with common medications including anticoagulants, aspirin, NSAIDs, platelet inhibitors, beta-adrenergic blockers, and verapamil.
		Use of ginger by patients who use increased alcohol may result in an increased risk for excretion of magnesium.
	Cannabinoids	Cannabinoids such as dronabinol and nabilone may be indicated for patients with chemotherapy-induced nausea and vomiting who are refractory to other conventional antiemetics. Smoking cannabis during pregnancy has been associated with babies with low birth weight.

[a]See National Center for Complementary and Integrative Health "Herbs at a glance" for more information at https://www.nccih.nih.gov/health/herbsataglance.
NSAIDs, Nonsteroidal antiinflammatory drugs.

and vomiting but may cause rectal irritation with regular use. Once nausea and vomiting are resolved, the patient may be switched to oral antiemetics. If symptoms persist, dehydration may occur, leading to hypokalemia and metabolic alkalosis. In these cases, patients should be referred to an urgent care or other acute care setting for appropriate intravenous (IV) fluid resuscitation, electrolyte replacement, and IV antiemetic agents.

As mentioned earlier, major classes of antiemetics include antihistamine and anticholinergic agents, dopamine antagonists, serotonin/5-HT$_3$ antagonists, and P/neurokinin 1 (NK$_1$) antagonists (Table 17.2). Differing classes of antiemetics affect different receptors. For example, dopamine antagonists block dopamine receptors in the CTZ, while antihistamines and anticholinergics block muscarinic cholinergic and histamine receptors in the vestibular medulla. Of note, certain corticosteroids and benzodiazepines may be administered as adjuncts to help manage anticipatory nausea/vomiting associated with cancer chemotherapy. These agents are discussed in Chapter 22 and Chapter 33, respectively.

Anticholinergics and Antihistamines

Anticholinergic antiemetics inhibit the action of acetylcholine at the muscarinic receptors in the neural pathway that connect the inner ear to the vomiting center. Antihistamines primarily block the action at the H$_1$ receptor. These drugs reduce stimulation of the vomiting center from the vestibular system.

TABLE 17.2   Antiemetics

Category/ Medication	Indication	Dosage	Considerations and Monitoring
Serotonin/5-HT$_3$ Antagonists			
Ondansetron	Treatment of nausea/ vomiting associated with acute gastroenteritis in infants, children, and adolescents	*Infants and children ≥6 months and 8–15 kg:* 2 mg orally as a single dose with rehydration. Alternatively, 0.2 mg/kg/dose orally every 8 hr for 3 doses. *Children 15–30 kg:* 4 mg orally as a single dose with rehydration or 0.2 mg/kg/dose every 8 hr for 3 doses. *Children and adolescents >30 kg:* 6–8 mg orally as a single dose with rehydration or 0.2 mg/kg/dose orally every 8 hr for 3 doses.	While routine use of antiemetics is not recommended for acute gastroenteritis in children and infants, guidelines from the AAP and the CDC suggest that single and multiple oral doses are safe and effective for reducing vomiting and increasing ability to tolerate oral rehydration.
	Also used in prophylaxis of CINV and RINV	Dosage varies with emetogenesis of specific therapy.	For patients with chemotherapy or radiotherapy, follow the most recent clinical practice guidelines and recommendations of specialty practitioners.

TABLE 17.2 Antiemetics—cont'd

Category/ Medication	Indication	Dosage	Considerations and Monitoring
Substance P/Neurokinin 1 (NK$_1$) Antagonists			
Aprepitant, fosaprepitant	Prophylaxis of CINV	Dosage varies according to emetogenic properties of chemotherapy agent. *Maximum dosages for children, adolescents, and adults ≥12 yr:* 125 mg/day orally (day 1) and 80 mg/day orally (days 2 and 3).	For patients with chemotherapy or radiotherapy, follow most recent clinical practice guidelines and recommendations of specialty practitioners.
Dopamine Receptor Antagonists			
Promethazine	Prevention of motion sickness	25 mg orally or rectally 30 minutes before departure and every 12 hr as needed. *For children and adolescents ≥2 yr:* 0.25–0.5 mg/kg/dose (maximum: 25 mg/dose) orally given 30–120 minutes prior to travel and every 6–12 hr as needed.	Because of risk of confusion and oversedation, older patients should be started on low doses and slowly increased as tolerated. Not recommended in infants and children <2 yr due to risk of fatal respiratory depression. For patients with motion sickness, recommend reserving for patients with moderate to severe symptoms.
	Treatment of active nausea/vomiting	*Adults:* 12.5–25 mg orally or rectally every 4–6 hr as needed. Maximum dosage: 100 mg/day. *Children and adolescents ≥2 yr:* 0.25–1.1 mg/kg/dose orally or rectally every 4–6 hr as needed. Maximum 25 mg/dose.	
Trimethobenzamide	Control of nausea and vomiting due to gastroenteritis	*Adults:* 300 mg orally three or four times daily as needed.	Rectal suppositories are not effective in adults and children. For older adults, reduce daily dose by increasing dosing interval.
Antihistamine-Anticholinergics			
Meclizine hydrochloride	Treatment and prevention of nausea/vomiting and dizziness due to motion sickness	*Adults, adolescents, and children ≥12 yr:* 25–50 mg orally 1 hr before travel; may repeat every 24 hr as needed.	Start at lowest dose for older adults as they may have more significant anticholinergic effects. For chewable tablets, chew or crush completely before swallowing (do not swallow whole). Oral disintegrating tablets: place tablet on the tongue; once dissolved, swallow the medication.
	Treatment of vertigo associated with vestibular system disease	*Adults:* 25–100 mg orally daily in divided doses.	

Continued

TABLE 17.2 Antiemetics—cont'd

Category/ Medication	Indication	Dosage	Considerations and Monitoring
Dimenhydrinate	Treatment of nausea/ vomiting, nausea/ vomiting prophylaxis, and vertigo associated with motion sickness	*Adults, adolescents, and children ≥12 yr:* 50 mg orally 30–60 minutes before starting the activity (e.g., travel), and then 50–100 mg orally every 4–6 hr as needed. Maximum dosage: 400 mg/day. *Children 6–11 yr:* 25–50 mg orally 30–60 minutes before starting the activity (e.g., travel), and then 25–50 mg every 6–8 hr as needed. Maximum dosage: 150 mg/day. *Children 2–5 yr:* 12.5–25 mg orally 30–60 minutes before starting the activity, and then 12.5–25 mg orally every 6–8 hr as needed. Maximum dosage: 75 mg/day.	May be given in IM form if needed and tolerated. Adult dose: 50 mg every 4 hr as needed. May increase to 100 mg IM every 4 hr (maximum: 400 mg). For children and adolescents ≥2 yr, 1.25 mg/kg/dose or 37.5 mg/m2/dose IM four times daily as needed. Do not exceed 300 mg/day IM.
Scopolamine	Prevention of nausea and vomiting due to motion sickness	Apply 1 patch (delivers approximately 1 mg over 3 days) at least 4 hr before antiemetic effects are needed.	Apply patch to a hairless area of the skin behind the ear. May be left in place for 3 days. If needed for more than 3 days, remove the first patch and apply a new patch to the hairless area behind the opposite ear.
Other			
Doxylamine/ pyridoxine	Treatment of pregnancy-induced nausea/vomiting unresponsive to conservative management	**Delayed-release 10 mg doxylamine/10 mg pyridoxine:** *Adult pregnant females:* 2 tablets orally at bedtime on day 1; if dose controls symptoms the next day, take 2 tablets daily at bedtime. If symptoms persist on the afternoon of day 2, take 2 tablets at bedtime, then 3 tablets starting on day 3 (1 tablet in the morning and 2 tablets at bedtime); if symptoms are controlled, continue regimen. If symptoms persist, on day 4 take 4 tablets (1 tablet in the morning, 1 tablet mid-afternoon, and 2 tablets at bedtime). Do not exceed 4 tablets/day. **Extended-release 12-hour multilayer bi-phasic tablets (doxylamine 20 mg with pyridoxine 20 mg):** *Adult pregnant females:* 1 tablet orally (on an empty stomach) at bedtime on day 1; if dose controls symptoms the next day, continue taking 1 tablet orally daily at bedtime only. If symptoms persist on day 2, increase the daily dose to 1 tablet in the morning and 1 tablet at bedtime, approximately 12 hours apart. Maximum dosage: 2 tablets/day orally.	Medication should be taken on an empty stomach with a full glass of water. Should be taken daily, not on an "as needed" basis. Must reassess need as pregnancy progresses. Safety and efficacy not established in pregnant adolescents. Doxylamine/pyridoxine is considered first-line in the treatment algorithm for nausea and vomiting due to pregnancy by the American College of Obstetricians and Gynecologists.

AAP, American Academy of Pediatrics; *CDC,* Centers for Disease Control and Prevention; *CINV,* chemotherapy-induced nausea and vomiting; *IM,* intramuscular; *RINV,* radiation-induced nausea and vomiting.

Scopolamine

Pharmacokinetics. Scopolamine is well absorbed after oral, subcutaneous, or transdermal administration and is distributed throughout the body. Scopolamine crosses the placenta and the blood–brain barrier. It is metabolized in the liver and excreted by the kidneys. The onset of action after oral and subcutaneous administration is approximately 15 to 30 minutes, and the elimination half-life is approximately 8 hours. The onset of action of the transdermal patch is approximately 4 hours after application, with a duration of 72 hours.

Indications. Scopolamine may be used in patch form to prevent nausea and vomiting in motion sickness. It may also be used in subcutaneous form for nausea and vomiting in adults and children.

Adverse Effects. The most common adverse effect of scopolamine is xerostomia (up to 67% of patients). Other common adverse effects include drowsiness (fewer than 17%), blurred vision, constipation, and xeropthalmia. Confusion or memory impairment occurs infrequently, with the greatest risk in older adults. Patients with preexisting hypertension may experience exaggerated orthostatic hypotension and tachycardia.

Contraindications. Scopolamine is contraindicated in patients with closed-angle glaucoma. It should be used cautiously in any patient who may be more sensitive to anticholinergic effects, such as patients with asthma, chronic obstructive pulmonary disease (COPD), a history of cardiac disease, or open-angle glaucoma. Patients with hyperthyroidism may be at greater risk for tachycardia. Of note, skin burns have been reported in patients wearing the aluminized transdermal system during a magnetic resonance imaging (MRI) scan. Use cautiously in patients with psychiatric disorders as scopolamine has been associated with exacerbation of psychotic symptoms.

Monitoring. No laboratory monitoring is required. Remind patients using the patch to wash their hands carefully with soap and water after application as contact with the eyes can result in temporary pupil dilation and blurred vision. Advise patients upon removing the patch to fold it in half with the sticky side together and then carefully discard it in the trash to prevent accidental contact or ingestion by children or pets.

Meclizine Hydrochloride

Pharmacokinetics. Meclizine is well absorbed after oral administration. It is metabolized by the liver, predominantly by cytochrome (CYP) 2D6. The onset of action is about 1 hour, with effects ranging from 8 to 24 hours. Peak is about 3 hours after dosing, and half-life is 5 to 6 hours. Excretion is via the urine and feces.

Indications. Meclizine can be used for the treatment of nausea and vomiting as well as dizziness with motion sickness. It also can be used to control vertigo in adults with vestibular system diseases.

Adverse Effects. The most common adverse effects are drowsiness (up to 31% of patients) and dry mouth (approximately 16%). Rarely, patients may experience blurred vision. Older adults are more likely to experience anticholinergic effects such as constipation, urinary retention, dry eye, and mydriasis. Patients with glaucoma are at greater risk of experiencing increases in intraocular effects.

Contraindications. Meclizine should be used cautiously in patients who are at risk of anticholinergic effects, such as those with benign prostatic hyperplasia (BPH), asthma, or closed-angle glaucoma. It is important to consider the sedating effect of meclizine and to advise patients to avoid driving or operating heavy machinery.

Monitoring. Laboratory monitoring is not needed for patients taking meclizine. Follow-up is needed, particularly for older adults, to determine the presence of adverse effects.

Dimenhydrinate

Pharmacokinetics. Dimenhydrinate is well absorbed following oral administration, with onset of action within 15 to 30 minutes. Duration of action ranges from 3 to 6 hours.

Indications. Dimenhydrinate is indicated for the prevention and treatment of nausea and vomiting as well as vertigo associated with motion sickness. It can be used in children as young as 2 years of age for motion sickness.

Adverse Effects. The majority of adverse effects are due to the inhibition of muscarinic receptors (i.e., anticholinergic effects) and include blurred vision, dry mouth, dry eyes, confusion, and drowsiness. Children (and occasionally adults) may experience paradoxical stimulation after taking dimenhydrinate.

Contraindications. Dimenhydrinate is contraindicated in neonates and in patients with benzyl alcohol or tartrazine dye hypersensitivity. It should be used cautiously in patients who are taking other anticholinergic medications or are at risk for anticholinergic side effects, such as those with COPD, asthma, urinary retention, or glaucoma. It may be used in pregnant patients to treat nausea and vomiting, and as premedication for travel. Dimenhydrinate should be used cautiously during breastfeeding.

Monitoring. Laboratory monitoring is not necessary in patients using dimenhydrinate. While this medication does cause sedation, tolerance to the CNS depressant effects usually occurs within a few days of treatment.

Dopamine Receptor Antagonists

Dopamine receptor antagonists, also known as antidopaminergic agents, block D2-dopamine receptors in the CTZ as well as other areas of the brain. They also typically have anticholinergic and antihistamine effects. Two subcategories of agents include phenothiazines and benzamides. Phenothiazines have a spectrum of dosing ranges and indications. Discussion in this chapter will be restricted to their use in nausea and vomiting. Use of phenothiazines in psychosis is discussed in Chapter 35.

Promethazine

Pharmacokinetics. Promethazine is widely distributed in body tissues and fluids and is metabolized by the liver and eliminated in the urine and feces. The half-life is 10 to 14 hours, and the onset of action after administration via oral or rectal routes is typically with 15 to 60 minutes. Antihistaminic and sedative effects last for 4 to 6 hours and 2 to 8 hours, respectively.

Indications. Promethazine can be used in the prevention of motion sickness as well as for the treatment of active nausea/vomiting. It may also be used in the prevention and treatment of PONV.

Adverse Effects. Adverse effects are generally dose related, with higher doses and chronic use increasing risk. For use in nausea and vomiting, adverse effects include drowsiness, dry mouth, dizziness, and mydriasis. Higher doses may result in significant neurological, respiratory, and cardiac adverse effects as discussed in Chapter 35.

BLACK BOX WARNING!

Promethazine

Promethazine is contraindicated for use in neonates, infants, and children younger than 2 years of age due to the risk of fatal respiratory depression. In addition, seizures and/or paradoxical CNS stimulation may also occur.

Contraindications. Promethazine is contraindicated in children younger than 2 years of age. It should not be used in patients with asthma or COPD due to associated anticholinergic effects.

Monitoring. Promethazine should be adjusted to the lowest effective dose to minimize risk of adverse effects.

Trimethobenzamide

Pharmacokinetics. Trimethobenzamide is administered orally and excreted in the urine and feces. Onset of action is within 10 to 40 minutes, with a duration of approximately 3 to 4 hours.

Indications. Trimethobenzamide is used for the control of a known etiology. It is not recommended for use in children.

Adverse Effects. Adverse effects are infrequent at usual doses. The most common adverse effect is drowsiness. Other effects included blurred vision, dizziness, headache, and diarrhea. Serious adverse effects such as depressed mood, extrapyramidal symptoms (EPS), and seizures have occurred, but these are very rare. Trimethobenzamide should

be discontinued at the first sign of angioedema, skin rash, or blood dyscrasias as these may be signs of hypersensitivity.

Contraindications. Trimethobenzamide is contraindicated in neonates, infants, and children due to the risk of EPS and other serious CNS effects. It should be used cautiously in patients with bone marrow suppression due to the risk of blood dyscrasias. There are limited data on the use of trimethobenzamide in pregnant and breastfeeding patients. Risks and benefits must be weighed carefully.

Monitoring. No laboratory monitoring is needed. Follow up with patients to determine effectiveness of doses.

Serotonin/5-HT$_3$ Antagonists

Serotonin/5-HT$_3$ receptor antagonists inhibit the 5-HT$_3$ receptors in the small intestine, the vagus nerve, and the CTZ of the brain. By inhibiting these receptors, the drug interrupts the vomiting reflex. Serotonin/5-HT$_3$ antagonists are widely used in the prevention and treatment of CINV, PONV, and RINV. Of note, while not for routine use, serotonin/5-HT$_3$ antagonists have been used off-label for the short-term treatment of nausea and vomiting associated with acute gastroenteritis to enhance patients' ability to tolerate oral rehydration.

Serotonin/5-HT$_3$ antagonists such as granisetron, dolasetron, and palonosetron are used to treat CINV, RINV, and PONV and are not commonly used in primary care, but rather in oncology and surgical settings.

Ondansetron

Pharmacokinetics. Oral ondansetron is well absorbed from the GI tract and undergoes first-pass metabolism. It may be given without regard to food. Absorption is not affected by antacids. Ondansetron is metabolized in the liver by multiple P450 (CYP 450) drug-metabolizing enzymes, including CYP 1A2, CYP 2D6, and CYP 3A4, with CYP 3A4 playing the largest role. While interactions with inhibitors or inducers of these enzymes have not been reported, the potential exists for these interactions to change the clearance and, hence, the half-life of ondansetron. Ondansetron is a substrate of P-glycoprotein. The inactive metabolites are eliminated in the urine.

Indications. Ondansetron is primarily used for CINV prophylaxis and RINV prophylaxis. Off-label uses include HG unresponsive to other antiemetics, and for acute, short-term treatment of nausea and vomiting associated with acute gastroenteritis. Follow current clinical guidelines for details.

Adverse Effects. The most common adverse effects are mild headache, diarrhea, drowsiness, and fatigue. From 6% to 11% of patients experience moderate constipation. Potential cardiovascular effects are infrequent to rare but may include severe bradycardia, angina, syncope, ventricular tachycardia, and other dysrhythmias. Serotonin syndrome has been reported with 5-HT$_3$ receptor antagonists, if used in addition to other medications that may increase CNS or peripheral serotonin levels.

Contraindications. Ondansetron should be used cautiously in patients with hepatic disorders because it is extensively metabolized in the liver. It increases the risk of developing QT prolongation in a dose-dependent manner. As a result, there is increased risk for significant, potentially fatal dysrhythmia. Avoid in patients with congenital long QT syndrome and in patients with increased risk for QT prolongation. Electrocardiogram (ECG) monitoring and cautious use are recommended in patients with hypokalemia, hypomagnesemia, congestive heart failure, and significant bradycardia, and in patients taking other medications known to prolong the QT interval. Data on the use of ondansetron during pregnancy are inconsistent, and it is only recommended in pregnancy in patients who are dehydrated, require IV fluid replacements, and have failed other therapies. It should be used cautiously in breastfeeding patients.

Monitoring. Monitor the patient's ECG, serum electrolytes, and liver function studies. Ensure adequate fluid balance to prevent dehydration.

Substance P/Neurokinin 1 (NK₁) Antagonists

Substance P/neurokinin receptor antagonists can prevent both peripheral and central stimulation of vomiting centers in the brain. They have been shown to cross the blood–brain barrier and are used primarily for nausea and vomiting associated with cancer chemotherapy. They can be effective in both acute and delayed nausea and vomiting.

Aprepitant
Pharmacokinetics. Aprepitant can be administered orally and is highly bound (95%) to plasma proteins. It crosses the blood–brain barrier and is primarily metabolized by CYP 3A4 enzymes, with minor metabolism via CYP 1A2 and CYP 2C19. Aprepitant is a moderate CYP 3A4 inhibitor after multiday dosing and a weak CYP 3A4 inhibitor after a single dose. Aprepitant is eliminated primarily through metabolism and is not renally excreted.

Indications. Aprepitant is used, often in combination with corticosteroids and serotonin/5-HT₃ inhibitors, for CINV prophylaxis. Differing protocols are used according to the emetogenicity of the chemotherapy.

Adverse Effects. The most common reactions to aprepitant are diarrhea (6% to 13% of patients) and fatigue (5% to 15%). Less common reactions include mild headache, weakness, and mild dizziness. GI effects include mild hiccoughs, dyspepsia, dry mouth, and flatulence. Bradycardia and severe dermatologic reactions are rare.

Contraindications. Aprepitant is contraindicated in any patient with known hypersensitivity to aprepitant or fosaprepitant. Use cautiously in patients with severe hepatic disease, as well as in patients taking warfarin for anticoagulation, as it may significantly decrease the international normalized ratio (INR). For females of childbearing age, aprepitant may reduce the efficacy of hormonal contraceptives. While there are insufficient data that show aprepitant is teratogenic, caution should be used in administering to pregnant patients. It should be avoided in those who are breastfeeding, unless the benefit to the mother outweighs the risk to the infant. Use with caution in older adults who may have decreased renal and liver function.

Use of aprepitant is contraindicated in patients using pimozide, as inhibition of CYP 3A4 by aprepitant could result in elevated plasma concentrations of pimozide, potentially causing serious reactions including QT prolongation, an adverse reaction of pimozide.

Monitoring. For maximum effectiveness, follow administration directions of liquid formulations carefully. Specific instructions for administration include that all doses be prepared by the health care provider. For patients on chronic warfarin therapy, monitor the INR following initiation of aprepitant with each antiemetic treatment, particularly at 7 to 10 days or as guided by specialty practitioners.

Remind females of childbearing age that efficacy of hormonal contraceptives may be reduced during administration of aprepitant 28 days after administration of the last dose. Advise females using any hormonal contraceptives to use an effective alternative or backup nonhormonal contraceptive during treatment with aprepitant and for 1 month following the last dose.

Other

Doxylamine/Pyridoxine
Pharmacokinetics. Doxylamine/pyridoxine is given orally. Doxylamine is biotransformed in the liver, and pyridoxine is a prodrug primarily metabolized in the liver. The half-lives of doxylamine and pyridoxine are 12.5 hours and 0.5 hours, respectively. Food delays absorption, so it should be administered on an empty stomach with a full glass of water for best effects.

Indications. Doxylamine is a sedating antihistamine (H₁ receptor antagonist) and pyridoxine is vitamin B₆. This combination drug is used to treat pregnancy-induced nausea/vomiting unresponsive to nonpharmacologic treatment.

Adverse Effects. The most common adverse effects are drowsiness and dry mouth (more than 10% of patients). Other adverse effects include those related to antihistamine and anticholinergic effects such as dry mouth, thickening of bronchial secretions, urinary retention, and constipation. This combination drug has rarely caused anxiety, insomnia, and nightmares.

Contraindications. Doxylamine has not be studied in pregnant patients with HG. It is contraindicated in patients taking monoamine oxidase inhibitors (MAOIs) due to the risk of increased anticholinergic effects. Doxylamine/pyridoxine may cause drowsiness, so it should be used cautiously when driving or operating heavy machinery. Use cautiously in patients with peptic ulcer disease, urinary tract obstruction, or urinary retention, and in patients who are taking any anticholinergic medications. Using alcohol may increase the risk of sedation.

Monitoring. Monitor for effectiveness in reducing nausea and vomiting during pregnancy. Advise patients to avoid over-the-counter (OTC) medications, alcohol, and drugs that increase the risk for anticholinergic or antihistamine effects.

Prescriber Considerations for Antiemetic Therapy

Clinical Practice Guidelines

In 2015, Furyk and colleagues conducted a systematic review of the efficacy and safety of antiemetic medications in the management of nausea and vomiting in adults. They concluded that there was no definitive evidence of the superiority of one antiemetic over another in the treatment of acute nausea. In fact, they suggested that, because even patients who received a placebo had decreased symptoms, the IV fluids may have been the most influential in reducing symptoms. They recommended that treatment be based on etiology, patient preference, adverse-effect profile, and cost of the medication.

Patients with severe or intractable nausea and vomiting resulting in dehydration or other significant complications are typically referred to specialty care. Patients with mild to moderate symptoms or who are using antiemetics for preventive reasons may be carefully assessed and monitored in primary care practices.

BOOKMARK THIS!

National Comprehensive Cancer Network

The National Comprehensive Cancer Network can be accessed to find the most recent clinical practice guidelines in the care of cancer patients. For example, antiemesis guidelines can be accessed at https://www.nccn.org/professionals/physician_gls/default.aspx#supportive.

Clinical Reasoning for Antiemetic Therapy

Consider the individual patient's health problem requiring antiemetic therapy. Accurate assessment of the patient's symptoms and determination of a working diagnosis will help to determine the need for nonpharmacologic vs. pharmacologic treatment. What strategies has the patient tried to manage the nausea and vomiting? What are the factors that contribute to the patient's nausea and vomiting? Which symptom is predominant? For example, if nausea is the predominant symptom, an oral agent may be effective while the underlying condition is being treated.

Determine the desired therapeutic outcome based on the degree of antiemetic effect needed for the patient's health problem. Is the goal prevention or treatment of nausea and vomiting? To prevent nausea associated with motion sickness, the patient may require a transdermal scopolamine patch or antihistamine such as meclizine. If the patient has nausea secondary to the introduction of an antidepressant, pharmacologic intervention may not be needed. Instead, treat the patient with nonpharmacologic interventions as these effects may dissipate after a few doses. For mild to moderate nausea in early pregnancy, doxylamine with pyridoxine may be prescribed, with referral to specialty practice for severe nausea and vomiting associated with HG.

Assess the antiemetic selected for its appropriateness for an individual patient by considering the medication's side effects and the patient's age, race/ethnicity, comorbidities, and genetic factors. Common antihistamines and anticholinergics may be effective in treating nausea and vomiting but are associated with a variety of adverse effects, particularly those related to anticholinergic actions. Older adults may be at greater risk for confusion, sedation, and dizziness, so begin at the lowest dose and monitor for effects. Patients with glaucoma are at greater risk for increased intraocular pressure.

Initiate the treatment plan with the selected medication by first providing adequate patient education to ensure the patient's understanding and promote full participation in the antiemetic therapy. Ensure that the patient has information regarding nonpharmacologic interventions for nausea and vomiting such as clear liquids or a bland diet (depending on the extent of symptoms), proper timing of the medication (e.g., the transdermal scopolamine patch should be placed 4 hours before the antiemetic effect is needed), and understanding of the potential adverse effects.

Ensure complete patient and family understanding about the medication prescribed for antiemetic therapy using a variety of education strategies. Carefully review the patient's use of herbal and OTC medications as well as the prescribed medications to determine the potential for adverse effects. These medications can only resolve the symptoms and are not curative for the underlying conditions. It is imperative to thoroughly educate the patient and family to improve adherence and prevent complications.

Conduct follow-up and monitoring of patient responses to antiemetic therapy. Instruct the patient to report any adverse effects associated with the medication, and provide an expected time frame for the nausea to be resolved. If the treatment is not effective or if symptoms exacerbate, determine the need for alternative actions at the level of primary care or referral to specialty care.

Teaching Points for Antiemetic Therapy

Health Promotion Strategies

- Instruct the patient to use good oral hygiene practices as well as good handwashing while experiencing nausea and vomiting.
- Remind patients that many of the antiemetics cause drowsiness as an adverse effect. Advise patients to avoid

driving, operating heavy or dangerous machinery, and making difficult decisions while taking these medications.

- Provide patients with information regarding bland diets and the importance of avoiding dehydration.
- Teach patients to avoid solid food until vomiting episodes pass, and to maintain intake of clear to bland liquids and oral rehydration solutions.
- Carefully review the patient's medication list to determine whether any medications can be discontinued temporarily.
- Dopamine antagonists may exacerbate preexisting mental illnesses.

Patient Education for Medication Safety

- Use oral rehydration solutions as instructed by your provider to decrease the risk of dehydration. These are typically available in grocery stores and pharmacies.
- Drink clear fluids, such as water, ice chips, low-calorie sports drinks, and diluted fruit juices, slowly and in small amounts.
- Avoid sugary drinks, such as fruit juices with added sugar, soda, and sports drinks.
- Avoid drinks with caffeine, such as coffee, teas, and energy drinks, as much as possible.
- Eat bland, easy-to-digest foods in small amounts. Examples of bland foods include low-fat or fat-free dairy, potatoes, refined hot cereals, eggs, lean tender meats, creamy peanut butter, refined white flour crackers, and bread.
- Avoid spicy or fatty foods.
- Contact your primary care provider if you experience increased vomiting, fever, light-headedness or dizziness, or muscle cramps.
- Do not delay accessing care if you have any severe symptoms such as headache, extreme pain or dizziness, chest pain, confusion, or trouble breathing.

Application Questions for Discussion

1. Differentiate between the major categories of antiemetics for use in the treatment of nausea and vomiting. How does the primary care provider determine the need for pharmacologic in addition to nonpharmacologic treatments?
2. A 28-year-old female presents with mild nausea and vomiting. She asks about using ginger instead of a prescription medication such as doxylamine/pyridoxine. You know that ginger is only recommended for off-label use in treating pregnancy-induced nausea and vomiting during the first trimester, and that while no evidence suggests that ginger causes harm to the mother or fetus, data are insufficient to recommend long-term use. How will you proceed? What resources will you use to proceed?

Selected Bibliography

Berger, M. J., Ettinger, D. S., Aston, J., Barbour, S., Bergsbaken, J., Bierman, P. J., ... Hughes, M. (2017). NCCN guidelines insights: Antiemesis, version 2.2017. *Journal of the National Comprehensive Cancer Network, 15*(7), 883–893. http://doi.org/10.6004/jnccn.2017.0117.

Flake, Z. A., Linn, B. S., & Hornecker, J. R. (2015). Practical selection of antiemetics in the ambulatory setting. *American Family Physician, 91*(5), 293–296.

Furyk, J. S., Meek, R. A., & Egerton-Warburton, D. (2015). Drugs for the treatment of nausea and vomiting in adults in the emergency department setting. *The Cochrane Database of Systematic Reviews, 2015*(9), Cd010106. http://doi.org/10.1002/14651858.CD010106.pub2.

Furyk, J. S., Meek, R., & McKenzie, S. (2014). Drug treatment of adults with nausea and vomiting in primary care. *BMJ, 349*, g4714. http://doi.org/10.1136/bmj.g4714.

Gravatt, L. A. H., Donohoe, K. L., & Gatesman, M. L. (2020). Nausea and vomiting. In J. T. DiPiro, G. C. Yee, L. M. Posey, S. T. Haines, T. D. Nolin, & V. Ellingrod (Eds.), *Pharmacotherapy: A Pathophysiologic Approach* (11e). New York: McGraw-Hill Education.

Greenlee, H., DuPont-Reyes, M. J., Balneaves, L. G., Carlson, L. E., Cohen, M. R., Deng, G., & Tripathy, D. (2017). Clinical practice guidelines on the evidence-based use of integrative therapies during and after breast cancer treatment. *CA: A Cancer Journal for Clinics, 67*(3), 194–232. http://doi.org/10.3322/caac.21397.

Ibrahim, M. A., & Preuss, C. V. (2020). Antiemetic neurokinin-1 receptor blockers. [Updated 2020 Apr 20]. In: StatPearls [Internet]. Treasure Island (FL): StatPearls Publishing. Jan-Available from. https://www.ncbi.nlm.nih.gov/books/NBK470394/.

McCance, K. L., & Huether, S. E. (2019). *Pathophysiology: The Biologic Basis for Disease in Adults and Children* (8th ed.). St. Louis: Elsevier.

McQuaid, K. R. (2017). Drugs used in the treatment of gastrointestinal diseases. In B. G. Katzung (Ed.), *Basic & Clinical Pharmacology* (14e). New York: McGraw-Hill Education.

Rosenthal, L. D., & Burchum, J. R. (2018). *Lehne's Pharmacotherapeutics for Advanced Practice Providers*. St. Louis: Elsevier.

Singh, P., Yoon, S. S., & Kuo, B. (2016). Nausea: A review of pathophysiology and therapeutics. *Therapeutic Advances in Gastroenterology, 9*(1), 98–112. http://doi.org/10.1177/1756283X15618131.

18

Male Genitourinary Medications

JUAN MANUEL GONZALEZ AND CONSTANCE G. VISOVSKY

Benign Prostatic Hypertrophy

Overview

Benign prostatic hypertrophy (BPH) is a benign neoplasm of the prostate gland that, if large enough, causes voiding dysfunction. BPH is extremely common in the aging male and occurs in fewer than 10% of males 31 to 40 years of age. However, by age 60 nearly half of males will develop BPH, and by age 85 more than 80% will have it. Prostatism has three components: histologic prostatic hyperplasia, an increase in outflow resistance, and response of the bladder (detrusor) muscle to obstruction.

Relevant Physiology

In an adult male, the prostate gland is a walnut-sized organ that surrounds the uppermost portion of the urethra starting at the bladder neck, and has ductal connections to the urethra. Its elliptical shape makes it slightly wider (4 cm) than its anteroposterior diameter (3 cm), and it normally weighs between 20 and 25 Gm. The location of the prostate deep within the pelvic cavity and close to the rectal wall allows relatively easy digital palpation for size and texture. The prostate is composed of fibrous, muscular, and glandular epithelial tissues loosely bound together and surrounded by a capsule-like layer of connective tissue. The gland is innervated and contains a network of blood vessels and capillaries.

Quiescent until puberty, the immature prostate, under the influence of the gonadotrophins and testosterone, enlarges to adult size and the epithelial tissues begin to secrete acid phosphatase, prostate-specific antigen, seminoprotein, and a variety of other substances as a thin, milky fluid. The epithelial tissues in fold-forming structures are surrounded by smooth and skeletal muscle bands. The function of the prostate is to provide fluid that contributes to the volume and composition of seminal fluid ejected during sexual climax. When stimulated during the sex act, the muscular bands contract and propel about 3 mL of prostatic fluid into the urethra, along with semen and fluids from the seminal vesicles and vas deferens.

Pathophysiology

The two major pathologic problems within the prostate are BPH and the development of prostate cancer. After about age 50, the prostate gland slowly begins to normally involute, causing epithelial cells to diminish in size and undergo *apoptosis* (programmed cell death). However, as the testes produce less testosterone, the epithelial cells increase their numbers of androgen receptors. The increased numbers of androgen receptors make the epithelial cells very sensitive to the presence of testosterone and any other androgens. Existing testosterone binds to these receptors, interferes with involution and apoptosis, and sends signals to cellular nuclei to increase the production of growth factors. In addition, nonepithelial support cells (*stromal cells*) hypertrophy. Both of these events result in the formation of widespread large nodules that can increase prostate weight to 100 Gm or more. As this tissue enlarges and tightens, the urethral structures are compressed, restricting outflow from the bladder and causing the associated symptoms of hesitancy, increased bladder fullness, reduced volume of the urine stream, and nocturia, among others.

Although the presence of testosterone and other androgens increases the size of the cells and the proliferation of certain cell types within the prostate, research does not demonstrate a clear *causative* role of the hormones with the development of prostatic cancer. Rather, these hormones appear to be important in the continuing growth and proliferation of prostate cells once they have become malignant. Thus, the actual cause(s) of prostate cancer is unknown, but it appears to be a complex mixture of genetic, environmental, and personal factors including age, race, and family history. Whatever the cause of malignant transformation into cancer cells, prostatic cancer growth is enhanced by the presence of androgens. The vast majority of prostate cancers are adenocarcinomas and are relatively slow growing.

Benign Prostatic Hypertrophy Therapy

Pharmacologic management of BPH includes alpha-1 adrenergic antagonists, 5-alpha-reductase inhibitors, anticholinergics, and phosphodiesterase inhibitors. The alpha-1 adrenergic receptor blockers, such as doxazosin and terazosin, are also indicated for hypertension. Tamsulosin (Flomax) is an alpha-adrenergic receptor blocker specific to the prostate and is indicated only for the treatment of symptoms of BPH. With finasteride, an androgen hormone inhibitor, months of therapy are required to achieve maximum benefit. Androgen hormone inhibitors such as alpha-reductase inhibitors not only improve the symptoms of BPH but also physically reduce the size of the prostate. While alpha-1 adrenergic receptor blockers result in immediate relief,

alpha-reductase inhibitors can support long-term management. Anticholinergics have a limited role in the management of lower urinary tract symptoms (LUTS) of patients with BPH, as they are reserved for patients who do not have elevated postvoid residual volumes. Phosphodiesterase inhibitors are medications traditionally used for pulmonary hypertension and erectile dysfunction (ED) but have received approval for management of BPH with a concomitant diagnosis of ED. It would be appropriate for the clinician to consider this medication for management of mild to moderate symptoms of BPH. Table 18.1 provides a summary of the pharmacologic treatment of BPH.

Classification of Adrenergic Antagonists

The nonspecific alpha-1 adrenergic antagonists (terazosin, doxazosin, and prazosin) reduce sympathetic tone and relax the urethral stricture that causes BPH symptoms. They block the dynamic component of bladder outlet obstruction

TABLE 18.1 Pharmacologic Treatment of BPH and ED

Category	Medication	Indication	Dosage	Considerations and Monitoring
Alpha-1 adrenergic Antagonist	Tamsulosin	BPH	0.4 mg orally daily	If no response after 2–4 weeks of therapy, dose can be increased to 0.8 mg orally, once daily.
5-Alpha-Reductase Inhibitor	Finasteride	BPH	5 mg orally once daily	Monitor PSA; monitor for urinary retention.
Phosphodiesterase Type 5 Enzyme Inhibitors	Tadalafil	ED	*For use as needed:* starting dose is 10 mg orally *For daily use:* 2.5 mg orally daily at same time each day	Dose may be increased to 20 mg or decreased to 5 mg based on individual efficacy and tolerability; maximum recommended dosing frequency is once daily in most patients. Monitor blood pressure for hypotension.
		Concurrent BPH and ED treatment	5 mg orally daily at same time each day	
	Sildenafil	ED	50 mg orally approximately 1 hr before sexual activity, up to once daily. *Older adults:* 25 mg orally once daily is recommended	Dose may be taken 0.5–4 hr before sexual activity. Increase up to 100 mg or decrease to 25 mg based on clinical response. Monitor blood pressure for hypotension.
Prostaglandin E1	Alprostadil	Intracavernous injection for ED	2.5 mcg initially, injected into corpus cavernosa; adjust dosage by 2.5-mcg increments, to 5 mcg, then by 5-mcg increments according to patient response. Maximum dose: 60 mcg/dose. Do not administer more than 3 times/week, with a minimum of 24 hr between doses.	Monitor for prolonged erection, signs of penile infection, pain, or penile fibrosis. Heart rate and blood pressure should be monitored as some patients may develop hypotension and increased heart rate.

BPH, Benign prostatic hypertrophy; *PSA*, prostate-specific antigen; *ED*, erectile dysfunction.

through the relaxation of smooth muscle in the neck of the bladder. Prazosin has a shorter duration of action than the other medications in this category and generally is not used as first-line therapy. These drugs also lower blood pressure by blocking alpha-1 adrenergic receptors on arterioles, causing vasodilation. Newer selective agents such as tamsulosin and alfuzosin are specific for the alpha-1A adrenergic in the prostate and have less effect on blood pressure. About 75% of alpha-1 adrenergic receptors in the prostate gland are of the alpha-1A adrenoreceptor subtype.

Tamsulosin

Pharmacokinetics. Tamsulosin is absorbed well at 90% bioavailability. It has a protein binding of 94% to 99%, mainly to the alpha-1 acid glycoprotein. This medication is metabolized by the liver extensively via the cytochrome (CYP) 450 isoenzymes 3A4 and 2D6. If taken on an empty stomach or while fasting, the bioavailability of the drug increases by 30%. The half-life of the medication is 9 to 13 hours and the recommended dosing is daily. The onset of action is 4 to 8 hours. This medication peaks in the blood in 4 to 5 hours when fasting or 6 to 7 hours if taken with food. It may take 2 to 4 weeks to see peak effect related to BPH. Excretion happens primarily in the urine (76%), with the remainder excreted in the stool (21%) or unchanged (less than 10%).

PHARMACOGENETICS

Tamsulosin Therapy

- CYP 2D6 is a highly polymorphic enzyme that accounts for fewer than 2% of all hepatic isoenzymes, but it metabolizes more than 25% of drugs used in clinical practice.
- CYP 2D6 genotype variant alleles increase the plasma concentration of tamsulosin in Asians. A lower dose is required for these individuals. Starting at 0.2 mg orally daily is common practice in Asia.

Indications. This medication is indicated for the management of signs and symptoms of BPH.

Adverse Effects. The main adverse reaction associated with tamsulosin is hypotension, especially during the first dose (6% to 19% of patients), which tends to decrease with chronic use of the medication (fewer than 1%). Headache, dizziness, ejaculation failure, and rhinitis or nasal congestion may occur. Other side effects are drowsiness, decreased libido, diarrhea, weakness, back pain, and blurred vision. There are also some postmarketing surveillance reports of intraoperative floppy iris syndrome during cataract surgery.

Contraindications. This medication is contraindicated if the patient is hypersensitive or allergic to any of the components in tamsulosin. Clinicians should avoid prescribing other medications that are inhibitors of CYP 450 3A4, such as ketoconazole. Interaction with phosphodiesterase inhibitors may lead to prolonged hypotension when the two medications are given together, so close monitoring is required. This synergistic hypotension is seen more often with medications such as terazosin and doxazosin, and is less likely seen with tamsulosin. Other medications or chemicals associated with hypotension are alcohol, alpha-adrenergic blockers, and cimetidine.

Monitoring. While taking this medication, patients should have their blood pressure monitored regularly. Do not open tamsulosin capsule; doing so can lead to a rapid drop in blood pressure. Additionally, the clinician must reevaluate the patient for improvement or worsening of the urinary symptoms, paying close attention to complications such as urinary obstruction. Using either the American Urological Association Symptom Score (AUASS) or the International Prostate Symptom Score (I-PSS) is beneficial to assess the effectiveness of the medication therapy and quality of life of a patient diagnosed with BPH. Patients should be asked about any adverse effects while taking the medication, and education should be provided. Monitor for side effects related to sexual activity.

PRACTICE PEARLS

Alpha-1 Adrenergic Blocking Therapy

- The medication should be taken 30 minutes after the same meal each day.
- The initial dose is 0.4 mg orally daily, and if needed, dosage may increase to 0.8 mg in 2 to 4 weeks.
- At the beginning of therapy, consider giving at night to decrease orthostasis.
- No dose adjustment is needed for renal impairment if creatinine clearance (CrCl) is equal to or greater than 10 mL/minute.
- No dose adjustment is needed for mild to moderate hepatic impairment.
- Sound-alike drugs may be confused with tamsulosin (Flomax), such as Flonase, Flovent, and Fosamax.
- Tamsulosin is pregnancy category B, according to the U.S. Food and Drug Administration (FDA), but there are currently no human data related to pregnancy category or lactation with this medication.

BLACK BOX WARNING!

Tamsulosin Therapy

- This medication should be discontinued if the patient develops angina or worsens from baseline.
- Development of floppy iris syndrome, an intraoperative complication involving a combination of flaccid iris, miosis, and potential prolapse of the iris, may occur.
- This medication can lead to significant orthostatic hypotension, especially during the first 4 to 8 hours of use. This is known as the *first use phenomenon*. Hypotension may worsen when combined with drugs that lower blood pressure, such as vasodilators or a phosphodiesterase type 5 (PDE 5) inhibitor.
- Patients should be warned about performing hazardous activities such as driving or operating heavy machinery when beginning therapy or after adjusting the dose.
- Patients should be educated about possible priapism and told to seek care if they have an erection that lasts more than 4 hours.
- This drug should be avoided in patients with a medical history of severe sulfonamide allergy.
- Patients with BPH and prostate cancer can have the same symptoms.

Other Drugs in Class

Drugs that are from the same category or subcategory are similar to the key drug except in the following ways:

- *Alfuzosin (Uroxatral) contraindications:* Moderate to severe hepatic impairment, concomitant use with potent 3A4 inhibitors (e.g., itraconazole, ketoconazole, ritonavir) or ED drugs.
- *Drug interactions:* Inhibitors of CYP 3A4; can increase serum levels; inducers of CYP 3A4 (e.g., carbamazepine, phenobarbital, phenytoin, rifamycin); can decrease serum levels and efficacy of alfuzosin.
- *Prazosin:* Because of first-dose syncope, high incidence of hypotension, and shorter duration of action, it is seldom used for BPH.
- *Doxazosin:* Use with caution in severe gastrointestinal (GI) narrowing, mild to moderate hepatic impairment (not recommended in severe hepatic impairment), congestive heart failure (CHF), and coronary artery disease (CAD); use with PDE 5 inhibitors (e.g., sildenafil).

5-Alpha-Reductase Inhibitors

The 5-alpha-reductase inhibitors are used alone or in combination with alpha-1 adrenergic blocking agents in the management of BPH. There are currently two medications in this class that have been approved in the United States and the United Kingdom: finasteride and dutasteride. Both medications have been shown to improve the symptoms of BPH and reduce the size of the prostate gland, but 6 to 12 months may be required for full effect. Finasteride, a synthetic 4-azasteroid, is a type II 5-alpha-reductase enzyme inhibitor that works by blocking the conversion of testosterone to dihydrotestosterone, the potent androgen upon which the development of the prostate gland is dependent. Dutasteride is a second-generation 5-alpha reductase inhibitor that inhibits both types I and II 5-alpha reductase.

Finasteride

Pharmacokinetics. Finasteride is 90% protein bound and is heavily metabolized by the liver through CYP 450 isoenzymes 3A4. The bioavailability of this medication is about 65% and it is not affected by the ingestion of food. The medication peaks in 1 to 2 hours in the serum with a half-life of 5 to 6 hours, although in patients 70 years of age and older, it may take about 8 hours. More than half of this drug (57%) is excreted in the stool and about 39% is excreted in the urine as metabolites. It may take 6 to 12 months to see peak efficacy of this drug with symptoms of BPH.

PHARMACOGENETICS

Finasteride Therapy

- Testosterone conversion is mediated by the androgen metabolizing enzymes steroid 5 (alpha) reductase types 1 and II in the tissue located in the prostate (encoded SRD5A1 and SRD5A2).
- Genetic mutations seen in the target enzyme SRD52 can affect how patients respond to this medication and their chances of developing complications such as prostate cancer.
- Mutations can happen as a single-point variant, compound heterozygotes, and haplotypes, also known as double mutants.
- Some of the genetic mutations seen in the target enzymes are P30L, P48R, F194L, R227Q, F234L, V89L-A49T, V89L-T187M, and V89L-F234L.
- Because finasteride is metabolized by CYP 450 3A4, the variant allele of this enzyme dictates how the medication affects the individual.
- CYP 3A4*1B variant frequency is seen more in the African American population than in Asian, Caucasian, and Hispanic populations.

Indications. Finasteride is recommended as a monotherapy or combination therapy with an alpha-blocker for the management and improvement of symptoms of BPH, to reduce the progression of the disease, and to decrease risk of acute urinary obstruction and retention.

Adverse Effects. The most common side effect reported with finasteride is impotence (5% to 19% of patients). Cardiovascular side effects such as orthostatic hypotension, peripheral edema, and hypotension have also been reported. Additionally, ejaculation disorders such as decreased ejaculate volume are experienced with this drug. Some patients report breast tenderness and nasal congestion or rhinitis with this medication.

Contraindications. Finasteride is contraindicated in individuals who are allergic or have a hypersensitivity to it or any of its components. Additionally, this medication is contraindicated for pregnancy and for females who are of childbearing age.

Monitoring. Patients should be monitored for any side effects associated with the medication, such as impotence and hypotension. Additionally, the AUASS or the I-PSS should be utilized to evaluate the effectiveness of the drug, keeping in mind that unlike the alpha-adrenergic blocking agents, this medication may take from 6 to 12 months to reach its maximum effectiveness. Monitor for signs and symptoms of relief, such as improvement of urine flow and a reduction in frequency, nocturia, urgency, and difficulty with urination. Patients should be monitored for urinary complications such as acute urinary retention and should be instructed to report these symptoms immediately to their health care provider. The prescribing clinician should establish a prostate-specific antigen (PSA) baseline at 6 months and monitor periodically after that.

PRACTICE PEARLS

Finasteride

- PSA should decrease in concentration by about 50% within months of finasteride use. If PSA increases during use of this medication, additional testing will be needed to rule out prostate cancer.
- Finasteride can be started and maintained at 5 mg orally once daily. This medication does not need titration.
- This medication is pregnancy category X.
- It is not well known whether this medication is present in breast milk, due to limited studies.
- Use with caution in patients with hepatic impairment as this medication is heavily metabolized by the liver.
- No dosage adjustment is needed with renal impairment.
- This product is marketed as Propecia to treat male pattern hair loss at 1 mg daily.

BLACK BOX WARNING!

Finasteride

- The FDA has issued a warning that there is an increased risk of being diagnosed with high-grade prostate cancer while taking 5-alpha reductase inhibitors.
- Patients with diminished urinary flow and with a large residual urinary volume may not be candidates for therapy with finasteride.
- Tablets must not be touched by females who may be pregnant, because the product may be absorbed through the skin and the medication is teratogenic.
- A pregnant female should not encounter the semen of a male who is taking finasteride.

Phosphodiesterase Type 5 Enzyme Inhibitors

PDE 5 is a group of medications that traditionally were used to treat arterial pulmonary hypertension and ED. For patients with BPH, these medications can be helpful in cases where the patient has mild to moderate symptoms with ED. The precise mechanism of action that helps with BPH is not yet fully understood, but it is strongly believed that it is a PDE 5 modulated decrease of smooth muscle and endothelial cell proliferation combined with smooth muscle relaxation and increased tissue perfusion of the prostate and bladder. In 2011, tadalafil received FDA approval in the United States for use in managing BPH. If this drug is combined with finasteride, it is recommended for no more than 26 weeks of use.

Tadalafil

Pharmacokinetics. Tadalafil is found to be 94% bound to protein, and the onset of action is within 1 hour of being administered. Peak effectiveness varies depending on the condition that it is being used for, but it usually occurs around 2 hours after administration. This medication is metabolized by the liver through CYP 450 isoenzyme 3A4. The half-life of this drug is 15 to 17.5 hours. Excretion occurs mainly through stool (61%) and urine (36%), and mainly as metabolites.

PHARMACOGENETICS

Tadalafil Therapy

Although the metabolism of tadalafil is mediated through the CYP 450 enzyme 3A4, from the same subfamily of 3A, enzyme 3A5 also plays a role, and allele variations (CYP 3A5*1/*1, 1/*3 OR *3/3) may change how the medication affects individuals and mean plasma concentrations of the drug.

Indications. This medication is indicated for the treatment of BPH with or without ED, pulmonary hypertension, and ED.

Adverse Effects. Reported side effects with this medication include flushing, headache, nausea, myalgia, respiratory tract infections, nasopharyngitis, and nasal congestion. Other, less commonly reported side effects include chest pain, facial edema, palpitations, hypotension, diarrhea, nausea, and prolonged erection.

Contraindications. This medication is contraindicated if the patient has hypersensitivity to tadalafil or any component that is part of the formulation of the drug. Additionally, it should not be used with nitrates as it may cause hypotension.

Monitoring. Patients should be monitored for improvement of urinary symptoms and for adverse effects. Patients should be instructed to report any chest pain, changes in vision that affect color discrimination, hearing loss, hypotension, priapism (painful erection longer than 4 to 6 hours), or visual loss.

Anticholinergics

Anticholinergics are medications that can be used as an alternative for patients with LUTS secondary to BPH as long as they do not demonstrate an elevated postvoid volume in the bladder. Data demonstrate that if used in conjunction with alpha-1 adrenergic blocking medications, anticholinergics can offer some benefit to patients with LUTS. Anticholinergics block acetylcholine centrally and peripherally in the nervous

system. Blocking acetylcholine decreases bladder spasm and LUTS in patients with BPH. According to the American Urological Association (AUA), three studies have been published, but there are not enough data to say how effective this group of drugs is with BPH. However, the AUA committee has recommended tolterodine as one more option for a select group of patients with LUTS secondary to BPH.

Prescriber Considerations for Benign Prostatic Hypertrophy Therapy

Clinical Practice Guidelines

- The Agency for Healthcare Research and Quality (AHRQ) Guideline on Benign Prostate Hyperplasia: Diagnosis and Treatment was developed in 1994 and continues as the seminal resource in this area. Guidelines on the management of benign prostatic hyperplasia (BPH) have been archived since 2016 due to a lack of federal funding.
- American Urological Association management of BPH (2021). The AUA has developed guidelines for the evaluation and treatment of patients with BPH.
- American Urological Association benign prostatic hyperplasia: Surgical management/lower urinary tract symptoms (2021) https://www.auanet.org/guidelines/benign-prostatic-hyperplasia-(bph)-guideline
- European Urological Association management of non-neurogenic male lower urinary tract symptoms (LUTS) (2020) https://uroweb.org/guideline/treatment-of-non-neurogenic-male-luts/

Evidence-Based Recommendations

- *Medications:* alpha-blockers, 5-alpha reductase inhibitors, and phosphodiesterase inhibitors are beneficial.
- *Surgery:* Transurethral microwave thermotherapy and transurethral resection are beneficial.
- *Herbal treatments:* β-Sitosterol plant extract and saw palmetto plant extracts are likely to be beneficial; *Pygeum africanum* and rye grass pollen extract have unknown effectiveness.

Clinical Reasoning for Benign Prostatic Hypertrophy Therapy

Consider the individual patient's health problem requiring BPH therapy. Urinary hesitance, urinary frequency, or urinary retention is the typical issue that results in a patient seeking therapy for BPH. Surgical removal of the prostate is the primary treatment for BPH. Watchful waiting is also a common treatment plan in which symptoms are monitored and treatment is initiated only when symptoms become problematic. A recent randomized, controlled study compared bipolar plasma vaporization of the prostate (TUVP) to transurethral resection of the prostate (TURP), and both groups had significantly lower international prostate symptom scores (49.7% and 70.6%, respectively) after the procedure (Christidis et al., 2017; Elsakka et al., 2016). Surgery is indicated when the patient has refractory urinary retention, recurrent urinary tract infections (UTIs), hematuria, bladder stones, or renal insufficiency.

Determine the desired therapeutic outcome of BPH therapy. The goals of BPH treatment are to alleviate symptoms and maintain kidney function. Pharmacologic treatment for BPH is designed to address the impact these symptoms have on the patient's quality of life and to provide treatment when the patient is reluctant or unable to have surgery or when the symptoms are mild enough that surgery is not warranted. Primary care providers often provide prescriptions and watchful waiting and would typically refer a symptomatic patient to a urologist to further discuss treatment options.

Assess the medication therapy selected for its appropriateness for an individual patient. All alpha-blockers used in the treatment of BPH (alfuzosin, doxazosin, tamsulosin, and terazosin) are considered equally efficacious in appropriate doses (American Urological Association, 2021). The selection of one medication over another was based largely on patient history and medication side-effect profiles. The selective alpha-blockers, tamsulosin and alfuzosin, were found to be better tolerated than their nonselective counterparts, as rates of discontinuation due to side effects were comparable with those of a placebo. In contrast, 8% to 20% of patients discontinued treatment with nonspecific alpha-blockers because of orthostatic hypotension and headache.

Even with similar effectiveness profiles, Roehrbonr et al. (2016) concluded that from the selective alpha-blockers, silodosin exhibited the highest selectivity and greatest reduction in bladder outlet obstruction when compared to other medications in the same class. In older adults, tamsulosin was found to have less effect on blood pressure than alfuzosin. Nonspecific alpha-blockers should be considered in patients with concomitant BPH and hypertension. If the patient does not have hypertension, tamsulosin is an appropriate first choice. These drugs have an onset of action of approximately 2 to 4 weeks. In another systematic review of randomized clinical trials, patients receiving alpha-blockers were more likely to complete the trial without the need for catheterization due to obstruction (56.8% versus 38.9%) (Guang-Jun et al., 2014). Although alpha-blockers are best for rapid symptom relief, the 5-alpha reductase inhibitor finasteride can prevent growth of the prostate over the long term. Treatment for 1 year led to a reduction in AUASS by 23% and has been shown to reduce the need for surgery by 55% in males treated for 5 years. In general, patients with larger prostates (more than 40 Gm) at presentation have been found to derive the greatest benefit from treatment with a 5-alpha reductase inhibitor. Dutasteride has shown to be efficacious and safe for the treatment of BPH and to have side effects comparable with those of finasteride.

Initiate the treatment plan with the selected medication by first providing adequate patient education. Patient education begins with the various options for treatment, which include watchful waiting, urology consult, and a discussion of the various pharmacologic treatment options. *First-line therapy* for patients with BPH consists of an alpha-1A selective antagonist for patients without hypertension or a long-acting alpha-1 antagonist for patients with hypertension. The goal of this treatment is the reduction of urinary symptoms. *Second-line therapy* for patients with BPH is a 5-alpha reductase inhibitor given to shrink the size of the prostate; however, 6 to 12 months of therapy is required to achieve maximum benefit. *Combination therapy* with an alpha-1 antagonist plus a 5-alpha reductase inhibitor can be utilized if a single agent is ineffective. *Consider a PDE 5 enzyme inhibitor,* such as tadalafil, for patients with mild to moderate BPH who also have erectile dysfunction.

Conduct follow-up and monitoring of patient responses to BPH therapy. The FDA has issued a warning that, despite resulting in an overall reduction in the number of patients diagnosed with prostate cancer, there is an increased risk of being diagnosed with *high-grade* prostate cancer while taking 5-alpha reductase inhibitors. Thus, the patient's PSA and other signs of prostate cancer should be monitored.

Treatment of BPH with 5-alpha reductase inhibitors results in about a 50% reduction in PSA after 6 months. Monitor sexual adverse effects in patients taking Proscar, as some sexual adverse effects persist after discontinuing treatment, although it remains effective and safe for approved indications.

Combination therapy with finasteride and doxazosin was shown to lower the risk of clinical progression of BPH by 66% in patients treated for more than 4 years.

Teaching Points for Benign Prostatic Hypertrophy Therapy

Health Promotion Strategies

Patient and family education is important when managing patients with BPH. The use of medications is recommended in conjunction with lifestyle modifications.

- Patients should decrease their intake of substances that can be bladder irritants, such as caffeine, alcohol, and spicy foods.
- Patients should avoid high intake of fluids before going to sleep at night.

Patient Education for Medication Safety

- When taking medications such as alpha-1 adrenergic blockers, change positions slowly and avoid stooping forward. Instead, dangle your feet on the side of the bed to decrease excessive lowering of your blood pressure.
- When first starting therapy with alpha-1 antagonists, take the dose at night to decrease some of the symptoms of hypotension as you will be in a recumbent position while in bed.
- You should avoid taking over-the-counter (OTC) medications such as antihistamines, sympathomimetics, and other drugs that may potentially have strong anticholinergic side effects and worsen urinary retention.

Erectile Dysfunction

Overview

Erectile dysfunction (ED) is a condition under the umbrella term "male sexual dysfunction" and is defined as the consistent inability to maintain an erect penis with sufficient rigidity to allow sexual intercourse. ED is a common condition and becomes more frequent with age. Erection and ejaculation involve complex interactions with psychologic, hormonal, neural, and vascular functions.

Relevant Physiology

Both parasympathetic and sympathetic pathways are involved in the erection and ejaculation process. *Parasympathetic* (cholinergic) stimulation controls erection of the penis. *Sympathetic* (adrenergic) pathways produce ejaculation by causing contraction of the prostate and seminal vesicles, as well as effects on the bulbocavernosus and ischiocavernosus muscles.

Pathophysiology

ED may result from a malfunction in one or more areas. Causes are categorized as psychologic or organic. Psychologic causes are usually abrupt in onset, and incidence varies with partner, position, or situation. This type occurs more commonly in younger males. Organic causes usually have a gradual onset and are consistent. New studies find that males with severe periodontal disease have a higher risk of erectile problems compared to males with healthy gums.

Neurologic causes for ED include diabetes, multiple sclerosis, spinal cord damage, nerve damage after a prostatectomy, decreased blood flow to the penis because of atherosclerosis, and vascular damage resulting from injury—for example, renal transplant, bypass procedures, hyperprolactinemia, or structural abnormalities. Chronic renal disease has also been associated with the development of ED. There are certain activities that, although controversial, have been linked to the development of ED. Bicycling for prolonged periods is one of those activities, as the pressure from sitting may decrease blood flow to the cavernosal artery and subsequently lead to ED. Numerous drugs may also be responsible (e.g., antihypertensives, opioids, antidepressants, antianxiety agents, antipsychotic agents, ethyl alcohol, chemotherapeutic agents, cimetidine, and estrogenic agents). In a report from the California Men's Health Study, the use of multiple medications was tied to a higher prevalence of ED, according to data on 37,712 participants. It is estimated that 25% of patients are experiencing ED because of medications. Eight out of the 12 most-prescribed drugs list ED as a side effect. Thus, an essential step in the evaluation of ED is to review the patient's current medications and their potential side effects.

Exercise has been associated with a decreased risk for the development of ED. Patients with obesity, tobacco use, and a sedentary lifestyle have a higher incidence of ED. While males who have cardiovascular disease may develop ED, current research suggests that males who have ED are at increased risk for cardiovascular disease (particularly silent CAD and myocardial infarction), stroke, and death. ED may not only contribute to cardiovascular disease risk prediction, but also serve as a potential target for cardiovascular disease prevention. Researchers are trying to determine whether ED is an independent risk factor for cardiovascular disease. Before starting a medication to help with ED, it is important to rule out cardiovascular disease, because sexual activity is associated with an increased cardiac risk.

ED in males with diabetes is often associated with diabetic neuropathy and peripheral vascular disease. ED occurs at an earlier age in males with diabetes than in males in the general population, and several studies have demonstrated that ED affects 35% to 75% of males with diabetes.

Erectile Dysfunction Therapy

Table 18.1 provides a summary of the pharmacologic treatment of ED.

Phosphodiesterase Type 5 Enzyme Inhibitors

An erection involves the release of nitric oxide in the corpus cavernosum in response to stimulation. Nitric acid increases the levels of cyclic guanosine monophosphate (cGMP), producing smooth muscle relaxation in the corpus cavernosum and allowing inflow of blood. PDE 5 is the enzyme that breaks down cGMP in the corpus cavernosum. PDE 5 inhibitors (e.g., sildenafil) inhibit cGMP and thus allow for increased blood flow into the penis, resulting in an erection.

The PDE 5 enzyme is very specific to receptors in the corpus cavernosum smooth muscle. It is also found in much lower concentrations in platelets, vascular and visceral smooth muscle, and skeletal muscle. PDE 3 is found in cardiac contractility; therefore, these drugs are not active in this condition. They are closely related to PDE 6, which may explain the abnormalities in color vision seen with PDE 5 inhibitors. Tadalafil has a different chemical structure than sildenafil and vardenafil. It has less affinity for PDE 6 (retina) but a greater affinity for PDE 11. PDE 11 is found in the skeletal muscle, testes, heart, prostate, kidney, liver, and pituitary.

PDE 5 inhibitors have been found to be beneficial and effective for the management of ED. In one study, 57% of patients who received sildenafil were able to have successful intercourse when compared to 21% in the placebo group. These results have been replicated in patients with other conditions, such as diabetes mellitus and postprostate removal. Vardenafil is very similar to the profile of sildenafil and is also very effective in the management of ED (65% versus 30% placebo). Tadalafil is chemically different from vardenafil and sildenafil and can be used for the management of BPH.

Sildenafil

Pharmacokinetics. This medication has an onset of action of about 60 minutes and peaks in the blood at about 1 to 2 hours. If the medication is taken with a fatty meal, absorption is slower; if taken on an empty stomach, absorption is rapid. In the adult population, this medication is found to be 96% protein bound. The main metabolism pathways are through the liver isoenzymes CYP 450 3A4 and 2C9. The mean bioavailability of oral administration is 41% and the half-life is 4 hours. Eighty percent of excretion occurs in the feces and roughly 13% in the urine.

PHARMACOGENETICS

Sildenafil Therapy

- Although sildenafil is metabolized mainly by CYP 450 3A4, 3A5 also plays a role.
- In one study, patients who carried CYP 3A5 5*3/*3 and 3A4 1/*1 variation had a higher mean plasma concentration of sildenafil after oral administration of a 100 mg dose.
- Polymorphisms in the NO-cGMP pathway have altered the effectiveness of PDE 5 inhibitors in different populations, helping to explain increased effectiveness in Asians when compared to Caucasians.

Indications. Sildenafil is indicated for the management of ED and pulmonary artery hypertension.

Adverse Effects. The most common side effects reported with this medication are flushing, headache, dyspepsia, visual disturbances, and epistaxis. Additionally, patients may report dizziness, nausea, diarrhea, myalgias, and nasal congestion. Some patients may also experience elevated liver enzymes when taking this drug.

Contraindications. Sildenafil is contraindicated in patients with hypersensitivity to the drug or any component in the formulation. The use of this medication with organic nitrates is also contraindicated. Although not included in the label contraindications in the United States, in Canada this medication is contraindicated for patients with a prior episode of nonarteritic anterior ischemic optic neuropathy. Careful evaluation of cardiovascular disease should be performed before starting management for ED as some patients may not be candidates due to underlying heart conditions.

Monitoring. Clinicians should monitor patients for improvement of sexual dysfunction symptoms. Additionally, if taking any other medications that could potentially lower blood pressure, either in-office or ambulatory blood pressure monitoring is recommended. Lung sounds should be monitored for the development of pulmonary edema. Patients need to be instructed to immediately report to their health care provider a prolonged erection of 4 to 6 hours (priapism), hypotension, hearing loss, trouble with color discrimination, hypersensitivity, or loss of vision.

PRACTICE PEARLS

Sildenafil Therapy

- When used for ED, this medication is taken 1 hour before sexual activity.
- Sildenafil dosing can be increased to 100 mg orally.
- With renal impairment, if CrCl is equal to or greater than 30 mL/minute, no dosage adjustment is needed.
- With mild to severe hepatic impairment, a starting dose of 25 mg orally should be considered.
- Limit alcohol use with sildenafil and other drugs in this class due to increased side effects or reduced efficacy of medication.

BLACK BOX WARNING!

Sildenafil

- Sildenafil should not be taken with organic nitrates.
- Report problems with color discrimination or vision loss immediately.
- Monitor for sudden decrease or loss of hearing.
- Hypersensitivity reactions may occur, such as hives, rash, and anaphylactic reactions.
- Hypotension may occur from vasodilation, especially in patients with decreased ejection fraction, left ventricle outflow problems, or those who are using other antihypertensive medications.
- Priapism can occur. Patients should report a painful erection lasting more than 4 to 6 hours.
- Sildenafil is a 3A4 and 2C9 substrate; inhibitors of these enzymes may reduce sildenafil clearance, causing an increase in plasma concentrations.
- Inducers will decrease sildenafil concentration.
- Use a lower dose of sildenafil when using with ritonavir, ketoconazole, itraconazole, or erythromycin.
- Sildenafil may add to the hypotensive effect of other antihypertensive drugs, especially alpha-adrenergic blocking agents.

Other Drugs in Class

Drugs that belong to the same category or subcategory are similar to the key drug except in the following ways:

- *Vardenafil (Levitra):* The manufacturer states that vardenafil has a shorter onset of action than sildenafil, but studies have not substantiated this claim. Vardenafil is about 10 times as potent as sildenafil.
- *Tadalafil (Cialis):* This drug's chemical structure is different from sildenafil and vardenafil. Tadalafil has a longer duration of action when compared to sildenafil and vardenafil and it has been more effective in patients with psychogenic ED. Tadalafil has been approved for use in patients with LUTS due to BPH.
- *Avanafil (Stendra):* This is a newer PDE 5 inhibitor that has been approved in the United States and Europe and has increased PDE 5 selectivity and more rapid onset of action as compared to other medications in this class. It should be taken 30 minutes before sexual activity (some doses as early as 15 minutes before sexual activity).

Warnings and Precautions

- Vardenafil can cause slight prolongation of the QT interval. Do not use with antiarrhythmic drugs or in patients with hepatic insufficiency. Concomitant use with potent 3A4 inhibitors could increase serum levels of vardenafil.

- Tadalafil (Cialis) has a longer duration of action than sildenafil or vardenafil; the period of effectiveness may last up to 36 hours. Visual changes have not been reported. Potent CYP 3A4 inhibitors increase the serum level of tadalafil. This agent does not interact with hypertensive drugs.

- Avanafil (Stendra), like sildenafil (Viagra), should be taken on an empty stomach, as a fatty meal may delay the absorption of the medication.

- Rare transient global amnesia is reported on all PDE 5 inhibitors labels. Transient global amnesia, or TGA, is a brief bout of amnesia lasting no longer than a day, without causing other problems.

Prostaglandin E1

Alprostadil is a prostaglandin that has many physiologic actions, including vasodilation and platelet inhibition. It induces erection by relaxing the trabecular smooth muscle and dilating the cavernosal arteries. This causes the expansion of lacunar spaces and entrapment of blood caused by compression of the venules against the tunica albuginea. This is called the *corporal venoocclusive mechanism.* This medication was approved for intracavernosal or intraurethral self-injection for the management of ED. Although highly effective in managing ED, administration of this medication requires training, and about half of patients, although satisfied with the management, reported pain as a result of the injection.

Alprostadil

Pharmacokinetics. This medication, when injected for ED, has an onset of action of 5 to 20 minutes and is found to be 81% bound to albumin, although systemic distribution is insignificant when injected directly into the penis. When injected intravenously for other conditions, metabolism happens mainly through lung oxidation (70% to 80%). The time to peak is 30 to 60 minutes, and excretion occurs 90% as metabolites through the urine.

Indications. This drug is recommended for the management of vasculogenic, neurogenic, psychologic, and mixed-etiology ED. Additionally, the medication can be used as an adjunct test in diagnosing ED.

Adverse Effects. Some common side effects experienced with this medication include penile pain, urethral burning sensation, dizziness, headache, testicular pain, urethral bleeding, hypertension, erection lasting longer than 4 hours (about 4% of patients), penile swelling, Peyronie's disease, local bruising, and the formation of a hematoma at the injection site.

Contraindications. This medication is contraindicated for patients who have hypersensitivity to alprostadil or any

component in the formulation. Also, this medication should not be used in individuals who have conditions that increase the chances of priapism, such as sickle cell disease or trait, multiple myeloma, leukemia, and anatomical deformities. It should not be used together with a penile implant. Careful evaluation of cardiovascular disease should be performed before starting this medication for management for ED. Concurrent use with PDE 5 inhibitors is not recommended as this may increase the chances of alprostadil side effects.

Monitoring. Patients should be monitored for improvement of ED symptoms. Additionally, they should be monitored for side effects of the medication such as a prolonged erection, signs of penile infection, pain, or penile fibrosis. Heart rate and blood pressure should be monitored as some patients may develop hypotension and increased heart rate.

Complementary Therapy

Yohimbine

Yohimbine is an alkaloid derived from the West African tree *Corynanthe yohimbine.* Similar to reserpine and exhibiting both sympatholytic and mydriatic properties, yohimbine is an alpha-2 adrenergic antagonist that affects erectile function by stimulating the release of presynaptic norepinephrine in the lower nerve centers. Yohimbine has a long history of use in treating ED; however, clinical effectiveness is lacking, and treatment is not without risk. In the treatment of males who have ED for psychologic reasons, yohimbine may have a role in therapy. Two clinical trials of 101 males found that yohimbine (5.4 mg three times daily) was shown to allow resumed

Alprostadil

- A 0.5-inch 29-or 30-gauge needle should be used, and the medication should be injected into the dorsolateral aspect of the most-proximal one-third of the penis. The patient should be instructed to avoid any visible veins and to rotate sides of the penis between injections. The injection site should be cleaned with an alcohol swab prior to injection and compressed with the same swab 5 minutes after the injection to decrease bruising and hematoma formation.

- Intraurethral placement of the prostaglandin alprostadil is another treatment alternative. Although this is less painful, research shows that it is less effective than injections and more costly, as many insurance plans will not cover the medication. A small pellet is placed into the urethra of the penis prior to anticipated sexual intercourse.

- There are no renal or hepatic impairment dosage-related adjustments recommended by the manufacturer.

- For older adults, use the lowest possible dose for effectiveness.

- The dose of the medication varies by manufacturer: for instance, Varveject is available in 10 mcg and 20 mcg doses; Edex is available in 10 mcg, 20 mcg, and 40 mcg doses.

sexual intercourse in 3 days to 3 weeks. Fifteen percent of males treated with a placebo had a similar response. Yohimbine has not been approved by the FDA for use in ED and should not be recommended to patients as a first-line treatment.

Pharmacokinetics. Data are not available on the pharmacokinetics of yohimbine.

Indications. Because of lack of data-driven evidence, yohimbine is not FDA approved for the management of ED.

Adverse Effects. Tachycardia and hypertension are possible side effect because of yohimbine's alpha-2-blocking effects; caution is advised in patients with heart disease. Yohimbine penetrates the central nervous system (CNS) to cause central excitation, including elevated blood pressure and heart rate, increased motor activity, nervousness, irritability, and tremor. Dizziness, headache, and skin flushing also have occurred.

Monitoring. Monitor patients for effectiveness and adverse reactions, especially priapism, chest pain, and bouts of amnesia.

Contraindications. Yohimbine is contraindicated with hypersensitivity and renal disease.

Prescriber Considerations for Erectile Dysfunction Therapy

Clinical Practice Guidelines

- American Urological Association Erectile Dysfunction guidelines (2018): https://www.auanet.org/guidelines/erectile-dysfunction-(ed)-guideline
- American Academy of Family Physicians (AAFP) Management of Erectile Dysfunction (2016): https://www.aafp.org/afp/2010/0201/p305.html
- European Association of Urology (EAU) Guidelines on erectile dysfunction, premature ejaculation, penile curvature, and priapism: https://uroweb.org/wp-content/uploads/EAU-Guidelines-Male-Sexual-Dysfunction-2016-3.pdf

Evidence-Based Recommendations

- Sildenafil improved erections and increased rates of successful intercourse compared with placebos. Adverse effects, including headaches, flushing, and dyspepsia, have been reported in up to 25% of males. Deaths have been reported in males on concomitant treatment with oral nitrates.
- Alprostadil increased the chances of a satisfactory erection compared with placebos.
- Some research suggests that vacuum devices were as effective as intracavernosal alprostadil injections for rigidity but not for orgasm.
- Some evidence suggests that intraurethral alprostadil increased the chances of successful sexual intercourse and at least one orgasm over 3 months compared with placebos. About 33% of males suffered penile ache.

Clinical Reasoning for ED Therapy

Consider the individual patient's health problem requiring ED therapy. There are several sexual problems in males, but the most common problem is an inability to acquire or maintain an erection satisfactorily for sexual intercourse. The most common conditions that limit blood flow to the penis include cigarette smoking, diabetes, high blood pressure, obesity, and medications. Evaluation of lifestyle modifications and medications that could lead to ED should be done prior to starting any therapy. PDE 5 inhibitors are safe and effective if used properly and are given as first-line therapy. The major risks associated with their use involve patients with cardiac conditions; these agents are contraindicated in patients who are taking nitrates because of excessive hypotension. Treatment with these drugs in controlled studies has shown that erectile function is improved regardless of patient age, duration of ED, or duration of diabetes. PDE 5 inhibitors are effective 50% to 80% of the time. Much controversy has arisen about the possible cardiovascular effects of PDE 5 inhibitors. Two consensus panels (Second Princeton and the ACC/AHA) have concluded that the use of PDE 5 inhibitors is safe and effective in males with stable CAD who are not receiving nitrates.

Determine the desired therapeutic outcome based on the patient's health problem. Assess the ED therapy selected for its appropriateness for an individual patient by considering the medication's side effects and the patient's age, race/ethnicity, comorbidities, and genetic factors. Certain medications (including erythromycin, ketoconazole, protease inhibitors, rifampin, and phenytoin) as well as grapefruit juice can alter the duration of time that sildenafil, vardenafil, and tadalafil remain in the bloodstream, which can cause additional side effects. Oral PDE 5 inhibitors (unless contraindicated) should be offered as first-line therapy for ED. Patients who have failed a trial with PDE 5 inhibitor therapy should be informed of the benefits and risks of other therapies, including the use of a different PDE 5 inhibitor, alprostadil intraurethral suppositories, intracavernous drug injection, vacuum constriction devices, and penile prostheses. The initial trial dose of alprostadil intraurethral suppositories and intracavernous injection therapy should be administered under supervision of the health care provider because of the risk of syncope.

Hormonal replacement with testosterone injections or topical patches can be used for males with documented androgen deficiency and no contraindications. This requires a thorough endocrine evaluation. Many nonpharmacologic treatments are available for ED. Vascular reconstruction may be appropriate in patients with decreased blood flow. Vacuum constriction devices are safe and effective. A wide variety of implanted penile prostheses have been devised.

Initiate the treatment plan with the selected medication by first providing adequate patient education to ensure the patient's understanding and promote full participation in ED therapy. Promote the understanding that all PDE 5 inhibitors are equally effective but have different durations of action. Tadalafil has a considerably longer period of effectiveness and is better absorbed in the presence of food. Males who are taking tadalafil are able to have an erection for a period of 36 hours versus 4 hours with sildenafil and vardenafil. Absorption of tadalafil is less affected by high-fat meals and alcohol. All three older drugs now list rare reports of transient global amnesia on their labels. Transient global amnesia, or TGA, is a brief bout of amnesia lasting no longer than 1 day, without causing other problems. Avanafil (Stendra) is a new drug, and it is not clear whether this warning will apply to this product.

There is an absolute contraindication for the use of any type of nitrates with PDE 5 inhibitors due to the risk of severe hypotension and potential for cardiovascular collapse and death. Common side effects to be expected with ED therapy include flushing and headaches. Blue hue vision changes can occur with sildenafil. Priapism is considered a medical emergency, and patients need to be instructed to go to the emergency room for an erection lasting 4 hours or longer. Educate patients about their expectations for ED therapy and potential side effects. Patients should be instructed to report any chest pain or discomfort during sexual activity.

Ensure complete patient and family understanding about the medication prescribed for ED therapy using a variety of education strategies. Provide instructions concerning the anatomic effect of blood flow to the penis in achieving an erection, and the role of ED therapy. Written instructions should be provided in addition to oral teaching to both the patient and partner regarding proper administration for optimal results, especially the importance of taking the medication exactly as prescribed and not exceeding recommended doses or frequency of use. In addition, a copy of the manufacturer's instructions should be provided to patients. Patients and their sexual partners need to understand the potential need for sexual stimulation to achieve an erection. Provide information regarding the risk for sexually transmitted infections and the need to use protective measures to guard against transmission of such diseases.

Conduct follow-up and monitoring of patient responses to ED therapy. Patients should schedule a follow-up appointment after 3 months of therapy to evaluate the effectiveness of treatment and any side effects that can be ameliorated with dose adjustment or change of medication. In each encounter, stress the importance of seeking immediate medical attention if an erection lasts longer than 4 hours or is painful. Monitor the medication usage regarding frequency and any adverse effects. If the prescribed therapy is effective and well tolerated, follow-up visits can be at 6-month intervals.

Teaching Points for ED Therapy

Health Promotion Strategies

- Discuss with patients the potential cardiac risk of sexual activity with preexisting cardiovascular disease.
- Advise patients who experience symptoms (e.g., angina pectoris, dizziness, nausea) upon initiation of sexual activity to refrain from further activity and discuss the episode with their provider.
- A number of Internet sources claim to sell medications such as Viagra, Cialis, Levitra, or herbal supplements for ED for a reduced cost, often without a prescription. These sources are not known to be safe or reliable, and it is not possible to know whether the pills from these sources contain the actual drug or are counterfeit.
- Priapism is an emergency. For any erections that last longer than 4 hours, patients should seek immediate medical assistance.
- Serious cardiovascular events, including myocardial infarction, sudden cardiac death, ventricular arrhythmia, cerebrovascular hemorrhage, transient ischemic attack, and hypertension, have been reported in temporal association with sildenafil.
- Use with caution in patients with anatomic deformation of the penis or with risk factors for priapism.
- Sildenafil has an effect on platelets but has shown no effect on bleeding time when taken alone or with aspirin.

Administer with caution in patients with bleeding disorders or active peptic ulceration.

- Mild, transient, dose-related impairment of blue or green color discrimination has been noted. Transient loss of vision has been reported, but no proof of cause and effect has been found.

Application Questions for Discussion

1. A 78-year-old patient with urinary symptoms believed to be originating from BPH states his symptoms are worsening. What other causes of urinary symptoms should be considered? What may be a first-line therapy for this patient?

2. A 65-year-old patient who presents to the clinic to discuss treatment options for ED states he had a heart attack approximately 6 years ago. What pharmacologic therapy would be appropriate for this patient?

Selected Bibliography

American Urological Association. (2021). *Management of benign prostatic hyperplasia.* Retrieved from https://www.auanet.org/guidelines/non-oncology-guidelines.

American Urological Association. (2018). *Erectile dysfunction: AUA guideline 2018.* Retrieved from https://www.auanet.org/guidelines/erectile-dysfunction-(ed)-guideline.

Burnett, A. L., Nehra, A., Breau, R. H., et al. (2018). Erectile Dysfunction: AUA Guideline. *The Journal of Urology, 200*(3), 633–641. http://doi.org/10.1016/j.juro.2018.05.004.

Choi, C., Bae, J., Jang, C., & Lee, S. (2014). Tamsulosin exposure is significantly increased by the CYP2D6*10/*10 genotype. *Journal of Clinical Pharmacology, 52*(12), 1934–1938. http://doi.org/10.1177/0091270011432168.

Christidis, D., McGrath, S., Perera, M., Manning, T., Bolton, D., & Lawrentschuk, N. (2017). Minimally invasive surgical therapies for benign prostatic hypertrophy: The rise in minimally invasive surgical therapies. *Prostate International, 5*(2), 41–46. http://doi.org/10.1016/j.prnil.2017.01.007.

Elsakka, A. M., Eltatawy, H. H., Almekaty, K. H., Ramadan, A. R., Gameel, T. A., & Farahat, Y. (2016). A prospective randomised controlled study comparing bipolar plasma vaporisation of the prostate to monopolar transurethral resection of the prostate. (Author Abstract). *Arab Journal of Urology, 14*(4), 280. http://doi.org/10.1016/j.aju.2016.09.005.

European Association of Urology. (2016). *Guidelines on erectile dysfunction, premature ejaculation, penile curvature and priapism.* Retrieved from https://uroweb.org/wp-content/uploads/EAU-Guidelines-Male-Sexual-Dysfunction-2016-3.pdf.

European Association of Urology. (2020). *Management of non-neurogenic male LUTS.* Retrieved from https://uroweb.org/guideline/treatment-of-non-neurogenic-male-luts/#1.

Guang-Jun, D., Feng-Bin, G., & Xun-Bo, J. (2015a). α1-blockers in the management of acute urinary retention secondary to benign prostatic hyperplasia: A systematic review and meta-analysis. Irish Journal of Medical Science *(1971 -),184*(1), 23–30. http://doi.org/10.1007/s11845-014-1094-3

Guang-Jun, D., Feng-Bin, G., & Xun-Bo, J. (2015b). α1-blockers in the management of acute urinary retention secondary to benign prostatic hyperplasia: A systematic review and meta-analysis. Irish Journal of Medical Science *(1971 -),184*(1), 23–30. http://doi.org/10.1007/s11845-014-1094-3

Lacchini, R., & Tanus-Santos, J. (2014). Pharmacogenetics of erectile dysfunction: Navigating into uncharted waters. (Report). *Pharmacogenomics, 15*(11), 1519. http://doi.org/10.2217/pgs.14.110.

Langan, R. C. (2019). Benign Prostatic Hyperplasia. *Primary Care: Clinics in Office Practice, 46*(2), 223–232. http://doi.org/10.1016/j.pop.2019.02.003.

Le, T. V., Tsambarlis, P., & Hellstrom, W. J. G. (2019). Pharmacodynamics of the agents used for the treatment of erectile dysfunction. *Expert Opinion on Drug Metabolism & Toxicology, 15*(2), 121–131. http://doi.org/10.1080/17425255.2019.1560421.

Mobley, D. F., Khera, M., & Baum, N. (2017). Recent advances in the treatment of erectile dysfunction. *Postgraduate Medical Journal, 93*(1105), 679–685. http://doi.org/10.1136/postgradmedj-2016-134073.

Pfizer. (2019). *Sildenafil.* Retrieved from http://labeling.pfizer.com/ShowLabeling.aspx?id=652.

Pfizer. (2020). *Alprostadil.* Retrieved from https://www.pfizermedicalinformation.com/en-us/caverject-impulse-alprostadil.

Roehrborn, C., Cruz, F., & Fusco, F. (2016). α1-blockers in men with lower urinary tract symptoms suggestive of benign prostatic obstruction: Is silodosin different? *Advances in Therapy, 33*(12), 2110–2121. http://doi.org/10.1007/s12325-016-0423-5.

Sanofi-Aventis. (2018). *Tamsulosin drug insert.* Retrieved from http://products.sanofi.us/Flomax/Flomax.pdf.

Skinder, D., Zacharia, I., Studin, J., & Covino, J. (2016). Benign prostatic hyperplasia: A clinical review. *JAAPA, 29*(8), 19–23. http://doi.org/10.1097/01.JAA.0000488689.58176.0a.

Van Asseldonk, B., Barkin, J., & Elterman, D. S. (2015). Medical therapy for benign prostatic hyperplasia: A review. *Canadian Journal of Urology, 22*(1), 7–17. Suppl.

Zurawin, J. L., Stewart, C. A., Anaissie, J. E., Yafi, F. A., & Hellstrom, W. J. (2016). Avanafil for the treatment of erectile dysfunction. *Expert Review of Clinical Pharmacology, 9*(9), 1163–1170. http://doi.org/10.1080/17512433.2016.1212655.

19

Urinary Incontinence Medications and Urinary Analgesics

STEPHEN McGHEE AND BEATRIZ VALDES

Overview

This chapter discusses genitourinary medications used to treat urinary incontinence, urinary retention, nocturnal enuresis in children, and urinary tract pain (*dysuria*). The anticholinergics/antispasmodics that are approved by the U.S. Food and Drug Administration (FDA) for urinary incontinence are discussed in detail in this chapter. A number of α-adrenergic agonists, α-adrenergic antagonists, tricyclic antidepressants, sympathomimetics, and estrogens are also used with varying success, and information about those medications may be found in the relevant chapters.

Relevant Physiology

Urinary incontinence is the unintentional leakage of urine. Causes of incontinence vary by gender. Four basic types of established incontinence are known: stress, urge, overflow, and mixed urinary incontinence.

Pathophysiology: Types of Urinary Incontinence

Stress incontinence is leakage of urine that results from a reduction in urethral resistance and increased abdominal pressure associated with physical exertion (e.g., exercise, coughing, and sneezing). Causative factors include weak pelvic floor muscles, prostatectomy, and obesity. Stress incontinence is the most common type of incontinence in females younger than age 60. It also occurs in males who have had prostate surgery.

Urge incontinence, or overactive bladder, is caused by a hyperactive detrusor muscle and is associated with an intense urge to void before the bladder is full. Urge incontinence is associated with localized conditions (e.g., infection, atrophic vaginitis, stones, calculi, or other obstruction), neurologic disorders (cerebral vascular accident, Parkinson's

disease, Alzheimer's disease), and metabolic conditions (diabetes, dehydration, vitamin B_{12} deficiency).

Overflow incontinence results from detrusor muscle underactivity and/or bladder outlet obstruction. Leakage of urine is small in volume and continual. Overflow incontinence is found in females with pelvic organ prolapse and in males with benign prostatic hyperplasia.

Mixed incontinence is defined as having symptoms of two or more types of incontinence, usually urge and stress incontinence. Urinary incontinence is a complex syndrome with multiple causes; it is not uncommon for individuals to experience more than one type of incontinence.

Treatment for urinary incontinence is specific to the type of incontinence being experienced and may include nonpharmacologic therapies, biofeedback, electrical stimulation, and surgical options. Nonpharmacologic approaches constitute the mainstay of treatment for urinary incontinence. These minimally invasive management techniques include fluid management, bladder training, bladder retraining, and pelvic floor muscle rehabilitation (Table 19.1).

Urinary Incontinence Therapy

In female stress incontinence, α-adrenergic agonists are used. The application of low-dose, topical estrogen in the form of a vaginal cream, or an estrogen-containing ring or a patch, may help rejuvenate deteriorating tissues in the vagina and urinary tract and relieve some incontinence symptoms.

For the treatment of urge incontinence, first-line pharmacotherapy consists of anticholinergic agents such as oxybutynin, darifenacin, solifenacin, tolterodine, trospium, and fesoterodine. Adverse effects include urinary retention, dry mouth, constipation, blurred vision, tachycardia, and sedation/confusion. These medications should be avoided with narrow-angle glaucoma and used cautiously with older adults due to the increased risk for cognitive impairment and falls (Wilson & Waghel, 2016). Propantheline and

TABLE 19.1	Common Contributors to Transient Urinary Incontinence
Cause	**Comment**
Delirium	Mental status changes; treat underlying medical condition
Infection	Irritated detrusor muscle
Atrophic urethritis or vaginitis	May present as dysuria, dyspareunia, burning on urination, urgency, and incontinence; requires a pelvic examination. Can treat with estrogen.
Pharmaceuticals	Side effect of numerous agents (diuretics, nonsteroidal antiinflammatory drugs [NSAIDs], antihypertensives). Sedatives may cause confusion and secondary incontinence.
Excessive urine output	Peripheral edema, hyperglycemia, congestive heart failure
Restricted mobility	Cognitive decline, physical weakness
Stool impaction	Requires rectal examination

From Gormley, E. A., & Kaufman, M. [2016]. *Medical student curriculum: Urinary incontinence.* American Urological Association. https://www.auanet.org/education/auauniversity/for-medical-students/medical-students-curriculum/medical-student-curriculum/urinary-incontinence.

flavoxate are older medications that are less often used for urinary incontinence. Propantheline has strong anticholinergic side effects and is now considered a third-line choice. The theoretical advantage of flavoxate with its direct action on smooth muscle has not been effective in trials.

A focused history with a careful physical examination is essential for determining the cause of incontinence. Transient or reversible causes should be ruled out. A bladder diary is a helpful diagnostic tool that reveals toileting habits, fluid intake, and leakage episodes. Urinalysis and post-void residual are essential laboratory tests. Further evaluation by specialists may involve urodynamic and imaging tests.

Anticholinergics

Anticholinergic medications have many actions. For one, they block muscarinic actions (a subset of the parasympathetic nervous system). The primary associated adverse effects are blurred vision, urinary retention, constipation, dry mouth, tachycardia, and sedation/confusion. Anticholinergic medications used for urge incontinence include those in this chapter, tricyclic antidepressants (TCAs), and dicyclomine (Bentyl®).

Anticholinergic medications also inhibit the action of acetylcholine on bladder smooth muscle. This blocks contraction of the bladder and decreases the urodynamic response of detrusor overactivity—the problem in urge incontinence. These actions result in increased bladder capacity, delayed desire to void, and diminished frequency of involuntary bladder contractions.

Oxybutynin

Oxybutynin has both direct antispasmodic effects and anticholinergic effects on smooth muscle. Its direct relaxant effect on smooth muscle is produced by way of phosphodiesterase inhibition (Aoki et al., 2017).

Pharmacokinetics. Oxybutynin is administered both topically as a transdermal patch or gel, and orally. The pharmacokinetics of oxybutynin are linear and dose dependent. The elimination half-life of oxybutynin is 2 to 5 hours. For the transdermal system, plasma concentrations increase for approximately 24 to 48 hours after patch application, with steady-state concentrations maintained for up to 96 hours. For the topical gel, steady-state concentrations are achieved within 3 to 7 days of continuous daily dosing. The oral formulation is rapidly absorbed, with peak concentrations occurring in 1 hour. Antispasmodic activity occurs within 30 to 60 minutes of administration and can last for 6 to 10 hours.

Indications. Oxybutynin is indicated for the treatment of overactive bladder with symptoms of urge urinary incontinence, urinary urgency, and urinary frequency, or incontinence due to involuntary detrusor muscle contractions.

Adverse Effects. The anticholinergic effect of oxybutynin results in xerostomia, regardless of formulation used. Gastrointestinal (GI) adverse effects include nausea, vomiting, diarrhea, dyspepsia, and flatulence. Dermatologic effects such as xerosis, pruritis, rash, and urticaria have been reported. The most common adverse effects associated with the use of the transdermal patch and topical gel are localized, application-site reactions. Central nervous system (CNS) adverse reactions of dizziness, drowsiness, headache, and flushing occur in 5% to 16% of patients. Psychiatric effects, including insomnia (3%) and confusion, were also reported in patients receiving extended-release oxybutynin.

Urinary hesitancy (8.5%), urinary tract infection (UTI) (6.5%), and urinary retention (6%) have been reported with both immediate and extended-release formulations. Cardiovascular effects of palpitations, sinus tachycardia, fluid retention, edema, peripheral edema, increased blood pressure, and decreased blood pressure have been reported in 1% to 5% of patients taking immediate-release oxybutynin.

Contraindications. All formulations of oxybutynin are contraindicated in patients with known hypersensitivity to oxybutynin. Due to its anticholinergic effects, oxybutynin is contraindicated in patients with urinary retention. Oxybutynin is also contraindicated in patients with uncontrolled narrow- or closed-angle glaucoma. Oxybutynin may increase intraocular pressure and aqueous outflow resistance in patients with closed-angle glaucoma. Oxybutynin is contraindicated for use in patients with gastroparesis, GI obstruction, and pyloric stenosis due to delayed gastric emptying.

Monitoring. Ocular hypertension can precipitate undiagnosed glaucoma. Ocular pain should be reported and evaluated.

PRACTICE PEARLS

Pediatric Considerations

- Oxybutynin is not indicated in children younger than 5 years of age; the safety and efficacy of other products in children younger than age 12 have not been established.
- Oxybutynin may cause hallucinations and agitation in children. Cholinergics are not indicated in children.
- Primary nocturnal enuresis is common in children; desmopressin may be used in children 6 years of age or older.

Darifenacin

Darifenacin is an oral competitive, selective M3 muscarinic receptor antagonist. Muscarinic receptors play an important role in contractions of the urinary bladder smooth muscle. Darifenacin is administered once daily and results in significant reductions in the frequency of urinary incontinence.

Pharmacokinetics. Darifenacin is administered orally. It is 98% protein bound to alpha-1-acid-glycoprotein. Darifenacin is extensively metabolized by the liver, mediated by cytochrome (CYP) 3A4 and CYP 2D6. After oral administration, peak plasma concentrations are reached in 7 hours and steady-state plasma concentrations are achieved by the sixth day of dosing. Approximately 60% of an orally administered dose is recovered in the urine and 40% in the feces, with 3% of the dose excreted in the urine as unchanged drug. The elimination half-life following chronic dosing is 13 to 19 hours.

Indications. Darifenacin is indicated for the treatment of overactive bladder with symptoms of urge urinary incontinence, urinary urgency, and urinary frequency.

Adverse Effects. The two most commonly reported adverse events are xerostomia and constipation. UTI was reported in 3.7% to 4.7% of darifenacin-treated patients. Angioedema of the face, lips, tongue, and larynx may occur shortly after the initiation of therapy.

Contraindications. Darifenacin is contraindicated in patients who have demonstrated darifenacin hypersensitivity or a history of angioedema. Due to its anticholinergic effects, darifenacin is contraindicated in patients with urinary retention. Darifenacin should be administered with caution to patients with GI obstructive disorders, because of the risk of delayed gastric emptying. Anticholinergics may in general aggravate conditions such as myasthenia gravis and autonomic neuropathy. Darifenacin is contraindicated in patients with uncontrolled narrow-angle or closed-angle glaucoma, as it may increase intraocular pressure and aqueous outflow resistance. Darifenacin is associated with CNS effects including headache, confusion, hallucinations, and somnolence.

Monitoring. Monitor for signs of hypersensitivity, urinary retention, and GI adverse effects.

Solifenacin

Solifenacin is a competitive M3 selective muscarinic receptor antagonist with effects on all muscarinic receptors. Antimuscarinic drugs depress both voluntary and involuntary bladder contractions and control secretion in the salivary glands, gastric ciliary muscle, and CNS.

Pharmacokinetics. Solifenacin is administered orally and is 98% protein bound to plasma proteins, principally to alpha-1-acid glycoprotein. Solifenacin is metabolized primarily in the liver by CYP 3A4. The elimination half-life of solifenacin at steady state is approximately 45 to 68 hours in adults and 26 hours in pediatric patients 2 to 17 years of age. Peak concentrations are attained in approximately 3 to 8 hours after administration of the oral tablet.

Indications. Solifenacin is indicated for the treatment of overactive bladder with symptoms of urge urinary incontinence, urinary urgency, and urinary frequency.

Adverse Effects. GI adverse events reported in at least 1% of adult patients receiving solifenacin are xerostomia, dyspepsia, nausea, vomiting, upper abdominal pain, and constipation. Ophthalmic adverse events reported include blurred vision, xerophthalmia, and glaucoma. Genitourinary effects such as UTI, cystitis, and urinary retention have been reported. Hypersensitivity reactions with solifenacin administration include angioedema, rash, pruritis, and urticaria.

Contraindications. Solifenacin is contraindicated in patients who have demonstrated solifenacin hypersensitivity or a history of angioedema with the drug. Solifenacin is also contraindicated in patients with urinary retention due to its anticholinergic effects, and in patients with uncontrolled narrow- or closed-angle glaucoma. Solifenacin may delay gastric emptying and is contraindicated in patients with gastric retention, GI obstruction, ileus, gastroparesis, and pyloric stenosis. Hepatic dysfunction can significantly alter the elimination of solifenacin, and thus, patients with moderately reduced hepatic function should have a dosage modification. Patients should be advised to use caution when driving or operating machinery while receiving solifenacin until the effects of the drug are known. Use solifenacin with caution in patients at increased risk of QT prolongation including congenital long QT syndrome, bradycardia, atrioventricular (AV) block, heart failure, cardiomyopathy, or myocardial infarction.

Monitoring. Patients should be monitored for signs of anticholinergic CNS effects, particularly after beginning treatment.

Trospium

Trospium is an oral nonspecific antimuscarinic agent indicated for the treatment of overactive bladder in adults. Trospium decreases the frequency of bladder contractions, resulting in a reduction in urinary frequency, urgency, and incontinence. Trospium is effective in patients with idiopathic or neurogenic detrusor overactivity, with symptoms of overactive bladder improving as early as 1 week following drug initiation. Trospium has been shown to be as effective as oxybutynin for overactive bladder, but with better tolerability.

Pharmacokinetics. After oral administration, less than 10% of the dose is absorbed. Protein binding ranges from 48% to 85% depending on formulation. Peak plasma concentration occurs after 6 hours, with a half-life of 20 hours. The pharmacokinetics of trospium are *not* dose dependent. Administration of the immediate or extended-release tablets with a high-fat meal results in reduced absorption. It is recommended, therefore, that trospium be administered at least 1 hour before meals or on an empty stomach. After oral administration, 85.2% of the dose is recovered in the feces. Of the proportion of trospium that is absorbed, 60% is excreted unchanged in the urine.

Indications. Trospium is indicated for the treatment of overactive bladder with symptoms of urge urinary incontinence, urinary urgency, and neurogenic bladder.

Adverse Effects. The most common adverse events reported by patients include both xerostomia (20% of patients) and constipation (9.6%). GI adverse reactions (1% to 1.5%) include upper abdominal pain, aggravation of constipation, dyspepsia, and flatulence. Antimuscarinic-related urinary adverse events include urinary retention, reported in 1.2% of patients. Trospium appears to have no effect on the QT interval in younger healthy volunteers; however, an increase in asymptomatic ST-T wave changes (nonspecific T wave inversions) was observed. Other cardiac effects such as palpitations, syncope, hypertension sometimes associated with hypertensive crisis, supraventricular tachycardia, and chest pain (unspecified) have been reported. Angioedema of the face, lips, tongue, and/or larynx has been reported with trospium.

Contraindications. Trospium is contraindicated in patients who have demonstrated hypersensitivity to the drug or its ingredients. Avoid ethanol ingestion within 2 hours of taking trospium extended-release capsules. Trospium is contraindicated in patients with urinary retention, and in patients with uncontrolled closed-angle glaucoma due to a potential for increased intraocular pressure. Trospium can delay gastric emptying and is contraindicated in patients with gastroparesis, GI obstruction, pyloric stenosis, ileus, toxic megacolon, or severe ulcerative colitis. Gastroesophageal reflux disease (GERD) may be aggravated with anticholinergic medications. Administer trospium cautiously to patients with moderate to severe hepatic disease. Anticholinergics in general may exacerbate the clinical symptoms of patients with myasthenia gravis or autonomic neuropathy.

Monitoring. Monitor serum creatinine before and throughout treatment. Monitor for adverse effects including constipation, urinary retention, cardiovascular issues, and hypersensitivity.

Fesoterodine

Fesoterodine is an oral selective muscarinic receptor antagonist (M3). The active metabolite of fesoterodine is responsible for the therapeutic actions of the drug. When using a bladder-specific antimuscarinic, use of extended-release oral formulations, such as fesoterodine, are preferred to immediate-release products as they may limit side effects such as dry mouth.

Pharmacokinetics. Fesoterodine is administered orally and is 50% bound to plasma proteins. The liver's two enzymes, CYP 2D6 and CYP 3A4, primarily metabolize fesoterodine. Following an oral dose, fesoterodine is rapidly hydrolyzed to its active metabolite, 5-hydroxymethyltolterodin. Fesoterodine is well absorbed, with maximum plasma levels reached at 5 hours and a half-life of 7 hours. The majority of the medication is excreted in the urine, with 7% excreted in the feces.

Indications. Fesoterodine is indicated for the treatment of overactive bladder with symptoms of urge urinary incontinence, urinary urgency, and urinary frequency.

Adverse Effects. The most common adverse effects are mild to moderate xerostomia and constipation, and are dose-related. Genitourinary adverse effects include UTI, dysuria, and urinary retention. Hypersensitivity reactions have been reported with fesoterodine. Angioedema of the face, lips, tongue, and/or larynx has also been reported with fesoterodine. In one case, angioedema occurred after the first dose.

Contraindications. Fesoterodine is contraindicated in patients who have demonstrated a hypersensitivity to the drug or its ingredients. The anticholinergic effects of fesoterodine make this medication contraindicated in patients with urinary retention. Fesoterodine is contraindicated for use in patients with gastric retention, gastroparesis, GI obstruction, and pyloric stenosis. Fesoterodine should be used cautiously in patients with decreased GI motility. Fesoterodine is contraindicated in patients with uncontrolled narrow- or closed-angle glaucoma, as it may increase intraocular pressure. Fesoterodine is not recommended for use in patients with severe hepatic impairment. Patients with mild to severe renal impairment can experience increased plasma levels of the active metabolite of fesoterodine. Dosage adjustments are required for those with renal failure or severe renal impairment (i.e., a creatine clearance [CrCl] less than 30 mL/minute).

Caution is advisable during use of fesoterodine in patients with myasthenia gravis, as anticholinergics may exacerbate the clinical symptoms of the disease. Safe and effective use of fesoterodine in children or infants has not been established. There are no data on the use of fesoterodine in pregnant patients. The drug should be avoided during pregnancy unless the benefit of therapy outweighs the potential risk to the fetus.

Monitoring. No laboratory monitoring is required. Monitor for anticholinergic-related adverse effects.

Antispasmodics

Antispasmodics have a direct action on smooth muscle, especially of the urinary tract. The administration of antispasmodic medications serves to relax the smooth muscles of the urinary tract (detrusor muscle), reducing the symptoms associated with bladder spasticity. These medications also increase urinary bladder capacity.

Flavoxate

Flavoxate acts as a direct smooth muscle relaxant. This effect causes relief of bladder spasticity and thereby produces increased bladder capacity. Flavoxate also exhibits local anesthetic and analgesic actions.

Pharmacokinetics. Flavoxate is administered orally, but the mechanism of metabolism is unknown. Once it is administered orally, the onset of flavoxate is 60 minutes, with peak plasma levels reached at 2 hours. Flavoxate is 57% excreted via the renal system (Paddock Laboratories, 2018; Prescriber's Drug Reference, 2020).

Indications. Flavoxate is indicated for the symptomatic relief of dysuria, urinary urgency, nocturia, suprapubic pain, urinary frequency, and urinary incontinence associated with cystitis, overactive bladder, prostatitis, urethritis, urethrocystitis, or urethrotrigonitis.

Adverse Effects. Flavoxate has anticholinergic effects including xerostomia, constipation, headache, dizziness, anxiety, vision changes, fatigue, dysuria, and somnolence. Ophthalmic adverse effects such as increased ocular tension, blurred vision, and disturbance in accommodation have been reported. CNS adverse effects include drowsiness, confusion and delirium, and hallucinations. Cardiovascular effects include tachycardia, arrhythmias, and anaphylaxis. Adverse allergic reactions to flavoxate include urticaria and other dermatoses, eosinophilia, and hyperpyrexia.

Contraindications. Flavoxate is contraindicated in patients with GI obstruction, pyloric or duodenal obstruction, obstructive intestinal lesions, ileus, urinary retention, or lower urinary tract obstruction. Flavoxate should be used with caution in patients with closed-angle glaucoma. Use flavoxate with caution in the older patient, due to the anticholinergic effects of the drug. The safe and effective use of flavoxate in neonates, infants, and children younger than 12 years of age has not been determined. It is not known whether flavoxate is excreted in breast milk.

Monitoring. Patients should be assessed periodically for medication effects on urinary incontinence as well as lower urinary tract symptoms and treatment tolerability. Careful dosing and close monitoring of clinical response and of tolerance of side effects is essential. Baseline and routine lab monitoring (complete blood count or CBC, chemistries, and renal and liver function) is recommended.

Propantheline

Propantheline, an older, less frequently utilized medication, is a synthetic quaternary ammonium antimuscarinic agent. Propantheline competes with acetylcholine at peripheral muscarinic and ganglionic nicotinic receptors in a dose-dependent fashion.

Pharmacokinetics. Propantheline reports 50% oral absorption with a 30- to 45-minute medication onset. Metabolized by the liver and GI tract, 70% of propantheline is excreted through the renal system. Propantheline maximum plasma levels are reached at 4 hours and have a half-life of 1.6 hours.

Indications. Propantheline is indicated for the treatment of urinary incontinence associated with overactive bladder or neurogenic bladder.

Adverse Effects. Anticholinergic effects such as dry mouth, constipation, diarrhea, headache, dizziness, anxiety, vision changes, fatigue, sinusitis, dysuria, and somnolence have occurred. Serious adverse effects include urinary retention, increased ophthalmic pressure, drowsiness, confusion and delirium, heatstroke, hallucinations, seizures, tachycardia, arrhythmias, hypertension, angioedema, and anaphylaxis.

Contraindications. Use propantheline bromide with caution in patients with known bromide hypersensitivity. Propantheline is contraindicated in patients with urinary tract obstruction or bladder obstruction, GI obstruction, myasthenia gravis, or closed-angle glaucoma. Propantheline should be used cautiously in patients with coronary artery disease (CAD) or heart failure because it can result in tachycardia, increasing oxygen demand on the heart.

Monitoring. Monitor serum creatinine/blood urea nitrogen (BUN) prior to and routinely throughout therapy. Monitor for adverse effects, and for exacerbated or new cardiac symptoms or tachycardia.

Cholinergic Agonists

Bethanechol is a synthetic muscarinic stimulant that exerts parasympathomimetic effects by a direct action on muscarinic or cholinergic receptors, all of which can be antagonized by atropine.

Bethanechol

Bethanechol has an effect that is opposite that of the anticholinergics in that it stimulates the parasympathetic nervous system, causing release of acetylcholine at parasympathetic nerve endings. This increases detrusor muscle tone. Increased tone causes a contraction that initiates voiding and bladder emptying, which is useful in some cases of overflow incontinence from urinary retention.

Pharmacokinetics. Bethanechol chloride is administered orally and subcutaneously. It has a poor absorption and both the metabolism and excretion remain unknown. Bethanechol has a half-life of 1 to 6 hours. The onset of action is 30 to 90 minutes and plasma levels are reached at 6 hours. Onset of action occurs within 5 to 15 minutes when given subcutaneously. The effects typically last 2 hours when taken subcutaneously.

Indications. Bethanechol, a urinary cholinergic, is indicated for the short-term treatment of urinary retention.

Adverse Effects. GI adverse effects include abdominal pain or cramps, colicky pain, belching, hypersalivation, diarrhea, flatulence, nausea, vomiting, and borborygmi, from increased tone and peristaltic activity. Bethanechol is a cholinergic agonist with the potential to cause bronchospasm. Urinary urgency and increased urinary frequency can occur. Cardiovascular adverse effects such as increases in blood pressure and sinus tachycardia have occurred. Bethanechol may induce dizziness or the potential for syncope, headache, and seizures.

Contraindications. Bethanechol is contraindicated for use in patients with GI obstruction, ileus, and bladder obstruction or urinary tract obstruction; in patients with inflammatory bowel disease, peritonitis, marked vagotonia, or who have undergone recent GI or bladder surgery; in patients with peptic ulcer disease; and in patients with pronounced bradycardia, hypotension, or CAD. Subcutaneously administered bethanechol can cause orthostatic hypotension and it should be used with caution in patients at risk for syncope. Bethanechol is contraindicated in patients with asthma, and it should be avoided in chronic obstructive pulmonary disease (COPD) because cholinergic stimulation constricts the airways. Bethanechol is also contraindicated in patients with hyperthyroidism, seizure disorder, or parkinsonism as it can exacerbate these conditions. Cholinergic drugs may precipitate atrial fibrillation in patients with hyperthyroidism.

Monitoring. Laboratory monitoring is not needed. Monitor for adverse effects, as well as for exacerbated or new cardiac symptoms or tachycardia.

Other Agents

Onabotulinumtoxin A

OnabotulinumtoxinA blocks neuromuscular conduction by binding to receptor sites on motor nerve terminals, entering nerve terminals, and inhibiting the release of acetylcholine. This toxin is used in urinary incontinence due to detrusor overactivity in patients with an inadequate response or intolerance to an anticholinergic medication. OnabotulinumtoxinA (formerly known as botulinum toxin type A) is an intramuscular toxin produced from fermentation of *Clostridium botulinum* type A. It is used when other agents for the treatment of urinary incontinence have failed, but it is expected to gain approval for more primary care conditions (Gormley & Kaufman, 2016).

Pharmacokinetics. OnabotulinumtoxinA is administered by local intramuscular injection. No systemic effects are expected to occur with this treatment. The onset and duration of action depend on the clinical use of the drug.

Indications. OnabotulinumtoxinA is indicated for the treatment of overactive bladder with symptoms of urge urinary incontinence, urgency, and frequency in adults who are intolerant to or with inadequate response from anticholinergic medications.

Adverse Effects. Adverse reactions typically occur within the first week following injection, and while they are usually transient, some have lasted several months. After using botulinum toxin types A and B, there have been reports of distant toxin effects, including respiratory arrest and death, that are suggestive of systemic botulism. Breathing difficulties may develop within hours to weeks after an injection. Patients with preexisting breathing difficulties may be more susceptible to respiratory complications following onabotulinumtoxinA injection. Serious and/or immediate hypersensitivity reactions have been reported following onabotulinumtoxinA injection, including anaphylactoid reactions, serum sickness, urticaria, soft tissue edema, and dyspnea.

UTI has occurred in 18% of patients, with a higher incidence observed in patients with diabetes. When onabotulinumtoxinA was given for overactive bladder and detrusor overactivity associated with a neurologic condition, the following genitourinary effects were reported within the first 12 weeks after injection: urinary retention, UTI, dysuria, and hematuria.

The formation of neutralizing antibodies to onabotulinumtoxinA may reduce the effectiveness of the toxin by inactivating the biologic activity of the toxin. Receiving injections at more frequent intervals or at higher doses may lead to a greater incidence of antibody formation.

Contraindications. OnabotulinumtoxinA is contraindicated in patients with infection at the injection site, UTI, or those with known hypersensitivity to any ingredient in the formulation. OnabotulinumtoxinA should be used cautiously in patients with cardiac disease as some effects including arrhythmia and myocardial infarction have been reported. The exact relationship of these events to the botulinum toxin injection has not been established. Antiplatelet therapy should be discontinued at least 3 days prior to onabotulinumtoxinA treatment in patients with detrusor overactivity associated with a neurologic condition.

It is not known whether onabotulinumtoxinA is excreted in breast milk, affects the breastfed infant, or affects milk production. The developmental and health benefits of breastfeeding should be considered along with the mother's clinical need for onabotulinumtoxinA and any potential adverse effects on the breastfed infant.

Monitoring. Due to the potential of systemic toxin effects, advise patients or caregivers to seek immediate medical care if swallowing, speech, or respiratory disorders occur. Monitor for skin reactions, reports of adverse cardiac effects, UTI, and infection.

Posterior Pituitary Hormones

The posterior lobe of the pituitary gland produces two hormones: vasopressin and oxytocin. These hormones are released when the hypothalamus sends messages to the pituitary gland through nerve cells. Vasopressin is also known as an antidiuretic hormone (ADH). It is secreted by the hypothalamus in response to physiologic responses such as hyperosmolarity, volume depletion, stress, and painful stimuli. Vasopressin also causes constriction of vascular smooth muscle and contraction of smooth muscle in the GI tract and uterus.

Desmopressin

Desmopressin (1-deamino-8-d-arginine vasopressin; DDAVP) is a synthetic analog of vasopressin that acts as an antidiuretic. Vasopressin is a naturally occurring antidiuretic hormone. Desmopressin is stronger as an antidiuretic than as a vasopressor in smooth muscle. It decreases urine output for about 6 hours in both intranasal and sublingual routes (Pfizer, 2020).

The pharmacologic treatment of primary nocturnal enuresis should be used as an adjunct to behavioral conditioning or other nonpharmacologic interventions. Desmopressin is effective in some cases that are refractory to conventional therapies. Desmopressin has been demonstrated to rapidly reduce the number of "wet nights" per week in children. However, this effect is not maintained after cessation of therapy.

Pharmacokinetics. Desmopressin can be administered by both oral and intranasal routes. The distribution of desmopressin is unknown. It is not clear whether desmopressin crosses the placenta, but desmopressin can be found in breast milk. It is not known how desmopressin is metabolized or excreted. However, desmopressin is primarily excreted in the urine, with a significant portion excreted as unchanged drug (65% after oral and 92% after intranasal administration). The half-life of the intranasal medication is 1.5 to 3 hours; the half-life of the sublingual medication is 2.8 hours. Onset of medication is 60 minutes for intranasal and 30 minutes for sublingual administration. Both routes reach plasma levels in 6 hours.

Indications. Desmopressin is indicated for primary nocturnal enuresis (intranasal), usually in children. However, desmopressin in the treatment of overactive bladder in adults is an unlabeled use. Desmopressin's sublingual administration safety and effectiveness has not been established for pediatric patients.

Adverse Effects. Hyponatremia can be serious and potentially fatal, and it requires prompt and adequate treatment. Due to the potent antidiuretic effects of desmopressin, hyponatremia leading to water intoxication, seizures, and/or coma can occur, especially in older adults or pediatric patients. A dose-related increase in von Willebrand factor VII and t-PA level decreases the activated partial thromboplastin time (aPTT) as well as bleeding time. Transient dose-related flushing, headache, rhinitis, nausea, abdominal pain, and dizziness have been reported. Nasal irritation and nosebleed can occur with intranasal administration.

Contraindications. Desmopressin should not be used in patients with known desmopressin hypersensitivity due to the potential for severe allergic reactions, including anaphylaxis. Desmopressin nasal spray for nocturia is contraindicated in patients with heart failure (New York Heart Association [NYHA] Class II to IV), and should be used with caution (monitoring of volume status) in patients with NYHA Class I heart failure. Both the nasal spray and sublingual tablets for nocturia are contraindicated in patients with uncontrolled hypertension. Desmopressin is contraindicated in patients with moderate to severe renal impairment (CrCl less than 50 mL/minute), in patients with hyponatremia, and in patients with a history of hyponatremia.

Monitoring. Monitor bleeding time, factor VIII concentrations, serum creatinine/BUN, serum sodium, and urine osmolality. Measure serum sodium within 7 days and approximately 1 month after initiating therapy or increasing the dose, and periodically during treatment.

Patients or caregivers should be alerted to monitor for symptoms that may indicate water intoxication. In pediatric patients, seizures are often preceded by headache, nausea, or vomiting that occur in the morning. All patients should be observed for signs and symptoms associated with hyponatremia (headaches, nausea, vomiting, lethargy, disorientation or confusion, altered thinking, and depressed reflexes). Patients with electrolyte or fluid balance abnormalities should be monitored carefully. Particular attention should be paid to the possibility of the rare occurrence of an extreme decrease in plasma osmolality that may result in seizures, leading to coma. Very young patients and older adults should be cautioned to drink only enough fluid to satisfy thirst to decrease the potential for water intoxication and hyponatremia. Children and infants require careful fluid intake restriction to prevent possible hyponatremia and water intoxication while on desmopressin.

Cardiovascular effects have been reported with high intranasal dosage, producing a slight elevation of blood pressure that disappears with dosage reduction. Use with caution in patients with coronary artery insufficiency or hypertensive cardiovascular disease.

Urinary Tract Analgesic Agents

Urinary tract analgesic agents, while not addressing the underlying problem of incontinence, are used for the symptomatic relief of pain, burning, urgency, frequency, and discomfort resulting from irritation of the lower urinary tract mucosa. Urinary tract analgesics are also useful for treating the symptomatic relief of UTI symptoms. The use of these medications for the relief of urinary symptoms should not replace the definitive diagnosis and treatment of the underlying condition.

Phenazopyridine

Phenazopyridine is an oral urinary tract analgesic azo dye that is excreted in the urine, resulting in urine that is orange/red in color, since it exerts a topical analgesic effect on the urinary tract mucosa. It is important to remember that phenazopyridine is only useful for the relief of pain associated with urinary tract conditions. Phenazopyridine is compatible with antibacterial therapy and should only be used short term (2 days) for treatment of UTI until antibiotic action reduces pain.

Pharmacokinetics. The pharmacokinetic profile of phenazopyridine is not fully understood. Phenazopyridine has a poor absorption. Metabolism of phenazopyridine probably occurs in the liver; phenazopyridine is rapidly excreted by the kidneys, with 65% of an oral dose excreted unchanged in the urine. The onset of action is 1 hour and the half-life is 7.35 hours. Serum plasma levels are maintained up to 24 hours. Trace amounts of phenazopyridine are thought to cross the placenta.

Indications. Phenazopyridine is used on a short-term basis for urinary analgesia, usually resulting from an acute UTI, including dysuria.

Adverse Effects. Methemoglobinemia and hemolytic anemia have been reported with the use of phenazopyridine, usually following an overdose. If a patient develops methemoglobinemia, methylene blue should be administered intravenously. Acute renal failure may occur rarely with use of phenazopyridine. Phenazopyridine can cause discoloration of body fluids, including urine. Other adverse effects include headache, rash, pruritus, anaphylactic reactions, and GI disturbances.

Contraindications. Phenazopyridine should not be used in patients who have previously exhibited phenazopyridine hypersensitivity. Phenazopyridine should not be used for more than 2 days in patients being treated for UTI. Phenazopyridine is contraindicated in patients with renal dysfunction, including renal failure. Glucose-6-phosphate dehydrogenase (G6PD) deficiency may predispose patients to hemolysis, so phenazopyridine should not be used in this patient population. There are no adequate and well-controlled studies of phenazopyridine use in pregnant patients; thus, treatment of females of child-bearing potential is not recommended unless negative pregnancy is confirmed.

Monitoring. Monitor for G6PD activity and urinalysis at baseline and throughout treatment (Tables 19.2 and 19.3).

Prescriber Considerations for Urinary Incontinence Therapy

Clinical Practice Guidelines

> **BOOKMARK THIS!**
>
> **Clinical Guidelines for Urinary Incontinence Therapy**
>
> - Brigham and Women's Hospital. Diagnosis, treatment, and prevention of urinary incontinence (available at https://www.brighamandwomens.org/obgyn/urogynecology/diagnosis-treatment-and-prevention-of-urinary-incontinence).
> - Nambian, A. K., Bosch, R., Cruz, F., et al. (2018). EAU guidelines on assessment and nonsurgical management of urinary incontinence. *European Urology, 73*(4), http://www.europeanurology.com/article/S0302-2838(18)30002-2/fulltext.

Clinical Reasoning for Urinary Incontinence Therapy

Consider the individual patient's health problem requiring urinary incontinence therapy. It is important to determine the type and severity of urinary incontinence the patient has before determining a pharmacologic treatment plan. This includes a thorough history and physical examination that focuses on the urinary system, as well as a urinalysis and post-void residual measurement. In addition, it is recommended that a diary be kept for several days that includes the total fluid intake for each day, the number of times the patient urinates, the total urine output daily, whether the patient experienced urinary urge, and the number of incontinence episodes.

Determine the desired therapeutic outcome based on the degree of urinary incontinence therapy needed for the patient's health problem. For patients with established urinary incontinence, the desired outcome is either a complete resolution of incontinence or a reduction in the number of incontinence episodes. Other important outcomes include pain relief and maintenance of skin integrity.

Assess the appropriateness of the urinary incontinence therapy by considering the medication's side effects and the patient's age, race/ethnicity, comorbidities, and genetic factors. Urinary incontinence occurs most frequently in females, with incidence ranging from 25% to 51% for one episode in the past year; 10% of females report weekly urinary leakage. The incidence of urinary incontinence in males is half that of females. While urinary incontinence is not considered part of normal aging, older adults experience more incidences of urinary incontinence. Comorbid illnesses such as neurologic impairment, glaucoma, mobility issues, prostate disease, and diabetes increase the risk for urinary incontinence. A review of current prescription and over-the-counter (OTC) medications is warranted before prescribing muscarinic medications.

TABLE 19.2 **Medications for Urinary Incontinence**

Drug Category/ Medications	Indication	Dosage	Considerations and Monitoring
Anticholinergics			
Oxybutynin	For the treatment of overactive bladder with symptoms of urge urinary incontinence, urgency frequency, or incontinence	**Immediate-release tablets:** *Adults:* 5 mg orally two or three times daily. *Older adults:* 5 mg orally two or three times daily. Maximum dosage: 20 mg daily. *Adolescents:* 5 mg orally two to four times daily. *Children 5–12 yr:* 5 mg orally twice daily. Maximum dosage: 15 mg daily. *Children 1–4 yr:* 0.2 mg/kg/day orally, given in divided doses. **Extended-release tablets:** *Adults:* 5–10 mg orally once daily initially. May adjust weekly by 5-mg increments. Maximum dosage: 30 mg/day. *Children and adolescents 6–17 yr:* 5 mg orally once daily initially. May adjust weekly by 5-mg increments. Maximum dosage: 20 mg/day.	Monitor for ocular pain and genitourinary, psychiatric, and cardiovascular effects.
Darifenacin	For the treatment of overactive bladder with symptoms of urge urinary incontinence, urgency frequency, or incontinence	**Extended-release formulation:** *Adults:* 7.5 mg orally once daily. May increase to 15 mg orally once daily after 2 weeks based on individual response. Maximum dosage: 15 mg/day orally. Do not exceed 7.5 mg/day orally in patients taking potent CYP 3A4 inhibitors.	Monitor for hypersensitivity reactions and urinary retention.
Solifenacin	For the treatment of overactive bladder with symptoms of urge urinary incontinence, urgency frequency, or incontinence	*Adults:* 5 mg orally daily. May increase to 10 mg orally once daily. Maximum dosage: 10 mg/day. In patients taking potent inhibitors of CYP 3A4, do not exceed 5 mg daily.	Monitor for hypersensitivity and ocular adverse events.
Trospium	For the treatment of overactive bladder with symptoms of urge urinary incontinence, urgency frequency, or incontinence	*Adults:* 20 mg orally twice daily. *Older adults:* 20 mg orally twice daily. *Children and adolescents ≥5 yr:* Dose not definitively established; however, dose range of 10–25 mg/day orally given in 2 divided doses has been suggested. **Extended-release formulation:** *Adults:* 60 mg orally once daily in the morning.	Monitor serum creatinine before and throughout treatment. Monitor for adverse effects including constipation, urinary retention, cardiovascular issues, and hypersensitivity.
Fesoterodine	For the treatment of overactive bladder with symptoms of urge urinary incontinence, urgency frequency, or incontinence	**Extended-release formulation:** *Adults:* 4 mg orally once daily initially. May increase to 8 mg orally once daily. Maximum dosage: 8 mg/day.	Monitor for anticholinergic-related adverse effects.

Continued

TABLE 19.2   Medications for Urinary Incontinence—cont'd

Drug Category/ Medications	Indication	Dosage	Considerations and Monitoring
Antispasmodics			
Flavoxate	For the symptomatic relief of dysuria, urinary urgency, nocturia, suprapubic pain, urinary frequency, and urinary incontinence	*Adults, adolescents, and children ≥12 yr:* 100–200 mg three or four times daily.	Monitor for urinary retention, increased ophthalmic pressure, drowsiness, confusion and delirium, seizures, tachycardia, arrhythmias, hypertension, angioedema, and anaphylaxis.
Propantheline	For the treatment of urinary incontinence	*Adults:* 7.5–30 mg orally three to five times daily.	Monitor serum creatinine/BUN. Monitor for adverse effects, including tachycardia.
Cholinergics			
Bethanechol	For the treatment of acute postoperative postpartum nonobstructive urinary retention and treatment of atonic neurogenic bladder	**Oral:** *Adults:* The usual dosage is 10–50 mg orally three or four times daily. *Children:* 0.6 mg/kg/day orally in 3–4 divided doses. **Subcutaneous:** *Adults:* The usual dose is 5 mg subcutaneously three or four times daily as needed. *Children:* Safety and efficacy not established.	Laboratory monitoring is not needed. Monitor for adverse effects, monitor for exacerbated or new cardiac symptoms or tachycardia.
Other Agents			
OnabotulinumtoxinA	For the treatment of symptoms associated with overactive bladder	**Intramuscular:** *Adults:* The recommended and maximum dose is 100 units IM per treatment injected into the detrusor muscle.	Monitor for skin reactions, reports of adverse cardiac effects, UTI, and infection.
Posterior Pituitary Hormones			
Desmopressin	For the treatment of primary nocturnal enuresis	**Intranasal:** *Adults:* 20 mcg (0.2 mL) intranasally of 0.01% nasal solution at bedtime; one-half of the dose is administered into each nostril. If no response after 3 days, adjust the dose upward to 40 mcg/day (20 mcg per nostril) intranasally at bedtime. Typical maintenance dose is 10–40 mcg/day (0.1–0.4 mL/day). **Oral:** *Adults:* 0.2 mg orally once daily at bedtime. Doses may be titrated up to 0.6 mg orally once daily at bedtime.	Desmopressin should not be administered in patients with a CrCl <50 mL/min. Monitor serum sodium with the first week and again at 1 month after initiating or resuming therapy. Monitor bleeding time, factor VIII concentrations, serum creatinine/BUN, and urine osmolality. Fluid restriction should be observed, and fluid intake should be limited to a minimum from 1 hour before administration until the next morning, or at least 8 hours after administration. Monitor for hyponatremia, water intoxication, and hypertension.

TABLE 19.2 Medications for Urinary Incontinence—cont'd

Drug Category/ Medications	Indication	Dosage	Considerations and Monitoring
Urinary Tract Analgesics			
Phenazopyridine	For the symptomatic relief of dysuria, urinary urgency, and irritation	200 mg orally three times daily after meals for 2 days.	Only use this medication for 2 days. Monitor for G6PD activity and urinalysis at baseline and throughout treatment.

BUN, Blood urea nitrogen; *CrCl*, creatine clearance; *G6PD*, glucose-6-phosphate dehydrogenase.

TABLE 19.3 Common Adverse Effects of Medications Used for Urinary Incontinence

Medication	Common Side Effects	Serious Adverse Effects
Anticholinergics	Dry mouth, constipation, headache, dizziness, anxiety, vision changes, fatigue, dysuria	Urinary retention, increased intraocular pressure, drowsiness, confusion and delirium, heatstroke, hallucinations, seizures, tachycardia, arrhythmias, hypertension, anaphylaxis, angioedema
Propantheline	Anticholinergic effects	Anaphylaxis
Flavoxate	Anticholinergic effects and antispasmodic effects (nausea, vomiting, nervousness, vertigo)	Tachycardia, leukopenia, confusion, respiratory distress
Bethanechol	Flushing, sweating, abdominal cramps, colicky pain, nausea, belching, diarrhea, borborygmi, salivation, lacrimation, malaise, urinary urgency, headache	Bronchial constriction, asthma, miosis, orthostatic hypotension, tachycardia, seizures
Desmopressin	Flushing, headache, rhinitis, nausea, abdominal pain, dizziness; nasal irritation, nosebleed when given intranasally	Severe fluid overload and hyponatremia, seizures, anaphylaxis, thrombosis
Phenazopyridine	Headache, rash, pruritus, nausea, vertigo, GI disturbances, discoloration of body fluids, staining of contact lenses	Anaphylaxis, anaphylactoid reaction, renal and hepatic toxicity, anemia

GI, Gastrointestinal.

Initiate the treatment plan with the selected medication by first providing adequate patient education to ensure the patient's understanding and promote full participation in the urinary incontinence therapy. The pharmacologic treatment plan should be instituted in accordance with the clinical guidelines for the specific type of UI. In addition to any planned pharmacologic treatment plan, teaching the patient/family behavioral therapy options should be included as appropriate to each specific patient and their type of urinary incontinence. Behavioral strategies include strengthening pelvic floor muscles, bladder training to lengthen the time between toileting to every 2.5 to 3.5 hours, double voiding, scheduled toileting, and fluid management. Along with pharmacologic agents, the assessment and treatment of vaginal atrophy may be needed to fully resolve urinary incontinence in females.

Ensure complete patient and family understanding about the medication prescribed for urinary incontinence therapy using a variety of education strategies. To promote understanding of the underlying cause, use pictorials of the urinary tract and bladder, reinforce medication regimens with teach-back strategies, and provide written instructions.

Conduct follow-up and monitoring of patient responses to urinary incontinence therapy. Follow-up is dependent on the type and underlying cause of the urinary incontinence. Refer patients to a specialist if they have abdominal or pelvic pain, or hematuria without an infectious cause. Refer patients to a gynecologist for a continence pessary. In general, patient follow-up can be monthly until the issue is resolved or the treatment goal is reached.

Teaching Points for Urinary Incontinence Therapy

Health Promotion Strategies

Treatment for urinary incontinence may be short or long term. The following strategies and practices should be presented to patients to help them become full partners in their health care.

- Maintain adequate hydration, especially if urinary stasis or infection is the underlying problem.
- Reduce caffeine intake, as caffeine-containing fluids have a diuretic effect that can contribute to incontinence.
- You may need to cut back on or avoid alcohol and acidic foods. Reducing liquid consumption, losing weight, or increasing physical activity also can ease the problem.
- Maintain adequate fluid and fiber intake to prevent constipation.
- Avoid hot environments (saunas, spas, hot tubs) to prevent suppression of sweat gland activity and increased risk for heatstroke. This is a particular problem for older adults because of age-related reduction in sweat gland activity.
- Institute a frequent toileting schedule. This strategy can be helpful even in patients who lack the cognitive ability to recognize the need to void.
- Do any recommended pelvic floor exercises in the morning.

Patient Education for Medication Safety

- Remember that urinary analgesic medications such as phenazopyridine can color body fluids orange or red and may stain clothing and contact lenses. These medications should not be used for more than 2 days.
- Avoid driving or participating in other hazardous activities until you know how the medication will affect you.
- Dry mouth may be relieved by sugar-free gum or hard candy.
- If you live in areas of high environmental temperature, your risk for heatstroke is increased because of suppression of sweat gland activity.
- Do not crush extended-release medications.
- Report any inability to urinate, retention of urine, or jaundice to your primary care provider right away.

Application Questions for Discussion

1. Since a focused history with a careful physical examination is essential for determining the cause of urinary incontinence, what are some transient or reversible causes that should be ruled out?
2. To ensure patient safety, what is some patient teaching regarding response and side effects of urinary incontinence medications?
3. As a health care provider, what are some safety concerns regarding posterior pituitary hormones for the treatment of urinary incontinence?

Selected Bibliography

Allergan, Inc. (2012). *Sanctura (trospium chloride): Prescribing information.* Retrieved from https://www.accessdata.fda.gov/drugsatfda_docs/label/2012/021595s009lbl.pdf.

ALZA Corporation. (2008). *Ditropan (oxybutynin chloride): Prescribing information.* Retrieved from https://www.accessdata.fda.gov/drugsatfda_docs/label/2008/017577s034,018211s017,020897s018lbl.pdf.

Aoki, Y., Brown, H. W., Brubaker, L., Cornu, J. N., Daly, J. O., & Cartwright, R. (2017). Urinary incontinence in women. *Nature Reviews Disease Primers, 3,* 17042. https://doi.org/10.1038/nrdp.2017.42.

Astellas Pharma US, Inc. (2019). *VESIcare-Solifenacin succinate: Prescribing information.* Retrieved from https://www.vesicare.com/.

Brigham and Women's Hospital (2020). *Diagnosis, treatment, and prevention of urinary incontinence.* Retrieved from https://www.brighamandwomens.org/obgyn/urogynecology/diagnosis-treatment-and-prevention-of-urinary-incontinence.

Demaagd, G. A., & Davenport, T. C. (2012). Management of urinary incontinence. *Pharmacy and Therapeutics, 37*(6), 345–361H. PMID: 22876096.

Drugbank. (2020). *Phenazopyridine.* Retrieved from https://www.drugbank.ca/drugs/DB01438.

ERFA Canada. (2015). *Pyridium (Phenazopyridine Hydrochloride: Product Monograph.)* Retrieved from https://reference.medscape.com/drug/azo-standard-pyridium-phenazopyridine-343349.

Gormley, E. A., & Kaufman, M. (2016). *Medical student curriculum: Urinary incontinence.* American Urological Association. Retrieved from https://www.auanet.org/education/auauniversity/for-medical-students/medical-students-curriculum/medical-student-curriculum/urinary-incontinence.

Novartis Pharmaceuticals. (2008). *Enablex (darifenacin): Prescribing information.* Retrieved from https://www.accessdata.fda.gov/drugsatfda_docs/label/2008/021513s005lbl.pdf.

Paladin Labs, Inc. (2009). *Duvoid (bethanechol chloride): Prescribing information.* Retrieved from https://www.paladin-labs.com/our_products/Duvoid_en.pdf.

Pfizer, Inc. (2020). *Desmopressin acetate: Ampul US physician prescribing information.* Retrieved from http://labeling.pfizer.com/ShowLabeling.aspx?id=4403.

Pfizer, Inc. (2012). *Toviaz (fesoterodine fumarate): Prescribing information.* Retrieved from https://www.accessdata.fda.gov/drugsatfda_docs/label/2012/022030s009lbl.pdf.

Prescriber's Digital Reference (PDR), LLC. (2020). *Flavoxate hydrochloride—Drug summary.* Retrieved from https://www.pdr.net/drug-summary/Flavoxate-Hydrochloride-flavoxate-hydrochloride-3592.

Prescriber's Digital Reference (PDR), LLC. (2020). *Oxybutynin chloride—Drug summary.* Retrieved from https://www.pdr.net/drug-summary/Oxybutynin-Chloride-Tablets-oxybutynin-chloride-2401.207.

Wilson, J. A., & Waghel, R. C. (2016). The management of urinary incontinence. *Urology/Nephrology, 42*(9), 22–26.

20

Contraceptive Medications

BRENDA GILMORE

Overview

Female reproduction is an intricate interplay of neuro-endocrine, ovarian, and uterine elements (Hall, 2019). A divergence in ovarian, uterine, and neuroendocrine function can significantly impact fertility. Fertility management is dynamic, complex, and continually evolving, with many contraceptive choices. Current prescription contraceptive options include hormonal contraceptives composed of both estrogen and progesterone and referred to as combination hormonal contraceptives (CHCs), and progestin-only contraceptive options. Long-acting reversible contraceptives (LARCs) encompass hormonal and nonhormonal intrauterine devices (IUDs). There are varying rates of effectiveness, indications for treatment, risks, and benefits for all the options available. Understanding patient characteristics and patient preferences as well as the effect of contraceptive agents on the reproductive system will assist in the decision-making process when prescribing contraception.

Relevant Physiology

Normal female reproduction encompasses repetitive menstrual cycles involving ovarian follicular development, ovulation, corpus luteum formation, and endometrium preparation for potential implantation. The neuroendocrine axis has a well-defined pattern throughout the menstrual cycle when ovulation occurs. The cyclic ovulatory pattern is propagated by precise hormonal integration among the hypothalamus, pituitary, and ovary. The first half of the cycle, the *follicular phase*, is dominated by increasing levels of estrogen secreted by the ovaries. Affected by the estrogen, the hypothalamus secretes gonadotropin-releasing hormone (GnRH) in a pulsatile fashion. This stimulates the release of the follicle-stimulating hormone (FSH) and luteinizing hormone (LH) by the anterior pituitary, resulting in recruitment and development of ovarian follicles and emergence of a dominant follicle. This midcycle surge of LH and FSH ultimately propels ovulation. The second half of the cycle, the *luteal phase*, is characterized by the formation of the corpus luteum. Progesterone produced by the corpus luteum dominates the luteal phase. However, the corpus luteum has a limited life span, and without conception and implantation, its function ceases, progesterone levels decline, and FSH levels rise to start a new cycle (Hall, 2019; Lessey & Young, 2019).

Ovarian function in the follicular phase progresses with the stimulation of FSH and LH, resulting in follicular recruitment and development. Ultimately, one dominant follicle emerges and produces the most estrogen. The other follicles undergo atresia. During the ovulation phase, the dominant follicle ruptures and the egg is released. In the luteal phase, the ruptured follicle becomes the corpus luteum. The corpus luteum produces large amounts of progesterone. Without fertilization, the corpus luteum rapidly deteriorates. The sharp decline in progesterone induces menstruation (Strauss & Williams, 2019).

The uterine lining, or endometrium, responds to the cyclic changes throughout the cycle as well. The first phase of the menstrual cycle for the uterus is the proliferative phase. Estrogen stimulates the endometrium to thicken and increase the number of progesterone receptors. The second phase of the menstrual cycle for the uterus is the secretory phase (Molina, 2018). Progesterone induces endometrial differentiation preparation for fertilization and implantation. Again, without pregnancy, the endometrium sloughs, resulting in menstruation (Lessey & Young, 2019).

There are significant changes to cervical mucus during ovulation. The cervical glands normally produce thick mucus that acts as a barrier to sperm and ascending infections. During ovulation, the elevated estrogen level changes the consistency of the cervical mucus, making it stretchy and thin. The cervical mucus serves as a direct conduit and reservoir for sperm, increasing the potential for fertilization for 24 to 72 hours (Hoffman et al., 2016).

Fertilization of the released egg leads to zygote formation. The zygote is propelled through the fallopian tube via cilia movement and smooth muscle contractions. The ruptured ovarian follicle reorganizes as the corpus luteum. The secretion of human chorionic gonadotropin (hCG) from the implanting embryo rescues the corpus luteum (Lessey

& Young, 2019; Strauss & Williams, 2019). The corpus luteum functions as a temporary endocrine gland, excreting estrogen and progesterone to maintain the early stages of pregnancy (Molina, 2018).

Pathophysiology

If ovulation does not occur during the menstrual cycle, this results in anovulation, the most common cause of menstrual irregularities. Anovulation frequently presents as *amenorrhea* or several months without menses, followed by irregular spotting and episodes of heavy, painless vaginal bleeding. Amenorrhea is differentiated as primary and secondary. *Primary amenorrhea* is defined as no menstrual cycle by age 16. *Secondary amenorrhea* is defined as a period of three to six months in a female who has a history of menstruation. Pregnancy, ovarian insufficiency, polycystic ovarian syndrome (PCOS), and hyperprolactinemia are some of the underlying causes for anovulation and amenorrhea (Wilson et al., 2017).

Dysmenorrhea, a common problem for menstruating females, is defined as painful abdominal cramps associated with menstruation. Dysmenorrhea can be mild, moderate, or severe. With severe symptoms, dysmenorrhea can be debilitating and significantly impact quality of life. Dysmenorrhea is differentiated as primary or secondary. *Primary dysmenorrhea*, the most common type, is related to excess prostaglandin release associated with ovulation. *Secondary dysmenorrhea* originates from underlying pathology other than just ovulation. Some common gynecologic causes include endometriosis, fibroids, and pelvic inflammatory disease (PID). Secondary dysmenorrhea tends to worsen over time (Zielinski & Lynne, 2017).

Endometriosis is a chronic condition in which endometrial glands and stroma migrate outside the uterine cavity. Common sites for endometriosis include the peritoneum, adnexa, and rectovaginal septum. However, any structure in the abdomen can potentially be affected. Cyclic hormonal stimulation of the endometrial glands causes inflammation and bleeding, potentially resulting in damage and scarring to the surrounding tissue. The most common sequelae of endometriosis are chronic pelvic pain and infertility (Laubach & Lorntson, 2013).

Premenstrual mood disorders include premenstrual syndrome (PMS) and premenstrual dysphoric disorder (PMDD). Both disorders encompass recurrent psychological and physical symptoms from the end of the luteal phase to menstruation (Leo et al., 2016). Common psychological symptoms include anxiety, sadness, sudden crying, irritability, and lack of mental focus. Physical symptoms include fatigue, breast swelling and tenderness, headache, and changes in eating behaviors (Kaiser et al., 2018). Variations in symptom expression are vast and patient specific. When symptoms are mild and self-managed, the syndrome is classified as *PMS*. When psychological symptoms interfere with everyday life and relationships, the syndrome is called *PMDD* (Leo et al., 2016).

Contraceptive Therapy

Prescribed contraception employs one or more synthetic steroid-based hormonal agents to affect female fertility by impacting ovarian and uterine function. These active agents include synthetic estrogen and progesterone. Exogenous estrogen formulations include a natural estrogen, estradiol valerate (EV2), and a synthetic derivative of estradiol (E2), ethinyl estradiol (EE) (Sitruk-Ware & Nath, 2013). EE is the most commonly used estrogen component for contraceptive agents in the United States (Mattison et al., 2014). Progestin agents were devised to mimic the actions of endogenous progesterone and are available in many forms that have been developed over more than 50 years. For contraceptive medications, they are employed either alone or in conjunction with an estrogen component.

Combination Hormonal Contraception

CHCs, composed of both a progestin and estrogen component, are well known for their cycle control and fertility management. With optimal use they are between 91% and 94% effective. The primary mechanisms of action include inhibiting pituitary secretion of FSH and LH and suppressing ovulation; however, both components have specific contributory pharmacodynamics. The progestin component inhibits ovulation by suppressing LH secretion, impedes sperm migration by thickening cervical mucus, and inhibits implantation by decreasing fallopian tube motility and thinning the endometrial lining (Chrousos, 2017). The estrogen component prevents ovulation with FSH suppression and provides endometrial stabilization. This endometrial support minimizes irregular or breakthrough bleeding and facilitates menstrual cycle management (Cunningham et al., 2018).

CHCs are available in several forms, including oral tablets, transdermal patches, and a vaginal ring. All forms have a similar mechanism of action. However, due to specific characteristics in delivery and absorption for each method, there are variations in pharmacokinetics, adverse effects, contraindications, and considerations for patient selection and management.

Combined Oral Contraceptives (COCs)

A variety of COCs are available. Mainstay COCs have 21 to 24 days of active hormone pills followed by 4 to 7 hormone-free days, either by omitting pills or taking placebo pills. Hormonal-withdrawal vaginal bleeding is expected during the hormone-free days. Extended-cycle formulations are also available that have hormone-free days only 0 to 4 times per year (Curtis et al., 2016a; Colquitt & Martin, 2017; Worly et al., 2018). There are numerous variations in hormonal composition of the COC options currently available. *Monophasic* options have fixed amounts of synthetic estrogen and progesterone for the entire cycle. *Multiphasic* options vary the amounts of synthetic hormones throughout the cycle to minimize dosages, reduce side effects, and more adequately mimic the natural menstrual cycle (Colquitt & Martin, 2017).

Pharmacokinetics. COCs are rapidly and completely absorbed. Synthetic estrogen agents bind primarily to albumin and, to some extent, sex hormone binding globulin (SHBG). Most of the first-, second-, and third-generation progestin agents bind primarily to SHBG, and fourth-generation progestins bind to albumin. Both hormonal agents in COCs are metabolized hepatically, typically through cytochrome (CYP) 3A4 pathways, subject to first-pass metabolism and enterohepatic circulation, and excreted as metabolites through urine and feces.

The primary synthetic estrogen used in COCs, EE, is a potent estrogenic agent due to the ability of the ethinyl chemical structure to inhibit first-pass hepatic metabolism. It has a longer half-life and increased tissue retention, and it exerts a stronger estrogen effect compared to natural estrogens (Sitruk-Ware & Nath, 2013; Mattison et al., 2014). EE peak plasma levels occur within 1 to 2 hours after ingestion, and a secondary peak can often be observed 10 to 14 hours later as a consequence of enterohepatic recirculation. The mean oral bioavailability of EE is approximately 45%, with significant variability in individual absorption in the range of 20% to 65% (Mattison et al., 2014). The EE dose ranges from 15 mcg to 50 mcg. Lower dosages are congruent with fewer side effects (Colquitt & Martin, 2017).

A natural estrogen used in COCs, E2V, is a 17b estradiol prodrug and it is quantitatively and qualitatively similar to E2. With oral administration, E2V is split to form 17b-estradiol and valeric acid both in the intestinal mucosa and via first-pass hepatic metabolism. The 17b-estradiol is further metabolized to active metabolites, estrone, estrone glucuronide, and estrone sulfate. E2V has a plasma peak of 6 hours and a half-life of 14 hours (Sitruk-Ware & Nath, 2013). The E2V dose is 1 to 3 mg and is currently only available in combination with dienogest.

Once absorbed, synthetic estrogens exert their effects through interaction with estrogen receptors (ERs). ERs are present in the reproductive system in the breast and the uterus, as well as in many nonreproductive system sites such as the central nervous system (CNS), including the hypothalamus and the pituitary gland, the liver, the kidneys, adipose tissue, the immune system, and the cardiovascular system.

The chemical structure of progestin agents currently available is similar to testosterone, progesterone, or spironolactone. There are four consecutive generations, and the goal for each new generation is for the progestin agents to act more specifically like endogenous progesterone (Toit et al., 2017). Absorption rates, bioavailability, and half-lives of oral progestin agents vary based on COC formulation and progestin type (Table 20.1).

Synthetic progestin agents affect their intracellular actions via the progesterone receptors (PRs) in reproductive tissue. Some progestins have a stronger agonistic PR impact than others. Most progestins have an antiestrogenic effect, but a few also bind with ERs with a mild additive effect. Many progestins also bind to other steroid receptors, such

as the glucocorticoid receptors (GR), androgen receptors (AR), and mineralocorticoid receptors (MRs), in nonreproductive tissues (Table 20.2). Progestin-related side effects are most likely due to binding to the other receptors in the steroid family in nonreproductive sites. The systemic effect of the COC components on steroid receptors informs the impact of these estrogen and progestin synthetic agents on multiple body systems (Table 20.3).

Indications. COCs are the most common contraceptive methods used in the United States (Cunningham et al., 2018). The primary indication is to prevent pregnancy. COCs are easy to initiate and they are readily reversible, allowing for autonomy and flexibility in family planning. However, patient adherence, proper agent administration, and self-management can be difficult for some patients (Leo et al., 2016).

COCs are also employed routinely to manage irregular cycles and heavy vaginal bleeding. The synergistic effects of the synthetic estrogen and progestin components suppress ovarian function and stabilize the endometrium, providing menstrual cycle management with reduced menstrual flow and shortened length of menses (Cunningham et al., 2018). The inherent reduction in endometrial thickness and the inhibition of prostaglandin production also renders COCs instrumental in the management of dysmenorrhea and endometriosis (Leo et al., 2016).

COCs have been used for PMS symptoms as treatment. PMS and PMDD are closely correlated with ovulatory cycles, and they may be managed by inhibiting ovulation. However, some of the known hormonal side effects of COCs are similar to the physical symptoms of PMS and PMDD, limiting the effectiveness of treatment in some patients (Cunningham et al., 2018; Leo et al., 2016). Lastly, COCs encompassing progestins with antiandrogenic properties have been shown to effectively treat hirsutism related to PCOS (Barrionuevo et al., 2018).

Adverse Effects. Common side effects can be specifically related to the estrogen or progestin components of the contraceptive agent. Typical estrogen-related side effects include breast tenderness, nausea, headache, and weight gain. Estrogenic effects also include potential water retention and elevated blood pressure; however, progestins with anti-MR properties can counteract these effects to some extent (Africander et al., 2011).

Progestin side effects are directly related to their chemical structure and steroid receptor propensity (see Table 20.2). Progestins with androgenic properties produce side effects such as acne and adverse changes in lipid metabolism. Progestins with antiandrogenic properties counteract these side effects but induce lower testosterone levels, potentially decreasing libido and increasing bone loss. Progestins that have an agonistic effect on GR receptors may also potentiate bone loss and alter immune function (Africander et al., 2011).

Known COC side effects can range from mild to moderate to severe. Mild symptoms include nausea, mastalgia, breakthrough bleeding, and mild headache. More significant

TABLE 20.1	Progestin Formulations				
Method Configuration	Progestin	Generation	Dosage	Bioavailability and Half-Life	Progestin Pharmacokinetics
Structurally Related to Testosterone					
COC with estradiol valerate	Dienogest (DNG)	4th	2–3 mg	91% 13 hr	Metabolized by CYP 3A4
COC with EE	Desogestrel (DSG)	3rd	0.1–0.15 mg	84% >38 hr	Converts to 3-keto-desogestrel; metabolized via CYP 2C9 and converts to etonogestrel, then metabolized by CYP 3A4
COC with EE	Ethynodiol diacetate	1st	1 mg	33%–55% 19–24 hr	Rapidly converted to norethindrone (active) and other metabolites
Vaginal ring with EE	Etonogestrel (ETG)	3rd	0.12 mg/day	100% 29 hr	Metabolite of desogestrel and metabolized hepatically via CYP 3A4
Subdermal implant			35 mcg/day	100% 25 hr	
COC with EE	Levonorgestrel (LNG)	2nd	0.05–0.15 mg	100% 22–49 hr	Forms conjugated and unconjugated metabolites
COC with EE	Norethindrone (NET)	1st	0.4–1.5 mg	33%–55% 19–24 hr	Undergoes hepatic reduction and conjugation
Progestin-only OC			0.35 mg		
COC with EE	Norgestimate (NORG)	3rd	0.18–0.25 mg	2 hr	Hepatic reduction to active metabolites norelgestromin and norgestrel
Transdermal patch with EE	Norelgestromin	2nd	0.15 mg	28 hr	Hepatic metabolism
Structure Similar to Progesterone					
Three-month injection	Medroxyprogesterone acetate (MPA)	1st	150 mg IM	10% 50 days	Metabolized extensively hepatically via hydroxylation and conjugation Does not bind with SHBG
Vaginal ring with EE	Segesterone acetate (nesterone/NES)	4th	0.15 mg/day	5 hr	Metabolized hepatically via CYP 3A4; does not bind with SHBG
Spironolactone Analogue					
COC with EE	Drospirenone (DSRP)	4th	3–4 mg	78% 30 hr	Metabolized hepatically via CYP 3A4; does not bind with SHBG

COC, Combined oral contraceptive; *EE,* ethinyl estradiol; *OC,* oral contraceptive; *SHBG,* sex hormone binding globulin.

or moderate effects encompass worsening migraine headaches, depression, persistent breakthrough bleeding, weight fluctuations, skin hyperpigmentation, and recurrent vaginal infections. Severe adverse effects have the potential to result in significant medical implications and can be life threatening, especially in patients with preexisting risk factors. These include cholestatic disease, hypertension, venous thromboembolic disease, myocardial infarction, and cerebrovascular disease (Chrousos, 2017).

Contraindications. Not every female who needs contraception is a candidate for COCs. The Centers for Disease Control and Prevention (CDC) offers specific medical

| TABLE 20.2 | Specific Progestin Steroid Receptor Properties |

Receptor						
Generation/ Progestin	Progesterone (PR)	Androgen (AR)	Anti-androgen (Anti-AR)	Anti-Mineralocorticoid (Anti-MR)	Glucocorticoid (GR)	Estrogen (ER)
1st MPA	++	+/-	-	-	+	-
NET	++	+	-	-	-	+/-
2nd LNG	++	+	-	+/-	-	+/-
3rd DSG	+	+	-	+/-	+/-	-
NORG	+	+/-	-	-	-	-
4th DNG	+	-	+	-	-	+/-
DSRP	++	-	+	+	-	-
NES	++	-	+	-	-	-

++ Strong effect.
+ Moderate effect.
+/- Weak effect.
- No effect.
DNG, Dienogest; *DSG*, desogestrel; *DSRP*, drospirenone; *LNG*, levonorgestrel; *MPA*, medroxyprogesterone acetate; *NES*, nesterone; *NET*, norethindrone; *NORG*, norgestimate;
From Africander, D., Verhoog, N., & Hapgood, J. P. [2011]. Molecular mechanisms of steroid receptor-mediated actions by synthetic progestins used in HRT and contraception. *Steroids, 76*[7], 638–652.

| TABLE 20.3 | Systemic Pharmacologic Effects of Combination Hormonal Contraceptives |

Reproductive System		Other Systems	
Endocrine	Ovulation suppression Changes in libido Increased sex hormone binding globulin Decreased testosterone	Central Nervous	Increased excitability that may cause: Moodiness Irritability Headaches
Ovarian	Decrease in ovary size Minimal follicular development	Hepatic	Altered drug metabolism Altered lipid and carbohydrate metabolism Changes in bile composition that may increase the risk of cholelithiasis
Uterus	Thickening of cervical mucus Endometrial thinning and glandular atrophy	Cardiovascular/ Hematologic	Increased heart rate and blood pressure Increase in certain clotting factors that may increase the risk of thromboembolic events
Breast	Mild stimulation that may cause: Tenderness Enlargement	Integumentary	Decreased sebum production and acne Increased pigmentation that may cause chloasma

From Chrousos, G. P. [2017]. The gonadal hormones and inhibitors. In B. G. Katzung (Ed.), *Basic & Clinical Pharmacology* [14th ed.]. New York: McGraw-Hill.

eligibility criteria for females with increased risk related to certain individual characteristics and medical conditions (Curtis et al., 2016b). These recommendations are based on an estradiol dose of 35 mcg. Patient conditions are classified into four categories. The first category includes conditions in which there is no restriction of use. The second category includes conditions in which the benefits of the hormonal contraceptive outweigh any inherent risk. The third category includes conditions in which the risks most likely outweigh the benefits, and the fourth category includes conditions that lead to unacceptable health risks should the contraceptive method be employed. Notable conditions that are classified as belonging in the fourth category and that exclude females from using CHCs include:

1. An increased risk of cardiovascular disease
   a. Females older than 35 years of age who smoke
   b. Hypertension
   c. Dyslipidemia
   d. Diabetes
   e. History of ischemic cardiovascular disease
2. Severe hepatic disease/cirrhosis
3. Breast cancer
4. Migraine with neurological sequelae such as aura
5. High risk for venous thromboembolism (VTE)
   a. History of a VTE
   b. Genetic predisposition to VTE
   c. Less than 21 days postpartum

PRACTICE PEARLS

COC Use and Obesity

Females with a body mass index (BMI) greater than 30 are classified as obese. There is limited research on the impact of COC use in obese females. Evidence suggests that obese females may have an increased risk of developing a VTE, but they are not at higher risk for acute myocardial infarction or stroke (Curtis et al., 2016). Evidence also does not support that obese females are more likely to gain weight (Curtis et al., 2016). There is inconsistent evidence that suggests there may be a small reduction in the effectiveness of some COC formulations related to increased basal metabolism, drug clearance, and steroid hormone storage in adipose tissue. In some cases, other contraceptive options may be considered superior to COCs for overweight and obese females (Patel & Carey, 2018).

Monitoring. With the initiation of COCs over the short term (3 months), follow-up can be helpful to assess adherence and tolerability of the prescribed agent, especially with adolescents or patients who have additional medical conditions. Adjustments in formulation may be warranted if there are significant side effects or irregular vaginal bleeding. Blood pressure and weight changes should be assessed during short-term follow-up and during all routine visits. Once the treatment plan has been established, contraceptive use and satisfaction with the method should be evaluated at subsequent routine visits (Curtis et al., 2016a). Additionally, based on medical eligibility criteria, changes in health status including medical conditions, medications, age, and smoking status that would affect the appropriateness and safety of combined hormonal contraceptive use should be evaluated at regular intervals, at least annually (Curtis et al., 2016b).

PRACTICE PEARLS

COC Use and Lactation

There is limited evidence on the impact of COCs on lactation. Some studies of poor to fair quality showed potential for increased formula supplementation and a shorter breastfeeding duration with the use of COCs. Some studies showed decreased infant weight gain if COCs were started before 6 weeks postpartum. There were no adverse effects on infant outcomes if COCs were initiated after 6 weeks postpartum (Tepper et al., 2016a). Other contraceptive methods should be considered for prior to 6 weeks postpartum to avoid any potential impact on the newborn, and to avoid added maternal VTE risk since it is the highest during this period (Curtis et al., 2016b).

Transdermal Patch

The transdermal contraceptive patch is an adhesive patch that releases 150 mcg of norelgestromin and 20 mcg of EE daily. One patch is applied to the skin on the abdomen, back, or upper arm weekly for 3 weeks. The fourth week is the hormone-free week when no patch is applied (Colquitt & Martin, 2017; Worly et al., 2018).

Pharmacokinetics. Because they are delivered transdermally, EE and norelgestromin are not subject to first-pass metabolism, are rapidly absorbed, and reach a peak response in 48 hours. EE steady-state concentrations are 60% higher using the topical patch when compared to COCs, rendering more consistent hormonal levels. EE binds mainly to albumin. Norelgestromin binds to albumin and its metabolite, norgestrel, binds to SHBG. Both EE and norelgestromin are hepatically metabolized and excreted in the urine and feces.

Indications. The indications for the transdermal contraception patch are consistent with those of COCs. Like COCs, this method is also easy to initiate and readily reversible, allowing for autonomy and flexibility in family planning. The transdermal method of CHC delivery allows for weekly instead of daily administration. Still, adherence, proper agent administration, and self-management can be difficult for some patients (Leo et al., 2016).

Adverse Effects. Adverse effects and bleeding profiles are comparable to COCs. Common adverse reactions reported for this method include irregular vaginal bleeding, nausea, breast tenderness, and headache. Additionally, problems with the patch adhesive including site irritation and patch nonadherence are common concerns with this method (Mylan Pharmaceuticals Inc., 2020).

Contraindications. The contraindications for use of the transdermal patch are consistent with the use of other CHC methods. The CDC medical eligibility criteria highlight females with increased risk related to certain individual characteristics and medical conditions (Curtis et al., 2016b). There is evidence that effectiveness of the contraceptive patch can be reduced in obese women (Dragoman et al.,

2017; Mylan Pharmaceuticals Inc., 2020). Additionally, the risk of venous thromboembolism is greater than with COCs but still very low (Galzote et al., 2017).

Monitoring. Follow-up with transdermal CHCs is consistent with the initiation and routine management of COCs. A change in contraceptive methods may be warranted if there are significant adverse effects or changes in weight, health status, age, or smoking status that would affect the appropriateness and safety of transdermal CHC use. These factors should be evaluated at regular intervals, at least annually (Curtis et al., 2016a).

Vaginal Ring

Flexible and nonbiodegradable, the vaginal ring is currently available in two versions. One version releases etonogestrel (ETG) 0.12 mg daily and EE 0.015 mg daily; the other releases segesterone acetate (NES) 0.15 mg daily and EE 0.013 mg daily for vaginal mucosal absorption. The version with ETG is a disposable ring that is changed once a month. The version containing NES is a vaginal ring that can be reused every month for up to 13 cycles. In both versions, the ring measures 54 cm in diameter and is easily compressed for vaginal insertion. Following insertion, the ring remains in the vagina for 3 weeks and then is removed for 1 week to allow for hormone-withdrawal bleeding (Merck Inc, 2020; Therapeutics MD, 2020).

Pharmacokinetics. Due to transmucosal delivery, all the components of both products are not subject to first-pass metabolism, are rapidly absorbed, and maintain consistent serum levels for 3 weeks. Both progestins are active agents that would be inactive if taken orally. ETG, an active metabolite of desogestrel (DSG), is structurally similar to testosterone. It binds to albumin and to SHBG (Merck Inc, 2020). NES is similar to progesterone and binds mainly to albumin but not to SHBG (TherapeuticsMD, 2020). EE in both systems binds mainly to albumin. For both products, EE and the progestin agents are hepatically metabolized through the CYP 3A4 pathway and are excreted in the urine, bile, and feces (Merck Inc., 2020; TherapeuticsMD, 2020).

Indications. The indications for the vaginal ring are consistent with those of other CHCs. Like other CHCs, this method is easy to initiate and readily reversible, allowing for autonomy and flexibility in family planning. The vaginal ring allows for monthly instead of either weekly or daily administration. Still, adherence, proper ring insertion, and self-management can be difficult for some patients (Merck Inc., 2020).

Adverse Effects. Adverse effects and bleeding profiles are comparable to COCs. Common adverse reactions reported for this method include vaginitis, vaginal discharge, headache, mood changes, and breast tenderness. Additionally, device issues such as a foreign-body sensation and unstable vaginal placement, partner discomfort with intercourse, and spontaneous expulsion have been reported (Merck Inc., 2020).

Contraindications. The contraindications for use of the vaginal ring are consistent with the use of other CHC methods. The CDC medical eligibility criteria highlight females with increased risk related to certain individual characteristics and medical conditions (Curtis et al., 2016b). Method-specific contraindications include the presence of hypersensitive reactions to the components of the vaginal ring and the presence of significant vaginal irritation, erosions, or ulcers (Merck Inc., 2020).

Monitoring. Follow-up with the vaginal ring CHCs is consistent with the initiation and routine management of COCs. A change in contraceptive methods may be warranted if there are undesirable alterations in vaginal health, significant adverse effects, or changes in weight, health status, age, or smoking status that would affect the appropriateness and safety of transvaginal CHC use. These factors should be evaluated at regular intervals, at least annually (Curtis et al., 2016a).

Progestin-Only Contraception

Progestin-only contraceptives (POCs) are composed of a specific synthetic progesterone without a synthetic estrogen. POCs have three primary mechanisms of action. The primary function of the synthetic progestins is the suppression of LH, inhibiting ovulation. The extent of ovulation suppression is dependent on the specific POC formulation. The two other effects include thickened cervical mucus, retarding sperm passage, and endometrial thinning and atrophy, inhibiting implantation.

Without the estrogen component to stabilize the endometrium, irregular vaginal bleeding is common with POCs. However, progestin agents are known for their protective, antiproliferative action on the endometrium. They are very effective in pregnancy prevention, with rates ranging from 91% to 99%, and they can be used by patients who have medical conditions or elevated VTE risk and who are not candidates for estrogen-containing contraceptives (Colquitt & Martin, 2017; Cunningham et al., 2018).

POCs are available in several forms, including the pill, 3-month injection, subdermal implant, and IUD. Though all forms have similar mechanisms of action, the higher dosing inherent in the injection and subdermal implant forms imposes a greater amount of ovarian suppression than lower-dose POC options (Jacobstien & Polis, 2014; Zigler & McNicholas, 2017). As with the various CHC options, specific characteristics in delivery and absorption for each POC method can impact the pharmacokinetics, adverse effects, contraindications, and considerations for patient selection and management.

Oral Progestin Contraceptives

Oral progestin contraception is available in a monophasic formulation. This option is a 28-day cycle of 35 mcg of norethindrone (NET) daily with no hormone-free week. Due to the short half-life and duration of action of oral NET, it is less effective in inhibiting ovulation than other POCs. Its mechanism of action is more reliant on thickening cervical mucus and endometrial atrophy. Consistently timed, daily use of oral progestin agents is imperative for effectiveness in pregnancy prevention (Zigler & McNicholas, 2017).

Pharmacokinetics. NET is rapidly absorbed after oral administration. Its bioavailability is 60%, its peak effect is in 2 hours, and its peak half-life is 8 to 9 hours. It binds to both albumin and SHBG and it is excreted as metabolites in the feces and urine.

Indications. Oral progestin therapy is employed in situations where estrogen-containing contraception is contraindicated. Its lower progestin dosage, its compatibility with breastfeeding, and the patient's ability to start and stop therapy independently make its use during the initial postpartum period common (Colquitt & Martin, 2017; Curtis et al., 2016a). Oral progestin contraception has not been shown to increase VTE risk or increase other cardiovascular risk factors such as high blood pressure (Tepper et al., 2016b).

Adverse Effects. Irregular bleeding is the most frequent side effect of progestin-only methods. It is also the most common reason for therapy discontinuation (Zigler & McNicholas, 2017). Progestin-only methods are also known to cause weight gain related to increased appetite and caloric intake and not the progestin agent itself (Dawson, 2019; Colquitt & Martin, 2017). Due to the short half-life and low bioavailability, without strict adherence to timed, daily use, pregnancy prevention failure is a common potential risk with oral progestin contraception (Zigler & McNicholas, 2017).

Contraindications. There are very few contraindications for progestin oral contraceptives. Breast cancer and pregnancy are considered absolute contraindications. In patients with extensive liver disease, cardiac disease, lupus, or unexplained vaginal bleeding, the risks may outweigh the benefits of use, according to the CDC (Curtis et al., 2016b).

Monitoring. With the initiation of progestin oral contraception, short-term follow-up should be planned to assess adherence of the prescribed agent, especially with adolescents or patients who have additional medical conditions. Ongoing assessment of bleeding patterns and tolerability may be warranted. Weight management related to appetite and diet changes should be assessed during short-term follow-up and during all routine visits. Once the treatment plan has been established, contraceptive use and satisfaction with the method should be evaluated at subsequent routine visits (Curtis et al., 2016a). Additionally, based on medical eligibility criteria, changes in the patient's health status, or changes in patient circumstance, the appropriateness and safety of oral progestin contraceptive use should be evaluated at regular intervals. More reliable methods may be indicated as a patient's life evolves (Curtis et al., 2016a).

Emergency Oral Contraceptives

Emergency contraception (ECP) is another oral progestin therapy option. The goal of ECP is to prevent unwanted pregnancy by initiating treatment within a specified time after unprotected sexual intercourse. Although this method does disrupt an implanted pregnancy, it is not considered an abortifacient. The modes of action include the inhibition or delay in ovulation and follicular maturation. It inhibits sperm migration, fertilization, and fallopian tube transport. Endometrial receptivity and corpus luteum sufficiency are also impaired.

Pharmacokinetics. The most common ECP regimen is 1 oral dose of the synthetic progestin, levonorgestrel (LNG) 1.5 mg, taken after unprotected sexual intercourse. LNG is rapidly absorbed after oral administration. Its peak effect is in 2 hours and its peak half-life is approximately 27 hours. It binds to both albumin and SHBG. It is metabolized hepatically via the CYP 3A4 pathway and excreted as metabolites in the feces and urine.

Indications. LNG has been shown to be effective when used within 72 hours after unprotected intercourse. However, optimal effectiveness occurs the earlier the treatment is initiated. The overall pregnancy prevention rate is 85%.Adverse Effects.

Adverse Effects. In general, most adverse effects are usually mild and transient. Fatigue, dizziness, and headache have been reported. Irregular or heavy bleeding can occur along with gastrointestinal (GI) upset, nausea, and vomiting (Upadhya, 2019).

Contraindications. Suspected pregnancy is a contraindication for this option. However, recent evidence suggests no association between using LNG as an ECP and an increased risk of congenital malformations or pregnancy complications (Matyanga & Dzingirai, 2018). Although there are no safety concerns, the use of ECP has been shown to be less effective in females with a BMI greater than 30 kg/m^2 (Curtis et al., 2016b). Additionally, a history of ectopic pregnancy is not a contraindication for use of ECP; the possibility of ectopic pregnancy should be considered, along with lower abdominal pain in association with missed menses and irregular vaginal bleeding (Curtis et al., 2016b).

Monitoring. The effect of LNG containing ECP is optimal within 72 hours of unprotected sex. However, there is evidence that suggests that use up to 120 hours after coitus may still prevent pregnancy (Upadhya, 2019). No physical exam or pregnancy testing is required to initiate therapy. Due to the possibility of delayed ovulation with this method, abstinence or another method of contraception is needed after the use of ECP. Subsequent unprotected sex after ECP is associated with a higher treatment failure rate. If no menses occurs within 3 weeks of treatment, evaluation for pregnancy must occur (Upadhya, 2019).

Three-Month Injection

Medroxyprogesterone acetate (MPA) is a derivative of progesterone and is the only progestin formulated as an injectable agent indicated for contraception (Colquitt & Martin, 2017). In the past, MPA was administered only via an intramuscular injection of 150 mg every 13 weeks. Now MPA can also be administered subcutaneously with a dosage of 104 mg every 13 weeks (Zigler & McNicholas, 2017). MPA prevents pregnancy by hindering the secretion of pituitary gonadotropins, which impedes follicular maturation, inhibits ovulation, and causes thinning and atrophy of endometrial tissue.

Pharmacokinetics. MPA absorption is slow following injection. Its peak effect is in 1 to 3 weeks and it has a peak half-life of approximately 45 to 50 days. It binds primarily to albumin and does not bind to SHBG. It is metabolized hepatically by P450 enzymes via hydroxylation and conjugation. It is excreted as metabolites in the urine.

Indications. The primary indication for MPA is pregnancy prevention. However, injectable MPA is also used in the treatment of endometriosis by suppressing new growth and implantation of endometrial tissue, reducing inflammatory factors, and decreasing pain associated with endometriosis (Gezer & Oral, 2015). Unlike estrogen containing contraceptive agents, MPA is compatible with breastfeeding once milk supply has been established (Colquitt & Martin, 2017; Curtis et al., 2016a).

Adverse Effects. The most common adverse effect of this method is menstrual irregularities (bleeding or spotting). This can stabilize over the time of use, with 57% of patients experiencing irregular bleeding at 12 months decreasing to 32% at 24 months. Weight gain of more than 10 pounds is another common adverse effect that can occur in more than one-third of females using this method. Other adverse effects include abdominal pain/discomfort, dizziness, headache, nervousness or anxiety, and decreased libido (Pfizer, 2017). There have been reports of increased anxiety and depression after the initiation of MPA; however, overwhelming evidence does not support this (Worly et al., 2018).

BLACK BOX WARNING!

MPA

The U.S. Food and Drug Administration (FDA) issued a black box warning for MPA. There is evidence that the use of the MPA injection may result in the loss of significant bone mineral density. Bone loss has been noted to be greater with increasing duration of use and may not be completely reversible (Pfizer, 2017). This has been supported by several studies (Babtunde & Forsyth, 2014; Modesto et al., 2015; Kyvernitakis et al., 2017). What is not known is the impact on bone health later in life when DMPA is used during critical bone growth, as in adolescence or early adulthood.

The FDA recommends that MPA should not be used longer than 2 years unless other birth control methods are considered inadequate (Pfizer, 2017).

Contraindications. Suspected pregnancy is a contraindication for this option. Other contraindications for use include active thrombophlebitis, current or past history of thromboembolic disorders, cerebral vascular disease, known or suspected malignancy of the breast, known hypersensitivity to MPA or any of its other ingredients, significant liver disease, and any undiagnosed vaginal bleeding (Pfizer, 2017).

Monitoring. With the initiation of MPA, 12-week follow-up is required for subsequent injection. However, continued support and education regarding irregular

bleeding patterns and tolerability may also be warranted. Weight management related to appetite and diet changes should be assessed during office visits for injections and during all routine visits (Curtis et al., 2016a). There is a risk for females who use MPA to experience a loss of bone mineral density. Bone loss is greater with increasing duration of use and may not be completely reversible. Additionally, it is not known whether the use of MPA during adolescence or early adulthood will reduce peak bone mass and increase the risk for osteoporotic fracture in later life. It is not recommended that MPA be used as a long-term birth control method unless other birth control methods are considered inadequate (Pfizer, 2017).

Subdermal Implant

The subdermal implant system currently available consists of a thin, pliable, progestin-containing cylinder that measures 4 cm in length and 2 mm in diameter and is surgically inserted subdermally in the medial surface of the upper arm aligned with the long axis of the arm. This single-rod implant contains 68 mg of ETG, an active metabolite of DNG, within an ethylene vinyl acetate copolymer cover that is designed to release hormone over time. This method is designed for continuous contraception use for a total of 3 years. This progestin method prevents pregnancy by suppressing ovulation, increasing the viscosity of cervical mucus, and inhibiting endometrial proliferation (Merck & Co. Inc., 2019).

Pharmacokinetics. Each implant maintains ETG levels sufficient to inhibit ovulation for 3 years. The rod releases ETG at a slowly declining rate over the 3-year period. Following removal of the rod, ETG levels decrease rapidly and are not detectable within 1 week. ETG binds mainly with albumin but it also binds with SHBG. It is metabolized hepatically via the CYP 3A4 pathway, forming metabolites of unknown activity. Excretion is primarily via urine but it also occurs through feces (Merck & Co. Inc., 2019).

Indications. The primary indication for this therapy is pregnancy prevention. However, for conditions that warrant ovarian suppression as treatment, such as dysmenorrhea and endometriosis, this method should be considered. Progestins are known to directly resolve endometriosis pain and dysmenorrhea not only by suppressing ovarian function but also by inducing endometrial atrophy, modulating antiinflammatory actions, and minimizing nerve fiber pain intensity (Gezer & Oral, 2015). Unlike estrogen containing contraceptive agents, progestin-only contraceptives are compatible with breastfeeding (Colquitt & Martin, 2017; Curtis et al., 2016).

Adverse Effects. The most commonly reported adverse effects are changes in the menstrual bleeding pattern, headache, vaginitis, weight gain, acne, breast pain, abdominal pain, and pharyngitis (Merck & Co. Inc., 2019).

Contraindications. Specific contraindications for this method include a known or suspected pregnancy, a current or past history of thrombosis or thromboembolic disorders, active liver disease or malignancy, undiagnosed vaginal bleeding, current or personal history of breast cancer, and an allergic reaction to any of the components of the contraceptive implant (Merck & Co. Inc., 2019).

Monitoring. Short-term follow-up can be offered to assess implant placement, and ongoing assessment of bleeding patterns and tolerability may be warranted. Weight management related to appetite and diet changes should be assessed during short-term follow-up and during all routine visits. Once the treatment plan has been established, contraceptive use and satisfaction with the method should be evaluated at subsequent routine visits (Curtis et al., 2016a). Additionally, based on the medical eligibility criteria, changes in health status that would affect the appropriateness and safety of progestin-only hormonal contraceptive use should be evaluated at regular intervals, at least annually (Curtis et al., 2016b).

PRACTICE PEARLS

LARCs

LARCs include the 3-month injection, subdermal implant, and IUD. With minimal chance for human error, the extended time of use (anywhere from 3 to 10 years), and an effective rate of 99%, these methods are considered the most effective contraception options currently available (Colquitt & Martin, 2017; Itriyeva, 2018; ACOG, 2016).

IUDs

One of the most common long-acting, reversible contraceptive options is the IUD. IUDs are small, T-shaped devices that are inserted by an experienced provider into the uterus via the cervix. All current IUDs are barium compounded for detection via X-ray and other imaging (Cunningham et al., 2018). The length of use of an IUD ranges from 3 to 10 years (Colquitt & Martin, 2017; Itriyeva, 2018). Nonhormonal and hormonal options are available.

The nonhormonal IUD is a T-shaped polyethylene device that is wrapped in copper and has a white IUD string extending from the end. This IUD is effective for 10 years (Cunningham et al., 2018). The hormonal IUD options are all T shaped and contain LNG. Several IUDs with varying dosages of LNG and sizes are currently available, and all have a duration of effectiveness ranging from 3 to 7 years. Table 20.4 provides an overview of the currently available IUD configurations. IUDs are highly effective and essentially omit human error. The risk of pregnancy is less than 1%, similar to that of permanent sterilization. There is no reduction in fertility with method discontinuation (Turner, 2019). Both the nonhormonal and hormonal IUDs prevent pregnancy by inhibiting sperm motility and preventing fertilization from occurring. IUDs containing LNG also thicken cervical mucus and thin the endometrial lining, further preventing the sperm from reaching a mature egg (Turner, 2019).

TABLE 20.4	IUD Configurations	
Type	**Progestin Type/Dose**	**Agent-Specific Considerations and Side Effects**
Hormonal	Levonorgestrel 52 mg	Irregular vaginal bleeding at 1 year 6%
	Levonorgestrel 19.5 mg	Irregular vaginal bleeding at 1 year 17%
	Levonorgestrel 13.5 g	Irregular vaginal bleeding at 1 year 23%

From Goldthwaite, L. M., & Creinin, M. D. [2019]. Comparing bleeding patterns for the levonorgestrel 52 mg, 19.5 mg, and 13.5 mg intrauterine systems. *Contraception, 100*(2), 128–131.

Pharmacokinetics. For the hormonal IUD, LNG is the active progestin agent. There is a higher release rate of LNG that is gradually reduced over 3 to 5 years, depending on the dose and time frame of the device (see Table 20.4). Low doses of LNG are administered into the uterine cavity with the hormonal IUD. A very low, stable serum concentration of LNG is maintained for the duration of IUD placement. LNG binds primarily to SHBG and, to a lesser extent, serum albumin. It is hepatically metabolized via the CYP 3A4 enzymatic pathway, forming inactive metabolites. LNG is excreted in both the urine and the feces.

Indications. The primary indication for IUD insertion is pregnancy prevention. With minimal systemic effects, IUDs are appropriate for patients who may be precluded from other contraceptive options. IUDs are considered top-tier options for females with comorbid medical conditions and obesity as well as for females in the perimenopausal period (Miller et al., 2018). IUDs also work well when avoidance of unplanned pregnancy is paramount, such as in the postpartum period and in the adolescent population (Apter, 2018; Itriyeva, 2018; Turner, 2019).

Treatment indications differ for nonhormonal and hormonal IUD options. The nonhormonal IUDs are extremely beneficial for pregnancy prevention when a prolonged contraceptive interval is desired (10 years). They can also be used for emergency contraception if IUD insertion occurs less than 5 days after unprotected sexual intercourse (Turner, 2019). The IUDs containing LNG also provide extended pregnancy prevention but for 3 to 5 years. The progestin effects of the hormonal IUD provide usefulness in other circumstances. Spencer et al. (2017) found that the LNG-containing IUDs were more cost effective and afforded better quality of life than hysterectomy and endometrial ablation for the treatment of heavy menstrual bleeding. There is also some evidence of symptomatic pain relief related to endometriosis, though LNG IUDs are not approved by the FDA as treatment for endometriosis (Gezer & Oral, 2015).

Adverse Effects. The procedure for IUD insertion can be uncomfortable, and significant postprocedural cramping is common. In general, the symptoms are self-limiting, easily managed with nonsteroidal antiinflammatory drugs (NSAIDs), and resolved shortly after the insertion is complete (Cunningham et al., 2018; Itriyeva, 2018; Miller et.al., 2018; Turner, 2019). Although there has been a theoretical concern regarding bacterial inoculation during IUD insertion, evidence does not support the need for antibiotic prophylaxis prior to the procedure (Curtis et al., 2016b). Menstrual irregularities are common but vary based on the IUD type and dose of LNG. There is also a 3% to 10% risk of IUD expulsion (Itriyeva, 2018; Miller et al., 2018). The most common reasons for IUD method discontinuation include pain, bleeding, and IUD expulsion (Itriyeva, 2018). After insertion of the hormonal IUD, other common adverse effects include abdominal/pelvic pain, amenorrhea, headache/migraine, genital discharge, and vulvovaginitis.

There are potentially serious complications with IUD use. These complications are rare and include uterine perforation, PID/infection, and ectopic pregnancy. A population cohort study done by Bosco-Levy, Gouvernuer, Langlade, and Pariente (2019) compared the risk of complications of the copper- and LNG-containing IUDs. Out of more than 10,000 females, the risk of uterine perforation, PID or infection, and ectopic pregnancy was 0.2%, 0.1%, and 0.2%, respectively. There was no significant difference in risk of complications between the copper- and LNG-containing IUDs.

Contraindications. Contraindications for any IUD insertion include known or highly suspected pregnancy, postpartum or post-pregnancy termination sepsis, current PID or other severe pelvic infection, current chlamydia or gonorrhea infection, the presence of uterine anatomical abnormalities, and evidence of or strong suspicion of uterine or cervical malignancy. In most cases, insertion can occur after treatment of and recovery from the infection or after treatment of cervical cancer (Curtis et al., 2016a).

There is a theoretical risk of LNG having an adverse effect in patients with breast cancer and patients with a history of ischemic heart or systemic lupus erythematosus. The nonhormonal IUD is recommended for use in these patients. Due to the potential risk of bleeding in patients with thrombocytopenia, the IUD with LNG is preferred (Curtis et al., 2016b).

Monitoring. There is limited evidence regarding appropriate follow-up post-IUD insertion. However, there is evidence that suggests that the incidence of PID is higher in the first 20 days post-IUD insertion. A follow-up visit in 4 to 6 weeks after IUD insertion is common to assess for the absence of infection, evaluate patient tolerance, and determine satisfaction with the IUD placement. Visualization of the IUD strings is done to verify appropriate placement at the follow-up visit and during routine gynecologic exams (Curtis et al., 2016a).

Subsequent gynecologic care should include discussion regarding any side effects or concerns related to the IUD that may affect patient well-being. Ongoing evaluation of health and lifestyle changes that may impact the appropriateness of the IUD should be assessed. Changes in family planning including plans for conception, IUD removal, reinsertion, or the use of other contraceptive options should also be discussed (Curtis et al., 2016a).

Prescriber Considerations for Contraception Therapy

In 2016, the CDC provided guidelines for selecting and prescribing contraceptive agents (Curtis et al., 2016a). The CDC also provides medical eligibility criteria for contraceptive use. These evidence-based guidelines are intended to facilitate informed decision-making when selecting and prescribing specific contraceptive methods for patients who have certain characteristics or medical conditions (Curtis et al., 2016b). The CDC summarizes current evidence regarding all current contraceptive methods, categorizes safety information, and makes recommendations for use with common medical conditions and health risks. These recommendations are communicated employing the medical eligibility criteria levels, which range from 1 (no restrictions) to 4 (the health risks outweigh the benefits of use) (Curtis et al., 2016b).

Clinical Reasoning for Contraception Therapy

Ensure complete patient and family understanding regarding contraceptive options using a shared decision-making approach. Available contraceptive options are as diverse and unique as the patients who use them. Patients look to their provider for guidance in making contraceptive choices. Developing a close and respectful relationship and establishing trust will allay fears and misconceptions regarding contraception, allowing for education and informed choice (Dehlendorf et al., 2014). With the shared decision-making approach, the patient becomes central in the selection process and the provider becomes the expert advisor. The provider imparts advanced and comprehensive knowledge about the contraceptive options and the patient brings individual values, perceptions, and preferences that are valid and integral to the decision-making process. Through partnership, the patient and provider can determine which contraceptive method would be most suitable for the patient's specific situation (Dehlendorf et al., 2014). Some evidence indicates that shared decision-making can improve patient satisfaction and increase adherence to treatment (Rivlin & Isley, 2017).

Provide comprehensive information on all available contraceptive options including mode of action, advantages, disadvantages, common risks, benefits, and side effects. To make an informed decision, patients need to be aware of all available contraceptive methods. This requires a knowledgeble provider well versed in all current contraceptive options. Elements to consider when choosing a contraceptive method include effectiveness, safety, availability, and acceptibility (Curtis et al., 2016a). Of highest concern for patients when selecting contraception is the degree of effectiveness, tolerability, and affordability (Rivlin & Isley, 2017). When reviewing contraception effectiveness, use plain language without confusing medical terms or overwhelming statistics. Since side effects are common reasons for method discontinuation, a discussion of tolerability with method-specific side effects is necessary to promote continuation of the selected contraceptive (Dehlendorf et al., 2014). Without a thorough explanation about and access to all available contraceptive methods, opportunities for optimal fertility management will be missed, resulting in patient dissatisfaction, lower adherence to therapy, and more unintended pregnancies (Kelly et al., 2017; Craig et al., 2019).

Assess the appropriateness of the contraceptive selected for an individual patient by assessing factors such as the patient's age, race/ethnicity, comorbidities, social factors, previous history with contraception, and genetic factors. Obtaining a thorough

PRACTICE PEARL

Drug–Drug Interactions

Certain drugs have the potential to decrease CHC effectiveness. In addition, there has been a misconception that the use of antibiotic therapy may impact CHC efficacy; however, evidence does not show an inhibitory effect. Rifampin is the only documented antimicrobial agent with reduced CHC efficacy. There is evidence to support that the antifungal griseofulvin and that anticonvulsants/sedatives including phenytoin, phenobarbital, primidone, carbamazepine, and ethosuximide may reduce CHC efficacy. These factors should be considered during medication review, patient counseling, and contraceptive method selection.

history to ascertain appropriate contraceptive options is paramount to minimize inherent risks related to therapy. Reviewing contraceptive method–specific characteristics, risks, and side effects and then corroborating them with the individual patient's medical conditions and social factors supports a safe and informed choice regarding contraception and fertility management (Curtis et al., 2016b). A medication review is imperative to assess for potential drug–drug interactions.

Initiate the treatment plan with the selected medication by first providing adequate patient education to ensure the patient's understanding and promote full participation in selecting contraception and managing family planning. To anticipate and address common barriers to consistent and appropriate use, a comprehensive review of the advantages and disadvantages of all the contraceptive methods should be conducted. Accurate information on risks, benefits, side effects, and effectiveness should be readily available to the patient (Dehlendorf et al., 2014). Written information should be offered when contraception is prescribed. Reliable resources that patients can review on their own should also

be provided (Rivlin & Isley, 2017). Method-specific administration, maintenance, and symptoms that require medical attention should also be discussed (Dehlendorf et al., 2014; Rivlin & Isley, 2017).

Conduct follow-up and monitoring of patient responses to contraception. Shared decision-making is ongoing after any contraceptive method is initiated. Patients should be encouraged to follow up whenever they have concerns regarding tolerability and side effects, a desire to change to a different contraceptive method, or a significant change in health status (Curtis et al., 2016a).

Teaching Points for Prescribing Contraception Therapy

Health Promotion Strategies

- Review the occurrence of side effects and overall tolerability of each contraceptive method.
- Have ongoing dialogue regarding current and future fertility plans.
- Routinely evaluate the appropriateness of the contraceptive method and tailor fertility management to the patient's evolving needs.
- Monitor for changes in health and encourage age-appropriate health screenings.
- Offer screening for sexually transmitted infections and encourage concurrent condom use.
- Encourage healthy lifestyle choices such as getting adequate exercise and avoiding smoking.
- Discuss weight changes that are attributed to contraception and provide counseling on weight management and dietary choices.

Patient Education for Medication Safety

The potential for patient harm is inherent with changes in personal risk factors, the occurrence of serious side effects, and the potential for unintended pregnancy related to incorrect or inconsistent medication administration. Ongoing evaluation for the development of contraindications for the use of contraception is imperative for patient safety. The new onset of smoking, recent discovery of a familial predisposition to VTE, or a development of breast cancer are excellent examples of situations when certain contraceptive methods should be discontinued and other methods should be considered (Curtis et al., 2016a).

Intolerance of contraceptive-specific side effects is a common reason for method discontinuation. Preparing patients for agent-specific side effects provides them with anticipatory guidance and realistic expectations, aiding them in the decision on what method would work best for them and what lies ahead (Dehlendorf et al., 2014). Additionally, educating patients on warning signs for potential serious side effects is essential to facilitate prompt medical treatment and avoid significant adverse events.

The primary goal of contraception is to avoid unintended pregnancy. Communication through follow-up visits,

TABLE 20.5 Patient Counseling for Method Interruption and Continuation

Combined Oral Contraception Missed Pills	Contraceptive Patch Delayed Patch Application or Detachment	Vaginal Ring Delayed Ring Insertion	Progestin-Only Oral Contraception Missed Pills
One pill more than 24 hours late: • Take the missed pill as soon as possible • Continue the current pill pack • No backup contraception is required Two or more consecutive pills are missed: • Take the most recently missed pill as soon as possible, discarding any other missed pills • Continue with the remaining pills in the current pill pack • If pills were missed in the last hormonal week (days 15–21), omit the hormone-free week and start a new pill pack • Use backup contraception for 7 days • Consider emergency contraception if the missed pills occurred with unprotected intercourse in the first week of pill use	Less than 48 hours: • Apply the patch as soon as possible • Maintain the same day for changing patches • No backup contraception is required Greater than 48 hours: • Apply a new patch as soon as possible • Maintain the same day for changing patches • If patch was missed in the last hormonal week (days 15–21), omit the hormone-free week and apply a patch immediately • Use backup contraception for 7 days • Consider emergency contraception if the delayed application or detachment occurred with unprotected intercourse in the first week of patch use	Less than 48 hours: • Insert the vaginal ring as soon as possible • Keep the ring in until the regularly scheduled day for removal • No backup contraception is required Greater than 48 hours: • Insert the ring as soon as possible • Maintain the same day for ring removal • If the ring removal was in the last hormonal week (days 15–21), omit the hormone-free week and insert a new vaginal ring immediately • Use backup contraception for 7 days • Consider emergency contraception if the delayed ring insertion occurred with unprotected intercourse in the first week of patch use	Less than 3 hours after the scheduled time: • Take 1 pill as soon as possible • Use backup contraception for 2 days • Emergency contraception should be considered if there was any unprotected intercourse during this time

Modified from Curtis, K. M., Jatlaoui, T. C., Tepper, N. K., Zapata, L. B., Horton, L. G., Jamieson, D. J., & Whiteman, M. K. (2016, July 29). US selected practice recommendation for contraceptive use. *Morbidity and Mortality Weekly Report, 65*(4), 1–66.

phone calls, and even patient portals can facilitate access to information and the ability to change methods if needed without unnecessary exposure to pregnancy. Strategies to promote consistent and appropriate administration of pre-scribed therapies are paramount in ensuring effectiveness. For non-LARC methods, initiation can be done at any time during the menstrual cycle as long as pregnancy has been ruled out. If the method is started more than 5 days after the start of the menstrual cycle, a backup method of pregnancy prevention is required for 7 days following method initia-tion (Curtis et al., 2016a). When prescribing a non-LARC method, provide a multiple-month supply of contraception to avoid delays in treatment and unnecessary pharmacy visits. Using online resources, text reminders, and calendar alarms prompts adherence to follow-up and method contin-uation (Dehlendorf et al., 2014). Providing a contingency plan by preparing patients for issues that might arise with certain methods empowers them to problem solve, main-tain consistent coverage, and avoid method discontinua-tion. One such plan is to be sure patients know what to do if they have a break or gap in their contraceptive therapy, as described in Table 20.5. Lastly, education on the use and provision of emergency contraception should be standard (Dehlendorf et al., 2014).

Application Questions for Discussion

1. As a health care provider, what are the patient safety fac-tors that should be considered before prescribing con-traception?
2. What should be included in the education plan for a pa-tient who has been prescribed a contraceptive method?
3. What role may lifestyle factors play in the adherence to some prescribed contraceptives?

Selected Bibliography

ACOG. (2016). Adolescents and long-acting reversible contracep-tion: Implants and intrauterine devices. *Obstetrics and Gynecology, 131*(5), 947–948.

Africander, D., Verhoog, N., & Hapgood, J. P. (2011). Molecular mechanisms of steroid receptor-mediated actions by synthetic progestins used in HRT and contraception. *Steroids, 76*(7), 638–652.

Apter, D. (2018). Contraception options: Aspects unique to the adolescent and the young adult. *Best Practice & Research: Clinical Obstetrics and Gynaecology, 48*(2018), 115–127.

Babtunde, O. O., & Forsyth, J. J. (2014). Association between depot medroxyprogesterone acetate (DMPA), physical activity and bone health. *Journal of Bone Mineral Metabolism, 32*(2014), 305–311.

Barrionuevo, P., Nabhan, M., Wang, Z., Erwin, P. J., Asi, N., Martin, K. A., & Murad, M. H. (2018). Treatment options for hirsutism: A systematic review. *Journal of Clinical Endocrinology Metabolism, 103*, 1258–1264.

Bosco-Levy, P., Gouvernuer, A., Langlade, C., & Pariente, A. (2019). Safety of 52 mg intrauterine system compared to copper intrauterine device: A population-based chort study. *Contraception, 99*(2019), 345–348.

Chrousos, G. P. (2017). The gonadal hormones and inhibitors. In B. G. Katzung (Ed.), *Basic & Clinical Pharmacology* (14th ed.). New York: McGraw-Hill.

Colquitt, C. W., & Martin, T. S. (2017). Contraceptive methods: A review of nonbarrier and barrier methods. *Journal of Pharmacy Practice, 30*(1), 130–135.

Craig, A. D., Steinauer, J., Kuppermann, M., Schmittdiel, J. A., & Dehlendorf, C. (2019). Pill, patch, or ring? A mixed methods analysis of provider counseling about combined hormonal contraception. *Contraception, 99*(2019), 104–110.

Cunningham, F., Leveno, K. J., Bloom, S. L., Hoffman, B. L., Casey, B. M., & Spong, C. Y (2018). Contraception. In F. Cunningham, K. J. Leveno, S. L. Bloom, J. S. Dashe, B. L. Hoffman, B. M. Casey, & C. Y. Spong (Eds.), *Williams Obstetrics* (25th ed.). New York: McGraw-Hill.

Curtis, K. M., Jatlaoui, T. C., Tepper, N. K., Zapata, L. B., Horton, L. G., Jamieson, D. J., & Whiteman, M. K. (2016a). US selected practice recommendation for contraceptive use. *Morbidity and Mortality Weekly Report, 65*(4), 1–66.

Curtis, K. M., Tepper, N. K., Jatlaoui, T. C., Berry-Bibee, E., Horton, L. G., Zapata, L. B., & Whiteman, M. K. (2016b). US medical eligibility criteria for contraceptive use. *Morbidity and Mortality Weekly Report, 65*(3).

Dawson, R. S. (2019). Birth control management for the primary care privider. *Pediatric Annuals, 48*(2), e51–e55.

Dehlendorf, C., Krajewski, C., & Borrero, S. (2014). Contraceptive counseling: Best practices to ensure quality communication and enable effective use. *Clinical Obstetrics and Gynecology, 57*(4), 659–673.

Dragoman, M. V., Simmons, K. B., Paulen, M. E., & Curtis, K. M. (2017). Combination hormonal contraceptive (CHC) use among obese women and contraceptive effectiveness: A systematic review. *Contraception, 95*, 117–129.

Galzote, R. M., Rafie, S., Teal, R., & Mody, S. K. (2017). Transdermal delivery of combined hormonal contraception: A review of the current literature. *International Journal of Women's Health, 9*, 315–320.

Gezer, A., & Oral, E. (2015). Progestin therapy in endometriosis. *Women's Health, 11*(5), 634–652.

Goldthwaite, L. M., & Creinin, M. D. (2019). Comparing bleeding patterns for the levonorgestrel 52 mg, 19.5 mg, and 13.5 mg intrauterine systems. *Contraception, 1*(2), 128–131.

Hall, J. E. (2019). Neuroendocrine control of the menstrual cycle. In J. F. Strauss & R. L. Barbieri (Eds.), *Yen & Jaffe's Reproductive Endocrinology: Physiology, Pathophysiology, and Clinical Management* (8th ed.). Philadelphia: Elsevier.

Hoffman, B. L., Schorge, J. O., Bradshaw, K. D., Halvorson, L. M., Schaffer, J. I., & Corton, M. M. (2016). Evaluation of the infertile couple. In B. L. Hoffman, J. O. Schorge, K. D. Bradshaw, L. M. Halvorson, J. I. Schaffer, & M. M. Corton (Eds.), *Williams Gynecology*. New York: McGraw-Hill.

Itriyeva, K. (2018). Use of long-acting reversible contraception (LARC) and the Depo-Provera shot in adolescents. *Current Problems in Pediatric and Adolescent Health Care, 48*, 321–332.

Jacobstien, R., & Polis, C. B. (2014). Progestin-only contraception: Injectable and implants. *Best Practice & Research: Clinical Obstetrics and Gynaecology, 28*(2014), 795–806.

Kaiser, G., Janda, C., Kleinstauber, M., & Weise, C. (2018). Clusters of premenstrual symptoms in women with PMDD: Appearance, stability and association with impairment. *Journal of Psychosomatic Research, 115*, 38–43.

Kelly, P. J., Cheng, A.-L., Carlson, K., & Witt, J. (2017). Advanced practice registered nurses and long-acting reversible contraception. *Journal of Midwifery & Women's Health, 62*(2), 190–195.

Kyvernitakis, I., Kostev, K., Nassour, T., Thomasius, F., & Hadji, P. (2017). The impact of depot medroxyprogesterone acetate on fracture risk: A case-control study from the UK. *Osteoporosis International, 28*(2017), 291–297.

Laubach, J. M., & Lorntson, R. P. (2013). Common gynecologic pelvic disorders. In E. Q. Youngkin, M. S. Davis, & D. M. Schadewald (Eds.), *Women's Health: A Primary Care Clinical Guide* (4th ed) (pp. 355–398). Upper Saddle River, NJ: Pearson.

Leo, V. D., Musacchio, M. C., Cappelli, V., Piomboni, P., & Morgante, G. (2016). Hormonal contraceptives: Pharmacology tailored to women's health. *Human Reproduction Update, 22*(5), 634–646.

Lessey, B. A., & Young, S. L. (2019). Structure, Function, and Evaluation of the Female Reproductive Tract. In J. F. Strauss, & R. L. Barbieri (Eds.), *Yen & Jaffe's Reproductive Endocrinology: Physiology, Pathophysiology, and Clinical Management* (8th ed) (pp. 206–247). Philadelphia: Elsevier.

Mattison, D. R., Karyakina, N., Goodman, M., & LaKind, J. S. (2014). Pharmaco-and toxicokinetics of selected exogenous and endogenous estrogens: A review of the data and identification of knowledge gaps. *Critical Reviews in Toxicology, 44*(8), 696–724.

Matyanga, C. M., & Dzingirai, B. (2018). Clinical pharmacology of hormonal emergency contraceptive pills. *International Journal of Reproductive Medicine, 2018*, 1–5.

Merck & Co. Inc. (2019). *Nexplanon (Etonogestrel Implant): Highlights of Prescribing Information*: Whitehouse Station: Merck & Co. Inc.

Merck Inc. (2020). *NuvaRing (etonogestrel/ethinyl estradiol vaginal ring)*: Merck Inc.

Miller, T. A., Allen, R. H., Kaunitz, A. M., & Cwiak, C. A. (2018). Contraception for midlife women: A review. *Menopause: The Journal of The North American Menopause Society, 25*(7), 817–827.

Modesto, W., Bahamondes, M. V., & Bahamondes, L. (2015). Prevalence of low bone mass and osteoporosis in long-term users of the injectable contraceptive depot medroxyprogesterone. *Journal of Women's Health, 24*(8), 636–640.

Molina, P. E. (2018). Female reproductive system. Editor. In P. E. Molina (Ed.), *Endocrine Physiology* (5th ed.). New York: McGraw-Hill.

Mylan Pharmaceuticals Inc. (2020). *Xulane-norelgestromin and Ethinyl Estradiol Patch*: Mylan Pharmaceuticals.

Patel, S., & Carey, L. (2018). Are hormonal contraceptives less effective in overweight and obese women? *Journal of the American Academy of Physician Assistants, 31*(1), 11–13.

Pfizer. (2017). *Depo Provera: Highlights of Prescribing Information*. New York: Pharmacia & Upjohn.

Rivlin, K., & Isley, M. (2017). Patient-centered contraceptive counseling and prescribing. *Clinical Obstetrics and Gynecology, 61*(1), 27–39.

Sitruk-Ware, R., & Nath, A. (2013). Characteristics and metabolic effects of estrogen and progestins in oral contraceptives. *Best Practice & Research: Clinical Endocrinology and Metabolism, 27*(2013), 13–24.

Spencer, J. C., Louie, M., Moulder, J. K., Ellis, V., Schiff, L. D., Troubia, T., & Wheeler, S. B. (2017). Cost-effectiveness of treatments for heavy menstrual bleeding. *American Journal of Obstetrics and Gynecology, 217*(5), 574.e1. 574.e9.

Strauss, J. F., & Williams, C. J (2019). Ovarian Life Cycle. In J. F. Strauss, & R. L. Barbieri (Eds.), *Yen & Jaffe's Reproductive Endocrinology: Physiology, Pathophysiology, and Clinical Management* (8th ed) (pp. 167–205). Philadelphia: Elseiver.

Tepper, N. K., Phillips, S. J., Knapp, N., Gaffield, M. E., & Curtis, K. M. (2016a). Combined hormonal contraceptive use among breastfeeding women: An updated systematic review. *Contraception, 94*, 262–274.

Tepper, N. K., Whiteman, M. K., Marchbanks, P. A., James, A. H., & Curtis, K. M. (2016b). Progestin-only contraception and thromboembolism: A systematic review. *Contraception, 94*(2016), 678–700.

TherapeuticsMD. (2020). *Annovera: Highlights of prescibing information*. Boca Raton, FL: TherapeuticsMD.

Toit, R. L., Storbeck, K.-H., Cartwright, M., Cabral, A., & Africander, D. (2017). Progestins used in endocrine therapy and implications for the biosynthesis and metabolism of endogenous steroid hormones. *Molecular and Cellular Endocrinology, 441*, 31–45.

Turner, J. H. (2019). Long-acting reversible contraceptives: Addressing adoloscents' barriers to use. *The Nurse Practitioner, 44*(5), 23–30.

Upadhya, K. K. (2019). Emergency contraception: Policy statement: American Academy of Pediatrics. *Pediatrics, 144*(6), 1–10.

Vricella, L. K., Gawron, L. M., & Louis, J. M. (2019). Immediate postpartum long-acting reversible contraception for women at high risk for medical complications. *The Society for Maternal-Fetal Medicine, 220*(5), B2–B12.

Wilson, C., McClure, R. A., & Kostas-Polston, E. A. (2017). Perimenstrual and pelvic symptoms and syndromes. In I. M. Alexander, V. Johnson-Mallard, E. A. Kostas-Polston, C. I. Fogel, & N. F. Woods (Ed.), *Women's Health Care in Advanced Practice Nursing* (2nd ed.). New York: Springer.

Worly, B. L., Gur, T. L., & Scaffir, J. (2018). The relationship between progestin hormonal contraception and depression: A systematic review. *Contraception, 97*(2018), 478–489.

Zielinski, R., & Lynne, S. (2017). Menstrual cycle pain and premenstrual conditions. In K. D. Scuiling, & F. E. Likis (Eds.), *Women's Gynecologic Health* (3rd ed) (pp. 549–573). Burlington, MA: Jones & Bartlett.

Zigler, R. E., & McNicholas, C. (2017). Unscheduled vaginal bleeding with progestin-only contraceptive use. *American Journal of Obstetrics & Gynecology*, 443–450.

21

Medications for the Menopausal Transition

BRENDA GILMORE

Overview

The menopausal transition is a natural biological process in females that marks the end of the childbearing years. It is characterized by physiologic changes in the hypothalamic-pituitary-ovarian axis resulting in a gradual decline of ovarian function and fertility. During the menopausal transition, changes to the menstrual cycle occur gradually over a 5- to 10-year period. The average age of menopause is 51, and it is operationally defined as amenorrhea for 12 consecutive months (Lobo, 2019; O'Neil & Eden, 2017).

In general, even though the timing of menopause is genetically determined, with notable familial concordance up to 87%, it varies significantly among females (Daan & Fauser, 2015; Lobo, 2019). Social, ethnic, and lifestyle factors can produce variability in the age of onset. Females of higher socioeconomic status and higher parity tend to go through the menopausal transition later. Females of lower socioeconomic status, lower body mass, and those who smoke become menopausal earlier. In the United States, African American and Hispanic females also experience menopause earlier than their Caucasian counterparts (Lobo, 2019).

When describing the menopausal transition, the Stages of Reproductive Aging Workshop, or STRAW, model offers universal nomenclature and a detailed staging system (Harlow et al., 2012). This model is illustrated in Table 21.1. Overall, female fertility is divided into three general categories—reproductive, menopausal transition, and postmenopausal. The reproductive stage has three stages: early, peak, and late; and the menopausal transition and postmenopausal categories each have an early and late stage. Physiologic and endocrinologic criteria and common symptomology are detailed for each stage.

Relevant Physiology

The hormonal changes inherent in the menopausal transition have significant effects on the reproductive system. For instance, ovarian function declines consistently over the female life span (Daan & Fauser, 2015). This process of reproductive aging is characterized by a gradual decline in the quality and quantity of primordial ovarian follicles. The greatest number of primordial follicles is present in utero at 20 weeks' gestation and undergoes a regular rate of atresia until around the age of 37. After age 37, the decline in primordial follicles becomes more rapid. By the time the menopausal transition ensues, fewer than 1000 follicles remain and they are primarily atretic in nature (Lobo, 2019). With advancing age, ovarian function declines and becomes unresponsive to gonadotropins, and menstrual cycles disappear (menopause) (Alford & Nurudeen, 2019).

As the number of primordial follicles declines, ovarian function is diminished and estrogen and progesterone levels fall (Alford & Nurudeen, 2019). As the negative feedback loop is altered, serum follicle stimulating hormone (FSH) and luteinizing hormone (LH) levels rise, anti-müllerian hormone (AMH) levels decline, and fertility is markedly reduced (Alford & Nurudeen, 2019; Lobo, 2019). These changes occur over time, with normal menstrual function up to 10 years before obvious endocrine deficiency ensues.

There is also a slow decline in testosterone levels throughout the menopausal transition (Lobo, 2019). As the menopausal transition progresses and the hormonal axis becomes less predictable, endometrial changes become apparent as well. In early menopausal transition, the endometrium may continue to reflect the monthly ovulatory cycles. As estrogen and progesterone become more discordant in later stages of the menopausal transition, anovulation is common, inducing disordered proliferative changes. After menopause, the endometrium becomes atrophic due to lack of estrogen stimulation (Hoffman et al., 2016a). Epithelial cells shrink in size, and the stroma becomes fibrotic (Lessey & Young, 2019).

Estrogen receptors are abundant throughout the female genitalia. During the menopausal transition, unstable and declining estrogen levels induce atrophic changes to the vagina and the vulva (O'Neil & Eden, 2017). The vagina loses collagen, adipose tissue, and the ability to retain water. Vaginal walls shrink, rugae flatten, and the vagina attains a smooth-walled, pale-pink appearance (Lobo, 2019). The vaginal surface epithelium thins and becomes friable and

TABLE 21.1	Genitourinary Syndrome of Menopause (GSM) Symptoms and Potential Complications: External Genital, Urologic, and Sexual Manifestations of GSM			
External Genital		**Urologic**		**Sexual**
Signs and Symptoms	**Complications**	**Signs and Symptoms**	**Complications**	**Signs and Symptoms**
Vaginal/pelvic pain and pressure	Labial atrophy	Frequency	Ischemia of vesical trigone	Loss of libido
Dryness	Vulvar atrophy and lesions	Urgency	Meatal stenosis	Loss of arousal and lack of lubrication
Irritation/burning	Atrophy of Bartholin glands	Postvoid dribbling	Cystocele and rectocele	Dyspareunia
Tenderness	Intravaginal retraction of urethra	Nocturia	Urethral prolapse	Dysorgasmia
Pruritus vulvae	Alkaline pH	Stress/urgency incontinence	Urethral atrophy	Pelvic pain
Decreased turgor and elasticity	Reduced vaginal and cervical secretions	Dysuria	Retraction of urethral meatus inside vagina associated with vaginal voiding	Bleeding or spotting during intercourse
Suprapubic pain	Pelvic organ prolapse	Hematuria		
Leukorrhea	Vaginal vault prolapse	Recurrent urinary tract infection	Uterine prolapse	
Ecchymosis	Vaginal stenosis and shortening		Urethral polyp or caruncle	
Erythema	Introital stenosis			
Thinning/graying pubic hair				
Thinning/pallor of vaginal epithelium				
Pale vaginal mucous membrane				
Fusion of labia minora				
Labial shrinking				
Leukoplakic patches on vaginal mucosa				
Presence of petechiae				
Fewer vaginal rugae				
Increased vaginal friability				

From Gandhi, J., Chen, A., Dagur, G., Suh, Y., Smith, N., & Cali, B. [2016, December]. Genitourinary syndrome of menopause: An overview of clinical manifestation, pathophysiology, etiology, evaluation, and management. *American Journal of Obstetrics & Gynecology*, 704–711.

prone to injury with minimal trauma. The vaginal walls narrow and lose elasticity and flexibility. The vaginal pH becomes more alkaline, creating an environment less conducive to lactobacilli growth and more susceptible to infection by urogenital and fecal pathogens (Hoffman et al., 2016a). The vulvar epithelium also atrophies with diminished secretions from sebaceous glands and lost subcutaneous fat in the labia majora. These changes lead to shrinkage and retraction of clitoral prepuce and the urethra, fusion of the labia minora, and introital narrowing (Hoffman et al., 2016a).

During the menopausal transition, the breast goes through a process of atrophy and involution (Karam, 2019). In premenopausal women, estrogen and progesterone exert proliferative effects on ductal and glandular structures of the breast (Hoffman et al., 2016a). Due to the hormonal withdrawal during the menopausal transition, the proliferation of glandular and ductal tissue is significantly reduced and replaced by adipose tissue. This results in a dramatic decrease in breast volume and tissue density (Hoffman et al., 2016a).

In addition to the changes to the reproductive system, the impact of menopause has far-reaching systemic effects that can have a profound impact on female aging and well-being. Naturally, bone loss is noted after bone maturity at age 25 to 30 at a steady rate of approximately 0.13% per year (Hoffman et al., 2016a). Estrogen is a major contributor to a bone formation and resorption imbalance, and estrogen deficiency has been well established as a cause of bone loss (Hoffman et al., 2016a). The rate of bone loss increases to an average of 2.5% per year during the menopausal transition (Lobo, 2019).

Prior to the menopausal transition, the overall female risk of cardiovascular disease is three times lower than a male of the same age. However, the risk of cardiovascular disease increases significantly for females as they enter the menopausal transition and as estrogen levels decline. By age 70, the risk of cardiovascular disease in females and males is equal (Hoffman et al., 2016a).

Estrogen has many powerful biochemical and neurophysiologic effects on brain structure and function which are mediated through specific receptors (Lobo, 2019). Reductions in estrogen levels during the menopausal transition are known to prompt significant changes in thermoregulation. These alterations are centrally mediated and attributed to a combination of hypothalamic dysfunction and altered neurotransmitter concentrations (O'Neil & Eden, 2017). There is also an increase in hypothalamic nor-epinephrine and serotonin release, which lowers the set-point in the thermoregulatory nucleus and allows heat loss mechanisms to be triggered by subtle changes in core body temperature (Lobo, 2019). These changes in thermoregulation propagate the most common and bothersome symptoms of menopause: vasomotor symptoms or hot flashes. Vasomotor symptoms, decreased estrogen levels, and normal aging changes can induce sleep disturbances, fatigue, moodiness, irritability, depressive symptoms, and cognitive decline (Hoffman et al., 2016a).

Pathophysiology

Changes in the hormonal axis related to the menopausal transition and aging can have a multisystem impact on overall health, well-being, and quality of life. Table 21.2 provides a summary of potential conditions related to estrogen deficiency and aging. Females can experience an array of common symptoms throughout the menopausal transition.

For example, vasomotor symptoms, also described as hot flashes and night sweats, are episodes of an abrupt sensation of heat and flushing of the upper body. These episodes are often followed by excessive perspiration or sweats and other associated symptoms such as clamminess, anxiety, and palpitations (O'Neil & Eden, 2017; Ward & Deneris, 2018). The occurrence of vasomotor symptoms can vary

TABLE 21.2	Potential Conditions Related to Estrogen Deficiency and Aging
System	Pathology Considerations
Breast	Breast cancer
Bone	Low bone mass / Osteopenia
Cardiovascular	Cardiovascular disease
Central Nervous	Insomnia/fatigue / Cognitive dysfunction / Depression
Endometrium	Endometrial cancer
Thermoregulation	Vasomotor symptoms
Urogenital	Dysuria / Frequent urinary tract infections / Urinary incontinence
Vulvovaginal	Genitourinary syndrome of menopause / Dyspareunia / Sexual dysfunction

From Hoffman, B. L., Schorge, J. O., Bradshaw, K. D., Halvorson, L. M., Schaffer, J. I., & Corton, M. M. [2016]. Menopausal Transition. In B. L. Hoffman, J. O. Schorge, K. D. Bradshaw, L. M. Halvorson, J. I. Schaffer, & M. M. Corton, *Williams Gynecology* [3rd ed.]. New York: McGraw-Hill.

greatly in frequency and length. Sleep disruption is a common complaint due to excessive diaphoresis (Lobo, 2019). This results in fatigue, irritability, and depressed mood (O'Neil & Eden, 2017). As many as 80% of females experience some vasomotor symptoms during the menopausal transition. Vasomotor symptoms usually occur after 2 years of estrogen deficiency and can persist for 10 years (Lobo, 2019). The average duration of symptom occurrence is 7.4 years. However, many females experience vasomotor symptoms well into their 70s (Ward & Deneris, 2018). Fifty percent of all females who experience vasomotor symptoms have them frequently enough to affect their quality of life, and 10% to 15% of females find these symptoms debilitating (Lobo, 2019).

With diminishing estrogen, most females in the menopausal transition will notice changes associated with genitourinary syndrome of menopause (GSM). This syndrome, formerly known as vulvovaginal atrophy or atrophic vaginitis, is a chronic and progressive condition that is caused by increased tissue friability, loss of tissue elasticity, and decreasing aperture and length of the vagina affecting vulvar-vaginal, urogenital, and sexual function (Gandhi et al., 2016; Ward & Deneris, 2018). Common vulvar-vaginal symptoms associated with GSM include dryness, burning, and irritation. Potential urinary symptoms include incontinence, urgency, dysuria, and recurrent urinary tract infections (UTIs). Common sexual symptoms of absent lubrication and dyspareunia prompt decreased arousal capacity, difficulty achieving orgasm, and decreased libido. Untreated symptoms associated with GSM worsen with age (Gandhi et al., 2016; Hoffman et al., 2016a; Ward & Deneris, 2018). See Fig. 21.1 for a comprehensive review of symptoms and potential complications of GSM.

Vasomotor symptoms, disturbed sleep patterns, interpersonal stress, anxiety, psychosocial and lifestyle factors, and other health-related issues can significantly affect mood and modulate depression risks (Hoffman et al., 2016a; Bhat et al. 2017). Menopausal females frequently report symptoms of mood instability, irritability, nervousness, and depression (O'Neil & Eden, 2017). The menopausal transition can be overwhelming, and mood disorders are more common in the late menopausal transition when compared with premenopausal and postmenopausal states. Females have long been recognized as having a higher lifetime risk of developing depression than males (Hoffman et al., 2016a). Additionally, the rate of primary depressive symptoms is notably higher in the late menopausal transition: females with no history of depression are 2.5 times more likely to report depressed mood during the menopausal transition compared to the premenopausal period. A history of depressive episodes prior to the menopausal transition remains the strongest indicator of depression reoccurrence during midlife (Hoffman et al., 2016a; Bhat et al., 2017). Females should be screened routinely for depression based on its prevalence during the menopausal transition (Hoffman et al., 2016a; Bhat et al., 2017).

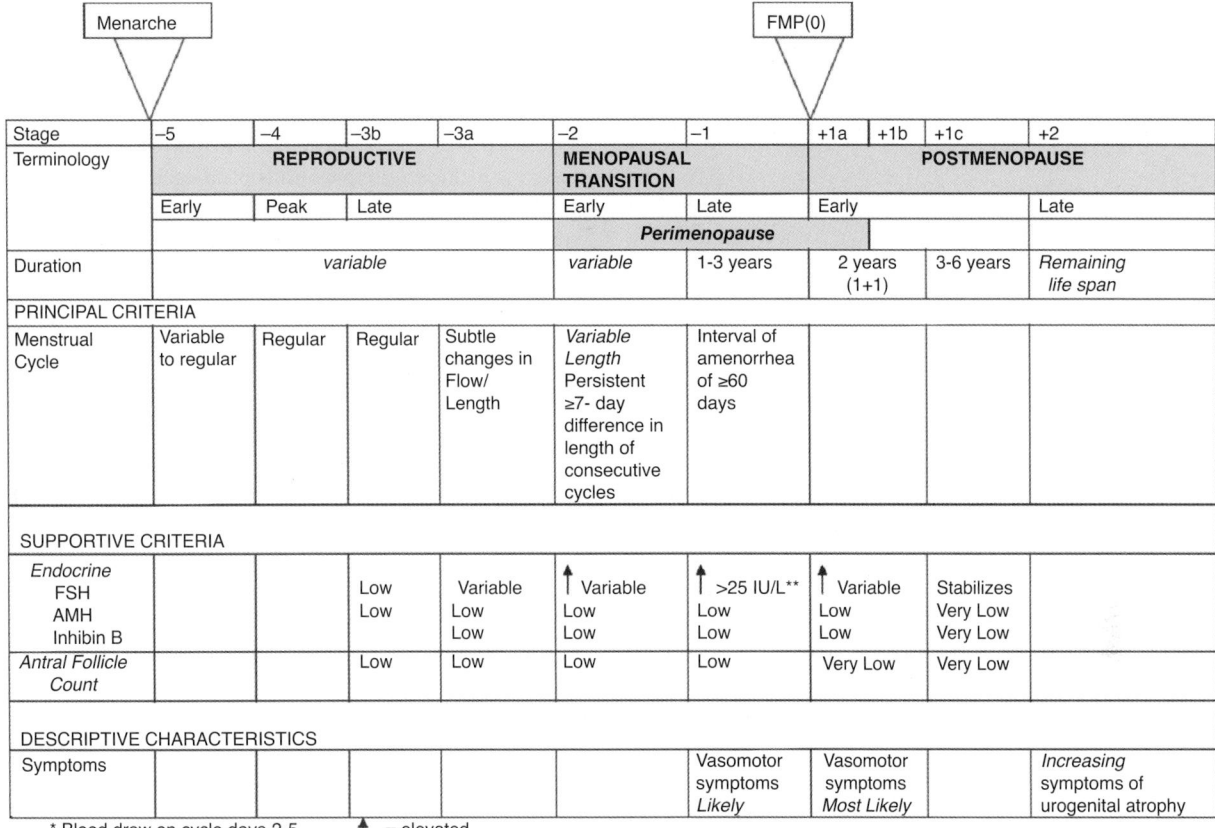

	Menarche						FMP(0)			
Stage	−5	−4	−3b	−3a	−2	−1	+1a	+1b	+1c	+2
Terminology	REPRODUCTIVE				MENOPAUSAL TRANSITION		POSTMENOPAUSE			
	Early	Peak	Late		Early	Late	Early			Late
					Perimenopause					
Duration	variable				variable	1-3 years	2 years (1+1)	3-6 years		Remaining life span
PRINCIPAL CRITERIA										
Menstrual Cycle	Variable to regular	Regular	Regular	Subtle changes in Flow/ Length	Variable Length Persistent ≥7- day difference in length of consecutive cycles	Interval of amenorrhea of ≥60 days				
SUPPORTIVE CRITERIA										
Endocrine FSH AMH Inhibin B			Low Low Low	Variable Low Low	↑ Variable Low Low	↑ >25 IU/L** Low Low	↑ Variable Low Low	Stabilizes Very Low Very Low		
Antral Follicle Count			Low	Low	Low	Low	Very Low	Very Low		
DESCRIPTIVE CHARACTERISTICS										
Symptoms						Vasomotor symptoms *Likely*	Vasomotor symptoms *Most Likely*			*Increasing symptoms of urogenital atrophy*

* Blood draw on cycle days 2-5   ↑ = elevated
**Approximate expected level based on assays using current international pituitary standards

• **Fig. 21.1** The Stages of Reproductive Aging Workshop + 10 staging system for reproductive aging in females. (From Harlow, S. D., Gass, M., Hall, J. E., Lobo, R., Maki, P., Rebar, R. W., . . . de Villiers, T. J. [2012]. Executive summary of the stages of the reproductive aging workshop +10: Addressing the unfinished agenda of staging reproductive aging. *Menopause: The Journal of The North American Menopause Society, 19*[4], 387–395.)

The changes to the hormonal axis, combined with the changes related to age during the menopausal transition, can have a synergistic effect on reproductive health. Age is the most prevalent risk factor for reproductive cancers including breast, ovarian, and endometrial cancers. Increased breast cancer risk is attributed to increasing age, elevated estrogen exposure, and genetic predisposing factors. Though ovarian cancer can occur at any age, it is more common in postmenopausal women. Endometrial, or uterine, cancer is the most common gynecologic cancer in the United States. It is much more common in females over the age of 50 and has been linked with increased estrogen exposure.

As estrogen levels decline, bone loss becomes more common. *Primary osteoporosis* is bone loss associated with aging and menopausal estrogen deficiency. *Osteoporosis* is defined as a skeletal disorder in which bone demineralization results in a porous and fragile bone structure that leads to a significant increase in fracture risk. The vertebrae, wrists, and femoral neck are common fracture sites. Fracture is associated with significant mortality and morbidity. The course of osteoporosis is silent and progressive, with no outward signs until fracture occurs.

The increased cardiovascular disease risk in menopausal females has been attributed to changes in the vasculature and lipid metabolism. Vascular changes include an increased presence of inflammatory markers, decreased vessel elasticity, and decreased blood flow in the vascular beds. Estrogen deficiency leads to declining high-density lipoproteins, increasing low-density lipoproteins, and increased total cholesterol levels resulting in increased risk of atherosclerotic plaque development (Lobo, 2019). Clotting features are also known to change with aging. Fibrinogen, plasminogen activator inhibitor-1, and Factor VII levels rise, increasing coagulability. These menopausal-related changes could potentially contribute to increases in cardiovascular disease and cerebrovascular disease rates in older females (Hoffman et al., 2016a). Aging changes such as increases in body weight, blood pressure, and glucose levels also contribute to the increase in cardiovascular disease risk (Lobo, 2019).

PRACTICE PEARLS

Examples of Increased Estrogen Exposure

- Early age at menarche
- Late age at menopause
- Low number of pregnancies
- No history of breastfeeding
- Obesity
- Polycystic ovarian syndrome (PCOS)

What are bioidentical hormone products?

Bioidentical hormone compounds have the same chemical composition as hormones produced within the human body. Many of the available hormone products approved by the U.S. Food and Drug Administration (FDA) are considered bioidentical, as indicated in Tables 21.2, 21.3, and 21.4.

What are compounded hormone products?

Compounded hormone products are prepared by a compounding pharmacy using a variety of hormone formulations that have not been controlled or tested for quality or efficacy. They are not tested or approved by the FDA. The hormone concentrations, pharmacokinetics, absorption, and patient response to these formulations are untested and unreliable. They are not currently recommended by the North American Menopause Society (NAMS) 2017 Hormone Therapy Position Statement Advisory Panel because insufficient guidelines for quality control have not been established (NAMS, 2017).

Menopausal Transition Therapy

Medications for common symptoms during the menopausal transition focus largely on alleviating vasomotor symptoms and symptoms related to GSM and improving quality of life. Options include systemic and topical agents. Hormonal therapy is the mainstay of menopausal symptom therapy and is specific to GSM; however, nonhormonal agents are also available.

Classification of Systemic Hormonal Therapy

Hormone replacement therapy (HRT) can include estrogen and progestin or estrogen alone. Estrogens affect many tissues and have many metabolic actions. Estrogen receptors are abundant in the female reproductive tract in the uterus, vagina, and ovaries. Estrogen receptors are also prominent in the mammary gland, the hypothalamus, endothelial cells, and vascular smooth muscle, with lower expression in lung, brain, bone, and vasculature (Levin et al., 2019). Table 21.3 provides a summary of actions on specific systems.

TABLE 21.3   Effects of Exogenous Estrogen (E2)

System	Action	Risk/Benefits
Breast	Stimulates E2 receptors in the breast	E2+P increases risk of breast cancer after 5 yr of use; E2 alone does not increase risk of breast cancer
Bone	Increases osteoblastic function and decreases osteoclast activity	Prevents bone loss
Cardiovascular	Reduces progression of atherosclerosis but does not affect regression of established atherosclerotic plaques	Cardiovascular disease risk: • Decreased risk <10 yr postmenopause at initiation of therapy • Increased risk >10 yr postmenopause at initiation of therapy
Coagulation	Increases both coagulation and fibrinolytic pathways, and creates an imbalance in these two opposing activities	Increased risk for venous thromboembolic events
Central Nervous System	Alleviates vasomotor symptoms Stimulates E2 receptors in the brain	Decreased sleep interruption Alzheimer's/dementia: • Decreased risk if no cognitive decline prior to initiation of therapy • Increased risk if cognitive decline present prior to initiation of therapy Mood: • Some evidence supports mood improvement • Depressive symptoms may occur with E2 discontinuation
Hepatic/Gallbladder	First-pass hepatic effect can: • Increase biliary cholesterol secretion • Promote bile precipitation/crystallization • Decrease gallbladder motility	Increased incidence of: • Cholelithiasis • Cholecystitis • Cholecystectomy
Endometrium	Endometrial stimulation	Increased risk of endometrial hyperplasia; mediated when used with a progestin
Thermoregulation	Stabilizes thermoregulatory dysfunction	Decreases vasomotor symptoms
Urogenital	Restores estrogen to the mucosal surfaces of the labia, vagina, urethra, and bladder	Alleviates genital and urinary symptoms of the genitourinary syndrome of menopause

From North American Menopause Society 2017 Hormone Therapy Position Statement Advisory Panel. (2017). The 2017 hormone therapy position statement of The North American Menopause Society. *Menopause* Jul;24(7), 728-753. doi: 10.1097/GME.0000000000000921. PMID: 28650869.

Estrogen therapy can be used alone in females posthysterectomy. However, combination therapy is indicated for females with an intact uterus. Combination HRT can be prescribed in a cyclic or continuous regimen. In the continuous regimen, which is more common, estrogen and progestogen dosing is the same every day. An example of a cyclic regimen is when estrogen is administered for 25 days each month and a progestin is added for the final 10 days. This is followed by a 5-day drug-free interval when withdrawal bleeding follows. Cyclic therapy is most often used by females in the perimenopausal period when there may still be sporadic menstrual cycles. Depending on patient risk, low-dose oral contraceptives can also be employed during this time (Bakour et al., 2017). Continuous therapy is usually selected for females following the menopausal transition (Hoffman et al., 2016b).

Estrogen

In general, current estrogen options are well absorbed due to their lipophilic nature. Daily oral agents are the most common and are available in many configurations. Several transdermal formulations deliver systemic estradiol therapy continuously. The three types of estrogen employed in HRT include 17β estradiol (E2), conjugated estrogens (CE), and ethinyl estradiol (EE). Due to differences in chemical configuration and variations in metabolism, the potency of these agents is very diverse (Levin et al., 2019).

Pharmacokinetics. All oral estrogen formulations are readily absorbed and metabolized in the liver, are converted to estrone and estriol, and are excreted via the urine and feces. E2 and CE formulations are used in sole estrogen therapy. EE, a semisynthetic estrogen, is more commonly used in combination HRT (Mattison et al., 2014). Bioavailability and metabolism vary among agents. Comparatively, E2 formulations, or endogenous estrogens, have very low bioavailability, at only 5%. Most E2 agents are micronized to improve bioavailability. They are metabolized in the liver via the cytochrome (CYP) 3A4 pathway, with circulates bound to albumin and sex hormone binding globulin (SHBG). Similar to E2, EE is metabolized via the CYP 3A4 pathway. However, EE is not bound to SHBG in the circulation and is considered more potent than E2. The bioavailability of EE is 45%, and it has a longer half-life due to enterohepatic recirculation and metabolism. CE is composed primarily of equine estrogen. CE is rapidly absorbed and undergoes extensive hepatic metabolism and recirculation, resulting in the highest bioavailability of 50%. It binds to SHBG and albumin in the circulation. A significant portion of the circulating estrogens exists as estrone sulfate, serving as a reservoir for the formation of more active estrogens (Mattison et al., 2014).

Transdermal estrogen formulations deliver nominal E2 doses when applied to the lower abdomen for 84 hours. Absorption is dose proportionate. E2 is widely distributed in the body and is generally found in higher concentrations in the sex hormone target organs. Similar to oral formulations, transdermal E2 circulates in the blood largely bound to SHBG and albumin. Although the transdermal delivery omits the enterohepatic first-pass effect, E2 is converted to estrone and estriol in the liver. Enterohepatic recirculation and reabsorption occur via hepatic sulfate and glucuronide conjugation, biliary secretion, and intestinal hydrolysis. The half-life of transdermal E2 ranges from 6 to 8 hours. Excretion is primarily in the urine (Drugs.com, 2020).

Indications. The FDA approves the use of systemic estrogen therapy during the menopausal transition for four primary indications: the alleviation of vasomotor symptoms, bone loss prevention, spontaneous or surgical premature hypoestrogenism, and genitourinary symptoms (North American Menopause Society, [NAMS], 2017). Amelioration of sleep disturbances, improvement of sexual function, decreased joint pain, and beneficial effects on skin and hair have also been demonstrated in some studies (NAMS, 2017).

Adverse Effects. Patients have reported mild side effects, such as breast tenderness, headaches, mood changes, and irregular vaginal bleeding, with HRT initiation. These symptoms usually resolve after several weeks of treatment. Systemic estrogen therapy affects a multitude of systems with the potential for more serious adverse events; these are summarized in Table 21.3 (Hoffman et al., 2016a). More common concerns about risk will be highlighted here.

Increased breast cancer risk is a common concern with HRT. Evidence suggests that estrogen-alone hormone therapy does not increase the risk, except with prolonged use at high doses. Estrogen in combination with a progestin does increase the risk, most notably after 5 years of use. However, even with the longer duration, many other endogenous risk factors pose a greater risk for breast cancer than combination HRT (NAMS, 2017).

Many studies have explored the relationship between HRT and cardiovascular disease. Current studies suggest that a lower risk of preexisting atherosclerotic changes is found in females who are within 10 years of menopause onset and are not at an increased risk of severe cardiovascular events (myocardial infarction or stroke). However, in females who are past 10 years of menopausal onset, HRT initiation has been shown to increase the risk of adverse cardiovascular events due to already having an increased propensity for congenital heart disease (NAMS, 2017; Mehta et al., 2019).

A similar relationship exists with cognitive function. HRT does not impact or decrease cognitive function in younger females within 10 years of menopause onset. However, in older females, where cognitive decline may already be present, the risk of Alzheimer's disease and dementia is increased (NAMS, 2017).

Unopposed estrogen therapy in menopausal females who have a uterus poses a significant risk for endometrial hyperplasia and, potentially, endometrial cancer. This risk can be mediated by adding a progestin agent to the hormone regimen (Hoffman et al., 2016a; NAMS, 2017). Other notable risks for estrogen alone and combination HRT include increased risk for a venous thromboembolism

(VTE), particularly in females who are more than 10 years postmenopausal onset, and increased risk of gallbladder and hepatic disease (NAMS, 2017).

Contraindications. Caution must be observed when prescribing HRT to menopausal females with preexisting medical conditions, and HRT initiation should be avoided in females 10 years postmenopausal onset. Smoking is not a contraindication for HRT. However, smoking should be considered in overall health status and cardiovascular disease risk prior to initiating HRT (NAMS, 2017). Absolute contraindications for estrogen therapy include current or suspected breast cancer, current endometrial cancer, untreated endometrial hyperplasia or undiagnosed vaginal bleeding, active ischemic heart disease, high risk of a VTE, cerebrovascular disease, and active hepatic disease (O'Neil & Eden, 2017; Shifren et al., 2019).

Monitoring. When initiating HRT, short-term follow-up should be considered to review common side effects, overall impact on symptom relief, and potential for dosage adjustments. Once therapy is established, annual gynecologic care is appropriate follow-up to determine whether continued therapy is desired. In general, there are minimal guidelines for HRT discontinuation (NAMS, 2017). Due to the potential for increased breast cancer risk and cardiac events with combination therapy, discontinuation should be considered after 5 years (Shifren et al., 2019). However, in females with persistent menopausal symptoms, quality-of-life considerations, or elevated risk for bone loss, extended use of HRT may be appropriate (NAMS, 2017).

PRACTICE PEARLS

When to Initiate and Discontinue HRT

Therapy Initiation
- Due to significant increased cardiovascular risk with increasing age, it is recommended that HRT be initiated only in females within 10 years of menopausal onset who are younger than age 60 (Shufelt & Manson, 2018; Mehta et al., 2019).
- A thorough disclosure of risks of HRT must be reviewed with patients prior to therapy initiation.
- Vaginal estrogen therapy and other nonhormonal treatments specifically for GSM can be initiated at any age (NAMS, 2017).

Therapy Discontinuation
- The optimal duration of HRT to manage menopausal symptoms and improve quality of life varies among females. Current recommendations suggest no more than 5 years. In the absence of contraindications, the preferred dose, formulation, and duration of HRT should be determined with ongoing evaluation of risks and benefits through shared decision-making with the patient and the clinician (Shifren et al., 2019).
- There is no evidence that tapering or "weaning" HRT prompts a better transition to therapy discontinuation than abruptly stopping treatment (NAMS, 2017). However, patients may be more reassured with the slower tapering transition.

Progestins

HRT formulations incorporating very low doses of progestins are given with estrogens to decrease estrogen-driven endometrial overgrowth. Common progestins used in HRT are listed in Table 21.4 and Table 21.5. Progestins are used in both oral and transdermal formulations.

Pharmacokinetics. Progestins used in hormone therapy are well absorbed through the skin, mucous membranes, and gastrointestinal (GI) tract. The most common progestin agents used in HRT formulations include MPA, drospirenone, norethindrone, and micronized progesterone. These agents are all strong in their progestogenic effects but vary in metabolism and bioavailability. MPA and drospirenone have peak concentrations within 1 to 3 hours and a bioavailability of 70% to 80%. Both of these agents bind to albumin and other proteins for circulation. Neither of these agents binds to sex hormone binding globulin (SHGB). Norethindrone reaches peak concentration in 2 hours, has a bioavailability of 33% to 55%, and binds to both albumin and SHGB in the circulation. Micronized progesterone is the least potent progesterone agent, with a peak concentration at 3 hours; bioavailability is unknown. Micronized progesterone binds to albumin and other proteins in the circulation. It does not bind to SHGB. All agents are metabolized via the liver and excreted primarily through the urine and feces (Africander et al., 2011).

Indications. The primary indication for the addition of a progestin in HRT is endometrial protection. HRT with estrogen only can lead to endometrial hyperplasia and an increased risk of endometrial cancer in females with an intact uterus. When progestin is included, endometrial proliferation is moderated and estrogen-related endometrial hyperplasia is avoided (Hoffman et al., 2016b; NAMS, 2017). Incidentally, the mild sedating effects and reduced wakefulness that occur when taking oral progestogens may provide added benefits if sleep disturbances are present. In addition, bedtime dosing may ameliorate insomnia (NAMS, 2017; Levin et al., 2019).

Adverse Effects. Evidence suggests that there may be an increased risk of breast cancer associated with estrogen-progestogen use in postmenopausal females, most notably after 5 years of therapy. The depressive central nervous system (CNS) effects of progestogens have been noted to have a negative impact on mood in some females (NAMS, 2017).

Contraindications. Females with untreated depression should avoid progestogen therapy alone as it may exacerbate depressive symptoms. As stated previously, due to the potential for increased breast cancer risk with combination therapy

---

PRACTICE PEARLS

Alternative to Progestin Therapy

Bazedoxifine is a selective ER modulator (SERM) that has been combined with estrogen to form an estrogen selective complex. This combination still has the same risk profile as estrogen-only HRT, but it negates the need for a progestogen for endometrial protection (NAMS, 2017).

TABLE 21.4	**Oral Hormonal Therapies**			
Category/Medication	Indication	Dosage (mg/day)		Considerations and Monitoring
Estrogen-Only Therapy				
17β-estradiol[a]	Hormonal therapy	**Tablets:** 0.5 mg, 1.0 mg, 2.0 mg		Women who are posthysterectomy may do estrogen-only therapy.
Conjugated estrogens (CE)	Hormonal therapy	**Tablets:** 0.3 mg, 0.45 mg, 0.625 mg, 0.9 mg, 1.25 mg		Progestin-only therapy may be considered when estrogen is contraindicated.
				Women with an intact uterus on estrogen require progestin therapy.
Progestin-Only Therapy				
Medroxyprogesterone acetate (MPA)	Hormonal therapy	5 mg, 10 mg		Progestin-only therapy may be considered when estrogen is contraindicated.
Micronized progesterone[a]	Hormonal therapy	200 mg		
Norethindrone acetate	Hormonal therapy	2.5 mg, 5 mg, 10 mg		
Estrogen (E) + Progestin (P) Combination Therapy				
Conjugated estrogen + medroxyprogesterone acetate	Hormonal therapy	0.625 mg CE + 5 mg MPA days 1–14 5 mg MPA Days 15–28		Women with an intact uterus on estrogen require progestin therapy.
17β-estradiol + norgestimate	Hormonal therapy	1 mg E + 0.09 mg P		
Conjugated estrogen + medroxyprogesterone acetate	Hormonal therapy	0.3 mg or 0.45 mg CE + 1.5 mg MPA 0.625 mg CE + 2.5 mg or 5 mg MPA		
Ethinyl estradiol + norethindrone acetate	Hormonal therapy	0.025 mg E + 0.5 mg P or 0.05 mg E + 1 mg P		
17β-estradiol + norethindrone acetate	Hormonal therapy	0.5 mg E + 0.1 mg P or 1 mg E + 0.5 mg P		
17β-estradiol + drospirenone	Hormonal therapy	1 mg E + 0.5 mg P or 0.5 mg E + 0.25 mg P or 1 mg E + 1 mg P		

[a]Considered bioidentical.

after 5 years, discontinuation at that time should be considered (Shifren et al., 2019). Menopausal females at high risk for developing breast cancer as well as those who currently have or previously have had breast cancer should not take estrogen-only or estrogen-progestogen HRT (NAMS, 2017; Shifren et al., 2019).

Monitoring. When initiating HRT, short-term follow-up should be considered to review common side effects, overall impact on symptom relief, and potential for dosage adjustments. Once therapy is established, annual gynecologic care is appropriate follow-up to determine whether continued therapy is desired. In general, there are minimal guidelines for HRT discontinuation (NAMS, 2017). Due to the potential for increased breast cancer risk with combination therapy after 5 years, discontinuation at that time should be considered (Shifren et al., 2019). However, in females with persistent menopausal symptoms,

quality-of-life considerations, or elevated risk for bone loss, extended use of HRT may be appropriate.

Nonhormonal Therapy

Paroxetine

Paroxetine is a selective serotonin reuptake inhibitor (SSRI), not an estrogen, and its mechanism of action for the treatment of vasomotor symptoms is unknown. However, several studies have shown a significant reduction in vasomotor symptoms compared to placebos.

Pharmacokinetics. Paroxetine is completely absorbed after oral ingestion, and peak concentrations are reached at 6 hours. The metabolism of paroxetine is accomplished primarily by the CYP 2D6 pathway. Steady-state concentrations are reached at 12 to 16 days of consistent use following

TABLE 21.5   Transdermal Hormonal Therapies

Category	Preparation	Delivery Form	Dosage Options (mg/day)	Considerations and Monitoring
Estrogen	17β-estradiol (generics available)	Patch/film	0.025, 0.05, 0.075, 0.1 Apply twice weekly	Women who are posthysterectomy may do estrogen-only therapy. Women with an intact uterus on estrogen require progestin therapy.
			0.025, 0.0375, 0.05, 0.06, 0.075, 0.1 Apply once weekly	
			0.05, 0.1 Apply twice weekly	
			0.025, 0.0375, 0.05, 0.075, 0.1 Apply twice weekly	
			0.025, 0.0375, 0.05, 0.075, 0.1 Apply twice weekly	
	17β-estradiol*	Gel	Foil packet dose: 0.25, 0.5, 1.0 daily	
			Metered-dose pump: 0.75 daily	
			Metered-dose pump: 0.52 daily	
	17β-estradiol*	Spray	1.53 Apply one spray daily	
Estrogen/ Progestogen	17β-estradiol (E)+ norethindrone acetate (P)	Patch/film	0.5 E + 0.14 P Apply twice weekly	Women with an intact uterus on estrogen require progestin therapy.
	17β-estradiol (E)+ levonorgestrel (P)	Patch/film	0.045 E + 0.015 P Apply once weekly	Continuous combined therapy.

CYP 2D6 pathway saturation. Paroxetine distribution is noted throughout the body, including in the CNS, with only 1% remaining in the plasma. Approximately 95% of paroxetine is bound to plasma protein. Alternative P450 isozymes govern paroxetine clearance with no evidence of saturation. Sixty-four percent of excretion is through the urine and 36% is through the feces via bile; this occurs gradually, over a 10-day period, after oral dosing (Sebela Pharmaceuticals, 2017).

Indications. Paroxetine is indicated for the treatment of moderate to severe vasomotor symptoms associated with menopause. This configuration and dosage of paroxetine is not indicated for psychological disorders (Sebela Pharmaceuticals, 2017).

Adverse Effects. The most common adverse reactions are headache, fatigue, and nausea/vomiting (Sebela Pharmaceuticals, 2017).

Contraindications. Paroxetine is contraindicated when used concurrently with monoamine oxidase inhibitors (MAOIs) or when used within 14 days of MAOI use. In addition, paroxetine is a strong CYP 2D6 inhibitor, altering concentrations of drugs metabolized in this pathway. Additional contraindications include thioridazine and pimozide. Efficacy may be reduced when administered concomitantly with tamoxifen. Concomitant use of non steroidal

antiinflammatory drugs (NSAIDs), aspirin, or other drugs that affect coagulation may cause abnormal bleeding. Angle closure glaucoma has occurred in patients who have untreated anatomically narrow angles and who are treated with antidepressants. Hyponatremia can occur in association with a syndrome of inappropriate antidiuretic hormone secretion. Epidemiological studies have reported an association between SSRI treatment and fractures. Paroxetine may cause activation of mania/hypomania; screen for bipolar disorder and monitor for mania/hypomania. Use cautiously in patients with a history of seizures or with conditions that potentially lower the seizure threshold. Akathisia can occur, most likely in the first few weeks of treatment. Paroxetine may cause cognitive impairment; patients should not operate machinery or motor vehicles until they are certain that paroxetine does not adversely affect them.

Monitoring. In addition to the risks and contraindications mentioned, all patients who initiate therapy should be monitored for suicidality or unusual changes in behavior. They should also be monitored for the development of serotonin syndrome, a potentially life-threatening condition that has been reported with SSRIs alone (including paroxetine), but particularly with concomitant use of serotonergic drugs and with drugs that impair metabolism of serotonin

(Sebela Pharmaceuticals, 2017). When initiating paroxetine therapy, short-term follow-up (1 to 2 weeks) should be considered to review common side effects and overall impact on symptom relief. Patients need to be aware that this treatment does not address GSM, which may continue to worsen over time. Adjuvant topical therapy for GSM may need to be considered. Once therapy is established, annual gynecologic care is appropriate follow-up to determine whether continued therapy is desired.

GSM-Specific Therapy

Many females choose not to initiate systemic hormonal therapy. However, to manage urogenital symptoms of GSM and maintain sexual function, specific therapy for GSM can be initiated. Currently available treatment is highlighted in Table 21.6 and Table 21.7.

Topical Estrogen

Topical vaginal nonsystemic estrogen products are used primarily for GSM (Gandhi et al., 2016). Topical vaginal estrogen replacement therapy rapidly restores vaginal epithelium and associated vasculature. This improves vaginal secretions, lowers vaginal pH, restores healthy vaginal flora, and alleviates overall symptoms of GSM (Gandhi et al., 2016). Topical estrogen preparations with minimal absorption are available for use intravaginally.

Pharmacokinetics. Estrogen drug products are well absorbed through the skin, mucous membranes, and GI tract. The vaginal delivery of estrogens circumvents first-pass metabolism but is metabolized and excreted similarly to oral and transdermal estrogen. However, systemic absorption of vaginal estrogen delivery systems is significantly lower and endometrial protection with concomitant progestin therapy is not indicated (Gandhi et al., 2016).

TABLE 21.6 Transvaginal Therapies

Formulation	Medication/Active Ingredients	Indication	Dosage	Considerations and Monitoring
Creams	17β-estradiol[a]	Vulvar and vaginal atrophy	0.1 mg/Gm: Initial 2–4 Gm/day for 1–2 weeks, then 1 Gm 1–3 times/week	Use for the shortest duration consistent with treatment goals and risks for the individual patient.
	Conjugated estrogen	Atrophic vaginitis, kraurosis vulvae	0.625 mg/Gm: 0.5–2 Gm/day for 21 days, then off 7 days	
		Moderate to severe dyspareunia	0.5 Gm twice weekly or for 21 days, then off 7 days	
Rings	17β-estradiol[a]	Moderate to severe vulvar and vaginal atrophy due to menopause	7.5 mcg/day: 2 mg/ring for 90 days	
	Estradiol acetate[a]	Moderate to severe vasomotor symptoms due to menopause	0.05 mg/day, 0.10 mg/day for 90 days	
		Moderate to severe vulvar and vaginal atrophy due to menopause		
Inserts	Estradiol hemihydrate[a]	Atrophic vaginitis due to menopause	10 mcg Initial 1 tab/day for 2 weeks, then 1 tab twice weekly	
	Estradiol[a]	Moderate to severe dyspareunia, a symptom of vulvar and vaginal atrophy, due to menopause	4 mcg, 10 mcg Initial 1 tab/day for 2 weeks, then 1 tab twice weekly	
	Prasterone	Moderate to severe dyspareunia, a symptom of vulvar and vaginal atrophy, due to menopause	6.5 mg Once daily at bedtime	

[a]Considered bioidentical.

TABLE 21.7	Other Oral Therapies		
Medication/Active Ingredients	Indication	Dosage	Considerations and Monitoring
Conjugated estrogens (E) + bazedoxifene	Moderate to severe vasomotor symptoms	0.45 (E) mg/day + 20 mg/day bazedoxifene	Use for the shortest duration consistent with treatment goals and risks for the individual patient.
Ospemifene	Moderate to severe dyspareunia due to genitourinary syndrome of menopause	60 mg/day	
Paroxetine	Moderate to severe vasomotor symptoms	7.5 mg/day	

Indications. Local estrogen therapy is the most accepted form of therapy for GSM for patients who do not want or are not candidates for systemic hormonal therapy. It offers the fastest and most effective symptomatic relief of GSM with minimal systemic absorption. A progestin is not necessary for endometrial protection, and hepatic metabolism is avoided. Topical treatment is best suited to patients who seek relief solely from vaginal atrophy symptoms and not for relief from other menopausal symptoms (Gandhi et al., 2016).

Adverse Effects. Some patients report that cream products can be messy and application can be difficult. Headache was also reported with some of the vaginal inserts (TherapeuticsMD, 2019).

Contraindications. Even though there is extremely limited systemic absorption with topical estrogen therapy, the contraindications are similar to systemic estrogen therapy. Contraindications include undiagnosed abnormal genital bleeding, current or history of breast cancer, known or previous estrogen-dependent neoplasia, active or previous history of VTE or known thrombophilic disorders, active or previous arterial thromboembolic disease (e.g., stroke and myocardial infarction), and liver impairment or disease (TherapeuticsMD, 2019).

Monitoring. When initiating topical estrogen therapy, short-term follow-up (4 to 6 weeks) should be considered to review common side effects, overall impact on symptom relief, and potential for dosage adjustments. Once therapy is established, annual gynecologic care is appropriate follow-up to determine whether continued therapy is desired.

Selective Receptor Estrogen Modulator: Ospemifene

Ospemifene, an oral agent, is an estrogen receptor agonist/antagonist with tissue-selective effects. Its biological actions are mediated through binding to estrogen receptors in the vulvovaginal tissues, improving vaginal structure and pH. This option can be used in some patients who are not candidates for estrogen therapy (Gandhi et al., 2016).

Pharmacokinetics. Ospemifene reaches peak serum concentration 2 hours after oral intake. Absolute bioavailability of this agent has not been determined. However, ingestion with food was noted to increase bioavailability and is recommended. Steady-state levels are reached after 9 days of therapy. Ospemifene enters the circulation highly bound to proteins and undergoes metabolism via CYP 3A4, CYP 2C9, and CYP 2C19. Drug excretion is accomplished primarily via feces and partially via urine (Duchesnay, 2019).

Indications. Ospemifene is indicated for the treatment of vulvovaginal atrophy and moderate to severe dyspareunia related to menopause (Duchesnay, 2019).

Adverse Effects. Adverse effects include hot flashes, vaginal discharge, muscle spasms, headache, hyperhidrosis, vaginal hemorrhage, and night sweats. Patients taking ospemifene are at increased risk for VTE (Duchesnay, 2019).

Contraindications. Although ospemifene is not an estrogen, the contraindications for use are very similar to those for systemic estrogen therapy. They include a current or previous history of VTE, current or previous history of arterial thromboembolic disease (e.g., stroke and myocardial infarction), undiagnosed abnormal genital bleeding, and known or suspected estrogen-dependent neoplasia (Duchesnay, 2019).

Monitoring. Studies show a significant improvement of symptom severity at 12 weeks. Patient follow-up at this point is warranted to consider therapy effectiveness, presence of side effects, and continued treatment plan. Ospemifene should be used for the shortest duration consistent with treatment goals and risks for the individual patient. After initial evaluation, postmenopausal females should be reevaluated at least annually, or more frequently if clinically appropriate, to determine therapy duration or to determine whether treatment is still necessary (Duchesnay, 2019).

Intravaginal Dehydroepiandrosterone: Prasterone

Prasterone is an inactive endogenous steroid and is converted into active androgens and/or estrogens intravaginally (AMAG Pharmaceutical, 2019). This increases superficial cell percentage and decreases parabasal cells in the vaginal epithelium, improving vaginal secretions, epithelial thickness, and color. The vaginal pH is decreased and there is a significant decrease in sexual pain (Gandhi et al., 2016).

Pharmacokinetics. In general, human steroidogenic enzymes such as hydroxysteroid dehydrogenases, 5-alpha-reductases, and aromatases metabolize prasterone into androgens and estrogens. Studies indicate that topical administration of the prasterone vaginal insert once daily for 7 days resulted in a mean prasterone serum level significantly higher than that in the group treated with a placebo. The serum levels of the metabolites testosterone and estradiol were also slightly higher in females treated with the prasterone vaginally compared to those receiving a placebo (AMAG Pharmaceutical, 2019).

Indications. Prasterone is indicated for the treatment of moderate to severe dyspareunia, a symptom of vulvar and vaginal atrophy, due to menopause (AMAG Pharmaceutical, 2019).

Adverse Effects. Increased vaginal discharge and some cases of abnormal Pap smear findings have been reported (AMAG Pharmaceutical, 2019).

Contraindications. The primary contraindication for prasterone use is undiagnosed abnormal genital bleeding. However, estrogen is a metabolite of prasterone, and exogenous estrogen therapy is contraindicated in females with current or previous breast cancer. Since the use of prasterone has not been studied in females with breast cancer, its use should be avoided in this population (AMAG Pharmaceutical, 2019).

Monitoring. Studies show a significant improvement of symptom severity at 12 weeks. Patient follow-up at this point is warranted to consider therapy effectiveness, presence of side effects, and continued treatment plan. After initial evaluation, regular gynecologic care including cervical cancer screenings should be encouraged. There is no evidence regarding treatment duration; long-term efficacy requires further study (Gandhi et al., 2016).

Prescriber Considerations for Menopausal Transition Therapy

Clinical Practice Guidelines

The 2017 Hormone Therapy Position Statement of the North American Menopause Society

The North American Menopause Society embedded clinical guidelines for HRT in its 2017 position statement. Graded levels were provided to support its recommendations. Level 1 was based on consistent scientific evidence, level 2 was based on limited evidence, and level 3 was based on consensus and expert opinion (NAMS, 2017).

Clinical Reasoning for Menopausal Transition Therapy

Consider the individual patient's prominent symptomology and health history when considering medications for the menopausal transition. Menopausal symptoms can vary significantly from person to person. Establishing treatment goals for the most prominent symptoms is imperative for an effective treatment plan. Obtaining a thorough history to ascertain appropriate treatment options is paramount to minimize inherent risks related to therapy. Many patients have strong feelings related to hormonal therapy and these must be considered during patient counseling.

Provide comprehensive information on all available therapies for menopausal symptoms including mode of action, advantages, disadvantages, common risks, benefits, and side effects. Myriad therapies, hormonal and nonhormonal, are available for menopausal symptoms. A detailed assessment of the patient's current knowledge and potential misinformation must be performed to allow for factual, effective planning, treatment, and follow-up. Accurate information on risks, benefits, side effects, and effectiveness should be readily available to the patient. Written information should be offered when menopausal therapies are prescribed. Reliable resources that patients can review on their own should also be provided.

Ensure complete patient understanding regarding options for menopausal symptoms using a shared decision-making approach. A shared decision-making approach should be employed when determining a treatment plan. Therapy options should be determined based on adverse-effect profiles, safety data, individual patient health risks, and personal preferences (NAMS, 2017).

Assess the agent selected for its appropriateness for an individual patient by considering the medication's side effects and the patient's age, race/ethnicity, comorbidities, and genetic factors. Management of menopausal symptoms should be individualized and should consider treatment goals, patient age, years since onset, and risk versus benefit balance. Hormonal versus nonhormonal options, timing of therapy (initial versus continuation), and treatment duration must be taken into account (NAMS, 2017).

Initiate the treatment plan with the selected medication by first providing adequate patient education to ensure the patient's understanding and promote full participation in therapy initiation and duration. A review of specific characteristics of menopausal symptom therapies, risks, and side effects along with corroboration with the individual patient's medical conditions and social factors supports a safe and informed choice regarding menopausal symptom management (NAMS, 2017).

Conduct follow-up and monitoring of patient responses to menopausal transition therapy. Appropriate treatment option formulation, route of administration, dosage, and treatment duration to meet treatment objectives can be obtained by incorporating ongoing input from the patient over time (NAMS, 2017; O'Neil & Eden, 2017).

Teaching Points for Menopausal Transition Therapy

Health Promotion Strategies

- Review the occurrence of therapy-specific side effects, risks, and overall tolerability.

- Conduct ongoing dialogue regarding changes in health history and the potential emergence of contraindications to continued treatment.
- Conduct routine evaluation of the appropriateness of the menopausal symptom therapy and planned duration of treatment.
- Encourage age-appropriate health screenings and health monitoring.
- Encourage healthy lifestyle choices including getting adequate exercise, maintaining a healthy diet, managing body weight, and avoiding smoking.

Patient Education for Medication Safety

The potential for patient harm is inherent with changes in personal risk factors, the occurrence of serious side effects, or the development of contraindications to treatment. Ongoing evaluation for the development of health risks that predispose patients to harm with the continued use of menopausal symptom therapy is imperative for patient safety. New onset of cardiovascular disease, development of breast cancer, or recent thromboembolic events are excellent examples of situations when certain menopausal therapies should be discontinued.

Application Questions for Discussion

1. As a health-care provider, what patient and safety factors should be considered before prescribing therapies for menopausal symptoms?
2. What should be included in the education plan for a patient who has been prescribed HRT?
3. What individual and lifestyle factors should be considered for the duration of HRT treatment?

Selected Bibliography

Africander, D., Verhoog, N., & Hapgood, J. P. (2011). Molecular mechanisms of steroid receptor-mediated actions by synthetic progestins used in HRT and contraception. *Steroids, 76*(2011), 636–652.

Alford, C., & Nurudeen, S. K. (2019). Physiology of reproduction in women. In A. H. DeCherney, L. Nathan, N. Laufer, & A. S. Roman (Eds.), *Current Diagnosis & Treatment: Obstetrics & Gynecology.* New York: McGraw-Hill.

AMAG Pharmaceutical. (2019, November). *Label: Intrarosa-prasterone insert.* U.S. National Library of Medicine: DailyMed. Retrieved December 2019 from https://dailymed.nlm.nih.gov/dailymed/drugInfo.cfm?setid=df731acd-7276-4fef-b037-bc7f30c112cb.

Bakour, S., Hatti, A., & Whalen, S. (2017). Contraceptive methods and issues around the menopause: An evidence update. *The Obstetrician & Gynaecologist, 2017*(19), 289–297.

Bhat, A., Reed, S. D., & Unutzer, J. (2017). The obstetrician-gynecologist's role in detecting, preventing, and treating depression. *Obstetrics and Gynecology, 129*(1), 157–163.

Curtis, K. M., Jatlaoui, T. C., Tepper, N. K., Zapata, L. B., Horton, L. G., Jamieson, D. J., & Whiteman, M. K. (2016a). US selected practice recommendation for contraceptive use. *Morbidity and Mortality Weekly Report, 65*(4), 1–66.

Curtis, K. M., Tepper, N. K., Jatlaoui, T. C., Berry-Bibee, E., Horton, L. G., Zapata, L. B., & Whiteman, M. K. (2016b). US Medical eligibility criteria for contraceptive use. *Morbidity and Mortality Weekly Report, 65*(3).

Daan, N. M., & Fauser, B. C. (2015). Menopause prediction and potential implications. *Maturitas, 82*(2015), 257–265.

Dehlendorf, C., Krajewski, C., & Borrero, S. (2014). Contraceptive counseling: Best practices to ensure quality communication and enable effective use. *Clinical Obstetrics and Gynecology, 57*(4), 659–673.

Dragoman, M. V., Simmons, K. B., Paulen, M. E., & Curtis, K. M. (2017). Combination hormonal contraceptive (CHC) use among obese women and contraceptive effectiveness: A systematic review. *Contraception, 95*, 117–129.

Drugs.com. (2020, 7 1). Estradiol patch. *FDA Product Information.*

Duchesnay. (2019). *Highlights of Prescribing Information: Osphena (ospemifine).* January: from Osphena (ospemifine) tablets 60 mg. Retrieved December 2019. https://files.duchesnay.com/duchesnay-usa/osphena/osphena-prescribing-information.pdf.

Gandhi, J., Chen, A., Dagur, G., Suh, Y., Smith, N., & Cali, B. (2016). Genitourinary syndrome of menopause: An overview of clinical manifestation, pathophysiology, etiology, evaluation, and management. *American Journal of Obstetrics & Gynecology, 215*(5), 704–711. https://doi.org/10.1016/j.ajog.2016.07.045.

Harlow, S. D., Gass, M., Hall, J. E., Lobo, R., Maki, P., Rebar, R. W., & de Villiers, T. J. (2012). Executive summary of the stages of the reproductive aging workshop +10: Addressing the unfinished agenda of staging reproductive aging. *Menopause: The Journal of The North American Menopause Society, 19*(4), 387–395. https://doi.org/10.1097/gme.0b013e31824d8f40.

Hoffman, B. L., Schorge, J. O., Bradshaw, K. D., Halvorson, L. M., Schaffer, J. I., & Corton, M. M. (2016a). Menopausal Transition. In B. L. Hoffman, J. O. Schorge, K. D. Bradshaw, L. M. Halvorson, J. I. Schaffer, & M. M. Corton (Eds.), *Williams Gynecology* (3rd ed.). New York: McGraw-Hill.

Hoffman, B. L., Schorge, J. O., Bradshaw, K. D., Halvorson, L. M., Schaffer, J. I., & Corton, M. M. (2016b). The Mature Women. In B. L. Hoffman, J. O. Schorge, K. D. Bradshaw, L. M. Halvorson, J. I. Schaffer, & M. M. Corton (Eds.), *Williams Gynecology* (3rd ed.). New York: McGraw-Hill.

Karam, A. (2019). Chapter 5: The Breast. In A. H. DeCherney, L. Nathan, N. Laufer, & A. S. Roman (Eds.), *Current Diagnosis & Treatment: Obstetric & Gynecology* (12th ed.). New York: McGraw-Hill.

Lessey, B. A., & Young, S. L. (2019). Structure, function, and evaluation of the female reproductive tract. In J. F. Steuass, & R. L. Barbieri (Eds.), *Yen & Jaffe's Reproductive Endocrinology: Physiology, Pathophysiology, and Clinical Management* (pp. 207–227). Philadelphia: Elsevier.

Levin, E. R., Vitek, W. S., & Hammes, S. R. (2019). Estrogens, progestins, and the female reproductive tract. In L. L. Brunton, R. Hilal-Dandan, & B. C. Knollman (Eds.), *Goodman & Gilman's: The Pharmacological Basis of Therapeutics.* New York: McGraw-Hill.

Lobo, R. A. (2019). Menopause and Aging. In J. F. Steuass, & R. L. Barbieri (Eds.), *Yen & Jaffe's Reproductive Endocrinology: Physiology, Pathophysiology, and Clinical Management* (8th ed.) (pp. 322–356). Philadelphia: Elsevier.

Mattison, D. R., Karyakina, N., Goodman, M., & Lakind, J. S. (2014). Pharmaco- and toxicokinetics of selected exogenous and endogenous estrogens: A review and identification of knowledge gaps. *Critical Review in Toxicology, 44*(8), 696–724. https://doi.org/10.3109/10408444.2014.930813.

Mehta, J. M., Chestor, R. C., & Kling, J. M. (2019). The timing hypothesis: Hormone therapy for treating symptomatic women during menopause and its relationship to cardiovascular disease. *Journal of Women's Health, 28*(5), 705–710. https://doi.org/10.1089/jwh.2018.7201.

North American Menopause Society 2017 Hormone Therapy Position Statement Advisory Panel (NAMS). (2017). The 2017 hormone therapy position statement of The North American *Menopause* Society. Menopause 24(7), 728–753. doi: 10.1097/GME.0000000000000921. PMID: 28650869.

O'Neil, S., & Eden, J. (2017). The pathophysiology of menopausal symptoms. *Obstetrics, Gynaecology, and Reproductive Medicine, 27*(10), 303–310. https://doi.org/10.1016/j.ogrm.2017.07.002.

Patel, S., & Carey, L. (2018). Are hormonal contraceptive less effective in overweight and obese women? *Journal of the American Academy of Physician Assistants, 31*(1), 11–13. https://doi.org/10.1097/01.JAA.0000527709.23569.dc.

Sebela Pharmaceuticals. (2017). *Highlights of Prescibing Information: Brisdelle (paroxetine) capsules.* April: from Brisdelle (paroxetine) 7.5 mg. Retrieved December 2019. https://brisdelle.com/pdf/Brisdelle_PI_0417.pdf.

Shifren, J. L., Crandall, C. J., & Manson, J. E. (2019). Menopausal Hormone Therapy. *JAMA, 321*(24), 2458–2459. https://doi.org/10.1001/jama.2019.5346.

Shufelt, C., & Manson, J. (2018). Managing menopause by combining evidence with clinical judgment. *Clinical Obstetrics and Gynecology, 61*(3), 470–479. https://doi.org/10.1097/grf.0000000000000378.

Soares, C. N. (2019). *Practice Pearl: Taking a Fresh Look at Mood, Hormone, and Menopause.* December 10: from Menopause.org. Retrieved December 2019. https://www.menopause.org/docs/default-source/professional/nams-practice-pearl-ht-and-depression.pdf.

TherapeuticsMD. (2019). *Highlight of Prescribing Information: Imvexxy.* November: from Imvexxy (estradiol vaginal inserts). Retrieved December 2019. https://www.imvexxy.com/pi.pdf?utm_medium=dir_org&utm_source=dir_org&utm_campaign=undefined&utm_content=undefined&utm_term=dir_org.

Ward, K., & Deneris, A. (2018). An update on menopause management. *Journal of Midwifery & Women's Health, 63*(2), 168–177. https://doi.org/10.1111/jmwh.12737.

22

Antiinflammatory Medications

DEBORAH ADELL

Overview

Inflammation is described as an adaptive local or systemic response to tissue injury caused by pathogen or antigen invasion, mechanical injury, tissue oxygen or nutrient deprivation, exposure to radiation or chemical agents, or temperature extremes. It essentially serves as a defense mechanism designed to protect the body from disease and promote healing of damaged tissue while also maintaining homeostasis. Inappropriate, chronic, or widespread inflammation can contribute to diseases such as asthma, inflammatory bowel disease, and atherosclerosis. Medications used to treat or control inflammation include corticosteroids and nonsteroidal antiinflammatory drugs (NSAIDs). It is important to remember that antiinflammatory medications do not treat the underlying cause of the inflammation but are palliative to manage the manifestations of the inflammatory process.

Relevant Physiology

Inflammation can be acute or chronic. *Acute inflammation* is designed to eliminate or inhibit pathogens, control tissue damage, and facilitate the healing process. Acute inflammation is characterized by erythema, swelling, pain, and increased temperature at the site of injury or infection. These manifestations of inflammation are the result of biochemical or cellular processes that are consistent but nonspecific to the type of insult. The processes are interdependent, with one process prompting the activation of other processes. The process is activated within seconds of insult. The duration of acute inflammation is short lived, resolving within 7 to 10 days with removal of the offending element (such as a splinter under the skin) or healing of the wound or injury. No matter what the cause, inflammation initiation follows a typical pattern:

- In response to tissue injury or pathogen invasion, activated plasma proteins induce vasodilation to increase blood flow to the site, causing erythema and heat.
- Leaking of plasma as a result of increased vascular permeability causes local edema and increases the concentration of red blood cells at the injury site.
- Enzymes within the clotting cascade prompt formation of fibrin strands to control the migration of infection.

- Degranulation of mast cells and release of histamine is prompted by specific complement products.
- Leucocytes arrive at the site, adhere to the endothelial cells, and prompt release of biochemical markers (e.g., histamine, leukotrienes, prostaglandins, cytokines) while also phagocytizing pathogens. Chemical mediators increase sensitivity of nociceptors and increase pain perception.
- Within hours, biochemical mediators attract neutrophils to the site, where they further phagocytize pathogens and release chemokines to attract macrophages. Macrophages arriving at the site induce vascular permeability and clotting and promote the action of leukocytes.
- Nociceptors are stimulated by several inflammatory mediators, such as bradykinins, prostaglandins, and TNF-α, resulting in pain.

The lymphatic system drains accumulated extravascular fluid and debris. Once in the system, pathogens drained from the injury site activate T and B lymphocytes. The lymphatic system is also subject to the inflammatory process, observed as swelling of glands or lymphangitis.

Chronic inflammation can result from failure to remove the offending causative agent of acute inflammation, continuous exposure to substances such as airborne allergens, autoimmune self-antigen response which continuously activates T-cells, repetitive injury, and cancers. In chronic inflammation, the actions of acute inflammation continue unchecked. Neutrophils are replaced by leukocytes and macrophages, creating the hallmark presentations of chronic inflammation: tissue damage and tissue overresponse of fibrosis and granuloma formation. Many chronic systemic diseases are recognized as having inflammatory components, such as diabetes, cardiovascular disease, allergies, and joint diseases.

Pathophysiology

While acute inflammation plays an important role in prompting tissue repair and preventing spread of infection, the biochemical and cellular activities involved in acute inflammation can contribute to the symptoms of local swelling and pain and the systemic reaction of fever. Additionally, the immune system can exhibit an exaggerated inflammatory response, or a hypersensitivity reaction to antigens. Antiinflammatory and immune-suppressing medications are used to mediate those effects.

Chronic, uncontrolled inflammation is considered pathologic. Uncontrolled local acute inflammation that extends past approximately 2 weeks can result from a wide variety of conditions, including unresolved infection, recurring exposure to allergens (e.g., inhaled pollen or mold), or repetitive reinjury such as tendonitis from overuse. Inflammatory mediators have been implicated in the pancreatic dysfunction of types 1 and 2 diabetes, inflammation and bronchial constriction of asthma, and endothelial dysfunction of atherosclerosis.

Inflammation Control Therapy

Glucocorticoids

Corticosteroids are adrenally produced hormones with multiple effects throughout the body. The class of corticosteroids is divided into *glucocorticoid hormones* (for their carbohydrate metabolism-regulating actions) and *mineralocorticoid hormones* (for their electrolyte balance-regulating actions). In practice, it is common for the terms *glucocorticoid* and *corticosteroid* to be used as synonyms. For the sake of clarity and specificity, the term *glucocorticoid* will be used in this chapter.

In addition to regulation of glucose, the endogenous role of glucocorticoids in the body includes blood pressure regulation; skeletal muscle function; mood and behavior regulation; electrolyte/water balance (although to a lesser extent than mineralocorticoid hormones like aldosterone); metabolism of proteins, lipids, and carbohydrates; bone resorption; and suppression of inflammation. Glucocorticoids, both endogenous and exogenous, exert their antiinflammatory and immunosuppressive actions through mediation or inhibition of leukocyte activity in addition to their suppression of cytokines, macrophages, fibroblasts, and lymphocytes.

Cortisol, the main glucocorticoid, is produced endogenously by the adrenal cortex. The adrenal cortex is under the control of the hypothalamic-pituitary-adrenal axis (HPAA) as a negative biofeedback loop. Receptors for cortisol are widely distributed throughout the body, affecting a variety of systems (Fig. 22.1). Endogenously produced cortisol is released in a diurnal pattern, peaking early in the morning with trough levels in the late afternoon. Related to normal secretion patterns, alterations in cortisol levels, either physiologic or through corticosteroid medication administration, can result in altered sleep patterns, arousal potential, and level of awareness.

PRACTICE PEARLS

Glucocorticoid Dosing Best Practice

Patients should be encouraged to take daily doses before 8 a.m. Doses administered twice daily should be taken before 8 a.m. and at approximately 4 p.m. in an attempt to mimic natural patterns of endogenously produced cortisol. This schedule assists in minimizing sleep disturbance.

Administered orally, all glucocorticoids are readily absorbed and can be administered intramuscularly in the primary care setting when prolonged release is desired. Glucocorticoids can also be used topically for local antiinflammatory action in the joints, lungs, conjunctival sac, and skin. Doses applied topically can have variable absorption depending on the application site. Use of corticosteroids in dermatologic, eye and ear, and pulmonary conditions can be found in Chapters 3 to 7.

Once absorbed into general circulation, glucocorticoids are bound to plasma proteins, including transcortin, which is specific to corticosteroids and, to a lesser extent, albumin. Only free, unbound drug is available for use. Drug metabolism is primarily hepatic, with some formulas (cortisone and prednisone) being metabolized to active compounds (hydrocortisone and prednisolone). Careful monitoring of liver function is advised if used in patients with a positive hepatitis B surface antigen. Excretion is via the kidney, with approximately 1% of the dose excreted unchanged. Caution is indicated in the use of any glucocorticoid medication in patients with renal insufficiency, acute glomerulonephritis, or chronic nephritis. Examples of common drug–drug interactions are listed in Table 22.1.

PRACTICE PEARLS

Management of Acute vs Chronic Inflammation

When glucocorticoids are prescribed to relieve inflammation associated with acute conditions, dosing is usually started at the high end of the scale, with the aim of prompt relief of symptoms. The dose is then adjusted to maintain control. For chronic conditions that may require long-term use, dosing is started at the lower end and titrated upward until control of unwanted symptoms is achieved.

Many of the adverse effects of glucocorticoid medications reflect exaggeration of normal cortisol function (Table 22.2), such as hyperglycemia, increased thirst or hunger, behavioral alterations, sleep pattern disturbance, increased blood pressure, and fluid retention. Long-term or high-dose usage can result in osteoporosis, myopathy, cataract formation, osteonecrosis of the femoral head, and deposition of adipose tissue in the face and neck. Use in children, even at relatively small doses, can result in growth suppression. When used concomitantly with NSAIDs, there is an increased risk of peptic ulcer formation. In the presence of infection, suppression of the immune system using glucocorticoid medications should include concomitant antimicrobial therapy; glucocorticoid medications should never be used in the presence of fungal infections. Glucocorticosteroids should be used cautiously in patients with latent tuberculosis, and the patient should be monitored for conversion to active disease. Suppression of the HPAA may mask signs or symptoms of new infection. Patients should monitor and report possible infections during treatment, such as sore throats or fever.

Live vaccines are contraindicated in patients taking high-dose or long-term steroid therapy. Short-course, low-dose

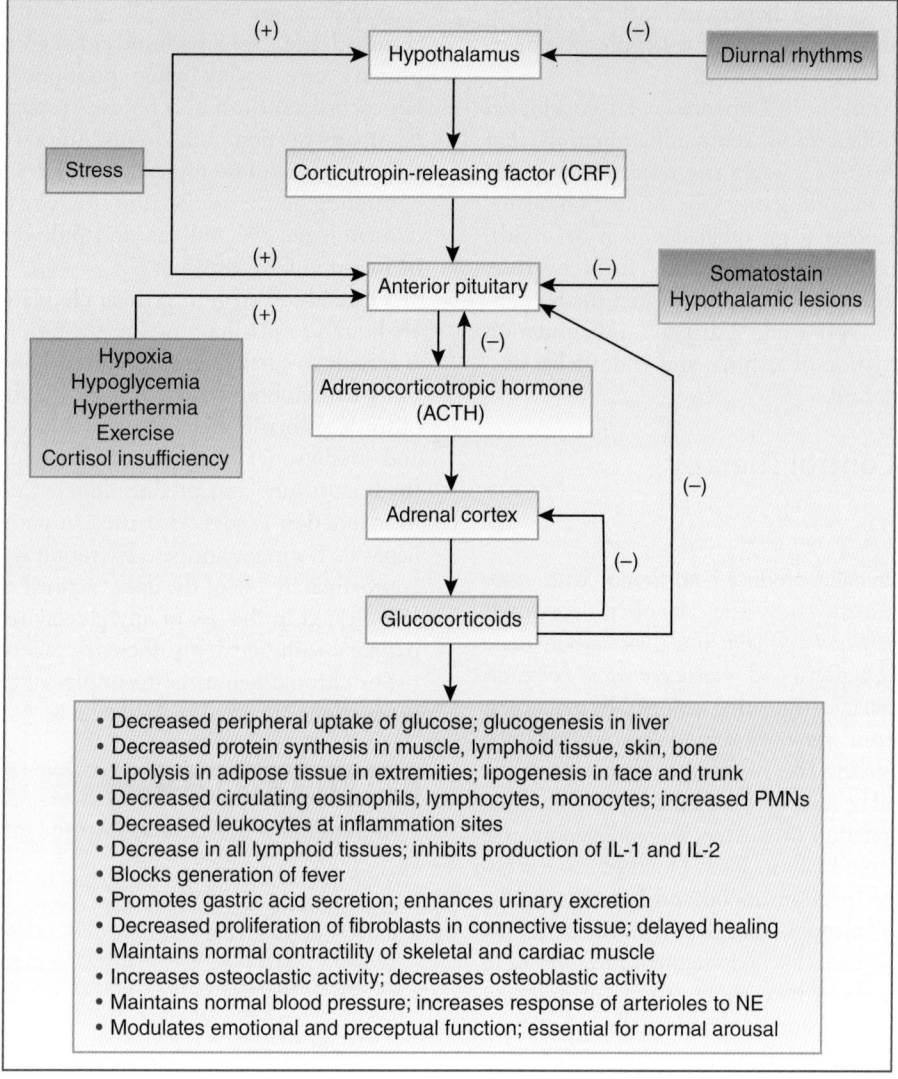

• **Fig. 22.1** HPA and cortisol systemic effects. (From Woo, T., & Robinson, M. [2020]. *Pharmacotherapeutics for advanced practice nurses.* Philadelphia: F.A. Davis.)

TABLE 22.1   Medications That Interact With Glucocorticoid Medications

Medication	Interacting Medication	Possible Effects
All corticosteroids and glucocorticoids	Salicylates, barbiturates, digoxin, isoniazid (INH), estrogen, ketoconazole, thiazide/loop diuretics, rifampin, hydantoins, piperacillin	Increased or decreased corticosteroid clearance or half-life, digitalis toxicity, hypokalemia, decreased risk of pharmacologic effects of corticosteroids
Betamethasone, cortisone, hydrocortisone	Insulin, oral hypoglycemics	Hyperglycemia
Methylprednisolone	Macrolide antibiotics	Decrease in methylprednisolone clearance
	Insulin, oral hypoglycemics	Hyperglycemia
Prednisone	NSAIDs	Increased risk for GI bleed
	Insulin, oral hypoglycemics	Hyperglycemia
Dexamethasone	Ephedrine	Decreased half-life and increased clearance of dexamethasone
	Insulin, oral hypoglycemia	Hyperglycemia

GI, gastrointestinal; *NSAIDs,* nonsteroidal antiinflammatory drugs.

TABLE 22.2 Adverse Effects of Corticosteroid Medications[a]

System	Effect	Action
Immune	Increased susceptibility to infection, activation of latent tuberculosis, Addisonian-like crisis with abrupt withdrawal after long-term use	Monitor for signs and symptoms of infection. Test for tuberculosis prior to initiation of long-term therapy. Avoid live vaccines.
Musculoskeletal	Myopathy and muscle weakness, which may be only partially reversible, osteoporosis, osteonecrosis	Monitor bone density, calcium, and vitamin D. Withdraw therapy for myopathy or weakness, use of concomitant bisphosphonates in long-term therapy.
Metabolic	Hyperglycemia, hunger, weight gain, fat redistribution, impaired wound healing, Cushing's-like syndrome	Monitor blood sugar.
Gastrointestinal	PUD, perforation, gastric bleed, alteration in liver enzymes	Monitor CBC, lipids, enzymes in long-term use, guaiac stool testing.
Behavioral	Nervousness, psychosis, insomnia, mood changes	Administer lowest dose for shortest time possible.
Eye	Cataract formation, glaucoma	Conduct periodic slit-lamp examination during long-term use.
Fluid and electrolytes	Hypokalemic alkalosis, hypertension	Monitor blood pressure and potassium in long-term use.
Growth and development	Growth retardation in children, subtle fetal abnormalities, adrenal insufficiency in babies born to mothers on large doses	Monitor growth in children, determine risk/benefit ratio when treating pregnant or nursing mothers.

[a]A single dose of glucocorticoid, even a large one, is virtually without harmful effects, and a short course of therapy (up to 1 week), in the absence of specific contraindications, is unlikely to be harmful. As the duration of glucocorticoid therapy is increased beyond 1 week, there are time- and dose-related increases in the incidence of disabling and potentially lethal effects. (Brunton et al., 2017. p. 855). Prolonged administration of physiologic replacement does not usually result in adverse effects.

CBC, complete blood count; *PUD,* peptic ulcer disease.

(2 weeks or less) therapy or administration of inhaled glucocorticoids is not a contraindication to the live vaccine. Inactivated vaccines may be administered during any course of steroid use; however, there is a theoretical possibility of decreased immune response to the vaccine.

Use of glucocorticoid medications at supraphysiologic doses for longer than 2 to 4 weeks can result in acute adrenal insufficiency if the medication is abruptly withdrawn related to suppression of the HPAA. Rebound or flare of the underlying disease for which the glucocorticoid was prescribed is also possible. Tapering of the medication instead of abrupt cessation should be implemented to avoid these effects. The length of taper is dependent upon the dose, duration of therapy, and disease state of the patient. Generally, the taper involves decreasing the dose by the equivalent of 2.5 to 5 mg of prednisone once or twice per week until a total dose of 5 mg is reached. Thereafter, decrease the dose by 1 mg per week until the medication is stopped. Short-term treatment (less than 2 weeks) does not require tapering.

An additional means that may be employed to minimize the potential for HPAA suppression is alternate-day therapy. The total weekly dose is divided and administered every other day. This can also be used for children in need of long-term therapy to assist with avoiding growth suppression.

Glucocorticoid medications readily cross the placental barrier. Although human studies are limited, animal studies have demonstrated fetal malformation and death. Use of glucocorticoid medications in pregnancy should involve careful risk/benefit analysis, especially in the first trimester, due to increased risk for cleft palate development. Glucocorticoid medications are excreted in breast milk and may have adverse effects on the infant, including interference with growth and HPAA suppression if given over long periods. Some studies indicate that doses of 20 mg daily or less of prednisone or prednisolone or 8 mg daily or less of methylprednisolone for short periods may pose low risk to the infant. Breastfeeding should be avoided for 4 hours after the maternal dose is administered.

The class of glucocorticoid medications is divided by time to onset of action and length of action. Glucocorticoid medications are further defined by potency, with higher-potency medications having a higher risk of adverse effects. Dosing is highly patient and disease state dependent. Common dosing schedules are illustrated in Table 22.3; however, individualization should be practiced. Potency can be compared across the class (Box 22.1). Principles to assist the primary care provider in guiding doses of glucocorticoids are provided in Box 22.2.

Hydrocortisone

Pharmacokinetics. Hydrocortisone is considered a parallel medication to endogenously secreted cortisone and one of the short-duration-of-action corticosteroids. Other corticosteroids have similar metabolism and excretion, and

| TABLE 22.3 | Glucocorticoids[a] | | | |

Category/ Medication	Indication	Dosage	Comments
Short Acting			
Cortisone (generic only)	Adjunctive, short-term therapy of rheumatic disorders, including acute gouty arthritis, AS, RA, JRA/JIA, posttraumatic OA, synovitis of OA, or psoriatic arthritis	*Adults:* 25–300 mg orally once daily or on alternate days. *Children:* 0.7–10 mg/kg/day or 20–300 mg/m²/day orally as single or divided dose.	Dosage is highly variable. Reduce dosage to the lowest possible for maintenance once a desired response has been achieved. Administer with meals. For once-a-day dosing, administer in the morning to mimic the body's normal cortisol secretion. Adjust dose according to patient response.
Hydrocortisone	Nonemergent treatment of hypersensitivity or allergic reactions As an adjunct in the treatment of rheumatic disorders, including acute gouty arthritis, AS, RA, JRA/JIA, posttraumatic OA, or psoriatic arthritis Acute episodes or exacerbation of non-rheumatic inflammation including acute and subacute bursitis, epicondylitis, and acute non-specific tenosynovitis	*Adults:* 20–240 mg orally daily in 2–4 divided doses. *Adolescents, children, and infants:* 0.56–8 mg/kg/day orally in 3–4 divided doses.	
	Relief of inflammation, pruritus ani, and swelling associated with hemorrhoids	**External topical dosage (hydrocortisone cream):** *Adults:* Apply a thin film to the external affected anal area 2–4 times per day (not for rectal use). **Rectal dosage (hydrocortisone acetate rectal suppositories):** *Adults:* Insert 1 suppository per rectum twice daily, morning and night, for 2 weeks.	
Intermediate Acting			
Triamcinolone	Acute episodes and exacerbations of AS, inflammation associated with acute gouty arthritis, acute and subacute bursitis, acute nonspecific tenosynovitis, epicondylitis, RA, JRA/JIA, psoriatic arthritis, and the synovitis of OA	**Intramuscular dosage (triamcinolone acetonide injectable suspension):** *Adults:* Begin with 60 mg IM and titrate to response. Usual dosage range is 40–80 mg daily. Some may be well controlled on less than 20 mg/day. *Children and adolescents:* 0.11–1.6 mg/kg/day (3.2–48 mg/m²/day) IM given as 3 or 4 divided doses.	IM injections should be administered deeply into a well-developed muscle. Rotate sites of injection. Titrate to lowest effective dose.
Prednisone	Rheumatic conditions, including RA, JRA/JIA, AS, acute and subacute bursitis, acute nonspecific tenosynovitis, acute gouty arthritis and gout, OA, or epicondylitis	*Adults:* Usual range 5–30 mg orally once daily. *Children and adolescents:* 0.05–2 mg/kg/day orally given in 1–4 divided doses.	Administer with food to minimize GI irritation. **NOTE:** Oral dose packs with tapered dosing are available.

TABLE 22.3	Glucocorticoids—cont'd			
Category/ Medication	**Indication**	**Dosage**	**Comments**	
Prednisolone	Adjunctive therapy in the treatment of rheumatic disorders, including AS, gout with gouty arthritis, JRA/JIA, posttraumatic OA, or RA Treatment of acute episodes or exacerbation of nonrheumatic inflammation, including acute and subacute bursitis, epicondylitis, and acute nonspecific tenosynovitis	*Adults:* 5–60 mg/day orally as a single dose or in divided doses. *Adolescents, children, and infants:* 0.14–2 mg/kg/day orally or 4–60 mg/m²/day in 3–4 divided doses.	Give with food to minimize indigestion or GI irritation. If oral dose is given once daily or every other day, give in the morning to coincide with the body's normal cortisol secretion. **NOTE:** Oral dose packs with tapered dosing are available.	
Methylprednisolone	Adjunctive medication in the treatment of rheumatic disorders, including acute gouty arthritis, AS, JRA/JIA, posttraumatic OA, psoriatic arthritis, or RA Treatment of acute episodes or exacerbation of nonrheumatic inflammatory conditions, including acute and subacute bursitis, epicondylitis, and acute nonspecific tenosynovitis	**Oral:** *Adults:* 4–48 mg/day orally in 4 divided doses. *Children and adolescents:* 0.5–1.7 mg/kg/day orally in divided doses every 6–12 hr. **IM dosage (methylprednisolone sodium succinate injection):** *Adults:* Initially, 10–40 mg IM. *Children and adolescents:* Initial dose range is 0.11–1.6 mg/kg/day IM in 3–4 divided doses (3.2–48 mg/m²/day). **IM dosage (methylprednisolone acetate injection suspension):** *Adults:* 10–120 mg IM. *Children and adolescents:* 0.5–1.7 mg/kg/day IM (a single injection during each 24-hr period equal to the total daily oral dose is usually sufficient).	Oral medication should be given with food to decrease gastric irritation. Give in the morning to mimic normal cortisol secretion. **NOTE:** Oral dose packs with tapered dosing are available. IM injections should be administered deeply into a well-developed muscle. Rotate sites of injection.	
Long Acting				
Dexamethasone	Adjunctive therapy in the treatment of rheumatic disorders, including acute gouty arthritis, AS, RA, JRA, posttraumatic OA, synovitis of OA, and for psoriatic arthritis Treatment of acute episodes or exacerbation of nonrheumatic inflammatory conditions, including acute and subacute bursitis, epicondylitis, acute nonspecific tenosynovitis, and cystic tumors of an aponeurosis tendon	**Oral dosage (dexamethasone):** *Adults:* 0.75–9 mg/day orally in 2–4 divided doses. *Infants, children, and adolescents:* 0.02–0.3 mg/kg/day or 0.6–9 mg/m²/day orally in 3–4 divided doses. **IM dosage (dexamethasone sodium phosphate injection solution):** *Adults:* 0.5–9 mg/day IM in 2–4 divided doses. *Adolescents, children, and infants:* 0.02–0.3 mg/kg/day or 0.6–9 mg/m²/day IM in 3–4 divided doses.	Dosage should be individualized and is variable depending on type and severity of disease as well as patient's response. **NOTE:** Oral dose packs with tapered dosing are available.	

ªSee Chapters 3–7 for common indications and doses of corticosteroids in integumentary, ocular, allergy, asthma, and other pulmonary conditions.

AS, Ankylosing spondylitis; *GI,* gastrointestinal; *IM,* intramuscular; *JIA,* juvenile idiopathic arthritis; *JRA,* juvenile rheumatoid arthritis; *OA,* osteoarthritis; *RA,* rheumatoid arthritis.

NOTE: Prolonged administration of physiologic replacement dosages of glucocorticoids does not usually cause adverse effects. The severity of the adverse effects associated with prolonged administration of pharmacologic dosages of corticosteroids, such as prednisone, increases with duration of therapy. Short-term administration of large doses typically does not cause adverse effects, but long-term administration can lead to adrenocortical atrophy and generalized protein depletion.

The following recommendations for withdrawal of corticosteroids based on the duration of therapy have been made: less than 2 weeks, may abruptly discontinue; 2–4 weeks, taper dose over 1 to 2 weeks; more than 4 weeks, taper slowly over 1–2 months to physiologic dose (approximately 2.5 mg/m²/day of prednisolone) and discontinue after assessment of adrenal function has demonstrated recovery.

• BOX 22.1 Glucocorticoid Potency Equivalency

Cortisone: 25 mg
Hydrocortisone: 20 mg
Prednisolone: 5 mg
Prednisone: 5 mg
Methylprednisolone: 4 mg
Triamcinolone: 4 mg
Dexamethasone: 0.75 mg
Betamethasone: 0.75 mg

From Elsevier. Clinical pharmacology powered by ClinicalKey®. (2019). [cited 2020 September] Retrieved from http://www.clinicalkey.com.

• BOX 22.2 Principles That Guide Dosing of Glucocorticoid Medications

- Dosing should be individualized to the patient and the disease being treated.
- Establish time frames for response. Reevaluate and refer if the desired response is not noted.
- For managing acute conditions, initial dose should be started at the high end of the dosing schedule. When the initial response is acceptable, reduce dose daily in small amounts until an adequate clinical response is attained or the medication is stopped. This may also be achieved by prescribing preformulated tapering such as with Medrol Dosepak.
- For chronic therapy, adjust dose upward in small amounts until the desired therapeutic response is attained. Once achieved, it is appropriate to slowly reduce the dose until the lowest possible dose to control the condition.
- For daily doses, administer prior to 9 a.m. to match endogenous patterns of secretion.
- For long-term use of intermediate-acting formulas, every-other-day dosing of twice the daily dose can be administered.

Adapted from Woo, T., & Robinson, M. (2020). *Pharmacotherapeutics for advanced practice nurses.* Philadelphia: F.A. Davis.

---

the activity of other corticosteroids is measured against hydrocortisone. When given orally, hydrocortisone is well absorbed in the jejunum, metabolized in the liver to inactive compounds, and excreted 1% unchanged in the urine. Onset of action of the oral dose is rapid, with a peak concentration in 1 hour. The plasma half-life is approximately 1.5 hours, with a biological half-life of 8 to 12 hours. Intramuscular administration results in a delayed onset of action of 4 to 8 hours.

Indications. Hydrocortisone has a wide array of uses in a variety of inflammatory conditions, as well as in patients with adrenocortical insufficiency.

Adverse Effects. Given the widespread effects of steroids in the body, adverse effects of hydrocortisone can manifest as excess secretion of natural cortisol, as observed in Cushing's disease. Additionally, suppression of the immune system can result in potential for uncontrolled infection without classic signs or symptoms, as well as interruption of the HPAA, resulting in Addisonian crisis. Typical adverse reactions are listed in Table 22.2.

Contraindications. Hydrocortisone should not be used in the presence of fungal infections and should not be used without concomitant treatment of other microbial infections. Reactivation of tuberculosis may occur in patients with latent tuberculosis, so these patients must be monitored carefully. Caution should be observed in prescribing corticosteroids to patients with conditions including hypertension, heart failure, osteoporosis, seizure disorder, and renal or hepatic disease. Hydrocortisone should also be used cautiously in patients with a history of psychosis or emotional lability.

Monitoring. Short-term use does not require laboratory monitoring. In long-term or high-dose use, patients should be monitored for adverse effects as listed in Table 22.2. Monitoring may include blood pressure, serum glucose and potassium levels, vitamin D levels, bone mineral density, and weight measurement. Children should be monitored for growth interruptions or delays.

Methylprednisolone

Pharmacokinetics. Methylprednisolone is considered an intermediate-acting steroid. To avoid HPAA suppression, it is recommended that this medication be administered once daily in the early morning. The medication is well absorbed in all forms. Onset of action is rapid, with peak concentration in 1 to 2 hours, a plasma half-life of approximately 2.5 hours, and a biological half-life of 18 to 36 hours. Intramuscular or intraarticular administration can delay both onset and duration of action.

Indications. Methylprednisolone is used primarily for treatment of inflammatory conditions and for use in patients who require immunosuppression.

Adverse Effects. In addition to the adverse effects for the glucocorticoid class, macrolide antibiotics may reduce clearance of methylprednisolone.

Contraindications. In addition to the cautions and contraindications for the glucocorticoid class, some formulas may contain sulfites or lactose.

Monitoring. All monitoring for adverse events or toxic levels of glucocorticoids as per the class should be observed.

Dexamethasone

Pharmacokinetics. Dexamethasone is considered a long-acting steroid. Absorption following oral administration is rapid, with peak concentration occurring in 1 to 2 hours. Plasma half-life is 3.5 hours, with a biological half-life of 36 to 57 hours. Intramuscular administration may delay onset of action. Related to the potency, prolonged administration or short-term high dosing requires taper due to the possibility of HPAA suppression.

Indications. Dexamethasone is used primarily for inflammation, such as acute allergy, and intra-articularly for joint inflammation, and immunosuppression.

Adverse Effects. All adverse effects for the glucocorticoid class apply to this medication.

Contraindications. All contraindications for the glucocorticoid class apply to this medication.

Monitoring. In addition to typical monitoring for the glucocorticoid class, the patient should be monitored for HPAA suppression during taper and following discontinuation of the medication.

Nonsteroidal Antiinflammatory Drugs (NSAIDs)

The NSAID class of medications is a large, chemically diverse group used to treat inflammation, pain, and fever through the indirect inhibition of the inflammatory mediator prostaglandin. Related to this action, this class of drugs is sometimes called *antiprostaglandin*. The chemical diversity of the group allows for varying degrees of antiinflammatory action and adverse-effect profiles. In general, the higher the antiinflammatory action, the higher the risk of adverse effects. This is attributed to the nonselective inhibition of the enzyme *cyclooxygenase (COX)*. COX is the first enzyme in the pathway responsible for the synthesis of the chemical mediators of inflammation: prostaglandins and thromboxane. Prostaglandins are powerful inducers of inflammation, pain, and fever but also serve important homeostatic functions, including stimulation of the goblet cells of the stomach to produce protective mucus. Inhibiting COX reduces circulating prostaglandins.

Cyclooxygenase exists in two forms: COX-1 and COX-2. Many tissues of the body contain COX-1, which affects platelet function, endothelial cells, the gastrointestinal (GI) tract, and renal microvasculature, glomeruli, and collecting ducts. COX-2 is induced by cytokines released by damaged tissue and is present at the site of inflammation (Fig. 22.2).

Nonselective NSAIDs inhibit COX-1 and COX-2, thereby affecting many systems. The side-effect profile related to inhibition of COX-1 and COX-2 includes effects on the GI, renal, cardiovascular, reproductive, neurologic, hepatic, and dermatologic systems. Effects are also noted on platelet aggregation, red and white blood cells, vision, and hearing. Hypersensitivity reactions can occur and may appear as cross-sensitivities within the class.

One NSAID that is selective for COX-2 inhibition, celecoxib, is available. Celecoxib targets only COX-2 inhibition at the site of inflammation to decrease continued prostaglandin production. Therefore, other systems that contain COX-1 are less affected. This results in a theoretical decreased potential for gastric bleeding and antiplatelet effects, although these adverse effects may still occur. Gastric rupture and bleed without warning have occurred with COX-2 inhibitor medications. An increased risk for cardiac events, including new-onset or worsening of existing hypertension and thromboembolism events resulting in myocardial infarction or stroke, resulted in several COX-2 inhibitor medications being removed from the market. Although COX-2 inhibitors have lower potential than nonselective NSAIDs for cardiac and GI risk, in 2005 the

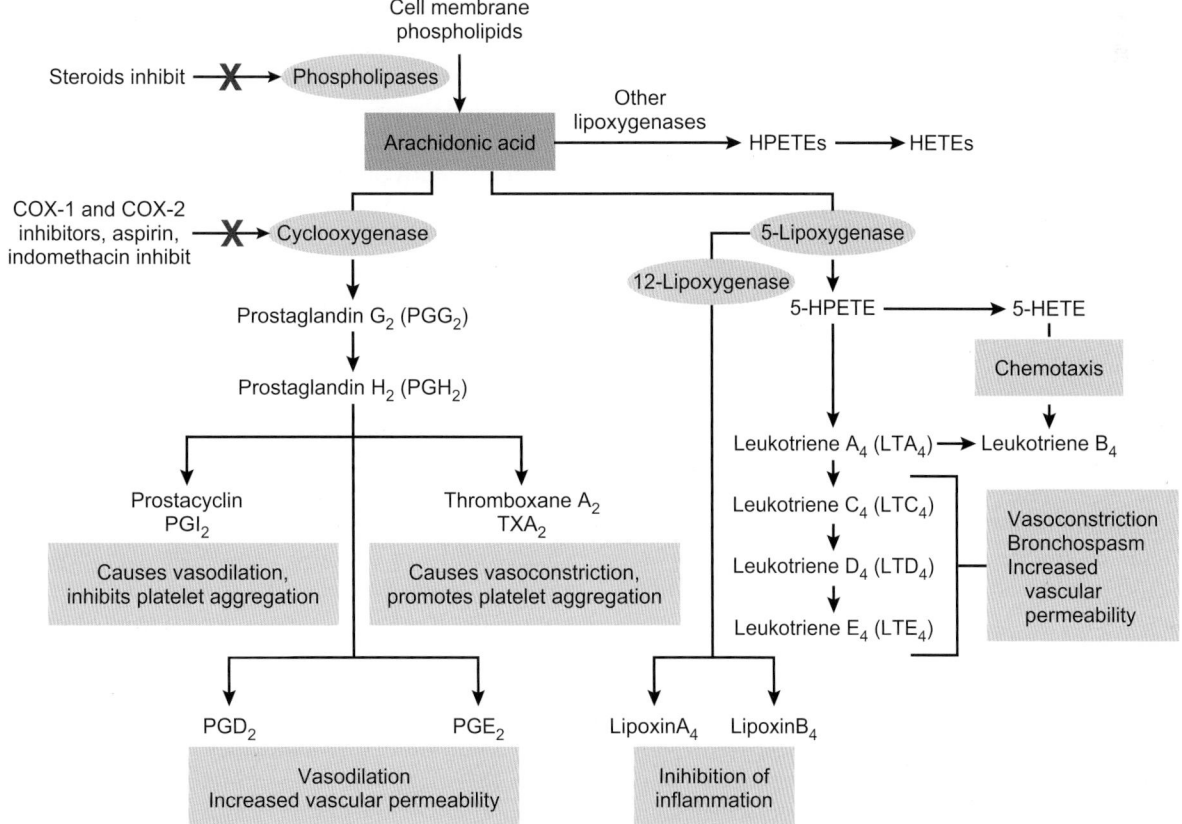

• **Fig. 22.2** Role of cyclooxygenase in inflammation. (From Banasik, J. [2021]. *Pathophysiology* [7th ed.]. St. Louis: Elsevier.)

U.S. Food and Drug Administration (FDA) required a black box warning on all NSAIDs, including celecoxib, stating the increased risk for thromboembolic events and GI bleed that can be fatal. Like nonselective NSAIDs, COX-2 inhibitors may cause or worsen renal failure and hepatic dysfunction, increase blood pressure, or exacerbate heart failure. These effects may be intensified in the older adult population.

The class of NSAIDs is further subdivided: *propionic acids* (ibuprofen), *indole and indene acetic acids* (indomethacin), *heteroaryl acetic acids* (ketorolac), *naphthylalanine* (nabumatone), *salicylic acids* (aspirin), *fenamates* (mefenamic acid), *oxicams* (meloxicam). One additional class, *para-aminophenol derivatives* (acetaminophen), can be included as an NSAID, as it inhibits prostaglandin synthesis through cyclooxygenase, but it does not have any significant antiinflammatory effects. Although the therapeutic action of each category is similar (a reduction in prostaglandin), significant differences are noted in efficacy related to the degree of effect on inflammation, pain, and fever, adverse-effect profile, and therapeutic dosing.

The antiinflammatory effect can vary from minimal (with little to no clinical efficacy, as in acetaminophen) to potent (indomethacin). Medications with higher antiinflammatory effects have higher side-effect profiles related to a greater effect on prostaglandin inhibition. The analgesic and antipyretic effect of NSAIDs can also vary across medications. For example, acetaminophen has little effect on inflammation, but it is an effective analgesic and antipyretic. Conversely, in addition to the antiprostaglandin effect, aspirin also blocks the effect of interleukin-1 on the hypothalamus, which is responsible for temperature control, making it a particularly effective antipyretic. Use of aspirin to reduce fever in children is contraindicated due to the risk of developing *Reye's syndrome*, a rare condition affecting the liver and brain. Reye's syndrome has been noted following salicylate administration in patients with viral illness, primarily influenza and chicken pox.

NSAIDs are chosen for relief of mild to moderate pain, especially pain caused by inflammation, but they also have important synergistic qualities when used in combination with opioid medications. The synergistic effect allows lower doses of opioids to be used, with pain relief similar to higher opioid doses if used alone. When choosing an NSAID for pain or fever control, consideration must be paid to the risk/benefit of the individual medications. Subclasses with potent antiinflammatory effects that may be chosen for serious, chronic conditions such as rheumatoid arthritis may possess a risk profile that would be unacceptable for treating mild pain or fever.

The antiprostaglandin effect of the class makes NSAIDs particularly effective for management of dysmenorrhea. Uterine cramping associated with dysmenorrhea is prompted by prostaglandins. Although medications with little or no antiinflammatory action, such as acetaminophen, are analgesic, NSAIDs with high antiprostaglandin activity, such as ibuprofen and naproxen, are effective interventions for menstrual pain.

Similarly, the effects of NSAIDs on platelet function vary across the class. The NSAID blockade of COX-1 causes inhibition of thromboxane, leading to reversible antiplatelet effects. The effect may also be observed with high-dose or long-term use of COX-2 selective inhibitors (e.g., celecoxib). Aspirin, a potent antiprostaglandin agent, is notable for its irreversible inhibition of platelet function. This aspect makes aspirin useful in patients for whom decreased platelet aggregation is desired, such as post-myocardial infarction cardiac patients, and is considered cardioprotective. Conversely, acetaminophen has the lowest effect on platelet function of the class, making it useful for patients taking anticoagulation therapy.

NSAID formulas can be administered orally, rectally, intramuscularly, and intravenously. Following oral administration, as a class they tend to be well absorbed but may cause direct irritation of the stomach, which can be mitigated by administering with food. The presence of food in the stomach can slightly delay absorption but has no effect on the total amount absorbed. Once it is absorbed, peak concentration occurs in 2 to 3 hours. Most NSAIDs are tightly and competitively bound to albumin. Administration concurrently with drugs that are also highly bound to albumin can result in competition for binding sites, resulting in excess free drug and the potential for adverse or toxic effects of either drug. Drug–drug interactions are described in Table 22.4. Conditions that result in lower plasma albumin levels can also result in excess free drug and increase the potential for toxicity.

NSAIDs are metabolized in the liver and excreted as inactivated metabolites via the kidney. The exceptions are sulindac and nabumatone, which are excreted as active metabolites. Acetaminophen, when taken over long periods or at high doses, can result in liver necrosis.

Caution should be exercised in prescribing NSAIDs to patients with preexisting renal or hepatic impairment. Concomitant use of alcohol can increase risk of liver damage, and use of NSAIDs concomitantly with anticoagulation medications can result in increased prothrombin times. Chronic alcoholism is a contraindication for acetaminophen use. With the exception of acetaminophen, which is pregnancy category B, adequate studies on humans for the use of NSAIDs in pregnancy are not evident. Across the class, NSAIDs range from B to D in pregnancy class. Use should balance the risk/benefit to both mother and fetus. Use of NSAIDs in the third trimester is contraindicated. Decreased prostaglandin synthesis can result in premature closure of the ductus arteriosus in the fetus. For preterm infants, indomethacin is used to facilitate closure of patent ductus arteriosus. NSAIDs are excreted in breast milk in small quantities. The American Academy of Pediatrics (AAP) considers NSAIDs compatible with breastfeeding at recommended doses for short periods. The need for the medication, alternative modalities, and risk/benefit potential to the infant should be considered. Doses should, ideally, be taken 4 hours prior to nursing.

The most common adverse effects of the class are listed in Table 22.5. Across the class, adverse effects may include gastric

TABLE 22.4 Medications That Interact With NSAIDs

Medication	Interacting Medication	Possible Effects
All NSAIDs	Loop diuretics	Decreased diuretic effect
	Lithium	Increased lithium levels except with sulindac
	Anticoagulants	Prolonged prothrombin time (except with acetaminophen)
	Beta-adrenergic blockers	Decreased effect on blood pressure
	Salicylates	Decreased plasma levels of NSAIDs
	Hydantoins	Hydantoin toxicity
	Probenecid	NSAID toxicity
	ACE inhibitors	Decreased ACE effect and hyperkalemia
		All NSAIDs may displace other highly protein bound drugs from binding sites
Acetaminophen	Oral contraceptives	Decreased half-life of acetaminophen
	Probenecid	Potentiates effect of acetaminophen
	Loop diuretics	Decreased effectiveness of diuretic
	Zidovudine	Decreased effect of zidovudine
	Alcohol	Increases potential for hepatotoxicity
	Propranolol	Increased effect of acetaminophen
	Anticholinergics	Delayed onset of action of anticholinergic
Indomethacin	Acyclovir	Increased risk for nephrotoxicity
	Dipyridamole	Increased risk for bleeding
Indomethacin, ibuprofen	Digoxin	Increases digoxin levels with potential for toxicity
Indomethacin, naproxen	Thiazide diuretics	Decreased antihypertensive and diuretic action

ACE, Angiotensin-converting enzyme; *NSAIDs*, nonsteroidal antiinflammatory drugs.

TABLE 22.5 Adverse Effects of NSAIDs

System	Adverse Effect	Action
Skin	Rash, pruritis	
Systemic	Stevens-Johnson syndrome, fever, toxic epidermal necrolysis, headache, anaphylaxis, cross-sensitivity to sulfa drugs (celecoxib), Reye's syndrome (aspirin)	Exercise caution. Cross-sensitivity to other NSAIDs may occur. Do not administer to children with viral infections (especially chicken pox and influenza). Avoid NSAID and aspirin combination.
Respiratory	Asthma, acute bronchospasm, respiratory alkalosis (aspirin)	Discontinue.
Gastrointestinal	Nausea, dyspepsia, vomiting, GI bleed; NSAID taken with aspirin may increase potential for GI bleed, may undermine cardioprotective action of aspirin, hepatoxicity	Monitor for bleeding, take with food.
Otic	Tinnitus (especially aspirin)	Discontinue.
Hematologic	Irreversible inhibition of platelet function and shortens erythrocyte survival time (aspirin); others inhibit platelet aggregation (reversible)	May be used therapeutically for inhibition of platelet function (cardioprotective). Avoid use with other medications that affect platelet function.
Renal	Decreased urate excretion, sodium/fluid retention, worsening of renal function in patients	Monitor weight, blood pressure.
Cardiovascular	Edema, hypertension	Monitor weight, blood pressure
Pregnancy	Premature closure of patent ductus arteriosus in fetus	Avoid all NSAIDs (except acetaminophen) in third trimester.

GI, Gastrointestinal; *NSAIDs*, nonsteroidal antiinflammatory drugs.

irritation, peptic ulcer disease (PUD), GI perforation or bleeding, and platelet dysfunction. A black box warning for the NSAID class, including the COX-2 selective celecoxib, indicates an increased risk of serious cardiovascular thrombotic events, myocardial infarction, and stroke. Renal effects include alteration in fluid balance and resultant hypertension related to fluid retention and increased extracellular fluid volume.

The risk for adverse effects can be affected by dose, duration of treatment, potency, and degree of COX-2 selectivity. Selection of medications should take these factors into consideration as well as the severity of illness, age of the patient, and concomitant acute or chronic conditions. Common dosing schedules are listed in Table 22.6. The risk of an adverse event appears to increase with age. Reduction

TABLE 22.6 Selective NSAID Dosing[a]

Category/ Medication	Indication	Dosage	Comments
Propionic Acid Derivatives			
Ibuprofen	OA, JRA, and RA	*Adults:* 300 mg orally four times daily or 400–800 mg orally three times daily. Maximum dosage: 3200 mg/day. *Children and adolescents:* 30–50 mg/kg/day in 3–4 divided doses. Maximum 800 mg/dose. Maximum dosage: 3200 mg/day.	For mild to moderate pain or fever, discontinue if no relief within 24 hr or if symptoms get worse or last more than 3 days. Administer oral forms with food or milk to decrease GI irritation. Shake liquid formulations well before using the calibrated measuring device in the packaging.
	Mild to moderate pain associated with headache, muscle pain, dental pain, strain/sprain, dysmenorrhea, fever	*Adults:* 200–400 mg orally every 4–6 hr as needed. Maximum dosage for prescription products: 3200 mg/day. Maximum dosage for OTC products: 1200 mg/day. *Children and adolescents 12–17 yr:* 200–400 mg every 6–8 hr as needed. Maximum dosage: 1200 mg/day. *Children 11 yr or weighing 72–95 pounds:* 300 mg orally every 6–8 hr as needed. Maximum dosage: 1200 mg/day. *Children 9–10 yr or weighing 60–71 pounds:* 250 mg orally every 6–8 hr as needed. Maximum dosage: 1000 mg/day. *Children 6–8 yr or weighing 48–59 pounds:* 200 mg orally every 6–8 hr as needed. *Children 4–5 yr or weighing 36–47 pounds:* 150 mg orally every 6–8 hr as needed. Maximum dosage: 600 mg/day. *Children 2–3 yr or weighing 24–35 pounds:* 100 mg orally every 6–8 hr as needed. Maximum dosage: 400 mg/day. **OTC concentrated drops:** *Children 12–23 months or weighing 18–23 pounds:* 75 mg orally every 6–8 hr as needed. Maximum dosage: 300 mg/day. *Infants 6–11 months or weighing 12–17 pounds:* 50 mg orally every 6–8 hr as needed. Maximum dosage: 200 mg/day. **Oral suspension:** *Infants and children 6 months to 2 yr:* 5–10 mg/kg/dose every 6–8 hr. Maximum dosage: 40 mg/kg/day.	

TABLE 22.6 Selective NSAID Dosing—cont'd

Category/ Medication	Indication	Dosage	Comments
Naproxen	OA, RA, AS, JRA	**Tablets or suspension:** *Adults:* 250–500 mg orally twice daily. Maximum dosage: 1500 mg/day for up to 6 months. *Children and adolescents 2–17 yr and weighing ≥50 kg:* 5 mg/kg/dose twice daily. Maximum dosage: 500 mg/day. **Delayed release:** *Adults:* 375–500 mg orally twice daily. Maximum dosage: 1500 mg/day for up to 6 months.	Delayed-release forms are not recommended for treatment of acute gout or for initial treatment of pain.
	Mild to moderate pain, dental pain, headache, bursitis, tendonitis, dysmenorrhea	**Tablets or suspension:** 500 mg orally once, then 250 mg every 6–8 hr. Maximum dosage: 1250 mg/day.	
	Acute gout	**Tablets or suspension:** *Adults:* 750 mg orally once, then 250 orally every 8 hr as needed until attack has subsided. **Controlled release:** *Adults:* 1000–1500 mg for one time only, then give 1000 mg once daily as needed until attack has subsided.	
Naproxen sodium	OA, RA, AS	**Tablets:** *Adults:* 275 or 550 mg orally twice daily. Maximum dosage: 1500 mg/day for up to 6 months. **Controlled release:** *Adults:* 750 or 1000 mg once daily. Maximum dosage: 1500 mg/day for limited periods.	Naproxen sodium is preferred to naproxen when fast-onset pain relief is required.
	Mild to moderate pain, dental pain, headache, backache, dysmenorrhea, bursitis, tendonitis	**Tablets:** *Adults:* 550 mg orally once, then 550 mg orally every 12 hr or 275 mg every 6–8 hr as needed. Maximum dosage: 1375 mg on day 1, then 1100 mg/day. **Controlled release:** *Adults:* 1000–1500 mg orally once daily. Usual maximum dosage: 1000 mg/day.	
	For OTC treatment of minor aches and pains, dental pain, headache	**OTC tablets or capsules:** *Adults, children, and adolescents 12–17 yr:* 440 mg orally once, then 220 mg orally every 8–12 hr. Maximum dosage: 660 mg/day. Discontinue use if pain worsens or lasts for more than 10 days.	
	OTC treatment of fever	**OTC tablets or capsules:** *Adults, children, and adolescents 12–17 yr:* 440 mg orally once, then 220 mg orally every 8–12 hr. Maximum dosage: 660 mg/day. Discontinue use if fever worsens or lasts for more than 3 days.	
Fenamates			
Mefenamic acid (Ponstel)	Acute mild to moderate pain	*Adults and adolescents ≥14 yr:* Begin with 500 mg orally followed by 250 mg every 6 hr for no longer than 7 days.	Give with food or milk to minimize GI upset.
	Primary dysmenorrhea	*Adults and adolescent females ≥14 yr:* Begin with 500 mg at the onset of menses followed by 250 mg every 6 hr as needed for 2–3 days.	

Continued

TABLE 22.6   Selective NSAID Dosing—cont'd

Category/ Medication	Indication	Dosage	Comments
Acetic Acid Derivative			
Nabumetone (Relafen)	OA, RA	Begin with 1000 mg orally once daily or in divided doses. Adjust to patient response. Maximum dosage: 2000 mg/day.	May be given without regard to meals. Use lowest effective dosage. Patients weighing less than 50 kg are less likely to require dosages greater than 1000 mg/day.
Indomethacin (Indocin)	Mild, moderate, or severe pain, such as arthralgia, myalgia, bursitis, or tendinitis	**Regular-release capsules:** *Mild to moderate pain:* 20 mg orally three times daily or 40 mg two or three times daily. *Moderate to severe pain:* 75–150 mg/day orally in 3–4 divided doses. **Extended-release capsules:** 75 mg orally once or twice daily. Usual length of therapy is 7–14 days.	Not recommended in older adults due to increased risk of adverse effects. If minor adverse effects develop with dosage increase, reduce dose and observe closely. Discontinue once signs and symptoms of inflammation have been controlled for several days.
	Acute gouty arthritis	**Regular-release forms:** 50 mg orally three times daily. Reduce dose and/or discontinue therapy as soon as possible.	For patients with acute gout, pain relief may occur within 2–4 hr. Tenderness and heat may decrease within 24–36 hr.
Salicylates			
Aspirin (Bayer)	Fever, pain, headache, dental pain, backache, dysmenorrhea, arthritis	*Adults, adolescents, and children ≥12 yr:* 325 or 650 mg orally every 4 hr as needed, or may give 975 mg every 6 hr as needed. Maximum dosage: 3900 mg/day. Discontinue use if pain worsens or lasts more than 10 days or if fever worsens or lasts more than 3 days.	Administer with food or at least 240 mL of water or milk to decrease gastric irritation/upset.
	Myocardial infarction prophylaxis, TIA	Use clinical practice guidelines and cardiovascular risk evaluation for correct doses of aspirin for primary and secondary prevention.	
Selective COX-2 Inhibitor			
Celecoxib (Celebrex)	Osteoarthritis	200 mg orally once daily or 100 mg twice daily.	For adults who are suspected or known as poor metabolizers of CYP2C9, begin therapy at half the lowest recommended dose. In all patients, use lowest effective dose. Begin with lower doses in older adults. Avoid using in children who are suspected or known as poor metabolizers of CYP2C9. Doses up to 200 mg twice daily may be given without regard to meals.
	JRA, RA	*Adults:* 100 or 200 mg orally twice daily. *Adolescents and children ≥2 yr and >25 kg:* 100 mg orally twice daily. *Children ≥2 yr and 10–25 kg:* 50 mg orally twice daily.	
	Acute, moderate, or severe pain associated with dysmenorrhea	*Adults:* Begin with 400 mg orally initially, followed by an additional 200 mg on the first day if needed. On subsequent days, 200 mg twice daily as needed.	
	Migraine with or without aura	*Adults:* 120 mg orally once daily for the fewest days of the month as needed. For known or suspected poor metabolizers of CYP2C9, begin with 60 mg.	

TABLE 22.6	Selective NSAID Dosing—cont'd			
Category/ Medication	Indication	Dosage		Comments
Para-Aminophenol				
Acetaminophen (Tylenol)	Fever, mild pain, or temporary relief of headache, myalgia, back pain, musculoskeletal pain, dental pain, dysmenorrhea, arthralgia, or minor aches and pains associated with the common cold or flu Not used for inflammatory processes	**Immediate-release formulations:** *Adults, adolescents, and children weighing ≥60 kg:* 325–650 mg orally every 4–6 hr as needed, or may give 1000 mg two to four times daily. Do not exceed 1 Gm/dose or 4 Gm/day. *Children and adolescents weighing <60 kg:* 10–15 mg/kg/dose orally every 4–6 hours as needed. Maximum single dose: 15 mg/kg/dose or 1000 mg/dose, whichever is less. Maximum dosage: 75 mg/kg/day or 4000 mg/day, whichever is less. **Extended-release formulations:** *Adults, adolescents, and children ≥12 yr:* 650–1300 mg orally every 8 hr as needed. Maximum single dose: 1300 mg/dose. Maximum dosage: 3900 mg/day.		Do not exceed maximum dosage limits for all routes of administration due to the risk of severe liver injury and even death.

ªDosing and choice of medication should be individualized to the specific patient (with history and comorbidities in mind) and the condition being treated.

AS, Ankylosing spondylitis; *COX-2,* cyclooxygenase-2; *GI,* gastrointestinal; *JIA,* juvenile idiopathic arthritis; *JRA,* juvenile rheumatoid arthritis; *OA,* osteoarthritis; *OTC,* over-the-counter; *RA,* rheumatoid arthritis; *TIA,* transient ischemic attack.

in doses and length of treatment in the older adult population would be prudent.

Aspirin (Acetylsalicylic Acid)

Pharmacokinetics. Administered orally, aspirin is rapidly absorbed from the stomach and small intestine. Aspirin may also be administered rectally. Aspirin is partially hydrolyzed by the liver, intestinal wall, and red blood cells to salicylic acid, which readily crosses the blood–brain barrier and placenta and is excreted in breast milk. Aspirin and salicylic acid are well distributed throughout the body. Aspirin has a half-life of 20 minutes, while the half-life of salicylic acid is 2 to 3 hours. Salicylic acid is protein bound in an inversely proportionate amount. At lower plasma levels, approximately 80% to 90% is protein bound. With increasing plasma levels, protein binding drops to approximately 76%. Salicylic acid binds competitively with many drugs, including penicillin, triiodothyronine, phenytoin, thyroxine, and other NSAIDs. Salicylic acid is excreted in the urine, and the amount that is excreted is dependent on urine pH. A more alkaline pH increases excretion. As a result, overdose of aspirin may be treated by alteration of pH to enhance excretion. Aspirin is contraindicated in the third trimester of pregnancy, although recent clinical practice guidelines indicate there may be some use for low-dose aspirin in patients at high risk for preeclampsia (Committee on Obstetric Practice Society for Maternal-Fetal Medicine, 2018). Aspirin is excreted in breast milk and so should be used with caution during breastfeeding.

Indications. Aspirin is used for analgesia of conditions associated with inflammation, such as osteoarthritis and rheumatoid arthritis, mild to moderate pain, fever, headache, tooth pain, coronary artery thrombosis prevention, and stroke prevention. The use of aspirin in platelet management is discussed in Chapter 14.

Adverse Effects. Salicylates should not be used in patients with known aspirin or NSAID sensitivity. The most common adverse effects of aspirin are related to its effect on the stomach, through either direct irritation or indirect effect on stomach mucosa related to prostaglandin inhibition, and include nausea, heartburn, GI bleeding (which may be painless), gastritis, and gastric ulcer. Systemic adverse effects include alteration in acid-base balance and electrolytes, retention of sodium and water, hepatic injury, decreased uric acid excretion leading to gout, respiratory alkalosis, and reversible ototoxicity. Irreversible inhibition of platelet function, while a desirable effect for cardio protection, increases the risk for bleeding. Reye's syndrome is associated with aspirin use in children with viral syndromes.

Contraindications. Cross-sensitivity to other NSAIDs has been noted. Caution is indicated in patients with a history of gout, previous GI bleed, gastritis or PUD, coagulopathy, or renal or hepatic impairment or failure, as well as in older adults. Aspirin is a category D medication and should be avoided in the third trimester of pregnancy. Children having known or suspected chicken pox or influenza should not take aspirin.

Monitoring. For patients on long-term or high-dose therapy, serum creatinine, salicylate levels, and liver function tests (LFTs) should be monitored. For patients with suspected GI bleeding, complete blood count (CBC) and fecal occult blood should be monitored. The patient should be aware of self-monitoring for GI bleeding. Patients undergoing surgery should stop taking aspirin 1 week prior to surgery or at their surgeon's recommendation.

Naproxen

Pharmacokinetics. Naproxen is available for oral use only. Naproxen and naproxen sodium are rapidly and completely absorbed. Pain relief begins in approximately 1 hour with naproxen and approximately 30 minutes with naproxen sodium. Analgesia can last up to 12 hours. Due to a half-life of 12 to 17 hours, the time to peak antiinflammatory action is 4 to 5 days. Protein binding is 99%. Unbound drug can be increased in older adults. Naproxen is heavily metabolized in the liver and excreted via the kidneys.

Indications. Naproxen is typically used for mild to moderately severe pain related to musculoskeletal inflammation, dental pain, headache, and dysmenorrhea.

Adverse Effects. These medications are contraindicated in patients with known NSAID or aspirin sensitivity. Due to its nonselective activity, naproxen's major adverse-event profile includes PUD, GI perforation or bleed, and gastritis. These can result from direct irritative action on the stomach as well as the loss of stomach protection due to decreased prostaglandin. Older adults are at higher risk of toxicity related to decreased renal function. Patients taking 3 or more doses, 5 or more days per week, for headache may experience rebound headache when stopping the medication.

Contraindications. Naproxen should be used cautiously in hepatic and renal disease. Use of naproxen with aspirin can interfere with aspirin's antiplatelet action. It should not be used long term in patients who use alcohol or smoke as both increase the risk for GI complications.

Monitoring. Monitoring of CBC, LFT, and serum creatinine/blood urea nitrogen (BUN) is reserved for long-term use. Patients should self-monitor for GI bleeding.

Celecoxib

Pharmacokinetics. Celecoxib is available for oral use only. It is absorbed slowly, but it is evenly distributed. Protein binding is approximately 97%, mostly to albumin. Half-life is 11 hours, but may be prolonged related to slow absorption. Metabolism is via the liver to inactive metabolites, with about half the dose excreted in the feces and the remaining via renal excretion.

Indications. Celecoxib is used to treat signs and symptoms associated with osteoarthritis and rheumatoid arthritis, ankylosing spondylitis, and postoperative orthopedic pain. It can also be used for relief of signs and symptoms of juvenile rheumatoid arthritis/juvenile idiopathic arthritis. Celecoxib may be used to treat moderate or severe pain for patients with dysmenorrhea. It can also be used to treat acute migraine with or without aura.

Adverse Effects. Despite COX-2 receptor selectivity, the adverse effects for celecoxib are similar to those of nonselective NSAIDs and include GI upset, gastritis, ulceration, or perforation, which may occur at any time during treatment. Perforation may occur as a sudden event, with no preceding pain or warning. A black box warning indicates an increased risk of cardiovascular events and GI bleed potential (as is the case for all nonselective NSAIDs). The medication may cause new-onset hypertension or aggravation of existing hypertension. Celecoxib is a sulfonamide, which may manifest as cross-sensitivity with other sulfa medications or may cause serious skin events including Stevens-Johnson syndrome and toxic epidermal necrolysis. Celecoxib should be discontinued if the patient reports a skin rash.

Contraindications. Celecoxib is contraindicated in patients with sulfa allergy or other NSAID sensitivity. Caution should be exercised, or alternative treatment considered, in patients with renal or hepatic impairment, hypertension, prior GI bleed or PUD, recent CABG, or congestive heart failure (CHF). Older patients are at increased risk for adverse events. Consider alternative therapy or start the dose at the low end of the dosing scale and monitor for fluid balance alteration or toxicity. No adequate safety studies are available in pregnant or nursing mothers. Alternative treatments should be considered.

Monitoring. For extended use or use in older adults, monitor blood pressure, LFTs, serum creatinine, BUN, and CBC. The patient should be aware of monitoring for symptoms of GI bleeding.

BLACK BOX WARNING!

Celecoxib

- Celecoxib is contraindicated to treat pain in patients 10 to 14 days post-coronary artery bypass graft (CABG) due to increased risk of myocardial infarction and stroke.
- Patients with a prior history of PUD and/or GI bleeding who use NSAIDs have a more than tenfold increased risk for developing a GI bleed compared to patients without risk factors.
- NSAIDs, including celecoxib, cause serious GI adverse events including inflammation, bleeding, ulceration, and GI perforation of the esophagus, stomach, small intestine, or large intestine, which can be fatal.
- Celecoxib, like all NSAIDs, may cause an increased risk of serious cardiovascular thromboembolism, including myocardial infarction or stroke, which can be fatal.

From Elsevier. Clinical pharmacology powered by ClinicalKey®. (2019). [cited 2020 September] Retrieved from http://www.clinicalkey.com.

Prescriber Considerations for Antiinflammatory Therapy

Clinical Practice Guidelines

Guidelines for the use of corticosteroids and NSAIDs are related to the specific underlying conditions being treated.

Both classes of medications are used to manage the symptoms of multiple disease processes and injuries. Unless they are being used for endogenous hormone replacement, corticosteroids and NSAIDs are not curative, but supportive. Guidance for the management of conditions such as acute back pain, tendonitis or bursitis, osteoarthritis or rheumatoid arthritis, dysmenorrhea, allergic reaction, or other conditions for which these medications are used should be sought from the appropriate guidelines.

Clinical Reasoning for Antiinflammatory Therapy

Consider the individual patient's health problem requiring antiinflammatory therapy. There are no clear, algorithmic, or evidence-based decision-making standards to guide therapeutic symptom management with corticosteroids or NSAIDs. Careful evaluation of the patient's condition, including medical and social history and physical examination, should guide prescribing. Medication, dose, and dosing schedule are highly dependent on the condition being managed, severity of symptoms, desired outcome, and patient-dependent factors. Therefore, an appropriate medication at the lowest effective dose should be used for the shortest length of time possible. Careful monitoring of the patient for symptom improvement, adverse effects, and adherence to treatment should be maintained.

Determine the desired therapeutic outcome based on the degree of inflammation control needed for the patient's health problem. Symptom management should be geared to specific patient needs and expectations. Working in concert with the patient, the primary care provider should develop a reasonable plan of action. Patients should be made aware of the limitations, adverse effects, and cost involved if medications are to be used for long-term symptom control of chronic conditions.

Assess the antiinflammatory selected for its appropriateness for an individual patient by considering the medication's side effects and the patient's age, race/ethnicity, comorbidities, and genetic factors. Most of the NSAID class of medications are heavily metabolized in the liver and excreted via the kidneys. Age-related changes to these symptoms can place older patients at increased risk for drug accumulation and adverse events. Lower doses or alternative therapies should be considered for this population. Corticosteroids and NSAIDs have limited or no human studies to confirm safety in pregnancy. Risk/benefit analysis should be performed for both mother and fetus. Race or ethnic factors related to metabolism should be considered. Even at the low daily dose of celecoxib 200 mg, the systolic and diastolic blood pressures of Hispanic and African American patients were raised in the presence of normal renal function.

Initiate the treatment plan with the selected medication by first providing adequate patient education to ensure the patient's understanding and promote full participation in the antiinflammatory therapy. It is important that patients understand that NSAIDs and corticosteroids will be used to manage symptoms of an underlying problem. This is especially important when using the medications to reduce pain as opposed to providing an ultimate "cure," such as in rheumatoid arthritis. Given the distressing nature of pain, patients must be made aware that more is not always better, to prevent patients from adjusting doses or frequency of doses upward without consulting with their primary care provider. The adverse-event profiles of these medications can have profound and life-threatening effects. Since many of the medications are available over the counter (e.g., aspirin, ibuprofen, Naprosyn), patients may believe these medications are "safe" and free from adverse effects. Education on adverse effects such as GI bleeding or perforation is important so that patients may identify potentially dangerous outcomes. Patients should be advised not to begin any other over-the-counter (OTC) medications that may contain an NSAID product without consulting with their primary care provider.

Although NSAIDs may be used for episodic discomfort management, such as an isolated headache, the importance of maintaining therapeutic blood levels of corticosteroids and NSAIDs for symptom management in acute injury or chronic disease should be stressed. Partially related to extended half-lives, antiinflammatory medications may take several days to 1 week to reach maximum therapeutic effect. Patients should be encouraged to adhere to dosing schedules as prescribed and not skip doses or days of doses.

Ensure complete patient and family understanding about the medication prescribed for antiinflammatory therapy using a variety of education strategies. The educational process should be tailored to the needs of the patient considering their education, language spoken, reading ability, previous experience with medical systems, and readiness to learn. Principles of therapeutic communication such as focusing and clarification by having patients restate instructions should be employed. Allowing patients time to express fears or concerns about the diagnosis is important. In addition to oral instruction, providing patients with written materials will assist with remembering instructions when arriving home. While giving oral instruction, simultaneously creating a table for medication administration that can be posted in the home is helpful. The patient's understanding of information should be verified using the teach-back method.

Conduct follow-up and monitoring of patient responses to antiinflammatory therapy. Acute, episodic use of antiinflammatory medications for the short term requires no specific follow-up or monitoring if symptoms abate. For patients on long-term corticosteroid medications or chronic NSAID use, monitoring consists of evaluation for adverse effects and medication adjustment needs. Additionally, assessment of the underlying pathology should be performed at appropriate intervals to adjust medication. Patients should be encouraged to take the medication with food; however, they should also be aware that this will not prevent the systemic effect of loss of stomach mucosal protection and potential gastric irritation.

Patients on long-term or high-dose corticosteroid medications should be monitored for signs or symptoms of underlying infection, metabolic disturbances such as elevated glucose levels, renal or hepatic dysfunction, signs or symptoms of gastric bleeding, osteoporosis, hypertension, weight gain, edema, and depression. An initial baseline of CBC, electrolytes, and glucose should be obtained. Yearly evaluation of those lab parameters should be instituted in addition to stool for guaiac and lipid measurement.

Patients using NSAIDs for long-term therapy should be routinely evaluated for gastric irritation or bleeding, and hypertension. In long-term use, yearly monitoring of CBC and serum creatinine is suggested.

Teaching Points for Antiinflammatory Therapy

Patient Education for Medication Safety

For corticosteroids:

- Remember that corticosteroids manage symptoms. Monitoring of the underlying condition must be continued.
- For once-daily dosing, the dose should be taken prior to 8 a.m.
- Take with food to reduce gastric distress.
- Do not stop this medication without consulting your primary care provider.
- If you are diabetic, monitor your blood sugar more frequently due to increased risk of hyperglycemia.
- Steroids may mask infection. While taking this medication, you should stay away from others with active infections, especially measles or chicken pox.
- Advise your health-care provider if you have a wound or sore that does not heal.
- If you are on this medication for a long time, talk to your health-care provider about bone health. Weight-bearing exercise and adequate calcium and vitamin D intake are important while on this medication.
- Do not take any other prescription or OTC medications, including vaccines, without consulting with the health-care provider who prescribed this medication.
- You may note weight gain, changes in mood, increased appetite, or difficulty sleeping.
- Notify your health-care provider if you note a change in vision, bright red or black/tarry stool or vomitus, fever or chills, muscle cramps or pain, excessive thirst and urination, or depression.
- If you miss a dose, take it as soon as you can. If it is almost time for your next dose, take only that dose. Do not take double or extra doses.
  For NSAIDs:
- NSAIDs may cause serious side effects including stomach irritation, bleeding, or ulcers. It is important to follow all directions.
- Eating a small amount of food with the medication will help prevent direct irritation of the stomach.
- Do not smoke or use alcohol while taking NSAID medication as this may increase stomach irritation.
- Do not take this medication in higher doses or more frequently than prescribed.

- If you miss a dose, take it as soon as you can. If it is almost time for your next dose, take only that dose. Do not take double or extra doses.
- Do not take additional pain medication, including aspirin, while taking this medication without the approval of your primary care provider.
- You should notify your primary care provider if you are or become pregnant while taking this medication.
- Notify your primary care provider of all medications, including OTC, herbal, natural, or holistic medications, that you are taking. Do not begin any new medications without consulting your primary care provider.
- Notify your primary care provider if you experience stomach pain, nausea, vomit or stool that contains tarry/black or bright red blood, skin rashes or blistering, yellowing of eyes or skin, chest pain, slurred speech, weakness on one side of the body, excessive fatigue, swelling of the legs, or weight gain.

Application Questions for Discussion

1. Your patient is on coumadin related to a previous deep vein thrombosis. If the patient needs to use an NSAID related to a sprain/strain, how would you prescribe for this patient?
2. Your patient requires long-term corticosteroid use. What specific patient conditions would need to be considered prior to beginning the steroid?
3. Discuss the main differences and similarities across the categories of NSAIDs and how those differences and similarities would guide prescribing.

Selected Bibliography

Bandoli, G., Palmsten, K., Forbess Smith, C., & Chambers, C (2017). A review of systemic corticosteroid use in pregnancy and the risk of select pregnancy and birth outcomes. *Rheumatic Disease Clinics of North America, 43*(3), 489–502. https://www.ncbi.nlm.nih.gov/pmc/articles/PMC5604866/.

Bello, A. E., & Holt, R. J. (2014). Cardiovascular risk with nonsteroidal anti-inflammatory drugs: Clinical implications. *Drug Safety, 37*, 897–902. https://doi.org/10.1007/s40264-014-0207-2.

Brunton, L. L., Hilal-Dandan, R., & Knollmann, B. C. (2017). *Goodman and Gilman's The Pharmacological Basis of Therapeutics* (13th ed.). New York: McGraw Hill Education.

Committee on Obstetric Practice Society for Maternal-Fetal Medicine. (2018). Low-dose aspirin use during pregnancy. *Obstetrics & Gynecology, 132*(1), e44–e52.

De-Kun, L., Ferber, J., Odouli, R., & Quesenberry, C. (2018). Use of nonsteroidal antiinflammatory drugs during pregnancy and the risk of miscarriage. *American Journal of Obstetrics & Gynecology, 219*(3), e1–e8. https://doi.org/10.1016/j.ajog.2018.06.002.

Prednisone. (2006). *Drugs and Lactation Database (LactMed) [Internet].* Bethesda (MD): National Library of Medicine (US. [Updated 2018 Oct 31]. Available from. https://www.ncbi.nlm.nih.gov/books/NBK501077/.

Elsevier. Clinical pharmacology powered by ClinicalKey®. (2019). [cited 2020 September] Retrieved from http://www.clinicalkey.com.

Iyalomhe, G. B., Iyalomhe, S. I., Enahoro, F. O., & Okhiai, O. (2012). Current trends in the prescription of non-steroidal anti-inflammatory drugs: A pharmacoepidemiological review. *International Research Journal of Pharmacy, 2*(9), 204–208. Retrieved from https://interesjournals.org/articles/current-trends-in-the-prescription-of-nonsteroidal-antiinflammatory-drugs-a-pharmacoepidemiological-review.pdf.

Kesanli, B. (n.d.) *Non-steroidal anti-inflammatory drugs (NSAIDs)*. Retrieved from http://docs.neu.edu.tr/staff/banu.kesanli/NEPH-AR%20305%20NSAIDs_15.pdf.

Kluckow, M., Jeffery, M., Gill, A. W., & Evans, N. (2014). A randomised placebo-controlled trial of early treatment of the patent ductus arteriosus. *Archives of Disease in Childhood, 99*(2), 99–104. Retrieved from https://fn.bmj.com/content/99/2/f99.long.

Lopez-Candales, A., Hernandez Burgos, P. M., Hernandez-Suarez, D. F., & Harris, D. (2017). Linking chronic inflammation with cardiovascular disease: From normal aging to the metabolic syndrome. *Journal of Natural Science, 3*(4), e341.

McCance, K., & Huether, S. (2018). *Pathophysiology: The Biological Basis for Disease in Adults and Children* (8th ed.). St. Louis: Elsevier Mosby.

National Institute of Neurological Disorders and Stroke. (2021). *Reye's syndrome information page*. Retrieved from https://www.ninds.nih.gov/disorders/All-Disorders/Reyes-Syndrome-Information-Page.

Pahwa, R., Goyal, A., Bansal, P., & Jialal, I. (2020). Chronic inflammation. [Updated 2020 Aug 10] *StatPearls [Internet]*. Treasure Island (FL): StatPearls Publishing. Retrieved from. https://www.ncbi.nlm.nih.gov/books/NBK493173/.

Porth, C., & Grossman, S. (2013). *Porth's Pathophysiology: Concepts of Altered Health States* (9th ed.). New York: Lippincott, Williams & Wilkens.

Tsalamandris, S., Antonopoulos, A., Oikonomou, E., Papamikroulis, G., Vogiatzi, G., Papaioannou, S., Deftereos, S., & Tousoulis, D. (2019). The role of inflammation in diabetes: Current concepts and future perspectives. *European Cardiology Review, 14*(1), 50–59. https://doi.org/10.15420/ecr.2018.33.1.

U.S. Food and Drug Administration. (2005). *Black box warning added to Celebrex label*. Retrieved from https://www.fdanews.com/articles/75244-black-box-warning-added-to-celebrex-labeling#:~:text=The%20FDA%20has%20approved%20a,events%20associated%20with%20the%20product.

Wongrakpanich, S., Wongrakpanich, A., Melhado, K., & Rangaswami, J. (2018). A comprehensive review of non-steroidal anti-inflammatory drug use in the elderly. *Aging and Disease, 9*(11), 143–150. http://doi.org/10.14336/AD.2017.0306.

Woo, T., & Robinson, M. (2020). *Pharmacotherapeutics for Advanced Practice Nurses*. Philadelphia: F.A. Davis.

23

Disease-Modifying and Immune Therapy Medications

MELISSA RUBLE AND JACLYN COLE

Overview

Rheumatoid arthritis (*RA*) is a chronic autoimmune disease in which the body provides an inappropriate immune response against healthy tissue. Damage to the bone, cartilage, joint, and synovium may occur, resulting in swelling of the bilateral symmetrical joints. Patients commonly experience morning stiffness or stiffness after periods of inactivity that last from 1 to several hours. While the most commonly affected joints include the small joints of the hands, wrists, and feet, many patients experience symptoms in the larger joints including ankles, knees, elbows, and shoulders. Additional flares may result in additional joint tenderness or swelling, as well as possible systemic symptoms such as fatigue or depression.

Patients are typically diagnosed in their 50s, although diagnosis can occur at any age and prevalence continues to increase with age. An exception is juvenile RA, which affects children 16 years of age or younger. Patients with RA have lower rates of employment, higher disability claims, and higher mortality rates. Life expectancy for RA patients has been reported to be 3 to 10 years less than that of the general population. In fact, when compared to the general population, patients with RA had a 54% higher mortality after adjustment for age, gender, and calendar year (van den Hoek et al., 2017). Mortality was higher for cardiovascular, respiratory, musculoskeletal, and digestive diseases.

Disease-modifying and immune agents are used to address disease progression and symptomatic relief for various autoimmune disease states. These medication classes include disease-modifying antirheumatic drugs (DMARDs), biologic agents, Janus kinase (JAK) inhibitors, and glucocorticoids. Therapy may transition between agents or require combination therapy, even within the same drug class, if treatment goals are not achieved with a specific medication. The agents used in these disease states focus on controlling inflammation to prevent disease state progression, as well as managing patient symptoms. Maintenance medications are typically continued long term, although additional agents may be added for acute management. Close monitoring for both therapeutic benefits and toxicities are required for the duration of therapy.

Relevant Physiology

There are two branches of the immune system: innate and adaptive. The *innate branch* is the part of the immune system that responds rapidly to any perceived threats, but lacks memory, whereas the *adaptive branch* does have a memory. The adaptive immune system produces B-cells and antibodies (*humoral immune system*), as well as T-cells and cytokines (*cell-mediated immune system*). The two components within the immune system that have the most direct impact on autoimmunity are the B-cells and T-cells in the adaptive immune system. Both are specialized white blood cells, or *lymphocytes*, that are named based on their location of maturity; B-cells in the bone marrow and T-cells in the thymus.

The main purpose of B-cells and T-cells is to identify dangers within the body and mount an appropriate response against them. B-cells create five different types of antibodies to neutralize threats: IgA, IgD, IgE, IgG, and IgM. Each antibody has a specific function: *IgA* is an antiviral; *IgD* is involved in B-cell differentiation; *IgE* responds to parasitic infections; *IgG* responds to toxins, activates the complement system, and targets the pathogen for destruction; and *IgM* activates the complement cascade. There are three types of T-cells: (1) *killer T-cells*, which trigger a target to it to kill itself; (2) *helper T-cells*, which create cytokines to signal and fight to destroy threats; and (3) *regulatory T-cells*, which help differentiate what is considered a threat in the body. The regulatory T-cells are the most notable in this case as their dysregulation is the cause of autoimmune disease, where the body inappropriately recognizes itself as a threat.

Pathophysiology

Rheumatoid Arthritis

Understanding the specific pathophysiology of RA is key to identifying appropriate treatment options (Fig. 23.1). In patients with RA, certain T-cell types play a significant role in cytokine release and inflammation within the joints. *T helper 1* (T_h1) cells produce large amounts of interferon gamma (IFN-γ) and promote cell-mediated immunity.

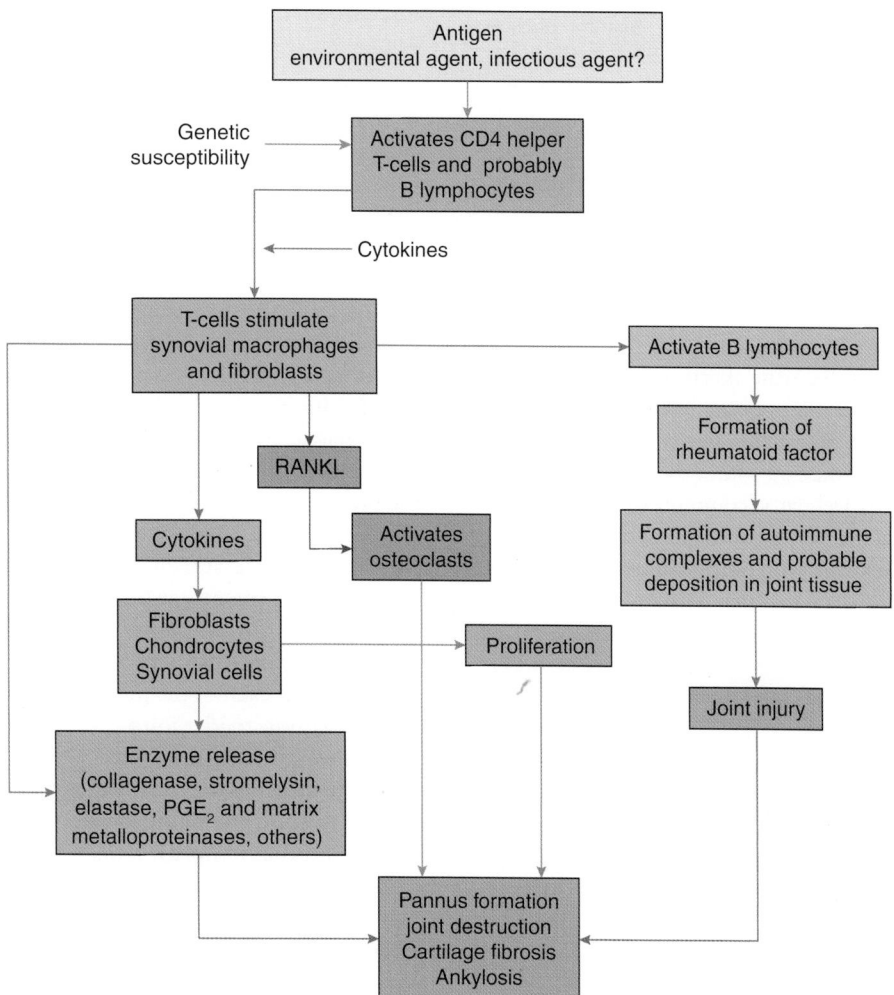

• **Fig. 23.1** Emerging model of pathogenesis of rheumatoid arthritis. Rheumatoid arthritis is an autoimmune disease of a genetically susceptible host triggered by an unknown antigenic agent. Chronic autoimmune reaction with activation of CD4+ helper T-cells and possibly other lymphocytes and the local release of inflammatory cytokines and mediators eventually destroy the joint. T-cells stimulate cells in the joint to produce cytokines that are key mediators of synovial damage. Apparently immune complex deposition also plays a role. Tumor necrosis factor (TNF) and interleukin-1 (IL-1), as well as some other cytokines, stimulate synovial cells to proliferate and produce other mediators of inflammation, such as prostaglandin E2 (PGE2), matrix metalloproteinases, and enzymes, all of which contribute to destruction of cartilage. Activated T-cells and synovial fibroblasts also produce receptor activator of nuclear factor κβ ligand (RANKL), which activates the osteoclasts and promotes bone destruction. Pannus is a mass of synovium and synovial stroma with inflammatory cells, granulation tissue, and fibroblasts that grows over the articular surface and causes its destruction. (From McCance, K. L., & Huether, S.E. [Eds.], [2019]. *Pathophysiology: The biologic basis for disease in adults and children* [8th ed.]. St. Louis: Elsevier.)

T helper 2 (T$_h$2) cells produce interleukins 4, 5, and 13 (IL-4, IL-5, IL-13) and contribute to the humoral immune system, or B-cell responses. *T helper 17* (T$_h$17) cells release interleukin-17 (IL-17), which has been detected in high levels within the joints of RA patients. The exposure of naïve T-cells to transforming growth factor beta (TGF-β) generates *regulatory T-cells* (T regs) to support immune response suppression. The type of T-cells activated will affect which interleukins are released, which explains why patient response to biologic therapy can be variable among individuals.

B-cells, which are responsible for autoantibody production, also play an important role in RA. The autoantibodies in this disease are rheumatoid factor (RF) and cyclic citrullinated peptide (CCP), which can both activate the complement system and trigger the creation of proinflammatory cytokines. The B-cells can also release cytokines directly, further contributing to inflammation, and they can co-stimulate the activation of T-cells. This all occurs within the *synovial membrane*, or *synovium*, which is located inside the synovial joint capsule and releases synovial fluid that lubricates and reduces friction between cartilage. The cytokines released by activated B-cells and T-cells contribute to joint tissue swelling and destruction. Inflammation within the synovium can be painful and eventually may damage the cartilage or bone, resulting in additional pain. Considering this process, cytokines serve as good targets for RA therapy.

Clinical Presentation

RA is the most prevalent autoimmune arthritis among adults, affecting about 1% of the general population, or approximately 1.3 million people in the United States, with an estimated annual cost of more than $120 billion (Helmick, 2008).

Risk factors include female gender, family history, obesity, smoking, and environmental factors (e.g., asbestos, silica).

General presentation includes joint swelling and tenderness, usually bilaterally and symmetrically, which results in synovial joint destruction, ultimately leading to significant disability and premature mortality. Rheumatoid nodules are extraarticular manifestations that occur in up to 30% of patients. They are commonly located on the arms and elbows but can also present at pressure points on the knees and feet. Although uncommon, nodules may arise in organs such as the heart, lungs, or sclera of the eye.

This chronic, progressive disease affects daily patient activities and quality of life, and it is associated with increased mortality. A limited number of patients (fewer than 10%) may experience spontaneous remission within the first 6 months of symptom onset. Alternatively, it is common to have flares or attacks followed by inactive periods throughout the early phases of the disease. However, this progressive disease will continue with persistent disease activity that may wax and wane.

PRACTICE PEARLS

RA Presentation

RA is an autoimmune disease characterized by inappropriate immune responses and inflammation that results in bilateral, symmetrical cartilage, bone, and synovium erosion.

Diagnosis and Disease Activity

Diagnosis of RA requires a combination of symptom duration history, detailed joint evaluation, at least one serologic test (e.g., RA; anticitrullinated protein antibodies [ACPA]), and at least one acute-phase response marker test (e.g., C-reactive protein [CRP]; erythrocyte sedimentation rate [ESR]). Criteria for the diagnosis of RA as defined by the American College of Rheumatology (ACR) can be found in Table 23.1.

RA can be further categorized based on duration, severity, and remission. *Early RA* involves disease diagnosis and/or symptoms for less than 6 months; more specifically, it is the duration of the disease/symptoms and not the time since diagnosis. *Established RA* can be identified as either duration of disease/symptoms for 6 months or longer, or the presence of at least four of the 1987 criteria for 6 weeks or more (Box 23.1). Disease activity can be classified as either low, moderate, or high and identified on various validated instruments, such as the Clinical Disease Activity Index (CDAI). *Remission of RA* is defined by either a low Simplified Disease Activity Scale (DAS) composite score or a low score on each of the following items in the DAS: swollen joint count, tender joint count, C-reactive protein level, and patient global assessment.

The treatment goal for RA therapy is to reach low disease activity or complete remission. It is important that patients understand that although remission is the ideal target, it is

TABLE 23.1	American College of Rheumatology Classification Criteria for RA
Classification Criteria for RA (sum of score from Categories A–D; a score of ≥6/10 classifies a patient as having definite RA)	
A. Joint involvement	
1 large joint	0
2–10 large joints	1
1–3 small joints (with or without involvement of large joints)	2
4–10 small joints (with or without involvement of large joints)	3
>10 joints (at least one small joint)	5
B. Serology (at least one test result is needed for classification)	
Negative RF *and* negative ACPA	0
Low-positive RF *or* low-positive ACPA	2
High-positive RF *or* high-positive ACPA	3
C. Acute-phase reactants (at least one test result is needed for classification)	
Normal CRP *and* normal ESR 0	0
Abnormal CRP *or* normal ESR 1	1
D. Duration of symptoms	
<6 weeks	0
≥6 weeks	1

ACPA, Anticitrullinated protein antibodies; *CRP,* C-reactive protein; *ESR,* erythrocyte sedimentation rate; *RF,* rheumatoid factor.

not always possible as no therapy will reverse joint damage that has already occurred. Pharmacologic therapy is usually needed to reduce inflammation within the body. This is especially important early in the disease when aggressive therapy may prevent irreversible joint damage. However, simultaneous nonpharmacologic therapy plays an equally important role in RA management. Examples include physical therapy, occupational therapy, weight loss, rest, and surgery.

PRACTICE PEARLS

RA Treatment Goals and Considerations

- Treatment goals focus on improving quality of life through low disease activity and/or remission.
- Drug therapy should be started by a rheumatoid-trained health care provider at the time of diagnosis.
- The level of disease activity, patient preference, comorbid conditions, and costs will guide treatment choice.

DMARDs have traditionally served as the backbone of RA therapy, but biologics and JAK inhibitors have also been proven to slow RA disease progression. Commonly used DMARDs include methotrexate, leflunomide, hydroxychloroquine, and sulfasalazine. Biologic medications include an array of therapies, such as tumor necrosis factor inhibitors (TNFi), abatacept, tocilizumab, and rituximab. The newer JAK inhibitors include tofacitinib, baricitinib, and upadacitinib. Additional agents with limited use due to reduced benefit and/or high toxicity include azathioprine, anakinra, cyclophosphamide, cyclosporine, gold, minocycline, and penicillamine. Supportive therapies for more rapid symptomatic relief include nonsteroidal antiinflammatory drugs (NSAIDs) and corticosteroids. Additional therapy not supported by guidelines due to their infrequent use in RA and/or lack of data include anakinra, azathioprine, cyclosporine, minocycline, and gold.

Early RA and Initial Treatment

DMARDs are the initial treatment choice for both early and established RA, regardless of the level of disease activity. Methotrexate is the preferred drug in this category. It is recommended to start with monotherapy DMARD treatment before moving on to double or triple therapy because it is

---

PRACTICE PEARLS

RA Therapy

- The mainstay of therapy includes DMARDs, with methotrexate being the preferred agent.
- Adjunctive therapies (NSAIDs, corticosteroids) may be initiated to assist with patient symptoms at the same time as DMARDs, which can take 3 to 6 weeks to begin showing patient benefits and up to 12 weeks for full effects.

BOX 23.1   ACR 1987 Criteria Used in Diagnosis of Established RA

1. At least 1 hour of morning stiffness in/around the joints
2. Physician-observed soft tissue swelling of at least 3 joints
3. Swelling of the wrist, proximal interphalangeal, or metacarpophalangeal joints
4. Symmetric swelling
5. Rheumatoid nodules
6. Positive rheumatoid factor
7. Periarticular osteopenia and/or radiographic erosion within the hand/wrist joints

---

easier to take, has better patient tolerability, and is lower in cost. Although these agents are effective in RA management, they can take a few weeks to reach their full benefit. It is recommended that short-term bridge therapy be used in the interim to assist with patient symptoms. These bridge therapies include low-dose steroids and NSAIDs, although additional analgesics such as acetaminophen may also be used. These agents are not typically used long term since corticosteroids have many side effects and NSAIDs do not affect disease state progression.

Established RA Treatment

Patients with established RA (6 months or longer) should still receive treatment with monotherapy DMARDs due to evidence of well-documented efficacy, safety profile, high level of clinical experience, low cost, and familiarity among rheumatologists. Should disease activity remain moderate or high, treatment may be adjusted based on current clinical practice guidelines and include therapies such as combination DMARDs, TNFi, other non-TNF biologics or JAK inhibitors with or without methotrexate. Due to various treatment options, it is important to work with a rheumatologist to evaluate the risks, benefits, and evidence for available therapies.

Treatment Failure

For patients who experience treatment failures with multiple TNFi or non-TNF biologic therapies, the treatment goal should be reframed to include the lowest disease activity over the goal of total remission. Remission is reasonable as an initial treatment goal but may need to be adjusted based on overall treatment effects and patient preferences.

Disease-Modifying and Immune Therapy

Traditional DMARDs

Methotrexate

Methotrexate remains the preferred DMARD for RA therapy based on its consistent evidence of clinical response, including steroid-sparing effects, over several decades. Methotrexate is a structural analog of (structurally similar to) folic acid. It works by inhibiting dihydrofolate reductase, an enzyme that converts dihydrofolic acid to its inactive metabolite, folinic acid. Methotrexate interferes with deoxyribonucleic acid (DNA) synthesis, DNA repair, and cellular replication, but its exact therapeutic mechanism on RA remains unknown.

Pharmacokinetics. Methotrexate dosing in RA is typically as an oral tablet or subcutaneous injection. The injectable formulation tends to have a lower risk of gastrointestinal (GI) side effects and is generally better tolerated by patients. Absorption of oral methotrexate appears to be dose dependent. Peak plasma levels typically occur within about 45 minutes to 6 hours after administration. It is approximately 50% protein bound. Methotrexate undergoes hepatic and intracellular metabolism and is primarily excreted by the kidneys. Therapeutic effects may take 3 to 6 weeks.

Indications. Methotrexate can be used to treat RA in adults. It may also be used to treat active juvenile rheumatoid arthritis (JRA)/juvenile idiopathic arthritis (JIA). The effects of methotrexate on articular tenderness and swelling can be seen in 3 to 6 weeks. It is important to educate patients that mistakenly taking RA dosing more often, such as daily, has resulted in fatal toxicities. Dosing needs to be carefully monitored, and in some cases adjusted, in renal impairment, ascites, or pleural effusions.

Adverse Effects. Because methotrexate is structurally similar to folic acid, it can cause folic acid deficiency. It may be beneficial to give methotrexate with 1 to 5 mg of folic acid daily to reduce the risk of fatigue, mouth sores, or anemia seen in folate deficiency. Other potential side effects include GI issues (e.g., diarrhea, perforation), hematologic changes (e.g., leukopenia, thrombocytopenia), hepatic toxicities (e.g., cirrhosis, elevated liver enzymes), infection, and pulmonary complications (e.g., respiratory fibrosis, chronic obstructive pulmonary disease [COPD]).

BLACK BOX WARNING!

Methotrexate

Methotrexate has multiple black box warnings that must be considered in assessing and monitoring patients. This medication should be prescribed only by an experienced clinician with expertise in antimetabolite therapy due to the risk for serious and even fatal adverse reactions.

Contraindications. Methotrexate is contraindicated in pregnancy due to its risk for teratogenicity and fetal death. Patients should not take methotrexate if they are breastfeeding or have chronic liver disease, alcoholic liver disease, alcoholism, blood disorders (leukopenia, thrombocytopenia, bone marrow hypoplasia, or significant anemia), or known hypersensitivity to any component of the medication. Possible toxic effects can be seen at any dose at any time during therapy, but may increase with dosing and frequency. Patients should be monitored closely, and dosing should be decreased or discontinued if toxicity occurs.

Additional drug-specific dosing and considerations are available in Table 23.2.

Monitoring. Baseline monitoring before starting methotrexate includes renal function, liver function enzymes (AST, ALT), and a complete blood count (CBC) with differential. Monitoring should continue every 2 to 4 weeks for 3 months after a dose initiation or increase, followed by every 8 to 12 weeks during months 3 to 6, and finally every 12 weeks after 6 months of treatment. Patients with underlying lung disease may benefit from a baseline chest X-ray prior to drug initiation. Baseline screenings for hepatitis B, hepatitis C, and tuberculosis (TB) should be done in high-risk patients.

Leflunomide

Leflunomide can be used either as monotherapy or in combination with other DMARDs for the treatment of RA. It works by inhibiting pyrimidine synthesis, which in turn suppresses the reaction of cells involved in the inflammatory process, ultimately reducing RA pain and swelling. Treatment with leflunomide has been effective at reducing RA symptoms, improving physical function, and inhibiting structural damage.

Pharmacokinetics. The active metabolite of leflunomide, teriflunomide, is more than 99% bound to plasma proteins. It affects several CYP450 enzymes and drug transporters. Peak teriflunomide concentrations occur between 6 and 12 hours after oral dosing. Due to the very long half-life of teriflunomide (18 to 19 days), an oral loading dose of 100 mg for 3 days may be used.

Leflunomide should be avoided in significant renal and hepatic impairment as both organs play a role in elimination of the medication. It may be given without regard to meals.

Indications. Leflunomide is indicated in the treatment of active RA. A risk/benefit assessment for each patient should be made due to the increased risk for adverse effects.

Adverse Effects. Adverse effects of leflunomide may include diarrhea, rash, elevated blood pressure, alopecia, and elevated liver enzymes. Patients taking leflunomide may be more susceptible to infections, including opportunistic infections and especially *Pneumocystis jiroveci* pneumonia; TB, including extrapulmonary TB; and aspergillosis.

Contraindications. Leflunomide is contraindicated in patients who are pregnant, are breastfeeding, have severe hepatic impairment, or have a known hypersensitivity to any component of the medication. It is not recommended in patient with severe immunodeficiency, severe infections, or bone marrow disorders. It has been shown to increase patient susceptibility to infections, and in some cases cause blood issues such as pancytopenia, thrombocytopenia, and agranulocytosis. It is also worth noting that, although rare, there have been reports of Stevens-Johnson syndrome and toxic epidermal necrolysis with use of leflunomide.

Monitoring. Before starting therapy, baseline monitoring should be completed for CBC with differential, liver function tests (LFTs) including AST and ALT, renal function, and screening for TB. This monitoring should continue

TABLE 23.2	Disease-Modifying and Immune Medications[a]			
Category/ Medication	**Starting Dose**	**Usual Dose**	**Consideration and Monitoring**	
DMARDs				
Methotrexate (Otrexup, Rasuvo, Trexall)	**Oral:** 7.5 mg once weekly. **Subcutaneous:** 7.5 mg once weekly.	**Oral or subcutaneous:** 7.5–15 mg weekly Maximum dosage: 20 mg/week.	Preferred DMARD. Addition of folic acid 1–5 mg/day may decrease side effects of folate deficiency (headache, fatigue, mouth ulcers). Contraindicated in pregnancy. Therapeutic response typically begins within 3–6 weeks.	
Leflunomide (LEF) (Arava)	**Oral loading dose:** 100 mg daily for 3 days (may omit loading dose if concerns for side effects, hepatic/ hematologic toxicities), then 20 mg orally daily.	**Oral:** 20 mg daily (consider 10 mg daily if not able to tolerate 20 mg dose).	Contraindicated in severe liver impairment (ALT >2 times ULN) and pregnancy. Discontinue if severe dermatologic reaction (i.e., Stevens-Johnson syndrome).	
Hydroxychloroquine (HCQ) (Plaquenil)	**Oral:** 400-600 mg once daily or in 2 divided doses.	**Oral:** 200 mg once daily or 400 mg once daily or in 2 divided doses.	Take with food. Caution in renal or hepatic impairment.	
Sulfasalazine (SSZ) (Azulfidine)	**Oral:** 500 mg once daily or 1 Gm/day in 2 divided doses; increase weekly to maintenance dose.	**Oral:** 1 Gm twice daily (if inadequate response after 12 weeks, may increase by 500 mg weekly to maximum dosage of 3 Gm/ day).	Caution in renal and hepatic impairment. Caution in G6PD deficiency (may cause hemolytic anemia). Caution in sulfa allergies. Used in patients who have responded inadequately to salicylates or other NSAIDs.	
TNF Inhibitor Biologics				
Adalimumab (Humira)		**Subcutaneous:** 40 mg every 2 weeks (may increase to weekly if not taking methotrexate).	Do not initiate in patients with active infection. Evaluate for risk and test for latent TB prior to starting. Malignancies such as lymphoma have been reported with use in children and adolescents.	
Certolizumab pegol (Cimzia)	**Subcutaneous:** 400 mg given as two 200-mg injections at weeks 0, 2, and 4.	**Subcutaneous:** 200 mg every other week (alternatively, 400 mg every 4 weeks).		
Etanercept (Enbrel)		**Subcutaneous:** 50 mg once weekly. Maximum dosage: 50 mg weekly.		
Golimumab (Simponi)		In combination with methotrexate. **IV:** 2 mg/kg at weeks 0 and 4, then every 8 weeks thereafter. **Subcutaneous:** 50 mg once monthly.		
Infliximab (Inflectra, Remicade, Renflexis)	In combination with methotrexate. **IV:** 3 mg/kg on weeks 0, 2, and 6.	In combination with methotrexate. **IV:** 3 mg/kg every 8 weeks after week 6 (can range from 3–10 mg/kg every 4–8 weeks).		

Continued

TABLE 23.2   Disease-Modifying and Immune Medications[a]—cont'd

Category/ Medication	Starting Dose	Usual Dose	Consideration and Monitoring
Non-TNF Biologics			
Abatacept (Orencia)	**IV:** Weight-based dose on weeks 0, 2, and 4. <60 kg: 500 mg. 60–100 kg: 750 mg. >100 kg: 1000 mg.	**Subcutaneous:** 125 mg once weekly (can start without IV loading dose). **IV:** weight-based dosing continues every 4 weeks.	COPD patients may experience higher rate of COPD-related adverse reactions. Should be administered only in settings with full resuscitation equipment available and by provider with experience in the administration of biologic therapies.
Sarilumab (Kevzara)		**Subcutaneous:** 200 mg every 2 weeks. May be used as monotherapy or in combination with nonbiologic DMARDs.	Do not start therapy if ANC is <2000/mm^3, platelets are <150,000/mm^3, or ALT or AST is >1.5 times ULN. Monitor for hepatotoxicity and hematologic toxicity. May increase risk of TB, malignancy, or infection.
Tocilizumab (Actemra, Actemra, ACTPen)	**Subcutaneous:** <100 kg: 162 mg once every other week.	**IV:** May be increased to 8 mg/kg once every 4 weeks based on clinical response (maximum dose: 800 mg). **Subcutaneous:** <100 kg: increase to 162 mg once weekly based on clinical response. ≥100 kg: 162 mg once weekly.	Due to concerns for severe or life-threatening cytokine release syndrome, do not initiate if ANC is <2000/mm^3, platelets are <100,000/mm^3, or ALT or AST is >1.5 times ULN. Interrupt therapy if AST/ALT is 3–5 times ULN; discontinue therapy if AST/ALT >5 times ULN for liver impairment. Do not initiate in patients with active infection. Evaluate for risk and test for latent TB prior to starting.
JAK Inhibitors			
Baricitinib (Olumiant)		Used as monotherapy or in combination with methotrexate or nonbiologic DMARDs. **Oral:** 2 mg daily.	Reserved for patients who have an inadequate response or intolerance to one or more TNF inhibitors. Do not use in combination with biologic DMARDs, azathioprine, or cyclosporine. Do not start therapy in patients with an absolute lymphocyte count <500 cells/mm^3, absolute neutrophil count <1000 cells/mm^3, or hemoglobin <8 Gm/dL. Renal dose adjustments for GFR <60 mL/min/1.73 m^2. Avoid in severe hepatic impairment. Do not initiate in patients with active infection. Evaluate for risk and test for latent TB prior to starting. May increase risks for malignancies such as lymphoma and thrombosis.

TABLE 23.2	Disease-Modifying and Immune Medications[a]—cont'd		
Category/ Medication	**Starting Dose**	**Usual Dose**	**Consideration and Monitoring**
Tofacitinib (Xeljanz)		Used as monotherapy or in combination with nonbiologic DMARDs. **Oral:** *Immediate release:* 5 mg twice daily. **Extended release:** 11 mg once daily.	Reserved for patients who have an inadequate response or intolerance to one or more TNF inhibitors. If transitioning from immediate release to extended release, begin extended release the day after the last dose of immediate release. Should not be used in combination with biologic DMARDs, azathioprine, tacrolimus, or cyclosporine. Do not initiate therapy in patients with an absolute lymphocyte count <500 cells/mm^3, ANC <1000 cells/mm^3, or hemoglobin <9 Gm/dL. Coadministration of certain drugs that inhibit or induce certain CYP isoenzymes may need to be avoided or dosage adjustments may be necessary; review drug interactions. Use with potent CYP3A4 inducers may result in loss of or reduced clinical response to tofacitinib. Renal and hepatic dose adjustments necessary. Do not initiate in patients with active infection. Evaluate for risk and test for latent TB prior to starting. May increase risks for malignancies such as lymphoma, thrombosis, all-cause mortality.
Upadacitinib (Rinvoq)		Used as monotherapy or in combination with methotrexate or other nonbiologic DMARDs. **Oral:** 15 mg daily.	Coadministration with certain drugs that inhibit or induce certain CYP isoenzymes may need to be avoided or dosage adjustments may be necessary; review drug interactions. Use with potent CYP3A4 inducers may result in loss of or reduced clinical response. Reserved for patients who have an inadequate response or intolerance to one or more TNF inhibitors. Do not use in combination with biologic DMARDs, azathioprine, or cyclosporine. Do not initiate therapy in patients with an absolute lymphocyte count <500/mm^3, ANC <1000/mm^3, or hemoglobin <8 Gm/dL. Avoid in severe hepatic impairment. Do not initiate in patients with active infection. Evaluate for risk and test for latent TB prior to starting. May increase risks for malignancies such as lymphoma and thrombosis.

ALT, Alanine transaminase; *ANC*, absolute neutrophil count; *AST*, Aspartate transaminase; *COPD*, chronic obstructive pulmonary disease; *CYP*, cytochrome; *DMARD*, disease-modifying antirheumatic drug; *G6PD*, glucose-6-phosphate dehydrogenase; *GFR*, glomerular filtration rate; *HBV*, hepatitis B virus; *NSAIDs*, nonsteroidal antiinflammatory drugs; *TB*, tuberculosis; *TNF*, tumor necrosis factor; *ULN*, upper limit of normal.

[a]**NOTE:** Although patients taking these medications may be cared for by primary care providers, they are typically managed by rheumatologists or specialists in rheumatoid arthritis.

every 2 to 4 weeks for the first 3 months of therapy initiation or dose adjustment, then every 8 to 12 weeks for months 3 to 6, followed by every 12 weeks after 6 months of continuous therapy on the same dose. If labs report ALT three times higher than the upper limit of normal (ULN), treatment should be discontinued.

Hydroxychloroquine

It is not fully understood how hydroxychloroquine works to manage RA. It may interfere with antigen processing in antigen-presenting cells such as macrophages, thereby providing antiinflammatory properties.

Pharmacokinetics. Hydroxychloroquine is administered orally and is widely distributed in body tissues. In RA patients, there is wide variability in absorption, with mean concentrations significantly higher in patients with less disease activity. Hydroxychloroquine is partially metabolized the liver and excreted in the kidney. Data suggest that it is primarily metabolized by CYP2C8, CYP3A4, and CYP2D6. It has been shown to be an inhibitor of the drug transporter P-glycoprotein. It should be administered with food or milk to decrease GI symptoms.

Indications. Hydroxychloroquine can be used as monotherapy in mild RA cases that lack poor prognostic factors. However, it is more commonly used in combination with other DMARDs for the management of moderate to severe disease, regardless of prognostic factors. There are no recommended dosing changes for renal or hepatic impairment.

Adverse Effects. GI issues are the most common side effects reported for hydroxychloroquine, including vomiting, nausea, diarrhea, and abdominal pain. Taking it with food or by using the twice daily dosing may limit these GI effects. More serious effects include irreversible QT interval prolongation and retinal damage. Risk factors for retinal issues include duration of use greater than 5 years, doses greater than 5 mg/kg/day, renal and hepatic impairment, and low body weight.

Contraindications. Therapy should be discontinued in patients who have suspected or confirmed ocular toxicity. These patients should then be closely monitored as the retinal changes may progress even after therapy has stopped. Hydroxychloroquine should not be given with other drugs that can cause QT interval prolongation. It should be used with caution in patients with a glucose-6-phosphate dehydrogenase (G6PD) deficiency due to risk for hemolytic anemia. Hydroxychloroquine appears to be safe in pregnancy as no increase in birth defects or fetal ocular toxicities has been reported. Caution should be taken in nursing mothers as this medication is excreted into breast milk.

Monitoring. One significant benefit of hydroxychloroquine is that it does not require the frequent laboratory monitoring that other DMARDs require since it has limited risk of infection or abnormalities in blood cells, renal function, or hepatic function as compared to other agents in this group. In light of concerns for retinal damage, an ophthalmologic examination should be done within the first year of therapy and then annually after 5 years of therapy. However,

if patients possess predisposing risk factors, eye examinations should be repeated annually while on hydroxychloroquine.

Sulfasalazine

Pharmacokinetics. The exact mechanism of action for sulfasalazine is unknown. The prodrug sulfasalazine is broken down into the active form 5-aminosalicyclic acid (5-ASA), which may modulate chemical mediators of the inflammatory response, such as leukotriene.

Indications. Sulfasalazine can be used either as monotherapy or in combination with other DMARDs. It is used in the treatment of patients with RA who have not responded well to salicylates or other nonsteroidal antiinflammatory drugs. Clinical benefit may take 4 to 12 weeks. No dose adjustments are provided in the package insert for renal or hepatic impairment, but caution should be used in these populations.

Adverse Effects. The most commonly reported side effects of sulfasalazine are rash and GI issues, such as nausea, vomiting, diarrhea, and anorexia. Less common but sometimes serious issues include blood cell abnormalities, photosensitivity, hypersensitivity (e.g., Stevens-Johnson syndrome), alopecia, and elevated liver enzymes. Patients should be informed that sulfasalazine may cause an orange/yellow discoloration of the skin and/or urine.

Contraindications. Since sulfasalazine contains sulfa, it should not be used in patients with a sulfonamide or salicylate allergy. It can be used in pregnant and nursing mothers with caution, although it does cross the placenta and is present in breast milk.

Monitoring. Baseline monitoring should be completed for renal function, ALT, AST, and a CBC with differential prior to initiating therapy with sulfasalazine. This monitoring should continue every 2 to 4 weeks for 3 months after starting therapy or a dose change, then every 8 to 12 weeks for months 3 to 6 of treatment, and then every 12 weeks after 6 months of continuous therapy. Patients should also be screened for G6PD deficiency as use of this medication can result in hemolytic anemia.

TNF Inhibitor Biologics

TNF inhibitor biologics include adalimumab, certolizumab, etanercept, golimumab, and infliximab. These medications work to block TNF-α, a proinflammatory cytokine present in elevated amounts in patients with rheumatic conditions such as RA. It can take weeks for their clinical benefit to begin, and up to 3 months before full effects are experienced.

These agents are typically reserved for patients who continue to experience moderate to high disease activity despite the use of DMARDs. One consideration is their high cost as compared to DMARDs. Their inherent risks also pose concerns and limit their use. These agents can cause new-onset or worsening heart failure. As a result, they should be avoided in patients diagnosed with New York Heart Association (NYHA) Class III or IV heart failure. In addition, they may increase the risk for malignancies and serious infections, or reactivation of serious infections such as TB and hepatitis B virus (HBV), by blocking TNF-medicated immune responses and interfering with innate immune responses. As a result, patients should be screened at baseline and continually for infections, malignancies, demyelinating disorders, and lab value abnormalities (i.e., pancytopenia). Baseline testing includes screenings for both TB and HBV, with negative patients continually screened throughout treatment and positive patients started on appropriate therapy prior to TNF initiation. Annual blood work should include a CBC with differential and complete metabolic panel (CMP) to evaluate the presence of cytopenias, hepatotoxicity, or other serious side effects. Therapeutic drug monitoring is not currently recommended for TNF agents in the management of RA, although this may be done in other disease states such as inflammatory bowel disease (IBD).

Non-TNF Biologics

A non-TNF biologic agent may be used in place of a biologic TNF inhibitor should a patient's disease severity remain uncontrolled while on the TNF inhibitor. Therapy changes from one non-TNF to another non-TNF may also occur if disease severity is not controlled. Finally, a non-TNF may be initiated in patients who have failed therapy on two TNF inhibitors. These medications have various mechanisms that target the inflammatory process. They include abatacept, rituximab, sarilumab, and tocilizumab.

JAK Inhibitors

JAK inhibitors inhibit intracellular enzymes that signal the stimulation of red blood cell production and immune cell function. JAK enzymes stimulate signal transducers and activators of transcription (STATs) when an inflammatory response is activated, which in turn regulates intracellular activity and gene expression. Blocking JAK enzymes prevents inflammatory response gene expression and the intracellular activity of immune cells, as well as reducing the circulation of immune system cells. As these are comparatively newer agents for the treatment of RA, tofacitinib is the only drug from this class that is referenced in current guidelines. These agents are indicated for moderate to severe disease activity in patients who failed therapy with DMARDs, and they can be used as monotherapy or in combination with nonbiologic DMARDs.

PRACTICE PEARLS

RA Treatment Evaluation and Monitoring

- Patient response to therapy is cumulatively evaluated through physical examinations, patient reports, imaging, and laboratory markers.
- Most RA therapies required extensive patient laboratory monitoring and screening at baseline and throughout treatment.

BOOKMARK THIS!

Clinical Guidelines for RA

- American College of Rheumatology guideline for the treatment of rheumatoid arthritis: https://www.rheumatology.org/Portals/0/Files/2021-ACR-Guideline-for-Treatment-Rheumatoid-Arthritis-Early-View.pdf

---

Prescriber Considerations for Disease-Modifying and Immune Therapy

The American College of Rheumatology most recently updated clinical practice guidelines for rheumatoid arthritis in March 2021 (Frankel et al, 2021). Although primary care providers typically do not initiate therapy, they will be partners in clinical management. Recognition of medication interactions and exacerbation of symptoms and management of comorbidities will require a basic understanding of medications and goals of therapy. Useful resources are available through the American College of Rheumatology (https://www.rheumatology.org/), European Alliance of Associations for Rheumatology (https://www.eular.org/index.cfm), and the Arthritis Foundation (https://www.arthritis.org/home.)

Clinical Reasoning for Disease-Modifying and Immune Therapy

Consider the individual patient's health problem requiring disease-modifying and immune therapy. Does the problem present as early RA and/or low disease activity or has the patient had persistently uncontrolled disease severity despite therapy? Early RA is defined as a symptom/disease duration of less than 6 months; not time from diagnosis. Disease activity or severity can vary between low, moderate, and high. DMARDs, notably methotrexate, are the preferred agents for treating early RA. It may be necessary to bridge with low-dose corticosteroids or NSAIDs during the first few weeks of therapy while waiting for the clinical benefit onset with DMARDs. Should disease severity remain moderate or high despite therapy, changes to medications may include combinations of DMARDs, TNF-inhibitors, and non-TNF biologics. JAK inhibitors may be used, but due to lack of longitudinal safety data, the current guidelines have lower recommendations for this drug class.

Established RA is defined as duration of disease/symptoms of 6 months or more, or a patient meeting at least four of the 1987 criteria for 6 weeks or more. Initial treatment with DMARDs is still recommended. However, progressive treatment for moderate to high disease severity will be more encompassing than early RA and will include additional combinations of DMARDs, TNF-inhibitors, non-TNF biologics, and JAK inhibitors. Additional considerations beyond disease severity include patient preference (e.g., route of administration, frequency, monitoring, side effects, etc.), comorbid health conditions, and cost.

Nonpharmacologic therapy plays an important supportive role for all RA patients. These treatments include physical and occupational therapy, mental health, coping mechanisms, weight management, and social work. Patients should also be actively involved in disease state and medication education. Surgical interventions are reserved for severe disease activity with significant loss of cartilage.

Determine the desired therapeutic outcome based on the degree of RA therapy needed for the patient's disease severity. The primary goal of RA therapy is to achieve low disease severity and/or disease remission to support higher quality of life. It is important to initiate drug therapy as soon as possible upon diagnosis. Patient participation in treatment evaluation is important to consider subjective assessment of symptoms, plus evaluation of physical exam and laboratory monitoring. It is important to education patients that there may be a few weeks of delayed onset for clinical benefit with agents such as DMARDs, so symptoms may be managed with NSAIDs or corticosteroids in the interim. Disease severity assessment and evaluation must also take into consideration that full clinical benefits may take months to appreciate.

Assess the disease-modifying and immune therapy selected for its appropriateness for an individual patient by considering the medication's side effects and the patient's comorbidities and genetic factors. Most RA therapies can increase the risk for infections, so it is important to screen and continually monitor for infections such as TB and HBV. Certain medications can also increase the risk for malignancies, organ dysfunction, and hematologic disorders. It is recommended to supplement folic acid while taking methotrexate as its mechanism of action may result in a deficiency. Patients should be screened for G6PD deficiency prior to starting sulfasalazine as use of this medication in this population can result in hemolytic anemia.

Initiate the treatment plan with the selected medication by first providing adequate patient education to ensure the patient's understanding, and promote full participation in the disease-modifying and immune therapy. Reinforce education at each visit to ensure full understanding. Assess for side and adverse effects and review challenges the patient may be having with adherence to therapy. In addition, reinforce the need for patients to follow-up with specialty providers on a regular basis. Refer to social services or pharmaceutical manufacturers if costs of medications are interfering with medication adherence. The Arthritis Foundation (https://www.arthritis.org/home) provides patients and families with additional strategies that may help reduce the financial burden.

Ensure complete patient and family understanding about the medication prescribed for disease-modifying and immune therapy using a variety of education strategies. The Arthritis Foundation (https://www.arthritis.org/home) provides multiple educational resources for patients and families as they manage their symptoms and slow progression of the illness. Topics include use of physical therapy, exercise, nutrition management, minimizing the risk for infection, and other topics. Although the majority of information is in written format, videos are available on select topics that may be of interest.

Conduct follow-up and monitoring of patient responses to disease-modifying and immune therapy. Regular assessment of the severity of joint involvement, pain level, and range of motion, as well as laboratory monitoring required for selected medications, is important. Regular communication with the rheumatologist will help ensure patient experiences best possible outcomes.

Patient Education for Medication Safety

Patients should be provided with realistic expectations for disease state goals and therapy. It is important to communicate that the ultimate goal of therapy is to improve quality of life by limiting disease activity and promoting remission. A rheumatology-trained care provider should guide management of the disease in conjunction with primary care to effectively meet treatment goals. Treatment should begin at the onset of diagnosis. Nonpharmacologic therapies may include physical therapy and support of mental health and wellness. Pharmacologic therapy will depend on level of disease activity, patient preferences, comorbid conditions, and cost.

Patient counseling on medications should include anticipated time to onset, or symptom relief. This is especially important for DMARDs as they can take weeks to months to provide their full effects based on their mechanisms of action. While patients are waiting for these drugs to take effect, they will likely be placed on NSAIDs and/or corticosteroids as a bridge to cover symptoms of pain and swelling. The patient's response to each therapy for RA will be holistically evaluated through subjective patient report, physical examination, imaging, and any relevant laboratory markers.

Monitoring should occur at baseline and intermittently every few weeks throughout treatment to avoid risks of toxicity (Table 23.3). The frequency of monitoring will decrease as stable drug dosing continues, but it will temporarily increase again if dosing is adjusted. These labs will typically include CBC with differential, liver enzymes (AST, ALT), and serum creatinine, which will provide insight on blood disorders, liver function, and renal function, respectively. The exception may be hydroxychloroquine, which does not require monitoring after baseline.

TABLE 23.3	Recommended Laboratory Monitoring for DMARDs[a]		
Therapeutic Agents[b]	**Monitoring Interval Based on Duration of Therapy[c]**		
	<3 Months	**3–6 Months**	**>6 Months**
Hydroxychloroquine	None after baseline[d]	None	None
Leflunomide	2–4 weeks	8–12 weeks	12 weeks
Methotrexate	2–4 weeks	8–12 weeks	12 weeks
Sulfasalazine	2–4 weeks	8–12 weeks	12 weeks

[a]More frequent monitoring is recommended within the first 3 months of therapy or after increasing the dose, and the outer bound of the monitoring interval is recommended beyond 6 months of therapy. Adapted from Saag, K. G., Teng, G. G., Patkar, N. M., Anuntiyo, J., Finney, C., Curtis, J. R., et al. (2008). American College of Rheumatology 2008 recommendations for the use of nonbiologic and biologic disease modifying antirheumatic drugs in rheumatoid arthritis. *Arthritis & Rheumatology, 59*, 762–784.
[b]Listed alphabetically.
[c]The panel indicated that patients with comorbidities, abnormal laboratory results, and/or multiple therapies may require more frequent laboratory testing than what is generally recommended laboratory monitoring for DMARDs in the table.
[d]See Saag, K. G., Teng, G. G., Patkar, N. M., Anuntiyo, J., Finney, C., Curtis, J. R., et al. (2008). American College of Rheumatology 2008 recommendations for the use of nonbiologic and biologic disease modifying antirheumatic drugs in rheumatoid arthritis. *Arthritis & Rheumatology, 59*, 762–784 for baseline monitoring recommendations.
From Singh, J. A., Saag, K. G., Bridges, S. L., et al. American College of Rheumatology [2016]. 2015 American College of Rheumatology guideline for the treatment of rheumatoid arthritis. *Arthritis Care & Research, 68*[1], 1–25. https://doi.org/10.1002/acr.22783.

Application Questions for Discussion

1. As a health care provider, what patient and safety factors should be considered before prescribing disease-modifying and immune therapy?
2. What should be included in the education plan for a patient and/or caregiver who has been prescribed methotrexate?
3. What role may monitoring play in the treatment choices for RA therapy?

Selected Bibliography

Abarientos, C., Sperber, K., Shapiro, D. L., et al. (2001). Hydroxychloroquine in systemic lupus erythematosus and rheumatoid arthritis and its safety in pregnancy. *Expert Opinion on Drug Safety, 10*(5), 705–714.

Abbas, A. K., Lichtman, A. H., & Pillai, S. (2012). *Leukocyte Migration into Tissues, Cellular and Molecular Immunology* (7th ed.). Philadelphia: Elsevier Saunders.

Actemra [package insert] (2018). South San Francisco: Genentech. https://www.gene.com/download/pdf/actemra_prescribing.pdf.

Aletaha, D., Neogi, T., Silman, A. J., et al. (2010). Rheumatoid arthritis classification criteria: An American College of Rheumatology/European League Against Rheumatism collaborative initiative. *Annals of the Rheumatic Diseases, 69*(9), 1580–1588.

Arava [package insert] (2011). Bridgewater, NJ: Sanofi-Aventis U.S. LLC. Available at https://www.accessdata.fda.gov/drugsatfda_docs/label/2011/020905s022lbl.pdf.

Arnett, F. C., Edworthy, S. M., Bloch, D. A., et al. (1988). The American Rheumatism Association 1987 revised criteria for the classification of rheumatoid arthritis. *Arthritis & Rheumatology, 31*, 315–324.

Azulfidine [package insert] (2012). New York: Pfizer. Available at https://www.accessdata.fda.gov/drugsatfda_docs/label/2012/007073s125lbl.pdf.

Bianchi, G., Caporali, R., Todoerti, M., et al. (2016). Methotrexate and rheumatoid arthritis: Current evidence regarding subcutaneous versus oral routes of administration. *Advances in Therapy, 33*, 369–378.

Carmona, L., Cross, M., Williams, B., et al. (2010). Rheumatoid arthritis. *Best Practice & Research: Clinical Rheumatology, 24*, 733–745.

Cimzia [package insert] (2018). Smyrna, GA: UCB. Available at https://www.cimzia.com/sites/default/files/docs/CIMZIA_full_prescribing_information.pdf.

Cooles, F. A., & Isaacs, J. D. (2011). Pathophysiology of rheumatoid arthritis. *Current Opinion in Rheumatology, 23*(3), 233–240.

Elsevier. Clinical pharmacology powered by ClinicalKey®. (2019). Retrieved from http://www.clinicalkey.com.

Enbrel [package insert] (2012). Thousand Oaks, CA: Immunex Corporation. December. Available at https://www.accessdata.fda.gov/drugsatfda_docs/label/2012/103795s5503lbl.pdf.

Fox, R. I. (1993). Mechanism of action of hydroxychloroquine as an antirheumatic drug. *Seminars in Arthritis and Rheumatism, 23*(2), 82–91. Suppl 1.

Fraenkel, L., Bathon, J. M., England, B. R., St.Clair, E. W., Arayssi, T., Carandang, K., Akl, ..., & E., A (2021). 2021 American College of Rheumatology Guideline for the Treatment of Rheumatoid Arthritis. *Arthritis & Rheumatology, 73*(7), 1108–1123. https://doi.org/10.1002/art.41752.

Gibofsky, A. (2012). Overview of epidemiology, pathophysiology, and diagnosis of rheumatoid arthritis. *The American Journal of Managed Care, 18*, S295–S302.

Harris, J., & Keane, J. (2010). How tumour necrosis factor blockers interfere with tuberculosis immunity. *Clinical & Experimental Immunology, 161*(1), 1–9. doi:10.1111/j.1365-2249.2010.04146.x.

Helmick, C. G., Felson, D. T., Lawrence, R. C., et al. (2008). Estimates of the prevalence of arthritis and other rheumatic conditions in the United States: Part I. *Arthritis & Rheumatology, 58*(1), 15–25.

Humira [package insert] (2018). North Chicago, IL: Abbvie. Available at https://www.rxabbvie.com/pdf/humira.pdf.

Joshi, P., & Dhaneshwar, S. S. (2014). An update on disease modifying antirheumatic drugs. *Inflammation & Allergy—Drug Targets, 13*(4), 249–261.

Kevzara [package insert] (2017). Bridgewater, NJ: Sanofi-Aventis U.S. May. Available at https://www.accessdata.fda.gov/drugsatfda_docs/label/2017/761037s000lbl.pdf.

Kirchner, E. (2017). Rheumatoid arthritis: Pathophysiology and safe administration of biologics. *Journal of Infusion Nursing, 40*(6), 364–366. http://doi.org/10.1097/NAN.0000000000000249.

Kremer, J. M., Alarcon, G. S., Lightfoot, R. W., Jr., et al. (1994). Methotrexate for rheumatoid arthritis. Suggested guidelines for monitoring liver toxicity. American College of Rheumatology. *Arthritis & Rheumatology, 37*(3), 316–328.

Kumar, V., Abbas, A. K., Fausto, N., & Aster, J. C. (2010). *Acute and Chronic InflammationRobbins and Cotran Pathologic Basis of Disease* (8th ed.). Philadelphia: Saunders Elsevier.

Martikainen, J. A., Kautiainen, H., Rantalaiho, V., & Puolakka., K (2016). Long-term work productivity costs due to absenteeism and permanent work disability in patients with early rheumatoid arthritis: A Nationwide Register Study of 7831 patients. *The Journal of Rheumatology, 34*(26), 2101–2015.

Methotrexate [package insert] (2016). Huntsville, AL: DAVA Pharmaceuticals, Inc. January. Available at https://www.accessdata.fda.gov/drugsatfda_docs/label/2016/008085s066lbl.pdf.

Myasoedova, E., Davis, J., III, Crowson, C., & Gabriel, S. (2010). Epidemiology of rheumatoid arthritis: Rheumatoid arthritis and mortality. *Current Rheumatology Reports, 12*, 379–385.

Olumiant [package insert] (2018). Indianapolis: Eli Lilly. Available at https://www.accessdata.fda.gov/drugsatfda_docs/label/2018/207924s000lbl.pdf.

Orencia [package insert] (2017). Princeton, NJ: Bristol-Myers Squibb. Available at https://packageinserts.bms.com/pi/pi_orencia.pdf.

Plaquenil [package insert] (2017). St. Michael, Barbados: Concordia Pharmaceuticals. Available at https://www.accessdata.fda.gov/drugsatfda_docs/label/2017/009768s037s045s047lbl.pdf.

Remicade [package insert] (2013). Horsham, PA: Janssen Biotech. November. Available at https://www.accessdata.fda.gov/drugsatfda_docs/label/2013/103772s5359lbl.pdf.

Rituxan [package insert] (2018). South San Francisco: Genentech. June. Available at https://www.gene.com/download/pdf/rituxan_prescribing.pdf.

Silman, A. J., & Hochberg, M. C. (2009). Descriptive Epidemiology of Rheumatoid Arthritis. In M. C. Hochberg, A. J. Silman, J. S. Smolen, M. E. Weinblatt, & M. H. Weisman (Eds.), *Rheumatoid Arthritis* (pp. 15–22). Philadelphia: Mosby Elsevier.

Silman, A. J., & Pearson, J. E. (2002). Epidemiology and genetics of rheumatoid arthritis. *Arthritis Research & Therapy, 4*(3), S265.

Simponi [package insert] (2011). Horsham, PA: Janssen Biotech. August. Available at https://www.accessdata.fda.gov/drugsatfda_docs/label/2011/125289s0064lbl.pdf.

Singh, J. A., Saag, K. G., Bridges, S. L., Jr., Akl, E. A., Bannuru, R. R., Sullivan, M. C., et al. (2015). American College of Rheumatology guideline for the treatment of rheumatoid arthritis. *Arthritis Care & Research, 68*, 1–25.

Smolen, J. S., Landewe, R., Bijlsma, J., et al. (2020). EULAR recommendations for the management of rheumatoid arthritis with synthetic and biological disease-modifying antirheumatic drugs: 2019 update. *Annals of the Rheumatic Diseases*. pii: annrheumdis-2019-216655. http://doi.org/10.1136/annrheumdis-2019-216655 [Epub ahead of print].

Sturgeon, J. A., Finan, P. H., & Zautra, A. J. (2016). Affective disturbance in rheumatoid arthritis: Psychological and disease-related pathways. *Nature Reviews Rheumatology, 12*(9), 532.

van den Hoek, J., Boshuizen, H. C., Roorda, L. D., et al. (2017). Mortality in patients with rheumatoid arthritis: A 15-year prospective cohort study. *Rheumatology International, 37*, 487–493. https://doi-org.ezproxy.hsc.usf.edu/10.1007/s00296-016-3638-5.

Warren, J. S., & Ward, P. A. (2020). The Inflammatory Response. In K. Kaushansky, M. A. Lichtman, J. T. Prchal, M. M. Levi, O. W. Pressz, L. J. Burns, & M. Caligiuri (Eds.), *Williams Hematology* (9th ed.). New York: McGraw-Hill http://accessmedicine.mhmedical.com/content.aspx?bookid=1581&sectionid=94302794 Accessed January 28.

Weinblatt, M. E. (1995). Efficacy of methotrexate in rheumatoid arthritis. *British Journal of Rheumatology, 34*(2), 43–48. Suppl.

Xeljanz [package insert] (2018). New York: Pfizer. May. Available at http://labeling.pfizer.com/ShowLabeling.aspx?id=959.

24

Antigout Medications

MELISSA RUBLE AND JACLYN COLE

Overview

Gout, one of the most common rheumatic diseases in adults, is caused by a buildup of uric acid crystals within the joints. Gout is a treatable disease whose prevalence and incidence have increased in recent years. Unfortunately, gout is often misdiagnosed, and even though effective treatments are available, management of the disease is suboptimal. Acute gout flares can have a detrimental impact on a patient's quality of life, both economically and socially, due to the pain and debilitation they cause. It is estimated that more than $1 billion is spent annually on gout in the ambulatory care setting, most of which is spent on prescription medications and treatment.

According to the 2015–2016 National Health and Nutrition Examination Survey (NHANES), the prevalence of gout in the United States was estimated at 3.9% of adults, or approximately 9.3 million people (Chen-Xu et al., 2019). While the prevalence of both hyperuricemia and gout in 2015–2016 was relatively stable compared to figures from the preceding (2007–2008) NHANES survey, only about one-third of patients met guidelines for target uric acid levels, suggesting a lack of progress in treatment efforts. Furthermore, adherence to gout treatment is poor compared to adherence to treatment for other common chronic illnesses (Briesacher et al., 2008).

Relevant Physiology

The most important risk factor for developing gout is high concentrations of serum urate. A linear relationship exists between the risk of an acute gout flare and serum urate concentration: the higher a patient's level of serum urate, the greater their chances for an acute gout flare. Gout and hyperuricemia are found more commonly in older adults, with the highest prevalence (12.6%) in those who are 80 years of age and older (compared to 0.4% in adults 20 to 29 years of age). Obese patients are twice as likely to develop gout than those who are at a healthy weight. In addition, gout is three times more likely to occur in males than in females, until females reach postmenopause, at which point their likelihood of developing gout equals that of males due to a loss of estrogen-influenced uricosuria. Lifestyle risk factors include consumption of alcohol (particularly beer and spirits) and sugar-sweetened drinks, heavy meals, and excessive intake of meat and seafood.

Over time, gout flares will increase if risk factors are not adequately addressed. Without treatment, acute flares can become chronic and can lead to joint damage, chronic arthritis, and tophi. Treatment is focused on both pain management and underlying inflammation.

Pathophysiology

Gout develops when there is precipitation of monosodium urate crystals in the synovial joints. The equilibrium of crystals in the joints and serum occurs slowly and is influenced by physical factors including temperature and blood flow. The proximal joints (toes and fingers) are cooler and have less blood flow than other areas of the body, which increases the risk for precipitation of crystals. Gout subsequently occurs when body fluids become saturated with uric acid (typically with serum levels greater than 7 mg/dL). Monosodium urate crystals are indicators of acute inflammatory processes that signal the activation of neutrophils. Uric acid is the end product of purine degradation and is a waste product with no physiologic purpose.

There is a delicate balance between the amount of urate that is created and excreted. Key players in the production of uric acid include hypoxanthine-guanine phosphoribosyl transferase (HPRT) and phosphoribosyl pyrophosphate (PRPP). These enzymes are highlighted in Fig. 24.1. Gout occurs when urate accumulates in the blood due to overproduction (10% of patients) or underexcretion (90% of patients) of uric acid. The intense inflammatory response that results will resolve spontaneously and completely over several days, even without therapy.

PRACTICE PEARLS

Conditions Associated With Hyperuricemia

- Obesity
- Congestive heart failure
- Starvation
- Chronic hemolytic anemia
- Diabetic ketoacidosis
- Impaired kidney disease
- Hypothyroidism
- Myeloproliferative disorders

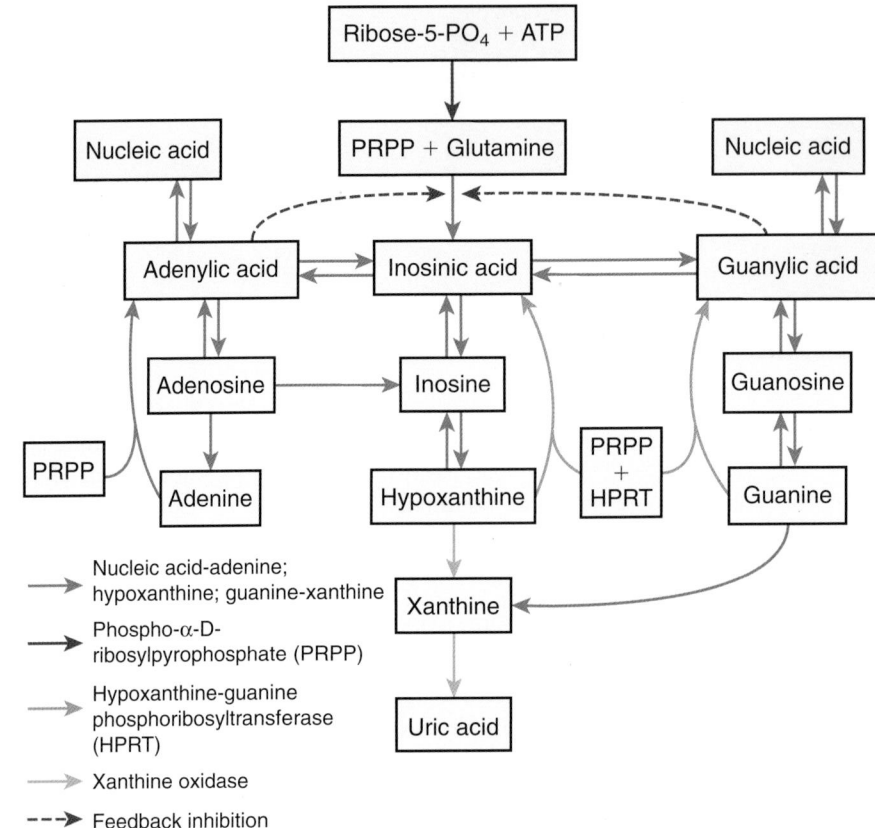

• **Fig. 24.1** Production of uric acid. The major pathways involved in purine nucleotide synthesis.
(Redrawn from Klippel, J. H., & Dieppe, P. A. [Eds.], [1998], *Rheumatology* [2nd ed.], Mosby-Wolfe. In McCance, K., & Huether, S. [2019]. *Pathophysiology* [8th ed.]. St. Louis: Elsevier.)

Overproduction and Underexcretion of Uric Acid

Uric acid is produced from purines originating from one of the following sources: dietary purines, conversion of tissue nucleic acid into purine nucleotides, or de novo synthesis of purine bases (Fig. 24.2). Purines lead to the production of either nucleic acid or uric acid.

Purine metabolism is regulated by several enzymes, and any changes or abnormalities in this process can lead to an overproduction of uric acid. For instance, conditions or medications that increase the breakdown of tissue nucleic acid or that increase the rate of cell turnover can result in uric acid overproduction due to lysis and breakdown of cells. Another cause of overproduction of uric acid is an increase in the production of PRPP due to an increase in the activity of PRPP synthetase. Additionally, a deficiency in HPRT, which converts guanine to guanylic acid and hypoxanthine to inosinic acid, causes guanine and hypoxanthine to metabolize to uric acid, which produces more PRPP to interact with glutamine in the purine pathway.

Under normal conditions, uric acid does not accumulate in the body: each day, two-thirds of the uric acid in the body is excreted in the urine, with the remainder excreted through the gastrointestinal (GI) tract. More than 90% of patients with gout experience a decrease in uric acid excretion for an unknown reason. Most of these cases are idiopathic in

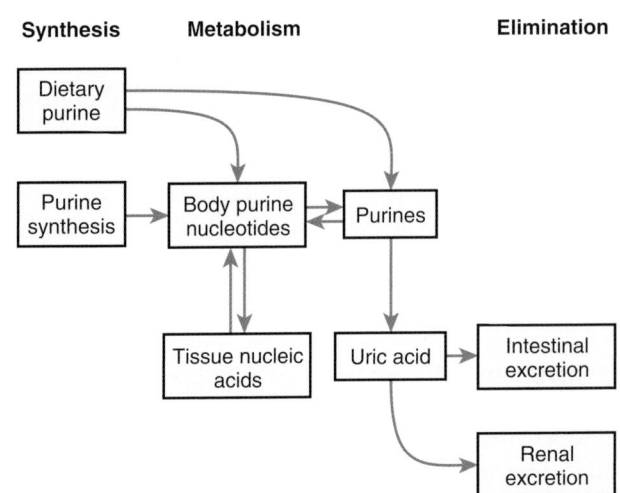

• **Fig. 24.2** Uric acid synthesis and elimination. Uric acid is derived from ingested purines or synthesized from ingested foods, as well as recycled following cell breakdown. Uric acid is then eliminated through the kidneys and gastrointestinal tract.
(Redrawn from Klippel, J. H., & Dieppe, P. A. [Eds.], [1998], *Rheumatology* [2nd ed.], Mosby-Wolfe. In McCance, K., & Huether, S. [2019]. *Pathophysiology* [8th ed.]. St. Louis: Elsevier.)

nature and are termed *primary idiopathic hyperuricemia*. A decline in urinary excretion of uric acid below the rate of production leads to hyperuricemia and sodium urate.

Differentiating between uric acid overproduction and underexcretion can be challenging. To better understand what has caused a patient to develop gout, the patient is placed on a purine-free diet for 3 to 5 days and then takes urine samples for 24 hours to measure the amount of uric acid that has been excreted. Sticking to a purine-free diet is difficult; thus, this test is rarely done in clinical practice. Individuals who excrete less than 600 mg of uric acid in 24 hours are classified as *underexcreters* of uric acid. Patients on a regular diet who excrete more than 1000 mg of uric acid in 24 hours are classified as *overproducers*.

PRACTICE PEARLS

Medications That Can Contribute to Hyperuricemia

- Diuretics (thiazide and loop diuretics)
- Nicotinic acid
- Salicylates
- Ethanol
- Pyrazinamide
- Levodopa
- Ethambutol
- Cytotoxic drugs
- Cyclosporine

Patients with gout typically present with *acute inflammatory monoarthritis*. The most common area where gout occurs is in the first metatarsophalangeal joint, also known as the podagra. Although this joint is the most common area, any joint in the lower extremity can be affected, even the wrist or finger. Gout can also manifest as chronic arthritis of one or more joints. An accumulation of uric acid around the joints, skin, or cartilage can cause a tophus to form. Tophi are mainly found in the articular, periarticular, bursal, bone, auricular, and cutaneous tissue and are detectable through physical examination, imaging, and/or pathology examination. Gout flares produce one of the most intense forms of inflammatory arthritis and can cause dramatic pain, redness, swelling, and warmth in the affected joints. Gout can occur in various areas, including the kidney, cartilage, tendons, and synovial membranes.

Diagnosis of gout is typically based on the presence of symptoms versus laboratory tests of uric acid. This is because many patients with elevated uric acid levels may never experience a gout attack and thus do not need to be treated. Patients with asymptomatic hyperuricemia do not require therapy but should be encouraged to make lifestyle modifications that will reduce urate concentrations. A definitive diagnosis of gout requires aspiration of synovial fluid from the affected joint(s) and identification of intracellular crystals of monosodium urate in synovial fluid leukocytes. These crystals are needle shaped and can also be observed during asymptomatic periods.

Types of Gout

Acute Gouty Arthritis

Acute gouty arthritis (*gout flare*) is identified as a rapid and localized onset of severe pain, swelling, and inflammation. More than 90% of patients with gout will experience podagra during their course of the disease. In older adults, gout can be confused with rheumatoid arthritis or osteoarthritis. Older females may present with gout in numerous small joints in the hands. The formation of crystals activates several chemical mediators that cause inflammation, increased vascular permeability, complement activation, and leukocyte activation. Untreated attacks may last from 3 to 14 days before resolving.

In addition to synovial fluid aspiration, health care providers can observe the clinical triad of inflammatory monoarthritis, elevated serum uric acid levels, and response to colchicine to help diagnose gout. Frequency of gout flares helps guide the need for urate-lowering therapy (ULT).

Uric Acid Nephrolithiasis

Nephrolithiasis occurs in 15% of patients with gout. The incidence of urolithiasis correlates with serum uric acid concentrations, acidity of the urine, and urinary uric acid concentrations. When urine is acidic, uric acid is primarily in the unionized, less soluble form. Normally, patients with nephrolithiasis have a urinary pH less than 5. When uric acid production increases and becomes saturated at a pH of 5, spontaneous precipitation of stones can occur.

Gouty Nephropathy

There are two types of gouty nephropathy: acute uric acid nephropathy and chronic urate nephropathy. In *acute uric acid nephropathy*, massive production of uric acid crystals will precipitate in the collecting ducts and ureters, leading to a blockage of urine flow. *Chronic urate nephropathy* occurs when there is a long-term deposition of urate crystals.

Tophaceous Gout

Tophi are uncommon in gout patients and are late complications of hyperuricemia. The most common sites for tophi are the base of the fingers, olecranon bursae, ulnar aspect of the forearm, Achilles tendon, knees, wrists, and hands. Resultant deformities can lead to soft tissue damage, joint destruction and pain, and/or carpal tunnel syndrome.

PRACTICE PEARLS

Goals of Therapy

- Terminate acute gout attack
- Prevent recurrent attacks of gouty arthritis
- Prevent complications associated with chronic deposition of urate crystals in tissues
- Limit adverse events associated with treatment

Gout Therapy

The 2020 American College of Rheumatology (ACR) guidelines outline general principles for the treatment of gout, including recommendations for nonpharmacologic treatment, initiation of ULT, duration and management of therapy, and approach to management of acute flares (FitzGerald et al., 2020). Similarly, the European League Against Rheumatism (EULAR) developed three overarching principles and 11 key recommendations to guide providers in choosing both pharmacologic and nonpharmacologic interventions for patients with gout (Richette et al., 2017). These guidelines emphasize that management of lifestyle factors should be encouraged for all patients regardless of the extent of their disease (Table 24.1).

Management of gout typically includes both nonpharmacologic and pharmacologic treatment approaches. Nonpharmacologic strategies focus on changing modifiable risk factors and include weight loss for patients who are overweight or obese and limiting intake of dietary purine. Pharmacologic agents focus on lowering urate levels and decreasing inflammation. Treatment is aimed at decreasing inflammatory cell activation and aggregation to the involved joints.

Nonpharmacologic therapy is recommended in addition to treatment with medications. General health, diet, and lifestyle measures for patients with gout include weight loss to achieve optimal body mass index (BMI), exercise, and adequate hydration. Patients should be instructed to avoid organ meats that are high in purine content, such as sweetbreads, liver, and kidneys, as well as cured meats such as salami. Patients should also avoid high-fructose corn syrup, which is found in sweetened sodas and foods. Limiting alcohol to no more than two servings daily for males and one serving daily for females is recommended for all gout patients. Avoidance of alcohol during periods of gout attacks or in cases of advanced gout is imperative. Patients with gout are encouraged to eat vegetables and low-fat or nonfat dairy products. Each of these recommendations aims to decrease the risk and frequency of acute gout attacks and lower serum urate levels. Recommendations emphasize the need for ideal health and the prevention and optimization of life-threatening comorbidities including coronary artery disease (CAD) and obesity, metabolic syndrome, diabetes mellitus, hyperlipidemia, and hypertension (Box 24.1).

The first step in managing an acute gout flare is to assess its severity. Providers should determine the patient's level of pain (mild, moderate, or severe) and the number of small and large joints that are affected. First-line agents used for monotherapy include low-dose colchicine, nonsteroidal antiinflammatory drugs (NSAIDs), and systemic corticosteroids (Fig. 24.3). Corticosteroids are discussed in detail in Chapter 22. Decisions regarding which of these first-line agents to use should be individualized based on patient factors and preferences. Interleukin-1 (IL-1) inhibitors are conditionally recommended only when patients are not responsive to first-line agents or when these agents are poorly tolerated or contraindicated.

During an acute gout flare, ice can be applied to the affected joint to reduce pain. Flaxseed, cherry, celery root, and vitamin C supplements are not recommended in the guidelines for treating gout as there is limited research to support their use.

NSAIDs

NSAIDs are the mainstay of treatment for gout due to their efficacy and minimal toxicity compared with other agents. Indomethacin, naproxen, and sulindac are approved by the U.S. Food and Drug Administration (FDA) for treating acute gout (Table 24.1). Indomethacin is the favored NSAID, but there is little evidence to support one NSAID over another. Therapy should be initiated within 24 hours of the onset of symptoms. The earlier the patient is able to start an NSAID, the more efficacious the medication will be. NSAIDs may need to be tapered, especially in patients with impaired hepatic or kidney function. Resolution generally occurs within 5 to 8 days after initiation. The provider may consider GI prophylaxis with an H2 antagonist or proton pump inhibitor with NSAID use.

All NSAIDs carry a black box warning stating that they may cause an increased risk of serious cardiovascular thrombotic events, myocardial infarction, or stroke, which can be fatal, and that the level of cardiovascular risk may increase with duration of use. Patients with a history of cardiovascular disease or risk factors for cardiovascular disease may be at the greatest risk. Therefore, caution should be taken to avoid these risks. NSAIDs can also cause an increased risk of serious GI adverse effects, including bleeding, ulceration, and perforation of the stomach or intestines, which can occur at any time during use and without warning symptoms. This risk is more serious in older adults.

Major adverse reactions that occur with the use of NSAIDs mainly affect the GI (gastritis, bleeding, perforation), kidney (reduced glomerular filtration rate through vasoconstriction), cardiovascular (sodium and fluid accumulation, vasoconstriction leading to increased blood pressure), and central nervous systems (impaired cognitive function, headache). Additional information regarding common NSAIDs is provided in Chapter 22.

Indomethacin

Pharmacokinetics. The onset of action for indomethacin is about 30 minutes, with a time to peak of 2 hours and duration of action of 4 to 6 hours. Indomethacin is highly protein bound (99%). The bioavailability of the oral formulation is 100% and the elimination from plasma appears to be biphasic, with the half-life about 1 hour in the first phase and 2.6 to 11.2 hours in the second phase. When indomethacin is taken with food, peak plasma concentration may be slightly decreased or delayed.

Indications. Indomethacin IR is indicated for the treatment of acute gout flares. It is also used off-label to treat tocolysis. Recommended dosing is 50 mg orally three times daily, and it should be initiated within 24 to 48 hours of the onset of a flare. Indomethacin should be discontinued 2 to

TABLE 24.1   Overarching Principles and Final Set of 11 Recommendations for the Treatment of Gout

Overarching Principles

A	Every person with gout should be fully informed about the pathophysiology of the disease, the existence of effective treatments, associated comorbidities, and the principles of managing acute attacks and eliminating urate crystals through lifelong lowering of serum uric acid levels below a target level.
B	Every person with gout should receive advice regarding lifestyle: weight loss if appropriate, and avoidance of alcohol (especially beer and spirits) and sugar-sweetened drinks, heavy meals, and excessive intake of meat and seafood. Low-fat dairy products should be encouraged. Regular exercise should be advised.
C	Every person with gout should be systematically screened for associated comorbidities and cardiovascular risk factors, including renal impairment, coronary heart disease, heart failure, stroke, peripheral arterial disease, obesity, hyperlipidemia, hypertension, diabetes, and smoking, which should be addressed as an integral part of the management of gout.

Final Set of 11 Recommendations

1	Acute flares of gout should be treated as early as possible. Fully informed patients should be educated to self-medicate at the first warning symptoms. The choice of drug(s) should be based on the presence of contraindications, the patient's previous experience with treatments, time of initiation after flare onset, and the number and type of joint(s) involved.
2	Recommended first-line options for acute flares are colchicine (within 12 hours of flare onset) at a loading dose of 1 mg followed 1 hour later by 0.5 mg on day 1 and/or an NSAID (plus proton pump inhibitors if appropriate), oral corticosteroid (30–35 mg/day of equivalent prednisolone for 3–5 days), or articular aspiration and injection of corticosteroids. Colchicine and NSAIDs should be avoided in patients with severe renal impairment. Colchicine should not be given to patients receiving strong P-glycoprotein and/or CYP 3A4 inhibitors such as cyclosporin or clarithromycin.
3	In patients with frequent flares and contraindications to colchicine, NSAIDs, and corticosteroid (oral and injectable), IL-1 blockers should be considered for treating flares. Current infection is a contraindication to the use of IL-1 blockers. ULT should be adjusted to achieve the uricaemia target following an IL-1 blocker treatment for flare.
4	Prophylaxis against flares should be fully explained and discussed with the patient. Prophylaxis is recommended during the first 6 months of ULT. Recommended prophylactic treatment is colchicine, 0.5–1 mg/day, a dose that should be reduced in patients with renal impairment. In cases of renal impairment or statin treatment, patients and physicians should be aware of potential neurotoxicity and/or muscular toxicity with prophylactic colchicine. Co-prescription of colchicine with strong P-glycoprotein and/or CYP 3A4 inhibitors should be avoided. If colchicine is not tolerated or is contraindicated, prophylaxis with NSAIDs at a low dosage, if not contraindicated, should be considered.
5	ULT should be considered and discussed with every patient with a definite diagnosis of gout from the first presentation. ULT is indicated in all patients with recurrent flares, tophi, urate arthropathy, and/or renal stones. Initiation of ULT is recommended close to the time of first diagnosis in patients presenting at a young age (<40 years) or with a very high SUA level (>8.0 mg/dL; 480 µmol/L), and/or comorbidities (renal impairment, hypertension, ischemic heart disease, heart failure). Patients with gout should receive full information and be fully involved in decision-making concerning the use of ULT.
6	For patients on ULT, SUA levels should be monitored and maintained to <6 mg/dL (360 µmol/L). A lower SUA target (<5 mg/dL; 300 µmol/L) to facilitate faster dissolution of crystals is recommended for patients with severe gout (tophi, chronic arthropathy, frequent attacks) until total crystal dissolution and resolution of gout. An SUA level <3 mg/dL is not recommended in the long term.
7	All ULTs should be started at a low dose and then titrated upward until the SUA target is reached. An SUA <6 mg/dL (360 µmol/L) should be maintained lifelong.
8	In patients with normal kidney function, allopurinol is recommended for first-line ULT, starting at a low dose (100 mg/day) and increasing by 100-mg increments every 2–4 weeks, if required, to reach the uricaemia target. If the SUA target cannot be reached by an appropriate dose of allopurinol, allopurinol should be switched to febuxostat or a uricosuric or combined with a uricosuric. Febuxostat or a uricosuric are also indicated if allopurinol cannot be tolerated.
9	In patients with renal impairment, the allopurinol maximum dosage should be adjusted to creatinine clearance. If the SUA target cannot be achieved at this dose, the patient should be switched to febuxostat or given benzbromarone with or without allopurinol, except in patients with estimated glomerular filtration rate <30 mL/min.
10	In patients with crystal-proven, severe debilitating chronic tophaceous gout and poor quality of life, in whom the SUA target cannot be reached with any other available drug at the maximal dosage (including combinations), pegloticase is indicated.
11	When gout occurs in a patient receiving loop or thiazide diuretics, substitute the diuretic if possible; for hypertension, consider losartan or calcium channel blockers; for hyperlipidemia, consider a statin or fenofibrate.

IL, Interleukin; *NSAID*, nonsteroidal antiinflammatory drug; *SUA*, serum uric acid; *ULT*, urate-lowering therapy.

From Richette, P., Doherty, M., Pascual, E., et al. (2017). 2016 updated EULAR evidence-based recommendations for the management of gout. *Annals of the Rheumatic Diseases, 76*, 29–42. http://doi.org/10.1136/annrheumdis-2016-209707.

The 2020 American College of Rheumatology guidelines (FitzGerald et al., 2020) strongly recommend beginning ULT for patients with any of the following:

- One or more subcutaneous tophi
- Radiographic damage (any modality) due to gout
- Two or more inflammatory gout flares per year

The guidelines initially conditionally recommend ULT for patients with:

- Fewer than two flares yearly
- First flare in presence of chronic kidney disease stage 3 or greater; serum urate level of 9 mg/dL or greater; or urolithiasis

The guidelines recommend against beginning ULT in patients with asymptomatic hyperuricemia or at first flare without the preceding conditions.

3 days after resolution of clinical signs and symptoms. The usual duration of therapy is between 5 and 7 days.

Adverse Effects. The main adverse effects include headache, vomiting, and central nervous system (CNS) effects such as dizziness, depression, drowsiness, and fatigue.

Contraindications. Indomethacin should be avoided in patients with a hypersensitivity reaction to the drug or any component of its formulation. This medication is contraindicated in the setting of coronary artery bypass graft (CABG) surgery due to the increased risk of myocardial infarction and stroke following this procedure.

Monitoring. Patients should be evaluated for cardiac risk and the potential for a GI bleed prior to starting indomethacin. Blood pressure should be monitored at the beginning of therapy and occasionally during use in patients with underlying hypertension. Patients started on indomethacin should obtain baseline renal function tests, a complete blood count (CBC) with differential, and liver function tests (LFTs).

Naproxen

Pharmacokinetics. Naproxen's onset of action is about 30 to 60 minutes, with a time to peak serum level of 1 to 2 hours. Oral absorption is almost 100%, and elimination half-life is 12 to 17 hours.

Indications. Naproxen tablets can be used in the treatment of acute gout flares. Delayed-release forms are not recommended because of absorption delay.

Adverse Effects. The main adverse reactions with naproxen include edema, palpitations, dizziness, drowsiness, and GI effects such as abdominal pain, constipation, nausea, heartburn, and dyspepsia.

Contraindications. Naproxen should be avoided in patients with a hypersensitivity to the medication or any component of its formulation. As with any NSAID, naproxen should be avoided in patients with a history of

For patients experiencing a gout flare

- Use colchicine, NSAIDs, or glucocorticoids (PO, IA, or IM) first-line over IL-1 inhibitors or ACTH.
  (The choice of colchicine, NSAIDs, or glucocorticoids is based on patient factors and preferences.)
- When using colchicine, use low-dose colchicine over high-dose colchicine.
- Use topical ice as adjuvant treatment.

For NPO patients

- Use glucocorticoids (IM, IV, IA) first-line over IL-1 inhibitors or ACTH.

For patients failing, contraindicated, or not tolerating other anti-inflammatory therapies

- Use IL-1 inhibition

LEGEND
- Strongly recommend
- Conditionally recommend
- Conditionally recommend against
- Strongly recommend against

• **Fig. 24.3** Management of gout flare. *ACTH,* Adrenocorticotropic hormone; *IA,* intraarticular; *IL,* interleukin; *IM,* intramuscular; *NPO,* nil per os; *NSAID,* nonsteroidal antiinflammatory drug. (From FitzGerald, J. D., Dalbeth, N., Mikuls, T., Brignardello-Peterson, R., Guyatt, G., Abeles, A. M., . . . Neogi, T. [2020]. 2020 American College of Rheumatology guideline for the management of gout. *Arthritis Care & Research [Hoboken], 72*[6], 744–760. http://doi.org/10.1002/acr.24180.)

myocardial infarction or other cardiovascular risk factors unless the benefit outweighs the risk. Naproxen can also cause serious GI inflammation, ulceration, bleeding, and perforation and therefore should be avoided, if possible, in older adults and in patients with a history of peptic ulcer disease and/or GI bleeding.

Monitoring. Baseline monitoring for patients taking naproxen includes a CBC with differential, LFTs, renal function tests, blood pressure, sign/symptoms of fluid retention, and signs of bleeding. All patients receiving an NSAID should be evaluated for cardiac risk and the potential for GI bleeding prior to starting this medication. Long-term use of naproxen can cause vision changes; thus, baseline and yearly ophthalmic exams should be encouraged to address any changes.

Sulindac

Pharmacokinetics. The time to peak concentration for sulindac is 3 to 4 hours, with the onset of therapeutic response taking up to 1 week. The elimination half-life of the parent drug is 7.8 hours; elimination half-life of the sulfide metabolite is 16.4 hours.

Indications. Sulindac is indicated for the relief of signs and symptoms of acute gouty arthritis. The lowest effective dose to get a satisfactory response is recommended.

Adverse Effects. The main adverse reactions with sulindac include edema, dizziness, headache, skin rash, GI pain, and constipation. This medication can cause several additional GI side effects including dyspepsia, nausea, abdominal cramps, and flatulence.

Contraindications. As with all NSAIDs, sulindac should be avoided in the setting of CABG surgery and in those with a history of asthma, urticaria, or allergic-type reactions after taking aspirin or other NSAIDs.

Monitoring. Baseline laboratory tests should include a CBC with differential, chemistry profile, and periodic LFTs. Additionally, the patient's blood pressure should be monitored, along with signs/symptoms of GI bleeding.

Colchicine

Colchicine is a highly effective medication for treating gout flares (Table 24.1). If used within the first 24 hours of symptom onset, colchicine produces a response within hours in two-thirds of patients. The longer the patient waits to take this medication, the less effective it is.

Pharmacokinetics. Colchicine is a major substrate of cytochrome (CYP) 450 3A4 and P-glycoprotein (P-gp). Caution should be taken in patients taking concomitant statin therapy or those with kidney dysfunction. Colchicine should be dose adjusted when taken with moderate/strong CYP 3A4 inhibitors due to accumulation and increased risk of toxicity. Time to peak serum concentration is 0.5 to 3 hours. The elimination half-life is 27 to 31 hours in young, healthy adults. Colchicine is about 45% bioavailable, with an onset of action for pain relief of about 18 to 24 hours.

Indications. Colchicine is indicated for the prevention and treatment of acute gout flares. Colchicine is not an analgesic and should not be used to treat pain from other causes.

Adverse Effects. There are several dose-limiting side effects with the use of colchicine, including nausea, vomiting, and diarrhea. Other significant side effects are neutropenia, neuromyopathy, and pharyngolaryngeal pain.

QUALITY AND SAFETY

Colchicine

Colchicine meets the Beers Criteria as a potentially inappropriate medication to use in older adults. Recommendations include reducing the dose of colchicine if the patient's creatinine clearance (CrCl) is less than 30 mL/minute. In addition, older adults may experience increased risk of GI and neuromuscular adverse effects as well as increased bone marrow toxicity.

Contraindications. Colchicine should be avoided in patients with renal or hepatic impairment who are also taking medications that are P-gp or strong CYP 3A4 inhibitors. This combination may lead to life-threatening and fatal toxicity even if taken at therapeutic doses.

Monitoring. Baseline monitoring before starting colchicine includes renal function, CBC with differential, and liver function enzymes. Long-term use can decrease vitamin B12 levels, resulting in the need to monitor these levels yearly where indicated. Practitioners should assess for GI symptoms and neuromuscular toxicity.

Treatment of Hyperuricemia in Gout

Once management of an acute attack is complete, primary care providers should focus on secondary prevention through maintenance of low uric acid concentrations using both nonpharmacologic and pharmacologic strategies. Patients should be counseled on the importance of adhering to both to reduce the risk of future attacks.

Nonpharmacologic Therapy

Revisiting risk factors for uricemia will be key in preventing and treating hyperuricemia. For instance, weight loss is encouraged in all overweight and obese patients with gout and hyperuricemia. Studies have researched the effects of the DASH (Dietary Approaches to Stop Hypertension) eating plan and demonstrate a serum uric acid lowering effect of about 1 mg/dL. In addition, restricting alcohol intake is crucial as there is a direct correlation between alcohol consumption and gout attacks. Acute ingestion of alcohol causes lactic acidosis, which decreases renal urate excretion; chronic alcohol intake promotes the production of purines. The ACR guidelines recommend limiting the use of alcohol, especially during periods of gout attacks, while the EULAR guidelines advise against the use of alcohol altogether in patients with gout. Patients should also limit their intake of foods containing high-fructose corn syrup as well as purine-rich foods such as organ meats and seafood. Finally, primary care providers should review and address any home medications that can cause hyperuricemia.

Pharmacologic Therapy

In general, initiating ULT is not recommended with the first acute flare unless the patient meets one of the following conditions: a diagnosis of chronic kidney disease stage 3 or greater; a serum urate level of 9 mg/dL or greater; or urolithiasis (FitzGerald et al., 2020). ULT is strongly recommended for patients who have two or more flares yearly and is conditionally recommended for patients who have infrequent flares. Allopurinol, a xanthine oxidase inhibitor, is the first-line agent for ULT. A combination of allopurinol and probenecid is conditionally recommended for those starting ULT (Fig. 24.4). If the patient has persistent inflammation, antiinflammatory prophylaxis is recommended for at least 3 to 6 months. The EULAR guidelines recommend ULT in patients with a first diagnosis of gout at less than 40 years of age, serum uric acid concentrations greater than 8 mg/dL, and/or high-risk comorbidities including hypertension, ischemic heart disease, or heart failure. For all patients, careful evaluation of all risk factors should be thoroughly addressed.

Pharmacologic therapy consists of a variety of agents, including xanthine oxidase inhibitors and uricosuric agents (Table 24.2). The ACR guidelines recommend a treat-to-target strategy that directs dose titration toward achieving and maintaining a serum urate level of less than 6 mg/dL. Lower targets may be warranted in patients with severe gout.

Xanthene Oxidase Inhibitors

Xanthene oxidase inhibitors reduce uric acid by inhibiting the activity of xanthine oxidase to convert hypoxanthine to xanthine. This then inhibits the conversion of xanthine to uric acid. This mechanism works for both underexcreters and overproducers of uric acid. Allopurinol and febuxostat are the two commercially available xanthine oxidase inhibitors.

Allopurinol

Allopurinol is an effective urate-lowering agent that is dosed once daily. Long-term adherence is challenging due to its significant adverse effects.

Pharmacokinetics. Allopurinol is 90% absorbed from the GI tract, with peak plasma levels occurring 1.5 to 4.5 hours after 1 dose. The plasma half-life of the parent drug is about 1 to 2 hours; its metabolites have a longer half-life of approximately 15 hours. This explains the xanthine oxidase inhibition of allopurinol of more than 24 hours. The onset of action is about 2 to 3 days, with a peak effect in 1 week or longer. Normal serum urate levels are achieved within 1 to 3 weeks.

PHARMACOGENETICS

Allopurinol

The 2020 ACR guidelines state that testing for the HLA–B*5801 allele prior to starting allopurinol is conditionally recommended for patients of Southeast Asian descent (e.g., Han Chinese, Korean, Thai) and for African American patients.

Indications. Allopurinol is indicated for the management of patients with signs and symptoms of primary or secondary gout. It is not recommended for the treatment of asymptomatic hyperuricemia due to the risk of adverse side effects. Allopurinol is also indicated for the management of patients with recurrent calcium oxalate calculi and high levels of daily uric acid excretion (more than 800 mg for males and more than 750 mg for females).

Adverse Effects. Common side effects include skin rash, leukopenia, GI effects, headache, and urticaria. Patients have also developed a more severe condition called allopurinol hypersensitivity syndrome. This condition manifests as a severe rash, hepatitis, interstitial nephritis, and eosinophilia and causes death in 20% to 25% of patients. Allopurinol should be discontinued at the first appearance of a skin rash or other signs that may indicate an allergic reaction. Due to the mechanism of action, there is an increased risk of acute attacks of gout during the early stages of administration. Maintenance doses of colchicine should be given prophylactically during initiation.

Contraindications. Allopurinol is contraindicated in patients who have developed a severe reaction to allopurinol in the past. Restarting this medication is not recommended.

Monitoring. Baseline monitoring before starting allopurinol includes CBC with differential, renal function, and liver function. A CBC with differential and serum uric acid levels should be obtained every 2 to 5 weeks during dose titration until a goal level is achieved. Monitoring should occur every 6 months thereafter. During titration, practitioners should monitor hydration status, LFTs, and signs/symptoms of hypersensitivity reactions.

Febuxostat

Febuxostat is similar to allopurinol in that it lowers serum urate concentrations in a dose-related manner. The EULAR guidelines recommend reserving febuxostat for use in patients who are unable to tolerate allopurinol due to cost. The ACR guidelines indicate a potential cardiovascular risk but suggest that further study is needed to determine the degree of risk.

Pharmacokinetics. Febuxostat is about 99% albumin bound, with a time to peak of 1 to 1.5 hours and elimination half-life of 5 to 8 hours. Concentrations—maximum concentration (Cmax) and area under the curve (AUC)—are found to be 30% and 14% higher, respectively, in females than in males.

Indications. Febuxostat is indicated for the chronic management of hyperuricemia in patients with gout who have an inadequate response to or are unable to take/tolerate allopurinol. This medication is not recommended for the treatment of asymptomatic hyperuricemia.

Adverse Effects. The most common adverse reactions include skin rash, nausea, hepatic insufficiency, and arthralgia. Due to the mechanism of action, this medication may precipitate an acute gout attack early in treatment. It is recommended to initiate colchicine or an NSAID for the first 3 to 6 months to help avoid an acute gout flare.

Choice of first-line ULT agent

- For all patients (including those with CKD ≥ 3), allopurinol is preferred first-line therapy
- For patients with CKD ≥ 3, XOI preferred over probenecid
- Pegloticase should not be a first-line agent

For those starting ULT

- Start with low dose and titrate up to target
for both   XOI   &   probenecid
- Use antiinflammatory prophylaxis for 3-6 months and longer if persistent active inflammatory disease
- For patients who present to their provider with an indication for ULT during a gout flare, ULT may be started during a flare rather than waiting until flare has resolved.

For all patients on ULT

- Use Treat-to-Target strategy that includes ULT dose titration to achieve and maintain SU target
- SU target <6 mg/dL
    (lower targets may be considered for patients with advanced disease)
- Continue ULT indefinitely
- Augmented protocol of ULT dose management to include patient education, shared decision-making, and treat-to-target protocol that can be delivered by allied health (e.g. nurse, pharmacist) providers where available

First XOI failure (SU > 6 and ongoing inflammatory/tophaceous disease despite maximum tolerated or FDA indicated dose)

Switch to 2nd XOI over adding a uricosuric agent.

XOI, uricosuric failures (SU > 6 and ongoing inflammatory/tophaceous disease despite maximum tolerated or FDA indicated dose)

with frequent flares or non-resolving tophi	with infrequent flares and no tophi
Switch to pegloticase	Against switching to pegloticase

LEGEND
- Strongly recommend
- Conditionally recommend
- Conditionally recommend against
- Strongly recommend against

• **Fig. 24.4** General management of urate-lowering therapy. *CKD,* Chronic kidney disease; *SU,* serum urate; *ULT,* urate-lowering therapy; *XOI,* xanthine oxidase inhibitor. (From FitzGerald, J. D., Dalbeth, N., Mikuls, T., Brignardello-Petersen, R., Guyatt, G., Abeles, A. M., . . . Neogi, T. [2020]. 2020 American College of Rheumatology guideline for the management of gout. *Arthritis Care & Research [Hoboken], 72*[6], 744–760. http://doi.org/10.1002/acr.24180.)

TABLE 24.2   **Gout Medication Management**

Category	Medication	Dosage: Initial Dosing	Dosage: Usual Range	Considerations and Monitoring
Acute Gout Flare				
NSAID	Ibuprofen	400 mg orally three times daily	400–800 mg three or four times daily	
	Indomethacin	50 mg orally three times daily	50 mg three times daily initially until attack resolves	Relief of pain may occur within 2–4 hours, and tenderness and heat usually decrease within 24–36 hours. Indomethacin is better tolerated than usual doses of colchicine.
	Naproxen	750 mg orally daily; 250 mg orally three times daily until attack subsides		Not recommended in patients with severe kidney dysfunction (CrCl <30 mL/min). Delayed-release is not recommended for patients with acute gout flares.
	Piroxicam	20 mg orally daily or in 2 divided doses		
	Sulindac	200 mg orally twice daily	200 mg orally twice daily until attack resolves	Decrease to the lowest effective dosage following satisfactory response. A treatment duration of 7–14 days is usually adequate.
Antigout/ antiinflammatory	Colchicine	1.2 mg orally daily; 0.6 mg 1 hr later	Do not exceed 1.8 mg in 1 hr or 2.4 mg/day	Dose adjustments required when used with select CYP 3A4 and P-glycoprotein inhibitors; dose to be repeated no earlier than 3 days; wait 12 hr after a treatment dose before resuming prophylaxis dosing.
Corticosteroids	Oral	Prednisone or equivalent 30–40 mg once daily or in 2 divided doses until flare resolution begins	After resolution of symptoms begin, taper dose typically over 7–10 days	Alternative may be an oral methylprednisolone dose pack.
Antiinflammatory Prophylaxis During Initiation of Urate-Lowering Therapy				
NSAIDs			Use at the lowest effective dose	
Antigout/ antiinflammatory	Colchicine (oral)	0.6 mg orally once or twice daily	0.6 mg orally once or twice daily; do not exceed 1.3 mg/day	CrCl <30 mL/min, decrease dose to 0.3 mg/day. Following an acute gout flare, guidelines state that prophylactic antiinflammatory treatment is recommended for at least 8 weeks and up to 6 months while uric acid–lowering therapy (ULT) is initiated.
Corticosteroid	Prednisone or prednisolone	≤10 mg orally daily		

TABLE 24.2   **Gout Medication Management—cont'd**

Category	Medication	Dosage: Initial Dosing	Dosage: Usual Range	Considerations and Monitoring
Urate-Lowering Therapy				
Xanthine oxidase inhibitors	Allopurinol	≤100 mg orally once daily initially, then increase by 100 mg/day weekly to titrate SUA level <6 mg/dL	Usual dose is 200–300 mg/day orally up to 400–800 in moderate to severe gout	Doses >300 mg/day should be given in divided doses. Lower doses should be given for patients with chronic kidney disease. SUA concentration should be used to indicate lowest effective dose.
	Febuxostat	≤40 mg orally daily	40–80 mg orally daily to reach goal SUA concentrations <6 mg/dL; max dose of 120 mg/day	No renal adjustments necessary; insufficient data in patients with CrCl <30 mL/min; use caution. Avoid using in patients with a history of CVD or new CV event. Gout flares may occur after initiation of febuxostat due to the mobilization of urate from tissue deposits. Flare prophylaxis with colchicine or an NSAID is recommended and may be beneficial for up to 6 months.
Uricosurics	Probenecid	250 mg twice daily for 1 week	500 orally twice daily. If necessary, may increase daily dose by 500 mg every 4 weeks to maximum dosage of 500 mg four times daily	Probenecid has been used in patients with some renal impairment. Use a reduced initial dosage in patients with renal impairment and titrate to response. Not recommended in patients with CrCl <50 mL/min.
	Lesinurad	200 mg orally daily in combination with xanthine oxidase inhibitor		Used as an adjunct in treatment of hyperuricemia due to gout in patients not achieving target SUA levels with xanthine oxidase inhibitor alone. Do not use as monotherapy. Not recommended in patients with CrCl <45 mL/min; not studied in patients with severe hepatic disease; contraindicated in patients with tumor lysis syndrome.
Combination therapy	Lesinurad/ Allopurinol	Lesinurad, 200 mg; allopurinol, 300 mg orally daily		Take in morning with food. Not recommended if CrCl <45 mL/min.
Other	Pegloticase	8 mg IV given over 2 hours every 2 weeks		Premedicate with an antihistamine and corticosteroid, plus/minus acetaminophen, before each dose. Optimal treatment duration has not yet been established; see black box warnings.

CrCl, Creatinine clearance; *CV(D)*, cardiovascular (disease); *GFR*, glomerular filtration rate; *IV*, intravenous; *NSAID*, nonsteroidal antiinflammatory drug; *SUA*, serum uric acid.

Contraindications. Febuxostat should not be used concurrently with azathioprine or mercaptopurine. This medication currently holds a black box warning for increased risk for cardiovascular events. Hypersensitivity and serious skin reactions have been reported as comparable to allopurinol.

Monitoring. Baseline LFTs, renal function, and serum uric acid levels should be obtained. Serum uric acid levels should be redrawn 2 weeks after initiation. Practitioners should monitor for signs/symptoms of cardiovascular events as well as hypersensitivity or severe skin reactions.

Uricosuric Drugs

Uricosuric drugs increase the renal clearance of uric acid by inhibiting reabsorption in the kidney. Two uricosuric medications are available: probenecid and lesinurad. These agents are generally limited to patients with a CrCl greater than 45 to 50 mL/minute due to their negative effects on the kidneys.

Probenecid

Pharmacokinetics. Probenecid is completely absorbed following oral administration. It is distributed throughout body tissues 75% to 95% protein bound. Probenecid undergoes metabolism in the liver, with the parent drug and resultant metabolites excreted in the urine. Half-life is dose dependent, with 500 mg at 3 to 8 hours and larger doses at 6 to 12 hours. Probenecid may not be effective in patients with a glomerular filtration rate of 30 mL/minute or less.

Indications. Probenecid is used for the treatment of hyperuricemia associated with chronic gout or gouty arthritis. It can also be used as an adjuvant to antibiotic therapy to increase and/or prolong antibiotic serum concentrations (including cefoxitin, aqueous procaine penicillin G, amoxicillin, and ampicillin).

Adverse Effects. Allergic reactions are rare but may occur with the use of probenecid. The patient may experience GI adverse effects including mild nausea, anorexia, and vomiting. Hepatic necrosis and hematologic adverse effects have occurred.

Contraindications. Probenecid is contraindicated in patients with hypersensitivity to any of its ingredients. It is also contraindicated in patients with uric acid kidney stones as renal excretion of uric acid can exacerbate this condition. Probenecid should not be used in patients with blood dyscrasias, or in neonates, infants, or children younger than 2 years of age. Use probenecid cautiously in patients with a glucose-6-phosphate dehydrogenase (G6PD) deficiency. Caution should also be used in patients with a sulfonamide history as there may be some increased risk for allergic reaction. Probenecid loses efficacy in patients with a CrCl less than 80 mL/minute and is ineffective in patients with a CrCl less than 30 mL/minute. There is a lack of adequate studies to recommend probenecid in patients who are pregnant or breastfeeding.

Monitoring. Baseline serum creatinine/BUN, uric acid, and urinalysis should be determined before therapy with probenecid. If indicated, assess creatinine clearance.

Lesinurad

Lesinurad is the first selective uric acid reabsorption inhibitor to be approved by the FDA. This medication works by inhibiting the urate transporter 1 (URAT1), which results in an increase in uric acid excretion. Due to its associated adverse effects on the kidney when used as monotherapy, this medication must be used in combination with xanthine oxidase inhibitors.

Pharmacokinetics. Lesinurad is rapidly absorbed, with a time to peak of 1 to 4 hours. The bioavailability is 100%, with an elimination half-life of 5 hours. Metabolism occurs mostly via CYP 2C9 and is 98% protein bound to albumin.

Indications. Lesinurad is indicated for the treatment of hyperuricemia associated with gout. This medication should be used in combination with a xanthine oxidase inhibitor to achieve target serum uric acid levels. Lesinurad is not indicated for the treatment of asymptomatic hyperuricemia and should not be used as monotherapy. Dosing for this medication is 200 mg orally daily, taken in the morning.

Adverse Effects. The main adverse reactions include headache, GERD, increased serum creatinine/renal failure, and influenza.

Contraindications. Lesinurad is contraindicated in patients with severe renal impairment (CrCl less than 30 mL/minute), end-stage renal disease (ESRD), dialysis, kidney transplant, tumor lysis syndrome, or Lesch-Nyhan syndrome.

Monitoring. Patients should have a baseline serum creatinine drawn to estimate CrCl prior to treatment initiation. Serum uric acid levels should be checked every 2 to 5 weeks during uric acid-lowering titration, then every 6 months. Patients should have their serum creatinine checked periodically to test for changes in renal function.

Pegloticase

Pegloticase is a pegylated recombinant uricase that reduces uric acid by converting it to allantoin, which is easily excreted. This medication is only available as an intravenous (IV) infusion and is given every 2 weeks. The pegylated nature of the drug can increase the risk for potential infusion-related allergic reactions. Pegloticase is expensive, therefore increasing the cost burden for the patient. The ideal duration of therapy is unknown, with the need for more studies to establish best practices. Pegloticase is not considered a first-line treatment for gout and should be reserved for patients who are unresponsive or unable to tolerate first-line treatments.

Pharmacokinetics. Pegloticase has an onset of action of about 24 hours following the first dose. The duration of action is 12.5 days, with a median elimination half-life of 14 days.

Indications. Pegloticase is indicated for the treatment of chronic gout in adults as refractory to conventional therapy. This medication should not be used to treat asymptomatic hyperuricemia. Dosing is 8 mg intravenously every 2 weeks.

Adverse Effects. The main adverse reactions include antibody development, urticaria, gout (acute flare within the first 3 months), nausea, bruising, and infusion-related reactions. Patients started on pegloticase should be given an NSAID or colchicine 1 week prior to the infusion, which should be continued for 6 months postinfusion to limit the chance of an acute gout flare.

Contraindications. Pegloticase is contraindicated in patients with a G6PD deficiency as these patients can develop a life-threatening hemolytic reaction and methemoglobinemia. Patients should be monitored and premedicated with antihistamines and steroids due to the increased risk of anaphylaxis, especially if they have a uric acid level greater than 6 mg/dL. This medication should not be used in combination with allopurinol, febuxostat, or probenecid due to the increased risk of anaphylaxis.

BLACK BOX WARNING!

Pegloticase

- Pegloticase is contraindicated in patients with G6PD deficiency or favism due to increased risk for life-threatening hemolysis. G6PD screening should be conducted prior to administration for patients of African, Mediterranean, or South Asian ancestry.
- Pegloticase is associated with anaphylaxis or severe hypersensitivity as well as infusion-related reactions. To decrease risk:
  - Pegloticase should be administered in a specialized clinical setting by experienced clinicians who have access to treatments if the patient has a severe reaction.
  - Clinicians should monitor patients' serum urate levels regularly; if levels are greater than 6 mg/dL after two treatments, the drug should be discontinued as it has lost its effectiveness.
  - Clinicians should premedicate all patients with antihistamines and corticosteroids.
  - Clinicians should monitor patients closely during infusion due to the increased risk for a reaction within 2 hours of infusion (patients may also have a delayed reaction).
  - Patients should not be taking oral urate-lowering medications while taking pegloticase.

Monitoring. Patients started on pegloticase should be screened for G6PD deficiency. Serum uric acid levels should be tested prior to infusions. Once the serum uric acid levels are greater than 6 mg/dL, providers should consider discontinuation due to increased risk of anaphylaxis and infusion reactions.

Antiinflammatory Prophylaxis During Initiation of ULT

Initiation of ULT can cause a rapid lowering of urate concentrations, which can precipitate an acute gout attack. Prophylactic antiinflammatory medications are recommended to prevent gout attacks and ensure patient adherence to the ULT. Agents should be continued for at least 3 to 6 months after achieving target serum uric acid levels (FitzGerald et al., 2020).

Interleukin-1 Inhibitors

During a gout attack, urate crystals trigger the production of interleukin-1 (IL-1), leading to inflammation. IL-1 inhibitors target the IL-1 receptor, leading to a decrease in inflammation and a decrease in symptoms. These agents are conditionally recommended only if the patient is not able to tolerate any other conventional alternatives. In addition, these agents are costly and so, if considered, patients should be referred to a specialty practice.

Prescriber Considerations for Gout Therapy

Clinical Practice Guidelines

Organizations including the ACR, American College of Physicians® (ACP), and EULAR have created several guidelines that provide recommendations on the management of gout. These guidelines have been published and updated to reflect changes in therapy.

Acute flares of gout should be treated as early as possible. It is important for patients to recognize the signs and symptoms and to self-medicate at the first warning symptoms. Early identification and management will decrease the risk of severe and chronic flares. Treatments should take into consideration comorbidities (e.g., hypertension, hyperlipidemia, or major organ transplant), contraindications, and the patient's previous experience with treatments. Other factors that should be considered include the time of initiation after the flare onset and the number and type of joint(s) involved.

BOOKMARK THIS!

Clinical Guidelines for Gout Management
- ACP: https://www.acponline.org/clinical-information/guidelines
- ACR: https://www.rheumatology.org/Practice-Quality/Clinical-Support/Clinical-Practice-Guidelines/Gout
- EULAR: https://www.eular.org/recommendations_management.cfm

Clinical Reasoning for Gout Therapy

Consider the individual patient's health problem requiring antigout therapy. One of the most important strategies when managing a patient with gout is to stress the importance of prevention. It is imperative to identify patients who are at risk for developing gout and to counsel them on nonpharmacologic therapies for prevention. These modifiable risk factors include obesity, excessive alcohol consumption, chronic kidney disease, and a diet consisting of organ meats and high-fructose corn syrup. Counseling patients on the importance of a well-balanced diet that includes low-fat dairy products and vegetables, along with weight control, regular physical activity, and a reduction or cessation of alcohol use, will help reduce the risk of gout flares.

Patients with asymptomatic hyperuricemia should not be treated with medications and should be monitored for trends in their uric acid levels. For patients with symptoms, carefully assess the frequency of gout flares, the presence of tophi, and any radiographic damage due to gout to determine the need for ULT.

Determine the desired therapeutic outcome based on the antigout medications needed for the patient's health problem. Remember that patients with hyperuricemia may never experience an attack of gout and thus do not need to be treated. Management goals are directed toward reducing symptoms with titration of ULT dosages to achieve serum urate levels of less than 6 mg/dL (levels may need to be lower in cases of advanced disease). When unable to reduce serum urate levels with first-line medications, clinical practice guidelines direct the overall plan of care. In patients who are not responsive to maximum doses of xanthine oxidase inhibitors and uricosuric therapy and who have frequent gout flares or debilitating tophi, pegloticase may be effective.

Assess the antigout therapy selected for its appropriateness for an individual patient by considering the medication's side effects and the patient's age, race/ethnicity, comorbidities, and genetic factors. Patients with cardiovascular disease should avoid febuxostat for ULT when possible due to an increased risk of cardiovascular events. Avoid prescribing colchicine in patients who are also taking strong P-glycoprotein and/or CYP 3A4 inhibitors due to the increased risk of colchicine toxicity. Dosages of allopurinol should be adjusted in patients with renal or liver impairment. For patients with hypertension, consider substituting thiazide or loop diuretics with other antihypertensive agents such as losartan or calcium channel blockers (CCBs). Patients taking HMG-CoA reductase inhibitors may have an increased risk for myopathy and rhabdomyolysis.

Patients of Southeast Asian descent and African American patients should be tested for the HLA-B*5801 gene variant before beginning allopurinol due to the risk of severe adverse effects. The ACR recommends that patients who are allergic to allopurinol and who cannot take other oral ULTs should undergo allopurinol desensitization.

Initiate the treatment plan with the selected medication by first providing adequate patient education to ensure the patient's understanding and promote full participation in the antigout therapy. Advise patients and families about the basic risk factors for gout and the need for risk-factor modification. For patients requiring ULT, begin treatment at the lower doses and titrate to achieve a serum urate level of 6 mg/dL (lower in patients with advanced disease). Achieving target serum urate levels requires a combination of risk-factor modification and medication therapy.

Ensure complete patient and family understanding about the medication prescribed for antigout therapy using a variety of education strategies. Provide patients with oral and written information regarding risk factors, medication side effects, and potential adverse effects as well as the need

to treat early. Websites like the one provided by the Arthritis Foundation (https://www.arthritis.org/diseases/gout) can provide health care information about living with gout, including medications, diet, and physical activity.

Conduct follow-up and monitoring of patient responses to antigout therapy. Monitoring and follow-up depend on the frequency and severity of attacks. Patients experiencing their first attack should be counseled on identifying signs and symptoms of another attack and have a plan in place to treat the condition as early as possible.

Teaching Points for Gout Management

Health Promotion Strategies

- Discuss strategies for weight loss with patients who are obese or overweight.
- Advise patients to avoid alcohol, including beer, wine, and spirits, to decrease the risk of gout flares.
- Recommend the use of topical ice as an adjuvant treatment during acute gout flares.
- The Arthritis Foundation (www.arthritis.org) provides resources that may be helpful to patients with gout.
- Advise patients to choose foods that are low in purines to help reduce the risk of gout flares.
  - Recommend a diet high in fruits and vegetables, low-fat or nonfat dairy, lean meats, and whole grains.
  - Avoid processed foods as well as those that contain high-fructose corn syrup and saturated fats.
  - Avoid meat-based sauces and gravy as well as canned and fresh fish including codfish, trout, haddock, scallops, tuna, and sardines, among others.
  - Avoid organ meats, bacon, and wild game as all are high in purines.
  - Avoid becoming dehydrated by drinking enough fluids to keep urine pale yellow to clear.
- Recommend that patients keep track of which foods seem to trigger gout flares so that they may more easily avoid flares in the future.

Patient Education for Medication Safety

- Colchicine should be taken with a full glass of water and may be taken with food if you experience mild nausea.
- Colchicine can be most effective in treating an acute gout flare if taken within 12 hours. Contact your primary care provider for specific directions for use in acute flares.
- You may be asked to return for laboratory work to monitor the effectiveness of your medication therapy to reduce your serum urate level. Dose adjustments may be required.
- Dietary intervention alone is less likely to effectively treat gout. Therefore, a combination of medication and carefully reducing your intake of high-purine foods is the best way to treat gout.
- Always remind your providers that you are taking medications for gout to decrease the risk of drug interactions.
- Avoid taking OTC medications as these may interact with your gout medications.
- Avoid grapefruit juice while taking colchicine.

Application Questions for Discussion

1. When first assessing your patient, what signs and symptoms may indicate an acute gout flare? What additional diagnoses must be considered?
2. What medication would you choose as a first-line treatment for an acute gout flare and why? What baseline labs are indicated with this agent?
3. Now that your patient's gout has been treated, what do you plan to institute as secondary prophylaxis?

Selected Bibliography

Briesacher, B. A., Andrade, S. E., Fouayzi, H., & Chan, K. A. (2008). Comparison of drug adherence rates among patients with seven different medical conditions. *Pharmacotherapy, 28*(4), 437–443. http://doi.org/10.1592/phco.28.4.437.

Burchum, J. R. R., & Rosenthal, L. D. (2018). *Lehne's Pharmacotherapeutics for Advanced Practice Providers.* St. Louis: Elsevier.

Chen-Xu, M., Yokose, C., Rai, S. K., Pillinger, M. H., & Choi, H. K. (2019). Contemporary prevalence of gout and hyperuricemia in the United States and decadal trends: The National Health and Nutrition Examination Survey, 2007–2016. *Arthritis & Rheumatology, 71*(6), 991–999. http://doi.org/10.1002/art.40807.

Colcrys [package insert]. Philadelphia: Mutual Pharmaceutical Company, Inc. July 2009. Available at. https://www.accessdata.fda.gov/drugsatfda_docs/label/2009/022351lbl.pdf.

Elsevier. Clinical pharmacology powered by ClinicalKey®. (2019). Retrieved from http://www.clinicalkey.com.

FitzGerald, J. D., Dalbeth, N., Mikuls, T., Brignardello-Petersen, R., Guyatt, G., Abeles, A. M., & Neogi, T. (2020). 2020 American College of Rheumatology guideline for the management of gout. *Arthritis Care & Research (Hoboken), 72*(6), 744–760. http://doi.org/10.1002/acr.24180.

Fravel, M. A., & Ernst, M. E. (2020). Gout and hyperuricemia. In J. T. DiPiro, G. C. Yee, L. Posey, S. T. Haines, T. D. Nolin, & V. Ellingrod (Eds.), *Pharmacotherapy: A Pathophysiologic Approach* (11th ed.). New York: McGraw-Hill.

Gelber, A. C., Levine, S. M., & Darrah, E. (2018). Inflammatory rheumatic diseases. In G. D. Hammer, & S. J. McPhee (Eds.), *Pathophysiology of Disease: An Introduction to Clinical Medicine* (8th ed.). New York: McGraw-Hill.

Indocin [package insert]. Philadelphia: Mylan Pharmaceuticals Inc. May 2016. Available at https://dailymed.nlm.nih.gov/dailymed/drugInfo.cfm?setid=568a1378-6dd4-49a5-a8b8-769972c1e0aa.

Kenalog [package insert]. Princeton, NJ: Bristol-Myers Squibb Company July 2014. Available at https://www.accessdata.fda.gov/drugsatfda_docs/label/2014/012041s042lbledt.pdf.

Khanna, D., FitzGerald, J. D., Khanna, P. P., et al. (2012) American College of Rheumatology guidelines for management of gout. Part 1: Systematic nonpharmacologic and pharmacologic therapeutic approaches to hyperuricemia. *Arthritis Care & Research (Hoboken), 64*, 1431–1446.

Khanna, P. P., Gladue, H. S., Singh, M. K., et al. Treatment of acute gout: A systematic review. Seminars in Arthritis and Rheumatism, *44*(1), 31–38. http://doi.org/10.1016/j.semarthrit.2014.02.003.

Khanna, D., Khanna, P. P., FitzGerald, J., et al. (2012). American College of Rheumatology guidelines for management of gout. Part 2: Therapy and antiinflammatory prophylaxis of acute gouty arthritis. *Arthritis Care & Research, 64*, 1447–1461.

Krystexxa [package insert]. East Brunswick, NJ: Savient Pharmaceuticals, Inc. April 2012. Available at. https://www.accessdata.fda.gov/drugsatfda_docs/label/2012/125293s034lbl.pdf.

McCance, K. L., & Huether, S. E. (2019). *Pathophysiology: The Biologic Basis for Disease in Adults and Children* (8th ed.). St. Louis: Elsevier.

Naprosyn [package insert]. Alpharetta, GA: Canton Laboratories, LLC August 2016. Available at https://www.accessdata.fda.gov/drugsatfda_docs/label/2017/017581s113,018164s063,020067s020lbl.pdf.

Neogi, T., Chen, C., Niu, J., Chaisson, C., Hunter, D. J., & Zhang, Y. (2014). Alcohol quantity and type on risk of recurrent gout attacks: An internet-based case-crossover study. *The American Journal of Medicine, 127*(4), 311–318. https://doi.org/10.1016/j.amjmed.2013.12.019.

Perez-Ruiz, F., & Dalbeth, N. (2019). Combination urate-lowering therapy in the treatment of gout: What is the evidence? *Seminars in Arthritis and Rheumatism, 48*(4), 658–668. https://doi.org/10.1016/j.semarthrit.2018.06.004.

Qaseem, A., Harris, R. P., & Forciea, M. A. (2017). Management of acute and recurrent gout: A clinical practice guideline from the American College of Physicians. *Annals of Internal Medicine, 166*(1), 58–68. http://doi.org/10.7326/M16-0570.

Rayos [package insert]. Deerfield, IL: Horizon Pharma USA, Inc. July 2012. Available at https://www.accessdata.fda.gov/drugsatfda_docs/label/2012/202020s000lbl.pdf.

Richette, P., Doherty, M., Pascual, E., et al. (2017). 2016 updated EULAR evidence-based recommendations for the management of gout. *Annals of the Rheumatic Diseases, 76*, 29–42. http://doi.org/10.1136/annrheumdis-2016-209707.

Roddy, E., Clarkson, K., Blagojevic-Bucknall, M., et al. (2020). Open-label randomized pragmatic trial (CONTACT) comparing naproxen and low-dose colchicine for the treatment of gout flares in primary care. *Annals of the Rheumatic Diseases, 79*, 276–284. http://doi.org/10.1136/annrheumdis-2019-216154.

Solu-Medrol [package insert]. New York: Pfizer October 2011. Available at https://www.accessdata.fda.gov/drugsatfda_docs/label/2011/011856s103s104lbl.pdf.

Uloric [package insert]. Deerfield, IL: Takeda Pharmaceuticals America, Inc. March 2013. Available at https://www.accessdata.fda.gov/drugsatfda_docs/label/2017/021856s011lbl.pdf.

Zurampic [package insert]. Wilmington: DE: AstraZeneca December 2015. Available at https://www.accessdata.fda.gov/drugsatfda_docs/label/2015/207988lbl.pdf.

Zyloprim [package insert]. East Brunswick, NJ: Casper Pharma LLC December 2018. Available at https://www.accessdata.fda.gov/drugsatfda_docs/label/2018/016084s044lbl.pdf.

25

Osteoporosis Medications

CHERYL H. ZAMBROSKI

Overview

Osteoporosis is a common and potentially devastating bone disease. Nearly 54 million Americans over the age of 50 have osteoporosis and low bone mass (Wright et al., 2014), placing them at substantially increased risk for bone fracture. In addition, patients with osteoporosis may experience significant pain, disability, placement in long-term care, and increased health care costs (Jeremiah et al., 2015). By gender, age-adjusted prevalence of osteoporosis of the lumbar spine or femur neck is higher among females (24.8%) than males (5.6%) (Looker & Frenk, 2015). In addition, females had lower bone mass than males at either skeletal site. While prevalence is higher in White and Asian females, Black females are more likely to die after hip fracture secondary to osteoporosis than White females (Cauley, 2011).

Medication therapy is directed toward prevention of osteoporosis for those at risk and treatment of osteoporosis for those who meet diagnostic criteria. Medications used include bisphosphonates, selective estrogen receptor modulators (SERMs), calcitonin, recombinant human parathyroid hormone (PTH), PTH-related protein analogs, and monoclonal antibodies. Estrogen therapy may be used in the prevention of postmenopausal osteoporosis but is not recommended for the treatment of patients with osteoporosis. Important to all medication therapy is the promotion of sufficient levels of calcium and vitamin D, regular physical activity, avoiding increased alcohol intake and smoking, and fall prevention.

Relevant Physiology

In general, the skeleton provides structural support for the body, protects vital organs, contributes to movement, and participates in mineral homeostasis and acid-base balance (Clarke, 2008). The skeleton is composed of four general categories of bones: long bones, short bones, flat bones, and irregular bones. These bones are composed of two types of tissue called *compact bone* (cortical bone) and *spongy bone* (cancellous bone). The majority of bone is compact bone (approximately 85%), with spongy bone comprising the remainder. Compact bone is dense and creates much of the hard shell that surrounds the spongy bone. Compact bone is

also highly organized, is very strong, and is the major component of long bones. With few exceptions, bones are composed of both types of tissue; however, the distribution of the tissue varies between bone sites. For example, the lumbar vertebrae are composed of approximately 66% spongy bone, while the femoral neck is about 75% compact bone (Langdahl et al., 2016).

Bone tissue is composed of a variety of elements, including bone cells (osteoblasts, osteocytes, and osteoclasts), bone matrix (collagen fibers, proteoglycans, and bone morphogenic proteins), various glycoproteins, and minerals (specifically, calcium and phosphate). Osteoblasts are the bone-forming cells. They synthesize collagen and proteoglycans, which contribute to the bone matrix. This matrix hardens with the deposit of calcium and phosphorus. Osteocytes help maintain the bone matrix and signal osteoblasts and osteoclasts to form and resorb bone. *Osteoclasts* are large, multinucleated cells that secrete a number of enzymes that dissolve collagen as well as inorganic calcium and phosphorus.

All bone cells undergo a continuous process of renewal and resorption to respond to mechanical loading, repair the bone from injury, strengthen the bone with growth and development, and release stored calcium levels in the blood. This is called *bone remodeling* (Fig. 25.1). Osteoclasts break down old bone (called *bone resorption*), releasing calcium and phosphate into the blood. Then they move to the resorption site and deposit osteoid, which undergoes calcification, thus creating new bone. The process of remodeling is signaled by a variety of factors, including receptor activator for nuclear factor κβ ligand (RANKL), interleukins-1 and -6 (IL-1 and IL-6), and tumor necrosis factor-alpha (TNF-α) for bone resorption. Factors for bone formation include estrogen as well as osteoprotegerin (OPG), and transforming growth factor-beta (TGF-β).

The body uses three major hormones to regulate calcium levels: PTH, calcitonin, and vitamin D. Each hormone plays a role in maintaining proper serum calcium levels in the blood. *PTH* is secreted by the parathyroid gland in response to a decrease in serum calcium, and it is then suppressed in conditions of increased serum calcium. Both actions help achieve a balance of calcium. PTH impacts the bone by increasing the activity of osteoclasts in breaking down

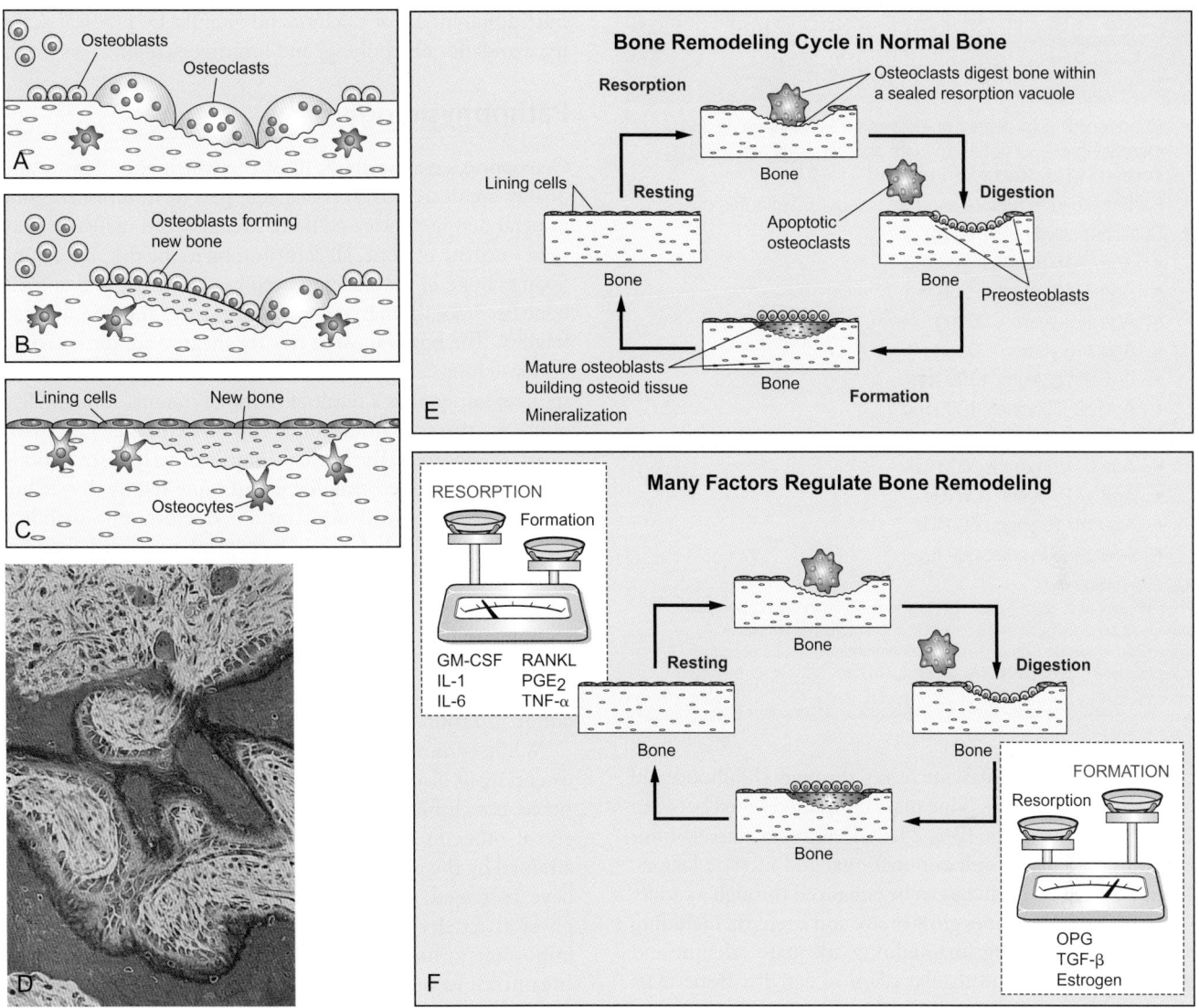

• **Fig. 25.1** Bone remodeling. All bone cells participate in bone remodeling. In the remodeling sequence, bone sections are removed by bone-resorbing cells (osteoclasts) and replaced with a new section laid down by bone-forming cells (osteoblasts). Bone remodeling is necessary because it allows the skeleton to respond to mechanical loading, maintains quality control (repairs and prevents microdamage), and allows the skeleton to release growth factors and minerals (calcium and phosphate) stored in the bone matrix to the circulation. The cells work in response to signals generated in the environment (F). Only the osteoclastic cells mediate the first phase of remodeling. They are activated, scoop out bone (A), and resorb it; then the work of the osteoblasts begins (B). They form new bone that replaces bone removed by the resorption process (C). The sequence takes 4 to 6 months. (D) Micrograph of active bone remodeling seen in the settings of primary or secondary hyperparathyroidism. Note the active osteoblasts surmounted on red-stained osteoid. Marrow fibrosis is present. (E) Bone remodeling cycle in normal bone. (F) Numerous signaling factors are necessary for remodeling. Factors most important for resorption include granulocyte-macrophage colony–stimulating factor (GM-CSF), interleukins-1 and -6 (IL-1 and IL-6), receptor activator for nuclear factor κβ ligand (RANKL), prostaglandin E2 (PGE2), and tumor necrosis factor-alpha (TNF-α). Important factors for bone formation include osteoprotegerin (OPG), transforming growth factor-beta (TGF-β), and estrogen.
(Adapted from Nucleus Medical Art. D from Damjananov, I., & Linder, J., Eds [2019]. *Anderson's pathology* [10th ed.], St. Louis: Mosby. In McCance, K. L., & Huether, S. E. [2019]. *Pathophysiology* [8th ed.]. St. Louis: Elsevier.)

bone tissue for release of calcium into the blood. It also increases resorption of calcium from the glomerulus and increases absorption of calcium from the gut via activation of vitamin D. *Calcitonin* is released from the thyroid gland when calcium levels are elevated. It lowers serum calcium by decreasing bone resorption and increasing calcium excretion from the kidney. Vitamin D enhances intestinal absorption of calcium. In general, the body prioritizes blood calcium over bone calcium, so if blood calcium is low, the body will acquire needed levels, even at the expense of bone health.

• **Box 25.1**   **National Osteoporosis Foundation Recommendations for Child and Adolescent Bone Health**

- Eat according to dietary guidelines for Americans, including increasing consumption of fruits and vegetables as well as consuming low-fat or fat-free dairy.
- Participate in moderate exercise at least 60 minutes daily.
- Sufficient calcium in the diet daily:
  - Age 0–16 months: 200 mg
  - Age 7–12 months: 260 mg
  - Age 1–3 years: 700 mg
  - Age 4–8 years: 1000 mg
  - Age 9–18 years: 1300 mg
  - Age 19–30 years: 1000 mg
- Sufficient vitamin D in the diet:
  - Age 0–12 months: 400 IUs
  - Age 1–13 years: 600 IUs
  - Age 14–18 years: 600 IUs
  - Age 19–30 years: 600 IUs

IUs, International units.
From Weaver et al. [2016]. National Osteoporosis Foundation's position statement on peak bone mass development and lifestyle factors: A systematic review and implementation recommendations. *Osteoporosis International 27*, 1281–1386. http://doi.org/10.1007/s00198-015-3440-3.

In general, bone mass increases through childhood and adolescence, with peak bone mass typically reached between 20 and 30 years of age (Box 25.1). Peak bone mass is influenced by genetics as well as nutritional and lifestyle factors. Achieving peak bone mass can be enhanced through a variety of health factors as bones grow in size and strength, including avoidance of smoking, maintaining adequate calcium and vitamin D intake, and regular physical activity. Bone mass begins to deteriorate as individuals age and bone resorption occurs more frequently than bone remodeling. Loss of bone mass accelerates in females at menopause and in males at around the age of 70. A variety of medical conditions and medications can contribute to bone loss (Box 25.2). Loss of bone mass may be slowed by factors including adequate nutritional intake of calcium and vitamin D, physical activity, avoidance of smoking, and limiting alcohol.

Pathophysiology

Osteoporosis is a metabolic disease in which bone density and quality are decreased. It is characterized by diminished bone mineral density, decreased bone strength, and reduced structural integrity of bone, all contributing to the risk of fracture. Spongy bone of the skeleton becomes less dense and cortical bone becomes thinner and more porous, leading to increased fragility. The bones most at risk for fracture are the vertebral bones, femur, and distal radius. Fractures may occur either spontaneously or as a result of minimal trauma. In fact, 90% of hip fractures are from simple falls (Osterhoff et al., 2016).

In osteoporosis, the normal coupling mechanism of bone remodeling—bone breakdown and bone regrowth—is not able to keep up with the constant microtrauma to bone, and either too little bone is formed or too much bone is removed. This results in a loss in bone amount and strength, with the bone appearing porous. In periods of rapid remodeling (e.g., after menopause), bone may be at an increased risk for fracture because newly produced bone is less densely mineralized, the resorption sites are temporarily unfilled, and maturation and isomerization of collagen are impaired.

While commonly associated with aging and menopause, osteoporosis also may be produced by long-term glucocorticoid use, lithium use, tamoxifen use, and use of a variety of other medications. If optimal bone strength is not attained by the time a person is in their 30s, the patient may have increased risk for osteoporosis. Good nutrition and physical activity help with bone strength and are extremely important to individuals during growth and development. In contrast to postmenopausal bone loss, the bone loss that accompanies aging is associated with a progressive decline in the supply of osteoblasts in proportion to the demand. Bone homeostasis is maintained by calcium, vitamin D, and PTH. Insufficient dietary calcium or impaired intestinal absorption of calcium due to aging or disease can lead to secondary hyperparathyroidism.

• **Box 25.2**   **Examples of Medications and Medical Conditions That May Cause Loss of Bone Mass and Osteoporosis**

- Glucocorticoids
- Lithium
- Proton pump inhibitors
- Tamoxifen
- Anticonvulsants
- Medroxyprogesterone acetate
- Aromatase inhibitors
- Selective serotonin reuptake inhibitors
- Serotonin and norepinephrine reuptake inhibitors
- Thiazolidinediones
- Calcineurin inhibitors

- Certain chemotherapy agents
- Cushing's disease
- Multiple myeloma
- Chronic obstructive pulmonary disease
- Diabetes
- Chronic kidney disease
- Chronic liver disease
- Hypogonadism
- Inflammatory bowel diseases
- Anorexia nervosa and/or bulimia nervosa
- Hyperparathyroidism

• Box 25.3 Risk of Osteoporosis in Black Females

- Although Black females typically have greater bone mineral density than White females, they still have risk factors that can lead to osteoporosis, including the following:
  - May have decreased calcium intake
  - More prone to lactose intolerance
  - Less likely to perceive osteoporosis as health risk
  - Less likely to be screened for osteoporosis
  - Less likely to receive an osteoporosis therapy when they are diagnosed

From National Institute of Arthritis and Musculoskeletal and Skin Diseases (2018). Osteoporosis and African American women. Washington, DC. https://www.bones.nih.gov/health-info/bone/osteoporosis/background/african-american-women.

Osteoporosis affects all races and genders. While it is generally considered that Whites and Asians are at highest risk for osteoporosis, recent National Health and Nutrition Examination Survey (NHANES) data showed that age-adjusted prevalence of osteoporosis was highest among Mexican-American adults (24.9%) and non-Hispanic White adults (15.7%). Prevalence was lowest among non-Hispanic Black adults, although this was still at a level of more than 10% (Looker & Frenk, 2015). Black females typically have a greater bone mineral density than White females but still have significant risk factors for osteoporosis (Box 25.3). Females have an increased risk for osteoporosis as bone loss is accelerated in the first few years after menopause and continues after menopause. While males are also at risk, the risk doesn't typically increase until after the age of 70 due to higher lifetime bone density. Additional risk factors are presented in Box 25.4. Evaluation of risk factors can be conducted using the Fracture Risk Assessment Tool (FRAX). FRAX is an evidence-based risk assessment tool housed with the University of Sheffield in the United Kingdom (Kanis et al., 2011). It is used to calculate the 10-year probability of fracture from population-based cohorts from North America, Asia, Europe, and Australia. Of note, it is a tool incorporated into the American Association of Clinical Endocrinology's clinical practice guidelines to diagnose osteoporosis in postmenopausal females.

BOOKMARK THIS!

Fracture Risk Assessment Tool (FRAX)

FRAX is readily available for calculating the 10-year probability of fracture from population-based cohorts from North America, Asia, Europe, and Australia. The tool for patients in the United States can be accessed at https://www.sheffield.ac.uk/FRAX/tool.aspx?country=9. U.S. scores take into account the patient's race/ethnicity, including White, Black, Asian, and Hispanic.

The U.S. Preventive Services Task Force (USPSTF) (2018) recommends screening for osteoporosis in females 65 years of age and older and in postmenopausal females younger than age 65 who are at increased risk. Of note, current evidence is not sufficient to recommend screening for osteoporosis to prevent fractures in males.

BOOKMARK THIS!

Screening for Osteoporosis

The U.S. Preventive Services Task Force continually updates practice guidelines, providing a searchable list of topics including those relating to osteoporosis: https://www.uspreventiveservicestaskforce.org/uspstf/topic_search_results?topic_status=P.

Bone loss typically does not show up on conventional radiographic films until significant bone mineral content is gone. As a result, conventional radiographic films are not adequate in measuring bone loss. The most commonly used technique for measuring bone loss is central dual-energy x-ray absorptiometry (DXA) to measure the spine and hip. It is the most sensitive test and provides the most precise T-scores. The *T-score* represents the number of standard deviations above or below the mean bone marrow density (BMD) for the young, healthy female population (i.e., females who are younger than 35 years of age). A T-score of –1 signifies a 10% to 12% loss of bone mass, compared with mean values for young, normal adults. According to recommendations of the WHO Task Force for Osteoporosis, osteoporosis is defined as a T-score of –2.5 in females without a history of fragility fractures (Table 25.1). Treatment generally is indicated if the patient is two or more standard

• Box 25.4 Examples of Risk Factors for Osteoporosis

- Female
- Age 50 or older
- Decreased intake of calcium and/or vitamin D
- Smoking
- Rheumatoid arthritis
- Sedentary lifestyle
- White or Asian race
- Positive family history

- Increased alcohol intake
- Low testosterone
- History of any previous fracture
- Increased caffeine intake
- Low body weight/small body frame
- Hyperthyroidism
- Early menopause (e.g., surgical)
- Cushing's syndrome

TABLE 25.1	WHO Criteria for Diagnosis of Osteoporosis for Postmenopausal Females and Males Aged 50 Years or Older

T-Score[a]	Classification
≥−1	Normal
≤−1 to −2.5	Osteopenia (low bone mass)
≤−2.5	Osteoporosis
≤−2.5 + fracture	Severe osteoporosis

[a]T-score indicates the number of standard deviations below the average peak bone mass in young adult females.

deviations below the normal premenopausal level. All treatments include attending to, addressing, and minimizing all risk factors as well as fall prevention.

Osteoporosis Therapy

Medication therapy for treating osteoporosis is primarily directed toward inhibiting bone resorption or stimulating bone formation (Table 25.2). The most commonly used category of therapy, bisphosphonates, inhibits bone resorption. Similarly, SERMs, calcitonin, and denosumab reduce bone resorption by osteoclasts. Medications including PTH analogs, PTH-related peptide analogs, and romosozumab are considered *anabolic agents*, as they stimulate bone formation. Medication therapy alone does not replace adequate calcium and vitamin D intake.

PRACTICE PEARLS

Optimize Calcium and Vitamin D Status

Optimization of calcium and vitamin D intake is foundational to all pharmacologic interventions. The International Osteoporosis Foundation provides an online calcium calculator that is available in seven languages for countries around the world, at https://www.iofbonehealth.org/calcium-calculator. In addition, the National Osteoporosis Foundation provides great resources for patients to learn about their calcium and vitamin D intake, at https://www.nof.org/patients/treatment/calciumvitamin-d.

Bisphosphonates

Bisphosphonates are considered first-line therapy for reducing the risk of vertebral, nonvertebral, and hip fractures in females with osteoporosis. They also have been shown to reduce the risk of vertebral fractures in males who are diagnosed with osteoporosis.

Bisphosphonates are nonhormonal agents that have an extremely high affinity for bone. They inhibit bone resorption by decreasing the activity of osteoclasts.

Alendronate

Pharmacokinetics. Alendronate is administered orally with an oral bioavailability of less than 1%. In fact, even

orange juice or coffee can reduce bioavailability by about 60%. To achieve maximum possible bioavailability, alendronate must be taken in the fasting state and at least 2 hours before a standard breakfast.

Approximately 80% is distributed protein bound and taken up by bone or excreted renally. There is no evidence that the drug is metabolized. Once alendronate is bound to bone, its half-life is estimated to be greater than 10 years; however, inhibition of bone resorption diminishes after treatment is complete. Because of the long half-life, once-weekly regimens have been found to inhibit bone resorption and provide similar benefits to bone mass and strength as daily regimens. It is believed to be excreted renally, so it should be avoided in patients with a creatinine clearance (CrCl) less than 35 mL/minute.

Indications. Alendronate is used for the prevention and treatment of osteoporosis. It can be used to treat postmenopausal females, patients with corticosteroid-induced osteoporosis, and osteoporosis in males. Of note, it can also be used to treat patients with Paget's disease.

Adverse Effects. Although generally mild, up to 18% of patients may experience hypocalcemia and hypophosphatemia. Gastrointestinal (GI) side effects associated with alendronate therapy include abdominal pain (up to 6.6% of patients), nausea, constipation, diarrhea, flatulence, and dyspepsia. Esophageal ulceration may occur in up to 1.5% of patients. Other adverse effects include headache, musculoskeletal pain, and even bone fracture. Rare ocular effects have occurred including uveitis, scleritis, and episcleritis. Alendronate may cause photosensitivity.

Although very rare, severe osteonecrosis of the jaw has been reported in postmarketing studies in patients receiving bisphosphonate therapy. Most cases have appeared after dental surgery; however, some have appeared spontaneously. The risk may increase with long-term use of bisphosphonates. If the patient exhibits symptoms, refer to specialty practitioners.

Contraindications. Alendronate is contraindicated in patients with achalasia, esophageal stricture, or the inability to sit or stand upright for at least 30 minutes after dose administration as the risk of esophagitis and esophageal ulceration/erosion appears to be greater in patients who lay flat after taking alendronate. It should be used cautiously in patients who are taking corticosteroids. Alendronate should be avoided in patients who have hypocalcemia or vitamin D deficiency. Precaution should be taken in patients with periodontal disease or dental disease, or who have upcoming dental procedures, due to risk of osteonecrosis of the jaw. Alendronate should be used during pregnancy only if the potential benefit justifies the use versus potential risks to the patient or fetus. It should be used cautiously in females who are breastfeeding.

Monitoring. Encourage dental evaluation prior to initiation of alendronate therapy and regular evaluation during the course of therapy. Prior to therapy and periodically throughout therapy, evaluate serum calcium, phosphate, creatinine, and serum 25-hydroxyvitamin D (25(OH)D) concentrations. Reassess the need for continued therapy

TABLE
25.2 **Osteoporosis Medications**

Category/Medication	Indication	Dosage	Considerations and Monitoring
Bisphosphonates			
Alendronate	Osteoporosis prevention or treatment	*For prevention of osteoporosis in postmenopausal females*: Using tablets for daily oral administration, give 5 mg orally daily. For weekly tablets, give 35 mg orally once a week. *For osteoporosis treatment in postmenopausal females and adult males:* Using daily dosage tablets, give 10 mg orally once daily. For once-weekly dosing regimens (including weekly tablets, solution, or effervescent tablets), give 70 mg orally once each week. *For prevention of glucocorticoid-induced osteoporosis in adults:* Take 5 mg orally once daily. *For prevention of glucocorticoid-induced osteoporosis in females not taking estrogen:* Dose is 10 mg daily.	For patients at low risk for fracture, consider stopping alendronate after 3–5 yr and continue to reassess for fracture risk. Administer in the morning. Patient must be able to sit or stand for at least 30 minutes after administration. Do not administer while patient is lying down. Administer with plain water only and at least 30 minutes before the first food, beverage, or other medications of the day. Ensure that patient is receiving adequate calcium and vitamin D.
Risedronate	Prevention and treatment of postmenopausal osteoporosis, osteoporosis in males, and glucocorticoid-induced osteoporosis in males and females	Available in tablets for daily (5 mg), weekly (35 mg), and monthly (150 mg) administration. *For prevention of osteoporosis in postmenopausal females:* 5 mg daily or 35 mg weekly or 150 mg monthly. *For treatment of osteoporosis in postmenopausal females:* 35 mg weekly or 150 mg monthly. *For prevention or treatment of glucocorticoid-induced osteoporosis in females and males:* 5 mg daily.	Ensure that patient is receiving adequate intake of calcium and vitamin D. Administration of immediate release is the same as alendronate. Delayed-release tablets may be given immediately after breakfast with at least 4 ounces of water. Do not chew or crush. Patient should be sitting or standing and should not lie down for at least 30 minutes. Calcium supplements, antacids, any magnesium-based supplements or laxatives, and iron preparations should be taken at a different time of the day as they interfere with the absorption. Consider discontinuing after 3–5 years for patients at low risk for fracture.
Ibandronate	Prevention and treatment of postmenopausal osteoporosis	*Prevention and treatment of osteoporosis:* 150 mg orally once monthly on the same date of each month. *Treatment of osteoporosis for postmenopausal females:* May use 3 mg IV (over 15–30 seconds) every 3 months. Do not administer more often than every 3 months.	For patients at low risk for fracture, consider stopping ibandronate after 3–5 yr and continue to periodically reassess fracture risk. Ensure adequate calcium and vitamin D intake. Administer with full glass of water 1 hr before first food, beverage, or medication of the day. Patient should remain sitting or standing at least 1 hr after taking oral medication. IV form available in prefilled syringes (3 mg/3 mL) must be administered slowly (over 15–30 seconds).

Continued

TABLE 25.2 Osteoporosis Medications—cont'd

Category/Medication	Indication	Dosage	Considerations and Monitoring
Zoledronate (Zoledronic acid)	Prevention of osteoporosis in postmenopausal females or prevention of glucocorticoid-induced osteoporosis Treatment of osteoporosis in males and postmenopausal females or for glucocorticoid-induced osteoporosis in males and females	*For prevention and treatment of glucocorticoid-induced osteoporosis in males and females:* 5 mg IV infusion once yearly. *For prevention of osteoporosis in postmenopausal females:* 5 mg IV once every other yr. *For treatment of osteoporosis in males and postmenopausal females:* 5 mg IV once yearly.	Concentrated form (4 mg/5 mL) must be diluted with 100 mL of 0.9% sodium chloride or 5% dextrose injection for infusion over at least 15 minutes. Ensure adequate levels of calcium and vitamin D. Consider stopping after 3–5 yr for patients at low risk for fracture, and continue to periodically reassess fracture risk. Follow packaging information carefully for administration and storage of solution. Assess serum creatinine and ensure proper hydration of the patient before each administration of the medication.
Selective Estrogen Receptor Modulators (SERMs)			
Raloxifene	Prevention or treatment of osteoporosis in postmenopausal females	60 mg orally once daily.	Should not be used in premenopausal females. Not a first-line therapy as it does not decrease risk of hip fracture or nonvertebral fracture. Has been found to reduce risk of vertebral fracture. Ensure adequate intake of calcium and vitamin D.
Calcitonin	Treatment of osteoporosis in females >5 yr postmenopause	100 IU intramuscularly or subcutaneously once daily, once every other day, or three times/week. OR 200 IU (1 spray) intranasally in 1 nostril once daily.	Ensure adequate calcium and vitamin D intake. Reserve use for patients >5 yr postmenopause in whom alternative treatments are not suitable. Should not be used in patients <5 yr postmenopause. Consider periodic nasal examination for signs of nasal trauma for those using the nasal route.
Parathyroid Hormone (PTH) Analog			
Teriparatide	Treatment of osteoporosis in postmenopausal females or in males with primary or hypogonadal osteoporosis Treatment of glucocorticoid-induced osteoporosis in males or females with high risk of fracture	20 mcg subcutaneously once daily.	Use of teriparatide or other parathyroid analogs >2 yr during a patient's lifetime is not recommended. Patients at high risk of fracture are defined as those with history of osteoporotic fracture, with multiple risk factors for fracture, or who have failed or are intolerant to other available osteoporosis therapy. Ensure adequate intake of calcium and vitamin D.
Parathyroid Hormone-Related Protein (PTHrp) Analog			
Abaloparatide	Treatment of postmenopausal osteoporosis in females with high risk of fracture	80 mcg subcutaneously once daily.	Use for >2 yr during a patient's lifetime is not recommended. High risk for fracture is defined as those with a history of osteoporotic fracture, with multiple risk factors for fracture, or who have failed or are intolerant to other available osteoporosis therapy. Ensure adequate calcium and vitamin D intake.

TABLE 25.2	Osteoporosis Medications—cont'd		
Category/Medication	Indication	Dosage	Considerations and Monitoring
Monoclonal Antibodies			
Denosumab (Prolia)	Treatment of osteoporosis in males and postmenopausal females at high risk for fracture, as well as for glucocorticoid-induced dosteoporosis	60 mg subcutaneously once every 6 months. Follow administration instructions on the package insert carefully.	Should only be administered by a health care professional. Denosumab is available in two different products: Prolia and Xgeva. Only Prolia is used for treatment and prevention of osteoporosis. All patients should receive 1000 mg of calcium and at least 400 IUs of vitamin D daily. Patients at high risk for fracture are considered those with a history of osteoporotic fracture, those with multiple risk factors for fracture, those who have failed or are intolerant to other available osteoporosis therapy, or those initiating or continuing systemic glucocorticoids.
Romosozumab	Treatment of osteoporosis in postmenopausal females at high risk for fracture	210 mg subcutaneously once monthly for 12 months. Not recommended for more than 12 doses.	Should be administered only by a health care provider. Full dose given in 2 separate injections (2 prefilled syringes) in 2 injection sites. May be given in thigh, abdomen, or outer area of the upper arm. Supplement with adequate calcium and vitamin D during therapy.

IU, International unit; *IV*, intravenously; *PTH*, parathyroid hormone, *PTHrp*, parathyroid hormone-related protein; *SERM*, selective estrogen receptor modulator.

after 3 to 5 years in patients with low risk of fractures. Continue to reassess for fracture risk after discontinuation of therapy.

Risedronate

Pharmacokinetics. Risedronate is absorbed orally throughout the GI tract. Approximately 60% of the drug is absorbed and distributed to the bone, with the remaining drug excreted in the urine. Drug that is not absorbed is eliminated in the feces. Risedronate is not metabolized in the liver. Bioavailability varies significantly if given with meals, so this must be considered in administration. Risedronate is considered effective when immediate-release tablets are given at least 30 minutes prior to breakfast and when delayed-release tablets are given after breakfast. Elimination of risedronate is biphasic with initial half-life of 1.5 hours and overall half-life of 220 hours.

Indications. Risedronate can be used for the prevention and treatment of postmenopausal osteoporosis in females, the treatment and prevention of corticosteroid-induced osteoporosis in males and females, and the treatment of osteoporosis in males. Risedronate can also be used in the treatment of Paget's disease.

Adverse Effects. Risedronate is generally well tolerated, with the majority of adverse effects not requiring discontinuance in clinical trials. The most common adverse effects were musculoskeletal and GI in nature. Mild arthralgia and back pain could occur in up to about 30% of patients. Moderate bone pain has been reported in up to 10% of patients. Up to 20% of patients may experience mild diarrhea. Constipation may occur in about 13% of patients. Other GI effects associated with bisphosphonate use include dysphagia, pyrosis (heartburn), esophagitis, and esophageal ulceration or gastric ulcers. It is important to note that esophageal ulcers and oral ulceration may also occur if risedronate tablets are chewed or dissolved in the mouth. Other adverse effects include headache (up to 20%), nausea, and/or vomiting (up to 13%).

Contraindications. Risedronate is contraindicated in patients with achalasia, esophageal stricture, or the inability to stand or sit upright. It is also contraindicated in patients with hypocalcemia. Risedronate should be used with caution in patients with other upper GI disease. Use of nonsteroidal antiinflammatory drugs (NSAIDs), aspirin, or corticosteroids may increase the potential for GI adverse effects. It should be avoided in patients with renal failure, particularly in patients with CrCl less than 30 mL/minute. Risedronate should be avoided in pregnant females unless the benefit to the patient outweighs the risk. It should not be used in breastfeeding females.

Monitoring. Monitor serum calcium, alkaline phosphatase, phosphate, and 25(OH)D concentration. Ensure that patients maintain adequate intake of calcium and vitamin D.

Selective Estrogen Receptor Modulators (SERMs)

SERMs produce estrogen-like effects on bone. They typically act by reducing resorption of bone and increasing bone mineral density in postmenopausal females. Raloxifene acts as an estrogen agonist/antagonist, activating estrogen in some pathways while blocking it in others. For example, raloxifene increases estrogen effects on bone, lipid metabolism, and clotting but blocks estrogen effects on the breast and endometrium. This has important implications, as raloxifene is associated with increased risk for significant thromboembolic events.

Raloxifene

Pharmacokinetics. Raloxifene is about 60% absorbed from the intestines and undergoes extensive first-pass metabolism. It is widely distributed throughout the body, metabolized by the liver, and excreted in the feces. Half-life is about 28 days.

Indications. Raloxifene can be used to prevent or treat osteoporosis in postmenopausal females. It is best used in females who are at risk for vertebral fracture. It has not been shown to reduce the risk of hip or nonvertebral fractures. Raloxifene is not considered first-line therapy in the prevention of osteoporosis due to increased risk for thromboembolic events.

> ## BLACK BOX WARNING!
>
> **Raloxifene**
>
> Raloxifene is contraindicated in patients with acute thromboembolism or a history of thromboembolic disease. It has been associated with an increased risk for mortality secondary to stroke in postmenopausal females with documented coronary heart disease or who are at increased risk for major coronary events.

Adverse Effects. The most common adverse effect associated with raloxifene is hot flashes, experienced by up to 29% of females. Other common effects include mild nausea, mild infection (such as sinusitis, influenza, or rhinitis), mild arthralgia, and moderate peripheral edema. Infrequently, patients may experience mild cough, abdominal pain, headache, or muscle ache. Approximately 9% of patients may experience weight gain. Severe adverse effects are related to the effect of raloxifene on blood clotting, including venous thromboembolism (deep vein thrombosis, pulmonary emboli). Cardiovascular adverse effects include chest pain, peripheral edema, and syncope. While severe, the incidence of stroke is rare, affecting about 0.1% of patients in clinical trials.

Contraindications. Raloxifene is contraindicated in patients with acute thromboembolism or a history of thromboembolic disease. It should be used cautiously in females with a history of cardiac disease or who have an increased risk of stroke. It should also be used cautiously in patients with liver disease or who have moderate or severe renal impairment. Raloxifene is contraindicated in females during pregnancy and in females who are breastfeeding.

Monitoring. Assess liver function and risk for thromboembolic disease prior to initiation of raloxifene therapy. Use of raloxifene is reserved for patients who cannot take first-line medications for osteoporosis. Evaluate patient risk factors for venous thromboembolism regularly.

Calcitonin

Calcitonin is a peptide hormone that is secreted by the thyroid gland and acts primarily on bone, with effects generally opposite of PTH to maintain calcium homeostasis. By directly inhibiting osteoclasts, calcitonin inhibits bone resorption, and the release of calcium and phosphate from bone is reduced. In addition, collagen breakdown is decreased. While it antagonizes PTH action, the therapy does not significantly increase PTH. Calcitonin is not recommended as first-line therapy for osteoporosis treatment but may be considered for women who cannot or will not take more effective agents; do not prescribe in early menopause, as the benefit and effectiveness have not been observed within the first 5 years of menopause onset. It has not been shown to prevent nonvertebral fractures. The increase in bone mineral density is less than that reported for other agents (e.g., bisphosphonates).

Pharmacokinetics. Calcitonin (salmon) is available in parenteral forms and intranasally. Both intramuscular and subcutaneous forms of calcitonin are absorbed directly into the systemic circulation, with onset of action typically within 15 minutes, peak about 4 hours, and duration about 8 to 24 hours. Intranasal absorption is rapid, with peak concentrations within 31 to 39 minutes. The metabolism of calcitonin is not well understood but is believed to be rapidly degraded by the kidneys, blood, and peripheral tissues into inactive fragments.

Indications. Calcitonin can be used to treat osteoporosis in females who are at least 5 years postmenopause. It should be reserved for females who cannot or will not take more effective agents. It should not be prescribed in early menopause. Of note, injections can be used for the treatment of moderate to severe Paget's disease.

Adverse Effects. Calcitonin has been associated with severe allergic reactions. Up to 10% of patients receiving injectable forms may experience nausea and vomiting. Antibody formation has been reported in patients receiving injectable or nasal spray forms. This may be the case in patients who respond early to treatment but stop responding later.

Contraindications. Calcitonin is a synthetic polypeptide similar to the natural calcitonin found in salmon. As a result, it is contraindicated in patients with hypersensitivity to fish. Use in those patients has resulted in serious hypersensitivity reactions.

Hypocalcemia with tetany and seizure activity has been associated with calcitonin therapy, so this medication should be used cautiously. Older adults had a higher incidence of adverse effects associated with nasal spray, such as rhinitis, irritation, and excoriation of the nares. Calcitonin-salmon should be used during pregnancy only if the potential benefit justifies the use versus potential risks to the patient or fetus. It should be used cautiously in females who are breastfeeding.

Monitoring. Consider periodic nasal examination for signs of nasal trauma for those using the nasal route. Monitor serum calcium, 25(OH)D concentrations, and alkaline phosphatase.

Parathyroid Hormone (PTH) Analog

Parathyroid analogs are used to treat patients with osteoporosis. While this may seem counterintuitive, the route of administration of teriparatide determines the impact on bone resorption and bone deposition. Normally, PTH increases bone resorption by osteoclasts to increase serum calcium. Parathyroid analogs such as teriparatide can increase or decrease bone mass depending on the route and administration. Intravenous (IV) infusions lead to persistent elevation of PTH and greater bone resorption. On the other hand, intermittent doses given subcutaneously increase serum PTH and preferentially stimulate osteoblastic activity over osteoclastic activity. This results in a net stimulation of new bone formation, resulting in an increase of bone remodeling and bone strength.

Teriparatide

Pharmacokinetics. Teriparatide is rapidly absorbed following subcutaneous injection. Peak levels are reached after approximately 30 minutes, with a half-life of about 1 hour. Metabolism occurs via the liver, with excretion by the kidneys.

Indications. Teriparatide is used for the treatment of osteoporosis in females with postmenopausal osteoporosis, males with primary or hypogonadal osteoporosis, and adults with glucocorticoid-induced osteoporosis. It should be reserved for patients who are at a high risk for fracture, including patients with a history of osteoporotic fracture, who have multiple risk factors for fracture, or who are intolerant to other medications for osteoporosis. Of note, teriparatide should not be used for more than 2 years during a patient's lifetime.

Adverse Effects. The most common adverse effects associated with teriparatide are arthralgia (about 10% of patients) and nausea (up to 14%). Less common adverse effects include mild dizziness, weakness, depression, headache, and rhinitis. Injection-site reactions may occur and include pain, swelling, and local bruising. Orthostatic hypotension has occurred in about 5% of patients receiving teriparatide. If it occurs, it is typically relieved with positioning and usually resolves after the first few doses.

Rarely, patients may have transient hypercalcemia or hypercalciuria within 4 to 6 hours of dosing. This is considered transient, however, as levels return to normal range without adverse effects. Severe allergic reactions are rare, occurring in fewer than 1% of patients.

> ## BLACK BOX WARNING!
>
> **Teriparatide**
>
> Teriparatide has been associated with the occurrence of osteosarcoma in animal studies. Use of the drug is not recommended for more than 2 years.

Contraindications. Teriparatide should not be used in patients with any underlying hypercalcemic disorders, such as primary hyperparathyroidism. Use cautiously in patients with a recent history of urolithiasis. Patients with a history of bone cancers or any metabolic bone disorders (besides osteoporosis) should not receive teriparatide. Teriparatide is not recommended for use in females who are pregnant or breastfeeding.

Monitoring. Monitor patient's response to initial doses for occurrence of orthostatic hypotension. Periodically assess serum calcium, alkaline phosphatase, uric acid levels, and bone mineral density.

Parathyroid Hormone-Related Protein (PTHrp) Analog

Parathyroid hormone-related protein analogs are a second-generation drug of the PTH analog similar to teriparatide. Adverse effects are similar to teriparatide, and the drug should not be used for more than 2 years. The main advantage of PTHrp analogs is that they have greater selectivity to the PTH1 receptor. They also increase bone mineral density faster than teriparatide and do not increase bone resorption. In addition, they can increase bone mineral density and bone strength at vertebral and/or nonvertebral sites.

Abaloparatide

Pharmacokinetics. Abaloparatide is administered subcutaneously with a mean time to peak concentration of about 30 minutes. Half-life is around 1 hour. Excretion is primarily through the kidneys.

Indications. Abaloparatide is indicated for postmenopausal females with a high risk for osteoporosis.

Adverse Effects. The most common adverse effect associated with abaloparatide is mild injection-site reactions including redness (58% of patients), edema (10%), and pain (9%). Other adverse effects include mild dizziness, nausea, headache, and fatigue as well as moderate hypercalciuria and hyperuricemia. Approximately 5% of patients experience palpitations. Orthostatic hypotension has been reported after administration of abaloparatide. Symptoms resolve after the patient lies down and may diminish over time.

Contraindications. Abalaparatide has a black box warning that it is not recommended for patients at increased risk for osteosarcoma. It should not be used in patients with Paget's disease, bone metastases, or a history of skeletal malignancy. It should be used with caution in patients with a history of orthostatic hypotension. It is not recommended in patients with preexisting hypercalcemia or hypercalciuria. Patients with severe renal impairment are more likely to experience adverse effects. Use beyond 2 years is not recommended. It should not be used in females who are pregnant or breastfeeding.

Monitoring. Monitor serum calcium and serum uric acid. Ensure that patients use proper techniques for administration and storage of abalaparatide. Teach patients that orthostatic hypotension may occur within 4 hours of injection.

Monoclonal Antibodies

Improved understanding of bone cell biology has led to increasing options for treatment of osteoporosis. The discovery of RANKL and sclerostin has led to development of monoclonal antibodies for treatment of osteoporosis. In general, in conjunction with macrophage colony stimulating factors, *RANKL* helps lead to the process of developing mature and active osteoclasts. Expression of RANKL is increased by the presence of glucocorticoids as well as other inflammatory cytokines, leading to greater osteoclastogenesis and ultimately bone resorption. *Sclerostin* is a small protein expressed by a gene in osteocytes that plays a role in bone remodeling by inhibiting osteoblastic bone formation. Denosumab is a subcutaneous, highly specific monoclonal antibody against RANKL, and romosozumab is a parenteral monoclonal antibody and sclerostin inhibitor; both have been used to improve health in patients with osteoporosis.

Denosumab

Pharmacokinetics. Denosumab (Prolia) is well absorbed after subcutaneous injection. Peak concentrations are achieved with a median time of 10 days (range: 3 to 21 days). Half-life is approximately 28 days.

Indications. Denosumab (Prolia) is used for the treatment of osteoporosis in males and postmenopausal females at high risk for fracture. In addition, it can be used to treat glucocorticoid-induced osteoporosis.

Adverse Effects. Patients receiving denosumab may experience an acute reaction including a flu-like syndrome of fever, chills, flushing, muscle and joint aches, and bone pain occurring within the first 3 days after dose administration. Other adverse effects include hypercholesterolemia, hypocalcemia, and hypophosphatemia. Patients taking denosumab are at increased risk for severe infection including cystitis, pneumonia, pharyngitis, and upper respiratory infections. Patients should be monitored carefully for new onset of primary malignancy. Osteonecrosis of the jaw has occurred in patients treated with denosumab.

Contraindications. Denosumab is contraindicated in patients with preexisting hypocalcemia due to the risk of sometimes fatal hypocalcemia. Denosumab may impair immune function and increase the risk of infection. Do not start denosumab therapy in any patient who has an active infection, whether chronic, localized, or systemic. Due to the risk of osteonecrosis of the jaw, a dental examination is recommended for patients who are receiving dental procedures or other dental work. Denosumab is contraindicated in females who are pregnant and should not be used in females who are breastfeeding.

Monitoring. Denosumab should only be administered by health care professionals via the subcutaneous route. Monitor serum calcium throughout therapy with denosumab, especially during the first weeks of therapy. If the patient is taking any additional medications that impact calcium, it may be necessary to monitor calcium levels frequently during administration of denosumab. In addition, monitor phosphate, magnesium, and serum creatinine/blood urea nitrogen (BUN). Ensure that patients are receiving adequate oral calcium, vitamin D, and magnesium. For patients who are predisposed to osteonecrosis of the jaw, ensure adequate follow-up with a dentist or oral surgeon.

Romosozumab

Pharmacokinetics. Romosozumab is administered by subcutaneous injection. Steady-state concentrations were achieved by month 3 after monthly administration of 210 mg to postmenopausal females. Medium time to peak concentration was reached in approximately 5 days, with a half-life of about 13 days.

Indications. Romosozumab is used for the treatment of osteoporosis in postmenopausal females who are at high risk for fracture. These include females with a history of osteoporotic fracture or multiple risk factors or those who are unable to tolerate other available medication therapies for osteoporosis.

Adverse Effects. The most common adverse reactions associated with romosozumab are arthralgia (about 13% of patients) and antibody formation (about 18%). Of note, antibodies formed did not change the efficacy or safety of romosozumab. Injection-site reaction occurred in about 5% of patients. Other adverse reactions include headache, paresthesias, and peripheral edema. While very rare, severe reactions can occur with romosozumab, including myocardial infarction, stroke, osteonecrosis of the jaw, and low-trauma bone fractures.

Contraindications. Romosozumab is contraindicated in patients with preexisting hypocalcemia. It should be avoided in any patient who may be predisposed to osteonecrosis of the jaw. Risk factors include anemia, cancer, radiation therapy, coagulopathy, preexisting dental disease or infection, and poor oral hygiene. Romosozumab should not be used in females who may become pregnant, who are pregnant, or who are breastfeeding.

BLACK BOX WARNING!

Romosozumab

Do not initiate treatment with romosozumab in patients who have experienced myocardial infarction or stroke within the preceding year. A higher incidence of major cardiac events including cardiovascular death, myocardial infarction, and stroke have occurred in patients taking romosozumab compared to those treated with alendronate during clinical trials.

Monitoring. Determine serum calcium prior to administration of romosozumab. Ensure that the patient maintains adequate calcium and vitamin D intake. Monitor carefully for adverse effects including symptoms of myocardial infarction or stroke. In clinical trials, atypical femoral fractures have occurred with minimal or no trauma. Patients reported dull, aching thigh pain prior to the complete fracture.

Prescriber Considerations for Osteoporosis Medication Therapy

Clinical Practice Guidelines

In 2020, the American Association of Clinical Endocrinology updated clinical practice guidelines for diagnosis and treatment of postmenopausal osteoporosis (Camacho, 2020). The guidelines emphasize that all postmenopausal females age 50 and older should be evaluated for osteoporosis risk using a careful history and physical examinations, as well as

a formal fracture risk assessment such as FRAX. The guidelines provide primary care providers direction for diagnosis and treatment for osteoporosis as well as lifestyle recommendations and fall prevention strategies.

BOOKMARK THIS!

Clinical Guidelines for Prevention and Treatment of Osteoporosis

Clinical practice guidelines for prevention and treatment of osteoporosis are available online from the National Osteoporosis Foundation (https://www.bonesource.org/clinical-guidelines) and the American Association of Clinical Endocrinology (https://www.aace.com/disease-state-resources/bone-and-parathyroid/clinical-practice-guidelines/clinical-practice)

Clinical Reasoning for Osteoporosis Therapy

Consider the individual patient's health problem requiring medications for osteoporosis. The first step for initiating treatment is thorough assessment of calcium and vitamin D intake. The International Osteoporosis Foundation online calcium calculator (https://www.iofbonehealth.org/calcium-calculator) is an excellent tool for determining calcium intake. Guidelines recommend calcium intake of 1000 mg/day for females 19 to 50 years of age. Similarly, 1000 mg/day is recommended for males 70 years of age or younger. For females 51 or older and males 71 or older, 1200 mg/day is recommended. In addition, guidelines recommend measurement of serum 25(OH) D in patients who are at risk for vitamin D insufficiency, particularly those with osteoporosis. Maintenance level of serum 25(OH)D should be at least 30 ng/mL in patients with osteoporosis (and preferably should be between 30 and 50 ng/mL). Based on the patient's risks, the provider can begin to select medication therapy to best impact bone health and minimize risk for medication side effects.

Determine the desired therapeutic outcome based on the degree of osteoporosis medication therapy needed for the patient's health problem. In general, medication therapies are directed toward reducing bone loss and/or increasing bone mineral density. Guidelines suggest that stable or increasing bone mineral density, with no evidence of new fractures or vertebral fracture progression, is a successful response to therapy for osteoporosis (Camacho et al., 2020). While a single fracture after initiation of therapy is not necessarily evidence of treatment failure, two or more fragility fractures are considered evidence of treatment failure. Foundational to achieving the desired outcome is the careful assessment and incorporation of adequate calcium and vitamin D intake. Should this not be achievable, supplementation may be required. In addition, fall prevention and lifestyle modification strategies are important to prevent fractures secondary to osteoporosis.

Assess the osteoporosis medication selected for its appropriateness for an individual patient by considering the medication's side effects and the patient's age, race/ethnicity, comorbidities, and genetic factors. The majority of the medications included in this chapter are directed toward postmenopausal females. However, since peak bone mass is achieved in one's late 20s and 30s, it is important to ensure adequate calcium and vitamin D intake across the life span to achieve optimal bone health. For patients taking bisphosphonates, it is important to follow specific medication administration instructions, including taking the oral medications with a full glass of water (not juice or milk) and being able to sit or stand for at least 30 minutes due to the risk of esophageal injury. Also, it is important to carefully assess dental health due to the risk of osteonecrosis of the jaw with several of the medications.

Initiate the treatment plan by first providing adequate patient education to ensure the patient's understanding and promote full participation in the osteoporosis medication therapy. Reinforce the importance of taking the medications exactly as directed to decrease the risk of adverse effects. For example, raloxifene should be discontinued at least 72 hours prior to and during prolonged immobilization and should be resumed only after the patient is fully ambulatory due to the risk of thromboembolic events. Patients should be advised to avoid prolonged restriction of movement during travel. Patients taking teriparatide should stand slowly as this medication may be associated with orthostatic hypotension, particularly early in therapy. Whatever the therapy, it is important to emphasize that medication therapy is not a substitute for sufficient intake of calcium and vitamin D, as well as lifestyle changes and fall prevention activities.

Ensure complete patient and family understanding about the medication prescribed for osteoporosis therapy using a variety of education strategies. Provide patients with specific administration directions for each medication, which will include techniques as well as directions for proper storage; abaloparatide, for example, should be stored in the refrigerator prior to the first dose. For medications requiring subcutaneous injection, use demonstration and return demonstration to ensure proper technique; for example, the patient should be taught to use the periumbilical region of the abdomen, avoiding the area within 2 inches of the navel or any areas of bruising, tenderness, scars, or stretch marks.

Conduct follow-up and monitoring of patient responses to osteoporosis medication therapy. Beyond monitoring for adverse effects essential to all medications used to treat osteoporosis, the length of therapy varies with the specific medication and the severity of the osteoporosis. For example, the AACE Clinical Practice Guidelines (Camacho et al., 2020) recommend that treatment with abaloparatide and teriparatide be limited to 2 years and followed with a bisphosphonate or denosumab. Drug holidays are recommended for patients taking oral bisphosphonates after 5 years of treatment if fracture risk is no longer high (such as when the T-score is greater than –2.5 or the patient has remained fracture free), but continued up to an additional 5 years if fracture risk remains high. Treatment is also monitored for effectiveness using DXA every 1 to 2 years until findings are stable. Then, guidelines recommend monitoring via follow-up DXA every 1 to 2 years or at a less-frequent interval, depending on clinical circumstances.

Teaching Points for Osteoporosis Therapy

Health Promotion Strategies

- Include strategies for fall prevention, including minimizing clutter, using nonskid rugs, adding handrails to showers or bathtubs, and encouraging proper, well-fitting shoes.
- Include the need for weight-bearing and resistance exercise to improve overall strength, balance, and posture. Refer to physical therapy as needed to teach exercises and proper body mechanics.
- Use evidence-based smoking cessation interventions as required to help the patient stop or reduce smoking.
- Assess the patient's medication profile for any medications that may impact mental status or increase risk for falls.
- Teach the patient to limit caffeine to fewer than 1 to 2 servings of caffeinated drinks per day. Caffeine can decrease absorption of intestinal calcium and increase excretion of calcium through the kidneys.
- Provide the patient with information to enhance calcium in the diet. If the patient is unable to incorporate adequate calcium into the diet, calcium supplementation may be necessary.
- Advise the patient to reduce alcohol intake to no more than two drinks daily for females or four drinks daily for males (one drink is equivalent to 120 mL of wine, 30 mL of liquor, or 260 mL of beer).
- Evaluate patient's need for supplemental vitamin D. This may be determined by measuring serum 25(OH)D levels.
- For patients requiring oral bisphosphonates, emphasize following administration directions carefully to avoid esophageal irritation. For example, both alendronate and risedronate require the patient to abstain from lying down for at least 30 minutes after the dose and until after the first food of the day. The medication can be taken with a full glass of plain water only (no juices, soft drinks, food, or other medications until after the 30-minute period).

Patient Education for Medication Safety

- It is imperative to take oral bisphosphonates on an empty stomach with a full glass of water only (no other food or drink). After taking the medication, make sure to stand or sit for at least 30 minutes before lying down to decrease the risk of esophageal injury.
- Follow administration for bisphosphonates carefully as food and drink significantly impact absorption. For example, alendronate should be taken 2 hours before a standard breakfast.
- Notify your primary care provider if you have a history of any dental disease or dental procedures while you are taking medications for osteoporosis.
- Do not chew risedronate as it may cause esophageal or oral ulcerations.
- Orthostatic hypotension has occurred in patients after taking teriparatide or abaloparatide. Symptoms typically resolve quickly with a change of position to sitting or lying down. Stand slowly and carefully at the beginning of therapy.
- If taking calcitonin-salmon nasal spray, you may require a periodic nasal examination to look for any signs of nasal trauma.

Application Questions for Discussion

1. A 75-year-old White female from the United States is evaluated for fracture risk using FRAX. Based on her weight of 61.2 kg, height of 167.6 cm, a T-score of –2.0, and a history of previous fracture, it is determined that she has an 18% chance of major osteoporosis-related fracture and a 4.7% chance of hip fracture. How would you proceed with determining the need for medication therapy?
2. Based on your decision in Question 1, what nonpharmacologic strategies would you incorporate in the patient's treatment plan?
3. Using the same data in Question 1, how would your treatment plan vary if the patient were Asian? Hispanic? Black?

Selected Bibliography

Aspray, T. J., & Hill, T. R. (2019). "Osteoporosis and the Ageing Skeleton." In J. R. Harris, & V. I. Korolchuk (Eds.), *Biochemistry and Cell Biology of Ageing: Part II Clinical Science* (pp. 453–476). Singapore: Springer Singapore.

Bhattacharyya, S., Pal, S., & Chattopadhyay, N. (2019). Abaloparatide, the second generation osteoanabolic drug: Molecular mechanisms underlying its advantages over the first-in-class teriparatide. *Biochemical Pharmacology, 166,* 185–191. http://doi.org/10.1016/j.bcp.2019.05.024.

Bijelic, R., Milicevic, S., & Balaban, J. (2017). Risk factors for osteoporosis in postmenopausal women. *Medical Archives, 71*(1), 25–28. http://doi.org/10.5455/medarh.2017.71.25-28.

Cauley, J. A. (2011). Defining ethnic and racial differences in osteoporosis and fragility fractures. *Clinical Orthopaedics and Related Research, 469*(7), 1891–1899. http://doi.org/10.1007/s11999-011-1863-5.

Camacho, P. M., Petak, S. M., Binkley, N., Diab, D. L., Eldeiry, L. S., Farooki, A., & Watts, N. B. (2020). American Association of Clinical Endocrinologists/American College of Endocrinology Clinical Practice Guidelines for the diagnosis and treatment of postmenopausal osteoporosis- 2020 Update Executive Summary. *Endocrine Practice, 26*(5), 564–570. doi:10.4158/gl-2020-0524.

Clarke, B. (2020). Normal bone anatomy and physiology. *Clinical journal of the American Society of Nephrology : CJASN, 3 Suppl 3,* (Suppl 3), S131–S139. doi:10.2215/CJN.04151206.

Cremers, S., Drake, M. T., Ebetino, F. H., Bilezikian, J. P., & Russell, R. G. G. (2019). Pharmacology of bisphosphonates. *British Journal of Clinical Pharmacology, 85*(6), 1052–1062. http://doi.org/10.1111/bcp.13867.

Faienza, M. F., Chiarito, M., D'Amato, G., Colaianni, G., Colucci, S., Grano, M., & Brunetti, G (2018). Monoclonal antibodies for treating osteoporosis. *Expert Opinion on Biological Therapy, 18*(2), 149–157. http://doi.org/10.1080/14712598.2018.1401607.

Felicilda-Reynaldo, R. F. D. (2019). First-line medications for osteoporosis. *MEDSURG Nursing, 28*(6), 381–386.

Jeremiah, M. P., Unwin, B. K., Greenawald, M. H., & Casiano, V. E. (2015). Diagnosis and management of osteoporosis. *American Family Physician, 92*(4), 261–268.

Kanis, J. A., Hans, D., Cooper, C., Baim, S., Bilezikian, J. P., Binkley, N., & McCloskey, E. V. (2011). Interpretation and use of FRAX in clinical practice. *Osteoporosis International, 22*(9), 2395–2411. doi:10.1007/s00198-011-1713-z.

Langdahl, B., Ferrari, S., & Dempster, D. W. (2016). Bone modeling and remodeling: Potential as therapeutic targets for the treatment of osteoporosis. *Therapeutic Advances in Musculoskeletal Disease, 8*(6), 225–235. http://doi.org/10.1177/1759720x16670154.

Lindsay, R., & Cosman, F. (2018). Osteoporosis. In J. L. Jameson, A. S. Fauci, D. L. Kasper, S. L. Hauser, D. L. Longo, & J. Loscalzo (Eds.), *Harrison's Principles of Internal Medicine* (20th ed.). New York: McGraw-Hill Education.

Looker, A. C., & Frenk, S. M. (2015). Percentage of adults aged 65 and over with osteoporosis or low bone mass at the femur neck or lumbar spine: United States, 2005–2010. Health E-Stat. *National Center for Health Statistics.* Retrieved from. https://www.cdc.gov/nchs/data/hestat/osteoporsis/osteoporosis2005_2010.htm.

McCance, K. L., & Huether, S. E. (2019). *Pathophysiology: The Biologic Basis for Disease in Adults and Children* (8th ed.). St. Louis: Elsevier.

Miller, P. D. (2016). Management of severe osteoporosis. *Expert Opinion on Pharmacotherapy, 17*(4), 473–488. http://doi.org/10.1517/14656566.2016.1124856.

National Institute of Arthritis and Musculoskeletal and Skin Diseases (2018), *Osteoporosis and African American women.* Washington, DC. Retrieved from https://www.bones.nih.gov/health-info/bone/osteoporosis/background/african-american-women.

O'Connell, M. B., Borchert, J. S., Slazak, E. M., & Fava, J. P. (2020). Osteoporosis. In J. T. DiPiro, G. C. Yee, L. M. Posey, S. T. Haines, T. D. Nolin, & V. Ellingrod (Eds.), *Pharmacotherapy: A Pathophysiologic Approach* (11th ed.). New York: McGraw-Hill Education.

Osterhoff, G., Morgan, E. F., Shefelbine, S. J., Karim, L., McNamara, L. M., & Augat, P. (2016). Bone mechanical properties and changes with osteoporosis. *Injury,* 47 Suppl 2(Suppl 2), S11–S20. https://doi.org/10.1016/S0020-1383(16)47003-8.

Qaseem, A., Forciea, M. A., McLean, R. M., & Denberg, T. D. (2017). Treatment of low bone density or osteoporosis to prevent fractures in men and women: A clinical practice guideline update from the American College of Physicians. *Annals of Internal Medicine, 166*(11), 818–839. http://doi.org/10.7326/m15-1361.

Rosenthal, L. D., & Rosenjack Burchum, J. (2018). *Lehne's Pharmacotherapeutics for Advanced Practice Providers*. St. Louis: Elsevier.

Russell, L. A. (2018). Management of difficult osteoporosis. *Best Practice & Research: Clinical Rheumatology, 32*(6), 835–847. http://doi.org/10.1016/j.berh.2019.04.002.

Shoback, D., Rosen, C. J., Black, D. M., Cheung, A. M., Murad, M. H., & Eastell, R. (2020). Pharmacological management of osteoporosis in postmenopausal women: An Endocrine Society Guideline update. *Journal of Clinical Endocrinology & Metabolism, 105*(3). N. PAG–N.PAG. http://doi.org/10.1210/clinem/dgaa048.

Weaver, C. M., Gordon, C. M., Janz, K. F., Kalkwarf, H. J., Lappe, J. M., Lewis, R., & Zemel, B. S. (2016). The National Osteoporosis Foundation's position statement on peak bone mass development and lifestyle factors: A systematic review and implementation recommendations. *Osteoporosis International, 27*(4), 1281–1386. http://doi.org/10.1007/s00198-015-3440-3.

Wright, N. C., Looker, A. C., Saag, K. G., Curtis, J. R., Delzell, E. S., Randall, S., & Dawson-Hughes, B. (2014). The recent prevalence of osteoporosis and low bone mass in the United States based on bone mineral density at the femoral neck or lumbar spine. *Journal of Bone and Mineral Research, 29*(11), 2520–2526. doi:10.1002/jbmr.2269.

26

Muscle Relaxant Medications

ANDREA J. EFRE AND KARLA L. MALDONADO

Overview

Skeletal muscle relaxant (SMR) medications are generally used to treat pain related to muscle spasms, tension, cramps, overuse, or spasticity. They are most often used to treat acute pain related to injury but may also be helpful for acute nontraumatic and postoperative pain management. Neck and back pain are the most common symptoms that muscle relaxant medications are used to treat, often in combination with nonsteroidal antiinflammatory drugs (NSAIDs) and additional analgesics if needed. With recent national concerns in prescribing opioids and studies evidencing negative side effects of NSAIDs, SMRs are commonly being considered in treating musculoskeletal pain.

Drugs that cause skeletal muscle relaxation are divided into two categories: antispasmodics and antispastics. As a general rule, *antispasmodic agents* are used to treat musculoskeletal pain and *antispastic medications* are used to treat chronic conditions such as cerebral palsy and upper motor neuron disorders. Skeletal muscle relaxants are used for their antispasmodic qualities, antispastic qualities, or a combination of both, as highlighted in Table 26.1. In general, centrally acting muscle relaxants are used to treat muscle spasm and are not effective in the treatment of spasticity. Likewise, agents used to treat spasticity do not usually relieve muscle spasm. However, some agents have both antispasmodic and antispastic properties, such as diazepam and tizanidine. Therefore, when selecting an SMR it is important to consider whether the underlying health problem will respond to either an antispasmodic therapy or an antispastic therapy, or whether both are needed. Selection criteria should largely be based on the risks versus benefits of using the SMR, and the patient's response to therapy.

Relevant Physiology

Skeletal muscles are composed of blood vessels, muscle fibers, and nerve fibers held together by connective tissue. The connective tissue and fascia protect the muscle fibers and provide support and structure to the body. Muscle fibers vary by number based on muscle type and by diameter based

on the required force needed to move the muscle. Muscle fibers bundle together into fascicles, which contain myofibrils. The myofibrils stimulate muscle contraction through the action of two cytoskeletal proteins: actin and myosin.

The peripheral nervous system controls skeletal muscle movement, and this movement is considered voluntary or controlled. Skeletal muscles produce movement by working in pairs—as one contracts (shortens) in response to a nerve stimulus, the other expands (lengthens). This process of contraction and relaxation causes movement of the bone and attached tissues.

Pathophysiology

Muscle spasms are involuntary, sudden, or convulsive muscle contractions. The spasms may be sustained (*tonic*), or they may alternate repetitively between contraction and relaxation (*clonic*). They involve smooth (*visceral*) muscle or skeletal (*striated*) muscle, and they may be characterized as strong, painful muscle cramping that interferes with muscle function. Muscle spasms result from a number of causes, including muscle fatigue, dehydration, electrolyte abnormalities, acute and chronic pain syndromes, and trauma or surgery.

Spasticity is associated with damage to higher motor centers and descending motor pathways. The damage results in increased flexor muscle tone and hyperexcitability of the stretch reflexes from overactivation of the alpha motor neurons in the spinal cord. Symptoms include increased muscle tone, hyperactive reflexes, sustained involuntary muscle contractions (*spasms*), and the spread of reflexes (*clonus*). Spasticity is often associated with cerebral palsy, multiple sclerosis, traumatic spinal cord injury, and stroke. Antispastic agents act on the central nervous system (CNS) or act directly on skeletal muscle to cause relaxation.

Antispasmodic Skeletal Muscle Relaxants

Antispasmodic SMRs are the most common SMRs used in the primary care setting and are highlighted throughout this section (Table 26.2). Antispasmodic drugs act on the CNS at the spinal cord level or brain stem to promote sedation

TABLE 26.1   Drug Overview for Subclassifications

Class	Subclass	Generic Name	Trade Name
Antispasmodics	Centrally acting sedatives/ CNS depressants	Carisoprodol	Soma, Vanadom
		Chlorzoxazone	Lorzone, Parafon Forte
		Metaxalone	Skelaxin
		Methocarbamol	Robaxin
	TCA relatives	Cyclobenzaprine	Fexmid, Amrix (Flexeril)
Antispastic agents	GABA receptor stimulants	Baclofen	Gablofen, Kemstro, Lioresal, Ozobax
	Muscle relaxant	Dantrolene	Dantrium
Agents with both antispasmodic and antispastic activity	Benzodiazepines	Diazepam	Valium
	β2-adrenergic agonists	Tizanidine	Zanaflex
Antispasmodic and neuromuscular blocker	Neurotoxin—Botulinum toxin	OnabotulinumtoxinA	Botox

CNS, Central nervous system; GABA, gamma-aminobutyric acid; TCA, tricyclic antidepressant.

TABLE 26.2   Antispasmodic Skeletal Muscle Relaxants

Medication	Indication	Dosage	Considerations and Monitoring
Carisoprodol	Muscle sprain, strain, and injury	**Tablet:** *Adults and adolescents ≥16 yr:* 250–350 mg orally, up to three times daily and at night, as needed. Maximum dosage: 1400 mg/day. Use should not exceed 2–3 weeks. Taper dose gradually.	Controlled substance Schedule IV. Avoid in substance abuse history. Beers Criteria = Avoid.
Chlorzoxazone	Musculoskeletal pain and spasm	**Tablet:** *Adults:* 250–750 mg orally up to four times daily as needed. Maximum dosage: 3000 mg/day.	Monitor LFTs. Not primary choice for back and neck pain. Beers Criteria = Avoid.
Cyclobenzaprine	Musculoskeletal pain and spasm	**Immediate release:** *Adults and adolescents ≥15 yr:* 5–10 mg orally three times daily as needed. Initial dose: 5 mg. Maximum dosage: 30 mg/day. Use should not exceed 2–3 weeks. **Extended release:** *Adults:* 15 mg orally once daily. May increase to 30 mg depending on response. Limit treatment to 3 weeks. Maximum dosage: 30 mg/day.	Be cautious of serotonin syndrome. Significant anticholinergic effects. Contraindicated in patients using MAOIs and TCAs. Beers Criteria = Avoid.
Metaxalone	Musculoskeletal pain and spasm	**Tablet:** *Adults and adolescents ≥12 yr:* 800 mg orally three to four times daily as needed. Maximum dosage: 3200 mg/day.	Fewer sedating side effects than other SMRs. Give on an empty stomach. Creatinine at baseline. Serial LFTs. Avoid in hepatic impairment. Beers Criteria = Avoid.
Methocarbamol	Musculoskeletal pain and spasm	**Tablet:** *Adults and adolescents ≥16 yr: Initial dose:* 1500 mg orally four times daily for 48–72 hr. Maximum dosage: 6000 mg/day. *Maintenance dosage:* Decrease to 1000 mg four times daily. Maximum dosage: 4500 mg/day. *Children:* Used intravenously for tetanus only.	Generally well tolerated. May be used intravenously or intramuscularly as an adjunct treatment in tetanus. Beers Criteria = Avoid.

LFTs, Liver function tests; MAOIs, monoamine oxidase inhibitors; TCAs, tricyclic antidepressants; SMRs, skeletal muscle relaxants.

and, thereby, muscle relaxation. The exact mechanism in relieving muscle spasm remains unknown; however, studies have suggested that the sedative effects cause a decrease in the neuronal activity, which reduces muscle reflexes and decreases spasm. Antispasmodics do not have antiinflammatory or analgesic properties. Drugs in this category include carisoprodol, cyclobenzaprine, metaxalone, chlorzoxazone, methocarbamol, and orphenadrine.

Carisoprodol

Carisoprodol is a Schedule IV drug and has a high potential for being abused. If prescribed, it should only be used for short periods, such as 2 to 3 weeks, and should not be used for chronic pain. It may cause significant drowsiness and dizziness and should not be used in patients over 65 years of age.

Carisoprodol blocks interneural activity and depresses neuronal transmission within the reticular formation and spinal cord. The resulting CNS depression leads to anxiolysis, euphoria, and decreased perception of pain. It is not recommended as first-line treatment for muscle spasms due to the potential to produce physical and psychological dependence following prolonged use. Additionally, its use should be limited to short periods (no more than 3 weeks).

Pharmacokinetics. Carisoprodol is administered orally, with an onset of action in about 30 minutes, and it lasts for 4 to 6 hours. It is renally excreted and has a half-life of 2.4 hours.

Indications. Carisoprodol is indicated for the relief of discomfort associated with muscle strain, sprains, and muscle injuries.

Adverse Effects. Sedation, dizziness, headache, gastrointestinal (GI) discomfort, vomiting, and rash are potential side effects. Cases of dependence, withdrawal, and abuse have been reported with prolonged use, most commonly in patients with a history of addiction and/or concomitant use of opioids or other drugs with potential abuse.

Contraindications. Carisoprodol is contraindicated in patients with a history of acute intermittent porphyria (abnormal heme production and metabolism) or a hypersensitivity to carbamate. It should be used with caution in patients with seizure disorders or potential for seizure activity.

Monitoring. No routine testing or monitoring is recommended. Due to its abuse potential, the duration of therapy should not exceed 2 to 3 weeks. If the patient has been using the medication long term, it will need to be tapered to discontinue. There are no data on the use of carisoprodol during pregnancy and no human studies on the incidence of congenital malformation in animal studies.

Cyclobenzaprine Hydrochloride

Cyclobenzaprine is a good first choice for SMR therapy and is very economical, but the side effect of significant drowsiness should be considered. It was previously known to many by the brand name Flexeril, but is no longer marketed under this name. Cyclobenzaprine releases local muscle spasm and hyperactivity

without acting directly on skeletal muscle. It is structurally related to the tricyclic antidepressants (TCAs) as a 5HT3 receptor antagonist in the CNS at the level of the brain stem. It has strong antimuscarinic effects and causes significant sedation in most patients. It also potentiates norepinephrine, which may cause mild to moderate increases in heart rate. Other side effects include confusion, hallucinations, and agitation; therefore, cyclobenzaprine should be avoided in older adults.

Pharmacokinetics. Cyclobenzaprine is metabolized by the cytochrome (CYP) 450, IA2, 2D6, and 3A4 substrates in the liver and is excreted as glucuronides by the kidney. It is eliminated slowly, with an effective half-life of 18 hours. The half-life of the extended-release form is 32 hours.

Indications. Cyclobenzaprine is used as an adjunct to rest and physical therapy for relief of muscle spasms and symptoms associated with acute, painful muscle skeletal disorders, including fibromyalgia. It has not been found effective in the treatment of spasticity associated with cerebral or spinal cord disease. Cyclobenzaprine should only be used for up to 2 to 3 weeks because prolonged use has not been proven effective.

Adverse Effects. CNS depression effects include drowsiness, dizziness, fatigue, headache, and confusion. Cyclobenzaprine lowers the seizure threshold and has strong serotonergic effects. Its anticholinergic effects include blurred vision, photosensitivity, dyspepsia, nausea, and constipation. Cyclobenzaprine may decrease urinary flow and cause urinary retention in older males.

Contraindications. Concurrent use of monoamine oxidase inhibitors (MAOIs) with cyclobenzaprine is contraindicated. Cyclobenzaprine and MAOIs should not be used within a 14-day window of each other due to the risk of hyperpyretic crisis, seizures, and death. Cyclobenzaprine should be avoided in patients with a hypersensitivity to the drug or its drug classification. The extended-release form should be avoided in older adults and in patients with hepatic impairment. It should also be avoided in patients with recent myocardial infarction, congestive heart failure, history of arrhythmias, heart block, or cardiac conduction disturbances. Use with caution in patients with a history of urinary retention, angle-closure glaucoma, or increased intraocular pressure. Cyclobenzaprine may enhance the effects of alcohol and other CNS depressants.

Monitoring. No routine testing or monitoring is recommended.

Metaxalone

Metaxalone has the fewest reported side effects of all the SMRs and has the lowest potential for sedation. It is a very well-tolerated muscle relaxant, but is not the most economical, even in generic form, and therefore some insurance companies may not encourage its use.

Pharmacokinetics. Metaxalone is metabolized in the liver by CYP 450 enzymes and is excreted in the urine as unidentified metabolites. The impact of hepatic and renal disease has not been determined; therefore, it should be used with caution in patients with renal and/or hepatic impairment.

Warnings and Precautions: Serotonin Syndrome

Serotonin syndrome, a potentially life-threatening condition, has been reported when cyclobenzaprine has been used with other drugs such as selective serotonin reuptake inhibitors (SSRIs), serotonin norepinephrine reuptake inhibitors (SNRIs), TCAs, tramadol, bupropion, meperidine, verapamil, or MAOIs.
Symptoms of serotonin syndrome include the following:

- Changes in mental status (hallucinations, agitation, and confusion)
- Autonomic instability (tachycardia, blood pressure instability, diaphoresis, and hyperthermia)
- Neuromuscular abnormalities (tremor, ataxia, hyperreflexia, clonus, and muscle rigidity)
- GI symptoms (nausea, vomiting, and diarrhea)
Treatment with cyclobenzaprine should be discontinued if any of these reactions occur.
Educate the patient on the drug interactions and risks for serotonin syndrome prior to initiating therapy with cyclobenzaprine.

Indications. Metaxalone is indicated as an adjunct to physical therapy and rest for the relief of acute, painful muscle spasms.

Adverse Effects. CNS adverse reactions to metaxalone include drowsiness, dizziness, headache, and irritability. Digestive effects are nausea, vomiting, and dyspepsia. Other adverse reactions include rash with or without pruritis, leukopenia, hemolytic anemia, and jaundice.

Contraindications. Metaxalone is contraindicated in patients with known hypersensitivity to the drug. It is also contraindicated in patients with a known tendency to drug-induced, hemolytic, or other anemias, and in those with impaired renal or hepatic function. Anaphylactoid reactions, while rare, have been reported.

Monitoring. Serial liver function tests (LFTs) should be performed.

Methocarbamol

Methocarbamol is widely used in the United States and is one of the only SMRs approved for use in parts of Europe. It is considered to be effective, it is fairly inexpensive, and it has relatively fewer sedating side effects than some other medications in this class. A recent European study determined it to be an efficient and well-tolerated therapeutic option for patients suffering from acute low back pain and the typical associated restrictions of mobility (Emrich et al., 2015).

Pharmacokinetics. Methocarbamol is metabolized in the liver by CYP450 enzymes and is excreted in the urine. Renal and hepatic impairment should be considered. Renal clearance is decreased by 40% in patients with severe renal insufficiency, and hepatic clearance is decreased by 70% (prolonged) in patients with hepatic impairment and cirrhosis.

Indications. Methocarbamol is indicated as an adjunct treatment of muscle spasm associated with acute, painful musculoskeletal conditions. It may also be used to treat tetanus, but benzodiazepines are more commonly used as first-line treatment.

Adverse Effects. Methocarbamol adverse reactions include hypersensitivity, anaphylaxis, seizures, leukopenia, syncope, bradycardia, and jaundice. More common reactions include drowsiness, dizziness, nausea, vomiting, rash, blurred vision, headache, nasal congestion, metallic taste, and hypotension.

Contraindications. Methocarbamol is contraindicated in patients with known hypersensitivity to the drug. It is also contraindicated in patients with a seizure disorder and in those with impaired renal or hepatic function. Use with caution in older adults or concurrent CNS depressant use or alcohol use.

Prescriber Safety Notes

- When prescribing a muscle relaxant, give the patient clear instructions about the side effects, including the potential for drowsiness.
- Caution patients in performing hazardous tasks, driving a motor vehicle, or operating machinery, especially when the muscle relaxant is used with alcohol or other CNS depressants.
- The sedative effects of CNS depressants (alcohol, benzodiazepines, opioids, tricyclic antidepressants) may be additive, and therefore caution should be used in patients who take more than one CNS depressant simultaneously.
- Concomitant use of SMRs, benzodiazepines, and opioids increases sedation significantly and can induce respiratory depression.

Life Span Considerations With Antispasmodic Skeletal Muscle Relaxants

Geriatrics

- The American Geriatrics Society (AGS) lists medications that are potentially inappropriate for use in older adults in The Beers Criteria. It is strongly recommended that the antispasmodic SMRs not be used in older adults as they are poorly tolerated, have anticholinergic adverse effects, cause sedation, and increase the risk of fractures (see Table 26.2).

Pediatrics

- Most of the SMRs have no well-controlled studies on safety and efficacy in pediatrics. For the most part, they are not generally indicated for use in children, as per the following recommendations.
  - Carisoprodol: dosing starts at 16 years of age.
  - Cyclobenzaprine: dosing starts at 15 years of age.
  - Metaxalone: safety and effectiveness in children younger than age 12 have not been established.
  - Methocarbamol and orphenadrine: these are not indicated in pediatric use.

Antispastic Skeletal Muscle Relaxants

Antispastic agents include baclofen and dantrolene (Table 26.3). They act as agonists at the gamma-aminobutyric acid (GABA) receptors in the CNS.

Baclofen

Baclofen is an antispastic SMR and is primarily used for upper motor neuron spasticity such as in multiple sclerosis, cerebral palsy, tetanus, stiff-person syndrome, and spinal cord injury patients (Shah, 2016). It is not the best option for neck or back muscle pain, and it can cause drowsiness. However, it is considered to be as effective as diazepam in reducing spasticity with less sedative effects. The precise mechanism of action is not fully known. It is a centrally acting SMR and is a structural analog of the inhibitory neurotransmitter GABA. It is also suggested that baclofen reduces pain associated with spasticity by inhibiting the release of substance P in the spinal cord. Baclofen may be used orally or intrathecally, and the effects, indications, and pharmacokinetics are a little different based on the route. The intrathecal route in single bolus test doses (via spinal catheter or lumbar puncture) may be used. For spasticity related to chronic disease, an implantable pump in the intrathecal space may be used.

Pharmacokinetics. Baclofen is rapidly and extensively absorbed. Peak plasma concentration can be reached with oral baclofen in 1 to 3 hours depending on oral preparation. Baclofen is primarily renally eliminated, with 85% of the dose being unchanged at excretion. The elimination half-life is 3 to 5 hours, and excretion is complete within 72 hours after administration. No dosage adjustment is necessary for hepatic impairment, but dose reductions are needed for renal impairment based on creatinine clearance (CrCl).

Indications. Baclofen is used to treat spasticity in patients with multiple sclerosis and other spinal cord lesions or injury, particularly for the relief of flexor spasms and concomitant pain, clonus, and muscular rigidity. In addition, it improves bowel and bladder function in some of these patients. It is also used in the treatment of dystonia, spasticity associated with cerebral palsy, and complex regional pain syndrome. Use baclofen with caution in patients with a history of autonomic dysreflexia. The use of baclofen in the treatment of hiccups, nystagmus, trigeminal neuralgia, tic disorders, gastroesophageal reflux disease (GERD), and cravings for cocaine, alcohol, and nicotine has been studied with various levels of evidence. It should be noted that these are currently off-label uses and have not been approved by the U.S. Food and Drug Administration (FDA). Baclofen is not indicated in the treatment of skeletal muscle spasm resulting from rheumatic disorders.

If antispastic medication is needed for the treatment of multiple sclerosis or spinal cord injuries, baclofen may be considered. Topical applications are less likely to affect the

TABLE 26.3	Antispastic Skeletal Muscle Relaxants			
Medication	**Indication**	**Dosage**	**Considerations and Monitoring**	
Baclofen	Spasticity, muscle spasm, myoclonus, muscle rigidity in multiple sclerosis, spinal cord injury, traumatic brain injury, and cerebral palsy	**Tablets, solution, oral granules:** *Adults, adolescents, and children ≥12 yr:* 5–20 mg orally three or four times daily. Maximum dosage: 80 mg/day. Taper dose gradually to discontinue. Taper oral dose over 2 weeks and intrathecal dose over 4 weeks. Guideline Use (off-label use for spinal cord injury, traumatic brain injury, and cerebral palsy): *Children 2-11 yr:* 10–80 mg/day dependent on age, divided three or four times daily.	Black box warning for intrathecal dose. Intrathecal dose requires special techniques and monitoring. It may be single bolus or designated intrathecal pump. Caution in renal insufficiency and consider renal dosing. Caution in diabetes, seizures, and psychiatric disorders. Not indicated for skeletal muscle spasm in rheumatic disorders.	
Dantrolene	Spasticity due to spinal cord injury, stroke, cerebral palsy, or multiple sclerosis	**Oral capsule:** *Adults:* 25–100 mg orally three or four times daily. Gradual dose titration once daily for 7 days. Maximum dosage: 400 mg/day for adults and children. *Adolescents and children 5–17 yr:* 0.5 mg/kg/dose to 100 mg depending on response. Use lowest dose possible. Discontinue after 45 days if inadequate response.	Black box warning of hepatotoxicity and absolute contraindication in hepatic disease. Monitor LFTs. Not indicated for skeletal muscle spasm in rheumatic disorders.	

nursing infant. Intrathecal administration (bolus or pump) is feasible but requires an invasive procedure.

Adverse Effects. Serious reactions include CNS depression, respiratory depression, ataxia, syncope, seizures, psychiatric disturbances, hallucinations, depression, and autonomic dysreflexia. Significant symptoms occur if baclofen is stopped abruptly (see the black box warning). Common reactions include dizziness, drowsiness, weakness, confusion, fatigue, hypotension, nausea, and vomiting. In addition, there are multiple drug–drug interactions between baclofen and many other medications, so review the medication list carefully prior to prescribing.

Contraindications. Use baclofen with caution in patients with diabetes as it may elevate blood sugar. Patients with preexisting psychiatric disorders (e.g., bipolar disorder, depression, psychosis, schizophrenia) are at increased risk for baclofen-induced psychiatric adverse reactions. Use baclofen with caution in patients with a history of autonomic dysreflexia (e.g., spinal cord injuries at T6 or above) as abrupt withdrawal or nociceptive stimuli may trigger autonomic dysreflexic episodes. Baclofen should not be used in patients who require some degree of spasticity to maintain upright posture and balance, such as those with cerebral palsy, head trauma, stroke, or intracranial bleed. Prescribe with caution in patients with any past seizure activity.

Monitoring. It is recommended that creatinine be checked at baseline as baclofen is primarily renally eliminated. Also, if the patient has an underlying history of epilepsy or has had a previous seizure, an electroencephalogram

---

BLACK BOX WARNING!

Baclofen

Abrupt discontinuation of intrathecal baclofen may cause severe reactions, including high fever, altered mental status, priapism, exaggerated rebound spasticity, and muscle rigidity, which, in rare cases, have advanced to rhabdomyolysis, multisystem organ failure, and death.

(EEG) is recommended prior to starting baclofen. Sudden discontinuation of oral baclofen is associated with confusion, hallucinations, other psychiatric disturbances, seizure(s), and exacerbations of spasticity or other neurologic events. Therefore, plan for gradual reduction of the oral dosage over a period of 2 weeks or more. Significant withdrawal symptoms may occur from oral or intrathecal baclofen and abrupt cessation should be avoided.

Dantrolene

Dantrolene is an antispastic SMR that causes muscle relaxation by binding to the ryanodine receptor, thereby inhibiting calcium release from the sarcoplasmic reticulum and thus interfering with normal excitation contraction in skeletal muscle. Cardiac muscle and smooth muscle are depressed only slightly. Dantrolene has a black box warning of hepatotoxicity (including hepatitis), and for this reason it is contraindicated in patients with active hepatic disease.

BLACK BOX WARNING!

Dantrolene

- Dantrolene may cause hepatotoxicity. Do not use in hepatic insufficiency or in combination with other hepatotoxic medication.
- Use only for recommended conditions at the lowest effective dose.
- Discontinue use if there is no observed benefit after 45 days.

PRACTICE PEARLS

Life Span Considerations with Antispastic Skeletal Muscle Relaxants

Pediatrics

- Baclofen has the most established pediatric dosing of all the SMRs, and it may be used in all ages to treat pediatric spasticity of cerebral origin. However, the safety and effectiveness of baclofen in children younger than age 12 have not been established. It is not recommended in oral form for children younger than 2 years of age, and the safe and effective use of intrathecal baclofen has not been established for children younger than 4 years of age. Baclofen can lower the seizure threshold, so use with caution in children with cerebral injury who may be at risk of seizures.
- Dantrolene may be used in children with a weight-based dose both orally and intravenously, depending on the clinical indication. Oral doses may be used in children over age 5 and are titrated up over 7 days.

Additionally, adverse effects include cardiovascular and pulmonary toxicity, visual disturbances, hallucinations, seizures, and depression. Dantrolene is used as an emergency treatment in malignant hyperthermia that can be triggered by volatile anesthetic agents and neuromuscular blocking medications such as succinylcholine. The antispastic effects of dantrolene are more often utilized in neurological disease processes managed by neurology rather than primary care.

Antispasmodic and Antispastic Skeletal Muscle Relaxants

Two medications have both antispasmodic and antispastic effects: tizanidine (Zanaflex) and diazepam (Valium) (Table 26.4). Choosing an antispastic agent can be difficult. Effectiveness versus side effects should be considered. Much work has been done in the area of multiple sclerosis. When comparing tizanidine to baclofen as an antispastic agent in the treatment of multiple sclerosis, the effects are equal, but tizanidine tends to have fewer side effects (Bass et al., 1988).

Tizanidine

Tizanidine has both antispastic and antispasmodic effects, and it is helpful in treating the muscle spasms and spasticity

TABLE 26.4 Antispasmodic and Antispastic Skeletal Muscle Relaxants

Medication	Indication	Dosage	Considerations and Monitoring
Tizanidine	Muscle spasm and muscle pain; spasticity related to multiple sclerosis or spinal cord injury	**Capsule:** *Adults:* 2–4 mg orally up to three times daily as needed. Maximum dosage: 36 mg/day.	May interact with antihypertensive medications. Blood pressure should be monitored for hypotension. Caution in renal or hepatic impairment. Creatinine and LFTs should be tested at baseline and 1 month after maintenance. May decrease urinary flow and cause urinary retention in older males. Beers Criteria = Avoid.
Diazepam	Muscle spasm, muscle pain, inflammation, or trauma; muscle spasm related to tetanus	**Tablet, oral solution:** *Adults:* 2–10 mg orally two to four times daily depending on severity of symptoms. Maximum dosage: 40 mg/day. *Older adults:* 2–2.5 mg once or twice daily. Use varies depending on regulation of facility. Observe Beers Criteria and federal regulations. *Adolescents, children, and infants ≥6 months–17 yr:* 1–2.5 mg orally three to four times daily depending on response.	Controlled substance Schedule IV. Very long elimination half-life of 20–70 hr. Monitor CBC and LFTs. Black box warning: absolute contraindications include closed-angle glaucoma, hepatic disease, myasthenia gravis, respiratory insufficiency, and sleep apnea. Beers Criteria = Avoid.

CBC, Complete blood count; *LFTs,* liver function tests.

of multiple sclerosis and cerebral palsy. It is not the best first-line option in treating neck and back pain. Tizanidine is an imidazoline derivative with significant alpha-2 adrenoceptor agonist effects at the brain stem and spinal cord, similar to clonidine. It also inhibits nociceptive transmission in the spinal cord. The antispasmodic activity causes less hypotension than clonidine. Studies have shown that tizanidine administration has benefited patients with spasticity and is more tolerable and comparable in efficacy to diazepam, baclofen, and dantrolene.

Pharmacokinetics. Tizanidine is metabolized extensively by the CYP 450–1A2 substrate. It is excreted 60% in the urine and 20% in the feces. The half-life is 2.5 hours.

Indications. Tizanidine is indicated for the management of spasticity by temporarily relaxing muscle tone. It may also be useful in the short-term relief of muscle spasm or muscle pain. Caution is recommended if activities require balance, muscle tone, or coordination. Tizanidine has a short duration of action but should not be used more than three times daily, so recommend its use during periods of peak discomfort.

Adverse Effects. Serious reactions include hepatotoxicity, hypotension, bradycardia, and syncope. Sedation, hallucinations, delusions, and psychosis-like symptoms have been reported. Other serious adverse effects include hypersensitivity reactions, anaphylaxis, Stevens-Johnson syndrome, and exfoliating dermatitis. Tizanidine may decrease urinary flow and cause urinary retention in older males.

Contraindications. Tizanidine should not be used with fluoroquinolones (such as ciprofloxacin), fluvoxamine, antiarrhythmics (including amiodarone), cimetidine, acyclovir, or oral contraceptives as they can cause hypotension, bradycardia, and increased sedation. Use decreased dosages in patients with renal or hepatic impairment.

Monitoring. Tizanidine is an alpha-2 adrenoceptor agonist that can produce hypotension. Possible interactions may occur with antihypertensive medications, so blood pressure should be monitored. Creatinine tests and LFTs should be conducted at baseline and 1 month after the maintenance dose is achieved.

BLACK BOX WARNING!

Diazepam

- Risks from concomitant use with opioids include abuse, misuse, addiction, dependence, and withdrawal reactions.
- As with most benzodiazepines, diazepam should not be used concomitantly with opioids as it may result in profound sedation, respiratory depression, coma, and death. For this reason, use only for patients in whom alternative treatment options are inadequate.
- Limit dosages and durations to the minimum required.
- Follow up with patients for signs and symptoms of respiratory depression and sedation.

Life Span Considerations With Antispasmodic and Antispastic Skeletal Muscle Relaxants

Older Adults

- Tizanidine may increase the risk for urinary retention and sedation (Beers Criteria).
- Diazepam may increase the risk of cognitive impairment, delirium, falls, fractures, and motor vehicle crashes in older adults (Beers Criteria).

Pediatrics

- Tizanidine may be used in patients 2 years of age and older.
- Diazepam may be used in children. Oral dosing starts at 6 months, and intravenous at 1 month for muscle spasm or spasticity. It may also be used in neonates intravenously if indicated for seizures. Review clinical guidelines for specific indication and dose.

SMR Therapy Use in Pregnancy and Lactation

Pregnancy

- Skeletal muscle relaxants are generally not recommended during pregnancy. The benefits of use should significantly outweigh the potential risks.
- Neonatal withdrawal symptoms from SMRs have been reported, starting hours to days after delivery.

Lactation

- As a general rule, avoid antispasmodic and antispastic agents in patients who are breastfeeding as properties of the drug may be excreted into breast milk. Consider an alternative therapy.

Diazepam

Diazepam is commonly used in the treatment of pain related to spasms. It can be beneficial when used intramuscularly in an acute care setting where the patient can be closely monitored. Like all benzodiazepines, diazepam has anxiolytic, sedative, hypnotic, amnestic, and anticonvulsant action in the CNS. It acts in both the brain and the spinal cord, and can be used in patients with any muscle spasm including local muscle trauma. However, the dose required to reduce muscle tone produces significant sedation in most patients. Due to the high possibility of abuse, dependence, and addiction, it is not recommended for long-term use. Therefore, it is not a medication used frequently in the primary care setting, and for this reason it is not expounded upon further in this chapter.

Muscle Relaxant and Neuromuscular Blocker

OnabotulinumtoxinA is a product of botulinum toxin that has both antispastic and antispasmodic qualities. It is an

acetylcholine release inhibitor and a neuromuscular blocking agent. It is indicated in the treatment of upper limb spasticity, chronic migraine, cervical dystonia, blepharospasm, strabismus, and primary axillary hyperhidrosis.

Although pediatric indications exist for some conditions, the age limit is dependent on the indication, so it should be used with caution. There are no adequate and well-controlled studies on the use of OnabotulinumtoxinA in pregnant patients, so it should be used during pregnancy only if the potential benefit justifies the potential risk to the fetus. It is not known whether this drug is excreted in breast milk, so caution should be exercised in administering to a patient who is nursing.

OnabotulinumtoxinA is administered by injection to the affected site by a provider who has specialty training in the use of the medication. Dosing is varied and specific to the indication and site (refer to manufacturer guidelines on use). The most serious concern in using this medication is the risk of botulinum toxin effects. These may include asthenia, generalized muscle weakness, diplopia, ptosis, dysphagia, dysphonia, dysarthria, urinary incontinence, and breathing or swallowing difficulties which may be life threatening. These symptoms have been reported hours to weeks after injection.

Prescriber Considerations for Skeletal Muscle Relaxant Therapy

Clinical Practice Guidelines

The use of SMRs is the first of three recommendations in the clinical guidelines for the noninvasive treatment of low back pain (Qaseem et al., 2017). Evidence shows that SMRs provided short-term relief of acute and subacute low back pain compared with placebo, but insufficient evidence is found for the treatment of chronic low back pain (Qaseem et al., 2017; Hauk, 2017). Some countries do not use benzodiazepines or muscle relaxants to treat back pain, and SMRs are not widely available in many parts of Europe (Schreijenberg et al., 2019). Studies have concluded that advanced practice nurses and physician assistants are more likely to utilize muscle relaxants along with nonnarcotic analgesics, whereas physicians are more likely to order narcotic analgesics (Roblin et al., 2017).

Clinical Reasoning for Skeletal Muscle Relaxant Therapy

Consider the individual patient's health problem requiring skeletal muscle relaxant therapy. Skeletal muscle relaxants are most useful in the short-term treatment of pain related to muscle spasm, soreness, or stiffness. They are most useful in the short-term treatment of acute and subacute low back pain. Use in chronic back pain is not recommended, and caution should be taken with long-term use as it can lead to dependence. However, some SMRs are used for long-term control of spasms and spasticity.

When selecting an SMR, consider whether the underlying health problem is spasmodic or spastic and if long- or short-term therapy is indicated. It is essential to review the side-effect profile and contraindications of the SMR and compare them to the patient's medical history. In general, SMRs are renally metabolized, and therefore they need adequate renal function or reduced renal dosing. Additional contraindications exist for each SMR that should be considered during the selection process. Most SMRs are available in generic preparations, which keeps the costs lower and similar to each other. However, insurance companies may favor select medications for their formulary, and this should be explored when prescribing.

Determine the desired therapeutic outcome based on the patient's health problem. Prior to starting SMR therapy, it is important to evaluate the specifics of the muscle problem and clarify whether an antispasmodic effect, an antispastic quality, or both are indicated in the treatment of the underlying problem. When treating muscle spasms, the combined drug therapy tends to include antiinflammatory, analgesic, and antispasmodic agents. In addition, general measures to reduce tension and promote muscle relaxation include muscle immobilization with orthopedic supports/braces, ice/heat therapy, massage, and physical therapy. Spasticity is primarily treated with medications and physical therapy.

The use of SMRs may be considered as a monotherapy, or in conjunction with other medication and therapies to treat the underlying health problem. A muscle relaxant added to acetaminophen or an NSAID is more effective than using either medication independently. However, when using SMRs in combined therapy, consider the effects and length of time needed for the medication, and plan for an end date with a follow-up evaluation. The combination of medications can enhance side effects, especially increased drowsiness. If the underlying health problem requires that the patient take the medication around the clock, consider whether a half dose would be sufficient for the daytime dose to prevent excessive sedative effects. In the treatment of low back pain, the choice between the use of NSAIDs and muscle relaxants should be made based on the risks associated with each and the patient's preference (Hauk, 2017). If the back pain is acute, SMR therapy may be a better choice. If the back pain becomes more chronic, an alternate long-term therapy should be considered.

Assess the SMR selected for its appropriateness for an individual patient by considering the medication's side effects and the patient's age, race/ethnicity, comorbidities, and genetic factors. Before initiating SMR therapy, the primary care provider must assess the risks versus benefits, particularly when considering the patient's age. Significant caution should be used if considering SMR use in an older adult. The Beers Criteria list SMRs as inappropriate for individuals over 65 years of age, primarily because of the anticholinergic effects, the sedation, and the increased risk of injuries, falls, and fractures. Skeletal muscle relaxants are also associated with an increased risk of ED visits and hospitalizations in older adults (Alvarez et al., 2015). With this in mind, primary care providers should look for opportunities to limit, wean, or discontinue SMRs in older patients. This family of medications is not usually used in children younger than 12 years of age, unless the medication is used in specialized cases with strict monitoring, most often in pediatric neurology. In general, race and ethnicity are not concerning criteria when prescribing SMRs.

Initiate the treatment plan with the selected medication by first providing adequate patient education to ensure the patient's understanding and promote full participation in the SMR therapy. It is important to discuss the therapeutic effects and side effects of the medication prior to initiating SMR therapy. Based on age, occupation, lifestyle, and activities of daily living, the patient may choose to accept or not accept SMR therapy. Discussing the risks and benefits of the medication with the patient is an important part of the shared decision-making process.

Patients should not drive or operate machinery while influenced by the SMR medication, which may affect their daily schedules or employment. Discuss the option of using SMR therapy at bedtime for pain relief without daytime drowsiness. If using SMRs at night, discuss nocturnal bathroom habits, and plan for measures to reduce risk of injury due to sedation. Factors such as advanced age, frailty, and concurrent disease processes should be considered. Evaluate whether bedside commodes or urinals may be needed if mobility is a concern.

If employment or daily activities may be affected by the use of the SMR, discuss how routines and activities could be adapted to accommodate. If a medical note is needed for employment, the duration of restriction and the limitations of activities should be clearly defined. If the patient does not receive pay for time away from work, they may choose not to take the medication.

Muscle relaxants have a high-risk potential for abuse and misuse. These risks should be discussed with the patient and family prior to initiating therapy. Diazepam is a benzodiazepine with a high risk of dependence and abuse. Carisoprodol is a Schedule IV-controlled substance with a long history of reported drug abuse. Baclofen, cyclobenzaprine, and chlorzoxazone all have reports of misuse.

Ensure complete patient and family understanding about SMR therapy using a variety of educational strategies. Educate the patient and family on the risks and benefits of using SMR therapy. Include the possible side effects of the chosen SMR, with specific signs and symptoms for them to observe. Counsel on potential sedation, interaction with other medications, contraindications, and the plan for weaning or discontinuation.

If SMRs are prescribed for the older adult, the patient, family, or caregiver should be instructed on injury prevention and fall potential. Discuss how to prepare the home, securing loose rugs, appropriate footwear, and use of a walker, bedside commode, or urinal. As SMRs are only indicated for short-term use, the family may choose to have the older patient stay with them for closer monitoring.

Conduct follow-up and monitoring of patient responses to SMR therapy. For most patients, the use of SMRs is a short-term plan for pain relief. A follow-up date for patient reevaluation should be planned after 2 to 3 weeks of use to determine whether the pain is resolved and whether the medications may be weaned or discontinued. If the pain is unresolved, the pain source may need further evaluation and diagnosis.

Muscle relaxants are not generally indicated for long-term chronic use, and they have the potential for abuse. If used long term for chronic disease processes such as multiple sclerosis, a baseline creatinine should be drawn to evaluate renal capacity, with regular creatinine monitoring moving forward. If there is preexisting hepatic dysfunction, it is recommended to monitor LFTs at baseline.

The use of SMRs in older adults is associated with a higher risk of injury and falls, and a higher frequency and severity of adverse effects. Therefore, the need for therapy should significantly outweigh the risks of adverse effects. Dosing should be slowly and carefully titrated, and the patient should be monitored regularly.

Teaching Points for Skeletal Muscle Relaxant Therapy

Health Promotion Strategies

Prior to prescribing SMR therapy, the primary care provider should discuss risks and benefits as part of the shared decision-making process. The patient should be aware that when SMR therapy is used for an acute condition, it should be taken as needed rather than routinely, which minimizes the side effects. Educate the patient on the additive effects of SMRs when used in combination with other CNS depressants, such as alcohol, opioids, sedating medications, antiepileptics, cannabis, and illicit drugs. The sedative effects of the SMR may be enhanced if used with other medications known to produce drowsiness, such as psychiatric drugs and cold and allergy medications.

Patient Education for Medication Safety

Antispasmodic SMR therapy is helpful in the short-term treatment of acute back and neck pain and localized muscle strain or spasm. Antispastic SMR therapy is more often used as a long-term treatment for spasticity as well as in many neurological conditions and CNS diseases. Teaching the patient why the medication is being used will help with adherence to therapy. The provider should encourage safe administration of the medication by emphasizing the following key points:

- Keep in mind that SMR therapy may cause mental and/or physical impairment, which may negatively affect the performance of daily activities of living and hazardous tasks such as driving a motor vehicle or operating machinery.
- Tell your primary care provider about your medication allergies and all medicines you are taking. This includes prescription medications, over-the-counter (OTC) products, herbal supplements, cannabis, and illicit drugs.
- Get emergency medical help if you exhibit signs of an allergic reaction, such as hives, difficulty breathing, or swelling of your face, lips, tongue, or throat.
- Call or visit your primary care provider immediately if you notice any behavioral changes, hallucinations, and/or psychiatric symptoms.

There are specific educational considerations for each individual medication. It is advisable to review the details of the medication and discuss the indications and adverse reactions with the patient prior to prescribing.

Application Questions for Discussion

1. Are there age-related considerations when prescribing SMR therapy?
2. What is the most common side effect for all SMR medications?
3. As a health care provider, what key points should be emphasized in the education plan for a patient and/or the caregiver of a patient who has been prescribed SMRs?

Selected Bibliography

2019 American Geriatrics Society Beers Criteria® Update Expert Panel. Fick, D. M., Semla, T. P., Steinman, M., Beizer, J., Brandt, N., … & Flanagan, N. (2019). American Geriatrics Society 2019 updated AGS Beers Criteria® for potentially inappropriate medication use in older adults. *Journal of the American Geriatrics Society, 67*(4), 674–694. https://doi.org/10.1111/jgs.15767.

Alvarez, C. A., Mortensen, E. M., Makris, U. E., Berlowitz, D. R., Copeland, L. A., Good, C. B., … & Pugh, M. J. V. (2015). Association of skeletal muscle relaxers and antihistamines on mortality, hospitalizations, and emergency department visits in elderly patients: A nationwide retrospective cohort study. *BMC Geriatrics, 15*(1), 2. https://doi.org/10.1186/1471-2318-15-2.

Bass, B., Weinshenker, B., Rice, G. P. A., Noseworthy, J. H., Cameron, M. G. P., Hader, W., … & Ebers, G. C. (1988). Tizanidine versus baclofen in the treatment of spasticity in patients with multiple sclerosis. *Canadian Journal of Neurological Sciences, 15*(1), 15–19. https://doi.org/10.1017/S0317167100027104.

Emrich, O. M., Milachowski, K. A., & Strohmeier, M. (2015). Methocarbamol in acute low back pain. A randomized double-blind controlled study. *MMW Fortschritte der Medizin, 157*, 9–16. https://doi.org/10.1007/s15006-015-3307-x.

Hauk, L. (2017). Low back pain: American College of Physicians practice guideline on noninvasive treatments. *American Family Physician, 96*(6), 407–408.

Katzung, B. G. (2018). *Basic and Clinical Pharmacology* (14th ed.). New York: McGraw Hill Education.

Otero-Romero, S., Sastre-Garriga, J., Comi, G., Hartung, H. P., Soelberg Sørensen, P., Thompson, A. J., … & Montalban, X. (2016). Pharmacological management of spasticity in multiple sclerosis: Systematic review and consensus paper. *Multiple Sclerosis Journal, 22*(11), 1386–1396. https://doi.org/10.11772/F1352458516643600.

Qaseem, A., Wilt, T. J., McLean, R. M., & Forciea, M. A. (2017). Noninvasive treatments for acute, subacute, and chronic low back pain: A clinical practice guideline from the American College of Physicians. *Annals of Internal Medicine, 166*(7), 514–530. https://doi.org/10.7326/M16-2367.

Roblin, D. W., Liu, H., Cromwell, L. F., Robbins, M., Robinson, B. E., Auerbach, D., & Mehrotra, A. (2017). Provider Type and Management of Common Visits in Primary Care. *The American Journal of Managed Care, 23*(4), 225–231.

Schreijenberg, M., Koes, B. W., & Lin, C. W. C. (2019). Guideline recommendations on the pharmacological management of nonspecific low back pain in primary care—is there a need to change? *Expert Review of Clinical Pharmacology, 12*(2), 145–157. https://doi.org/10.1080/17512433.2019.1565992.

Shah, M. U. (2016). "Neuromuscular Blocking Agents and Skeletal Muscle Relaxants." In *Side Effects of Drugs Annual* (Vol. 38. pp. 105–113): Elsevier. https://doi.org/10.1016/bs.seda.2016.07.012.

27

Migraine Headache Medications

CONSTANCE G. VISOVSKY

Overview

Migraine headaches are a common neurological disorder that occurs in about 18% of females, 6% of males, and 10% of children in the United States. Migraine headaches are most commonly present in adults 25 to 55 years of age (Boss & Huether, 2019; Gilmore & Michael, 2011). Migraines can be classified as *migraine with aura* (visual, sensory, or motor symptoms), *migraine without aura*, or *chronic migraine*.

Migraine headaches are diagnosed when at least two of the following features are present—unilateral head pain, throbbing pain, or pain that worsens with physical activity—and at least one of the following symptoms is present: nausea/vomiting, photophobia, or intolerance to loud noise. Imaging and electroencephalogram (EEG) can be used to confirm the diagnosis. Treatment strategies for patients with migraine headache fall into two categories: preventive therapies and treatment of acute migraine. Preventive therapies aim to reduce the frequency and severity of migraine headache, while acute treatments aim to stop a migraine headache attack already in progress (Table 27.1).

Relevant Physiology

Under normal conditions, total blood flow to the brain remains constant at approximately 750 mL/min, or 15% of the cardiac output. The heart pumps blood up to the brain through two sets of arteries: the carotid arteries and the vertebral arteries. Receptors control blood flow in the brain, so under normal conditions there is no excess dilation or abnormal vasoconstriction. Both neuronal and chemical changes autoregulate cerebral blood flow.

All neuronal tissues have a high metabolic demand that requires coordination between neuronal activity and blood flow within the brain parenchyma. *Autoregulation* is a process that results from the ability of an organism to adapt to stimuli. In cerebral blood flow, autoregulation permits the brain to maintain relatively constant blood flow despite changes in perfusion pressure. The exact mechanisms that underlie autoregulation of blood flow in the brain are not completely understood. It is believed that nitric acid and byproducts of metabolism may have a role in cerebral autoregulation. The supratentorial dura mater membrane is supplied by small meningeal branches of the trigeminal nerve (V1, V2, and V3). Sensory stimulation from the periphery can also stimulate blood vessels in the brain. An interaction between trigeminal nerve paths and the vascular system within the brain is seen with patients who have migraine headache. There are several known or suspected pathways for migraine pain that are abnormal, and some may be more common in patients with a familial pattern of migraines.

Pathophysiology

The pathophysiology underlying migraine headache is not fully understood. In human models of migraine development, a number of signaling pathways involving the trigeminal vascular system, cortical spreading depression, central and peripheral pain, and neuropeptide receptors have been implicated. Nitric oxide released from endothelial cells stimulates cyclic guanosine monophosphate (cGMP) synthesis, resulting in relaxation of smooth muscle and vasodilation. Studies show that cGMP accumulation can induce a migraine attack. A nitric oxide mechanism is also involved in stimulating the release of histamine, which is implicated in migraine development.

A spontaneous wave of glial and neuronal depolarization induces hyperactivity, beginning in the occipital area and spreading across the cortex. This action initiates migraine by stimulating the release of neurotransmitters, stimulating vasodilation of blood vessels in the dura, activating inflammation in the peripheral and central pain receptors. *Neuropeptides* are neurotransmitters released from nerve fibers that innervate intracranial blood vessels and play a role in migraine development. The neuropeptide calcitonin gene-related peptide (CGRP) is a strong vasodilator; elevated levels of CGRP have been found in 75% of patients experiencing migraine without aura and in 57% of patients experiencing migraine with aura (Ashina et al., 2017).

TABLE 27.1   Characteristics of Migraine Headache

	Migraine With Aura	Migraine Without Aura
Age	From childhood to middle-aged adult	From childhood to middle-aged adult
Gender	Higher prevalence in females	Higher prevalence in females
Family history	Yes	Yes
Onset	Slow to rapid onset	Slow to rapid onset
Timing	Intermittent	Intermittent
Quality	Throbbing	Throbbing
Location	Unilateral to bilateral	Unilateral to bilateral
Characteristics	Visual, sensory, or motor disturbance	Nausea/vomiting

Adapted from Boss, B., & Huether, S. [2019]. Disorders of the central and peripheral nervous system. In McCance & Huether (Eds.), *Pathophysiology: The biologic basis for disease in adults and children* (8th ed.). St. Louis: Elsevier.

Migraine-specific triggers induce brain stem center dysfunction, leading to dilation of cranial blood vessels innervated by sensory fibers of the trigeminal nerve. Prostaglandins work to mediate pain by stimulating nociceptors of sensory nerves. Prostaglandins also have vasodilation properties. Prostaglandin D_2, prostaglandin I_2, and prostaglandin E_2 have been shown to induce headache in healthy persons. Finally, the brain stem and spinal cord centers receiving the pain impulses from the trigeminal nerve become sensitized, worsening headache pain and increasing sensitivity to light and sound (Durham, 2006; Ashina et al., 2017). Migraine headaches have been shown to have a definitive genetic component. Familial patterns of CGRP and vasoactive peptides have been noted in persons with migraines with aura. A rare genetic disorder known as *familial hemiplegic migraine* (FHM) is an inherited migraine subtype characterized by hemiplegia during the aura phase. In a 2016 meta-analysis, a 22 genome-wide association of more than 59,000 patients identified that a single nucleotide polymorphism (SNP) in 38 genomic loci had significant association with risk for migraine (Gormley et al., 2016).

Migraine headaches are categorized into four phases. In the *premonitory phase,* one-third of individuals report having symptoms hours to days before the onset of a migraine headache. These premonitory symptoms include tiredness, difficulty concentrating, irritability, and food cravings. In the *migraine aura phase*, visual, motor, or sensory symptoms are present. In the *headache phase*, throbbing head pain begins, first unilaterally and then spreading to bilateral involvement. The headache phase may also include symptoms of nausea, vomiting, fatigue, and dizziness lasting 4 to 72 hours. Lastly, in the *recovery phase*, any symptoms that are still present begin to resolve, which can take hours to days to reach complete relief (Boss & Huether, 2019; Table 27.2).

While this text will concentrate on pharmacologic treatments for migraine headache, other strategies such as avoidance of known migraine triggers are important to convey to

TABLE 27.2   Phases of Migraine Headache

Phase	Symptoms
Premonitory phase	Tiredness, difficulty concentrating, irritability, and food cravings
Migraine aura phase	Visual, motor, or sensory symptoms
Headache phase	Unilateral to bilateral throbbing head pain, nausea, vomiting, fatigue, and dizziness lasting 4–72 hours
Recovery phase	Symptoms begin to resolve (hours to days)

patients diagnosed with migraines. Evidence-based preventive pharmacologic and nonpharmacologic therapies can be recommended depending on the frequency and severity of migraine headaches obtained from the patient history. Both a transcutaneous electrical neurostimulation device and botulism toxin A have been approved for the prevention of chronic migraine headache. Sleeping in a darkened room and applying ice to the head can provide a degree of relief from acute migraine.

PRACTICE PEARLS

Clinical Features of Pediatric Migraine Variants

- Normal neurological exam
- Occurs periodically
- Clinically evolves into classic migraine types
- Variants include abdominal migraine, benign paroxysmal vertigo, cyclic vomiting, and paroxysmal torticollis
- Vestibular migraine is the most common cause of vertigo in children

Migraine Headache Therapy

Acute Migraine Treatment

Serotonin-Receptor 1$_B$ and 1$_D$ Agonists (a.k.a. Triptans)

Selective serotonin agonists, also known as *triptans*, are indicated as first-line treatment of moderate to severe acute migraines and for mild migraines resistant to nonsteroidal antiinflammatory drugs (NSAIDs) or other combination analgesics. Most triptan medications are administered orally, but several are available in intranasal formulations (e.g., sumatriptan and zolmitriptan); sumatriptan also can be administered subcutaneously. Triptans are contraindicated in patients with coronary artery disease (CAD), peripheral vascular disease, cerebrovascular disease, and uncontrolled hypertension because of their propensity to cause vasoconstriction. They are also contraindicated for use in patients with basilar or hemiplegic migraine. Triptan medications are available in several formulations that share similar side-effect profiles. Individualizing migraine treatment with triptans includes consideration of the best evidence, patient preference, characteristics of the patient's migraine attacks, and patient sensitivity to side effects. For example, while subcutaneous sumatriptan has the fewest number of doses to a 2-hour pain-free treatment interval, most patients will prefer an oral formulation. Two-hour pain-free rates are best for eletriptan 40-mg and rizatriptan 10-mg doses, while almotriptan and naratriptan have the lowest rates of adverse effects. Patients allergic to sulfonamides would be prescribed rizatriptan, frovatriptan, or zolmitriptan as these agents do not have sulfa as part of their formulation. There is little evidence for the use of opioids in the treatment of acute migraine. Opioid preparations are linked to a high incidence of adverse events and a risk of addiction tolerance and withdrawal.

Sumatriptan

Sumatriptan can be used for the treatment of acute migraine headaches that occur with or without aura. Sumatriptan is not indicated for long-term prevention of migraines. This medication can be administered orally, subcutaneously, or intranasally. Sumatriptan is the only triptan available for subcutaneous injection. Sumatriptan stimulates presynaptic 5-HT$_1$D receptors, inhibiting both dural vasodilation and inflammation. It directly inhibits trigeminal nociceptive neurotransmission within the trigeminocervical complex of the brain stem and upper spinal cord. The vascular 5-HT$_1$B receptor agonist effects result in vasoconstriction of dilated intracranial blood vessels.

Pharmacokinetics. Sumatriptan is widely distributed throughout the body. Protein binding ranges from 14% to 21%. Approximately 80% of any dose is metabolized by the liver. Once it is metabolized, an inactive metabolite and its glucuronide conjugate are produced. Renal clearance is by tubular secretion and glomerular filtration. The elimination half-life of sumatriptan is approximately 2 hours.

Indications. Sumatriptan is indicated for the treatment of moderate to severe migraine with or without aura. It is not indicated for hemiplegic or basilar migraine.

Adverse Effects. Serious cardiac adverse events may occur during sumatriptan administration and are more likely to occur in patients with risk factors for CAD. These include cerebrovascular events and even death secondary to vasospasm. Abdominal aortic aneurysm, angina, and transient myocardial ischemia are rare, occurring in fewer than 0.1% of patients, but they have been reported. Life-threatening arrhythmias, including ventricular tachycardia and ventricular fibrillation leading to death, have been reported within a few hours following administration of 5-HT1 agonists.

Contraindications. Sumatriptan may cause coronary vasospasm and is contraindicated in patients with known or suspected CAD, angina, vasospastic angina such as Prinzmetal's variant angina (PVA), arteriosclerosis, silent myocardial ischemia, acute myocardial infarction, history of myocardial infarction, and uncontrolled hypertension. Patients with CAD risk factors (e.g., high blood pressure, diabetes, hypercholesterolemia) should not be given sumatriptan without a cardiac evaluation. The sumatriptan iontophoretic transdermal system should not be applied in areas near or over electrically active implantable or other medical devices (e.g., implantable cardiac pacemaker, body-worn insulin pump, implantable deep brain stimulator). The needle shield of the prefilled syringe contains dry natural rubber (a latex derivative) and may cause allergic reactions in patients with latex hypersensitivity.

Monitoring. Laboratory monitoring is not needed. However, the primary care provider should review the patient's medical history at each medication renewal to determine whether any new-onset risk factors or signs and symptoms of CAD and cerebrovascular disease are present.

PRACTICE PEARLS

Triptan Use in Pregnancy and Lactation

- The incidence of major birth defects during any trimester exposure was 4.2%.
- There are no adequate studies of pregnant patients taking almotriptan, and it is not known whether this medication crosses the placenta.
- Triptans are excreted in breast milk. Avoid breastfeeding 12 hours after migraine treatment, or express breast milk and discard it up to 8 hours after a treatment dose to minimize exposure.

Zolmitriptan

Zolmitriptan is used to treat acute migraine headache occurring with or without aura. Zolmitriptan has actions similar to those of sumatriptan, but unlike sumatriptan, zolmitriptan can penetrate the blood–brain barrier to act centrally within the trigeminovascular system. Zolmitriptan is available in an oral preparation, in an oral disintegrating tablet, and as an intranasal spray.

Pharmacokinetics. Zolmitriptan's peak plasma concentration occurs in 2 hours. The mean absolute bioavailability is approximately 40%; food has no effect on bioavailability. Zolmitriptan is metabolized by cytochrome (CYP) 1A2 and CYP 3A to one *active* N-desmethyl metabolite and two *inactive* metabolites: an acetic acid metabolite and an N-oxide metabolite. The active metabolite is about two to six times more potent than the parent compound and contributes to the overall effects of zolmitriptan. One-sixth of the total plasma clearance is through the kidneys. The mean elimination half-life of zolmitriptan and the active N-desmethyl metabolite is 3 hours.

Indications. Zolmitriptan is indicated for the treatment of moderate to severe migraine with or without aura. It is not indicated for hemiplegic or basilar migraine.

Adverse Effects. Zolmitriptan may cause coronary vasospasm or ischemia. Rare but serious cardiac events include coronary vasospasm, ventricular tachycardia, ventricular fibrillation, abdominal aortic aneurysm, angina, transient myocardial ischemia, myocardial infarction, cardiac arrest, and death. These events have been reported primarily in patients with risk factors for CAD.

Adverse gastrointestinal (GI) effects were reported in at least 2% of patients receiving zolmitriptan. Xerostomia (3% to 5%), dyspepsia (1% to 3%), and nausea (4%) were also reported. Dysgeusia (unusual taste) was frequently reported. Adverse events suggestive of GI vasospastic events, such as ischemic colitis, GI infarction, splenic rupture (infarction), and bowel necrosis, have been rarely reported.

Contraindications. Zolmitriptan is contraindicated in patients with known ischemic bowel disease and in patients with uncontrolled hypertension.

Monitoring. Patients who experience signs or symptoms suggestive of ischemic bowel syndrome (cramping, abdominal pain, bloody diarrhea) should be further evaluated. Patients with coronary disease risk factors should have an electrocardiogram (ECG) prior to and throughout therapy.

Almotriptan

Almotriptan is administered orally and acts therapeutically as an agonist at central serotonin 5-HT$_1$ type B and D receptors. By stimulating 5-HT$_1$D receptors, both dural vasodilation and inflammation are inhibited. They directly inhibit trigeminal nuclei cell nociceptive neurotransmission via 5-HT$_1$B/D receptor agonism within the trigeminocervical complex of the brain stem and upper spinal cord.

Pharmacokinetics. Almotriptan is well absorbed, with a bioavailability of approximately 70% and reaching peak plasma levels in 1 to 3 hours. It is metabolized by the monoamine oxidase (MAO) mediated pathway and by CYP P450. The mean elimination half-life of almotriptan is 3 to 4 hours. Almotriptan is primarily eliminated by the kidneys (75%), and 40% of the dose is excreted unchanged in the urine while approximately 13% is excreted in the feces.

Indications. Almotriptan is indicated for the treatment of moderate to severe migraine with or without aura. It is not indicated for migraine headache prevention or for hemiplegic or basilar migraine.

Adverse Events. Increases in blood pressure have been associated with significant clinical events in rare instances. Adverse cardiovascular effects reported in about 1% of patients include flushing, palpitations, chest pain, and sinus tachycardia. Acute myocardial infarction, coronary vasospasm, angina pectoris, and sinus tachycardia have been reported. Common GI adverse events associated with almotriptan therapy (6.25–12.5 mg) included nausea (1% to 2%) and dry mouth or xerostomia (1%). In pediatric patients 12 to 17 years of age, nausea (1% to 3%) and vomiting (2%) were reported. Almotriptan may cause vasospastic reactions including GI vascular ischemia. Other GI adverse effects including cramping, bowel ischemia, and ischemic colitis have been reported following administration of almotriptan. Patients who experience signs or symptoms suggestive of ischemic bowel syndrome (e.g., cramping, abdominal pain, bloody diarrhea) should be further evaluated. Overuse of drugs for treating acute migraines may lead to headache exacerbation (medication overuse headache).

Serotonin syndrome may occur with serotonin receptor agonists such as almotriptan, especially with concurrent use of selective serotonin reuptake inhibitors (SSRIs) or serotonin norepinephrine reuptake inhibitors (SNRIs). Symptoms of serotonin syndrome may include agitation or restlessness, muscle rigidity, headache, tremors, nausea, vomiting or diarrhea, sweating, hyperthermia, high blood pressure, and rapid heart rate.

Contraindications. Almotriptan is contraindicated in patients with known ischemic bowel disease.

Monitoring. Patients with coronary disease risk factors should have an ECG prior to and throughout therapy. The exact timing for ECG monitoring throughout therapy has not been established and can vary among patients. Patients who experience signs or symptoms suggestive of ischemic bowel syndrome (cramping, abdominal pain, bloody diarrhea) should be further evaluated.

PRACTICE PEARLS

Serotonin Receptor Agonists and Cardiac Events

- Patients with CAD risk factors should have a cardiac evaluation prior to beginning a serotonin receptor agonist.
- Patients who are long-term users of serotonin receptor agonists and who acquire risk factors predictive of CAD should undergo periodic cardiac evaluation.
- For patients with risk factors predictive of CAD who have had a satisfactory cardiac evaluation, the first dose of a serotonin receptor agonist should be given in a controlled setting such as a clinic or medical office. ECG monitoring is recommended due to possible asymptomatic cardiac ischemia during the time immediately following administration in patients with risk factors.

Eletriptan

Eletriptan is a central serotonin 5-HT 1_B, 1_D, and 1_F receptor agonist. All triptan medications stimulate HT_{1D} receptors, inhibiting both dural vasodilation and inflammation and directly inhibiting trigeminal nuclei cell nociceptive neurotransmission via 5-$HT_{1B/D}$ receptors within the trigeminocervical complex of the brain stem and upper spinal cord.

Pharmacokinetics. Eletriptan is administered orally and is rapidly absorbed. It is metabolized primarily by the CYP P450 hepatic enzyme 3A4. Eletriptan has a bioavailability of 50% compared to sumatriptan at 15%, accounting for the faster absorption and more rapid onset of action. The parent compound is converted to an active metabolite, with a half-life of 13 hours. Ten percent of the medication is cleared by the kidneys. When taken with a high-fat meal, eletriptan's area under the curve (AUC) and maximum peak serum concentration (Cmax) increases 20% to 30%, and can be higher in patients with moderate hepatic impairment. The time to peak plasma concentration is 1.5 hours.

Indications. Eletriptan is indicated for the treatment of moderate to severe migraine with or without aura.

Adverse Effects. Life-threatening disturbances of cardiac rhythm, including ventricular tachycardia and ventricular fibrillation leading to death, have been reported within a few hours following the administration of 5-HT1 agonists. Serious cardiac events include coronary vasospasm, transient myocardial ischemia, myocardial infarction, and atrial fibrillation. These events are rare and have been reported primarily in patients with risk factors for CAD.

GI adverse effects are dose related and include xerostomia (24% of patients), dyspepsia (1% to 2%), dysphagia (1% to 2%), nausea (4% to 8%), and abdominal pain/discomfort/stomach pain/cramps/pressure sensations (1% to 2%). Due to a higher incidence of adverse events, an 80-mg dose of eletriptan is not recommended. Vasospastic effects associated with eletriptan include peripheral vascular ischemia and bowel ischemia. Stomach pain, bloody diarrhea, and cramping have been associated with ischemic colitis and can occur with a median time to onset of 48 hours. Serotonin syndrome has been reported during administration of eletriptan. Serotonin syndrome may occur particularly during concurrent use of serotonergic agents such as SSRIs or SNRIs. Dermatologic effects observed in fewer than 1% of patients include pruritus and rash. Anaphylaxis and hypersensitivity reactions have been reported in patients taking eletriptan. Such reactions are more likely to occur in patients with a history of sensitivity to multiple allergens. Increased alkaline phosphatase and creatinine phosphokinase have been reported.

Contraindications. Eletriptan is contraindicated for patients with moderate to severe hepatic impairment. Eletriptan should not be used within 24 hours of an ergot-based medication or 72 hours of treatment with any known potent CYP 3A4 inhibitors.

Monitoring. Patients who experience signs or symptoms suggestive of decreased arterial flow, such as ischemic bowel syndrome, while receiving eletriptan should be further evaluated. Patients with coronary disease risk factors should have an ECG prior to and throughout therapy. Monitor liver function tests (LFTs).

Frovatriptan

Frovatriptan is a selective agonist of vascular serotonin, specifically of 5-hydroxytryptamine 1_B/1_D (5-HT_{1B}/$_D$) receptors. This action inhibits dural vasodilation and directly inhibits trigeminal nuclei cell nociceptive neurotransmission via receptor agonism within the trigeminocervical complex of the brain stem and upper spinal cord. Second-generation triptans such as zolmitriptan and rizatriptan are less likely to aggravate the coronary 5-HT_{1B} receptor than sumatriptan, which should reduce the incidence of chest pain or other cardiac effects in patients with normal coronary circulation, but these events are still possible.

Pharmacokinetics. Frovatriptan is administered orally and has a relatively low bioavailability. Peak plasma levels are achieved 2 to 4 hours after oral administration, and the half-life of this medication is 26 hours. Frovatriptan is primarily metabolized by CYP P450 1A2. Unlike most other 5-HT1 agonists, it is not an inhibitor of MAO or hepatic CYP P450. Significant interactions with CYP 1A2 inhibitors are not likely because of a wide therapeutic range and partial renal elimination.

Indications. Frovatriptan is indicated for the treatment of moderate to severe migraine with or without aura. It is not indicated for migraine headache prevention or for hemiplegic or basilar migraine.

Adverse Events. As with other serotonin agonists, frovatriptan may cause coronary or cerebral vasospasm, although the risk is lower with this medication. Life-threatening arrhythmias, including ventricular tachycardia and ventricular fibrillation leading to death, can occur within a few hours of administration. Significant increases in blood pressure occurred after single doses of 80-mg frovatriptan; however, the rise in blood pressure was transient and not clinically significant. GI effects such as xerostomia, dyspepsia, nausea/vomiting, and diarrhea have been reported in 1% to 3% of patients. Serotonin syndrome may occur with serotonin receptor agonists such as frovatriptan, particularly during concurrent use of serotonergic agents such as SSRIs or SNRIs.

Contraindications. Frovatriptan is contraindicated in patients with uncontrolled hypertension. Frovatriptan, like other 5-HT agonists, may cause coronary vasospasm, and therefore is contraindicated in patients with CAD, angina, Prinzmetal's variant angina, arteriosclerosis, silent myocardial ischemia, history of myocardial infarction, acute myocardial infarction, or other significant cardiac disease.

Monitoring. Patients with coronary disease risk factors should have an ECG prior to and throughout therapy.

Naratriptan

Naratriptan is a potent agonist at serotonin 5-HT_{1B} and 5HD_{1D} receptors. Stimulation of HT_{1D} receptors inhibits both dural vasodilation and inflammation, and it directly inhibits trigeminal nuclei cell nociceptive neurotransmission via $5\text{-HT}_{1B/D}$ receptors within the trigeminocervical complex of the brain stem and upper spinal cord.

Pharmacokinetics. Naratriptan is administered orally and is well absorbed after administration, with peak plasma levels occurring in 2 to 3 hours. It is metabolized by various CYP P450 isozymes into several inactive metabolites. Naratriptan does not inhibit MAO and is not a significant inhibitor of CYP P450. It is eliminated by the kidneys, with 50% being excreted unchanged and 30% as metabolites. The mean half-life of naratriptan is 6 hours.

Indications. Naratriptan is indicated for the treatment of moderate to severe migraine with or without aura. It is not indicated for migraine headache prevention or for hemiplegic or basilar migraine.

Adverse Events. Life-threatening disturbances of cardiac rhythm, including ventricular tachycardia and ventricular fibrillation leading to death, have been reported within a few hours following the administration of 5-HT1 agonists. Serious cardiac events include coronary vasospasm, transient myocardial ischemia, myocardial infarction, and atrial fibrillation. These events are rare and have been reported primarily in patients with risk factors for CAD. Anaphylaxis and hypersensitivity reactions, including angioedema, have been reported.

GI symptoms were reported in 2% to 7% of patients and included nausea, dyspepsia, diarrhea, constipation, and GI discomfort. Ischemic colitis has been reported and may be associated with cramping, abdominal pain, and bloody diarrhea, with a median time to onset of 48 hours following administration. Naratriptan can cause dizziness or drowsiness.

Contraindications. Naratriptan is contraindicated in patients with a history of hypersensitivity reaction to naratriptan. Naratriptan is contraindicated in patients with Wolff-Parkinson-White syndrome or cardiac arrhythmias associated with conduction pathway disorders. Patients with CAD risk factors should not be prescribed naratriptan without a thorough cardiac evaluation prior to taking naratriptan, and routinely during long-term therapy.

Monitoring. Patients with coronary disease risk factors should have an ECG prior to and routinely throughout therapy based on patient-specific risk factors and medical history.

Rizatriptan

Rizatriptan is a selective 5-hydroxytryptamine $1_B/1_D$ receptor agonist. It has very weak activity at other 5-HT receptors, and no activity at alpha, beta, dopaminergic, histaminergic, muscarinic, or benzodiazepine receptors. Rizatriptan inhibits both dural vasodilation and inflammation, and directly inhibits trigeminal nuclei cell nociceptive neurotransmission via $5\text{-HT}_{1B/D}$ receptors within the trigeminocervical complex of the brain stem and upper spinal cord. Rizatriptan activation of coronary 5-HT_{1B} receptors could result in clinically significant cardiac events in patients with cardiac disease or risk factors for cardiac disease. However, the cardiac effects of rizatriptan appear to be less frequent.

Pharmacokinetics. Rizatriptan is administered orally as a tablet and as a disintegrating tablet. This medication has a high level of bioavailability. The time to peak serum concentration is 1 to 2 hours. Rizatriptan is metabolized via oxidative deamination by monoamine oxidase-A (MAO-A). Rizatriptan undergoes significant first-pass metabolism, with 14% of the dose excreted as unchanged drug and 51% excreted as an inactive metabolite. The half-life of rizatriptan is 2 to 3 hours. Rizatriptan is a competitive inhibitor of CYP P450 2D6 at high dosages.

Indications. Rizatriptan is indicated for the treatment of moderate to severe migraine with or without aura. It is not indicated for migraine headache prevention or for hemiplegic or basilar migraine.

Adverse Events. Dose-related central nervous system (CNS) effects such as dizziness and drowsiness (4% to 9% of patients) have been reported. Rarer CNS effects such as vertigo, insomnia, ataxia gait abnormality, and hyperesthesia were noted in 0.1% to 1% of patients. Euphoria has been observed in at least 1% of patients receiving rizatriptan. Other psychiatric effects reported include nervousness, anxiety, depression, disorientation, confusion, irritability, memory impairment, and agitation (0.1% to 1%), but the cause in relation to rizatriptan is unknown.

Serotonin syndrome may occur with serotonin receptor agonists, particularly during concurrent use of serotonergic agents such as SSRIs or SNRIs. Chest pressure syndrome with symptoms of chest pain, tightness, heaviness, and jaw pain has been reported. Serious adverse cardiac events, including myocardial ischemia and myocardial infarction, can occur within a few hours following the administration of rizatriptan, but these are extremely rare and have been primarily reported in patients with risk factors predictive of CAD. Cerebral ischemia, increased intracranial pressure, cerebral hemorrhage or intracranial bleeding, subarachnoid hemorrhage, and stroke are among the reported events associated with rizatriptan and other 5-HT1 agonists. Other rare effects such as dyspnea, flushing, dermatologic effects, and hypersensitivity reactions were reported in 1% of patients receiving rizatriptan.

Contraindications. Rizatriptan should be given cautiously to patients with peripheral vascular disease including Raynaud's phenomenon or colitis due to the vasospastic reactions that can lead to ischemia. Rizatriptan and other 5-HT agonists may cause coronary vasospasm and therefore are contraindicated in patients with CAD, angina, Prinzmetal's variant angina, arteriosclerosis, myocardial infarction, or other significant cardiac disease. Patients with CAD risk factors should not be prescribed rizatriptan without a thorough cardiac evaluation prior to and routinely during long-term therapy. For patients with risk factors predictive of CAD and with a satisfactory cardiac evaluation, the first dose of rizatriptan should be given in a controlled setting such as a clinic or physician's office. ECG monitoring is strongly encouraged due to the possibility of asymptomatic cardiac ischemia during the time immediately following rizatriptan administration in patients with risk factors. Rizatriptan is

TABLE 27.3	Triptan Safety Issues						
Safety Issue	Sumatriptan	Zolmitriptan	Almotriptan	Eletriptan	Frovatriptan	Naratriptan	Rizatriptan
MI	X	X		X	X	X	X
Angina	X	X	X	X	X	X	X
Arteriosclerosis	X	X		X	X	X	X
Cardiac disease	X	X	X	X	X	X	X
Cerebrovascular disease	X	X	X	X	X	X	
CAD	X	X	X	X	X	X	X
Hepatic disease	X					X	
Hypertension	X	X		X	X		X
MAOI therapy	X	X				X	X
PVD	X	X	X	X	X	X	
Renal failure						X	
Stroke	X	X	X	X	X	X	
Hypersensitivity	X						
Vasospastic angina	X	X	X	X	X	X	X
Wolff-Parkinson-White syndrome	X			X	X	X	

CAD, Coronary artery disease; MAOI, monoamine oxidase inhibitor; MI, myocardial infarction; PVD, peripheral vascular disease.
From Elsevier. Clinical pharmacology powered by ClinicalKey®. [2019]. http://www.clinicalkey.com.

also contraindicated in patients with uncontrolled hypertension. Rizatriptan should be used with extreme caution in patients with cerebrovascular and renal disease. Rizatriptan is contraindicated in patients concurrently receiving or recently discontinuing MAOI agents. Patients with phenylketonuria should be warned that Maxalt-MLT® (rizatriptan) disintegrating tablets contain phenylalanine.

Monitoring. Patients with coronary disease risk factors should have an ECG prior to and throughout therapy (Table 27.3).

Preventive Migraine Treatment

The rationale for the preventive treatment of migraine headaches is to reduce the frequency, severity, and duration of the headache in patients who have four or more migraine headaches per month. Although preventive treatments may be prescribed, patients may not adhere to a preventive regimen (Hepp et al., 2015). Females of childbearing age prescribed preventive migraine medication will require education concerning the potential for fetal teratogenicity associated with these agents and the need for careful birth control. Preventive agents such as topiramate, valproic acid, propranolol, and timolol can be useful in some patients. Medications with off-label indications for migraine prevention will not be covered in this text, as the level of evidence to support their use is low to very low. Gabapentin as a preventive agent has conflicting data supporting its efficacy in migraine prevention. According to *Clinical Pharmacology*, the evidence for use of metoprolol, amitriptyline, riboflavin, and coenzyme Q10 is low, and therefore not recommended. Candesartan and lisinopril are classified as Level C (possibly effective) agents in migraine prevention. Oral ergotamine, while approved for migraine prevention, is seldom used due to its poor bioavailability, side effects (nausea), and lower efficacy as compared to the triptans.

PRACTICE PEARLS
Use of Preventive Migraine Medications

- Begin with the lowest possible dose; slowly titrate upward until efficacy or target dose is reached.
- A 2- to 3-month trial is needed to determine the efficacy of treatment. Consider that a 6-month period may be needed to see maximal response.
- Discuss the need for family planning in females of childbearing age to avoid adverse effects on the fetus of migraine medications.
- Discuss potential adverse effects that may occur. Some adverse events can be dose related and self-limiting.

TABLE 27.4	Migraine Triggers		
Foods	**Environment**	**Medications**	**Other**
Aged cheese	Travel	Antihypertensives	Sleep disturbance
Wine	Flashing, bright, or fluorescent lights	Oral contraceptives	Caffeine withdrawal
Chocolate	Weather changes	Antibiotics	Fasting
Nuts	Strong odors	Nitrates	Menopause
Caffeine	Pollution	HRT	Menstruation
MSG	High altitude	SSRIs	Stress
Aspartame	Barometric changes	Vasodilators	Inflammation

HRT, Hormone replacement therapy; *MSG*, Monosodium glutamate; *SSRIs*, selective serotonin reuptake inhibitors.

Nonpharmacologic preventive treatments include avoidance of potential migraine triggers. Behavioral therapies such as biofeedback and cognitive behavioral therapy are also helpful for those who cannot tolerate medication or who are pregnant or lactating (Table 27.4).

Anticonvulsants

Topiramate

Several of the effects of topiramate are thought to provide prophylaxis of migraines. Migraines are characterized by neuronal hyperexcitability involving several receptors and ion channels at the cerebral cortex, the trigeminovascular system, and brain stem nuclei. Topiramate inhibits the excitatory effect of glutamate and voltage-gated sodium channels and subtypes of the enzyme carbonic anhydrase–reducing cortical hyperexcitability. These effects result in reduction of cortical spreading depression, glutamatergic signaling by trigeminal afferent nerves, or modulating nociceptive signaling through gamma-aminobutyric acid (GABA) receptors in the trigeminal nucleus.

Pharmacokinetics. Administered orally, topiramate is absorbed rapidly, with peak plasma concentrations occurring 2 hours after administration of the immediate-release tablet and 24 hours following a 200-mg dose of extended-release capsules. Seventy percent of the dose is eliminated unchanged in the urine. Elimination half-life is 21 hours, with a steady state reached in 4 to 8 days. Topiramate pharmacokinetics may be affected by both renal and hepatic impairment, reducing clearance.

Indications. Topiramate is indicated for migraine prophylaxis.

Adverse Effects. CNS effects such as paresthesia, dizziness, hypoesthesia, involuntary movements/muscle contractions, ataxia, speech problems such as dysarthria, drowsiness, depression, agitation, and insomnia have been reported, and may be dose related.

In January 2008, the U.S. Food and Drug Administration (FDA) alerted health care professionals of an increased risk of suicidal ideation and behavior in patients receiving anticonvulsants to treat epilepsy, psychiatric disorders, or migraine. An analysis by the FDA showed that patients receiving anticonvulsants had approximately twice the risk of suicidal behavior or ideation compared with those receiving placebo between 1 and 24 weeks after therapy initiation.

GI effects such as nausea, diarrhea, abdominal pain, constipation, dyspepsia, xerostomia, vomiting, dysgeusia, taste changes, anorexia, and gastroenteritis have occurred. Increased serum ammonia levels higher than 50% of normal can occur without encephalopathy and may be dose related. Topiramate is associated with an increased risk for bleeding, ranging from mild epistaxis, ecchymosis, and increased menstrual bleeding to hemorrhage in those with increased risk for bleeding. The increased risk for bleeding with topiramate may be due to modulation of voltage-gated L-type calcium ion channels located on vascular smooth muscle and noncontractile tissues such as platelets.

A syndrome consisting of acute myopia associated with secondary angle-closure glaucoma has been reported in patients receiving topiramate without any history of visual conditions. Symptoms include acute onset of visual impairment including diplopia, myopia, blurred vision, and/or ocular pain. Mydriasis may or may not be present. Symptoms typically occur within 1 month of initiating topiramate therapy and are usually reversible with discontinuance of treatment.

Respiratory infections such as pneumonia and asthma (bronchospasm) were reported in more than 1% of patients. Topiramate has weak carbonic anhydrase inhibitor activity, which can promote renal calculi formation by reducing urinary citrate excretion and increasing urinary pH. Topiramate has been associated with metabolic acidosis in adult and pediatric patients. Those with renal impairment are at higher risk for metabolic acidosis.

Contraindications. Topiramate should be used with caution in patients with a history of thrombocytopenia, glaucoma, or ocular disease, renal calculi, and in those with renal or hepatic impairment. Dosage adjustments may be required.

Monitoring. Monitor serum ammonia concentrations in patients who develop unexplained lethargy, vomiting, changes in mental status, or hypothermia. Measure baseline and serum bicarbonate periodically throughout treatment. Evaluate platelets in patients at high risk for bleeding. Rapidly evaluate any patient with symptoms of visual disturbance.

PRACTICE PEARLS

Topiramate Use in Pregnancy and Lactation

- Topiramate is excreted in breast milk.
- Diarrhea and somnolence have been observed in breast-fed infants whose mothers received topiramate.
- Teratogenesis is a serious complication of valproic acid use during pregnancy as it readily crosses the placenta.

Valproic Acid/Divalproex Sodium

It is thought that migraine prevention occurs through increased brain concentrations of the inhibitory neurotransmitter GABA, which inhibits enzymes that catabolize or block the uptake of GABA, or by suppressing repetitive neuronal firing through inhibition of voltage-sensitive sodium channels.

Pharmacokinetics. Valproic acid is administered orally with almost 100% bioavailability. Peak plasma concentrations are achieved within 3 to 5 hours for divalproex delayed-release tablets and within 4 to 17 hours for divalproex extended-release tablets. Hepatic and renal impairment can influence pharmacokinetics with a prolonged half-life and elevated concentrations of valproic acid.

Indications. Valproic acid is indicated for migraine headache prophylaxis.

Adverse Effects. Anticonvulsants, including valproic acid, are thought to carry an increased risk of suicidal ideation and behavior, occurring mostly between 1 and 24 weeks of therapy. Five percent of patients report abnormal dreams, agitation, amnesia, anxiety, confusion, depression, emotional lability, hallucinations, nervousness, personality disorder, and thinking abnormalities.

Rare anaphylactic reactions and other allergic reactions have been reported with valproic acid, divalproex, and valproate.

Cardiovascular effects such as blood pressure alterations, palpitations, unspecified chest pain, and arrhythmias are experienced in 1% to 5% of patients. Minor elevations in LFTs are frequent, but fewer than 1% of patients have more serious GI effects such as hepatic dysfunction or pancreatitis. Hematologic effects have been reported in 1% to 5% of patients and include ecchymosis and petechiae. Hypothermia (body temperature <35°C) with or without hyperammonemia has been reported. Valproic acid has been reported to cause abnormal coagulation studies. Musculoskeletal effects (8%), respiratory symptoms (1% to 5%), diplopia (16%), and genitourinary effects (1% to 5%) can occur.

Contraindications. Valproic acid is contraindicated in patients with known *urea cycle disorders,* a genetic enzyme defect that impairs the production of urea. Valproic acid is contraindicated in patients with mitochondrial disease caused by mutations in mitochondrial deoxyribonucleic acid (DNA) polymerase gamma (POLG; Alpers-Huttenlocher syndrome). It is also contraindicated in patients with hepatic dysfunction, or symptoms indicative of pancreatitis.

Monitoring. Closely monitor all patients beginning treatment with anticonvulsants or currently receiving such treatment for emerging or worsening suicidal thoughts/behaviors, unusual moods or behaviors, or depression. Inform patients and caregivers of the increased risk of suicidal thoughts and behaviors and advise them to immediately report the emergence or worsening of depression, the emergence of suicidal thoughts or behaviors, thoughts of self-harm, or other unusual changes in mood or behavior. It is recommended that patients receiving valproate be monitored for complete blood count (CBC) and coagulation parameters prior to planned surgery and if the patient is pregnant. Evidence of bleeding, bruising, or a disorder of hemostasis/coagulation is an indication for reduction of the dosage or withdrawal of therapy. Monitor serum plasma drug levels periodically.

Beta-Blockers

Propranolol

Propranolol is a nonselective, beta-adrenergic receptor antagonist thought to prevent migraine headaches through beta-blockade, preventing arterial dilation, inhibiting renin secretion, and possibly decreasing catecholamine-induced lipolysis. Decreased lipolysis in turn decreases arachidonic acid synthesis and prostaglandin production.

Pharmacokinetics. Propranolol is administered orally for migraine prevention and undergoes first-pass metabolism through the liver. Metabolism is prolonged in patients with hepatic impairment. Peak plasma concentration is achieved within 1 to 4 hours with immediate-release preparations and 6 hours for capsules. Propranolol crosses the blood–brain barrier and can be found in breast milk. Excretion is through the kidneys and consists of active metabolites. The elimination half-life of propranolol ranges from 2 to 6 hours, with chronic dosing increasing the half-life possibly due to saturation of liver binding sites. The half-life of propranolol is reduced in patients with renal impairment.

Indications. Immediate-release tablets or extended-release capsules are available for use in migraine prophylaxis.

Adverse Events. Cardiac effects such as sinus bradycardia and hypotension are rarely serious. Heart failure in patients with preexisting left ventricular dysfunction can occur, and it usually responds to discontinuation of propranolol. Arterial insufficiency, usually of the Raynaud type, also has been reported.

Adverse CNS effects of propranolol include dizziness, lethargy, fatigue, weakness, self-reported visual impairment, hallucinations, short-term memory impairment, emotional lability, slight confusion, nightmares, and even catatonia. With immediate-release formulations, fatigue, lethargy, and nightmares can be dose related.

Respiratory effects are common in patients with preexisting bronchospasm conditions. Exacerbation of asthma and bronchospasm can occur with propranolol. GI adverse effects reported include nausea, vomiting, diarrhea, constipation, abdominal cramping, epigastric distress, mesenteric arterial thrombosis, and ischemic colitis. Propranolol can prolong or enhance hypoglycemia, and the beta effects can mask signs of hypoglycemia, especially tachycardia, palpitations, sweating, and tremors. Rare but severe hematologic side effects, such as agranulocytosis, have been reported with propranolol therapy. Nonthrombocytopenic purpura and thrombotic thrombocytopenic purpura (TTP) also have been reported.

Contraindications. Propranolol is contraindicated in patients with bronchial asthma or a history of bronchospasm. Beta-blockers should be used with caution in patients with hyperthyroidism or thyrotoxicosis. Beta-blockers are contraindicated in patients with severe bradycardia, sick sinus syndrome, or advanced atrioventricular (AV) block, unless a functioning pacemaker is present. Propranolol should be used with caution in patients with cerebrovascular disease or stroke because of the effects of beta-blockade on blood pressure and pulse. Propranolol should be prescribed with caution in patients with hepatic or renal disease due to decreased clearance. Avoid propranolol in patients with Raynaud's phenomenon or peripheral vascular disease as symptoms can be exacerbated during therapy. CNS effects suggest that propranolol should be avoided in patients with major depression.

Monitoring. Carefully monitor vital signs and blood glucose concentration during drug initiation and dosage escalation, and routinely thereafter based on the patient's condition, comorbidities, symptoms, and medication tolerance.

PRACTICE PEARLS

Beta-blockers for Migraine Prophylaxis

- Abrupt discontinuance of beta-blockers is contraindicated, especially in patients with preexisting cardiac conditions. Myocardial ischemia, angina, and ventricular arrhythmias can result.
- Beta-blockers should be used with caution in patients with hyperthyroidism or thyrotoxicosis. Beta-blockers can mask tachycardia. Abrupt withdrawal of beta-blockers in a patient with hyperthyroidism can precipitate thyroid storm.
- If prophylactic oral beta-blockers are to be discontinued, the dosage should be gradually decreased over a minimum of 2 weeks.
- There are no adequate and well-controlled studies in pregnant patients, so beta-blockers should be avoided.
- Timolol has been found in breast milk.

Timolol

Timolol is a nonselective, beta-adrenergic receptor antagonist with several mechanisms that may help to prevent migraine headaches. Similar to propranolol, beta-blockade with timolol can prevent arterial dilation, inhibit renin secretion, and block catecholamine-induced lipolysis. Blocking lipolysis decreases arachidonic acid synthesis and subsequent prostaglandin production.

Pharmacokinetics. Timolol is administered orally and is rapidly absorbed after administration. After oral administration, medication onset of action is 30 minutes, with peak plasma concentrations achieved within 1 to 2 hours and a dose-dependent duration of activity of 12 to 24 hours. There is extensive first-pass metabolism by the liver, with timolol metabolized to inactive metabolites. Both the parent drug (15%) and metabolites are excreted in the urine. The plasma half-life of timolol is 4 hours.

Indications. Timolol is indicated for migraine headache prophylaxis.

Adverse Effects. Cardiovascular effects such as bradycardia and hypotension are rarely serious and can be alleviated by decreasing the dose. Arrhythmia exacerbation, syncope, unspecified chest pain, and arterial insufficiency, usually of the Raynaud type, also have been reported. Heart failure is more likely to occur in patients with preexisting left ventricular dysfunction and usually responds to discontinuation of timolol.

Adverse CNS effects during timolol therapy include dizziness, fatigue, asthenia, and depression, and are more common with lipophilic beta-blockers such as timolol. Adverse CNS effects of propranolol include dizziness, lethargy, fatigue, weakness, self-reported visual impairment, hallucinations, short-term memory impairment, emotional lability, slight confusion, nightmares, and even catatonia. With immediate-release formulations, fatigue, lethargy, and nightmares can be dose related.

GI effects such as nausea, vomiting, diarrhea, and GI distress are common. Timolol exerts effects on bronchial smooth muscle; therefore patients with preexisting bronchospasm are at high risk for exacerbation of asthma. Rare but severe hematologic effects, such as agranulocytosis, nonthrombocytopenic purpura, and thrombocytopenic purpura, have been reported. Myalgia, arthralgia, and musculoskeletal pain can occur with timolol therapy. Timolol has been associated with elevated hepatic enzymes and electrolyte abnormalities.

Contraindications. Timolol should be used with caution in patients with hyperthyroidism or thyrotoxicosis as tachycardia can be masked. Abrupt withdrawal of beta-blockers in a patient with hyperthyroidism can precipitate thyroid storm. Timolol is contraindicated in patients with bronchial asthma or a history of bronchospasm. Timolol is also contraindicated in patients with severe bradycardia, sick sinus syndrome, or advanced AV block, unless a functioning pacemaker is present. Timolol should be used with caution in patients with cerebrovascular disease or stroke because of the effects of beta-blockade on blood pressure and pulse.

Use timolol with caution in patients with hepatic or renal disease due to decreased clearance. Avoid timolol in patients with Raynaud's phenomenon or peripheral vascular disease as symptoms can be exacerbated during therapy. Timolol should be avoided in patients with major depression.

Monitoring. Carefully monitor vital signs and blood glucose concentration during drug initiation and dosage escalation, and routinely thereafter based on the patient's condition, comorbidities, symptoms, and medication tolerance.

Toxins

OnabotulinumtoxinA

OnabotulinumtoxinA (formerly known as botulinum toxin type A) is an intramuscular toxin produced from fermentation of *Clostridium botulinum* type A. Originally, onabotulinumtoxinA was approved for use in treating cervical dystonia in adults, but additional approvals for several other conditions, including migraine headache prevention, have been granted. It is thought that onabotulinumtoxinA works for prevention of chronic migraine by blocking binding to receptor sites on motor nerve terminals, cleaving synaptosomal-associated protein, and inhibiting the release of acetylcholine, thereby blocking neuromuscular conduction. This multistep process disrupts pain neurotransmission.

Pharmacokinetics. The pharmacokinetics of onabotulinumtoxinA have not been studied due to the neurotoxic nature of the medication. Little systemic absorption is believed to occur following intramuscular injection. OnabotulinumtoxinA is thought to be metabolized by proteases.

Indications. OnabotulinumtoxinA injection is indicated for the prophylaxis of headaches in adult patients with chronic migraine (15 or more days per month, with headache lasting 4 or more hours each day).

Adverse Effects. Adverse events typically occur within 1 week of the injection and are temporary in nature but may last several months. Ophthalmic reactions such as eyelid edema (blepharedema), diplopia, and ptosis have been reported, even in patients not treated for cosmetic purposes.

Respiratory difficulties may develop within hours to weeks after an injection. Patients with preexisting respiratory ailments may be more susceptible to respiratory complications following onabotulinumtoxinA injection. Bronchitis (3% of patients) and ocular infection (fewer than 1%) were reported. Hypertension occurred in 2% of patients receiving onabotulinumtoxinA for chronic migraines. Rarely, serious cardiac effects including arrhythmia and myocardial infarction, some with fatal outcomes, have occurred. The exact relationship of these events to the onabotulinumtoxinA injection has not been established.

Dysphagia can occur with onabotulinumtoxinA, with an incidence of less than 1%. Dysphagia and symptomatic general weakness may be attributable to an extension of the pharmacology of onabotulinumtoxinA resulting from the spread of the toxin outside the injected muscles.

Serious and/or immediate hypersensitivity reactions have been reported after onabotulinumtoxinA injection and include anaphylactoid reactions, serum sickness, urticaria, soft tissue edema, and dyspnea.

Musculoskeletal effects such as neck pain (9%), musculoskeletal stiffness (4%), myasthenia (4%), myalgia (3%), musculoskeletal pain (3%), and muscle spasms (2%) have also been reported.

Contraindications. OnabotulinumtoxinA contains albumin and should be used cautiously in patients with albumin hypersensitivity. There are no human data on the risk associated with the use of onabotulinumtoxinA during pregnancy. Use onabotulinumtoxinA cautiously in patients with myopathy associated with neuromuscular disease (e.g., amyotrophic lateral sclerosis [ALS], motor neuropathy [autonomic neuropathy], myasthenia gravis, or Lambert-Eaton syndrome) as significant effects such as weakness, diplopia, ptosis, dysphonia, dysarthria, severe dysphagia, and respiratory distress can occur. Clinicians should use onabotulinumtoxinA with caution in patients with cardiovascular, respiratory, or ocular disease.

Monitoring. No specific laboratory monitoring is required (Table 27.5).

BOOKMARK THIS!

Clinical Practice Guidelines

- Practice guideline update summary: Acute treatment of migraine in children and adolescents: Report of the Guideline Development, Dissemination, and Implementation Subcommittee of the American Academy of Neurology and the American Headache Society: https://www.ncbi.nlm.nih.gov/pubmed/31413171
- The American Headache Society Position Statement on Integrating New Migraine Treatments into Clinical Practice (2018): https://onlinelibrary.wiley.com/doi/10.1111/head.13456

Prescriber Considerations for Migraine Headache Therapy

Clinical Practice Guidelines

- Determine the type (episodic or chronic) of migraine headache based on its frequency (Box 27.1).
- Treatment plans are individualized based on many factors, including patient preference, pregnancy and lactation status, frequency and severity of migraines, prior treatment response, comorbid illnesses, contraindications (cardiovascular disease), and the use of concomitant medications.
- Institute both preventive and acute treatment goals with the patient.
- NSAIDs, nonopioid analgesics, acetaminophen, or caffeinated analgesic combinations may be used for mild to moderate migraine headache acute attacks.
- Start with the lowest oral dose and titrate up slowly until response is achieved.

TABLE 27.5	**Migraine Medications**			

Category/ Medication	Indication	Dosage	Considerations and Monitoring
Acute Migraine Treatments			
Serotonin-receptor 1_B and 1_D Agonists (Triptans)			
Sumatriptan	Moderate to severe migraine headache	*Adults:* 5–20 mg intranasally into one nostril once; may be repeated after 2 hours if needed. *Adults:* 6 mg subcutaneously; may be repeated once if needed. *Adults:* 25–100 mg orally once; may be repeated once if needed. Safety and efficacy have not been established in infants and children.	Monitor patients for new-onset signs and symptoms of cerebrovascular or cardiac disease which may be cause to discontinue this medication.
Zolmitriptan	Moderate to severe migraine headache	*Adults:* 1.25 or 2.5 mg orally once. May repeat dose once after at least 2 hr. *Adults:* 2.5 mg oral tablet or disintegrating tablet. *Adults and children <12 yr:* Maximum single dose: 5 mg intranasally administered as 2.5 mg in each naris.	Patients with symptoms of ischemic bowel syndrome (e.g., cramping, abdominal pain, bloody diarrhea) should be further evaluated.
Almotriptan	Moderate to severe migraine headache	*Adults:* 12.5 mg orally. *Children and adolescents 12–17 yr:* 6.25–12.5 mg orally.	Monitor ECG prior to and during treatment.
Eletriptan	Moderate to severe migraine headache	*Adults:* 20–40 mg orally. Safety and efficacy have not been established in children and adolescents.	Monitor ECG and LFTs prior to and during treatment.
Frovatriptan	Moderate to severe migraine headache	*Adults:* 2.5 mg as a single dose at migraine onset. Safety and efficacy have not been established in infants and children.	Monitor ECG prior to and during treatment.
Naratriptan	Moderate to severe migraine headache	*Adults:* 1 mg or 2.5 mg orally once. A second dose can be administered after 4 hr.	Monitor ECG prior to and during treatment.
Rizatriptan	Moderate to severe migraine headache	*Adults:* 5–10 mg orally. May be repeated in 2 hr. *Children and adolescents ≥6 yr, ≥40 kg:* 10 mg orally as a single dose. *For those <40 kg:* 5 mg as a single dose.	Monitor ECG prior to and during treatment.
Migraine Prevention Treatments			
Anticonvulsants			
Topiramate	Migraine prevention	*Adults, adolescents, and children 12–17 yr (immediate release):* Dose is 25 mg orally for 1 week. *Adults, adolescents, and children 12–17 yr (extended release):* 25 mg orally once daily for 1 week, then 50 mg orally once daily for 1 week, then 75 mg orally once daily for 1 week, and then 100 mg orally once daily. Adjust dose and titration according to clinical outcome.	Monitor baseline and serum ammonia levels and serum bicarbonate periodically. Evaluate platelets in patients at high risk for bleeding.
Valproic Acid	Migraine prevention	*Adults (delayed release):* 250 mg orally twice daily. Titrate as needed up to a maximum of 500 mg twice daily. *Children and adolescents 7–17 yr (delayed release):* 10–45 mg/kg/day orally in divided doses twice daily.	Monitor for suicidal thoughts/ behaviors, unusual moods or behaviors, or depression. Monitor serum plasma levels and coagulation parameters periodically. LFT monitoring is recommended until a stable therapeutic level is found.

TABLE 27.5 **Migraine Medications—cont'd**

Category/ Medication	Indication	Dosage	Considerations and Monitoring
Beta-Blockers			
Propranolol	Migraine prevention	**Immediate-release tablets:** *Adults:* 80 mg/day orally, in divided doses. *Children and adolescents weight >35 kg:* 0.6–3 mg/kg/day orally in 2–3 divided doses. Maximum dosage: 120 mg/day. *Children and adolescents weight <35 kg:* 0.6–3 mg/kg/day orally given in 2–3 divided doses. Maximum dosage: 60 mg/day. **Extended-release tablets:** *Adults:* 80 mg orally daily.	Monitor vital signs and glucose levels throughout treatment.
Timolol	Migraine prevention	*Adults:* 10 mg orally twice daily. May increase to maintenance dose of 20 mg once daily.	Monitor heart rate, blood pressure, kidney function.
Toxins			
Onabotulinum- toxinA	Migraine prevention	*Adults:* 155 units intramuscularly as 5 units/ injection divided across 7 specific head and neck muscle areas. See drug information for specific sites/dosages Repeat every 12 weeks.	No specific laboratory monitoring needed.

ECG, Electrocardiogram; *LFTs,* liver function tests.

• BOX 27.1 **International Classification of Head-ache Disorders**

Episodic Migraine

A. At least 5 attacks fulfilling criteria B–D
B. Headache attacks lasting 4 to 72 hours (when untreated or unsuccessfully treated)
C. Headache has at least 2 of the following 4 characteristics:
 1. Unilateral location
 2. Pulsating quality
 3. Moderate or severe pain intensity
 4. Aggravation by or causing avoidance of routine physical activity (e.g., walking or climbing stairs)
D. During headache at least 1 of the following:
 1. Nausea and/or vomiting
 2. Photophobia and phonophobia

Chronic Migraine

A. Migraine-like or tension-type-like headache on ≥15 days/ month for >3 months that fulfill criteria B and C
B. Occurring in a patient who has had at least 5 attacks fulfilling criteria B–D for migraine without aura and/or criteria B and C for migraine with aura
C. On ≥8 days/month for >3 months, fulfilling any of the following:
 1. Criteria C and D migraine without aura
 2. Criteria B and C for migraine with aura
D. Believed by the patient to be migraine at onset and relieved by a triptan or ergot medication

- It is important to understand that trial and error may be necessary before the optimum treatment is instituted.
- Ensure an adequate medication trial time of at least 8 weeks at the target dose before determining a lack of response.
- Patients who have medication overuse may require an escalation in dose, a change in therapy, and/or the addition of biobehavioral approaches to migraine management.
- If migraine is accompanied by severe nausea and/or vomiting, consider using a subcutaneous or intranasal formulation instead of an oral formulation.
- Preventive treatments should be considered for those who have attacks that interfere with daily activities despite therapy, have frequent attacks, or failed prior therapies.
- Avoid preventive treatments for pregnant or breastfeeding patients and in patients planning to conceive in the near future.
- Develop a plan to maximize adherence to preventive therapy that considers patient preferences, adequate patient education, and understanding of treatment expectations.
- Develop realistic goals that include a reduction in migraine frequency and attack duration, and improved functioning and quality of life.

Clinical Reasoning for Migraine Headache Therapy

Consider the individual patient's health problem requiring migraine headache therapy. It is necessary to determine the frequency, duration, and pattern of migraine headache to confirm a diagnosis of acute versus chronic migraine headache. Determine the potential triggers of migraine headache and create a plan for migraine prevention.

Determine the desired therapeutic outcome based on the degree of migraine headache relief needed for the patient's health problem. For patients suffering from migraine headache, the desired therapeutic outcome is migraine prevention, with secondary outcomes of reduction in migraine frequency and severity and improved functioning and quality of life. Choose a therapy based on the type of migraine (episodic or chronic), the route (considering patient preference), and timeliness of migraine relief, while adding biobehavioral strategies for managing headache prevention and migraine triggers.

Assess the migraine headache therapy selected for its appropriateness for an individual patient by considering the medication's side effects and the patient's age, race/ethnicity, comorbidities, and genetic factors. The treatment of migraine headache in older patients may be more complex as a result of comorbidities, polypharmacy, and age-related changes in organ function that can affect efficacy and potentially increase toxicity. Some migraine medications are strictly contraindicated in patients with cardiovascular disease. Polypharmacy increases the risk for drug–drug interactions. Decreased hepatic and renal function affect medication metabolism and elimination. In younger patients, the potential effects of migraine therapy on pregnancy and lactation must be discussed and considered. In children and adolescents, use over-the-counter (OTC) pain relievers such as acetaminophen and ibuprofen first to see whether these are effective for migraine relief with the addition of other nonpharmacologic strategies. Triptans can be given to children older than 6 years of age for migraines not relieved by OTC medications.

In terms of genetics, patients who have homozygous C677T mutation in the 5,10-methylenetetrahydrofolate reductase (*MTHFR*) gene and associated increased serum homocysteine levels are at risk for cerebrovascular disorders, including migraine headaches.

Initiate the treatment plan with the selected medication by first providing adequate patient education to ensure the patient's understanding and promote full participation in migraine headache therapy. Once a migraine headache medication is selected, it is important for the patient to understand its purpose, route, frequency of use, and adverse effects. Since overuse of migraine medications can render them ineffective or predispose the patient to more severe adverse effects, advise specifically on the dose to be taken, dosage intervals, and maximum daily dosage. Encourage the patient to keep a migraine headache log to document frequency, duration, and effectiveness of treatments. This log should be brought to all primary care appointments. Patients should be instructed to inform the primary care provider if they develop conditions such as cardiovascular disease that preclude the use of specific migraine headache therapies.

Ensure complete patient and family understanding about the medication prescribed for migraine headache therapy using a variety of education strategies. Important medication information to provide includes expected therapeutic effects, side effects, adverse effects, and any follow-up needed. Instructions can be provided in verbal and written forms, along with reliable migraine headache websites that can offer self-management strategies to patients. Instruct the patient to consult their primary care provider if migraine headache frequency, duration, or severity worsens. Information should be verbalized in a way that the patient can understand, and reinforced with written materials or instructions.

Conduct follow-up and monitoring of patient responses to migraine headache therapy. Assess the effectiveness of treatment and determine whether additional or changes in the treatment plan are warranted. Timing of follow-up appointments with the primary care provider is dependent upon the effectiveness of the migraine medication selected in relieving the migraine in a timely manner, and reducing the duration and severity of the headache. In the case of chronic migraine therapy, more frequent follow-up may be desired due to the potential adverse effects of those medications, such as elevations in blood pressure and glucose. Since medication adherence is an issue for patients treated for chronic migraines, patient knowledge about the selected medication should be reassessed for education reinforcement. Ensure that the patient has an adequate supply of medication to last until the next follow-up appointment.

Teaching Points for Migraine Headache Therapy

Health Promotion Strategies

- Resting or sleeping in a dark, quiet room may help with migraine headache pain relief.
- Apply ice to the head to help decrease pain. Apply it for 15 to 20 minutes every hour.
- Keep a migraine log by writing down when your migraines start and stop, treatments you used, and any other symptoms you experience, such as nausea. Bring the migraine log with you to visits with your health care provider.
- Overuse of drugs indicated for the management of acute migraine attacks may make migraine headaches more frequent.
- Inform your primary care provider if you are or plan to become pregnant, or if you plan to breastfeed.
- Get regular exercise. Exercise may help reduce migraine frequency. Get at least 30 minutes of exercise on most days.

- Develop a plan to manage your stress. Stress may trigger a migraine. Learn new ways to relax, such as deep breathing.
- Create a sleep schedule. Go to bed and get up at the same time each day. Turn off all electronic devices 1 hour prior to bedtime.
- Eat healthy foods such as fruits, vegetables, whole-grain breads, low-fat dairy products, beans, lean meat, and fish. Avoid foods or drinks that trigger your migraines.
- Do not abruptly discontinue medications for chronic migraine headache without consulting your primary care provider.

Patient Education for Medication Safety

While migraine headaches are a relatively common ailment, some medications can have the potential for adverse effects when used inappropriately, or in patients with specific risk factors. Primary care providers should stress the following points for safe migraine medication management:

- Take your medication as prescribed by your primary care provider.
- Be sure to review your medical history with the primary care provider who is treating you for migraine headaches. Some medications cannot be taken by patients who have preexisting hypertension, cardiovascular disease, or stroke history.
- Notify your primary care provider if the medication prescribed fails to relieve migraine headaches when used as prescribed, or if you experience unacceptable side effects.
- Inform your primary care provider if you are pregnant, planning to become pregnant, or breastfeeding, as your migraine medication may need to be discontinued or changed.
- Your medication for migraines may interfere with other medication or supplements you are taking. Always tell your primary care provider all the medications and supplements you are taking.
- If you are using a transdermal medication applied to the skin, do not apply it to areas near or over any type of electrically active implantable or other medical device such as an implantable cardiac pacemaker, body-worn insulin pump, or implantable deep brain stimulator.
- If you have been prescribed an anticonvulsant for chronic migraine treatment, you may be at an increased risk of suicidal ideation and behavior. Inform your primary care

provider immediately if you are experiencing depression or suicidal thoughts, or go directly to an emergency room.

Application Questions for Discussion

1. When would it be appropriate to switch from episodic treatment to medication for the treatment for chronic migraines?
2. What would your advice be to a newly pregnant patient who reports experiencing frequent migraines?
3. What should be included in the assessment of migraine headache in children?

Selected Bibliography

American Headache Society. (2019). AHS Consensus Statement: The American Headache Society position statement on integrating new migraine treatments into clinical practice. *Headache, 59*, 1–18.

Ashina, M., Moller Hansen, J., Oladottir a Dunga, B., & Olsen, J. (2017). Human models of migraine: Short-term pain for long-term gain. *Nature Reviews Neurology, 33*, 713–724.

Boss, B., & Huether, S. (2019). Disorders of the central and peripheral nervous system. In McCance, & Huether (Eds.), *Pathophysiology: The Biologic Basis for Disease in Adults and Children* (8th ed.). St. Louis: Elsevier.

Dieterich, M., Obermann, M., & Clelbisoy, N. (2016). Vestibular migraine: The most frequent entity of episodic vertigo. *Journal of Neurology, 263*(Suppl), S82–S89.

Dodick, D. W. (2018). Migraine. *The Lancet, 391*, 1315–1330.

Durham, P. (2006). Emerging neural theories of migraine pathogenesis. *Headache, 246*(Suppl1), S3–S8.

Gilmore B, & Michael M. (2011). Treatment of acute migraine headache. *Am Fam Physician,* Feb 1;83(3):271-80. Erratum in: *Am Fam Physician.* 2011 Oct 1;84(7):738. PMID: 21302868.

Gormley, P., et al. (2016). Meta-analysis of individuals identifies 38 susceptibility loci for migraine. *Nature Genetics, 48*, 856–866.

Hepp, Z., Dodick, D. W., Varon, S. F., Gilliard, P., Hansen, R. N., & Devine, E. B. (2015). Adherence to oral migraine preventative medications among patients with chronic migraine. *Cephalalgia, 35*, 478–488.

Lagman-Bartolome, A. M., & Lay, C. (2015). Pediatric migraine variants: A review of epidemiology, diagnosis, treatment & outcome. *Current Neurology and Neuroscience Reports, 15*, 34.

Marmura, M., Silberstein, S. D., & Schwedt, T. J. (2015). The treatment of migraine in adults: The American Headache Society evidence assessment of migraine pharmacotherapies. *Headache, 55*, 3–20.

28

Attention-Deficit/Hyperactivity Disorder Medications

CONSTANCE G. VISOVSKY

Overview

Attention deficit hyperactivity disorder (ADHD) is considered a common neurobiologic disorder of childhood, affecting up to 10% of children in the United States (French, 2015). ADHD is also considered a chronic condition that is frequently seen in the primary care setting. Assessment for ADHD requires screening for symptoms of inattention, impulsivity, and hyperactivity during regular office visits. Primary care providers should be careful not to mistake normal challenges of self-regulation in childhood as symptoms of ADHD. Symptoms begin to manifest themselves most frequently in the early school years, but even with treatment, some level of impairment may persist or remain until adulthood. If ADHD goes untreated, children are at higher risk for health-related issues including substance abuse and motor vehicle accidents. Males are two to three times more likely to have ADHD than females and are more likely to have trouble controlling impulsivity and/or hyperactivity behaviors. Females with ADHD are more likely to present with inattention as opposed to overactivity and impulsive behaviors, leading to underdiagnosis of ADHD (Biederman et al., 2002; Groenewald et al., 2009). While there is a balance to be achieved between under- and overdiagnosis of ADHD, the cumulative effects of poor academic performance and altered social functioning can lead to a risk for low self-esteem, depression, poor employability, and substance abuse. There is evidence that early identification and treatment of ADHD may be able to protect against some of these risks.

Relevant Physiology

The neurobiologic processes involved in attention and inhibition necessitate coordination of cortical and subcortical functioning; the most critical structure for maintaining alertness and attention is the reticular activating system, whereas the ability to inhibit distractions is cortically mediated at the prefrontal cortex. Circuits that connect these areas help control how the brain both sustains and filters attention in response to stimuli. Executive functions are major tasks of the frontal lobes. Executive tasks are the major neurologic dysfunction impaired by neurotransmitter imbalance noted in persons with ADHD. Executive tasks such as organization, flexibility, planning, problem-solving, working memory, and inhibition and regulation of verbal and motor actions can be affected by ADHD. The catecholamines are the main neurotransmitters with frontal-lobe function. Dopamine and norepinephrine neurotransmitters appear to be important in linking subcortical areas to the frontal lobes (Fig. 28.1).

Pathophysiology

Genetic predisposition and environmental factors that can affect neurodevelopment are thought to play a role in the development of ADHD. Studies involving twins estimate that ADHD may be inheritable in up to 76% of cases, many of which had multiple genes involved (Feldman & Reiff, 2014). Earlier studies of potential candidate genes revealed preliminary evidence of dysregulation of the neurotransmitter systems that involve the dopamine norepinephrine, as well as serotonin pathways (Faraone & Mick, 2010). To date, genome-wide association studies (GWAS) have been unable to determine the exact variants in deoxyribonucleic acid (DNA) which increase a person's risk of developing ADHD, but FOXP2 and others have been implicated. Environmental factors such as prenatal and early developmental stress resulting from prenatal exposure to certain neurotoxins such as tobacco smoke or lead, poor nutrition during pregnancy, or severe early deprivation, have been found to increase the risk of ADHD (Box 28.1).

BOOKMARK THIS!

DSM-5 Diagnostic Criteria for ADHD

Team ADHD: https://www.team-adhd.com/complex-adhd/diagnosis-adhd

CDC: https://www.cdc.gov/ncbddd/adhd/diagnosis.html

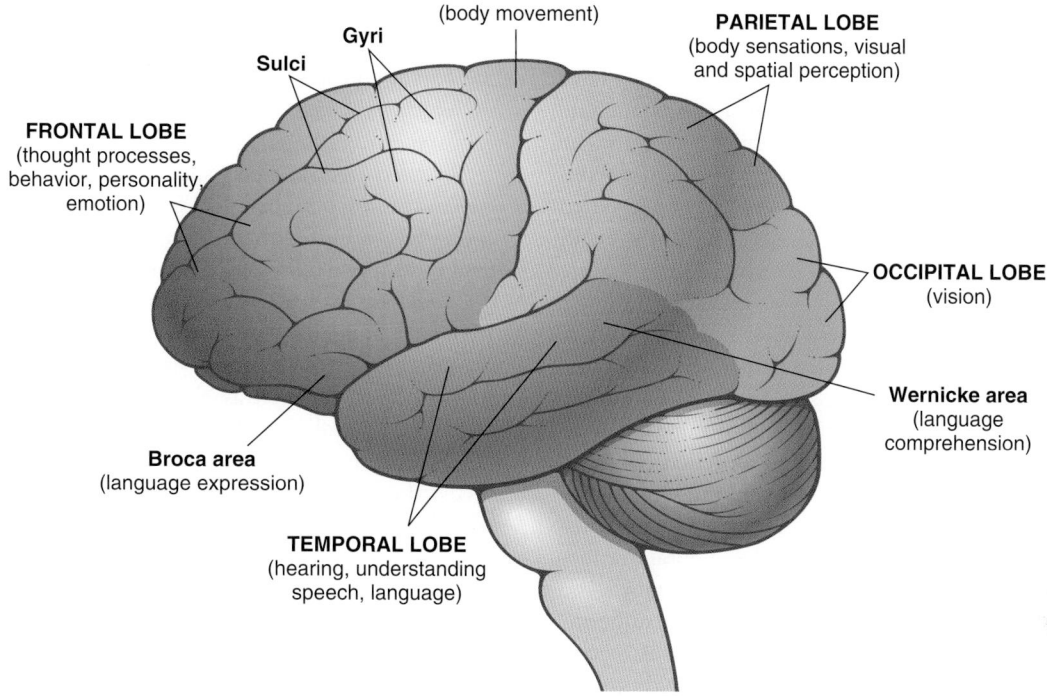

• **Fig. 28.1** Lobes of the brain. (From Chabner, D. [2021]. *The language of medicine* [12th ed.]. St. Louis: Elsevier.)

• BOX 28.1 Environmental and Genetic Factors in ADHD Development

Environmental Factors

- Prenatal and early developmental stress caused by exposure to neurotoxins (lead, maternal smoking while pregnant)
- Poor nutrition during pregnancy
- Perinatal complications (toxemia or fetal traumatic brain injury)
- Severe early deprivation

Genetic Factors

Findings from studies of twins estimated the heritability of ADHD at 70% to 80% throughout the lifespan.

- A total of 12 independent genome-wide significant loci are associated with ADHD.
- FOXP2 encodes a transcription factor and has a role in synapse formation and neural mechanisms that mediate speech and learning development.
- SORCS3 encodes a brain-expressed transmembrane receptor linked to neuronal development and plasticity.

Attention Deficit Hyperactivity Disorder Therapy

Central Nervous System Stimulants

Central nervous system (CNS) stimulants are among the most effective medications for ADHD. Stimulants are considered Schedule II controlled substances that have the potential for abuse, and therefore patients must be closely monitored for signs of misuse or abuse of these medications. Stimulants have been associated with sudden death in pediatric patients who have a history of structural cardiac abnormalities, cardiomyopathy, or arrythmias.

Methylphenidate

Methylphenidate is a CNS stimulant that resembles that of amphetamines indicated for use in ADHD. Methylphenidate is believed to work by increasing brain levels of dopamine and has been shown to assist with increasing attention while decreasing distractibility, impulsivity, and disruptive social and classroom behavior. Methylphenidate preparations are available under many brand names (Concerta, Ritalin, Metadate) and in regular, immediate-release, extended-release, and combination (immediate- and extended-release) formulations. Suggested dosage ranges for children are based on age. Methylphenidate is available in various oral formulations including a chewable tablet, and as a transdermal patch.

Pharmacokinetics. Methylphenidate can be administered orally or transdermally. While the exact distribution of methylphenidate is unknown, it does cross the blood–brain barrier. The low degree of protein binding and high lipid solubility is an indication of high penetrance into the CNS. Peak serum concentrations are achieved in about 1.9 hours for immediate-release formulations and 4.7 hours for extended-release forms. The duration of action ranges from 3 to 6 hours with regular tablets and about 8 hours with extended-release tablets. Since the transdermal form of methylphenidate does not go through first-pass metabolism, higher serum concentrations with lower initial doses result.

Indications. Methylphenidate has been approved for the treatment of ADHD in both children and adults.

Adverse Effects. Methylphenidate preparations have numerous potential adverse effects. *CNS* effects include nervousness and insomnia (2% of patients); these are the most common adverse reactions to methylphenidate and may occur with all formulations. Insomnia is believed to occur in 6% of pediatric patients 12 to 17 years of age and in 16% of adult patients when given less than 6 hours before bedtime. Continued interrupted sleep patterns may indicate a need for dosage reduction or may resolve with once-daily extended-release dosing. Drowsiness, lethargy, and fatigue occur with all methylphenidate dosage forms, although the exact incidence is unknown. Seizures can occur (less than 1%), and reversible ischemic neurological deficit has been reported, although again the incidence and cause related to the medication are unknown. Mild headaches are a common complaint. If headaches do not resolve, a dosage reduction may be helpful in decreasing headache frequency.

Gastrointestinal (GI) adverse effects such as abdominal pain, nausea, vomiting, xerostomia, dyspepsia, and decreased appetite are commonly associated with methylphenidate use. Appetite changes such as anorexia are more commonly reported in children as compared to adult patients. In adults, adverse GI effects were found more commonly among those receiving 70-mg and/or 100-mg doses.

Mental health effects such as anxiety, depression, agitation, decreased libido, confusion, and mood changes (anger, hypervigilance, panic attacks) have been reported in 20% of treated patients. Methylphenidate may increase the risk of adverse mental health effects in patients with preexisting anxiety, tension, and agitation. Stimulants can cause new-onset psychotic or manic symptoms (hallucinations, psychosis, delusional thinking, or mania). These symptoms occurred in approximately 0.1% of patients treated with stimulants. Minor dyskinesia has been reported with methylphenidate. These include minor, rapid, abnormal movements that are often patterned. Exacerbation of dyskinesia may respond to dosage reduction.

Respiratory system effects include upper respiratory tract infection (2%) in adults. In children, respiratory system adverse effects include pharyngitis (3%), streptococcal pharyngitis (3%), cough (2%), upper respiratory tract infection (17%), and oropharyngeal pain (1.2%).

Cardiovascular and cerebrovascular adverse effects such as hypertension, tachycardia, cardiac murmur, palpitations, angina, nonspecific chest pain, and cardiac arrhythmias including supraventricular tachycardia, sinus tachycardia, bradycardia, extrasystole, myocardial infarction (adults), and stroke (adults) have occurred. Cardiovascular events, including sudden death, have been associated with stimulant use in pediatric patients with structural cardiac abnormalities or other serious heart problems.

Skin effects known as chemical leukoderma, a condition in which the skin loses color from repeated exposure to specific chemical compounds, may occur with use of the methylphenidate patch. The onset of chemical leukoderma can range from 2 months to 4 years after starting the patch. Skin hypopigmentation has occurred under and around the patch, and less frequently on parts of the body where the patch is placed. Chemical leukoderma can mimic the appearance of vitiligo.

Vascular adverse effects such as peripheral vasoconstriction, including peripheral coldness and Raynaud's phenomenon, have been reported. Symptoms are usually mild and tend to improve following dosage reduction.

Hematologic adverse effects including anemia, thrombocytopenia, and leukopenia with methylphenidate treatment can occur rarely; no causality has been identified.

Hepatic effects such as elevated liver enzymes, alkaline phosphatase, and hyperbilirubinemia have been reported. Acute liver failure and hepatocellular injury have also occurred during treatment with methylphenidate, but causality has not been established.

Ocular disturbances including blurred vision and diplopia have been reported in 2% of pediatric and 1.7% of adult patients treated with methylphenidate formulations. Sympathetic stimulation resulting from methylphenidate can block aqueous outflow, raising intraocular pressure and consequently exacerbating ocular hypertension or glaucoma.

Sexual adverse effects such as decreased libido and priapism have occurred, often following a dose increase. Priapism has also been reported during periods of drug withdrawal. Priapism can occur in males of any age, with a median age of patients who experienced priapism being 12.5 years (range: 8 to 33 years).

Contraindications. Methylphenidate is contraindicated in patients with known *hypersensitivity* to methylphenidate. A cross-sensitivity with dexmethylphenidate also occurs. Life-threatening hypersensitivity reactions, including angioedema and anaphylaxis, have been reported. Skin sensitization can occur with use of the transdermal patch. Some formulations are contraindicated in patients with *symptomatic anxiety, tension, or agitation* as methylphenidate can further exacerbate these symptoms. Methylphenidate should be prescribed with caution in patients with *bipolar disorder and/or mania*, as an increase in manic episodes can occur. Methylphenidate is contraindicated in patients with *Tourette's syndrome* or those with a family history of Tourette's syndrome, as motor or verbal tics can be precipitated. Some methylphenidate products are contraindicated in patients with *glaucoma* due to the increased sympathetic stimulation that raises intraocular pressure. Methylphenidate has a high potential for *substance abuse* so should be prescribed very cautiously in patients with a history of substance abuse. Methylphenidate should not be prescribed for patients with *cardiac problems* such as serious structural cardiac abnormalities, aortic stenosis, prosthetic heart valves, valvular heart disease, cardiomyopathy, ventricular dysfunction or heart failure, serious cardiac arrhythmias, coronary artery disease (CAD), cerebrovascular disease, or advanced arteriosclerosis. Methylphenidate is contraindicated in patients who have received *monoamine oxidase inhibitor (MAOI) therapy* within the past 14 days as it may precipitate a hypertensive crisis. Methylphenidate may lower the seizure threshold and should be used cautiously in patients with a *history of a seizure disorder* or electroencephalogram (EEG) abnormalities.

Monitoring. A thorough cardiac assessment is warranted prior to the start of treatment. Monitor blood pressure and heart rate at baseline, after dosage increases, and regularly for any significant changes throughout methylphenidate therapy.

Monitor height and weight in children as there have been some concerns about potential growth issues related to methylphenidate therapy. Because of effects on the peripheral vascular system, carefully monitor all patients for changes to the digits of the hands and feet during treatment, especially those with preexisting circulation problems. Periodically monitor complete blood count (CBC) with differential and platelet counts.

PRACTICE PEARLS

Stimulant Therapy in Pregnancy and Lactation

- The safety of stimulants during pregnancy has not been established.
- Stimulants can cause vasoconstriction that may decrease placental perfusion. Neonates who had in utero exposure to stimulants may experience withdrawal after delivery, so monitor the newborn for symptoms of feeding difficulty, irritability, agitation, and excessive drowsiness.
- Methylphenidate has a low molecular weight and is excreted in human breast milk, but rigorous studies of human lactation are lacking.
- Consider registering pregnant patients taking stimulants for ADHD with the National Pregnancy Registry for ADHD Medications at 1-866-961-2388 or https://womensmentalhealth.org/adhd-medications.

Dextroamphetamine

Dextroamphetamine is an orally administered CNS agent (amphetamine) that stimulates the release of several low molecular weight organic bases from storage sites in the nerve terminal. At typical doses, amphetamines stimulate the release of norepinephrine, and at higher doses, dopamine is released from its storage sites. These actions account for the behavioral changes seen with amphetamine use in ADHD. The primary sites of activity in the CNS are the cerebral cortex and the reticular activating system. When administered, amphetamine-induced CNS stimulation produces decreased fatigue, increased motor activity, and increased mental alertness.

Pharmacokinetics. Dextroamphetamine is distributed to most body tissues, with highest concentrations found in the CNS. Metabolism occurs in the liver and excretion is by the renal system. Acidification of the urine speeds amphetamine elimination. The plasma half-life is 10 to 12 hours in adults. Following oral administration of regular-release tablets, dextroamphetamine is absorbed from the GI tract, achieving peak plasma concentrations in 2 hours. After administration of extended-release capsules, peak plasma concentrations were achieved within 8 to 10 hours.

Indications. Dextroamphetamine is indicated for the treatment of ADHD in children and adults.

Adverse Effects. Effects such as insomnia and anorexia (reported as loss or decrease of appetite) occur in most patients in the first few days of therapy, occasionally accompanied by dyspepsia or, rarely, nausea/vomiting. *GI effects* that occur include abdominal pain or cramping and headache. Abdominal pain or headache may respond to a dosage reduction. Most side effects disappear within a few weeks of continued dextroamphetamine use. *Growth and development* inhibition in children is a potential long-term side effect of dextroamphetamine and may be the result of suppression of appetite or an alteration in growth hormone secretion. *Cardiovascular adverse effects* such as increases in both systolic and diastolic blood pressure can occur, exacerbating hypertension. Sudden cardiac death has been reported in association with CNS stimulant treatment at usual doses in children, adolescents, and adults with structural cardiac abnormalities and other serious heart conditions. *Psychiatric effects* such as psychotic or manic symptoms (i.e., hallucinations, delusional thinking, or mania) in children and adolescents without a prior history of psychosis or mania occurred in approximately 0.1% of patients. As with methylphenidate, dyskinesia and tics have been reported with amphetamine use. Prolonged use of amphetamines, including dextroamphetamine, may lead to psychologic/physiologic dependence. *Skin adverse reactions* are rare; however, serious events such as angioedema, anaphylactoid reactions, Stevens-Johnson syndrome, and toxic epidermal necrolysis have all been reported. *Ocular adverse effects* occur as a result of sympathetic stimulation from amphetamines that blocks aqueous outflow and raises intraocular pressure, exacerbating ocular hypertension or glaucoma. Visual impairment such as blurred vision, mydriasis, and visual accommodation have been reported with stimulant use.

Contraindications. Dextroamphetamine is contraindicated for use in patients with known hypersensitivity to the medication. Dextroamphetamine is contraindicated in patients with a history of substance abuse due to its ability to cause dependence. Dextroamphetamine should be used cautiously in those with bipolar disorder and/or mania due to the potential for manic episodes to occur. Dextroamphetamine is contraindicated in patients with moderate to severe hypertension, advanced atherosclerosis, and symptomatic cardiovascular disease, and must be used very cautiously in patients with preexisting hypertension or tachycardia. Dextroamphetamine is contraindicated in patients with glaucoma due to the ability of sympathetic stimulation to block aqueous outflow and raise intraocular pressure. Dextroamphetamine is contraindicated for use in patients with hyperthyroidism, including thyrotoxicosis, as sympathomimetic stimulation may induce cardiac arrhythmias. Use dextroamphetamine with caution in patients with seizures or a history of a seizure disorder as the seizure threshold can be reduced. Dextroamphetamine may cause hypercortisolism as amphetamines can cause elevations in plasma corticosteroid concentrations. The potential for growth inhibition in pediatric patients should be monitored during stimulant therapy.

Monitoring. Monitor height and weight in children as there have been some concerns about potential growth issues related to dextroamphetamine therapy. Because of effects on the peripheral vascular system, carefully monitor all patients for changes to the digits of the hands and feet during treatment, especially those with preexisting circulation problems. Monitor blood pressure and heart rate at baseline, after dosage increases, and periodically throughout therapy.

Alpha-2 Adrenergic Agonists

Clonidine

Clonidine is a centrally acting alpha-2 adrenergic agonist that is available in immediate- and extended-release tablet and transdermal formulations for the treatment of ADHD in children and adolescents. It is important to note that clonidine is not considered a first-line agent for ADHD due to the potential for toxic cardiac effects. When clonidine is used for the treatment of ADHD, the American Heart Association (AHA) recommends careful cardiovascular screening and monitoring of patients. The mechanism of action of clonidine is unknown for its use in treating ADHD.

Pharmacokinetics. Fifty percent of a clonidine dose is metabolized in the liver and changed into inactive compounds. The remaining unchanged drug and its metabolites are excreted in the urine and feces. The half-life of clonidine is approximately 12 to 16 hours. Following administration of the immediate-release tablets, peak plasma concentrations are reached in approximately 1 to 5 hours. After administration of the extended-release tablets, peak concentrations occur in approximately 5 hours. The clonidine transdermal patch releases the medication at a constant rate over 7 days, with a bioavailability of 60%. Steady-state clonidine plasma concentrations are reached within 3 days.

Indications. Clonidine is used in the treatment of ADHD in pediatric patients either as monotherapy or as adjunctive therapy to a prescribed stimulant.

Adverse Effects. *CNS adverse effects* are common. Headache, drowsiness, somnolence, fatigue, and sedation are more common, with hallucinations, delirium, insomnia, mental depression, and other behavioral changes occurring less frequently. The CNS effects tend to subside with time and/or dose reduction. There are less severe CNS effects associated with transdermal therapy. *Adverse cardiovascular effects* include heart failure, electrocardiogram (ECG) abnormalities such as bradycardia, sinus node arrest, junctional bradycardia, AV block, and other arrhythmias. Severe rebound hypertension can occur if clonidine is abruptly discontinued regardless of route of administration. *Hypersensitivity reactions*, including generalized rash, urticaria, and angioedema, have occurred with oral clonidine. Localized, temporary skin effects have occurred following administration of clonidine patches, with the most common reactions being

erythema (26%), pruritus (26%), contact dermatitis (5%), and a vesicular rash (7%). *Sexual adverse effects* such as erectile dysfunction and decreased libido have been reported in about 3% of patients on clonidine therapy. More rarely, urinary retention (0.1%), difficulty in micturition (0.2%), and nocturia (1%) have also occurred.

GI adverse effects common in adults associated with clonidine therapy include constipation (10%); xerostomia (13% to 40%); ileus, abdominal pain, and anorexia (1%); mild liver function abnormalities (1%); nausea (1% to 13%); vomiting (5% to 10.5%); dysgeusia (1%); and mildly elevated hepatic enzymes (1%). In pediatric patients receiving extended-release clonidine, the most common GI adverse effects were upper abdominal pain (15%), nausea (5%), constipation (1% to 6%), xerostomia (5%), and anorexia (4%).

Contraindications. Clonidine is contraindicated in patients with a known hypersensitivity to clonidine. Clonidine should be used with caution in patients with a history of hypotension, AV block, bradycardia, or cardiovascular disease. Clinical trials are lacking to determine the safety of clonidine use during pregnancy, and it must be administered cautiously to breastfeeding women as clonidine is excreted in human breast milk.

Monitoring. Monitor heart rate and blood pressure at baseline and regularly throughout treatment for any significant changes that would require dosage adjustment or would indicate that the medication was withdrawn abruptly. For pediatric patients, the AHA recommends a thorough family history, physical exam, and ECG prior to the start of treatment, as well as monitoring for changes in blood pressure at treatment initiation, periodically during treatment, and when tapering the drug.

Guanfacine

Guanfacine is an oral, centrally acting alpha-2 adrenergic receptor agonist. The extended-release formula treats ADHD symptoms by targeting central alpha-2 adrenergic receptor activity in the prefrontal cortex. Guanfacine inhibits sympathetic nervous system outflow, reducing peripheral vascular resistance and lowering blood pressure.

Pharmacokinetics. The guanfacine immediate-release formulation is 80% bioavailable, and the extended-release formulation is 58% bioavailable. Peak plasma concentrations occur 1 to 4 hours following administration of immediate-release tablets and 5 hours following administration of extended-release tablets. Guanfacine is primarily metabolized by cytochrome (CYP) 3A4, and its plasma concentrations can be significantly affected by moderate to strong CYP 3A4 inhibitors and inducers. The elimination half-life of the immediate-release tablet is age dependent, ranging from 10 to 30 hours. The half-life of the extended-release tablet is approximately 18 hours. Since guanfacine is cleared by the liver and kidney, a reduced dose may be needed in patients with hepatic or renal impairment.

Indications. Guanfacine is indicated for the treatment of ADHD in adults, adolescents, and children either as monotherapy or as adjunctive therapy to a psychostimulant.

Adverse Effects. Cardiovascular adverse effects including dose-dependent decreases in blood pressure, bradycardia, orthostatic hypotension, and syncope can occur. Nonspecific chest pain, palpitations, and sinus tachycardia have been reported. *CNS effects* are mostly dose related and can lead to depression, sedation, drowsiness or somnolence, fatigue, dizziness, lethargy, headache, irritability, emotional lability, and insomnia. Asthenia and seizures were reported during other clinical trial evaluations. *GI side effects* of guanfacine are relatively common and include xerostomia, abdominal pain, and constipation. Alterations in taste and blurred vision have been reported during use of extended-release guanfacine. *Dermatologic effects* such as pruritus, rash, dermatitis, and hypersensitivity reactions (pruritus, rash) have been reported.

Contraindications. Guanfacine is contraindicated in patients with a hypersensitivity to the medication. Use cautiously in patients with a history of hypotension and in those with cardiac conduction abnormalities. Dose-dependent declines in blood pressure and heart rate can be experienced, so dosage increases should be done slowly. The sympathetic action of guanfacine may worsen sinus node dysfunction and AV block. Use guanfacine with caution in patients with hepatic disease or renal disease.

Monitoring. Monitor blood pressure and pulse rate at baseline, after dose adjustments, and throughout therapy.

Selective Norepinephrine Reuptake Inhibitors

Atomoxetine

Atomoxetine is a selective norepinephrine reuptake inhibitor (sNRI) and the first nonstimulant medication approved for the treatment of ADHD. Atomoxetine has been shown to be a safe and effective treatment for ADHD in adults and children 6 years of age and older to treat inattentive subtype and both inattentive and hyperactive/impulsive subtypes of the disorder. Atomoxetine may be considered an alternative ADHD therapy in patients for whom psychostimulants are not an option, or when preferred by the provider or patient.

Pharmacokinetics. Atomoxetine is administered orally and is rapidly absorbed from the GI tract, with peak plasma levels in 1 to 2 hours and an elimination half-life of 6 to 8 hours. Atomoxetine is excreted primarily in the urine (more than 80%). With once-daily dosing, plasma drug concentrations are low in most patients by late afternoon (half-life of 4 hours in extensive metabolizers). Patients who are poor metabolizers of CYP 2D6 metabolized drugs (7% of Caucasians; 2% of African Americans) have elevated levels of atomoxetine and an increased half-life of 19 hours due to reduced pathway activity.

Indications. Atomoxetine is indicated for the treatment of ADHD in children at least 6 years of age, adolescents, and adults.

Adverse Effects. *CNS effects* are common with atomoxetine use in adult and pediatric populations, with dizziness, drowsiness, feeling nervous or jittery, tremors, and insomnia being reported. These adverse effects are more pronounced in patients who are CYP 2D6 poor metabolizers. Psychiatric effects experienced by children and adolescents including mood swings, agitation, and restlessness were reported with atomoxetine. Psychotic or manic symptoms (hallucinations, delusional thinking, or mania) were reported in 0.2% of pediatric patients with no prior history of a psychotic or bipolar disorder. Suicidal ideation has been reported more frequently in children with a comorbid condition. Some psychiatric adverse effects such as depression are more frequent in adolescents who are CYP 2D6 poor metabolizers. *Neurologic adverse effects* including seizures occurred in 0.1% to 0.2% of adults and children, respectively. Seizure risk among children was greater among CYP 2D6 poor metabolizers. *GI effects* that can frequently occur in adults include xerostomia (20%), nausea (26%), constipation (8%), abdominal pain (7%), dyspepsia (4%), and vomiting (4%). In pediatric patients, GI effects include abdominal pain (18%), vomiting (11%), nausea (13%), and constipation (2%). Rare cases of severe liver injury, including jaundice, hepatitis, hepatic fibrosis, and hepatic necrosis, are possible, but the cause is unknown. Adults, children, and adolescents have experienced weight loss, decreased appetite, and anorexia, with the potential for growth inhibition in children during continued therapy with atomoxetine.

Genitourinary and reproductive system effects such as urinary retention/hesitancy (6%), dysuria (2%), and dysmenorrhea (3%) have been reported. Prostatitis, testicular pain, and urinary retention (0.4%) were among the most common reasons for medication discontinuation. *Sexual adverse effects* such as impotence, impaired ejaculation, priapism, and decreased libido have occurred. *Cardiovascular adverse effects* in adults include elevations in both systolic and diastolic blood pressure and an increase in heart rate of at least 20 beats/minute. Orthostatic hypotension and syncope have also occurred. Cardiovascular events, including sudden death, have occurred with atomoxetine use in pediatric patients with structural cardiac abnormalities or other serious cardiac disorders. QT prolongation has been reported with atomoxetine use. *Ophthalmic adverse events* occurred in at least 2% of children and adolescents who are CYP 2D6 poor metabolizers and include conjunctivitis and mydriasis. Blurred vision was more frequently found in adults who are CYP 2D6 poor metabolizers.

Contraindications. Atomoxetine is contraindicated in patients with severe cardiac conditions that would be expected to deteriorate from potentially significant increases in blood pressure. Atomoxetine should be used with caution in patients with a predisposition to hypotension or other conditions associated with abrupt heart rate or blood pressure changes. Atomoxetine carries a possible risk of torsade de pointes, and it is recommended to avoid use of atomoxetine in patients with confirmed or suspected long QT syndrome.

Atomoxetine is contraindicated for concomitant use in patients receiving MAOI therapy or anyone with a known hypersensitivity to atomoxetine. Atomoxetine is contraindicated in patients with pheochromocytoma or a history of pheochromocytoma due to potential serious elevations in blood pressure and tachyarrhythmia. Atomoxetine is contraindicated in patients with closed-angle glaucoma due to an increased risk for mydriasis.

Monitoring. Blood pressure measurements should be obtained at baseline, following dose increases, and periodically throughout atomoxetine therapy. Monitor height and weight at atomoxetine initiation and periodically thereafter. Monitor liver enzymes at baseline and intermittently during treatment. Prior to initiating treatment with atomoxetine, patients with comorbid depressive symptoms should be screened for suicidal ideation and bipolar disorder and monitored for increased depressive symptoms (Table 28.1).

Prescriber Considerations for Attention Deficit Hyperactivity Disorder Therapy

The AHA recommends careful screening, including a detailed patient and family history as well as physical examination for all children and adolescents prior to initiating pharmacologic therapy for ADHD. The presence of any serious heart rate increase, blood pressure increase, or cardiovascular event requires evaluation and consideration of drug discontinuation. Pediatric patients who develop symptoms such as exertional chest pain (unspecified), unexplained syncope, or other symptoms suggestive of cardiac disease during treatment should undergo a prompt cardiac evaluation.

BOOKMARK THIS!

American Academy of Pediatrics Subcommittee on Attention-Deficit/Hyperactivity Disorder and Steering Committee on Quality Improvement and Management. (2011). ADHD: Clinical Practice Guideline for the Diagnosis, Evaluation, and Treatment of Attention-Deficit/Hyperactivity Disorder in Children and Adolescents. *Pediatrics, 128*(5), 1007–1022. https://doi.org/10.1542/peds.2011-2654

Clinical Reasoning for Attention Deficit Hyperactivity Disorder Therapy

Consider the individual patient's health problem requiring ADHD therapy. One of the first considerations is to ensure that an age-appropriate diagnosis of ADHD was obtained. Treatment decisions also are affected by the patient's age and the ability of the patient/family to follow through with the prescribed therapy and follow-up to monitor treatment. Understanding the nature of the patient's behaviors such as poor emotional control, inattention, impulsivity, and hyperactivity will also provide insight into the need for adjunctive treatment, such as behavioral therapy.

Determine the desired therapeutic outcome based on the degree of ADHD therapy needed for the patient's health problem. The desired therapeutic outcome may vary slightly for each patient dependent upon age and maturation. However, common outcomes include an increased ability to concentrate, decreased hyperactivity and impulsivity behaviors, and more self-control. For children, self-control early in life is associated with lower rates of substance abuse, divorce, and incarceration, as well as higher rates of college graduation. Lastly, the criteria for a diagnosis of ADHD rely heavily on the number of symptoms/behaviors but do not take into account the severity of those symptoms/behaviors. Therefore, the desired outcome of therapy needs to be discussed with the patient and/or family.

Assess the ADHD therapy selected for its appropriateness for an individual patient by considering the side effects of the medication and the patient's age, race/ethnicity, comorbidities, and genetic factors. Children and adolescents with ADHD are coping with a chronic disorder and will need careful monitoring of the selected medication and other adjunctive treatments for effectiveness and adverse effects, such as growth inhibition. Pharmacologic therapy is likely to be maintained into adulthood. Despite this fact, the primary care provider should be aware that insufficient data are available on the long-term effectiveness of pharmacologic treatment for ADHD. In addition, adverse effects on sleep, appetite, growth, and potential long-term adverse effects on the cardiovascular system in children must be considered.

While it is important to consider the potentially serious side effects of medications for ADHD, it is most important to consider the potential for addiction and substance abuse behaviors that can result. Other medications such as atomoxetine or a tricyclic antidepressant may be useful instead of a stimulant/amphetamine in those with a history of substance abuse. While there are genetic influences in ADHD development, there are currently no pharmacogenomic targets for treatment. The genetic overlap of ADHD with other disorders has also been studied. Correlations between ADHD and major depressive disorder, anorexia nervosa, obesity, and insomnia have been found.

Comorbid conditions, especially structural heart conditions in children, are particularly concerning and require a full cardiac workup prior to initiation of therapy. Patient and family history should be acquired before stimulant therapy is started. The history should include questions about the following: history of fainting or dizziness, high blood pressure, heart murmur, rheumatic fever, chest pain or shortness of breath with exercise, any changes in exercise tolerance, palpitations, extra or skipped beats, or seizures. Family history should include questions about the following: sudden or unexplained death in a young person, other sudden cardiac death, heart attack or event requiring resuscitation in persons younger than 35 years of age, family members who died during exercise, and family history of cardiomyopathy, QT syndrome, Brugada syndrome, Wolff-Parkinson-White syndrome, and Marfan syndrome.

When changing medications for ADHD, follow medication conversion formulas approved by the U.S. Food and Drug Administration (FDA). The ratio for conversion between medications is complex and must consider ADHD

TABLE 28.1	ADHD Medications		
Category/ Medication	Indication	Dosage	Considerations and Monitoring
CNS Stimulants			
Methylphenidate	Treatment of ADHD in adults, adolescents, and children	*Adults:* 20–30 mg orally daily in 2 to 3 divided doses 30 min before meals. *Children ≥6 yr and adolescents:* 5 mg orally twice daily before meals. Dose may be increased by 5–10 mg/day at weekly intervals. Maximum dosage: 60 mg/day.	Several severe adverse effects are associated with methylphenidate, including the risk for hemato-logic effects, growth abnormalities, seizures, dependence, psychiatric effects, GI effects, cerebral vascular events, and cardiovascular events including sudden death. Monitor blood pressure, pulse rate, CBC with differential, and platelet count. In children, monitor growth rate and weight.
Methylphenidate SR		*Adults ≤65 yr:* 18–36 mg orally once daily in the morning. Dose may be increased by 18-mg increments at weekly intervals. Maximum dosage: 72 mg/day. *Children ≥6 yr and adolescents:* 18 mg orally once daily in the morning. Dose may be increased by 18–mg increments at weekly intervals.	
Methylphenidate trans-dermal patch		Initially, apply a 10-mg/9-hr patch topically once daily in the morning. After 1 week, may titrate patch strength in weekly intervals.	
Dextroamphetamine		*Adults:* 5 mg orally once or twice daily. *Children ≥6 yr and adolescents:* 5 mg orally once or twice daily. *Children 3–5 yr:* Initially, 2.5 mg orally once daily in the morning. May titrate daily dose in 2.5-mg increments at weekly intervals to the minimum effective dose. Maximum dose not established.	
Mixed Amphetamine Salts			
Amphetamine/dextroam-phetamine	Treatment of ADHD in adults, adolescents, and children	**Immediate release:** *Adults:* 5 mg orally once or twice daily. *Children ≥6 yr and adolescents:* 5 mg orally once or twice daily. *Children 3–5 yr:* 2.5 mg orally once daily.	Same as for methylphenidate. Monitor blood pressure, pulse rate, CBC with differential, and platelet count. In children, monitor growth rate and weight.
Alpha-2 Adrenergic Agonists			
Clonidine IR	Treatment of ADHD in children and adoles-cents as monother-apy or as adjunctive therapy to a psycho-stimulant	*Children ≥6 yr and adolescents:* 0.1 mg orally at bedtime. Can titrate up by 0.1 mg/day to 0.1 mg orally twice daily, up to four times daily. Maxi-mum dosage: 0.4 mg/day.	Monitor for CNS effects (fatigue, somnolence, sedation, depression, hallucinations), GI effects (nausea, anorexia), cardiac effects (ECG abnormalities), and hypersensitivity reactions. Monitor blood pressure.

Continued

TABLE 28.1   ADHD Medications—cont'd

Category/ Medication	Indication	Dosage	Considerations and Monitoring
Clonidine ER (Kapvay ER)		*Children ≥6 yr and adolescents:* Initially, 0.1 mg/day orally at bedtime. Increase by 0.1-mg/day increments weekly as needed to attain the desired response. Maximum dosage: 0.4 mg/day.	
Clonidine transdermal patch		Once stabilized on an oral dose, convert to the transdermal patch that provides an equivalent daily dose (e.g., 0.1, 0.2, or 0.3 mg/day).	Due to variable absorption in pediatric patients, patches may need to be changed every 5 days, as opposed to every 7 days for adults.
Guanfacine IR tablets	Treatment of ADHD as monotherapy or as adjunctive therapy to a psychostimulant	*Adults:* 0.25–2 mg/day orally given in divided doses. *Children and adolescents 4–17 yr:* 0.5 mg orally at bedtime initially, then titrated to 0.5 mg orally four times daily if weight <45 kg or 1 mg orally at bedtime initially, then titrated to 1 mg orally four times daily if weight ≥45 kg.	Do not abruptly discontinue. Taper the daily dose by no more than 1 mg every 3–7 days to avoid rebound hypertension; monitor blood pressure and pulse with dose reduction or discontinuation. Check for weight-based target dosages.
Guanfacine ER		*Adults:* Guanfacine ER: 1 mg orally once daily. Maximum dosage: 6 mg orally once daily. *Children and adolescents 6–17 yr:* 1 mg orally once daily.	Monitor blood pressure, pulse rate, CBC with differential, and platelet count. In children, monitor growth rate and weight.
Select Norepinephrine Reuptake Inhibitors			
Atomoxetine	Treatment of ADHD in adults, adolescents, and children	*Adults, children and adolescents 6–17 yr weighing >70 kg:* Initial dose 40 mg/day orally. After 3 days, titrate to the target dose of 80 mg/day orally given in divided doses. After 2–4 weeks, dose may be titrated up to 100 mg/day orally in patients with suboptimal response. Maximum dosage: 100 mg/day. *Children and adolescents 6–17 yr weighing ≤70 kg:* 0.5 mg/kg/day orally initially. Dose may be increased after a minimum of 3 days to a target dose of 1.2 mg/kg/day. Maximum dosage: 1.4 mg/kg/day (not to exceed 100 mg/day).	Monitor for CNS effects (drowsiness, dizziness, tremors), psychiatric effects (mood swings, agitation, restlessness, manic episodes), neurologic effects (seizures), ophthalmic effects (blurred vision), GI effects (xerostomia, nausea, vomiting, constipation, abdominal pain, weight loss, anorexia, decreased growth), and cardiac effects (increased blood pressure and pulse rate, sudden death).

CBC, Complete blood count; *CNS*, central nervous system; *ECG*, electrocardiogram; *ER*, extended release; *GI*, gastrointestinal; *IR*, immediate release; *SR*, sustained release.

symptoms, comorbid conditions, and adverse effects. Conversion among extended-release preparations should follow the serum concentration curves.

Initiate the treatment plan with the selected medication by first providing adequate patient education to ensure the patient's understanding and promote full participation in ADHD therapy. Methylphenidate is typically the first-line therapy for ADHD. When initiating treatment for ADHD in children, it is recommended that the parents provide consent to the therapy due to the significant number and

potential severity of possible adverse effects. Appropriate counseling regarding the selected medication is necessary. Consider whether the child being treated can take medication multiple times daily, or whether an extended-release formulation would be the best choice. The primary care provider is responsible for providing comprehensive education concerning the adverse effects to be monitored for and reported to the primary care provider. Engage the patient and family in reporting new-onset or exacerbation of symptoms or concerning thoughts or behaviors. The importance of keeping regularly scheduled follow-up appointments should be stressed.

Ensure complete patient and family understanding about the medication prescribed for ADHD therapy using a variety of education strategies. Important medication information to provide includes expected therapeutic effects, side effects, adverse effects, and the importance of monitoring or follow-up appointments. Instruct the patient and family concerning the critical symptoms, behaviors, or thoughts to be reported to the health care provider, and to seek emergency care for symptoms of cardiovascular, cerebral, or psychiatric illness. Instructions and educational materials should be given both verbally and in writing and be leveled to the patient's age and family's ability to understand the variety and complexity of adverse effects that can occur with ADHD treatment.

Conduct follow-up and monitoring of patient responses to ADHD therapy. Recommendations by the AHA for cardiac monitoring when using ADHD medications in children with heart disease (Cortese et al., 2013) determined that these medications should not be used in children with structural cardiac abnormalities due to the high risk of sympathomimetic effects. Prior to initiating therapy with stimulant agents, a baseline ECG should be obtained, although data are lacking as to whether this step will prevent sudden cardiac death. Blood pressure and pulse should be evaluated within 1 to 3 months of initiating treatment with any medication and then every 6 to 12 months. This should be done more often during titration of doses or weaning of alpha agonists. Periodic blood counts and platelet counts should be performed. When converting from one medication to another, close follow-up is recommended as dose titration may be needed. Follow-up to assess for new-onset or exacerbated psychiatric conditions, psychosis, aggression, depression, or suicidal thoughts. Once stabilized, follow-up can be at either 6- or 12-month intervals.

Teaching Points for ADHD Therapy

Health Promotion Strategies

The following strategies and practices should be presented to patients to help them become full partners in their health care:

- There is evidence to suggest that poor nutrition may play a part in the development and exacerbation of ADHD. Encourage patients to consume a healthy diet, limiting processed foods, sweet snacks, and alcohol during treatment. A diet high in sugar, salt, and saturated and total fat, and low in whole grains, fish, fruits, and vegetables, is associated with increased ADHD symptoms.
- For patients experiencing decreased appetite, eating small, frequent meals or snacks may help limit appetite problems.
- Regular physical activity should be encouraged as there are positive associations between physical activity and the reduction of ADHD symptoms of hyperactivity and inattention.

- While rare in occurrence, inform male patients and their families to make sure that they know the signs and symptoms of priapism, and stress the need for immediate medical treatment should it occur. Younger males may not recognize the problem or may be embarrassed to tell anyone.
- Encourage healthy sleep habits of 6 to 8 hours of sleep nightly.

Patient Education for Medication Safety

Due to the number of potentially serious medication adverse effects, safety considerations must be included in the education plan for patients and families.

- Advise patients and their families to promptly report any changes in mood or behaviors. If suicide-related events emerge during treatment, consider dose reduction or drug discontinuation, especially if symptoms are severe, are abrupt in onset, or were not part of the presenting symptoms.
  - When using transdermal ADHD medications, patients and families should be advised to assess for new areas of lighter skin, especially under the patch, and immediately report these changes to the primary care provider.
  - Patients are encouraged to promptly report any unusual changes in vision for evaluation.
  - Prolonged erections in male patients should be promptly reported, as immediate diagnosis and treatment are essential to avoid tissue damage.
  - For patients with a history of seizures, methylphenidate can lower the seizure threshold, so education of the patient and family for monitoring of seizure activity is warranted.
  - Avoid alcohol use during treatment for ADHD as alcohol can potentiate the effects of stimulants.
  - Instruct the patient and family to promptly report any adverse effects of the prescribed ADHD medication.
  - Instruct patients to avoid adding any herbal remedies or supplements to their medication regimen before checking with their primary care provider due to potential adverse interactions.

Application Questions for Discussion

1. Describe the differences in considerations for therapy for ADHD between a child or adolescent and an adult.
2. What criteria would prompt a consideration for a change in therapeutic agents for ADHD treatment?
3. How can the primary care provider prevent substance abuse among patients treated for ADHD?

Selected Bibliography

Biederman, J., Mick, E., Faraone, S. V., et al. (2002). Influence of gender on attention deficit hyperactivity disorder in children referred to a psychiatric clinic. *American Journal of Psychiatry, 159*(1), 36–42.

Biederman, J., & Faraone, S. V. (2005). Attention-deficit hyperactivity disorder. *Lancet, 366*, 237–248.

Christakis, D. A. (2016). Rethinking attention-deficit/hyperactivity disorder. *JAMA Pediatrics, 170*(2), 109–110.

Cortese S., Holtmann M., Banaschewski T., et al. European ADHD Guidelines Group. Practitioner review: current best practice in the management of adverse events during treatment with ADHD medications in children and adolescents. *Journal of Child Psychology and Psychiatry*. Mar;54(3):227-246, 2013. doi: 10.1111/jcpp.12036. Epub 2013 Jan 7. PMID: 23294014.

Demontis, D., Walters, R. K., Martin, J., et al. (2019). Discovery of the first genome-wide significant risk loci for attention deficit/hyperactivity disorder. *Nature Genetics, 51*, 63–75.

Faraone, S. V., & Mick, E. (2010). Molecular genetics of attention deficit hyperactivity disorder. *Psychiatric Clinics of North America, 33*(1), 159–180.

Feldman, H. M., & Reiff, M. I. (2014). Clinical practice: Attention deficit-hyperactivity disorder in children and adolescents. *New England Journal of Medicine, 370*(9), 838–846.

French, W. (2015). Assessment and treatment of attention-deficit/hyperactivity disorder: Part 1. *Pediatric Annals, 44*(3), 114–120.

Groenewald, C., Emond, A., & Sayal, K. (2009). Recognition and referral of girls with attention deficit hyperactivity disorder: Case vignette study. *Child: Care, Health and Development, 35*(6), 767–777.

Hoekstra, P. J., & Dietrich, A. (2014). Attention-deficit/hyperactivity disorder: Seeking the right balance between over- and undertreatment. *European Child & Adolescent Psychiatry, 23*, 623–625.

29

Antiepileptic Medications

CONSTANCE G. VISOVSKY

Overview

Epilepsy is defined by the International League Against Epilepsy (ILAE) as two or more unprovoked seizures that occur more than 24 hours apart, or a single unprovoked seizure with a more than 60% risk of recurrence (Fisher et al., 2014). The prevalence of epilepsy is 1% in developed countries, with approximately 50 million people affected with epilepsy worldwide. The response to antiepileptic medications for seizure control and adverse effects can vary among individuals depending on seizure type, risk factors, genetics, and underlying causation. In addition, epilepsy treatment is complicated due to the many different syndrome and seizure types.

Relevant Physiology

Seizures are invoked by high-frequency discharge from hyperexcitable neurons. The specific causation of this hyperexcitability can be due to brain trauma or insult, inflammation, or genetics, resulting in seemingly normal neurons discharging in an abnormal fashion. In the brain, signals from nerves are transmitted by action potentials that spread the impulse along the nerve fiber membrane to the nerve fiber end. The stages of inducing action potentials are the resting stage, depolarization stage, and repolarization stage.

In the *resting stage*, before an action potential begins, the nerve membrane is considered "polarized." The *depolarization stage* is characterized by permeability of the membrane to positively charged sodium ions that rapidly diffuse to the interior of the axon. This allows the polarized state to become neutralized, closing the sodium channels and opening the potassium channels. The influx of potassium ions to the exterior returns the membrane to the normal resting state and is known as *repolarization* of the membrane. Thus, both the sodium and potassium voltage-gated channels and the Na-K$^+$ pump play a role in increasing the speed of membrane repolarization for both sensory and motor transmissions to the brain. An action potential will occur only when the proportion of sodium ions entering the nerve fiber is greater than the number of potassium ions leaving the fiber. The sudden rise in membrane potential results in the development of an action potential (Fig. 29.1).

Pathophysiology

Epilepsy is a chronic condition characterized by the recurrence of unprovoked seizures. Acquired epilepsy results from a known lesion or acute insult that establishes a series of alterations in cellular, molecular, and physiological properties that give rise to seizures.

Seizures occur in epilepsy when the basal level of excitability in the nervous system rises above the seizure threshold. When nervous system excitability remains below this critical threshold, no seizures occur. Epilepsy is classified into three major types: grand mal epilepsy, petit mal epilepsy, and focal epilepsy. *Grand mal epilepsy* is characterized by extreme neuronal impulse discharge from all areas of the brain. In *petit mal (absence seizures) epilepsy*, the thalamocortical brain–activating system stimulates repetitive abnormal electrical impulses from the neurons of the brain. *Focal epilepsy* can involve almost any area of the brain, usually from a localized lesion of functional abnormality. These lesions provoke extremely rapid electrical discharges in local neurons.

Most individuals with grand mal epilepsy have a genetic predisposition that is present in one of every 50 to 100 persons. For dominant transmission of epilepsy, a mutation in one of the two alleles is sufficient to cause disease, as seen in the known familial epilepsy syndromes, such as genetic/

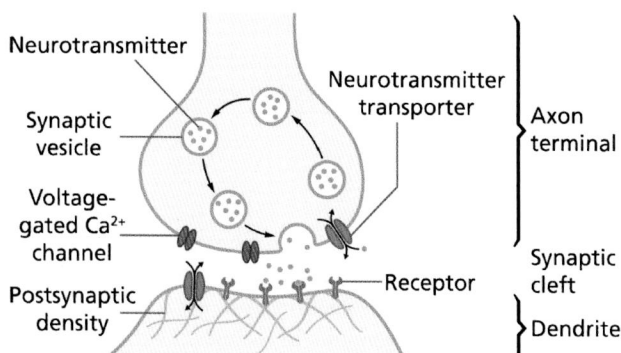

• **Fig. 29.1** The presynaptic neuron (top) releases a neurotransmitter, which activates receptors on the nearby postsynaptic cell (bottom). (From Zhang, J. [2019]. Basic neural units of the brain: Neurons, synapses and action potential. Retrieved March 22, 2021, from https://arxiv.org/abs/1906.01703.)

generalized epilepsy with febrile seizures due to mutations in *SCN1A* or *SCN1B*. Frontal lobe epilepsy is the result of mutations in *CHRNA4*, *CHRNB2*, or *CHRNA2*, while familial neonatal and infantile epilepsies are due to mutations in *KCNQ2*, *KCNQ3*, *SCN2A*, or *PRRT2*.

Recessive epilepsies are caused by mutations in both alleles of a gene. These alleles can be affected through homozygous mutations, in which an identical mutation is inherited from each parent, or through compound heterozygous mutations, in which the specific mutation affecting the same gene from father and mother differ. Several genes for familial temporal lobe epilepsies have been identified (*LGI1*, *DEPDC5*, *RELN*, and *VPS13A*). Mutations in these genes have been found mainly in patients with familial focal epilepsies. There is little evidence to suggest that these known genes play a major role in sporadic, nonfamilial cases.

Antiepileptic Therapy

The decision regarding initiation of antiepileptic medication is largely based on the potential and consequences of seizure recurrence for the individual and is typically made in consultation with the primary care provider, the neurologist, and the patient and family. Another important factor is the choice of antiepileptic medication based on the type of seizure the patient experienced. The goal of therapy is the control of seizure activity. Ideally, a single medication is used at a low beginning dose that is gradually increased until the seizures are controlled. A second medication can be added if the patient continues to experience seizures at the maximum tolerated dose. Discontinuation of antiepileptics can be considered after the patient has been seizure free for more than two years. Seizures can return following medication discontinuance, and tend to occur within the first year for 40% of patients.

BOOKMARK THIS!

Clinical Guidelines for Epilepsy Treatment
- American Epilepsy Society: https://www.aesnet.org/clinical-care/clinical-guidance
- American Academy of Neurology: https://www.aan.com/Guidelines/home/ByTopic?topicId=23

Hydantoins

Hydantoins block sodium channels from recovering from an inactivated state and thus inhibit neuronal firing by slowing synaptic transmission. This action stops the repeated excitation of neural cells that results in seizures. Hydantoin anticonvulsants are used to treat a wide range of seizures types.

Phenytoin
Pharmacokinetics. Phenytoin can be administered orally or parenterally. Oral formulations of phenytoin are generally considered to be 90% to 100% bioavailable. Phenytoin is highly protein bound and exhibits a nonlinear pharmacokinetic profile. Metabolism is highly variable, with extensive metabolization occurring in the liver via cytochrome (CYP) 2C9 and CYP 2C19. Phenytoin's half-life varies extensively from 7 to 60 hours. Small dosage increases can result in a large increase in plasma concentration. Immediate-release products reach peak concentrations in 1.5 to 3 hours, and extended-release capsules reach peak concentrations in 4 to 12 hours. The maximal elimination rate (Vmax) is higher and more variable in children than in adults, so children require higher doses on an mg/kg basis than adults to achieve the same serum concentrations.

Indications. Intravenous (IV) phenytoin is used in the treatment of status epilepticus, while the oral formulation is used in the treatment of tonic-clonic seizures or partial seizures or for maintenance dosing to treat tonic-clonic or complex partial seizures.

Adverse Effects. Anticonvulsants, including phenytoin, are thought to carry an increased risk of suicidal ideation and behavior that occurs from 1 to 24 weeks after therapy initiation. Dose-related adverse central nervous system (CNS) effects can include nystagmus, ataxia, slurred speech, decreased coordination, drowsiness, and mental confusion. Peripheral neuropathy (sensory), usually occurring weeks to months after drug initiation, has also been reported. Adverse gastrointestinal (GI) effects include nausea/vomiting, constipation, and abdominal pain. Taking the drug with food may reduce some symptoms. Gingival hyperplasia can occur, especially with long-term therapy.

Contraindications. Phenytoin is contraindicated in patients with a hydantoin hypersensitivity as hypersensitivity reactions (fever, sore throat, skin rash, periorbital or facial edema, angioedema, myalgia, arthralgia, easy bruising, lymphadenopathy, and petechial or purpuric hemorrhage) to anticonvulsants may be severe and sometimes fatal. Phenytoin can cause liver dysfunction, blood dyscrasias, and serious skin rashes, requiring discontinuation of treatment. Phenytoin is contraindicated in patients with a history of prior acute hepatotoxicity attributable to phenytoin. Phenytoin injection is contraindicated in patients with sinus bradycardia, sinoatrial block, second- or third-degree AV block, and Adams-Stokes syndrome because of the effects of the drug on ventricular automaticity. Do not abruptly discontinue phenytoin, as this may precipitate acute seizures/status epilepticus.

Monitoring. All patients beginning treatment or currently receiving treatment with anticonvulsants should be closely monitored for emerging or worsening suicidal thoughts/behaviors or depression, and be advised to immediately report to their primary care provider the emergence or worsening of depression, the emergence of suicidal thoughts or behaviors, thoughts of self-harm, or other unusual changes in mood or behavior. Nystagmus is an early manifestation of phenytoin toxicity (>20 mcg/mL), while ataxia and confusion generally occur when plasma concentrations exceed 30 mcg/mL. Patients with renal disease, renal impairment, or renal failure leading to uremia should be monitored for phenytoin toxicity. Blood sugar should be monitored closely in patients with diabetes mellitus as phenytoin can stimulate glucagon secretion and can impair insulin secretion, causing hyperglycemia. Patients with hypothyroidism should be monitored for signs of underactive thyroid. Phenytoin may cause an increased degradation of circulating concentrations of thyroid hormone (T3 and T4). Monitor liver function tests (LFTs).

PRACTICE PEARLS

Phenytoin Use in Pregnancy and Lactation

- Phenytoin is a known teratogen and poses a reproductive risk.
- Discuss contraception requirements with females of childbearing years.
- Phenytoin is secreted in low concentrations in human milk, so breastfeeding is not recommended for females taking phenytoin.

PRACTICE PEARLS

Phenytoin Therapy for the Older Adult

- Use phenytoin cautiously in older adults as they may have reduced hepatic biotransformation and subsequent drug toxicity.
- Phenytoin serum concentration monitoring may be necessary to achieve optimal dosage adjustments. Anticonvulsants can produce ataxia, impaired psychomotor function, syncope, and falls.

BLACK BOX WARNING!

Antiepileptic Therapy

- In January 2008, the U.S. Food and Drug Administration (FDA) issued an alert related to an increased risk of suicidal ideation and behaviors in patients receiving anticonvulsants to treat epilepsy, psychiatric disorders, or other conditions (e.g., migraine, neuropathic pain).
- In the analysis, patients receiving anticonvulsants had approximately twice the risk of suicidal behavior or ideation (0.43%) as patients receiving placebo (0.22%).
- All patients beginning treatment with anticonvulsants or currently receiving such treatment should be closely monitored for emerging or worsening suicidal thoughts/behaviors or depression.

GABA Analogs

A GABA analog is a derivative of the amino acid gamma-aminobutyric acid (GABA). GABA is one of the most important neurotransmitters (chemical messengers) in the

CNS. It is essential for maintaining the balance between nerve cell excitation and nerve cell inhibition.

Valproic Acid

Pharmacokinetics. Valproic acid is administered orally. After administration, the bioavailability is nearly 100%. Peak plasma concentrations are achieved within 1 to 4 hours after oral administration of immediate-release, within 3 to 5 hours of delayed-release, and within 4 to 17 hours of extended-release tablets. Magnesium-aluminum antacids can increase the area under the curve (AUC) by 12%. The half-life is prolonged in patients with hepatic impairment, and valproic acid clearance may be decreased by 50% in patients with cirrhosis.

Indications. Valproic acid is available as an oral capsule in delayed- and extended-release formulations. Rectal formulations are available for refractory status epilepticus. Valproic acid is indicated for patients with simple absence seizures, complex absence seizures, or complex partial seizures, and adjunctively for other seizure types that include absence or partial complex seizures.

Adverse Effects. Psychiatric adverse effects such as depression, behavior changes, and agitation have been reported. There is an increased risk of suicidal ideation and behavior with valproic acid use; this occurs most commonly from 1 to 24 weeks after therapy initiation, but can occur after longer periods as well.

GI adverse effects such as nausea and vomiting are common, especially at the initiation of treatment. From 1% to 5% of patients report increased appetite, constipation, dysgeusia, fecal incontinence, flatulence, gastroenteritis, glossitis, hematemesis, and xerostomia. Hepatotoxicity is most likely to occur within the first 6 months of treatment, especially in children younger than 2 years of age, patients with mitochondrial disease, and patients receiving multiple anticonvulsants. The most serious adverse reaction is hepatic failure. Hyperammonemia can be present despite normal LFTs.

Hematologic adverse effects include ecchymosis and petechiae, occurring in 1% to 5% of patients. Abnormal coagulation tests and thrombocytopenia have also been reported and occur more frequently in patients receiving higher doses. CNS adverse effects such as drowsiness can also occur with higher dosages. Reversible and irreversible cerebral and cerebellar atrophy, dementia, and behavioral changes (apathy or irritability) have occurred. Dermatologic effects such as rash, pruritis, and alopecia erythema multiforme, Stevens-Johnson syndrome, cutaneous vasculitis, and nail or nail bed disorders have been reported.

Cardiovascular adverse effects include hypertension, hypotension, palpitations, orthostatic hypotension, sinus tachycardia, peripheral vasodilation, and chest pain (unspecified). In addition, arrhythmia exacerbation has been reported. Drug rash with eosinophilia and systemic symptoms (DRESS), also known as multiorgan hypersensitivity, has been reported in patients taking valproic acid and its analogs. Cases of life-threatening pancreatitis have been reported in both pediatric and adult patients receiving valproic acid or its analogs.

Contraindications. Valproic acid and its analogs are contraindicated in patients with known urea cycle disorders due to a genetic enzyme defect. This can lead to an impaired ability to produce urea, thereby causing hyperammonemic encephalopathy. Valproic acid and its analogs are contraindicated in patients known to have a mitochondrial disease caused by mutations in mitochondrial DNA polymerase gamma. Valproic acid is contraindicated in patients with hepatic disease or significant hepatic dysfunction. It should be used with caution in patients with severe renal impairment or renal failure, because uremia can cause increased free drug, resulting in possible toxicity. Valproic acid is associated with reproductive risk, so it may be contraindicated in pregnancy.

Monitoring. Close monitoring of valproic acid serum concentrations may be warranted in those with hepatic impairment to limit toxicity. Closely monitor all patients beginning treatment with anticonvulsants or currently receiving such treatment for emerging or worsening suicidal thoughts/behaviors, unusual moods or behaviors, or depression. Monitor the patient's motor and cognitive functions routinely while on valproate therapy. Patients should be warned about the possibility of drowsiness and the inability to perform tasks requiring mental acuity. Clinical signs of urea cycle disorders include hyperammonemia, encephalopathy, and respiratory alkalosis. Patients who develop signs and symptoms consistent with urea cycle disorders should be promptly evaluated, with discontinuation of valproate therapy. Abdominal pain, nausea, vomiting, and/or anorexia can be symptoms of pancreatitis that require prompt medical evaluation.

PRACTICE PEARLS

Valproic Acid and DRESS Syndrome

- DRESS may be fatal or life threatening.
- Common symptoms of DRESS are fever, serious rash, and/or lymphadenopathy, in association with other organ system involvement such as hepatitis, nephritis, hematological abnormalities, myocarditis, or myositis sometimes resembling an acute viral infection. Eosinophilia is often present. If DRESS is suspected, the patient should be evaluated immediately, and valproate should be discontinued.

Gabapentin

Pharmacokinetics. Gabapentin is administered orally. The bioavailability of immediate-release gabapentin is 60% for a 300-mg dose and 35% for a 1600-mg dose. Less than 3% of gabapentin is bound to proteins. Gabapentin has a high level of lipid solubility, and thus is readily distributed into the CNS. Gabapentin is not metabolized, and is excreted intact in the urine. The elimination half-life in patients with normal renal function taking a dose range

of 1200 to 3000 mg/day of immediate-release gabapentin ranges from 5 to 7 hours.

Indications. Gabapentin is indicated as an adjunctive treatment for partial seizures with or without secondary generalized tonic-clonic seizures.

Adverse Effects. Fatigue, lethargy, and asthenia are the most commonly reported adverse effects of gabapentin, occurring in about 10% of patients. Less common were dizziness, headache, and confusion. In children 3 to 12 years of age, weight gain and dehydration have been reported. As with other anticonvulsants, gabapentin is thought to carry an increased risk of suicidal ideation and behavior, occurring largely between 1 and 24 weeks after therapy initiation. But as with other anticonvulsants, this can occur at any point in therapy. Depression occurred in 1% to 2% of patients receiving gabapentin in either immediate- or extended-release formulations.

Contraindications. Gabapentin is contraindicated in patients who have demonstrated hypersensitivity to gabapentin or any of its components. Gralise and Horizant extended-release tablets are *not* interchangeable with each other or other gabapentin products due to differing chemical and pharmacokinetic profiles. Gabapentin is known to be substantially excreted by the kidney. While not contraindicated, the dose of gabapentin in patients with renal impairment or renal failure needs adjustment. Avoid abrupt discontinuation of gabapentin to limit drug withdrawal and the possibility of increasing seizure frequency. Gradually discontinue gabapentin over a minimum of 1 week or longer. Patients receiving gabapentin encarbil (Horizant) 600 mg or less may discontinue the drug without tapering.

Monitoring. All patients should be closely monitored for emerging or worsening suicide thoughts/behaviors and depression. Monitor pediatric patients closely for CNS side effects such as emotional lability, behavioral problems, aggressive behaviors, problems with concentration, impaired cognition, restlessness, and hyperactivity. Advise patients against driving or operating machinery until tolerance for somnolence develops, as gabapentin impairs the ability to perform such tasks. Carefully evaluate patients for a history of substance abuse, and monitor for signs and symptoms of gabapentin misuse or abuse (development of tolerance, self-dose escalation, and drug-seeking behavior).

PRACTICE PEARLS

Gabapentin Use in Pregnancy and Lactation

- There are no adequate and well-controlled studies of gabapentin in pregnant patients. Gabapentin actively crosses the placenta.
- Gabapentin is excreted in breast milk, so a breastfeeding infant could be exposed to a maximum gabapentin dosage of approximately 1 mg/kg/day.

Barbiturates

Phenobarbital is the oldest and longest acting of the common anticonvulsants and is available in both oral and parenteral formulations. As a barbiturate, phenobarbital has both anticonvulsant and sedative hypnotic properties. In general, phenobarbital is effective in all seizure disorders except absence (petit mal) seizures.

Phenobarbital

Pharmacokinetics. Phenobarbital can be administered orally, or by intramuscular (IM) or IV injection. The distribution of phenobarbital is less rapid than that of other barbiturates because it is less lipid soluble. Bioavailability of the oral formulation is approximately 70% to 90%. Phenobarbital is the longest-acting barbiturate, with a half-life in adults ranging from 50 to 120 hours and a mean of 96 hours. Peak serum concentrations are achieved 8 to 12 hours after oral dosing. For anticonvulsant activity, the therapeutic plasma concentration is 10 to 40 mcg/mL. Plasma concentrations greater than 50 mcg/mL may produce coma or respiratory depression. Concentrations greater than 80 mcg/mL are potentially fatal. Twenty-five percent of phenobarbital is eliminated in the urine, with the remainder inactivated by the liver via CYP 2C9.

Indications. Phenobarbital is indicated for the maintenance treatment of all seizure types, including partial seizures, myoclonic seizures, tonic-clonic seizures, and neonatal seizures not responding to other anticonvulsants. The IV formulation is used in status epilepticus.

Adverse Events. As with all anticonvulsants, phenobarbital carries an increased risk for suicidal ideation and behaviors. This increased risk occurred from 1 to 24 weeks after therapy initiation; however, the risk can exceed 24 weeks. CNS depressant effects including drowsiness, dizziness, lethargy, headache, vertigo, and irritability can develop during therapy with phenobarbital. Hypnotic doses may produce residual sedation, emotional lability, and impaired cognition. Children and older adults may experience a higher incidence of CNS effects.

Hypersensitivity reactions to barbiturates like phenobarbital may present as various organ system problems, including blood, liver, renal, and skin disorders. Blood dyscrasias such as agranulocytosis, aplastic anemia, neutropenia, and thrombocytopenia are rare, but can occur during therapy. Cutaneous reactions occur in roughly 1% to 2% of patients and include scarlatiniform or morbilliform maculopapular rash. While rash or urticaria may not appear to be a serious side effect, such a reaction can precede more serious effects and may be accompanied by other indicators of drug allergy.

GI adverse effects such as nausea and vomiting occurring with initial dosing are usually mild and attenuate with continued administration. Administration with food and/or sufficient fluid may help alleviate these symptoms. Phenobarbital is associated with vitamin A, vitamin D, and folic acid deficiencies with long-term use, and can result in megaloblastic anemia, osteopenia, or osteomalacia. Unusual fatigue, weight loss, bone pain, or tenderness should be investigated.

Symptoms of sexual dysfunction including erectile dysfunction and loss of libido have been reported with long-term use. Prolonged use of barbiturates can produce physiological dependence with or without a psychological dependence. Abrupt withdrawal of phenobarbital can result in anxiety, muscle twitching, tremor of hands, progressive weakness, dizziness, distortion of vision, insomnia, nausea, vomiting, and postural hypotension. Major manifestations of withdrawal include hallucinations, delirium, and seizures. Sudden withdrawal of phenobarbital can precipitate status epilepticus. To maintain seizure control, phenobarbital should be withdrawn gradually.

Contraindications. Avoid the use of phenobarbital in patients with a history of barbiturate hypersensitivity. A history of hypersensitivity reactions should be obtained for the patient and their immediate family members. Hypersensitivity reactions have been reported in patients who previously experienced hydantoin hypersensitivity (phenytoin) or carbamazepine hypersensitivity. IV administration of phenobarbital sodium should generally be reserved for emergency settings; close supervision is necessary in a monitored unit.

Administration of phenobarbital is contraindicated in patients with pulmonary disease with dyspnea or obstruction, as phenobarbital can cause dose-dependent respiratory depression. Phenobarbital should be prescribed with caution to patients with known substance abuse due to the potential for psychological/physical dependence on the drug. Alcoholic beverages should be avoided due to the potential for additive CNS depressant effects. The lethal dose of a barbiturate is significantly less if alcohol is also ingested. Additionally, alcohol use may reduce seizure control.

According to the Beers Criteria, barbiturates are considered potentially inappropriate medications in older adults, especially for those with a history of falls or fractures due to phenobarbital's effects on gait and balance, and the CNS adverse effects. Phenobarbital is also contraindicated in patients with severe hepatic dysfunction due to the increased risk for drug toxicity.

Monitoring. All patients beginning treatment with anticonvulsants or currently receiving such treatment should be closely monitored for emerging or worsening suicidal thoughts/behaviors or worsening depression. Monitor for hypersensitivity reactions through periodic complete blood counts (CBCs) if phenobarbital is used for long-term therapy. Patients should be taught to report unusual sore throat, fever, or tiredness for etiology. Monitor LFTs and renal function as phenobarbital has been reported to cause interstitial nephritis and drug-induced liver problems such as hepatitis and jaundice with accompanying elevated hepatic enzymes. Monitor phenobarbital concentration levels throughout treatment (Table 29.1).

TABLE 29.1	Serum Phenobarbital Concentrations		
Type of Level		Traditional Units	Scientific International Units
Therapeutic concentration		15–40 mcg/mL	65–172 µmol/L
Toxic concentration, slowness, ataxia, nystagmus		>30 mcg/mL	>129 µmol/L
Toxic concentration, coma with reflexes		>50 mcg/mL	>15 µmol/L
Toxic concentration, coma without reflexes		>100 mcg/mL	> 431 µmol/L

Iminostilbenes

Carbamazepine

Carbamazepine is an oral antiepileptic structurally similar to tricyclic antidepressants.

Pharmacokinetics. Carbamazepine absorption from the GI tract is variable, with approximately 85% bioavailability. Carbamazepine is metabolized in the liver to active metabolites and is considered a potent inducer of CYP 3A4. Plasma concentrations peak within 4 to 5 hours after administration of the immediate-release tablets and within 1.5 hours after administration of the suspension. The plasma half-life of carbamazepine is 25 to 65 hours initially but decreases to 12 to 17 hours with repeated dosing. Serum concentrations of 4 to 12 mcg/mL are considered to be therapeutic in the treatment of seizure disorders, and it may take several days to reach a steady state. Carbamazepine is excreted in the urine—72% as metabolites, with 3% as unchanged drug—and the remainder is excreted in the feces. The effects of renal and hepatic impairment on pharmacokinetics are unknown.

Indications. Carbamazepine is used for the treatment of simple and complex partial seizures, and for generalized tonic-clonic seizures.

Adverse Effects. The most frequent adverse reactions to carbamazepine are nausea and vomiting, which are most frequent in the beginning phases of treatment. Dermatologic effects of carbamazepine may cause serious/life-threatening rash, including Stevens-Johnson syndrome and toxic epidermal necrolysis.

Psychiatric adverse effects include suicidal ideation and suicidal behaviors. As with other antiepileptics, this adverse effect is most often observed between 1 and 24 weeks of therapy. CNS effects such as dizziness, drowsiness, confusion, fatigue, unsteady gait, and ataxia have been observed. Hepatic effects such as asymptomatic elevations in liver enzymes and, more rarely, hepatitis, cholestasis, and hepatocellular jaundice have occurred with carbamazepine. Hematologic toxicity is relatively uncommon, but transient leukopenia, neutropenia, thrombocytopenia, or more severe reactions such as agranulocytosis or aplastic anemia have been reported. Cardiovascular adverse effects such as hypertension have been reported in 3% of patients taking carbamazepine. Other cardiovascular effects including AV block, cardiac arrhythmias, heart failure, edema, and coronary artery disease (CAD) have also occurred.

Genitourinary adverse effects of carbamazepine have included increased urinary frequency, urinary retention, oliguria with elevated blood pressure, azotemia, and renal failure. Albuminuria, glycosuria, elevated blood urea nitrogen (BUN), proteinuria, and microscopic deposits in the urine have also occurred. Vitamin deficiencies occur as anticonvulsants enhance the hepatic breakdown of vitamin D into inactive metabolites, and also impair folate metabolism. Patients receiving carbamazepine for more than 6 months should be monitored for vitamin D and folate deficiency, and receive supplementation as needed. Hyponatremia can occur, especially within the first 3 months or later. Normalization of sodium levels usually occurs within a few days of discontinuing the drug.

Contraindications. Carbamazepine is not recommended for use in absence seizures, atonic seizures, or myoclonic seizures because it can exacerbate these conditions. Abrupt discontinuation of carbamazepine therapy is contradicted and the medication should be withdrawn gradually to minimize the potential of increased seizure frequency. Carbamazepine is contraindicated in patients with carbamazepine or tricyclic hypersensitivity. Carbamazepine is also contraindicated in patients with a history of bone marrow suppression. Carbamazepine should be used with caution in any patient with cardiac disease, cardiac arrhythmias, or heart failure because symptoms may be potentiated or exacerbated. Females of child-bearing potential should be informed of the potential risk to the fetus, and patients should be instructed to contact their health care provider immediately if they become pregnant or intend to become pregnant. Carbamazepine is contraindicated in patients who are receiving monoamine oxidase inhibitor (MAOI) therapy or who have received an MAOI in the last 14 days.

Monitoring. Monitor patients for increased risk of suicidal thoughts and behaviors. Patients should be advised to immediately report to their health care provider the emergence or worsening of depression, thoughts of self-harm, or other unusual changes in mood or behavior. Monitor patients for signs of hypersensitivity or rash. Consider discontinuation of carbamazepine in patients who develop signs or symptoms of symptomatic hyponatremia (headache, new or increased seizure frequency, concentration difficulty, memory impairment, confusion, weakness, or unsteadiness). Monitor patients for evidence of bone marrow depression, such as fever, difficulty breathing on exertion, fatigue, easy bruising, petechiae, epistaxis, gingival bleeding, and heavy menses.

Carbamazepine Use in Pregnancy and Lactation

- There is a risk for teratogenesis when carbamazepine therapy is used in pregnant patients; therefore, the relative risks should be weighed carefully.
- Carbamazepine accumulates in the fetus after crossing the placenta and is found in breast milk.

Oxcarbazepine

Oxcarbazepine is an oral anticonvulsant that is an analog of carbamazepine.

Pharmacokinetics. Oxcarbazepine is administered orally and is almost completely absorbed from the GI tract. Following absorption, it undergoes rapid reduction in the liver. Plasma levels are reached in 4 to 6 hours, with steady-state levels reached within 2 to 3 days of twice-daily dosing. Ninety-five percent of the dose is excreted renally, with less than 1% unchanged. Almost one-half of a dose is eliminated as metabolites. Less than 4% of a dose is excreted in the feces.

Indications. Oxcarbazepine is indicated for the treatment of partial-onset seizures.

Adverse Effects. CNS effects include headache (13% to 31% of patients), dizziness (25%), drowsiness (19%), ataxia (6%), insomnia (6%), and incoordination (3%). Psychiatric effects include anxiety (7%), confusion (7%), nervousness (6%), amnesia (5%), and emotional lability (3%). As with all anticonvulsants, use of oxcarbazepine is thought to carry an increased risk of new or worsened depression, suicidal ideation, and suicidal behavior. GI effects include nausea (16%), vomiting (7% to 14%), diarrhea (7%), dyspepsia (6%), anorexia (5%), abdominal pain (5%), xerostomia (3%), and rectal hemorrhage (2%). Similar to carbamazepine, genitourinary effects also occur. Clinically significant hyponatremia (sodium <125 mmol/L) may develop during treatment with oxcarbazepine. This typically occurs during the first 3 months; however, cases of symptomatic hyponatremia beginning more than 1 year after treatment initiation have been observed. Normalization of sodium levels usually occurs within a few days of discontinuing the drug.

Contraindications. Oxcarbazepine should not be used in patients with a known hypersensitivity reaction to the drug or any of its components.

Monitoring. Monitor patients for the increased risk of suicidal thoughts and behaviors. Patients should be advised to immediately report to their health care provider the emergence or worsening of depression, thoughts of self-harm, or other unusual changes in mood or behavior. Monitor patients for signs of hypersensitivity or rash. Consider discontinuation of carbamazepine in patients who develop signs or symptoms of symptomatic hyponatremia (headache, new or increased seizure frequency, concentration difficulty, memory impairment, confusion, weakness, or unsteadiness). Monitor patients for evidence of bone marrow depression, such as fever, difficulty breathing on exertion, fatigue, easy bruising, petechiae, epistaxis, gingival bleeding, and heavy menses.

Carbamazepine and Oxcarbazepine

- Carbamazepine and oxcarbazepine may cause serious and potentially life-threatening dermatologic adverse reactions such as Stevens-Johnson syndrome and toxic epidermal necrolysis.
- The risk is about 1 to 6 per 10,000 new users in countries with mainly Caucasian populations.
- The risk of these reactions in countries with primarily Asian patients may be 10 times higher because of variants found in the immune system gene HLA-B 1502, which occur at a higher rate in Asian patients.
- It is recommended that Asian patients undergo a genetic blood test prior to initiation of treatment.

Miscellaneous Anticonvulsants

Topiramate

Topiramate is derived from the naturally occurring monosaccharide D-fructose and is structurally different from other antiepileptics. Instead of raising the seizure threshold, topiramate appears to block the spread of seizures. Due to its several mechanisms of action, topiramate can be effective in patients with various seizures that are refractory to other agents.

Pharmacokinetics. Topiramate is administered orally. Human plasma protein binding ranges from 15% to 41%. Topiramate is absorbed rapidly, with peak plasma concentrations occurring approximately 2 hours after oral administration of a 400-mg immediate-release preparation. Peak plasma concentrations of topiramate are reached approximately 24 hours after a 200-mg dose of extended-release capsules. The relative bioavailability from the tablets is about 80%. Steady-state concentrations are reached in 4 to 8 days in adult patients with normal renal function. The mean plasma elimination half-life is 21 hours following single or multiple doses. About 70% of an administered dose is eliminated unchanged in the urine. Pharmacokinetics may be affected by renal or hepatic impairment, reducing medication clearance. With the same mg/kg dose, plasma concentrations may be lower in children.

Indications. Topiramate is an oral antiepileptic used as monotherapy or adjunctive therapy in adults, adolescents, and children with partial onset, generalized primary tonic-clonic seizures, and as an adjunct therapy in Lennox-Gastaut syndrome.

Adverse Effects. Serious rash (Stevens-Johnson syndrome and toxic epidermal necrolysis) has been reported in patients receiving topiramate. Topiramate is associated with an increased risk of bleeding. CNS adverse effects of topiramate include paresthesia, dizziness, hypoesthesia, ataxia, drowsiness, and insomnia. In pediatric patients 6 to 15 years of age, paresthesia, involuntary movements/muscle contractions, and vertigo occurred.

Emerging or worsening suicidal thoughts/behaviors, depression, or other changes in mood/behavior are associated with antiepileptic therapy. Dose-related hyper-ammonemia with and without encephalopathy has been reported with topiramate use. GI effects reported are constipation, gastritis, xerostomia, dysgeusia, gastroesophageal reflux, anorexia, and weight loss . In pediatric patients 6 to 15 years of age, both diarrhea and weight loss occurred.

Contraindications. Topiramate is contraindicated in patients with known hypersensitivity to the drug or any of the product's components. Exfoliative dermatologic reactions have been reported that were serious and potentially fatal. There may be a cross-reactivity to antibiotic sulfonamides and nonantibiotic sulfonamides, such as topiramate in predisposed patients. Extended-release topiramate is contraindicated in patients with metabolic acidosis who are taking concomitant metformin. Topiramate can cause hyperchloremic nonanion gap metabolic acidosis. As topiramate is a CNS depressant, avoid alcohol while taking topiramate. Closely monitor patients (especially neonates, infants, and children) treated with topiramate for evidence of decreased sweating and increased body temperature, especially in hot weather. Use caution when topiramate is given with other drugs that predispose patients to heat-related disorders. Patients with inborn errors of metabolism or reduced hepatic mitochondrial activity (mitochondrial disease) may be at an increased risk for hyperammonemia with or without encephalopathy. Anticonvulsants may be contraindicated in older adults with a history of falls or fractures, since anticonvulsants can produce ataxia, impaired psychomotor function, syncope, and additional falls.

Monitoring. Monitor all patients treated with topiramate closely for emerging or worsening depression or suicidal ideation. Advise patients and caregivers of the increased risk of suicidal thoughts and behaviors and to immediately report the emergence of new or worsening depression, suicidal thoughts, or behaviors. In patients with or without a history of seizures or epilepsy, withdraw topiramate gradually to minimize the potential for seizures or increased seizure frequency. Monitoring of baseline and periodic serum bicarbonate during topiramate treatment is recommended. If metabolic acidosis develops and persists, consider reducing the dose or discontinuing topiramate (using dose tapering).

Felbamate

Pharmacokinetics. Felbamate is administered orally. While the therapeutic range has not been established, plasma protein binding ranges from 25% to 35%. Absorption of oral felbamate is approximately 90% and is not affected by food. It is similar for both the tablet and suspension formulations. Time to peak serum concentration is 1 to 6 hours. About 45% of the administered dose is present in the urine unchanged, and 40% is present as metabolites and conjugates. Less than 5% of an orally administered dose is present in the feces. The plasma half-life of felbamate is 13 to 25 hours.

Indications. Felbamate is indicated for the treatment of partial seizures, and partial and generalized seizures associated with Lennox-Gastaut syndrome in children.

Adverse Effects. Psychiatric adverse effects include anxiety (5.2% of patients) nervousness (7%), and depression (5.3%). Agitation, aggression, and hallucinations were reported in fewer than 1% of patients. Anticonvulsants are thought to carry an increased risk of suicidal ideation and behavior. GI adverse effects with felbamate as monotherapy include dyspepsia (8.6%), vomiting (8.6%), constipation (6.9%), diarrhea (5.2%), and weight loss (3.4%). These effects increase in frequency when felbamate is used as adjunctive therapy. In children prescribed felbamate for Lennox-Gastaut syndrome, anorexia (54.8%), vomiting (38.7%), constipation (12.9%), hiccups (9.7%), nausea (6.5%), dyspepsia (6.5%), and weight loss (6.5%) were present. Elevated hepatic enzymes, hepatitis, hepatic failure, and jaundice have been reported. Dermatologic effects such as rash (3.4%) and Stevens-Johnson syndrome were reported rarely (<0.1%). CNS effects include insomnia (8.6%), headache (6.9%), drowsiness (19%), dizziness (18.4%), tremor (6.1%), abnormal gait (5.3%), and stupor (2.6%). In adults, hyperphosphatemia was reported in 3.4% of patients receiving felbamate. Adverse cardiovascular effects including palpitations and sinus tachycardia were reported in at least 1% of patients. Hematologic adverse effects such as an increase in the incidence of aplastic anemia also occurred.

Contraindications. Felbamate is contraindicated in patients with felbamate or carbamate hypersensitivity. Do not discontinue felbamate abruptly as this can precipitate seizures. Felbamate is contraindicated in breastfeeding mothers.

Monitoring. Patients receiving felbamate should be monitored for signs of hepatotoxicity, including periodic assessment of serum transaminase concentrations at baseline and regular intervals. Monitor CBC with differential, LFTs, platelet count, and serum iron.

PRACTICE PEARLS

Felbamate Use in Pregnancy and Lactation

- There are no studies in pregnant females to determine the effect of felbamate on the fetus.
- Physicians are advised to recommend that pregnant patients receiving felbamate enroll in the North American Antiepileptic Drug (NAAED) Pregnancy Registry to provide information about the effects of in utero exposure to the drug.
- Felbamate is excreted into breast milk, but its effects on the infant are unknown. Breastfeeding should generally be avoided during treatment with felbamate.

Levetiracetam

Levetiracetam is a pyrrolidine derivative antiepileptic medication that is used for the treatment of certain types of partial, myoclonic, and generalized tonic-clonic seizures. Levetiracetam is available in oral (immediate and extended release) and IV preparations.

Pharmacokinetics. The bioavailability of the oral preparation is similar (100%) for both the immediate- and extended-release formulations. The immediate-release fast-melting tablets disintegrate in about 11 seconds when taken with a sip of water. Absorption is rapid, with a peak plasma concentration reached 1 hour after administration in adult and pediatric patients.

Indications. Levetiracetam is indicated for the treatment of partial, myoclonic, and generalized tonic-clonic seizures.

Adverse Effects. Adverse effects of levetiracetam occurring in fewer than 10% of patients are hypertension, anorexia, asthenia, cough, drowsiness, fatigue, and headache. Psychological adverse effects such as irritability, hallucinations, and psychosis have been reported. Depressive symptoms, agitation, anxiety, confusion, emotional lability, and insomnia are less frequent, occurring in 1% to 10% of patients. Suicidal ideation, Stevens-Johnson syndrome, and toxic epidermal necrolysis are rare occurrences (fewer than 1%).

Contraindications. There are no absolute contraindications for the use of levetiracetam. However, this medication should be used with caution in the geriatric, infant, child, and pregnant and breastfeeding patient populations. Levetiracetam should also be used cautiously in patients with preexisting suicidal ideation, psychosis, depression, or renal impairment. Do not discontinue levetiracetam abruptly.

Monitoring. Due to potential adverse effects on the kidney, patients with renal impairment or risk for renal impairment should have their BUN and creatinine monitored at baseline and routinely throughout treatment (Table 29.2).

Prescriber Considerations for Antiepileptic Therapy

Clinical Reasoning for Antiepileptic Therapy

Consider the individual patient's health problem requiring antiepileptic therapy. One of the first considerations in initiating antiepileptic therapy is to accurately determine the type of seizure that is to be treated. Treatment of seizures may be delayed if a seizure is a one-time event, as opposed to a history of more than one seizure. Once a definitive diagnosis is determined, treatment choice is largely dependent upon the adverse-effect profile of the medication in consideration of the specific patient's history. In addition, consider whether the patient has had a history or episode of status epilepticus requiring treatment with IV antiepileptics, as this will require consideration of acute seizure therapy with a benzodiazepine.

Determine the desired therapeutic outcome based on the degree of antiepileptic needed for the patient's health problem. The desired therapeutic outcome is an increase in the seizure threshold that results in a reduction of seizure activity. There are many different epilepsy syndromes, and all have different outcomes and treatment responses. Early response to

treatment is an important predictor of the long-term prognosis of newly diagnosed epilepsy.

Assess the antiepileptic therapy selected for its appropriateness for an individual patient by considering the medication's side effects and the patient's age, race/ethnicity, comorbidities, and genetic factors. Adults with an unprovoked first seizure have the highest seizure recurrence risk within the first 2 years (21% to 45%) (Krumholtz et al., 2015). Prior brain insult, an electroencephalogram (EEG) with epileptiform abnormalities, brain-imaging abnormality, and nocturnal seizures are associated with increased seizure recurrence risk. Instituting immediate antiepileptic drug therapy, as compared with delay of treatment pending a second seizure, is likely to reduce recurrence risk within the first 2 years but may not improve quality of life. Also consider the age of the patient; for example, carbamazepine is preferred over phenobarbital for children because it has fewer adverse effects on behavior and alertness. Initiate therapy at the lowest recommended dose and monitor for symptoms of respiratory depression and sedation in older adults, patients with underlying pulmonary disease such as COPD, and during coadministration with other CNS depressants. Asian patients should undergo genetic testing prior to treatment if an iminostilbene is being considered.

Initiate the treatment plan with the selected medication by first providing adequate patient education to ensure the patient's understanding and promote full participation in antiepileptic therapy. A complete understanding of the potential risks and benefits of antiepileptic treatment is advised, especially due to the serious dermatologic, hematologic, psychiatric, cardiovascular, and fetal risks involved. Advise patients that if adverse reactions are of such severity that therapy must be discontinued, the therapy should be gradually withdrawn. Abrupt discontinuation of any anticonvulsant drug may lead to drug withdrawal seizures or even status epilepticus, which may be life-threatening.

Ensure complete patient and family understanding about the medication(s) prescribed for antiepileptic therapy using a variety of education strategies. The treatment of epilepsy may involve more than one prescribed therapy, so steps that ensure the patient's and family's understanding of the illness and the medications are imperative. Education strategies that incorporate verbal, written, and web-based resources and support groups are very helpful in assisting in the understanding of planned therapy and necessary follow-up. A detailed explanation of the serious adverse effects that need to be reported to the provider, with accompanying pictorials, is advised.

Conduct follow-up and monitoring of patient responses to antiepileptic therapy. Follow-up and monitoring should include a patient diary of seizure activity, and information as to when the emergency room is appropriate and when to call the provider. Patient response to the therapy is directly related to a reduction in seizure activity, severity, and duration. The potential seriousness of some adverse events requires the provider to assess the patient for signs and symptoms of all potential serious

TABLE 29.2 **Antiepileptic Medications**

Category/ Medication	Indication	Dosage	Considerations and Monitoring
GABA Analogs			
Valproic acid	Monotherapy or adjunct treatment of simple, complex, or complex partial seizures, and adjunctively for other seizure types, such as tonic-clonic or myoclonic seizures	**Delayed release:** *Adults, children, and adolescents 10–17 yr:* 10–15 mg/kg/day orally. Titrate in 5–10 mg/kg/day increments at weekly intervals until seizures are controlled.	Monitor CBC, LFTs, and plasma ammonia concentrations.
Gabapentin	Adjunctive treatment of partial seizures with or without secondary generalized tonic clonic seizures	*Adults and adolescents:* 300 mg orally three times daily. Effective dose is 900–1800 mg/day, but up to 2400 mg/day has been used long term. *Children 3–12 yr:* 10–15 mg/kg/day orally in 3 divided doses. Can be titrated upward over 3 days. If >5 yr, the effective dose is 25–35 mg/kg/day orally.	Monitor serum creatinine/BUN and WBC.
Barbiturates			
Phenobarbital	Maintenance treatment of partial seizures, myoclonic seizures, tonic-clonic seizures, or neonatal seizures not responding to other anticonvulsants	*Adults:* 1–3 mg/kg/day orally in 1–2 divided doses. Gradually titrate dosage based on patient response and serum concentrations. Can also be given by IM or IV. *Children and adolescents ≥7 yr:* 3–6 mg/kg/day orally in 1–2 divided doses. Gradually titrate dosage based on patient response and serum concentrations. *Infants and children ≤6 yr:* 4–8 mg/kg/day orally in 1–2 divided doses. *Neonates:* 3–4 mg/kg orally once daily initially; titrate dose based on patient response and therapeutic concentration. May increase to 5 mg/kg/day.	Monitor CBC, LFTs, serum creatinine/ BUN, and serum phenobarbital concentrations.
Iminostilbenes			
Carbamazepine	Management of generalized tonic-clonic seizures, or for partial seizures, either simple or complex	*Adults and adolescents:* 200 mg orally twice daily initially. Increase in weekly increments of 200 mg/day, as needed, up to 1600 mg orally (adults) or 1000–1200 mg (adolescents) daily in 3 or 4 divided doses. *Children 6–11 yr:* 100 mg orally twice daily initially. Increase in weekly increments of 100 mg/day, as needed, up to 1000 mg orally daily in 3 or 4 divided doses. *Children <6 yr:* 10–20 mg/kg/day orally initially, in 2 or 3 divided doses. Increase weekly, as needed, up to 35 mg/kg/day given in 3 or 4 divided doses.	Monitor CBC, LFTs, reticulocyte count, serum carbamazepine concentrations, serum creatinine/ BUN, serum iron, and urinalysis.

TABLE 29.2   Antiepileptic Medications—cont'd

Category/Medication	Indication	Dosage	Considerations and Monitoring
Oxcarbazepine	Monotherapy or adjunct treatment of partial seizures	*Adults and adolescents ≥17 yr:* 300 mg orally twice daily initially. Titrate by 300 mg/day every third day or 600 mg/day every week as indicated and tolerated. Maximum dosage: 2400 mg/day in 2 divided doses. *Children and adolescents 4–16 yr:* 8–10 mg/kg/day orally initially, in 2 divided doses. Increase by 5 mg/kg/day every third day to the recommended manufacturer weight-based daily maintenance dosage. **Extended-release formula:** *Adults and adolescents ≥17 yr:* 600 mg orally once daily initially for 1 week. Increase dose weekly in 600 mg/day increments to achieve the recommended dose of 1200–2400 mg once daily. *Children and adolescents 6–16 yr:* 8–10 mg/kg orally once in the first week initially. Titrate by 8–10 mg/kg/day increments (not to exceed 600 mg/day).	Laboratory monitoring not necessary.
Miscellaneous Agents			
Topiramate	Monotherapy or adjunct treatment of partial seizures	*Adults, adolescents, and children ≥10 yr:* 50 mg/day initially, in 2 divided doses. Increase daily dose by 50 mg once weekly. *Children 2–9 yr and >38 kg:* 25 mg orally once daily initially in the evening. If tolerated, may increase dosage to 25 mg orally twice daily during week 2 of therapy. *Children 2–9 yr:* Dosages vary by weight.	Monitor serum bicarbonate, serum creatinine/BUN, and serum electrolytes.
Felbamate	Treatment of partial seizures with or without generalization in adults and adolescents and for partial and generalized seizures associated with Lennox-Gastaut syndrome in children	*Adults and adolescents >14 yr:* 1200 mg/day orally in 3–4 divided doses. Increase dose in 600 mg increments every 2 weeks to 2400 mg/day orally based on clinical response. *Adolescents and children 2-14 yr:* 15 mg/kg/day orally in 3–4 divided doses while reducing dosages of other antiepileptics by 20%–30%. Increase felbamate dosage by 15 mg/kg/day increments at weekly intervals to 45 mg/kg/day orally. Maximum dosage: 3600 mg/day.	Monitor CBC with differential, LFTs, platelet count, and serum iron.
Levetiracetam	Treatment of partial seizure and adjunctive treatment of myoclonic seizures with juvenile myoclonic epilepsy	*Adults and adolescents 16–17 yr:* 500 mg orally twice daily initially. Increase dose every 2 weeks by 500 mg/dose, to a maximum dosage of 1500 mg orally twice daily. *Children and adolescents 4–15 yr:* 10 mg/kg/dose orally twice daily initially. Increase dose every 2 weeks by 10 mg/kg/dose increments to the recommended dose of 30 mg/kg/dose orally twice daily. *Infants and children 6 months to 3 yr:* 10 mg/kg/dose orally twice daily initially. Increase dose every 2 weeks by 10 mg/kg/dose increments to the recommended dose of 25 mg/kg/dose orally twice daily. *Infants 1–5 months:* 7 mg/kg/dose orally twice daily initially. Increase dose every 2 weeks by 7 mg/kg/dose increments to the recommended dose of 21 mg/kg/dose orally twice daily.	Monitor serum creatinine/BUN.

BUN, Blood urea nitrogen; *CBC,* complete blood count; *IM,* intramuscular; *IV,* intravenous; *LFT,* liver function test; *WBC,* white blood cell.

adverse effects that are specific to the patient's prescribed treatment. The follow-up period is not specified and is dependent upon each patient's seizure history, but clinic visits should be more frequent at the start of treatment to determine efficacy and/or the need for additional adjunctive medications.

Teaching Points for Antiepileptic Therapy

Health Promotion Strategies

- Take your seizure medication exactly as prescribed. If your seizures seem to increase in frequency or severity, consult with your primary care provider before making any dose adjustments.
- Avoid alcohol while taking antiepileptic medications as alcohol can increase feelings of drowsiness.
- Keep a diary of your seizure activity, noting the type, duration, and severity of each seizure, especially if the seizure is witnessed.
- Keep all scheduled laboratory appointments if your medication requires blood-level monitoring.
- Wear a Medic Alert bracelet in the event a seizure occurs and emergent health care is needed.

Patient Education for Medication Safety

Primary care providers need to stress the following points and actions to patients for safe medication management:

- To achieve the best seizure control, take your antiepileptic medication as prescribed. Do not discontinue your antiepileptic without consulting with your primary care provider.
- Missing medication doses can result in loss of seizure control. Refill your medication in a timely manner.
- If you are planning to be out of town, take additional medication with you to prevent missing doses due to travel delays.
- Avoid driving or operating hazardous machinery until your seizures are under control.
- Report any changes in mood, depression, or thoughts of self-harm to your health care provider immediately.

Application Questions for Discussion

1. As a health care provider, what are the patient and safety factors that should be considered before prescribing an antiepileptic?

2. What should be included in the education plan for a patient and/or caregiver who has been prescribed antiepileptics?
3. What role may genetics play in the treatment response to some antiepileptics?

Selected Bibliography

Balestrini, S., & Sisodiyaa, S. M. (2018). Pharmacogenomics in epilepsy. *Neuroscience Letters, 667,* 27–39.

Barker-Haliski, M. L., Löscher, W., White, H. S., & Galanopoulou, A. S. (2017). Neuroinflammation in epileptogenesis: Insights and translational perspectives from new models of epilepsies. *Epilepsia, 58* (Suppl 3), 39–47. http://doi.org/10.1111/epi.13785.

Beghi, E., Giussani, G., & Sander, J. W. (2015). The natural history and prognosis of epilepsy. *Epileptic Disorders, 17*(3), 243–253.

Ferlazzoa, E., Trenitec, Kasteleijn-Nolst, D., de Haane, G., J., Nitschkef, F., Ahonenf, S., Gasparinia, S., & Minassian, B. A (2017). Update on pharmacological treatment of progressive myoclonus epilepsies. *Current Pharmaceutical Design, 23*(37), 5662–5666. http://doi.org/10.2174/1381612823666170809114654.

Fisher R.S., Acevedo C., Arzimanoglou A., Bogacz A., Cross J. H., Elger C. E., Engel J. Jr, Forsgren L., French J. A., Glynn M., Hesdorffer D. C., Lee B. I., Mathern G. W., Moshé S. L., Perucca E., Scheffer I. E., Tomson T., Watanabe M., Wiebe S. ILAE official report: a practical clinical definition of epilepsy. *Epilepsia*, Apr;55(4):475-482, 2014. doi: 10.1111/epi.12550. Epub 2014 Apr 14. PMID: 24730690.

Gaston, T. E., & Szaflarski, J. P. (2018). Cannabis for the treatment of epilepsy: An update. *Current Neurology and Neuroscience Reports, 18,* 73.

Jacob, L., Hamer, H., & Kostev, K. (2017). Adherence to antiepileptic drugs in children and adolescents: A retrospective study in primary care settings in Germany. *Epilepsy & Behavior, 75,* 36–41.

Krumholz., A., et al. (2015). Evidence-based guideline: Management of an unprovoked first seizure in adults: Report of the Guideline Development Subcommittee of the American Academy of Neurology and the American Epilepsy Society. *Neurology, 84,* 1705–1713.

Maguire, M. (2019). The psychopharmacology of epilepsy. *Handbook of Clinical Neurology*, Vol. 165 (3rd series). In *Psychopharmacology of Neurologic Disease*, V. I. Reus and D. Lindqvist (Eds.). https://doi.org/10.1016/B978-0-444-64012-3.00012-5

Manford, M. (2017). Recent advances in epilepsy. *Journal of Neurology, 264,* 1811–1824. http://doi.org/10.1007/s00415-017-8394-2.

Nabbout, R., et al. (2017). Treatment issues for children with epilepsy transitioning to adult care. *Epilepsy & Behavior, 69,* 153–160.

Patel, D. C., Tewari, B. P., Chaunsali, L., & Sontheimer, H. (2019). Neuron–glia interactions in the pathophysiology of epilepsy. *Nature, 20,* 282–297.

30

Parkinson's Disease Medications

MARCIA JOHANSSON AND CONSTANCE G. VISOVSKY

Overview

Parkinson's disease (PD) is the most common neurodegenerative disorder after Alzheimer's disease. The array of pharmacologic and surgical treatments available for the treatment of PD is broader than for any other degenerative disease of the central nervous system (CNS). Dr. James Parkinson first described paralysis agitans or shaking palsy in 1817. Today we know this condition as PD, Parkinson's syndrome, or parkinsonism. Age at onset of signs and symptoms varies; however, most patients first experience symptoms between the ages of 50 and 69. In up to 30% of patients, symptoms occur before the age of 50. Patients present with one or more of four typical clinical symptoms: tremor at rest, bradykinesia, rigidity, and postural instability. Some patients with PD may present with only a resting tremor of 4 to 7 cycles/second as the principal symptom. These patients usually experience a slower progression of disease and little mental status change. Patients who present with postural instability and gait difficulty, however, often have a more rapid disease progression that includes dementia and bradykinesia.

Management of individual patients requires careful consideration of a number of factors, including the patient's symptoms and signs, age, stage of disease, degree of functional disability, and level of physical activity and productivity. The prevalence and incidence rates of PD increase with age, and the incidence in males is 1.5 times higher than in females. Parkinson's disease is not curable; symptoms progress and worsen over time. A neuroprotective treatment that can slow or halt disease progression has not yet been established. The treatment of PD is complex, owing to the array of motor and nonmotor features combined with early- and late-treatment adverse effects. Treatment for patients with PD is highly individualized and can be divided into pharmacologic, nonpharmacologic, and surgical therapies.

Correct diagnosis is fundamental to the appropriate therapy of PD, although the same menu of drugs is used to treat all of the various parkinsonian syndromes. The decision to initiate symptomatic medical therapy in patients with PD is determined by the degree to which symptoms interfere with functioning or impair quality of life. The timing of this decision varies greatly among patients but is influenced by a number of factors, including the effect of disease on the dominant hand, the presence of significant bradykinesia or gait disturbance, the degree to which the disease interferes with work and activities of daily living, including social and leisure function, and the patient's values and preferences regarding the use of medications.

Relevant Physiology

The neurotransmitters acetylcholine and dopamine, and others in the neurons of the substantia nigra, modulate movement. Damage to these neurons caused by amyloid results in excess acetylcholine and diminished dopamine in the basal ganglia. Replacement and regulation of the neurotransmitters with exogenous medications represent the hallmark of PD management; however, to improve symptoms and avoid side effects, these medications must be able to cross the blood–brain barrier without being metabolized in the periphery.

Tyrosine is converted to levodopa (L-dopa) by tyrosine hydroxylase. L-dopa then is enzymatically decarboxylated by L-amino acid decarboxylase (L-AAD) to form dopamine. Dopamine is stored in synaptic vesicles until needed and then is released into the synapse, where it activates dopamine (D) receptors. The action of dopamine is terminated by reuptake into presynaptic vesicles or metabolism via monoamine oxidase-B (MAO-B) or catechol-O-methyltransferase (COMT). This results in the formation of hydrogen peroxide, which then is metabolized to water by glutathione. If glutathione is deficient, or if a surplus of hydrogen peroxide exists, hydroxyl free radicals are formed, causing lipid peroxidation and cell membrane damage.

Pathophysiology

Parkinsonism is a chronic, debilitating disease with no known cure. The goals of treatment are to relieve the symptoms of the disease and help the patient maintain independence and mobility. By origin, PD is categorized as primary or idiopathic, secondary or acquired, heritable, or multisystem. For purposes of this text, only idiopathic PD is discussed. Practitioners are urged to consult differential diagnostic references to distinguish among the types of parkinsonism, including drug-induced cases.

Parkinson's disease results from a relative excess of cholinergic activity and a deficiency of dopaminergic activity in the basal ganglia. Lewy bodies (amyloid inclusion bodies) in the neurons of the pars compacta region of the substantia nigra are common in the pathophysiology of parkinsonism. Damage to these dopaminergic neurons causes loss of dopamine at their terminal projections in the caudate nucleus and putamen. Dopamine normally inhibits the action of acetylcholine in the striatum; therefore, decreased concentrations of dopamine caused by neuronal degeneration result in unopposed acetylcholine. This manifests as tremors in the patient. Clinical signs and symptoms of parkinsonism develop after approximately 80% of dopaminergic neurons are lost.

Some understanding of the origin of PD was gained when several intravenous (IV) drug abusers developed PD after injecting a meperidine analog known as methyl phenyl tetrahydropyridine (MPTP). The MPP ion that was formed after oxidative metabolism of MPTP by MAO-B was found to be neurotoxic to melanin-containing neurons in the substantia nigra. Inhibition of MAO-B by selegiline prevented the formation of MPP. Epidemiologic studies have shown an increased risk of developing PD with rural living and exposure to well water, pesticides, herbicides, and wood pulp mills. Discovery of a gene that could be responsible for a certain type of familial PD has brought hope for further research into the mechanism and prevention of the disease, perhaps through the use of stem cells. Stem cells represent only a very small portion of all the neuroprotection trials and other work currently underway (Table 30.1).

Parkinson's Disease Therapy

The decision to initiate symptomatic medical therapy in patients with PD is determined by the degree to which symptoms interfere with functioning or impair quality of life. Over the past decade, a paradigm shift has been noted from initiating symptomatic therapy with levodopa, the gold standard of PD treatment, to beginning treatment with a dopamine agonist (in particular, for young-onset patients

who are at high risk of developing motor complications) and adding levodopa as a supplement when dopamine agonist monotherapy can no longer provide satisfactory clinical control. Long-term levodopa treatment is associated with the development of motor complications that probably are initiated by abnormal pulsatile stimulation of dopamine receptors via intermittent administration of agents with short half-lives (such as levodopa). Dopamine agonists with longer half-lives can provide relatively continuous stimulation and thus can possibly diminish motor response complications. However, treatment initiation with levodopa is still preferred in patients with PD with cognitive impairment, in older adults, and in those with atypical parkinsonism. The choice among available treatment options depends on clinical characteristics such as patient age, disease severity, and the presence of comorbidities, as well as the patient's lifestyle characteristics and preferences, costs of different medications, awareness and perception of available treatment options, and educational background of the treating health care provider.

Drug treatment for PD has centered on increasing the availability of dopamine in the CNS, inhibiting the effects of acetylcholine, and attempting to prevent further cell membrane damage through neuroprotective trials. The D_2-receptor subtype is the primary modulator of both clinical improvement and adverse reactions such as dystonia and hallucinations. Increased levodopa precursors and synthesis cofactors usually are not effective.

The first category of drugs used for PD include those that work directly or indirectly to increase the level of dopamine in the brain. The drugs most commonly used for PD are dopamine precursors, or substances such as levodopa, that cross the blood–brain barrier and then are changed into dopamine. Other drugs mimic dopamine or prevent or slow its breakdown (Fig. 30.1).

Dopamine Precursors

Levodopa and Levodopa/Carbidopa
Levodopa is administered orally and as an oral inhalation. Levodopa has been the single most important drug in the antiparkinson armamentarium. Levodopa (L-dopa) is an aromatic amine that is metabolized to dopamine.

Pharmacokinetics. Levodopa/carbidopa administered orally enters the blood after it is absorbed from the

TABLE 30.1	Stages of Parkinson's Disease			
Stage 1	**Stage 2**	**Stage 3**	**Stage 4**	**Stage 5**
Mild symptoms	Moderate symptoms with facial modifications	Progression of disease is observed	Drastic change is observed	Advanced stage with aggressive symptoms
Tremors on one side of the body and postural changes are observed	Tremors on both sides of the body are observed	Imbalance of body and improper reflexes are observed	Personal assistance is required, even in simple tasks	Hallucination and spasm occur

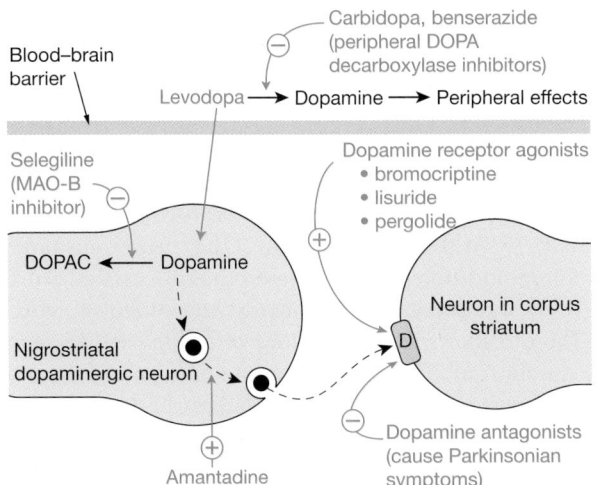

• **Fig. 30.1** Mechanisms of Parkinson's disease medications. (From Page, C., & Pitchford, S. [2021]. *Dale's pharmacology condensed* [3rd ed.]. Philadelphia: Elsevier.)

gastrointestinal (GI) tract; 95% of levodopa is converted to dopamine by L-AAD. The action of this enzyme can be blocked by the antagonist carbidopa, which does not cross the blood–brain barrier; therefore, levodopa in the CNS follows the synthetic path to dopamine formation and storage. Combining carbidopa with levodopa results in increased concentrations of levodopa in the CNS and decreased conversion of L-dopa to dopamine in the periphery, where it causes adverse effects. The plasma half-life of oral levodopa is about 50 minutes. When levodopa is administered with carbidopa, the half-life is increased to 1.5 hours. The half-life of levodopa following a single orally inhaled dose (84 mg) is 2.3 hours. High-protein or high-fat foods may interfere with oral levodopa absorption.

Indications. Levodopa is available in an oral inhalation formulation (Inbrija) that is used as needed up to five times daily for off episodes in Parkinson's patients receiving levodopa/carbidopa. Oral levodopa formulas are combined with carbidopa (Sinemet, Sinemet CR, Duopa) for treating motor symptoms associated with Parkinson's disease or parkinsonism.

Adverse Effects. Dyskinesia, a hyperkinetic movement disorder, is the most common of the serious effects of levodopa therapy and includes abnormal involuntary movements such as chorea, myoclonia, tics, akathisia, and dystonic reaction. Peak-dose dyskinesia accounts for more than 80% of dyskinesias, followed by off-period dystonia which affects 30% of patients and diphasic dyskinesia which affects 20% of patients. Bradykinetic episodes, or on-off phenomena, including akinesia and akinesia paradoxica, can occur during levodopa therapy and are likely due to both disease progression and excessive levodopa dosage.

Hypersensitivity reactions to levodopa have included angioedema, urticaria, pruritus, Henoch-Schönlein purpura, and bullous rash. Psychiatric adverse effects include agitation, anxiety, depression, suicidal ideation, dementia, toxic delirium, hallucinations, psychosis, paranoia, delusions, confusion, euphoria, decreased mental acuity, memory impairment, nervousness, nightmares, abnormal dreams, restlessness, and disorientation. GI adverse effects that are common and occur frequently include nausea/vomiting, anorexia, and weight loss. The incidence of GI adverse effects is elevated at the initiation of therapy. It is recommended that oral levodopa is administered with food until tolerance develops, and then it can be given within 30 minutes of meals. Rare episodes of GI bleeding and peptic ulcer have been reported with oral levodopa.

Laboratory abnormalities such as elevated hepatic enzymes, bilirubin levels, serum creatinine, uric acid, proteinuria, positive direct antibody test (Coombs' test), glycosuria, and decreased serum potassium have been reported. Cardiac abnormalities such as orthostatic hypotension are a frequent adverse effect, especially in older adults, and some patients may require a dosage reduction. Cardiac arrhythmias or rate disturbances, usually sinus tachycardia, can occur. Adverse respiratory effects include dyspnea, pharyngeal pain, cough, bizarre breathing patterns, upper respiratory infection, and hoarseness.

Adverse hematologic effects include agranulocytosis, leukopenia, nonhemolytic and hemolytic anemia, thrombocytopenia, decreased white blood cell count, and decreased hemoglobin or hematocrit. Adverse genitourinary effects include urinary retention, increased urinary frequency, urinary tract infection (URI), urinary incontinence, priapism, leukocyturia, hematuria, and bacteriuria. Sleep disturbances that include sudden sleep onset have been reported in patients receiving levodopa. Prior to initiating treatment with levodopa, patients should be advised of the potential to develop somnolence and specifically asked about factors that may increase the risk of sudden sleep episodes, such as coadministration with other CNS depressants.

Adverse ophthalmic effects include increased intraocular pressure in patients with closed-angle glaucoma diplopia, blurred vision, mydriasis, and blepharospasm, an indication of possible toxicity. Neurologic adverse effects resembling neuroleptic malignant syndrome can develop following abrupt discontinuation or dose reduction of levodopa, especially in patients receiving antipsychotic agents concomitantly. Patients should be monitored closely for fever or hyperthermia. Other neurologic findings, including muscle rigidity, involuntary movements, altered consciousness, and mental status changes, can occur.

Contraindications. Levodopa use is contraindicated in patients currently taking nonselective monoamine oxidase inhibitor (MAOI) therapy, or who have taken a nonselective MAOI within the previous 2 weeks. Hypertension can occur if these drugs are used concurrently. Nonselective MAOIs should be discontinued at least 2 weeks before initiation of oral or inhalational levodopa therapy.

Monitoring. Laboratory monitoring of complete blood count (CBC), liver function tests (LFTs), and assessment of neurologic functioning should be completed prior to and throughout treatment.

Levodopa Management Problems

- As PD progresses, neurons lose their storage capabilities for dopamine, and patients are dependent on the rate of levodopa administration for a therapeutic response.

- Approximately 50% of patients treated with levodopa will experience fluctuations in their response to the drug within 5 years. These fluctuations include wearing off, also called end-of-dose failure, as well as on-off effects, dyskinesias, and dystonias.

- Patients who experience choreiform dyskinesias during their peak levodopa effect may benefit from substituting an immediate-release for a sustained-release product, or the opposite.

- Patients in whom dystonias occur at the end of the dosing cycle may benefit from more frequent doses of levodopa/carbidopa or from addition of or increase in the dose of a dopamine agonist. Restriction of levodopa/carbidopa to several early to midday doses also may be of benefit.

- Early-morning foot dystonias may improve as the result of nocturnal administration of sustained-release levodopa/carbidopa. If this is not successful, a nocturnal dopamine agonist or an early-morning levodopa/carbidopa or paracopa could be used. Patients with dystonias that occur at peak dose time may benefit from lowering the dose of levodopa/carbidopa or from addition of or increase in the dopamine agonist dose.

- Patients may experience wearing off of therapeutic effect after 1.5 to 2 hours with some products.

- On-off effect is a sudden loss of therapeutic effect that may be alleviated by more frequent doses of levodopa or a sustained-release formulation.

- If onset of action is delayed, levodopa may be given on an empty stomach before meals, and crushed or chewed and taken with a full glass of water.

Diet and Levodopa

Levodopa competes directly with amino acids for absorption across the GI membrane and with amino acid transport mechanisms into the CNS. Patients should take levodopa initially with food to avoid GI adverse effects; then they should move dosing to 30 minutes before meals. Tolerance to these effects usually develops. Patients may eat 15 minutes after taking levodopa if they can tolerate the GI effects. Patients who experience suboptimal response or fluctuations with levodopa should limit protein intake at the morning and noon meals to enhance absorption and bioavailability of the drug.

Selective MAO-B Inhibitors

Selective MAO-B inhibitors irreversibly block the metabolism of dopamine in the brain, where MAO-B is the major subtype and extends the duration of action of L-dopa. Three MAO-B inhibitors are available to use in patients with PD: selegiline, rasagiline, and safinamide. These three medications inhibit the enzyme MAO-B, which breaks down dopamine in the brain. MAO-B inhibitors cause dopamine to accumulate in surviving nerve cells and reduce the symptoms of PD.

Selegiline

Selegiline (also called deprenyl), an MAO-B inhibitor, is used with other drugs early in the management of PD. Selegiline is an irreversible inhibitor of the monoamine oxidase (MAO) enzyme system. The neurotransmitters serotonin and norepinephrine are primarily catabolized by MAO-A and dopamine is primarily catabolized by MAO-B. The use allows dose reductions of L-dopa and increases the duration of effect by 1 or more hours in patients who experience wearing-off effects. Selegiline can delay the need for levodopa therapy by 1 year or longer. When selegiline or rasagiline is given with levodopa, it appears to enhance and prolong the response to levodopa and thus may reduce the wearing-off effect.

Pharmacokinetics. Selegiline is available as an oral tablet, oral capsule, orally disintegrating tablet, and transdermal patch. Selegiline is readily absorbed from the GI tract and rapidly penetrates the blood–brain barrier, reaching peak serum concentrations in 0.5 to 2 hours. The bioavailability of selegiline is increased three to four times when it is taken with food. Using the transdermal route, 25% to 30% of the selegiline dose is delivered systemically over a 24-hour period, with steady-state plasma concentrations reached within 5 days. The elimination half-life of selegiline after an oral or disintegrating tablet dose is 10 hours once steady state is reached. In vitro studies have demonstrated that selegiline is not an inhibitor of cytochrome (CYP) 450 enzymes.

Indications. Selegiline is used in the treatment of Parkinson's disease or parkinsonism in combination with levodopa or levodopa/carbidopa.

Adverse Effects. GI adverse effects denote nausea (11% of patients) as the most common adverse effect of selegiline therapy. Constipation (4%), diarrhea (2%), dysphagia (2%), dyspepsia (5%), stomatitis (5%), vomiting (3%), and xerostomia (4%) have been reported.

CNS adverse effects of ataxia (3%), dizziness (11%), dyskinesia (6%), hallucinations (4%), headache (7%), insomnia (7%), drowsiness/somnolence (3%), and tremor (3%) have been reported. In clinical trials, many other CNS–mediated adverse effects were noted, including abnormal gait, agitation, akinesia, anxiety, apathy, aphasia, bradykinesia, chorea, delusions, disorientation, dystonic reaction, and emotional lability, among others.

Cardiac adverse effects of selegiline include the potential for hypertensive crisis due to the inhibition of monoamine oxidase-A (MAO-A), the enzyme responsible for the catabolism of dietary amines such as tyramine. Hypertensive crisis, which can be fatal, may manifest as occipital headache, fever, chest pain, neck stiffness, nausea, and tachycardia or bradycardia. Significant inhibition of intestinal MAO-A activity can result in cardiovascular adverse effects following the ingestion of tyramine-rich foods or beverages (e.g., aged cheese, yeast extract, protein extract, and soy sauce).

Serotonin syndrome has been reported when selegiline is given with other medications known to increase central serotonin levels, such as selective serotonin reuptake inhibitors (SSRIs).

Vision and hearing adverse effects include visual impairment, blurred vision, cataracts, conjunctivitis, diplopia, xerophthalmia, ocular hemorrhage, glaucoma, retinal artery occlusion, retinal detachment, hearing loss, otitis, and tinnitus; however, the frequency is unknown.

Contraindications. Selegiline is contraindicated in patients receiving any other MAOI therapy due to the risk for hypertensive crisis. Selegiline transdermal system is contraindicated with SSRIs, serotonin and norepinephrine reuptake inhibitors (SNRIs), St. John's wort, the tricyclic antidepressants, cyclobenzaprine, meperidine, tramadol, and other opiate agonists, and dextromethorphan because of a risk of serotonin syndrome. Transdermal selegiline is contraindicated in patients with pheochromocytoma due to the secretion of norepinephrine by the tumor, potentially cause a hypertensive crisis. The safety and efficacy of oral selegiline have not been established in patients younger than 18 years of age.

Monitoring. Monitor patients for the presence of severe or continuing headache and any other symptoms of hypertension, or hypertensive crisis. Monitor patients for new-onset hypertension or exacerbation of preexisting hypertension. Monitor heart rate, LFTs, and serum creatinine/blood urea nitrogen (BUN).

Rasagiline

Rasagiline may delay the use of levodopa/carbidopa in the early stages of PD. Rasagiline is classified into two major molecular species, A and B, and is localized in the mitochondrial membranes throughout the body in nerve terminals, brain, liver, and intestinal mucosa. MAO regulates the metabolic degradation of catecholamines and serotonin in the CNS and peripheral tissues. Blockade of MAO-B reduces the metabolism of dopamine, but not that of norepinephrine or serotonin, and inhibits MAO-B in the human brain. The exact mechanism whereby it causes an increase in extracellular levels of dopamine in the striatum is not known.

Pharmacokinetics. Rasagiline is administered orally, with plasma protein binding ranging from 88% to 94%. Rasagiline is rapidly absorbed from the GI tract, reaching peak plasma concentration in 1 hour. The bioavailability of rasagiline is approximately 36% and it can be administered with or without food. Rasagiline is extensively metabolized in the liver and is affected by CYP 450 isoenzymes and drug transporters, CYP 1A2, and CYP 2C8/9.

The half-life of rasagiline is approximately 3 hours. Elimination occurs primarily via urine and secondarily via feces (7%), with less than 1% excreted in the urine as unchanged drug.

Indications. Rasagiline is used for the treatment of Parkinson's disease, or as adjunctive therapy with levodopa with or without other Parkinson's disease drugs.

Adverse Effects. The most common adverse effects seen with the use of rasagiline were weight loss (2% to 9% of patients), dose-related orthostatic or postural hypotension (13%), dry mouth, abnormal involuntary movement (18%), drowsiness (6%), and hallucinations (1.3%). CNS adverse effects may be potentiated when rasagiline is used as an adjunct to levodopa, resulting in dopaminergic side effects, and may exacerbate preexisting dyskinesia, involuntary movements, or hallucinations. When used alone, rasagiline can result in headache (14%), depression (5%), paresthesias (2%), and vertigo (2%). Older adults may be at greater risk for adverse psychiatric effects, thereby requiring dose reduction. Respiratory system adverse effects have occurred in at least 2% of patients receiving rasagiline and include influenza (5%), fever (3%), and rhinitis (3%). Rasagiline selectively inhibits MAO-B and at recommended dosages does not affect MAO-A, so patients taking rasagiline can consume most foods containing tyramine with less risk of uncontrolled hypertension. Serotonin syndrome with the use of rasagiline in combination with antidepressants has been reported.

Contraindications. Contraindications of rasagiline are similar to those of other MAOIs. While less common, rasagiline still may cause hypertension, exacerbate preexisting hypertension, or cause hypertensive crisis. Caution is advisable during use of rasagiline in patients with hypertension or other cardiovascular conditions. Medication interactions with rasagiline can be serious. Review potential medication interactions carefully prior to prescription of rasagiline. Concurrent use of rasagiline with other MAOI therapy or other drugs that are potent inhibitors of monoamine oxidase, including linezolid, is contraindicated due to the risk for hypertensive crisis.

There are contraindications for certain medication use with rasagiline due to the potential risk for serotonin syndrome and hypertensive crisis. This list includes, but is not limited to, meperidine and selected other opioid drugs, SNRIs, SSRIs, tricyclic antidepressants, cyclobenzaprine, and stimulants such methylphenidate, amphetamines, St. John's wort, and dextromethorphan.

Rasagiline should be used with caution in patients with a history of psychosis or psychotic disorders due to the risk for hallucinations and exacerbation of the psychotic disorder. Do not use rasagiline in patients with moderate to severe hepatic disease.

Monitoring. Monitor patients on rasagiline for somnolence because some of the events occur well after initiation of treatment. Monitoring of LFTs before and during rasagiline therapy is recommended if patients have hepatic impairment. Assess neurologic functioning before and during treatment.

Safinamide

Safinamide is an oral selective and reversible inhibitor of MAO-B. MAO exists as two catabolic isoenzymes: MAO-A and MAO-B. Serotonin and norepinephrine are primarily catabolized by MAO-A, and dopamine is primarily catabolized by MAO-B. Safinamide has selective MAO-B inhibitory effects, so it can be used without severe dietary tyramine restrictions.

Pharmacokinetics. Following oral administration, safinamide has a bioavailability of 95%. The time to maximum concentration (Tmax) occurs between 2 and 3 hours after a dose, with a half-life of 20 to 26 hours. Safinamide is extensively metabolized in the liver, and about 5% of the drug is eliminated unchanged in the urine and 76% as inactive metabolites.

Indications. Safinamide is indicated in the adjunctive treatment to levodopa/carbidopa therapy in patients with Parkinson's disease experiencing off episodes.

Adverse Effects. The most frequently reported adverse reaction is dyskinesia, occurring in more than 10% of patients. Patients may experience new or worsening mental status and behavioral changes, which may be severe, including psychotic-like behaviors, psychosis, and hallucinations. In cases of dyskinesia or psychotic hallucinations, dose reduction or discontinuation may be warranted. Drowsiness can occur, so patients should be advised to use caution when driving or performing tasks that require mental alertness. Foods that contain very high amounts of tyramine could potentially cause a hypertensive reaction, even though safinamide is a highly selective MAO inhibitor. In clinical trials, 5% of patients developed increases in hepatic enzymes. Neuroleptic malignant syndrome (frequency unknown) can occur and is associated with rapid dose reduction, withdrawal, or changes in drugs that increase dopaminergic tone.

Contraindications. Safinamide may cause hypertension, exacerbate preexisting hypertension, or cause hypertensive crisis. Drug interactions with safinamide can be serious. Review drug interactions carefully prior to prescribing safinamide.

Monitoring. Monitor LFTs before and throughout treatment at regular intervals. Monitor patients for new-onset hypertension or hypertension that is not adequately controlled after starting safinamide.

Dopamine Agonists

Dopamine agonists include pramipexole, ropinirole, and apomorphine. They mimic the role of dopamine in the brain and can be given alone or in conjunction with levodopa. They may be used in the early stages of the disease, or later to lengthen the duration of response to levodopa in patients who experience wearing-off or on-off effects. They generally are less effective than levodopa in controlling rigidity and bradykinesia.

Dopamine agonists are used in the treatment of patients with PD to increase the availability of dopamine in the CNS. These drugs work at postsynaptic dopamine receptors in the nigrostriatal system by stimulating dopamine receptors. They are being used more frequently in early parkinsonism to avoid using high doses of levodopa and in late stages of the disease to aid in the management of levodopa dose-response fluctuations.

Pramipexole

Pramipexole is a non-ergot dopamine agonist with specificity for the D_2 dopamine receptors. It binds with lower-affinity D_3- and D_4-receptor subtypes. The relevance of D_3-receptor binding in PD is unknown. According to treatment guidelines, non-ergot dopamine agonists are first-line pharmacologic options for early Parkinson's disease.

Pharmacokinetics. Pramipexole is administered orally as immediate-release and extended-release tablets, with a bioavailability greater than 90%. Peak serum concentrations of the immediate-release formula occur 2 hours after a dose, while the average time to peak of the extended-release tablets is 6 hours after a dose. Pramipexole is secreted by the renal tubules, with approximately 90% of a dose eliminated as unchanged drug. Renal clearance of immediate-release pramipexole is about 60% to 75% lower in patients with moderate to severe renal impairment.

Indications. Pramipexole is recommended for the treatment of the signs and symptoms of idiopathic Parkinson's disease.

Adverse Effects. The most common adverse effects reported are mild dizziness (3% to 26% of patients), drowsiness (6% to 36%), headache (4% to 16%), and insomnia (4% to 27%). Moderate dyskinesia (fewer than 47%), hallucinations (5% to 17%), and orthostatic hypotension (up to 53%) were also reported. The relative risk of hallucinations is increased in older adults with Parkinson's disease. Drowsiness can occur, so patients should be advised to use caution when driving or performing tasks that require mental alertness. Sudden sleep onset has been reported during the use of dopamine agonists, including pramipexole. Although relatively rare, heart failure has been reported with the use of pramipexole. In September 2012, the U.S. Food and Drug Administration (FDA) warned patients and health care professionals that pramipexole may be associated with an increased risk of heart failure. Patients should report symptoms of heart failure to their health care provider.

Contraindications. Extended-release pramipexole is not recommended in patients with severe renal impairment (creatinine clearance [CrCl] less than 30 mL/minute) or in patients on dialysis. Pramipexole should be used with caution in patients with cardiac disease or hypotension. Due to the risk of exacerbation of psychosis, patients with psychotic disorders should generally not receive treatment with dopamine agonists. Avoid abrupt discontinuation or rapid dose reduction of pramipexole, as neuroleptic malignant syndrome has been reported in association with rapid dose reduction of, changes in, or withdrawal of dopaminergic therapy.

Monitoring. Assessment for somnolence is necessary throughout pramipexole therapy because patients may not acknowledge drowsiness or sleepiness until directly questioned about drowsiness or sleepiness during specific activities. Monitor neurologic status and the occurrence of behavioral alterations throughout therapy.

Ropinirole

Ropinirole is an oral immediate- or extended-release preparation that is a non-ergot alkaloid dopamine agonist used as early monotherapy and in combination with levodopa. Use of ropinirole early in the disease may delay the need for levodopa therapy.

Pharmacokinetics. Ropinirole is widely distributed and rapidly absorbed, with a peak plasma concentration occurring in approximately 1 to 2 hours. Food does not affect the extent of absorption. It is metabolized to form inactive metabolites. Less than 10% of the administered drug is excreted unchanged in the urine. The elimination half-life of ropinirole is roughly 6 hours. Steady-state concentrations of immediate-release and extended-release ropinirole are expected to be achieved within 2 days and 4 days of dosing, respectively.

Indications. Ropinirole is indicated in the treatment of Parkinson's disease.

Adverse Effects. Cardiovascular adverse reactions have been reported in patients receiving ropinirole alone and in combination with levodopa and include atrial fibrillation (2% of patients), arrythmia (2%), hypertension (up to 15%), hypotension (2%), orthostatic hypotension (6%), palpitations (3%), sinus tachycardia (2%), and syncope (12%). The most common CNS effects included dizziness (40%), hyperkinesis (2%), hyperesthesia (4%), headache (5% to 15%), and vertigo (2%). Ropinirole commonly causes somnolence, and sudden sleep onset has been reported during the use of dopamine agonists. Psychiatric adverse effects include amnesia (3% to 5 %), impaired concentration (2%), anxiety (2% to 6%), confusion (5% to 9%), abnormal dreams (3%), hallucinations (8% to 10%), and nervousness (5%). Some patients receiving medications that increase dopaminergic tone have reported intense and uncontrollable urges to gamble, increased sexual urges, or other intense urges. Genitourinary adverse effects that are most common are erectile dysfunction (3%), pyuria (2%), and urinary incontinence (2%).

Contraindications. Ropinirole is contraindicated in patients with a known hypersensitivity to the medication or its ingredients (including urticaria, angioedema, rash, pruritus). Caution is advised in the use of ropinirole in patients with severe cardiac disease. Ropinirole should be used cautiously in patients with preexisting psychosis, as

hallucinations, paranoia, or aggressive behaviors have been reported in patients receiving ropinirole alone or in combination with L-dopa. Ropinirole may be contraindicated in patients with sleep disorders (narcolepsy, sleep apnea) due to sudden somnolence that can occur. Abrupt discontinuation or rapid dose reduction of immediate-release and extended-release ropinirole is contraindicated due to neuroleptic malignant syndrome-type effects experienced with abrupt withdrawal.

Monitoring. Patients receiving ropinirole should be monitored for signs and symptoms of orthostatic hypotension, particularly during dosage increases, and should be advised of the risk for syncope and hypotension. Due to variable hepatic effects, LFTs should be monitored before and during treatment (Table 30.2).

Apomorphine

Apomorphine, a nonnarcotic derivative of morphine, is similar to the neurotransmitter dopamine that may contribute to its central dopamine receptor agonist properties. The exact mechanism by which apomorphine exerts its therapeutic effects in Parkinson's disease is unknown but is thought to occur via activation at postsynaptic dopamine (D_2) receptors in the caudate nucleus and putamen areas of the brain that are both involved in executing movement.

Pharmacokinetics. Apomorphine is administered in a sublingual film, as a high first-pass metabolism prohibits an oral formulation. Apomorphine is 85% to 90% bound to plasma proteins, primarily albumin. Metabolism is thought to occur in the liver through several pathways including glucuronidation, sulfation, and N-demethylation. Subcutaneous apomorphine has a mean elimination half-life of approximately 40 minutes, and sublingual apomorphine has a mean elimination half-life of about 1.7 hours. A reduction in the starting dose of subcutaneous apomorphine is recommended in patients with mild to moderate renal impairment. The effects of subcutaneous apomorphine in severe renal impairment or renal failure have not been evaluated.

Indications. Apomorphine is approved as a sublingual film for the treatment of acute, intermittent off episodes associated with Parkinson's disease and as a subcutaneous

---

TABLE 30.2 Ropinirole Conversion

Ropinirole Conversion From Immediate-Release (IR) to Extended-Release (ER) Tablet

- Adults taking an oral dose of 0.75–2.25 mg/day of IR: Give 2 mg/day ER.
- Adults taking an oral dose of 3–4.5 mg/day IR: Give 4 mg/day ER.
- Adults taking an oral dose of 6 mg/day IR: Give 6 mg/day ER.
- Adults taking an oral dose of 7.5–9 mg/day IR: Give 8 mg/day ER.
- Adults taking an oral dose of 12 mg/day IR: Give 12 mg/day ER.
- Adults taking an oral dose of 15–18 mg/day IR: Give 16 mg/day ER.
- Adults taking an oral dose of 21 mg/day IR: Give 20 mg/day ER.
- Adults taking an oral dose of 24 mg/day IR: Give 24 mg/day ER.

injection for use in patients with advanced Parkinson's disease.

Adverse Effects. CNS adverse effects of apomorphine included drowsiness and somnolence in about 35% of patients receiving the subcutaneous formulation of the medication. The risk of sudden sleepiness is also present.

GI adverse effects of apomorphine include severe nausea and vomiting at recommended doses due to stimulation in the chemoreceptor trigger zone (CTZ). Nausea and vomiting are extremely likely when apomorphine is not given with an antiemetic and usually occurs within 5 to 10 minutes of a parenteral dose. Cardiovascular adverse effects such as dose-related hypotension have occurred and can exacerbate coronary and cerebral ischemia. If patients are taking concomitant antihypertensives or vasodilators, hypotension can increase the risk of serious falls. QT prolongation of 10 msec has also been observed. Although the extent of exposure of sublingual apomorphine is lower than subcutaneous apomorphine, QT prolongation with sublingual apomorphine cannot be excluded. QT prolongation carries a risk of torsade de pointes, with palpitations and syncopal episodes often preceding serious cardiac adverse events.

Hypersensitivity reactions such as contact dermatitis, rash, urticaria, and pruritus can occur with exposure to or contact with the solution or powder of subcutaneous apomorphine. Patients and their caregivers should be instructed on the proper handling of the medication. Psychiatric effects in about 5% of patients receiving subcutaneous apomorphine include depression and anxiety. With sublingual apomorphine, hallucinations, delusions, disorientation, or confusion have been reported in 6% of patients. Impulse control disorder including intense and uncontrollable urges to gamble can occur. Although uncommon, painful erections and priapism can occur in 1% of patients receiving subcutaneous apomorphine.

Contraindications. Apomorphine is contraindicated in patients with sulfite hypersensitivity. The concomitant use of drugs of the 5-HT$_3$ antagonist class (ondansetron, granisetron, dolasetron, palonosetron) is contraindicated for the treatment of nausea due to the profound hypotension that can occur. The coadministration with other CNS depressants and the presence of sleep disorders (narcolepsy, sleep apnea) can increase the risk for somnolence.

Apomorphine should be avoided in patients with major psychotic disorders such as psychosis or schizophrenia and in patients with cardiovascular or cerebrovascular disease due to the risk of exacerbating those illnesses. Apomorphine should be used cautiously in patients with mild to moderate hepatic disease. In patients with mild to moderate renal impairment, dosages should be titrated accordingly. Symptoms of neuroleptic malignant syndrome can occur with abrupt discontinuation of apomorphine.

Monitoring. Monitor the patient's blood pressure and neurologic function over the course of therapy.

Other PD Medications

There are additional categories of PD drugs that affect neurotransmitters in the body to ease some symptoms of the disease. For example, anticholinergic drugs interfere with production or uptake of the neurotransmitter acetylcholine. These drugs help to reduce tremors and muscle stiffness, which can result from the presence of more acetylcholine than dopamine. Anticholinergic agents are used to control tremors caused by excessive, unopposed acetylcholine. They suppress central cholinergic activity and may inhibit reuptake and storage of dopamine in the CNS, thus prolonging the action of dopamine. They also reduce the incidence and severity of akinesia, rigidity, and tremor by about 20%, and may reduce drooling.

COMT inhibitors are central and/or peripheral blockers of dopamine metabolism. COMT is another enzyme that helps break down dopamine. Two COMT inhibitors have been approved to treat PD in the United States: entacapone and tolcapone. These drugs, which prolong the effects of levodopa by preventing the breakdown of dopamine, are used as adjuvants with levodopa to extend the therapeutic effect in patients who experience breakthrough tremors prior to their next dose. The mechanism of action of entacapone probably is related to its ability to inhibit COMT and alter the plasma pharmacokinetics of levodopa. The administration of entacapone in conjunction with levodopa and carbidopa produces more sustained plasma levels of levodopa than does the administration of levodopa and carbidopa alone. These sustained plasma levels may result in increased therapeutic effects on the symptoms of PD, as well as increased adverse effects. A decrease in the levodopa dose may be required.

Amantadine, a glutamate antagonist (antiviral), has been used for many years and appears to potentiate CNS dopaminergic responses. It may release dopamine and norepinephrine from storage sites and inhibit the reuptake of dopamine and norepinephrine. It is clearly less effective than levodopa but can offer additional benefit in patients experiencing maximal or waning effects from levodopa. It has also been used for the treatment of Sinemet-associated dyskinesia.

Rivastigmine is a cholinesterase inhibitor available in oral formulation or as a transdermal system (Exelon Patch) for the treatment of patients with mild to moderate dementia associated with PD (Table 30.3).

BLACK BOX WARNING!

Antipsychotics for the Treatment of PD

- All antipsychotics (especially newer drugs such as Seroquel and Abilify) should not be used in patients with Parkinson's because these drugs appear to increase the risk of death in older dementia patients.

TABLE 30.3   Medications for Parkinson's Disease

Drug Category/ Medication	Indication	Dosage	Considerations and Monitoring
Dopamine Precursors			
Levodopa oral inhalation	For intermittent treatment for PD off episodes in patients treated with levodopa/carbidopa	Inhale the contents of two 42-mg capsules (total 84 mg) via oral inhalation with the provided inhaler as needed for off symptoms up to five times daily.	DO NOT swallow the capsules. Use only with the inhaler provided by the manufacturer. Monitor CBC, LFTs, serum glucose, creatinine, uric acid, urine protein, and neurologic function.
Levodopa/carbidopa	For the treatment of idiopathic Parkinson's disease	*Adults, immediate release:* Typical dose is carbidopa 25-mg/levodopa 100-mg tablet orally three times daily. Dosage may be increased by 1 tablet every day or every other day to a maximum of 8 tablets daily. *Adults, extended release (Sinemet CR):* Typical dose is carbidopa 50-mg/ levodopa 200-mg tablet orally twice daily. *Adults, extended release (Rytary):* One 23.75 mg/95 mg tablet orally three times daily for the first 3 days. On day 4, may increase dose to one 36.25 mg/145 mg three times daily. Maximum dosage: 97.5 mg/390 mg three times daily.	Monitor CBC, LFTs, serum glucose, creatinine, uric acid, urine protein, and neurologic function.
Selective MAO-B Inhibitors			
Selegiline	For the treatment of Parkinson's disease or parkinsonism in combination with levodopa or levodopa/carbidopa	**Oral dose:** *Adults:* 5 mg orally twice daily, administered with breakfast and lunch. **Oral disintegrating tablets (Zelapar ODT):** *Adults:* 1.25 mg orally once daily in the morning before breakfast for at least 6 weeks. After 6 weeks, dose may be increased to 2.5 mg orally once daily in the morning.	Monitor heart rate, blood pressure LFTs, serum creatinine/BUN, and thyroid function tests.
Rasagiline	For the treatment of Parkinson's disease as monotherapy or as adjunct therapy	*Adults:* 0.5–1 mg orally once daily. Maximum dose: 1 mg/day.	Monitor LFTs and neurologic function.
Safinamide		*Adults:* 50 mg orally once daily initially. After 2 weeks, may increase to 100 mg orally once daily, based on individual need and tolerability. Maximum dosage: 100 mg/day.	
Dopamine Agonists			
Pramipexole	For the treatment of signs and symptoms of idiopathic Parkinson's disease	*Adults, immediate release:* 0.125 mg orally three times daily. Gradually increase by 0.125–0.25 mg/dose every 5–7 days. Maximum dosage: 1.5 mg orally three times daily. *Adults, extended release:* 0.375 mg orally once daily initially. May increase up to 0.75 mg orally once daily after a minimum of 5 days. May then increase by 0.75 mg daily no more frequently than every 5–7 days.	No laboratory monitoring is needed. Monitor neurologic function.

Continued

TABLE 30.3 Medications for Parkinson's Disease—cont'd

Drug Category/ Medication	Indication	Dosage	Considerations and Monitoring
Ropinirole	For the treatment of Parkinson's disease	*Adults, immediate release (IR):* 0.25 mg orally three times daily initially for the first week. Gradually titrate at weekly intervals as follows: Week 2: 0.5 mg three times daily. Week 3: 0.75 mg three times daily. Week 4: 1 mg three times daily. Maximum dosage: 24 mg/day. *Adults, extended release (ER):* 2 mg orally once daily initially for 1–2 weeks. Subsequent increases of 2 mg/day at 1-week intervals. Maximum dosage: 24 mg/day.	No laboratory monitoring is needed. Monitor neurologic function.
Apomorphine	For the treatment of acute, intermittent of off episodes associated with Parkinson's disease and advanced Parkinson's disease	*Adults, sublingual (film) dose:* 10 mg sublingually for the off state. Given with provider monitoring of pulse and blood pressure. If tolerated, can be used as needed up to five times daily. Dose range: 10–30 mg sublingually. Maximum single dose: 30 mg sublingually.	Monitor pulse, blood pressure, and neurologic function.
COMT Inhibitors			
Entacapone	For use as an adjunct to levodopa and carbidopa to treat end-of-dose wearing off in patients with Parkinson's disease	*Adults:* 200 mg orally administered with each levodopa/carbidopa, with a maximum of 8 times daily.	Monitor blood pressure and neurologic function. To discontinue, withdraw entacapone therapy slowly.
Tolcapone	For use as adjunctive treatment to levodopa and carbidopa for the treatment of idiopathic Parkinson's disease	*Adults:* 100 mg orally three times daily. Maximum dosage: 600 mg/day.	Monitor LFTs and neurologic function.
Dopamine Release			
Amantadine	For the treatment of idiopathic parkinsonism or Parkinson's disease	*Adults, immediate release:* 100 mg once or twice daily. Maximum dosage: 300–400 mg orally per day in divided doses. For patients unable to tolerate more than 100 mg/day of immediate-release amantadine, there is no equivalent dose/ regimen of amantadine extended-release tablets. *Adults, extended release:* 129 mg orally once daily in the morning. May be increased at weekly intervals. Maximum dosage: 322 mg/day. Do not discontinue extended-release tablets abruptly. Reduce the dose gradually from higher doses to 129 mg/day for 1–2 weeks before discontinuing.	Monitor LFTs and neurologic function.

BUN, Blood urea nitrogen; *CBC,* complete blood count; *COMT,* catechol-O-methyltransferase; *LFTs,* liver function tests; *MAO-B,* monoamine oxidase-B.

PRACTICE PEARLS

Medication Treatment of PD Off Time

- Entacapone and rasagiline should be offered to reduce off time.
- Pergolide, pramipexole, ropinirole, and tolcapone should be considered to reduce off time.
- Selegiline, rasagiline, pramipexole, ropinirole, tolcapone, cabergoline, and entacapone may be considered to reduce off time and so are used when the action of other drugs is wearing off. Apomorphine is used primarily to treat freezing.
- Available evidence does not establish the superiority of one medicine over another in reducing off time.
- Amantadine may be considered to reduce levodopa-associated dyskinesia (level C).
- Deep brain stimulation (DBS) of the subthalamic nuclei (STN) may be considered to improve motor function and reduce off time, dyskinesia, and medication usage.
- Evidence is insufficient to support or refute the efficacy of DBS of the globus pallidus pars interna (GPi) or ventral intermediate (VIM) nucleus of the thalamus in reducing off time, dyskinesia, or medication usage, or in improving motor function.
- Preoperative response to levodopa predicts better outcome after DBS of the STN (level B).

PRACTICE PEARLS

Parkinson's Disease Medication Use in Pregnancy and Lactation

- Most antiparkinsonian medications are categorized as pregnancy category C or unknown.
- Excretion in breast milk is unknown or does occur; therefore, avoid using any antiparkinson medications during pregnancy or lactation.

Prescriber Considerations for Parkinson's Disease Therapy

Clinical Practice Guidelines

The American Academy of Neurology has published guidelines for the treatment of patients with Parkinson's disease. The clinical guidelines cover initial medication selection, management of motor fluctuations, and neuroprotection.

BOOKMARK THIS!

American Academy of Neurology Clinical Practice Guidelines

https://www.aan.com/Guidelines/Home/Search

Clinical Reasoning for Parkinson's Disease Therapy

Consider the individual patient's health problem requiring antiparkinsonian therapy. Parkinson's disease is a progressive neurological disorder that can present with symptomatology ranging from early, mild symptoms to severe motor impairment, tremors, gait and balance abnormalities, impaired sense of smell, and dysphagia. The therapeutic goal of therapy would address the patient's specific disease stage to control symptoms of PD and optimize quality of life.

Determine the desired therapeutic outcome based on the degree of antiparkinsonian therapy needed for the patient's health problem. The overall therapeutic goal is to control or minimize symptoms of PD. There are no therapeutic treatments to reverse neurological damage or prevent further degeneration; thus, supportive care is the cornerstone of treatment. The selection of the appropriate antiparkinsonian medication is dependent upon the extent to which PD is interfering with activities and quality of life. Dosages can be adjusted as needed to control symptoms.

Assess the PD therapy selected for its appropriateness for an individual patient by considering the medication's side effects and the patient's age, race/ethnicity, comorbidities, and genetic factors. For initial therapy for patients with mild PD, a selective MAO-B inhibitor such as selegiline or rasagiline would be an appropriate choice. For patients with more advanced PD, treatment with levodopa, levodopa/carbidopa, or a dopamine agonist such as pramipexole can be given with levodopa therapy or as monotherapy. Long-term effects of levodopa include severe dyskinesia, so monitoring of motor function and worsening symptoms is a consideration in choosing therapy. Older adult patients have been shown to take more time to achieve peak concentration for extended-release tablets as compared to immediate-release tablets.

Comorbid cardiovascular and psychiatric conditions can adversely affect patients receiving PD therapy; therefore, close monitoring for worsening of symptoms related to the comorbidity is required. Prescriptions should be written for the smallest quantity needed. Regularly assess the following: facial appearance, salivation, seborrhea, speech, tremor, rigidity/dyskinesia, finger/foot tapping, rapid alternating movement, standing up from the chair without assistance of arms/hands, posture, stability, gait, handwriting, and intellectual and psychiatric assessment.

Off times exhibited as less-than-desired symptom control can be managed with either dopamine agonists, COMT inhibitors, or MAO-B inhibitors. Istradefylline (Nourianz) is a newer medication that may be used to treat motor symptoms that can happen when levodopa wears off. It was approved in 2019, but additional studies are needed to understand the risks and benefits relative to other medications. Amantadine can be prescribed for dyskinesia resulting from levodopa treatment.

Initiate the treatment plan with the selected medication by first providing adequate patient education to ensure their understanding and promote full participation in the antiparkinsonian therapy. For best results, teach patients to take PD medication at the same time each day. A medication diary can help patients recall side effects of medication and what to report to the primary care provider. Patients should be informed that a smartphone can help with disease management and symptom tracking using available applications. Other important points of patient education are to keep a list of all medications and to plan for obtaining refills of the prescription for PD medication so as not to run out. The primary care provider should be notified if the patient has difficulty swallowing pills. Also stress to the patient never to change the dosage or stop taking the PD medications without talking to their health care provider.

Ensure complete patient and family understanding about the medication prescribed for antiparkinsonian therapy using a variety of education strategies. Because patients with Parkinson's disease may develop impaired cognitive ability, communication problems, and/or depression, provide them with both oral and written communication throughout the course of the disease. Information should be individually tailored and reinforced as necessary, along with consistent communication from the primary care provider.

Conduct follow-up and monitoring of patient responses to antiparkinsonian therapy. At regular intervals of 6 to 12 months, a review of the diagnosis, symptoms, and treatment planning is recommended. More frequent follow-up is recommended for patients with cardiovascular and/or psychiatric comorbidities that require closer monitoring.

Teaching Points for Parkinson's Disease Therapy

Health Promotion Strategies

Since treatment for Parkinson's disease occurs over a lengthy time, the following strategies and practices should be presented to patients to help them become full partners in their health care:

- Eat a balanced diet. Nerves and muscles govern the functioning of the GI system and may be adversely affected by PD. To prevent constipation and gastroparesis, a diet high in fiber and taking adequate hydration with water is recommended.
- If you develop problems swallowing, consult your primary care provider. You may need to have some testing done to determine the extent of the problem. Consultation with a dietitian may help you manage your diet to help with difficulty swallowing.
- Speech or mobility problems can improve with rehabilitation, so engage in regular physical activity and exercise to maintain and improve mobility, flexibility, strength, and walking and to prevent falls. Strengthening exercises can improve muscle weakness.

- Speech therapy may help to improve your voice and speech function.
- Occupational therapy may help to improve your fine motor skills.
- Talk to your primary care provider if you are having feelings of depression or anxiety. Available treatments can help you manage those symptoms and improve your quality of life.
- Do a home safety check to minimize the risk of falls and injury. Make sure areas are well lit, throw rugs are removed or secured, and safety bars and nonslip mats are installed in the bath or shower.
- You may experience symptoms of low blood pressure, such as dizziness upon standing.

There are several ways to reduce this symptom:

- Avoid large meals, as they divert blood to the digestive system.
- Increase the amount of salt in your diet.
- Reduce alcohol consumption.
- Drink 1.5 to 2 quarts of water daily.

Patient Education for Medication Safety

- Take your medications on time for optimum effectiveness.
- Tell your primary care provider all the medications you are taking, including over-the-counter (OTC) medications and any vitamins or supplements, as some of these can interfere with your medication for PD.
- Report symptoms of heat or cold intolerance and excessive sweating that can occur when Parkinson's medications are not as effective.
- If you are taking levodopa (Sinemet), your medication may become less effective if it is taken with a high-protein meal. To address this, try taking your levodopa 30 minutes before or 60 minutes after you eat.

Application Questions for Discussion

1. As a health care provider, what are the patient and safety factors that should be considered before prescribing a treatment for PD?
2. What should be included in the education plan for a patient who has been prescribed levodopa/carbidopa for PD?
3. What role may comorbid conditions play in the treatment response to medication for PD?

Selected Bibliography

Bloem, B. R., Henderson, E. J., Dorsey, E. R., et al. (2020). Integrated and patient-centered management of Parkinson's disease: A network model for reshaping chronic neurological care. *Lancet Neurology, 19*, 623.

Bressman, S., & Saunders-Pullman, R. (2019). When to start levodopa therapy for Parkinson's disease. *New England Journal of Medicine, 380*, 389.

Connolly, B. S., & Lang, A. E. (2014). Pharmacological treatment of Parkinson's disease: A review. *JAMA, 311*, 1670.

Grimes, D., Fitzpatrick, M., Gordon, J., et al. (2019). Canadian guideline for Parkinson's disease. *Canadian Medical Association Journal, 191*, E989.

Katz, M., Goto, Y., Kluger, B. M., et al. (2018). Top ten tips palliative care clinicians should know about Parkinson's disease and related disorders. *Journal of Palliative Medicine, 21*, 1507.

Kluger, B. M., Miyasaki, J., Katz, M., et al. (2020). Comparison of integrated outpatient palliative care with standard care in patients with Parkinson's disease and related disorders: A randomized clinical trial. *JAMA Neurology, 77*, 551.

Postuma, R. B., Berg, D., Stern, M., et al. (2015). MDS clinical diagnostic criteria for Parkinson's disease. *Movement Disorders, 30*, 1591.

Rogers, G., Davies, D., Pink, J., & Cooper, P. (2017). Parkinson's disease: Summary of updated NICE guidance. *BMJ, 358*, j1951.

Seppi, K., Ray Chaudhuri, K., Coelho, M., et al. (2019). Update on treatments for nonmotor symptoms of Parkinson's disease—An evidence-based medicine review. *Movement Disorders, 34*, 180.

Suchowersky, O., Gronseth, G., Perlmutter, J., et al. (2006). Practice parameter: Neuroprotective strategies and alternative therapies for Parkinson's disease (an evidence-based review): Report of the Quality Standards Subcommittee of the American Academy of Neurology. *Neurology, 66*, 976.

Verschuur, C. V. M., Suwijn, S. R., Boel, J. A., et al. (2019). Randomized delayed-start trial of levodopa in Parkinson's disease. *New England Journal of Medicine, 380*, 315.

WHO. Definition of palliative care. (n.d.). Accessed January 10, 2020, at www.who.int/cancer/palliative/definition/en.

31

Dementia and Alzheimer's Disease Medications

MARCIA JOHANSSON AND AND CONSTANCE G. VISOVSKY

Overview

Dementia is a disorder characterized by a decline in cognitive function that also impairs one or more of the cognitive domains of learning and memory, language, executive function, complex attention, perceptual-motor function, and social cognition. Generally, dementia should be considered an acquired syndrome that has multiple possible causes rather than a definite disease itself.

Alzheimer's disease (the most common type of dementia) and vascular dementia often coexist and share common risk factors, many of which are modifiable before disease development (Figs. 31.1 and 31.2). Global estimates suggest that dementia affects up to 7% of individuals over age 65, with an even higher prevalence (8% to 10%) in developed countries due to higher life expectancy. As the population ages, the overall burden of dementia and Alzheimer's disease (AD) is increasing. The most common form of dementia in older adults is Alzheimer's disease, accounting for 60% to 70% of cases (GBD 2016 Neurology Collaborators, 2019). Although dementia mainly affects older people, it is not a normal part of the aging process and is one of the major causes of disability and dependency among older people worldwide.

Relevant Physiology

While there is no common physiology regarding dementia, a common way to conceptualize the causes of dementia is to consider the two different categories of the disease: those that are neurodegenerative or potentially irreversible, and those that are non-neurodegenerative or potentially reversible (Table 31.1). While this contrast is helpful for understanding the disease, it is limited by its simplicity as the cause may be multifactorial. For example, patients with dementia can, and often do, have numerous diseases that can be neurodegenerative (e.g., Lewy body dementia) and non-neurodegenerative (e.g., cerebrovascular disease), which cumulatively account for the impairment. Diseases can also impair cognition without leading to a decline in daily functioning, either at diagnosis or subsequently.

Most cases of dementia in older adults are caused by some degree of neurodegeneration. Some common degenerative dementias in older adults are Alzheimer's disease, Lewy body dementia, vascular dementia, frontotemporal lobar degeneration, and Parkinson's disease. Common causes of non-neurodegenerative dementia that can occur across the life span include vitamin deficiencies (B_{12}, thiamine), hypothyroidism, normal pressure hydrocephalus, chronic alcohol abuse, chemotherapy-related cognitive dysfunction, infections (human immunodeficiency virus or HIV, syphilis), intracranial masses (subdural hematomas, brain tumors), traumatic brain injury, and psychiatric illness (profound depression/anxiety). These non-neurodegenerative dementias may be reversible, or their progression may be slowed or halted, if the underlying cause can be identified and adequately treated (Table 31.1).

Pathophysiology

Alzheimer's disease and vascular dementia are the most common causes of dementia. In patients with Alzheimer's, pathologic changes include a loss of neurons in the nucleus basalis of Meynert, which is the origin of the cholinergic neurons. A decrease in cholinergic activity results from neuronal loss and from a decrease in the activity of choline acetyl transferase, the enzyme responsible for acetylcholine synthesis. The brain of a patient with Alzheimer's disease often shows marked atrophy, with widened sulci and shrinkage of the gyri. In most cases, every part of the cerebral cortex is involved, except for the occipital pole, which is often relatively spared. The cortical ribbon may be thinned and ventricular dilation may be apparent, especially in the temporal horn, as the result of atrophy of the amygdala and hippocampus. Microscopically, significant loss of neurons is apparent, in addition to shrinkage of large cortical neurons. Many researchers believe that a loss of synapses, in association with shrinkage of the dendritic arbor of large neurons, is the critical pathologic substrate in cases of Alzheimer's. The neuropathologic hallmarks of Alzheimer's are neuritic plaques and neurofibrillary tangles. Classic neuritic plaques are spherical structures that consist of a central core of fibrous protein known as *amyloid* that is surrounded

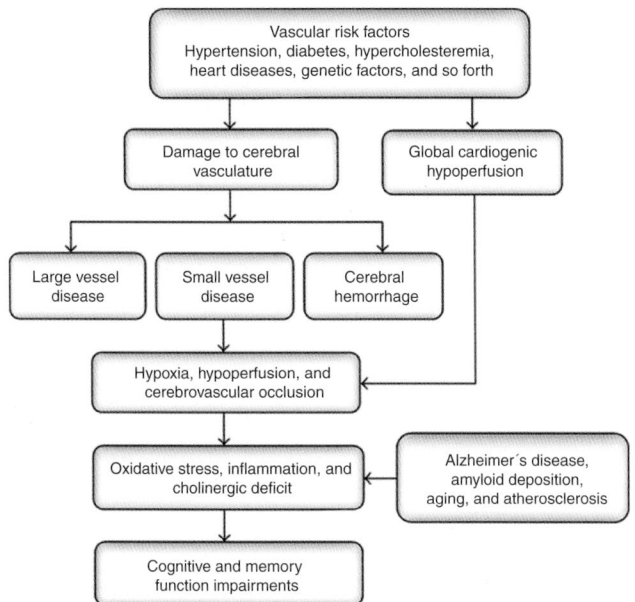

• **Fig. 31.1** Pathophysiology of dementia. (From Chang, D., Liu, J., Bilinski, K., Xu, L. Steiner, G. Z., Seto, S. W., & Bensoussan, A. [2016]. Herbal medicine for the treatment of vascular dementia: An overview of scientific evidence. *Evidence-Based Complementary and Alternative Medicine*, *2016*, 7293626. https://doi.org/10.1155/2016/7293626.)

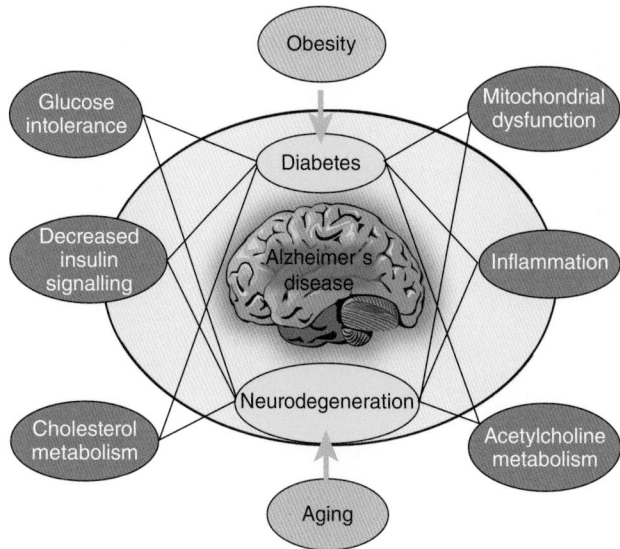

• **Fig. 31.2** Factors contributing to the development of Alzheimer's disease. (From Folch, J., Ettcheto, M., Petrov, D., Abad, S., Pedrós, I., Marin, M., et al. [2018]. Una revisión de los avances en la terapéuticade la enfermedad de Alzheimer: Estrategia frente a la proteína -amiloide. *Neurología*,*33*,47–58. http://doi.org/10.1016/j.nrleng.2015.03.019.)

by degenerating or dystrophic nerve endings (neurites). Two other types of amyloid-related plaques are recognized in the brains of patients with Alzheimer's: diffuse plaques, which contain poorly defined amyloid but no well-circumscribed amyloid core, and "burnt-out" plaques, which consist of an isolated dense amyloid core.

Dementia Therapy

Cholinesterase Inhibitors

Cholinesterase inhibitors, also known as acetylcholinesterase inhibitors, are chemical compounds that prevent acetylcholinesterase enzymes from breaking down acetylcholine, an important neurotransmitter. This action increases the availability of acetylcholine, which results in more acetylcholine in the synaptic cleft, enhancing cholinergic transmission. Currently, cholinesterase inhibitors are the standard therapy for Alzheimer's disease. Examples of cholinesterase inhibitors include donepezil (Aricept), galantamine (Reminyl), and rivastigmine (Exelon). All three medications are currently available for the treatment of mild to moderate dementia of the Alzheimer's type, while donepezil is also approved for severe Alzheimer's disease. These medications may modestly improve daily function; however, no evidence suggests that cholinesterase inhibitors alter the disease process or cure the disease. The efficacy of medications for dementia decreases as neuronal loss continues with disease progression. These medications are often initiated by primary care providers for patients who meet the criteria for mild to moderate Alzheimer's-type dementia, or they may be initiated after consultation with a provider who specializes in geriatrics, neurology, or neuropsychiatry.

Donepezil

Donepezil is a reversible cholinesterase inhibitor that is approved for the symptomatic management of mild to severe Alzheimer's disease. While treatment with cholinesterase inhibitors may result in small improvements in cognition and the ability to engage in activities of daily living, cholinesterase inhibitors do not prevent progression of the disease. Current data indicate that donepezil does not improve agitation associated with Alzheimer's disease.

Pharmacokinetics. Donepezil is administered orally and reaches peak levels in 3 to 4 hours, with a steady state reached in 15 days. The half-life is about 70 hours. Neither food nor time of administration influences the rate or extent of absorption. Ninety-six percent of the medication is protein bound. Seventeen percent is excreted in urine intact. The drug is extensively metabolized in the liver by the P450 2D6 and 3A4 enzyme systems. Donepezil may decrease the effects of anticholinergic medications.

Indications. Donepezil is indicated for the treatment of dementia of the Alzheimer's type. Efficacy has been demonstrated in patients with mild, moderate, and severe Alzheimer's disease. Donepezil is considered first-line therapy with only once-daily dosing. Treatment should be started at 5 mg orally daily; if this dose is tolerated after 4 weeks, the dose may be increased to 10 mg daily. Donepezil may be better tolerated than the other cholinesterase inhibitors.

Adverse Effects. Gastrointestinal (GI) effects are the most common adverse effects noted with donepezil, with nausea, vomiting, diarrhea, anorexia, and weight loss

TABLE 31.1	Medications for Dementia		
Category/ Medication	**Indication**	**Dosage**	**Considerations and Monitoring**
Cholinesterase Inhibitors			
Donepezil	For the treatment of moderate to severe Alzheimer's disease	*Adults:* Initial dose 5 mg orally once daily. Can increase to 10 mg orally once daily after 4–6 weeks.	No laboratory monitoring is necessary. Monitor neurologic function and weight. Because of the numerous and common GI effects, it is advised to take these medications with food.
Rivastigmine	For the treatment of mild to moderate Alzheimer's disease	*Adults:* 1.5 mg orally twice daily with food. If tolerated, may increase to 3 mg orally twice daily after 2 weeks. Subsequent increases to 4.5 mg and then 6 mg orally twice daily are based on tolerance after 2-week intervals. Typical maintenance dosage is 3–6 mg orally twice daily. *Transdermal dosage:* Apply one 4.6-mg/24 hr patch once daily. After 4 weeks, may increase to 9.5 mg/24 hr patch if tolerated.	Monitor LFTs, neurologic function, and weight.
Galantamine	For the treatment of mild to moderate vascular dementia or Alzheimer's disease	*Adults:* Initial dose of 4 mg orally twice daily with food. If tolerated after minimum of 4 weeks, dose may be increased to 8 mg orally twice daily. *Extended-release tablets:* 8 mg orally once daily in the morning with food. Dose may be increased to 16 mg orally once daily in the morning after 4 weeks. Another dosage increase may be given after 4 weeks of the previous dose, if well tolerated. Maximum dosage: 24 mg orally once daily.	Monitor neurologic function and weight.
NMDA Receptor Antagonist			
Memantine	For the treatment of symptoms of moderate to severe Alzheimer's disease	*Adults:* 5 mg orally once daily. Increase dose by 5 mg/week over 3-week period to target dose of 10 mg orally twice daily at week 4. *Extended-release tablets:* 7 mg orally once daily. Titrate in 7-mg increments at no sooner than 1-week intervals up to recommended target dose of 28 mg orally once daily.	Monitor serum creatinine and neurologic function.

GI, Gastrointestinal; *LFTs,* liver function tests; *NMDA,* N-methyl-D-aspartate.

reported. Musculoskeletal effects include muscle cramps (6% of patients), arthralgia (2%), unspecified pain (3% to 9%), and back pain (3%). Central nervous system (CNS) adverse effects such as headache (4% to 10%), insomnia (5% to 9%), dizziness (2% to 8%), abnormal dreams (3%), somnolence/drowsiness (2%), and depression (2% to 3%) have been reported. Most adverse effects are correlated to dose titration. Cardiovascular effects such as hypertension (3%), unspecified chest pain (2%), hyperlipidemia (2%), and syncope (2%), along with QT prolongation and torsades de pointes, have been reported during postmarketing use of donepezil. If accidental overdosage occurs, cholinergic crisis may occur. Symptoms include severe nausea,

vomiting, bradycardia, sweating, convulsions, collapse, and death, if respiratory muscles are involved. Atropine is used as an antidote.

Contraindications. Donepezil is contraindicated in patients with known hypersensitivity. Avoid abrupt discontinuation of therapy where possible to limit sudden decline in cognitive function or increase in behavioral disturbances. Donepezil is considered a drug with a known risk of torsades de pointes, and it is recommended to avoid use in patients with confirmed or suspected long QT syndrome. Special care should be exercised in those at risk for developing ulcers as donepezil can result in symptoms of active or occult GI bleeding.

Monitoring. Laboratory monitoring is not necessary. Monitor neurologic function and weight throughout treatment.

Rivastigmine

Rivastigmine is a cholinesterase inhibitor available in both oral and transdermal formulations and approved for the symptomatic management of mild to moderate Alzheimer's disease.

Pharmacokinetics. Following oral administration, rivastigmine is completely absorbed and peak plasma concentrations are reached in approximately 1 hour. Absolute bioavailability after a 3-mg oral dose is 36%, indicating a significant first-pass effect. Renal elimination (greater than 90%) is completed within 24 hours. Less than 1% of the administered dose is excreted in the feces. Following transdermal application, absorption begins within 30 minutes to 1 hour and peak plasma concentrations are typically reached in 8 hours. With transdermal application, trough levels are about 60% to 80% of peak levels at steady state. Approximately 50% of the drug load is released from the transdermal system over 24 hours.

Indications. Rivastigmine has demonstrated a benefit for patients with Lewy body dementia and for those with dementia associated with Parkinson's disease.

Adverse Effects. GI adverse effects commonly experienced by those taking rivastigmine include diarrhea (7% to 19% of patients), anorexia (6% to 17%), abdominal pain (13%), dyspepsia (9%), and weight loss (3%). If severe GI adverse effects occur, treatment with rivastigmine can be withheld for several doses. Therapy should then be reinitiated at the lowest daily dose and titrated slowly back to the maintenance dose as prescribed. CNS effects include dizziness (6% to 21%), headache (4% to17%), syncope (3%), insomnia (3% to 9%), restlessness (1% to 3%), and somnolence/drowsiness (5%). Falls were reported in 6% to 10% of patients receiving active treatment. Psychiatric effects include confusion (8%), depression (6%), anxiety (5%), hallucinations (4%), and aggressive behaviors (3%). These effects are often hard to distinguish from behavioral changes due to the progressive nature of the disease process. Cardiovascular adverse effects include unspecified chest pain, hypotension, orthostatic hypotension, atrial fibrillation, bradycardia, angina, myocardial infarction, and palpitations.

Contraindications. Rivastigmine, a carbamate derivative, is contraindicated in patients with carbamate hypersensitivity or a history of hypersensitivity to rivastigmine. The rivastigmine patch is contraindicated in patients who have a history of application site reactions suggestive of allergic contact dermatitis. GI disorders such as nausea and vomiting may occur, particularly when initiating treatment and/or increasing the rivastigmine dose. These adverse events occur more commonly in females. Patients with active peptic ulcer disease or those who are at high risk for peptic ulcers should be treated with caution. Rivastigmine should be used cautiously in patients with mild to moderate hepatic disease and in patients with asthma or chronic obstructive pulmonary disease (COPD). Rivastigmine has a weak affinity for peripheral cholinesterase, which may increase bronchoconstriction and bronchial secretion. Use rivastigmine with caution in patients with certain types of cardiac disease, such as sick sinus syndrome, severe cardiac arrhythmias, or cardiac conduction disturbances.

Monitoring. Monitor respiratory status in those with pulmonary disease as safety has not been demonstrated. Monitor liver function tests (LFTs), neurologic function, and weight.

Galantamine

Galantamine is a reversible cholinesterase inhibitor and natural alkaloid originating from the bulbs of the daffodil. Galantamine is approved for the symptomatic management of mild to moderate Alzheimer's disease.

Pharmacokinetics. Following oral administration, galantamine is completely and rapidly absorbed. Peak concentration levels are achieved in about 1 hour, with 90% bioavailability. Galantamine is a significant inhibitor of hepatic cytochrome (CYP) 450 enzymes, specifically by CYP 3A4 and CYP 2D6. No single dominant pathway has been identified for medication elimination, but 20% of the dose is excreted renally.

Indications. Galantamine is indicated in the treatment of mild to moderate Alzheimer's disease, Lewy body dementia, and vascular dementia.

Adverse Effects. Nausea and vomiting are common adverse reactions seen in fewer than 10% of patients. Other, less frequent adverse effects include abdominal pain, diarrhea, dyspepsia, depression, fatigue, headache, and lethargy.

Contraindications. There are no absolute contraindications, but galantamine should be used with caution in patients with COPD, asthma, cardiac disease, GI bleeding, peptic ulcer disease, renal impairment, seizure disorder, urinary tract obstruction, or history of serious rash.

Monitoring. Because the liver metabolizes these drugs, periodic monitoring of hepatic function may be justified, particularly in those receiving multiple medications and in those with weight loss, anorexia, or nausea, vomiting, and

---

PRACTICE PEARLS

Cholinesterase Inhibitors

- Vagotonic effects on heart rate may be provoked, causing bradycardia. Use with caution in patients with conduction abnormalities.

- Because of their cholinergic activity, cholinesterase inhibitors may increase gastric acid secretion. Use with caution in patients who are at increased risk for developing ulcers or who have a history of ulcer disease, as well as in patients who are taking nonsteroidal antiinflammatory drugs (NSAIDs).

- If the patient cannot tolerate a cholinesterase inhibitor because of GI or cardiac effects, the sole N-methyl-d-aspartate (NMDA) receptor antagonist can be used alone.

abdominal pain as these are signs and symptoms that suggest hepatic dysfunction. Monitor heart rate and blood pressure, particularly in patients with cardiovascular disease. Monitor for signs and symptoms of toxicity, such as vomiting and diarrhea, diaphoresis, urinary incontinence, psychosis (including hallucinations, nervousness, and behavioral changes), tremor, and weight loss. If exacerbations occur, consider adjusting the medications or looking for other potential causes of delirium. It is important to note that visual hallucinations are a hallmark feature of Lewy body dementia.

Memantine

Memantine hydrochloride is approved for treatment of moderate to severe dementia and is used in combination with a cholinesterase inhibitor. It is the first *N*-methyl-d-aspartate (NMDA) receptor antagonist, a subclass of medications that have a different mechanism of action from the cholinesterase inhibitors. The NMDA receptor is linked to learning and memory and is stimulated by glutamic acid, the principal excitatory neurotransmitter. Excessive stimulation of the NMDA receptor, however, leads to excitotoxicity. Blocking of this receptor is thought to prevent cognitive damage in patients with vascular dementia. Memantine blocks the excitotoxic effects associated with abnormal transmission of glutamate. It may improve overall patient function slightly, but no evidence indicates that it prevents or slows neurodegeneration.

Memantine may slightly improve function, reduce care dependency, and slow clinical decline in patients with moderate to severe dementia (those in stages 5 through 7 on the Global Deterioration Scale or who have achieved a Mini-Mental State Exam score less than 10). It may be given in addition to the cholinesterase inhibitors or as monotherapy.

Pharmacokinetics. Memantine is well absorbed. It has a half-life of 60 to 80 hours and is excreted unchanged in the urine. The CYP system plays no significant role.

Indications. Memantine is indicated in the treatment of mild to moderate Alzheimer's disease as monotherapy or with donepezil.

Adverse Effects. Adverse effects include hypertension, tachycardia, dizziness, headache, back pain, gait abnormalities, arthralgia, confusion, somnolence, hallucination, cough, weight gain or loss, sweating, nausea, vomiting, diarrhea, constipation, anorexia, and urinary incontinence. Use cautiously in patients with impairment or a history of seizures.

PRACTICE PEARLS

Memantine

- Seizures have occurred in a small number of patients.
- Reduce dose in patients with severe renal impairment.
- Genitourinary conditions, drugs, and diets that raise urine pH will increase plasma levels of memantine.
- Observe caution with concomitant use of other NMDA receptor antagonists.

Contraindications. There are no absolute contraindications, but memantine should be used cautiously in patients with hepatic dysfunction and any renal impairment.

Monitoring. Monitor serum creatinine and neurologic function at each visit.

Prescriber Considerations for Dementia Therapy

Clinical Practice Guidelines

Clinical practice guidelines for mild cognitive impairment and dementia can be found at the links in the box below.

BOOKMARK THIS!

- American Academy of Neurology: Practice Guideline Update Summary: Mild Cognitive Impairment: https://www.aan.com/Guidelines/home/GuidelineDetail/881
- Indian Journal of Psychiatry: Clinical Practice Guidelines for Management of Dementia: https://www.ncbi.nlm.nih.gov/pmc/articles/PMC5840907/

Clinical Reasoning for Dementia Therapy

Consider the individual patient's health problem requiring dementia therapy. The institution of pharmacologic therapy for dementia is highly dependent on the type of dementia, the stage of mental impairment, and the amount of interference with daily life. An accurate diagnosis of dementia type (Alzheimer's disease, vascular dementia, Lewy body dementia) is critical to therapy initiation and ongoing treatment.

Determine the desired therapeutic outcome based on the degree of dementia therapy needed for the patient's health problem. Initiating treatment as early as possible may help the patient maintain independence longer, delaying progressive disease symptoms. Typically, the goal of dementia therapy is to slow the progression of mental impairment and control of behavioral symptoms in order to maximize quality of life and functioning. Pharmacologic and nonpharmacologic therapies such as psychotherapy and environmental modifications are often used together.

Assess the dementia therapy selected for its appropriateness for an individual patient by considering the medication's side effects and the patient's age, race/ethnicity, comorbidities, and genetic factors. While dementia can occur in younger adults (41 to 60 years of age), it is fairly rare. Most commonly, dementia affects individuals after age 60. In addition to difficulty with memory, individuals must experience one additional impairment that significantly interferes with daily life, such as language or communication, ability to focus, and alterations in mood. Individuals with a history of depression, vascular disease, increased plasma homocysteine, head injury, genetics/family history, smoking/alcohol use, hearing loss, or diabetes have a high risk for dementia.

Initiate the treatment plan with the selected medication by first providing adequate patient and family education to ensure understanding and promote full participation in the dementia therapy. Educational strategies for medication teaching should focus on simple information, including pictures and easy reminders for medication adherence. Families and caregivers need to fully understand the medication that has been selected, how and when to administer it, and how to promote compliance. Patients are always included in the discussion of medication, and written instructions should also be given to assist the family in promoting adherence. It is important for the primary care provider to elicit understanding (as appropriate) from the patient as well as family/caregivers.

Ensure complete patient and family understanding about the medication prescribed for dementia therapy using a variety of education strategies. The altered mental state of the patient will determine the type and length of educational instruction provided. Educational strategies may be primarily for the family/caregiver. Educate the family/caregiver regarding behavioral and environmental management, and recommend family/caregiver support groups and the use of community resources, including respite care. Teach the family/caregiver that behavioral issues such as delusions, hallucinations, depression, agitation, aggression, and sleep disturbances can occur and may require further treatment and/or dose adjustment. Other teaching should include safety around the topics of medication administration, driving, cooking, falls, and wandering behaviors.

Conduct follow-up and monitoring of patient responses to dementia therapy. It is important that patients, families, and caregivers understand that the medication will not provide a "cure" or reversal of the dementia process, but it will slow the progressive nature of the disease. A one-month postinitiation follow-up to determine any side effects and tolerability to the medication is warranted. The follow-up should also include a clinical test of mentation (Global Deterioration Scale or Mini-Mental State Exam) to track progression at each visit, as well as a discussion of fall history, ability to engage in activities of daily living, and mood. After the first month, a clinic visit every 3 to 6 months can be instituted.

Teaching Points for Dementia Therapy

Health Promotion Strategies

- Inadequate nutrition is common in patients with dementia and is associated with increased morbidity and mortality. Possible causes include a decreased sense of smell which adds to poor appetite and weight loss, ongoing eating problems, and issues related to feeding problems.
- Oral nutrition supplements may improve weight and fat-free mass and should be implemented in patients with dementia.

- Cognitive rehabilitation may help patients in the early stages of dementia to maintain memory and higher cognitive function. Strategies to compensate for declining function should also be addressed.
- Exercise programs may improve physical functioning or at least help to slow the progression of functional decline.
- Occupational therapy may help to maintain activities of daily living and motor and processing skills.

Patient Education for Medication Safety

- Teach the patient and their family/caregiver to administer the prescribed medication safely through measures that promote safe self-administration (a.m./p.m. medication boxes, alarms, etc.) or family/caregiver administration.
- Check with the patient's pharmacist before crushing any pills or adding them to food for ease of administration. Extended-release preparations may not be crushed.
- Use simple language and instructions.
- If the patient refuses to take the medication, stop and try again later.
- If swallowing is a problem, check with your health care provider to see whether the medication is available in another form.

Application Questions for Discussion

1. How is the rate of absorption of cholinesterase inhibitors affected by ingestion of food?
2. Cognitive assessment tools are critical for patients with Alzheimer's disease. Discuss the assessment tools and when they would be best implemented for these patients.

Selected Bibliography

Birks, J., & Flicker, L. Selegiline for Alzheimer's disease. Cochrane Database Syst Rev. 2000;(2):CD000442. doi: 10.1002/14651858. CD000442. Update in: Cochrane Database Syst Rev. 2003;(1):CD000442. PMID: 10796544.

Brauner, D. J., Muir, J. C., & Sachs, G. A. (2000). Treating non-dementia illnesses in patients with dementia. *JAMA, 283*(24), 3230.

Chen, R., Chan, P. T., Chu, H., et al. (2017). Treatment effects between monotherapy of donepezil versus combination with memantine for Alzheimer disease: A meta-analysis. *PLoS One, 12*(8): e0183586. http://doi.org/10.1371/journal.pone.0183586.

GBD 2016 Neurology Collaborators. (2019). Global, regional, and national burden of neurological disorders, 1990-2016: a systematic analysis for the Global Burden of Disease Study 2016. *The Lancet. Neurology, 18*(5), 459-480. doi: 10.1016/S1474-4422(18)30499-X.

Howard, R., McShane, R., Lindesay, J., et al. (2012). Donepezil and memantine for moderate-to-severe Alzheimer's disease. *New England Journal of Medicine, 366*, 893. http://doi.org/10.1056/NEJMoa1106668.

McShane R, Areosa Sastre A, Minakaran N. (2006). Memantine for dementia. Cochrane Database Syst Rev. Apr 19;(2):CD003154. doi: 10.1002/14651858. CD003154.pub5. Update in: Cochrane Database Syst Rev. 2019 Mar 20;3:CD003154. PMID: 16625572.

Qaseem, A., Snow, V., Cross, J. T., Jr, et al. (2008). Current pharmacologic treatment of dementia: A clinical practice guideline from the American College of Physicians and the American Academy of Family Physicians. *Annals of Internal Medicine, 148*, 370.

Raina, P., Santaguida, P., Ismaila, A., et al. (2008). Effectiveness of cholinesterase inhibitors and memantine for treating dementia: Evidence review for a clinical practice guideline. *Annals of Internal Medicine, 148*, 379.

Reisberg, B., Doody, R., Stöffler, A., et al. (2003). Memantine in moderate-to-severe Alzheimer's disease. *New England Journal of Medicine, 348*, 1333.

Woods, B, Aguirre, E, Spector, AE, & Orrell, M. (2012). Cognitive stimulation to improve cognitive functioning in people with dementia. *Cochrane Database Syst Rev.* Feb 15;(2):CD005562. CD005562. doi: 10.1002/14651858.pub2. PMID: 22336813.

32

Pain Management Medications and Substance Abuse

MARCIA JOHANSSON AND CONSTANCE G. VISOVSKY

Overview

Pain is described as "an unpleasant sensory and emotional experience associated with, or resembling that associated with, actual or potential tissue damage" (Raja et al., 2020). Pain is a subjective sensation that may or may not have correlating objective findings. Pain is described as being *acute* or *chronic* in nature. Acute pain is of short duration and occurs as the body's response to tissue damage. Chronic pain is described as ongoing or recurrent pain, lasting beyond the usual course of acute illness or injury or more than 3 to 6 months, and which adversely affects the individual's well-being (Raja et al., 2020). Currently, chronic pain is estimated to occur in 20.4% of adults in the United States, negatively impacting their mobility and daily activities and potentially leading to opioid dependance, anxiety, depression, poor health, and decreased quality of life (Dahlhammer et al., 2018). The location, duration, and intensity of pain; characteristics of the illness or trauma; and prior exposure to certain pain medications all influence the type of medication needed for pain relief. Chronic pain is one of the most common reasons patients seek medical attention from their provider. Patients with chronic pain can more easily develop tolerance to analgesics as compared with patients with acute pain.

Pain can be classified as *nociceptive* or *neuropathic*. Nociceptive pain is further divided into two categories: *somatic* and *visceral*. Nociceptive pain arises from the direct stimulation of afferent nerves in cutaneous or deep musculoskeletal tissues and occurs in response to tissue injury or disease infiltration of the skin, soft tissue, or viscera. Somatic pain is well localized in skin and subcutaneous tissues but not in bone, muscle, blood vessels, or connective tissue and is often described as dull or aching. Visceral pain is poorly localized and often is described as a continual aching, or a deep, crampy, or sharp, squeezing pain. Visceral pain occurs in response to stretching, distention, compression, or infiltration of organs such as the liver. Neuropathic pain results from injury to peripheral nerves or the central nervous system (CNS) and is described as episodes of shooting or stabbing pain superimposed over a background of aching and burning. Because it originates from peripheral nerves, the spinal cord, or the brain, it is poorly localized and often is associated with paresthesias and dysesthesias (Table 32.1).

Relevant Physiology

The sensation of pain is a protective mechanism in response to tissue damage. Pain is generally classified as *fast* or *slow*. With fast pain, the painful sensation is felt about 0.1 second after a stimulus is applied, while with slow pain it is felt at least 1 second after the stimulus is applied. Fast pain is often described as a sharp, prickling, acute, or electric shock type of pain; the sensation is transmitted from the peripheral nerves to the spinal cord by small nerve fibers. Slow pain is often described as burning, aching, or chronic; the sensation is transmitted to the spinal cord via type C nerve fibers. A series of sensory events are required for the brain to detect the sensation of pain. The first event is pain sensitivity. This is followed by the pain signal being transmitted from the periphery to the dorsal horn in the spinal cord via the peripheral nervous system. Finally, the pain signal is transmitted to the brain via the CNS. Typically, pain signals are transmitted via two routes: ascending and descending pathways. The ascending pathway carries sensory information from the body via the spinal cord and toward the brain. The descending pathway carries sensory information from the brain via the spinal cord to the reflex organs. Chemicals such as bradykinin, serotonin, histamine, potassium ions, and acetylcholine excite chemical pain. Substance P and prostaglandins act to enhance sensitization of pain nerve endings.

Pathophysiology

Four processes are required for pain to occur: transduction, transmission, modulation, and perception. Sensory receptors, or nociceptors, that are sensitive to painful or tissue-damaging (noxious) stimuli are present in the skin, bone, muscle, connective tissue, and thoracic, abdominal, and pelvic viscera. *Transduction* occurs when a noxious stimulus depolarizes peripheral nerve endings and sets off electrical activity. The nerve endings that transduce the noxious stimuli conduct electrical signals to the spinal cord through two

TABLE 32.1	**Classification of Pain**	
Category	**Characteristics**	**Examples**
Nociceptive		
Somatic	Well localized	Laceration, fracture, cellulitis, arthritis
	Dull, aching, or throbbing	
Visceral	Poorly localized	Subscapular pain arising from diaphragmatic irritation
	Continual aching	Right upper quadrant pain arising from stretching of the liver capsule
	Referred to dermatomal sites that are distant from the source of pain	
Neuropathic		
	Shooting or stabbing pain superimposed over a background of aching and burning	Postherpetic neuralgia, postthoracotomy neuralgia, poststroke pain, trigeminal neuralgia, diabetic polyneuropathy
	Pain not well localized	

types of nerve fibers: A delta fibers and C fibers. The A delta fibers are myelinated, and their activation is associated with sharp, stinging sensations. The C fibers are unmyelinated, and their activation is associated with vaguely localized pain that may be dull or burning.

Next, *transmission* occurs, whereby electrical impulses are carried throughout the peripheral and central nervous systems. *Modulation* is the central neural activity that controls the transmission of pain impulses. Finally, during *perception*, the neural activities involved in transmission and modulation result in a subjective correlate of pain that includes behavioral, psychological, and emotional factors.

All of these lead to one end result, and the pathway of pain has been initiated and completed, thus allowing us to feel the painful sensation triggered by the stimulus (Fig. 32.1).

Pain Management Therapy

Opioid Analgesics

Opiate receptors in the CNS mediate analgesic activity. Opioid agonists occupy the same receptors as endogenous opioid peptides, and both alter the central release of neurotransmitters from afferent nerves sensitive to noxious stimuli. The actions of opioid analgesics can be defined by their activity at three specific receptor types: mu, kappa, and delta. The mu receptors mediate morphine-like supraspinal analgesia, miosis, respiratory depression, euphoria, physical dependence, and opiate withdrawal suppression. The kappa receptors mediate spinal analgesia, respiratory depression, and sedation. The delta receptors mediate antagonist activity. Morphine-like agonists have activity at the mu, kappa, and delta receptors. Mixed agonist-antagonist drugs, such as pentazocine, have agonist activity at some receptors and antagonist activity at other receptors. The opioid antagonist naloxone does not have agonist activity at any opioid receptors.

The mechanism by which opioids produce euphoria is not fully understood, but it is thought to alter hypothalamic heat regulation that slightly decreases body temperature. Opioids also affect the hypothalamus by causing decreased levels of testosterone, cortisol, adrenocorticotropic hormone (ACTH), and β-endorphin. With long-term use, these effects are diminished. CNS effects in the limbic system can include dysphoric mood, especially with long-term use, intense and unusual dreams, and hallucinations. Pupillary miosis results from excitatory effects on the parasympathetic nerves that cause constriction of the pupil. The respiratory depression associated with opioids is caused by a direct effect on the brain stem respiratory centers by which the brain stem becomes less responsive to carbon dioxide. Death from morphine overdose is usually the result of respiratory arrest.

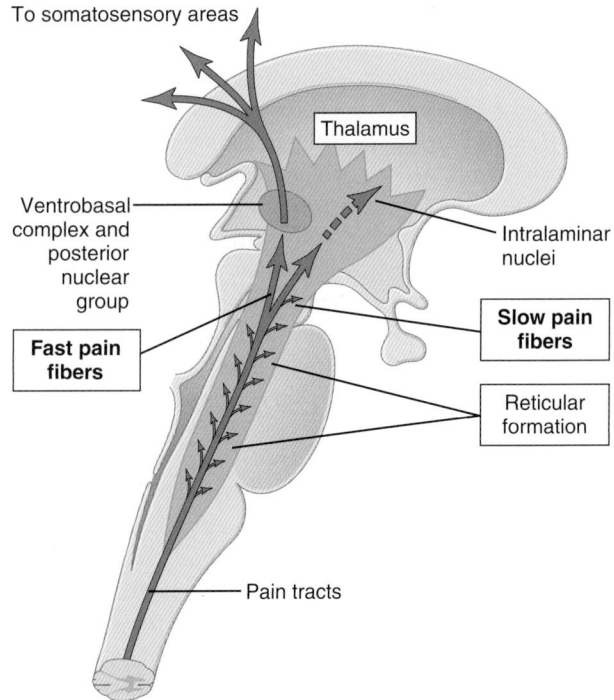

• **Fig. 32.1** Transmission of pain signals into the brain stem, thalamus, and cerebral cortex (From Hall, J. E., & Hall, M. E. [2021]. *Guyton & Hall textbook of medical physiology* [14th ed.]. Philadelphia: Elsevier.)

Opioids produce nausea and vomiting through direct stimulation of the chemoreceptor trigger zone (CTZ) for emesis in the medulla. A vestibular component is part of the effect, in that nausea and vomiting are more common in ambulatory patients than in those on bed rest. Opioids produce peripheral vasodilation, reduce peripheral vascular resistance, and inhibit baroreceptor reflexes, causing orthostatic hypotension. The effects of opioids on the gastrointestinal (GI) system include decreased gastric motility and diminished biliary, pancreatic, and intestinal secretions. The sphincter of Oddi constricts and causes increased pressure in the common bile duct, leading to biliary colic. Opioids delay the digestion of food in the small intestine. Propulsive peristaltic waves in the colon are diminished and tone is increased to the point of spasm. This delays the passage of stool and leads to constipation. Opioids also inhibit the urinary voiding reflex and may cause urinary retention. Some opioids such as morphine and meperidine, but not methadone or fentanyl, cause histamine release, leading to pruritus, sweating, and urticaria.

Opioids are highly addictive, and overdose can lead to respiratory depression that can result in permanent brain damage, coma, or death. Naloxone is a medication that can reverse opioid overdose when administered right away. Primary care providers should be familiar with regulations regarding the use and dispensing of narcotic analgesics. Methadone is prescribed chiefly for the treatment of opiate detoxification and may be dispensed only by pharmacies and maintenance programs approved by the U.S. Food and Drug Administration (FDA) and state authorities, according to federal methadone regulations. Methadone is also used for pain management; it may be prescribed by any provider with a U.S. Drug Enforcement Administration (DEA) license to prescribe Schedule II drugs and be dispensed by any licensed pharmacy. Because of the potential for abuse, the primary care provider must justify the use of opioid analgesics for ambulatory patients.

Providers need to be aware of the issues and measures to help prevent overdose and misuse of pain medications. Some risk factors identified for prescription opioid abuse and overdose include receiving overlapping prescriptions from multiple primary care providers and pharmacies, high daily opioid dosage, mental health disorders or history of substance abuse, low income, and rural settings. Many states have implemented Prescription Drug Monitoring Programs (PDMPs) and mandates.

All opioid drugs cause tolerance and dependence. This is not the same as abuse. *Tolerance* is a pharmacologic phenomenon characterized by decreasing drug effect over time. More drug is needed to produce the same effect. *Dependence* is the physiologic development of abstinence syndrome or withdrawal symptoms when a drug is discontinued, or an antagonist is given. Slowly tapering the medication can eliminate withdrawal symptoms. Psychologic dependence, or *addiction,* is the overwhelming obsession with obtaining and using a drug for a nonmedical purpose.

PRACTICE PEARLS

Signs and Symptoms of Opioid Overdosage

- *Acute overdose:* Profound respiratory depression, a respiratory rate of fewer than 12 breaths per minute, irregular and shallow respirations, deep sleep, stupor or coma, miosis, cyanosis, gradually decreasing blood pressure, oliguria, clammy skin, hypothermia
- *Chronic abuse:* Constricted pupils, skin infection, mood changes, depressed level of consciousness, itching, needle scars, abscesses

Opioid Agonists: Phenanthrenes

Synthetic opiates are structural analogs of morphine. These include heroin, hydromorphone, hydrocodone, and oxycodone. Methylmorphine (codeine) is also found in nature but is produced commercially by adding a methyl group to the morphine base. Morphine is the prototypical opioid against which all other opioids are compared for equianalgesic potency. Morphine is hydrophilic and thus remains in the blood until it is eliminated. Currently available forms of morphine include short- and long-acting preparations.

Morphine

Morphine is the primary opioid analgesic used for relief of severe pain. It is classified as a Schedule II controlled substance. Morphine is more effective against dull, continuous pain than sharp, spasmodic pain.

Pharmacokinetics. Morphine sulfate is administered orally, parenterally, intrathecally, epidurally, and rectally. When morphine is administered orally, bioavailability is approximately 20% to 40%. It is readily absorbed from the gut and has a more rapid absorption with rectal administration. Peak analgesia is obtained after about 60 minutes following immediate-release oral administration and in 8 hours following administration of sustained-release formulations. Morphine is metabolized primarily by the liver and by P-glycoprotein which is present on the absorptive cells of the intestine (enterocytes) and hepatocytes. Opioid analgesics are metabolized in the liver through glucuronidation and, to a lesser extent, by the cytochrome (CYP) P450 2D6 enzyme system. They are excreted through the kidney in a conjugated form. Genetic variability produces wide differences in how quickly opioids are metabolized. All opioids are excreted in urine; some are excreted to a small extent in feces.

After intravenous (IV) administration, peak analgesia is obtained within 20 minutes and the duration of analgesia is approximately 3 to 6 hours. Peak analgesia is obtained about 30 to 60 minutes after intramuscular (IM) injections and the duration of analgesia is approximately 3 to 6 hours. Following rectal administration, peak analgesia is achieved in 20 to 60 minutes. After epidural administration, morphine is rapidly absorbed and analgesia is achieved within 15 to 30 minutes, with a duration of 4 to 24 hours. Excretion of morphine is largely in the urine and bile as the morphine 3-glucuronide and 6-glucuronide metabolites. Between 7% and 10% is excreted in the feces, mainly via the bile. The elimination half-life of oral morphine is about 1 to 2 hours, and 2 to 4 hours after IV administration.

Indications. Morphine is indicated for the relief of acute and chronic moderate to severe pain. Morphine is also used to manage chronic, severe pain in patients who require daily, around-the-clock, long-term opioid treatment.

Adverse Effects. Respiratory depression is the most significant adverse effect associated with an opiate agonist, occurring in 2% to 5% of patients. Respiratory arrest and apnea also occur, due to a decreased sensitivity to carbon dioxide in the brain stem. Respiratory depression is more common in older adults, debilitated patients, and non–opioid-tolerant patients and when opioids are given with other agents that cause CNS depression. Respiratory depression is most significant after IV administration. Fatal overdose may result if the extended-release form is chewed, crushed, or diluted. These agents may produce drowsiness or dizziness; advise patients to observe caution while driving or performing other tasks that require alertness or physical activity. Symptomatic respiratory depression should be treated cautiously with an opioid antagonist such as naloxone.

Opioid tolerance to the analgesic effects of opiate agonists has been reported. Tolerance is the need for increasing opioid doses to maintain initial pain relief. Tolerance presents as a decrease in the duration of analgesia and is managed by increasing the opioid dose or frequency. GI adverse effects such as nausea (more than 10% of patients), vomiting (3% to at least 10%), and constipation (9% to at least 10%) are common. Nausea and vomiting are most commonly seen at the initiation of therapy or when switching agents. Treatment with an antiemetic during the first 1 to 2 days, then as needed during opiate therapy, will usually control these symptoms until tolerance develops. To avoid constipation, patients require a bowel regimen consisting of a stool softener and mild stimulant throughout opioid therapy.

While rare, anaphylactoid reactions have been reported. Evidence of histamine release such as urticaria, wheals, and local tissue irritation may occur with parenteral morphine administration; urticaria (fewer than 5%) has also been reported with other formulations. CNS depression, including drowsiness (2% to 19%), confusion (fewer than 10%), and dizziness (more than 5%), can occur.

Contraindications. Caution needs to be employed in patients with chronic obstructive pulmonary disease (COPD), decreased pulmonary reserve, or cardiovascular disease; in patients taking other CNS depressants; and in patients who have hypersensitivity to opioids. Bronchospasm has been reported in patients receiving extended-release morphine and should be used cautiously in patients with preexisting airway resistance, CNS depression, increased intracranial pressure, acute alcohol intoxication, convulsive disorders, heart failure secondary to chronic lung disease, and cardiac arrhythmias. Morphine is contraindicated for use in patients taking

monoamine oxidase inhibitors (MAOIs) or who have received MAOIs within 14 days. When given to patients with renal or hepatic dysfunction, morphine may have a prolonged duration and a cumulative effect, requiring reduced dosage and longer intervals between doses.

Monitoring Monitor respiratory status due to the ability of morphine to depress respiratory drive. Monitor blood pressure as morphine may cause severe hypotension, especially in patients at risk for orthostatic hypotension. Monitor for opioid abuse and dependence.

PRACTICE PEARLS

Opiate Use in Pregnancy and Birth

- Routine use of opioid agonists by an expectant mother can lead to depressed respiration in the newborn and neonatal opioid withdrawal syndrome.
- Neonatal opioid withdrawal syndrome is estimated to occur in up to 50% of neonates born to opioid-dependent mothers.
- Withdrawal symptoms may include irritability, hyperactivity, abnormal sleep pattern, tremor, high-pitched crying, vomiting, diarrhea, poor feeding, failure to gain weight, rigidity, and seizures.

Hydrocodone

Hydrocodone is a Schedule III semisynthetic opioid whose primary actions, analgesia and sedation, affect the CNS and smooth muscle organs. Hydrocodone is used to treat moderate to severe pain of an acute nature, or as an antitussive. It is available in combination only with acetaminophen, aspirin, or ibuprofen and with antihistamines, decongestants, and expectorants for cough suppression.

Pharmacokinetics. Hydrocodone is administered orally and is metabolized through CYP 3A4 mediated N-demethylation to norhydrocodone as the primary metabolic pathway. Hydrocodone and its metabolites are eliminated primarily in the kidneys. The mean half-life of hydrocodone extended-release capsules and tablets ranges from 7 to 12 hours, and peak plasma concentrations are reached approximately 5 hours after administration. Food has no significant effect on the extent of absorption.

Indications. Hydrocodone is indicated for the treatment of chronic, severe pain in patients who require daily, around-the-clock, long-term opioid treatment.

Adverse Effects. CNS-related adverse reactions reported with hydrocodone extended-release capsules include drowsiness (1% to 5% of patients), headache (4% or fewer), dizziness (2% to 3%), and tremor (3%). Pharmacologic tolerance to the analgesic effects of codeine may occur and presents as a decrease in the duration of analgesia. As with other opiate agonists, there is potential for abuse. GI-related effects reported in clinical trials of hydrocodone extended-release capsules include constipation (8% to 11%), nausea (7% to 10%), xerostomia (3% or fewer), vomiting (3% to 5%), and abdominal pain (fewer than 10%). Abdominal discomfort and gastroesophageal reflux disease (GERD) were reported in 1% to 10% of patients. Routine use of opiate agonists by an expectant mother can lead to depressed respiration in the newborn and neonatal opioid withdrawal syndrome. Respiratory depression can occur following large initial doses in non–opioid-tolerant patients, or when opioids are given with other agents that cause CNS depression. Respiratory depression is most common in older adults and debilitated patients and may lead to respiratory arrest and death if not immediately treated.

Hydrocodone can cause cardiovascular adverse reactions due to its anticholinergic effects and its ability to release histamine. QT prolongation has been observed with some extended-release formulations at higher doses. Hydrocodone has the potential to cause severe hypotension and syncope. Dehydration and hypokalemia were reported in clinical trials of hydrocodone extended-release capsules at an incidence of 1% to less than 10%. While pruritus can occur (fewer than 5%) rash, hyperhidrosis, and flushing were each reported in 1% to 5% of patients. However, true drug hypersensitivity was observed in fewer than 1% of patients. Chronic use of opioids may influence the hypothalamic-pituitary-gonadal axis, leading to hormonal changes that may manifest as hypogonadism (gonadal suppression), libido decrease, erectile dysfunction, amenorrhea, or infertility. Serotonin syndrome has been reported in patients taking opioids at recommended doses. Patients taking opioids concomitantly with a serotonergic medication should seek immediate medical attention if they develop symptoms such as agitation, hallucinations, tachycardia, fever, excessive sweating, shivering or shaking, muscle twitching or stiffness, trouble with coordination, nausea, vomiting, or diarrhea.

Contraindications. Hydrocodone is contraindicated for use in patients with significant respiratory depression and in patients with acute or severe asthma or COPD. Use with caution in patients with obesity as this is a risk factor for obstructive sleep-apnea syndrome and/or decreased respiratory reserve. Opioids increase the risk of central sleep apnea and sleep-related hypoxemia in a dose-dependent fashion. Hydrocodone extended-release capsules and tablets are contraindicated in patients with known or suspected GI obstruction or paralytic ileus. Hydrocodone should be used with caution in patients with biliary tract disease, including acute pancreatitis. Use hydrocodone with caution in geriatric or debilitated patients as these patients are more susceptible to adverse reactions, especially sedation and respiratory depression. Use hydrocodone with caution in patients with CNS depression, head trauma, intracranial mass, increased intracranial pressure, adrenal insufficiency, hypothyroidism, or myxedema.

Monitoring. Monitor patients closely for signs or symptoms of respiratory depression or sedation. Assess patients for risks of addiction, abuse, or misuse before drug initiation, and monitor patients who receive opioids routinely for development of these behaviors or conditions.

PRACTICE PEARL

Opioids and Serotonin Syndrome

- Advise patients taking opioids concomitantly with a serotonergic medication to seek immediate medical attention if they develop symptoms such as agitation, hallucinations, tachycardia, fever, excessive sweating, shivering or shaking, muscle twitching or stiffness, or trouble with coordination.

- Symptoms of serotonin syndrome generally present within hours to days of taking an opioid with another serotonergic agent, but they may also occur later, particularly after a dosage increase.

- If serotonin syndrome is suspected, the opioid and/or the other agent should be discontinued.

Tramadol

Tramadol is an oral opioid agonist indicated for the treatment of pain severe enough to require an opioid analgesic and for which alternate treatments are inadequate. The analgesic effect of tramadol is from both binding to mu-opioid receptors and through weak inhibition of reuptake of norepinephrine and serotonin.

Pharmacokinetics. Tramadol is administered orally and undergoes significant first-pass metabolism. Sixty percent of a tramadol dose is metabolized by the liver through two metabolic pathways to form N- and O-demethylated tramadol. Patients with impaired CYP 2D6 activity or those receiving concurrent medications that affect CYP 2D6 or CYP 3A4 enzymes may experience an altered response to tramadol. The mean peak plasma concentration of tramadol occurs after 2 to 3 hours. The half-life of tramadol is about 7 hours after administration of the immediate-release formulation, 8 hours after administration of coated extended-release tablets, 7.5 hours after administration of dual-matrix extended-release tablets, and 10 hours after administration of extended-release capsules. Excretion of tramadol and its metabolites is mostly renal. Approximately 30% of the dose is excreted in the urine as unchanged drug, whereas 60% of the dose is excreted as metabolites.

Indications. Tramadol is indicated for the treatment of severe pain requiring an opioid analgesic and for which alternative treatments are inadequate.

Adverse Effects. Serious, life-threatening, or fatal respiratory depression has been reported with the use of opioids, even when used as recommended. Respiratory depression may lead to respiratory arrest and death if not immediately treated. As with other opioid agonists, tramadol presents the potential for abuse or psychological dependence.

Somnolence, dizziness, and vertigo are among the most common adverse reactions associated with tramadol use, occurring in 26% to 33% of patients. GI adverse effects of dry mouth, dyspepsia, nausea and vomiting, constipation, and diarrhea are common. Dermatologic effects such as pruritus may be a common adverse reaction associated with tramadol use; this effect may occur independently or may indicate a hypersensitivity reaction. Serious but rarely fatal anaphylactoid reactions have been reported in patients receiving tramadol. Other allergic manifestations associated with tramadol include urticaria (fewer than 1%), bronchospasm, angioedema rash, Stevens-Johnson syndrome (fewer than 1%), and toxic epidermal necrolysis (fewer than 1%).

Serotonin syndrome (fewer than 1%) may occur with tramadol within the recommended doses, especially when used with serotonergic drugs. CNS adverse effects such as nervousness, anxiety, agitation, tremor, spasticity, euphoria, emotional lability, and hallucinations have been reported in 7% to 14% of patients. Tramadol may cause severe hypotension, including orthostatic hypotension and syncope. Risk of seizure may also increase in patients with a seizure disorder, history of seizures, or recognized risk for seizures.

Contraindications. Tramadol is contraindicated in patients with known tramadol hypersensitivity, opiate agonist hypersensitivity, or hypersensitivity to any other component. Tramadol is contraindicated in patients with suicidal ideation and must be used with caution in patients with a history of prior substance abuse or misuse. The use of tramadol is also contraindicated in patients who are receiving or have received MAOI therapy within the past 14 days. The safety and efficacy of tramadol in pediatric patients have not been established. Tramadol is contraindicated in neonates, infants, and children younger than 12 years of age, and for postoperative pain management in pediatric patients younger than 18 years of age after a tonsillectomy and/or adenoidectomy. Tramadol is also contraindicated in patients with significant respiratory depression or with acute or severe asthma in an unmonitored setting or in the absence of resuscitative equipment. Patients with COPD, cor pulmonale, respiratory insufficiency, hypoxemia, hypercapnia, or preexisting respiratory depression are at increased risk of decreased respiratory drive, even at recommended doses. Tramadol is contraindicated in patients with GI obstruction, including paralytic ileus.

Monitoring. Patients will require both counseling about the risks and proper use of tramadol and intensive monitoring for signs of addiction, abuse, and misuse. Monitor patients for signs of hypotension after initiating or titrating the opioid dosage. Monitor for the presence of serious adverse effects such as serotonin syndrome, acute hypersensitivity reactions, and increased or new-onset seizure activity.

Codeine

Codeine is a Schedule II–III opioid agonist that has analgesic and antitussive therapeutic effects. Ten percent of codeine is metabolized to morphine. Codeine is less potent than morphine and does not have the abuse potential of morphine. However, codeine is more likely than other opioids to cause both constipation and nausea. When used for analgesia purposes, codeine preparations are often combined with nonopioid analgesics, centrally acting muscle relaxants, antihistamines, and decongestants. Noncombination forms of codeine are classified as Schedule II controlled substances. Oral codeine is as effective as the parenteral form.

Pharmacokinetics. Codeine is administered orally and is known to have an extensive volume of distribution into the body's tissues. It is well absorbed after oral administration, with an onset of action within 30 to 60 minutes, and it is slightly bound to plasma proteins. Plasma half-lives of codeine and its metabolites have been reported to be approximately 3 hours. Approximately 90% of the total dose of codeine is excreted through the kidneys, of which approximately 10% is unchanged codeine. Codeine passes through both the blood–brain barrier and the placental barrier. Small amounts of codeine and its metabolite, morphine, are transferred to human breast milk.

Indications. Codeine can be used in the treatment of mild to moderate pain and for cough.

Adverse Effects. Pharmacologic tolerance to the analgesic effects of codeine may occur and presents as a decrease in the duration of analgesia. As with other opiate agonists, use of codeine presents the potential for abuse. Routine use of opiate agonists by an expectant mother can lead to depressed respiration in the newborn and neonatal opioid withdrawal syndrome. Codeine produces dose-related respiratory depression. Respiratory depression is most common in older adults and debilitated patients and may lead to respiratory arrest and death if not immediately treated. Drowsiness, light-headedness, and dizziness are common reactions with codeine. Codeine's effect on opiate receptors produces sedation. Patients should be warned that activity requiring mental alertness can be affected because CNS depression can occur. Hallucinations (especially of bugs and spiders) and seizures have been reported in patients receiving high doses of opiate agonists. Serotonin syndrome has been reported in patients taking opioids at recommended doses. Patients taking opioids concomitantly with a serotonergic medication should seek immediate medical attention if they develop symptoms such as agitation, hallucinations, tachycardia, fever, excessive sweating, shivering or shaking, muscle twitching or stiffness, trouble with coordination, nausea, vomiting, or diarrhea.

GI adverse effects of codeine include nausea, vomiting, and constipation. Nausea and vomiting are most common at the initiation of therapy or when switching agents. Codeine and other opiate agonists are known to cause pruritus. Opiate agonist–induced pruritus is thought to be mediated through stimulation of central opiate receptors. Codeine, like morphine, can cause miosis. Therapeutic doses can increase accommodation and sensitivity to light reflex and decrease intraocular tension.

Contraindications. Codeine is contraindicated in patients with known or suspected GI obstruction, including paralytic ileus. It is contraindicated for use in patients with a history of respiratory depression, or acute or severe bronchial asthma or COPD. Patients with head trauma or with increased intracranial pressure should not be given codeine unless the benefits outweigh the risks, because it can compromise the evaluation of neurologic parameters. Codeine should be used with caution in patients with cardiac arrhythmias, hypotension, or hypovolemia. Patients with severe hepatic disease can experience increased toxicity and reduced analgesic effects from codeine. Codeine is contraindicated in neonates, infants, and children younger than 12 years of age, and for postoperative pain management in pediatric patients younger than 18 years of age after a tonsillectomy and/or adenoidectomy. Use codeine with caution in patients with adrenal insufficiency (e.g., Addison's disease), hypothyroidism, or myxedema due to an increased risk of adverse events. Use of codeine is contraindicated in patients who are receiving or have received MAOI therapy within the past 14 days because of additive CNS depression, drowsiness, dizziness, or hypotension.

Monitoring. Monitor patients closely for respiratory depression, especially within the first 24 to 72 hours after initiation and dose escalation. Assess patients for risks of addiction, abuse, or misuse before drug initiation, and monitor patients who receive opioids routinely for development of these behaviors or conditions.

PRACTICE PEARLS

Prescribing Oral Opiates

- Assess the patient for prior use and response to opiates.
- Assess for a history of substance use or abuse.
- Prescribe pain medication that is appropriate to the cause and level of pain experienced.
- Prescribe the lowest effective dose for the shortest time required.
- If converting from one opioid to another, use an equianalgesic dose.
- Adjust the dosage to achieve pain relief with acceptable levels of adverse effects.
- When titrating opioids, consider the half-life of the prescribed opioid in determining the titration plan.

PRACTICE PEARLS

Steps to Changing Opioids

1. Calculate the 24-hour dose of the current opioids, including around-the-clock and rescue doses.
2. Use an equianalgesic table to convert the dosage of the current drug to the equivalent dosage of the new drug.
3. Adjust the dosage of the new drug to accommodate patient variability and to account for incomplete cross-tolerance.
4. Determine the dosing interval according to the duration of action of the new opioid.
5. Calculate rescue doses.
6. When converting from extended-release morphine, give the same 24-hour total as a divided regimen given at appropriate intervals.

Oxycodone and Hydromorphone

Similar to hydrocodone, oxycodone and hydromorphone are used to treat chronic, severe pain in patients who require daily, around-the-clock, long-term opioid treatment. Oxycodone is administered orally, while hydromorphone can be administered via an oral, parenteral, or rectal route. The adverse effects and contraindications are essentially the same for both medications.

Oxycodone is a Schedule II medication that is a semisynthetic opioid. It is similar to codeine in that, in oral form, it retains at least one-half of its analgesic activity. The immediate-release form is used to treat moderate to severe pain, and the controlled-release form is indicated only for chronic pain that requires continuous analgesia for an extended period.

Controlled-release tablets are not to be broken, crushed, or chewed, because this allows rapid release and absorption of a potentially lethal dose of oxycodone, particularly with the 80- and 160-mg tablets. Oxycodone is also available in combination with aspirin or acetaminophen.

Hydromorphone is a potent Schedule II opioid of the phenanthrene class used to treat moderate to severe pain. Hydromorphone has approximately five times the potency of morphine. It produces less sedation, nausea, vomiting, and constipation than its counterpart. The incidence of associated respiratory depression is marked, requiring close observation. It is recommended to use the lowest dose possible to prevent respiratory depression.

Hydromorphone is indicated for moderate to severe chronic pain in opioid-tolerant patients. The product comes in immediate-release, extended-release, parenteral, and rectal suppository formulations. Rectal suppositories are particularly useful for producing a prolonged effect. Higher-than-usual doses may be required when hydromorphone is used in patients tolerant to opioid agonists. Careful titration of hydromorphone in opioid-naïve patients is required until tolerance develops to prevent drowsiness and respiratory depression (Table 32.2).

TABLE 32.2	Benefits and Limitations of Immediate- and Controlled-Release Opioids	
Controlled-Release Opioids	**Immediate-Release Opioids**	
Benefits		
Treat chronic pain effectively	Treat acute pain effectively	
Produce more stable blood levels	Have quick onset of action	
Reduce risk for adverse effects and euphoria	Useful for dose finding at treatment	
Better patient compliance	Effective in treating breakthrough pain	
Limitations		
Less effective for treating breakthrough pain	Increased risk of side effects such as euphoria	
	Less effective in treating chronic pain due to frequent fluctuations in peak and trough levels	

Methadone

Methadone hydrochloride is a potent mu-opiate receptor agonist and opioid analgesic used primarily in the detoxification, treatment, and maintenance of persons with opiate addiction. It may be used orally to manage severe and chronic pain in patients unable to tolerate other narcotics. When it is used for persons with heroin and other opiate addiction for longer than 3 months, methadone use moves from a treatment phase to a maintenance phase. Regulations for its use for narcotic detoxification and maintenance are complicated.

Pharmacokinetics. Methadone may be administered orally, intravenously, subcutaneously, or intramuscularly. IV methadone should only be used on a temporary basis, usually for hospitalized patients who cannot take oral medications. Methadone is 85% to 90% bound to alpha-1-acid-glycoprotein and has a half-life of 2 to 3 hours. Methadone is widely distributed into tissues due to its basic and lipophilic properties, and it is secreted into breast milk. Methadone undergoes N-demethylation in the liver by CYP 450 microsomal isoenzymes, primarily by CYP 3A4 to an inactive metabolite. Fecal elimination accounts for most methadone excretion. The elimination half-life in adults varies widely, from 8 to 150 hours. With repeated dosing, methadone is retained in the liver and slowly released, extending the duration of potential toxicity. Steady-state plasma concentrations and full analgesic effects are usually not obtained until days 3 to 5 of dosing.

Indications. Methadone is indicated for the treatment of opiate agonist withdrawal during detoxification treatment, and for maintenance treatment of opiate agonist dependence.

Adverse Effects. The most significant adverse effects associated with methadone use are respiratory depression, respiratory arrest, dyspnea, and apnea. The peak respiratory depressant effects of methadone occur later and persist longer than the peak analgesic effect, making the drug particularly hazardous during the early stages of treatment. When methadone is appropriately titrated, the risk of respiratory depression is generally small as tolerance rapidly develops to this effect. Sedation is a common effect of methadone, and patients should be warned that activity requiring mental alertness can be affected. GI adverse effects are common with methadone therapy and include nausea, vomiting, and constipation. Nausea and vomiting are most commonly seen at the initiation of therapy. For constipation, a bowel regimen consisting of a stool softener and mild stimulant will be needed throughout therapy. The administration of IM or subcutaneous methadone may cause injection site reactions such as pain, erythema, or swelling. Cardiovascular effects of methadone include peripheral vasodilation resulting in severe hypotension including orthostatic hypotension and syncope, arrhythmias, bigeminal rhythms, extrasystoles, electrocardiogram (ECG) abnormalities, T-wave inversion, sinus tachycardia, sinus bradycardia, palpitations, ventricular fibrillation, ventricular tachycardia, and prolongation of the QT interval.

Contraindications. Methadone should be used cautiously in patients with cardiac arrhythmias, hypokalemia, hypomagnesemia, hypotension, hypovolemia, or orthostatic hypotension. Methadone is associated with an increased risk for QT prolongation and torsade de pointes, mostly occurring in patients receiving large doses for pain management (more than 100 mg/day). However, smaller doses of methadone for maintenance of opiate addiction have also been implicated. As with other opiate agonists, methadone is contraindicated in GI obstruction and paralytic ileus, and in patients with a risk for respiratory failure (acute asthma) in unmonitored settings. Careful monitoring is also required with concomitant use of medications that may inhibit or induce the metabolism of methadone or that increase methadone concentrations, resulting in potentially fatal respiratory depression.

Monitoring. Monitor ECGs as appropriate, especially at initiation of therapy and dose increases due to the potential for prolongation of the QT interval. Monitor for respiratory depression. Monitor patients for hypotension at the initiation of therapy and during dose titration.

False-positive urine drug screens for methadone have been reported for several drugs including diphenhydramine, doxylamine, clomipramine, chlorpromazine, thioridazine, quetiapine, and verapamil.

Phenylpiperidines

Meperidine hydrochloride and fentanyl are synthetic opiate agonists that may be used in primary care. There are other medications in this class, but they are not used for pain control in the primary care setting.

Meperidine

Meperidine is a Schedule II synthetic opioid analgesic that has less potency than morphine and is available in both oral and parenteral forms. It is used to relieve moderate to severe pain, for preoperative sedation, for postoperative analgesia, for obstetric anesthesia, and, when given intravenously, for supportive anesthesia. Due to a short duration of action and a risk of seizures associated with the metabolite normeperidine, meperidine is not recommended for the treatment of chronic pain.

Pharmacokinetics. When administered orally, meperidine undergoes extensive first-pass metabolism. It also undergoes N-demethylation to normeperidine, an active metabolite. Meperidine is less than half as effective when given orally as opposed to parenterally. However, parenteral meperidine is not recommended in the primary care setting. After oral administration, the onset of analgesia is within 15 minutes and peak effects occur in 60 to 90 minutes.

In patients with normal hepatic and renal function, meperidine half-life is 3 to 5 hours. Oral bioavailability increases to approximately 90% in patients with hepatic impairment as compared with 50% to 60% in patients with normal hepatic function. The protein binding to albumin of meperidine is 65% to 75%. Patients with a normal urine pH excrete about 30% as the active metabolite and about 5% as unchanged parent drug. Acidification of the urine greatly enhances excretion of both meperidine and normeperidine. Meperidine is distributed widely, crossing the placenta and distributing into breast milk.

Indications. Meperidine is prescribed for the treatment of severe pain requiring an opioid analgesic and for which alternative treatments are inadequate.

Adverse Effects. The most significant adverse effect associated with the use of opioid agonists such as meperidine is respiratory depression, resulting from a decreased sensitivity to carbon dioxide in the brain stem. The toxic metabolite of meperidine (normeperidine) has serotonergic properties, which correlates with an increased risk of serotonin syndrome and seizure. This correlation has led to the removal of meperidine from the World Health Organization's list of essential medicines—the list of most effective and safe medicines in the health system—in 2003. Respiratory depression is more common in older or debilitated patients, following large initial doses in non–opioid-tolerant patients, or when opioids are given with other agents that cause CNS depression.

As with other opioid agonists, tolerance to meperidine can develop, requiring increasing opioid doses to maintain pain relief. However, increasing the meperidine dosage may result in accumulation of its neurotoxic metabolite, normeperidine, which limits the usefulness of meperidine in persistent pain. There remains the potential for abuse or psychological dependence with meperidine as with other opioid agonists.

Diaphoresis, dizziness, light-headedness, drowsiness, and sedation are the most frequently observed adverse reactions noted with meperidine. The most frequently observed GI adverse reactions included constipation, nausea, and vomiting. Meperidine may cause spasm of the sphincter of Oddi. Biliary tract spasm has been reported with meperidine. Biliary effects due to opioid agonists have resulted in hyperamylasemia. Prolonged meperidine use may increase the risk of seizures from the accumulation of normeperidine.

Cardiovascular adverse effects include flushing of the face, sinus tachycardia, bradycardia, palpitations, hypotension, and syncope. Anaphylaxis and hypersensitivity reactions have been reported in patients treated with meperidine and include symptoms of pruritus, urticaria, and rash as well as histamine release leading to flushing.

Contraindications. Meperidine is contraindicated in patients with known hypersensitivity. It may be possible to use an opioid agonist from the diphenylheptane subclass (methadone) or the phenanthrene subclass (codeine, hydromorphone, or oxycodone). Due to its effects on the GI system, meperidine is contraindicated in patients with known or suspected GI obstruction or paralytic ileus. Use meperidine with caution in patients with a history of ulcerative colitis or other inflammatory bowel diseases, as they may be more sensitive to constipation caused by opioid agonists.

Caution must be employed in patients with COPD, decreased pulmonary reserve, or cardiovascular disease, and in those who are taking other CNS depressants, due to the risk for respiratory depression. Meperidine should be used with caution in patients with obesity due to the risk for obstructive sleep-apnea syndrome and/or decreased respiratory reserve. Seizure activity can be increased with the use of meperidine over time, so it is not recommended for patients with a history of seizure activity.

Monitoring. Since meperidine can cause spasm of the sphincter of Oddi, monitor patients for increased serum amylase concentrations or acute pancreatitis in those with preexisting biliary disease (Table 32.3).

Fentanyl

Fentanyl is a potent synthetic opiate agonist. It is a phenylpiperidine derivative and is structurally similar to meperidine. Fentanyl is a strong agonist at mu- and kappa-opiate receptors. The exact mechanism for how opioid agonists cause both inhibitory and stimulatory processes is not known. It is available as a transmucosal lozenge, transmucosal film, buccal tablet, sublingual tablet, nasal spray, sublingual spray, and iontophoretic transdermal system. These products are not interchangeable on a dose-per-dose basis.

Pharmacokinetics. Fentanyl is administered via transmucosal, parenteral, transdermal, and intranasal routes. The analgesic effect of fentanyl is related to the fentanyl blood concentration. Fentanyl is approximately 80% protein bound, mainly to alpha-1-acid glycoprotein. Fentanyl is

TABLE 32.3	Management of Opioid-Induced Side Effects	
Side Effect	**Treatment**
Confusion	Eliminate other nonessential medications that may have CNS effects; titrate the opioid dose downward; consider switching to another opioid.
Constipation	Increase fluid intake; increase dietary fiber; consider using a stool softener; may add an osmotic laxative or a cathartic lactulose, polyethylene glycol, or sorbitol agent.
Dizziness	Try meclizine for dizziness or vertigo.
Nausea or vomiting	Add antiemetic medication; may require switching to another opioid.
Pruritus (itching)	Use an antihistamine; consider switching to another opioid.
Respiratory depression	Gradually titrate the opioid dose downward; for patients who are minimally responsive, consider adding naloxone carefully so that withdrawal symptoms are not provoked.
Sedation	Eliminate other nonessential drugs that may be sedating or have CNS effects; lower opioid dose; consider using a mild stimulant.

CNS, Central nervous system.

metabolized in the liver and intestinal mucosa via CYP 450 3A4 to an inactive metabolite. Approximately 75% of an administered fentanyl dose is excreted in the urine as metabolites, with less than 10% as unchanged drug. Less than 10% of the administered dose is recovered in the feces as metabolites. For transdermal patches, peak fentanyl concentrations occur 24 to 72 hours after the first patch is applied.

Indications. Fentanyl is used to treat moderate to severe chronic pain in opioid-tolerant patients or breakthrough pain in opioid-tolerant cancer patients.

Adverse Effects. The most significant adverse effects associated with opioid agonist use are respiratory depression, respiratory arrest, and apnea. Fentanyl can potentially cause hypoventilation (fewer than 4% of patients using the transdermal patch) or respiratory depression (1% or fewer), apnea, or dyspnea, regardless of administration route. Fentanyl transdermal patches can cause hypoventilation 1 to 3 days after the initial application or after a dose increase. Life-threatening hypoventilation resulting in apnea or respiratory arrest may occur at any dose of available nonparenteral fentanyl products in patients not taking chronic opioids and not tolerant to opioids.

CNS depression including sedation (at least 1%), drowsiness/somnolence (at least 1%), or fatigue (at least 1%); confusion or disorientation (at least 1%); impaired cognition; asthenia (at least 1%); and dizziness (at least 1%) can occur. Pharmacologic tolerance to the analgesic and toxic effects of fentanyl varies widely among individual patients. As with other opiates, the use of fentanyl presents the potential for abuse.

GI adverse effects of nausea (up to 45%) and vomiting (up to 33%) are common. Constipation (20%) and fecal impaction (fewer than 1%) that occur are due to a decrease in GI motility. Therefore, patients require a bowel regimen consisting of a stool softener and mild stimulant throughout opioid therapy. Fentanyl can result in cardiovascular adverse effects such as orthostatic hypotension, arrhythmia exacerbation, myocardial infarction, and atrial fibrillation. As with other opiates, fentanyl can cause pruritus (at least 1%) with intranasal or transmucosal use and 3% to 10% with transdermal use. Anticholinergic effects with fentanyl include xerostomia, flushing, and blurred vision. Urinary retention has also been reported (2%).

Application site reactions and other mucosal or dermal adverse effects have been reported with fentanyl and include skin reactions such as irritation or localized erythema (14% to 60%), papules, pustules, diaphoresis, vesicular rash, and urticaria. Hematologic abnormalities such as anemia, leukopenia, neutropenia, thrombocytopenia, and pancytopenia have also occurred.

Contraindications. The fentanyl iontophoretic transdermal system (Ionsys) is contraindicated in patients with cetylpyridinium chloride hypersensitivity (e.g., Cepacol) as this is an inactive ingredient of the preparation. Fentanyl transdermal patches and the Ionsys iontophoretic transdermal system are contraindicated for use in patients with known or suspected paralytic ileus or with known or suspected GI obstruction.

Nonparenteral fentanyl products are contraindicated for use in patients with acute or severe bronchial asthma in an unmonitored setting or in the absence of resuscitative equipment. Accidental exposure to fentanyl can occur; advise patients and caregivers to wash hands after handling any fentanyl product or packaging and to seek immediate medical help if an accidental exposure occurs. The use of fentanyl in patients who have received MAOI therapy within 14 days is not recommended. Opiate agonists may be used in children with moderate to severe pain; however, all forms of fentanyl should be used cautiously in children. The age of inclusion of pediatric patients in safety and efficacy studies has varied by fentanyl product. Use fentanyl with caution in patients with adrenal insufficiency, hypothyroidism, or myxedema due to the increased risk of adverse events.

Monitoring. Monitor patients for respiratory depression, particularly during the first 24 to 72 hours after therapy initiation or a dose increase. Monitor for the presence of severe adverse events, opioid misuse, and/or abuse.

Mixed Agonist-Antagonists

The mixed agonist-antagonists produce potent analgesic effects by stimulating the kappa receptor and blocking the mu receptor. Thus, they may produce withdrawal symptoms in patients with opioid dependency but are also less likely to be abused when compared with pure opioid agonists.

Pentazocine

Pentazocine is a synthetic opiate agonist-antagonist analgesic used to treat moderate to severe pain. It is considered to be one-sixth to one-third as potent as morphine. At therapeutic doses, pentazocine has less respiratory depression than pure opiate agonists. Pentazocine is an agonist at kappa receptors but is a weak antagonist or partial agonist at mu receptors. Actions at kappa receptors are believed to produce alterations in the perception of pain and in the emotional

TABLE 32.4   Equagesic Opioid Analgesic Doses Equivalent to Morphine 10 mg IM

Medication	Oral Dose	Subcutaneous Dose
Morphine	30 mg	10 mg
MS Contin	30 mg	ND
Hydromorphone	7.5 mg	1.5 mg
Fentanyl (Duragesic patch)[a]	ND	ND
Codeine	200 mg	120 mg
Hydrocodone	30 mg	ND
Oxycodone	20–30 mg	ND
Meperidine	300 mg	75–100 mg
Methadone	20 mg	10 mg

[a]100 mcg/hr = morphine 10 mg IM q4h.
IM, Intramuscular; *ND*, not determined.

PRACTICE PEARLS

Fentanyl Transdermal System

Initial Dose Selection

- If the patient is opioid naïve, start with the lowest dose (25 mcg/hour).
- The fentanyl patch should be used only in those with chronic pain whose condition cannot be managed with short-acting narcotics.
- To convert the patient from oral opioids to the transdermal systems:
  - Calculate the previous 24-hour analgesic requirement.
  - Convert this amount to the equianalgesic oral morphine dose (Table 32.4).
  - Convert from the 24-hour morphine dose to the transdermal fentanyl dose (Janssen Pharmaceutical Company provides a dosage conversion calculator).

Application of Fentanyl Patch

- Apply to nonirritated skin on a flat surface of the upper torso.
- Clip, but do not shave, hair in the application areas.
- Clean the skin with clear water; do not use soaps, oils, lotions, alcohol, or other agents that might irritate the skin or alter its characteristics.
- Allow the skin to dry completely before applying the patch.
- Apply the patch immediately upon its removal from the sealed package. Press firmly with the palm of the hand for 10 to 20 seconds, making sure contact is complete, especially around the edges.
- Each system works continuously for 72 hours. However, occasionally patients may find that they need to replace the system every 48 hours.
- Remove the old patch and apply the new patch to a different skin site.
- Dispose of the old system carefully.
- Wash hands after applying the patch and following patch disposal.

Wearing the First System

- Peak serum levels are not reached for 24 hours; thus, the patient may need short-acting analgesics.
- After 24 hours, assess the efficacy of the system by counting the number of times the patient needs a rescue dose of short-acting analgesic.

Titrating Fentanyl Dosage

- Titrate the dose upward, if necessary, after the use of the initial 3-day system.
- Because the conversion system from morphine to fentanyl is conservative, about half of patients will need upward titration.
- If the patient uses rescue doses of analgesic equivalent to 90 mg/24 hours of morphine, increase the fentanyl system dose by 25 mcg/hour.
- After the first titration, titrate upward every 6 days.
- For delivery rates in excess of 100 mcg/hour, multiple systems may be used.

To Discontinue Fentanyl Patches

- If the patient requires more than 300 mcg/hour, change the patient to another method of opioid administration.
- It takes about 18 hours for the fentanyl concentration to decrease by 50% after the system has been removed.
- A fentanyl patch can be used to discontinue opioids by wearing the patch, then simply removing it, and allowing the concentration to gradually decrease over time.

response to pain. Pentazocine is given parenterally via IV, IM, or subcutaneous injection. In the primary care setting, the subcutaneous or IM route may be used. The subcutaneous route should be used only when necessary, because of the possibility of severe tissue damage at injection sites.

Pharmacokinetics. Following subcutaneous or IM injection of pentazocine, the onset of analgesia occurs in approximately 15 to 20 minutes, with an analgesia duration of 2 to 3 hours.

Indications. Pentazocine is indicated for the treatment of moderate to severe pain.

Adverse Effects. Acute CNS adverse reactions with pentazocine limit its clinical utility. Patients receiving therapeutic doses of pentazocine have experienced confusion, disorientation, and visual hallucinations lasting several hours. The exact mechanism responsible is unknown but may be associated with activity at the sigma-opiate receptor.

GI effects include nausea or vomiting, anorexia, constipation, abdominal pain or cramps, diarrhea, xerostomia, altered taste, and biliary tract spasm. Cardiovascular adverse effects such as hypotension, hypertension, sinus tachycardia, circulatory depression, and syncope have occurred. Dermatologic reactions include flushing, plethora, pruritus, urticaria, angioedema, and anaphylactic shock. Injection site reactions such as skin ulcers and scleral induration involving subcutaneous tissues and underlying muscle have occurred in patients receiving multiple IM injections of pentazocine. It is important to rotate injection sites and avoid subcutaneous injections.

Leukopenia, especially neutropenia, and transient eosinophilia have been reported with pentazocine. Ocular effects associated with pentazocine include blurred vision or difficulty focusing, diplopia, nystagmus, and miosis. As noted with opiates, pharmacologic tolerance to the analgesic effects of pentazocine may occur with extended use.

Contraindications. Alcohol consumption is contraindicated with pentazocine and will result in additive CNS depressant effects. Pentazocine is contraindicated for use in patients with significant respiratory depression and in those with acute or severe asthma in care settings or in the absence of resuscitative equipment. Pentazocine is contraindicated in patients with known or suspected GI obstruction, including paralytic ileus. Due to the effects of opiate agonists on the GI tract, pentazocine should be used cautiously in patients with diseases such as ulcerative colitis.

Monitoring. No laboratory monitoring is needed. Monitor for adverse dermatologic and hematologic effects. Monitor for respiratory depression.

Buprenorphine

Buprenorphine is a semisynthetic mixed opiate agonist-antagonist. A partial mu receptor agonist, buprenorphine exhibits a ceiling to its pharmacologic effects, so the danger of overdose, abuse lability, and toxicity from buprenorphine may be less than with full opioid agonists. Buprenorphine is available in an immediate-release parenteral formulation for moderate to severe pain, and in transdermal and buccal formulations for the management of chronic, severe pain in patients who require daily, around-the-clock, long-term opioid treatment. A sublingual formulation (Subutex), a 6-month subdermal implant (Probuphine), and an extended-release monthly subcutaneous injection (Sublocade) are used for the treatment of opioid dependence. Buprenorphine was the first medication approved for in-office treatment of opioid dependence under the federal Drug Addiction Treatment Act.

Pharmacokinetics. Within the systemic circulation, buprenorphine is approximately 96% protein bound, primarily to alpha and beta globulin. The drug undergoes N-dealkylation metabolism by CYP 3A4 isozymes to an active metabolite, norbuprenorphine. Buprenorphine is primarily eliminated in the feces (69%), with 31% eliminated in the urine. There are specific pharmacokinetics that vary by the route used.

Indications. Buprenorphine is indicated for the treatment of moderate or severe pain, or for the treatment of chronic, severe pain in patients who require daily, around-the-clock, long-term opioid treatment. It is also indicated for the treatment of opiate agonist dependence, including opiate agonist withdrawal symptoms, and the prevention of undue symptoms of opiate agonist withdrawal during induction of opiate agonist dependence treatment.

Adverse Effects. Clinically significant respiratory depression may occur following administration of therapeutic doses of buprenorphine in about 1% of patients. Buprenorphine-induced respiratory depression may not be fully reversed by the administration of naloxone in the event of an overdose, and supportive measures may be needed to maintain adequate ventilation.

The use of buprenorphine is associated with various neurologic and psychiatric effects including agitation, anxiety, weakness, confusion, dizziness, drowsiness, somnolence, emotional lability, and hallucinations. The use of buprenorphine in any dosage form may lower the seizure threshold and induce seizures. Buprenorphine is associated with cardiovascular effects, with parenteral or transdermal formulations inducing more cardiovascular adverse events than sublingual buprenorphine. Hypertension or hypotension (1% to 5%), angina pectoris, atrial fibrillation (no more than 0.2%), second-degree AV block (fewer than 1%), bradycardia (fewer than 1%), and unspecified chest pain (no more than 0.2%) have also been reported. Buprenorphine use has been associated with QT prolongation (fewer than 1%).

GI adverse effects include abdominal pain (11.7%), anorexia (1% to 5%), constipation (4% to 11%), diarrhea (1% to 5%), nausea (6% to 23%), and vomiting (5.5% to 9.4%). Cases of elevated hepatic enzymes (no more than 5%), hepatitis, and jaundice have been reported.

Although uncommon, cases of anaphylactic shock, bronchospasm, and anaphylactoid reactions such as angioedema (fewer than 1%) have been reported. Pruritus, urticaria, or rash (fewer than 5%) were observed in patients who received parenteral or transdermal buprenorphine.

Contraindications. Buprenorphine use is contraindicated in patients with buprenorphine hypersensitivity. Buprenorphine subdermal implant is also contraindicated in patients with a history of hypersensitivity to ethylene vinyl acetate. When buprenorphine is used in the treatment of opioid dependence, it is not appropriate as an analgesic for pain management. These products are not appropriate for use in patients who are opiate naïve. Buprenorphine subdermal implants should be initiated only in patients who have achieved clinical stability on low to moderate doses of a transmucosal buprenorphine-containing product; they should be used with caution in patients with compromised respiratory function (COPD, cor pulmonale, decreased respiratory reserve, or preexisting respiratory depression). Keep buprenorphine products out of the reach of pediatric patients and pets, as accidental exposure can cause serious injury or death. Avoid abrupt discontinuation of buprenorphine as serious withdrawal symptoms, uncontrolled pain, suicide, and drug-seeking behaviors can occur. Buprenorphine should not be used in patients with GI obstruction or paralytic ileus.

Monitoring. Baseline and periodic liver function tests (LFTs) are recommended in patients receiving sublingual buprenorphine or buprenorphine subdermal implants and in patients receiving transdermal or buccal buprenorphine who are at increased risk of hepatotoxicity. Monitor for signs of respiratory depression, cardiac effects, or abuse or misuse (Table 32.5).

Norepinephrine Reuptake Inhibitor

Tapentadol

Tapentadol is a new, synthetically derived, centrally acting oral analgesic. It is available in both immediate- and extended-release formulations. In addition to central opiate receptor agonist activity, it activates the mu-opioid receptor and inhibits norepinephrine synaptic reuptake. Norepinephrine reuptake inhibition appears to have an additive analgesic effect to that of the drug's opioid activity.

Pharmacokinetics. Tapentadol is administered orally and is widely distributed throughout the body. It is extensively metabolized to inactive compounds, with only 3% excreted as unchanged drug after oral administration. Metabolism occurs by methylation through CYP 2C9 and CYP 2C19 (approximately 13%), and by hydroxylation via CYP 2D6. Approximately 99% of tapentadol and metabolites are eliminated in the urine, with 1% in the feces. The half-life of tapentadol is approximately 4 hours with immediate-release tablets and approximately 5 hours with extended-release tablets.

Indications. Tapentadol is indicated for the management of chronic, severe pain, including severe neuropathic pain associated with diabetic peripheral neuropathy, in patients who require daily, around-the-clock, long-term opioid treatment.

TABLE 32.5 Adverse Effects of Opioid Analgesics

Body System	Adverse Effects
Body, general	Interference with thermal regulation, paresthesia, pain at injection site, local tissue irritation and induration after injection, facial flushing, chills, faintness, and pruritus
Hypersensitivity	Pruritus, urticaria, rash, diaphoresis, laryngospasm, edema, hemorrhagic urticaria, and anaphylactoid reactions after intravenous administration
Respiratory	Bronchospasm, depression of cough reflex, laryngospasm, respiratory depression, and respiratory arrest
Cardiovascular	Peripheral circulatory collapse, tachycardia, bradycardia, arrhythmia, palpitations, hypertension, hypotension, orthostatic hypotension,[a] syncope, asystole, shock, and coma
Gastrointestinal	Nausea,[a] vomiting, diarrhea, cramps, abdominal pain, taste alterations, dry mouth, anorexia, constipation,[a] biliary tract spasm, and exacerbation of ulcerative colitis
Musculoskeletal	Muscular rigidity and weakness
Central nervous system	Euphoria, dysphoria, delirium, insomnia, agitation, anxiety, fear, hallucination, disorientation, drowsiness,[a] sedation,[a] lethargy, impairment of mental and physical performance, skeletal or uncoordinated movement, mood changes, weakness, headache, mental cloudiness, tremor, convulsions, dependence, toxic psychoses, depression, increased intracranial pressure, miosis, sweating headache, dizziness, light-headedness, and coma
Vision	Blurred vision, visual disturbances, diplopia, miosis, and hydromorphone nystagmus
Hepatic	Jaundice and elevated liver enzymes
Genitourinary	Ureteral and spasm of vesical sphincters, urinary retention or hesitancy, oliguria, antidiuretic effect, and reduced libido or potency

[a]Very common.

Adverse Effects. Pharmacologic tolerance to the analgesic effects of opioid agonists including tapentadol has been reported in some patients. Tapentadol presents the potential for abuse or psychological dependence. Accidental and nonaccidental overdose of this medication may occur. Patients taking immediate-release or extended-release preparations experienced nausea (21% to 30%), vomiting (8% to 18%), xerostomia (4% to 7%), anorexia (2% to 6%), impaired gastric emptying (fewer than 1%), dyspepsia (1% to 3%), and diarrhea (7%, extended release). Constipation has been reported in 8% to 17% of study patients who received the immediate-release and extended-release tablets. CNS effects of sedation, drowsiness, or somnolence (15%) have been reported for both immediate-release and extended-release tablets. Patients should be warned that activity requiring mental alertness can be affected due to opioid-induced CNS depression. As with other opioid agonists, the most significant adverse effect associated with tapentadol is respiratory depression, reported in fewer than 1% of patients. Older adults and debilitated patients and those who are opioid naïve are most at risk. Tapentadol can cause cardiovascular adverse reactions, specifically tachycardia and labile blood pressure. Tapentadol and other opioid agonists are known to cause adverse dermatologic effects; generalized pruritus was reported in 3% of patients with immediate-release tablets and 1% of patients with extended-release tablets. Serotonin syndrome has been reported in patients taking opioids at recommended doses. Patients taking opioids concomitantly with a serotonergic medication should seek immediate medical attention if they develop symptoms such as agitation, hallucinations, tachycardia, fever, excessive sweating, shivering or shaking, muscle twitching or stiffness, trouble with coordination, nausea, vomiting, or diarrhea.

Contraindications. Tapentadol is contraindicated for use in patients with a known hypersensitivity to the drug or any of its ingredients. Tapentadol use is associated with a significant potential for overdose, so careful patient selection and counseling are recommended. The extended-release formulation is not intended for use in the management of acute pain or on an as-needed basis, but only for patients requiring continuous, around-the-clock opioid analgesia for an extended period of time. Drinking alcohol while taking tapentadol will result in additive CNS depressant effects, and use with extended-release tablets will result in increased drug exposure that may cause a fatal overdose. Tapentadol is contraindicated in patients with significant respiratory depression and in those with acute or severe asthma or COPD. Tapentadol use is also contraindicated in patients who are receiving or have received MAOI therapy within the past 14 days due to the risk for additive CNS depression, drowsiness, dizziness, or hypotension. Abrupt discontinuation of prolonged tapentadol can result in withdrawal symptoms; gradually taper patients off prolonged tapentadol to avoid a withdrawal reaction. Tapentadol should not be used in patients with preexisting severe renal impairment or renal failure due to accumulation of glucuronidation, a metabolite formed during tapentadol use.

Monitoring. Monitor respiratory function, especially at higher dosages, and cardiovascular and neurologic function. Monitor for signs of tolerance, misuse, or abuse (Table 32.6).

PRACTICE PEARLS

Considerations in Pain Management

- The primary care provider must follow federal and state regulations and commonly accepted guidelines when prescribing opioids.
- Chronic pain requires routine administration of pain medication. Long-acting preparations should be considered for patients with chronic pain.
- Complex pain syndromes may be relieved by combining pain management medications and therapies.
- Patients with chronic pain may have multiple problems, including psychological responses to chronic pain and other comorbid conditions, that may require a comprehensive pain management program.
- Primary care providers may have to refer patients to pain management clinics for evaluation and specialized treatment, such as nerve block. Hospice referral must be considered for terminal conditions.

PRACTICE PEARLS

Methadone Treatment

- For the treatment of narcotic addiction in detoxification programs, methadone may be dispensed only by pharmacies and clinics approved by the FDA and state authorities according to treatment requirements stipulated in the Federal Methadone Regulations.
- Patients need to show withdrawal symptoms but no signs of sedation or intoxication.
- Detoxification shall not exceed 21 days or be repeated earlier than 4 weeks after completion of a preceding course.
- Loss of opioid tolerance should be considered for a patient who has not taken opioids for more than 5 days.
- An ECG should be performed 2 to 4 weeks after methadone initiation and after any significant dose increase.
- Clinical practice guidelines for methadone safety recommend that an ECG also be obtained when the methadone dose reaches an adult equivalent of 30 to 40 mg/day in patients started at lower doses and again at 100 mg/day.
- In utero methadone exposure can result in the risk for low birth weight in the neonate.

TABLE 32.6 **Selected Opioid Medications**

Drug Category/ Medication	Indication	Dosage	Considerations and Monitoring
Phenanthrenes			
Morphine	Relief of acute and chronic moderate or severe pain	**Immediate release:** *Adults (regular release):* 15–30 mg orally every 4 hr as needed in opioid-naïve patients. *Children and adolescents ≥50 kg:* 15 mg orally every 4 hr as needed. Maximum initial dose: 30 mg. *Children and adolescents <50 kg:* 0.15–0.3 mg/kg/dose orally every 3–6 hr as needed. Maximum initial dose: 5 mg. General weight-based dosing for pediatric patients is 0.15–0.3 mg/kg/dose orally. Morphine is also available in oral solution, Dose varies by age and opioid tolerance. **Extended release:** *Adults:* 15 mg orally every 8 or 12 hr (Arymo ER, Morphabond, or MS Contin) or 30 mg orally every 24 hr. *Children and adolescents:* Limit pediatric use to opioid-tolerant patients. Limited data are available. Doses of 0.2–2.3 mg/kg/dose orally every 12 hr have been used in patients with cancer and sickle cell disease.	Monitor respirations, and blood pressure. Monitor for opioid abuse and dependence.

TABLE 32.6   Selected Opioid Medications—cont'd

Drug Category/ Medication	Indication	Dosage	Considerations and Monitoring
Hydrocodone	Treatment of chronic, severe pain in patients requiring daily, around-the-clock, long-term opioid treatment	*Adults (non–opioid tolerant):* • Zohydro ER[a] 10 mg orally every 12 hr. • Hysingla ER[a] 20 mg orally every 24 hr. • Vantrela ER[a] 15 mg orally every 12 hr.	Monitor for respiratory depression or sedation. Assess patients for risks of addiction, abuse, or misuse before drug initiation, and monitor for these behaviors throughout treatment. When discontinuing hydrocodone therapy in opioid-dependent patients, taper gradually by 10–25% every 2–4 weeks.
Tramadol	Treatment of severe pain	*Adults:* 25 mg orally once daily. Can titrate to 50–100 mg every 4–6 hr as needed. Maximum dosage: 400 mg. *Extended release:* 100 mg orally once daily.	Monitor for respiratory depression, especially within the first 24–72 hr after initiation and dose escalation. When discontinuing tramadol therapy in opioid-dependent patients, taper the dose gradually by 10–25% every 2–4 weeks.
Codeine	Treatment of mild to moderate pain	*Adults:* 15–60 mg orally every 4 hr as needed. Do not exceed 360 mg/24 hr. Maximum dosage: 60 mg/dose. *Children and adolescents 12–17 yr:* 0.5 to 1 mg/kg/dose orally every 4 hr as needed. Maximum dosage: 60 mg/dose.	Monitor for respiratory depression, especially within the first 24–72 hr after initiation and dose escalation. When discontinuing codeine therapy in opioid-dependent patients, taper the dose gradually by 10–25% every 2–4 weeks.
Oxycodone	Treatment of severe pain, or for management of chronic, severe pain in patients who require daily, around-the-clock, long-term opioid treatment	*Adults (immediate-release tablets, oral solution):* 5–15 mg orally every 4–6 hr as needed for pain for opioid-naïve patients. *Children and adolescents 12–17 yr:* 0.2 mg/kg orally given 30 minutes before procedure to reduce pain associated with wound care in children 5–14 yr.	Monitor for respiratory depression and blood pressure. Monitor for opioid abuse and dependence.
Hydromorphone	Relief of acute and chronic moderate pain or severe pain	*Adults:* 2.5–10 mg orally every 3–6 hr (oral solution) or 2–4 mg orally every 46 hr (tablets). *Children adolescents ≥50 kg:* 2–4 mg orally every 3–4 hr in opioid-naïve patients. *Infants ≥6 months and children and adolescents <50 kg:* 0.04–0.08 mg/kg orally every 3–4 hr in opioid-naïve patients.	Assess patients for risks of addiction, abuse, or misuse before drug initiation, and monitor for these behaviors throughout treatment.
Methadone	Treatment of chronic, severe pain in patients who require daily, around-the-clock, long-term opioid treatment	*Adults[a]:* Initially, 2.5 mg orally every 8–12 hr in the opioid-naive patient. In opioid-tolerant patients, convert the total daily dose of all opioids to an oral morphine equivalent dose, then multiply the morphine equivalent dose by the corresponding percentage in the dose conversion table provided in the FDA-approved labeling.	Monitor ECG, especially at initiation of therapy. Monitor for respiratory depression. Monitor patients for hypotension at the initiation of therapy and during dose titration.
Phenylpiperidines			
Meperidine	Treatment of severe pain requiring an opioid analgesic and for which alternative treatments are inadequate	*Adults:* 50–150 mg orally every 3–4 hr as needed. *Adolescents and children:* 1.1–1.8 mg/kg orally every 3–4 hr as needed. Maximum dosage: 150 mg/dose.	Monitor patients frequently for respiratory depression, particularly during the first 24–72 hr after initiation or dose escalation. When discontinuing meperidine therapy, reduce by 25–50% every 2–4 days.

Continued

TABLE 32.6   Selected Opioid Medications—cont'd

Drug Category/ Medication	Indication	Dosage	Considerations and Monitoring
Fentanyl	Control of moderate pain or severe pain or management of chronic, severe pain in opioid-tolerant patients who require daily, around-the-clock, long-term opioid treatment	*Adults (transdermal dosage, Ionsys iontophoretic transdermal system):* 1 dose activation delivers 40 mcg transdermally over 10 minutes up to 24 hr or 80 doses. Maximum total duration of treatment should not exceed 3 days (72 hr). *Transdermal (Duragesic)*[a]*:* Apply at minimum a 25-mcg/hr transdermal patch for patients receiving at least 60 mg/day oral morphine equivalents. *Children ≥2 yr:* apply at minimum a 25-mcg/hr transdermal patch for patients receiving at least 60 mg/day oral morphine equivalents.	Monitor patients frequently for respiratory depression, particularly during the first 24–72 hr after initiation or dose escalation. Change patch every 72 hr. Each subsequent system is applied to a different skin site. Follow the FDA-approved conversion chart in the product label to convert 24-hr oral morphine equivalents dose to the corresponding transdermal fentanyl system dose. Discontinue all other around-the-clock opioid drugs upon transdermal fentanyl initiation. When discontinuing fentanyl therapy, slow withdrawal is recommended, especially in patients receiving higher doses or long-term therapy.
Mixed Agonist/Antagonist			
Pentazocine	Treatment of moderate to severe pain	*Adults:* 30 mg IM or subcutaneously every 3–4 hr as needed.	Monitor for adverse effects such as dermatologic and hematologic effects. Monitor for respiratory depression.
Buprenorphine	Treatment of moderate or severe pain, or treatment of chronic, severe pain in patients who require daily, around-the-clock, long-term opioid treatment	*Adults:* 0.3 mg IM. May be repeated once if needed 30–60 minutes after the initial dose and then every 6–8 hr as needed. *Children ≥2 yr:* 2–6 mcg/kg/dose IM every 4–8 hr as needed. *Adults: Transdermal dosage for use as the first opioid analgesic (Butrans):* 5 mcg/hr applied topically to intact skin, every 7 days. *Adults: Transmucosal dosage for use as the first opioid analgesic (Belbuca):* 75 mcg transmucosally once daily, or every 12 hr, placed against the inside of the cheek. After 4 days, increase dosage to 150 mcg every 12 hr.	Monitor patients frequently for respiratory depression, particularly during the first 24–72 hr after initiation and dose escalation. When discontinuing buprenorphine therapy, slow withdrawal is recommended, especially in patients receiving higher doses or long-term therapy. For the transdermal buprenorphine patch, gradually decrease the dose every 7 days.
	Treatment of opiate agonist dependence, including opiate agonist withdrawal symptoms, and for maintenance treatment of opiate agonist dependence	*Adults: Sublingual:* Target dose of 16 mg sublingually once daily is suggested; however, doses may range from 4–24 mg/day. Initiate treatment with supervised administration.	

TABLE 32.6	Selected Opioid Medications—cont'd			
Drug Category/ Medication	**Indication**	**Dosage**		**Considerations and Monitoring**
Norepinephrine Reuptake Inhibitor				
Tapentadol	Treatment of pain severe enough to require an opioid analgesic and for which alternative treatments are inadequate	*Adults (regular release):* 50–100 mg orally every 4–6 hr as needed; a second dose may be administered as soon as 1 hr after the first dose. *Oral dosage (extended-release tablet):* For use as the first opioid analgesic or in patients who are not opioid tolerant: initially, 50 mg orally twice daily every 12 hr.		Monitor patients frequently for respiratory depression, particularly during the first 24–72 hr after initiation or dose escalation. When discontinuing tapentadol therapy, slow withdrawal is recommended, especially in patients receiving higher doses or long-term therapy. Tapentadol therapy can be decreased by 25%–50% every 2–4 days with careful monitoring.

ªSee manufacturer's instructions for titration and conversion information. *ECG,* Electrocardiogram; *FDA,* U.S. Food and Drug Administration; *IM,* intramuscular.

Prescriber Considerations for Pain Management Therapy

When considering possible pain management strategies, first review the most up-to-date guidelines available from sources such as the American Pain Society or other professional, peer-reviewed resources. Limited evidence suggests that there is very little difference between hydromorphone

PRACTICE PEARLS

Pain Management

- For mild to moderate pain, begin pharmacologic pain management with acetaminophen on an around-the-clock schedule, taking care to determine the maximum daily dose for the specific patient's pain and hepatic function.
- If acetaminophen around the clock is not effective, a nonsteroidal antiinflammatory drug (NSAID) can be used. The combined use of NSAIDs and acetaminophen is unlikely to improve pain relief.
- NSAIDs can cause GI bleeding and may elevate blood pressure, cause fluid retention, or provoke renal failure, particularly in older adults.
- Adjuvant medications are particularly useful for neuropathic pain when given alone or in combination with NSAIDs or opioids. Gabapentin and other, newer anticonvulsants are good first-line choices and have fewer side effects than the older tricyclic antidepressants. Serotonin-norepinephrine reuptake inhibitors (SNRIs) such as duloxetine (Cymbalta) may also be effective.
- If nonopioid medications are not effective or are not tolerated, opiates can be given alone or with acetaminophen for nonmalignant and malignant pain.
- When prescribing opioids, prophylactically treat constipation.

BOOKMARK THIS!

Clinical Practice Guidelines for Acute Musculoskeletal Injury

- Clinical Practice Guidelines for Pain Management in Acute Musculoskeletal Injury: https://journals.lww.com/jorthotrauma/fulltext/2019/05000/clinical_practice_guidelines_for_pain_management.11.aspx
- Pain Management Best Practices Inter-Agency Task Force Report: https://www.hhs.gov/sites/default/files/pain-mgmt-best-practices-draft-final-report-05062019.pdf

and other opioids in terms of analgesic efficacy, adverse effects, and patient preference.

Clinical Practice Guidelines

The Pain Management Best Practices Inter-Agency Task Force was convened by the U.S. Department of Health and Human Services (HHS), the Department of Defense (DOD), the Veterans Administration (VA), and the Office of National Drug Control Policy (ONDCP) to address the treatment of acute and chronic pain in the ongoing opioid crisis. The Task Force emphasizes the importance of individualized, patient-centered care in the diagnosis and treatment of acute and chronic pain. An effective pain treatment plan should be established after a thorough evaluation to determine a diagnosis, with a focus on improvements in quality of life, physical improved functioning, and the ability to engage in activities of daily living.

The Agency for Health Care Policy and Research (AHCPR) clinical practice guidelines include the following classic principles of pain assessment (A-A-B-C-D-E-E):

- Ask about pain at every office visit or phone call.
- Assess pain systematically using the same pain intensity scale for pain measurement.
- Believe the patient and family regarding their reports of pain and what relieves it.
- Choose pain control options that are appropriate for the patient, family, and setting.
- Delivery of pharmacologic or nonpharmacologic interventions should be made in a timely, logical, and coordinated fashion.
- Empower patients and their families.
- Enable them to control their course to the greatest extent possible.

Clinical Reasoning for Pain Management Therapy

Consider the individual patient's health problem requiring pain management. The first step is to determine the type and etiology of the patient's pain to form an appropriate pain treatment plan. Consideration must also be given to the patient's past medical and surgical history, experience with pain medications, history of substance misuse and abuse, and comorbid conditions.

A thorough pain assessment should include a detailed history and physical examination, functional and psychosocial evaluation, and diagnostic evaluation as indicated. Associated acute pain findings can include facial grimacing, tachycardia, hypertension, pallor, diaphoresis, mydriasis, and nausea. Chronic pain may be accompanied by fatigue, depression, sleep disturbance, decreased appetite, increased irritability, and decreased libido.

Because pain is a subjective experience, the assessment must include patient self-report, which includes a description of pain and its onset, duration, and diurnal variation, as well as information on the location and radiation of pain, its intensity or severity, aggravating and relieving factors, and the patient's goal for pain control. A variety of common pain assessment tools can be used to help grade pain severity in children and adults.

Determine the desired therapeutic outcome based on the degree of pain management needed for the patient's health problem. The therapeutic outcome depends upon the type of pain (acute or chronic) and the etiology of the pain as to whether the pain can be completely relieved or greatly reduced to allow the patient to have an improved quality of life and the ability to perform activities of daily living. In addition to pharmacologic management, consider referring the patient to appropriate specialists and members of the interdisciplinary team, such as orthopedists, neurosurgeons, pain management specialists, physical and occupational therapists, or hospice staff, for further evaluation and additional interventions. Provide the patient with education regarding the nature of pain and assessment tools. Encourage the patient to keep a pain diary and to use a daily pain rating scale. To reduce anxiety, allow the patient to have some control over the situation and to make decisions when possible.

Assess the pain management therapy selected for its appropriateness for an individual patient by considering the medication's side effects and the patient's age, race/ethnicity, comorbidities, and genetic factors. Discuss goals, expectations, potential risks, and alternative therapies. The goal of therapy must be clearly stated and that to be completely pain free may not be an attainable goal. For patients coping with chronic pain, the comorbid condition of depression can accompany chronic pain syndromes, so assessment of depression using a valid scale such as the Beck Depression Inventory or the Patient Health Questionnaire 9 (PHQ9) is recommended. If the patient is depressed, appropriate measures such as counseling referral and antidepressants should be initiated. Assess hepatic and hematopoietic function prior to prescribing opioids for pain, especially in the older patient. Assess females of childbearing age for potential pregnancy to prevent adverse effects of opioids on the fetus. If longer-term NSAIDs are prescribed, renal functioning should be monitored. Patients should also be assessed for a history of substance abuse as opioids can be highly addictive. Patients with a substance abuse history require careful monitoring; tools such as the Addiction Behavior Checklist can be used to determine risk.

The pain management therapy selected is highly dependent on the etiology of pain. Opioids are reserved for more severe pain, while NSAIDs are appropriate for inflammatory pain. Adjunctive pain medications such as tricyclic antidepressants, muscle relaxants, anticonvulsants, and selective serotonin reuptake inhibitors (SSRIs) are also helpful for control of chronic pain.

Perform a medication reconciliation before prescribing any Schedule II pain medications for drug interactions and consideration of expected side effects such as constipation. A thorough medical history should be obtained to prevent respiratory and cardiovascular adverse events. Lastly, pain therapy should include nonpharmacologic approaches in addition to medication. Nonpharmacologic approaches can include physiotherapy, cognitive behavioral training, music therapy, progressive relaxation, and massage, among others.

Initiate the treatment plan with the selected medication by first providing adequate patient education to ensure the patient's understanding and promote full participation in pain management. Effective pain management requires the level of pain to be measured and described. Teach patients about the type of pain they are experiencing, such as acute or chronic, musculoskeletal, neuropathic, etc. Provide patients and family members with a pain assessment tool appropriate to their age and level of understanding that can be completed daily along with a pain diary so that trends in pain, pain triggers, and management strategies can be evaluated. Provide time for both instruction and questions in the teaching session. Assist the patient in identifying the expected side effects and potential adverse effects of the pain therapy selected, with instructions to address the issues, including when to notify the primary care provider. Patient and family education should also address opioid use and misuse issues and address any concerns regarding addiction.

Ensure complete patient and family understanding about the medication prescribed for pain management using a variety of education strategies. When the source of pain (acute or chronic) has been identified, provide teaching about the condition using pictorials for better understanding. Ensure that the patient and family clearly understand the instructions for taking the prescribed pain medication, as well as how to use breakthrough pain treatments, as appropriate, by providing written and verbal instructions with feedback from the patient. Demonstrate the use of the pain assessment tool and diary. Provide a printed list of circumstances for which the primary care provider should be notified.

Conduct follow-up and monitoring of patient responses to pain management to determine the effectiveness of the pain management therapy, manage side effects, and prevent adverse events. A follow-up assessment of the outcome of pain management is required to assess the effectiveness of the intervention. Changes in pain pattern or new pain development should trigger reassessment, diagnostic evaluation, and modification of the treatment plan. Documentation of the patient's adherence to the prescribed plan with regard to dosing and duration of prescriptions is essential for all pain management. The primary care provider should assess physical and emotional functioning, ability to engage in daily activities, and level of pain relief at each encounter. Frequent follow-up is needed to assess patient outcomes and side effects, provide reassurance, and reestablish goals. Concurrent problems such as depression, anxiety, and insomnia augment the perception of pain in many patients and will need to be addressed.

The patient for whom opioids are prescribed should be prescribed a bowel regimen and should be seen at least weekly until pain is controlled. Side effects of opioids should be assessed and monitored. Monitor for nausea, especially when the patient is starting to take opioids. Monitor for behaviors that may indicate misuse or abuse, such as unsanctioned dose escalations, losing prescriptions, and resisting change to a medication regimen.

Teaching Points for Pain Management

Health Promotion Strategies

Whether the need for pain management is short term (acute pain) or long term (chronic pain), patients can potentially decrease their need for the medication and increase functioning through adjunctive therapies. The following strategies and practices should be presented to patients to help them become full partners in their health care:

- Treatment of pain should be multidimensional and not solely focused on pain medication alone.
- Try mild exercises, stretching, walking, yoga, or tai chi.
- Start any increase in activity slowly, and be prepared that it may take several weeks to reach a level that is comfortable.
- Use stress-relieving strategies such as meditation and progressive muscle relaxation.

PRACTICE PEARLS

Life Span Considerations With Opioids

Geriatric Patients

- Older patients are more susceptible to the CNS and GI effects of opioids.
- Prescribe a prophylactic bowel regimen whenever opioids are prescribed.
- Prescribe the lowest effective dose of opioids.
- In older patients, avoid propoxyphene, tramadol, and methadone when possible.

Pediatric Patients

- Children may experience greater difficulty communicating pain sensations. A pain scale that uses smiling or frowning faces may facilitate the assessment of pain.
- For prescribing opioids in pediatric patients, use morphine, codeine, or meperidine. Do not use oxycodone, propoxyphene, methadone, or pentazocine. The safety of hydromorphone in children has not been established.

Pregnancy and Lactation

- The use of codeine in the first trimester has been associated with the development of congenital defects.
- When morphine is administered just prior to delivery, the neonate may exhibit respiratory depression due to a more immature blood–brain barrier.
- Opioids cross the placental barrier and are excreted in breast milk.

- Guided imagery, breathing techniques, and relaxation techniques are often very effective, particularly when feeling anxious.
- Consider acupuncture to help with pain relief, or physical therapy to increase function.
- Apply heat/cold to a painful area for 20 to 30 minutes several times daily.
- Consider applying topical agents such as capsaicin three to four times daily to reduce pain. Topical 5% lidocaine or diclofenac patches may also help.
- Stay well hydrated throughout treatment to prevent constipation.

Patient Education for Medication Safety

- Take the prescribed pain medications *exactly* as prescribed.
- Take a stool softener/laxative daily to prevent constipation from opioids.
- Keep a pain dairy that includes a pain scale (level of pain) and when the medication was last taken to prevent overdose.
- Do not add other pain-relieving or sedating medications without informing your primary care provider.
- Inform your health care provider of all prescribed, over-the-counter (OTC), and herbal medications that you are taking.

- Do not drink alcoholic beverages while taking pain medications.
- Report to your primary care provider any new or troublesome symptoms that occur after beginning your pain medication treatment.
- The common side effects that you may experience include constipation, drowsiness, dizziness, nausea, sweating, and flushing.
- After you have taken your pain medication, avoid operating heavy machinery, driving, or performing tasks that require alertness.
- Rise slowly from a lying or sitting position to minimize feelings of light-headedness.
- During initial doses, lie down for short periods to avoid developing nausea.
- Family members should alert the primary care provider of the following symptoms: shallow, slow respirations; shortness of breath; pupil constriction; deep sleep; vomiting; abdominal pain; chest pain; palpitations; or skin rash.
- Keep your medication out of the reach of children and all others for whom it is not prescribed.
- Dispose at your pharmacy all extra prescription medication when they are no longer needed. Do not save opioids for another pain-related illness.
- Do not share your medication with any other person.
- Used fentanyl patches still may contain enough fentanyl to cause a fatal overdose in a child, adult, or pet. Proper disposal of the used patch out of the reach of children or pets is essential.
- Wash your hands after handling fentanyl patches.

Application Questions for Discussion

1. As a health care provider, what patient factors should be considered before prescribing an opioid?
2. What should be included in the education plan for a patient and/or caregiver who has been prescribed opioids for chronic pain?
3. What role would comorbid conditions play in the treatment response to opioids?

Selected Bibliography

Boté, S. H. (2019). U.S. opioid epidemic: Impact on public health and review of prescription drug monitoring programs (PDMPs). *Online Journal of Public Health Informatics, 11*(2), e18. https://doi.org/10.5210/ojphi.v11i2.10113.

Dowell, D., Haegerich, T. M., & Chou, R. (2016). CDC guideline for prescribing opioids for chronic pain–United States, 2016. *Morbidity and Mortality Weekly Report Recommendations and Reports, 65* (No. RR-1), 1–49. https://www.cdc.gov/mmwr/volumes/65/rr/rr6501e1.htm?CDC_AA_refVal=https%3A%2F%2Fwww.cdc.gov%2Fmmwr%2Fvolumes%2F65%2Frr%2Frr6501e1er.htm.

Dahlhamer J., Lucas J., Zelaya C., Nahin R., Mackey S., DeBar L., Kerns R., Von Korff M., Porter L., Helmick C. (2018). Prevalence of chronic pain and high-impact chronic pain among adults: United States, 2016. *MMWR Morbity and Mortality Weekly Report* Sep 14;67(36):1001-1006. doi: 10.15585/mmwr.mm6736a2. PMID: 30212442; PMCID: PMC6146950.

Ehrlich, A. T., & Darcq, E. (2019). Recommending buprenorphine for pain management. *Pain Management, 9*(1), 13–16. http://doi.org/10.2217/pmt-2018-0069.

Goesling, J., Lin, L. A., & Clauw, D. J. (2018). Psychiatry and pain management: At the intersection of chronic pain and mental health. *Current Psychiatry Reports, 20*(2), 12. http://doi.org/10.1007/s11920-018-0872-4. PMID: 29504088.

Jones, L. K., Lussier, M. E., Brar, J., Byrne, M. C., & Greskovic, G. (2019). Current interventions to promote safe and appropriate pain management. *American Journal of Health-System Pharmacy, 76*(11), 829–834. http://doi.org/10.1093/ajhp/zxz063.

Koller, G., Schwarzer, A., Halfter, K., & Soyka, M. (2019). Pain management in opioid maintenance treatment. *Expert Opinion on Pharmacotherapy, 20*(16), 1993–2005. http://doi.org/10.1080/14656566.2019.1652270.

Morrone, L. A., Scuteri, D., Rombolà, L., Mizoguchi, H., & Bagetta, G. (2017). Opioids resistance in chronic pain management. *Current Neuropharmacology, 15*(3), 444–456. http://doi.org/10.2174/1570159x14666161101092822.

Raja S. N., Carr D.B., Cohen M., Finnerup N.B., Flor H., Gibson S., Keefe F.J., Mogil J.S., Ringkamp M., Sluka K.A., Song X.J., Stevens B., Sullivan M.D., Tutelman P.R., Ushida T., Vader K. (2020). The revised International Association for the Study of Pain definition of pain: concepts, challenges, and compromises. *Pain* Sep 1;161(9):1976-1982. doi: 10.1097/j.pain.0000000000001939. PMID: 32694387; PMCID: PMC7680716.

Subedi, M., Bajaj, S., Kumar, M. S., & Yc, M. (2019). An overview of tramadol and its usage in pain management and future perspective. *Biomedicine & Pharmacotherapy, 111*, 443–451. http://doi.org/10.1016/j.biopha.2018.12.085.

Tompkins, D. A., Hobelmann, J. G., & Compton, P. (2017). Providing chronic pain management in the "fifth vital sign" era: Historical and treatment perspectives on a modern-day medical dilemma. *Drug and Alcohol Dependence, 173*(Suppl 1), S11–S21. Suppl 1. http://doi.org/10.1016/j.drugalcdep.2016.12.002.

Yam, M. F., Loh, Y. C., Tan, C. S., Adam, S. K., Manan, N. A., & Basir, R. (2018). General pathways of pain sensation and the major neurotransmitters involved in pain regulation. *International Journal of Molecular Sciences, 19*, 2164. http://doi.org/10.3390/ijms19082164.

33

Antianxiety and Insomnia Medications

DEBORAH ADELL

Overview

Anxiety is characterized by excessive fear or apprehension, often related to an event that is unfamiliar or that may have an unknown outcome. It is a normal reaction, and it can be a positive protective factor in some situations as it heightens one's awareness and sharpens one's learning abilities. Anxiety becomes a problem when it interferes with everyday personal, social, and/or occupational functions, or when it develops into panic attacks or compulsive behavior. This can lead to symptoms and psychological distress that can become incapacitating. Conditions that manifest as or encompass components of anxiety include panic disorders, phobic disorders such as social anxiety disorder and generalized anxiety disorder, obsessive-compulsive disorder, and posttraumatic stress disorder.

Panic Disorder

A *panic attack* is an unexpected severe, acute onset of symptoms of anxiety accompanied by intense fear. It starts abruptly and reaches a peak within 10 minutes, with at least four of the following symptoms: palpitations, tachycardia, sweating, shaking or trembling, shortness of breath, choking, chest pain or discomfort, nausea or abdominal distress, dizziness or faintness, feeling unreal or detached from oneself, fear of going crazy, fear of dying, paresthesias, and chills or hot flashes. A panic attack becomes a *panic disorder* when the patient consistently worries excessively about having another attack and about what will happen if that should occur.

Phobic Disorders

A patient who has a *phobia* displays a persistent and irrational fear of a clearly definable situation, object, or activity. Exposure to the feared stimulus results in intense anxiety and avoidance that interfere with the patient's life. Three main groups of phobic disorders have been identified:

- *Agoraphobia* is the fear of being in a place or situation that would elicit symptoms of a panic attack and that would cause the patient to have difficulty leaving or to be embarrassed. This often occurs in concert with a panic attack.
- *Social phobia* is a fear of social situations, such as public speaking.
- *Specific phobia* is a fear of specific objects or situations, which may include animals, insects, heights, water, needles, and so forth.

Obsessive-Compulsive Disorder

Obsessive-compulsive disorder (OCD) is a preoccupation with thoughts or acts that occur despite the patient's efforts at resistance. *Obsessions* are persistent thoughts, ideas, or images that intrude into conscious awareness. *Compulsions* are urges or impulses for repetitive intentional behaviors that are performed in a stereotyped manner in an attempt to reduce anxiety. The patient realizes these are senseless and intrusive but is unable to stop. Insight and resistance may not be present in children who have OCD.

Posttraumatic Stress Disorder

Patients with *posttraumatic stress disorder* (PTSD) have recurrent anxiety precipitated by exposure to or memory of some past traumatic situation. They may have recurrent dreams or suddenly may act or feel as though the event is recurring, and they will have increased arousal and hypervigilance, leading to flashbacks and severe anxiety with an enhanced startle reaction. These patients have experienced a catastrophic event that would be distressing to anyone. Onset follows the trauma after a latency period of a few weeks to months, but not longer than 6 months, and the condition lasts for at least 1 month. More than four times as many females as males develop PTSD. Traumatic events reported in females include molestation and physical assault.

Sleep Disorders

An estimated 90 million people in the United States suffer from sleep disorders (Colten & Altevogt, 2006) that can lead to poor health outcomes and social and relationship difficulties, as well as affect longevity. Effects of poor sleep on health can encompass many systems and disease states, such as hypertension and cardiovascular disease, depression, obesity, and diabetes. Sleep disorders have many causes: physical, such as restless leg syndrome or chronic illness; a disturbance in circadian rhythm; psychiatric or mental health issues causing hypo- or hypersomnia; ineffective sleep hygiene; or causes related to other health conditions. With aging, the quality and quantity of sleep naturally diminish. It is not uncommon for patients in their 70s to require up to an hour less sleep per night. Although several classes of medications are available to treat sleep disorders, the underlying conditions that contribute to poor sleep should be investigated and managed. Medications used to treat sleep disorders are often the same as those used for anxiety (benzodiazepines) but also include nonbenzodiazepine gamma-aminobutyric acid type A ($GABA_A$) receptor modulators (zolpidem, eszopiclone); melatonin, a naturally occurring hormone that regulates sleep cycles; and ramelteon, a melatonin receptor agonist.

Relevant Physiology

Anxiety

The manifestations of anxiety are similar to the normal physiologic effects of "fight or flight," highlighted in Box 33.1. Activation of the sympathetic nervous system (SNS) in emergency situations results in a flood of epinephrine, norepinephrine, and cortisol to prepare for facing the emergency (fight) or escaping the situation (flight). At the same time, the parasympathetic system, responsible for the "rest and digest" response, is inhibited. The result is increased

---

• BOX 33.1 Physiologic "Fight or Flight" Response

1. Epinephrine, norepinephrine, and cortisol are released into the blood.
2. The liver releases stored sugar into the blood to meet energy needs.
3. Digestion slows, allowing blood to be shifted to the brain and the muscles.
4. Breathing becomes rapid to allow for greater oxygen supply to the muscles.
5. Heart rate and blood pressure increase.
6. Perspiration increases to cool the body.
7. Muscles tense in preparation for action.
8. Pupils dilate.
9. All senses become more acute.
10. Blood flow to the extremities becomes constricted to protect the body from bleeding from injury.

---

heart rate; pupil dilation; constriction of blood vessels, except for coronary arteries, which dilate; increased blood pressure; increased respiratory rate; and decreased motility of the large bowel. Subjective sensations of fear, loss of control, and the need to escape or run away are described by the patient. In response to an emergency such as a fire in the kitchen or a physical threat of danger from an assailant, the response provides the heightened sensory response necessary for quick, astute reaction. Once the danger is past or controlled, stimulation to the sympathetic nervous system ceases and physiology returns to normal, homeostatic function.

This response is protective in nature and appropriate when safety is threatened. However, it would be harmful if every stressful situation in everyday life produced such an exaggerated response.

Sleep

Following a diurnal pattern, humans experience a natural sleep–wake cycle. *Sleep* is described as a time of diminished consciousness for renewal of mental and physical function. Tissue repair, restoration of energy, integration of activities into permanent memory, and reestablishing communication between different parts of the brain are accomplished during sleep. Two types of sleep that alternate in 90 to 110 cycles are recognized: rapid eye movement (REM) and non-rapid eye movement (non-REM). People will move back and forth through the stages during sleep, with varying lengths of time spent in each stage.

Non-REM sleep is divided into four stages, which total approximately 80% of sleep. The stages are characterized by changes in brain waves and become progressively deeper:

- *Stage 1* is brief, lasting up to about 7 minutes, and is the lightest stage from which people are easily awakened. Brain waves are low-voltage, mixed-frequency alpha waves. If undisturbed, the person will enter stage 2.
- *Stage 2* lasts up to 25 minutes and is characterized by the person being more difficult to awaken and a transition to theta brain waves with bursts of high-frequency waves. It is theorized that during this stage, integration of new memories into long-term memory occurs.
- *Stage 3* serves as the transition to deeper sleep and lasts only a few seconds to minutes.
- *Stage 4* is a deep sleep from which is it difficult to awaken the person. The person's muscles relax, and their heart rate, blood pressure, and gastrointestinal (GI) activity decrease.

Stages 3 and 4 are characterized by high-voltage, low-frequency delta brain waves. After 20 to 40 minutes, the person enters REM sleep.

Accounting for 20% to 25% of sleep time, REM sleep is characterized by cessation of muscle movement and tone, vivid dreams, rapid eye movement, and an increase in blood pressure, heart rate, and respiration. Brain activity and metabolism are high in REM sleep. A lack of REM sleep is often noted in patients suffering from depression.

Induction of sleep is a complex process regulated by the circadian rhythm in response to hormones. Melatonin, a hormone produced by the pineal gland in response to decreasing light levels, prompts sleepiness in the evening hours. Cortisol rises during the night, peaks at daybreak, and prompts wakefulness. During the day, adenosine levels rise in the brain, which signals the need for sleep. During sleep, the adenosine is broken down and eliminated from the brain.

Pathophysiology

Anxiety

In some individuals, the heightened state of "fight or flight" can occur in a dramatic, sudden onset known as a panic attack, may exist at the level of an intermittent, situational anxiety (such as when facing a public-speaking event), or may manifest as a generalized anxiety disorder in which a constant low level of arousal and pathological worry is maintained. Anxiety can coexist with a depressive state and heighten the potential for suicide. Fear of the unknown, especially an unknown outcome of a new or unfamiliar situation, may prompt an anxiety reaction. In some cases, even in the face of familiar, low-threat, or benign situations, the patient is unable to sufficiently overcome their fear. This is common in posttraumatic stress conditions in which the original, frightening event is no longer present but the reaction is triggered by similar stimuli.

It is unclear why some people are able to process and overcome stressful situations and others continue to have the sympathetic nervous system response. A hypothesis is that some people exhibit the presence of a highly sensitive "fear network" in the amygdala. Other causes are attributed to abnormal fear processing, intolerance of uncertainty, or emotional hyperarousal. A genetic component to anxiety disorders must also be considered, with studies of twins demonstrating a heritable potential.

Both the constant, low-level state of anxiety and the intense, sudden, episodic state of a panic attack expose the body to heightened levels of cortisol, norepinephrine, epinephrine, catecholamines, and cytokines. Over time, this continued maladaptive stress response can result in disrupted sleep patterns, elevated insulin and blood glucose levels, increased blood pressure, intraabdominal fat storage, compromised immune function, increased caloric intake related to changes in appetite, and alterations in social patterns, including isolation.

Multiple medical conditions can have symptoms that mimic anxiety, including cardiovascular disease, hyperthyroidism, Cushing's disease, asthma, hypoglycemia, and neurological disorders. Medications may prompt symptoms similar to anxiety, including caffeine, beta agonists, excess thyroid hormone, and sympathomimetic agents. Illegal substances such as cocaine, methamphetamine, and cannabis can also prompt symptoms.

While medication management is appropriate, investigation and treatment of underlying causes are necessary for successful intervention.

Insomnia

Insomnia can take the form of difficulty falling asleep, awakening too early with an inability to fall back to sleep, difficulty maintaining sleep through the night, or sleep that chronically leaves the patient feeling unrefreshed. Accompanying criteria for a diagnosis of insomnia include daytime fatigue or sleepiness; inability to concentrate; disturbance of mood; decreased academic and social relationships or work performance; GI disturbance or headache; and worry about sleep.

Insomnia can take a chronic form or can be acute and situational, which lasts from days to a few weeks. Personal stressors such as work, relationships, finances, family disturbances, or illness can result in acute insomnia. Other causes are an unfamiliar or uncomfortable environment, jet lag, and hospitalization related to noise and hospital routine. Use of over-the-counter (OTC) medications such as pseudoephedrine, alcohol, nicotine, and caffeine can delay onset of sleep or interrupt the sleep cycle. *Chronic insomnia*, identified as lasting more than 30 days, is frequently associated with mental health or physical illness.

Older adults report more difficulty falling asleep, more early-morning awakening from which they cannot fall back to sleep, and more awakening due to environmental noise or light. Females of menopausal age complain more about insomnia than males. A cumulative loss of sleep due to these factors can result in daytime sleepiness and further disruption of the sleep cycle if napping occurs during the day. Additionally, older adults may experience sleep difficulty due to chronic illness and medication use.

To correctly treat insomnia, a complete health history and physical exam as well as a sleep history should be obtained to address underlying physical or mental health problems. In addition to medications, behavioral strategies such as relaxation therapy, sleep restriction therapy, stimulus control therapy, and cognitive therapy should be instituted. Good sleep hygiene practices (Box 33.2) should be encouraged. Medications to promote sleep are usually restricted to short-term time frames.

Antianxiety and Insomnia Therapy

Medications to manage anxiety include benzodiazepines (alprazolam, clonazepam, diazepam, lorazepam, temazepam) and serotonergic anxiolytics (buspirone). Although a mainstay treatment of anxiety and sleep disorders in the past, barbiturates such as secobarbital and phenobarbital are seldom used due to very high abuse and overdose potential. Note that some antidepressant medications (serotonin reuptake inhibitors, nonselective norepinephrine-serotonin reuptake inhibitors, and serotonin-norepinephrine reuptake inhibitors) are also approved for management of anxiety. These classes of medications are discussed in Chapter 34.

Medication management can be effective in handling the symptoms of anxiety. However, multidisciplinary management including psychotherapy, teaching coping skills, and

Quick Sleep Tips

Follow these tips to establish healthy sleep habits:
1. Keep a consistent sleep schedule. Get up at the same time every day, even on weekends or during vacations.
2. Set a bedtime that is early enough for you to get at least 7 hours of sleep.
3. Don't go to bed unless you are sleepy.
4. If you don't fall asleep after 20 minutes, get out of bed.
5. Establish a relaxing bedtime routine.
6. Use your bed only for sleep and sex.
7. Make your bedroom quiet and relaxing. Keep the room at a comfortable, cool temperature.
8. Limit exposure to bright light in the evenings.
9. Turn off electronic devices at least 30 minutes before bedtime.
10. Don't eat a large meal before bedtime. If you are hungry at night, eat a light, healthy snack.
11. Exercise regularly and maintain a healthy diet.
12. Avoid consuming caffeine in the late afternoon or evening.
13. Avoid consuming alcohol before bedtime.
14. Reduce your fluid intake before bedtime.

From American Alliance for Health Sleep. [2017]. *Healthy sleep habits*. http://sleepeducation.org/essentials-in-sleep/healthy-sleep-habits.

alternative modalities such as meditation, essential oil therapy, massage, and pet therapy are useful adjunctive treatments.

Benzodiazepines

Although the exact mechanism by which benzodiazepines inhibit anxiety is unclear, it is known that they act in the CNS, binding to $GABA_A$ receptors. The result is an inhibitory effect on the firing of neurons responsible for promoting behavioral arousal and known to be mediators of the inhibitory effects of fear. This causes sedation, decreased anxiety, antiseizure activity, and difficulty retaining new information. Physiologic effects are muscle relaxation, coronary vasodilation, and when administered in large doses, neuromuscular blockade. Some benzodiazepines are more sedating (triazolam, lorazepam) than others (alprazolam, oxazepam, diazepam) while some excel at muscle relaxation for use in spasticity. Antiseizure activity varies across the class.

Benzodiazepines are considered short-term treatment for newly diagnosed anxiety disorders and for intermittent use in flares of controlled anxiety conditions. Regular, long-term monotherapy with benzodiazepine medication is discouraged due to potential for tolerance and physiologic dependence, even in the absence of abuse or misuse. The abuse potential for these medications is intensified by concomitant use of alcohol or other substances. Psychological dependence is possible. The class should be avoided in people who are at risk for or have a history of substance abuse. Although at doses used for anxiety and hypnotic effects, benzodiazepines do not cause respiratory depression in adults, caution should be used in people with chronic obstructive pulmonary disease (COPD) or sleep-related disorders such as sleep apnea. Decreased tone in the upper airway may result in apneic episodes. At higher doses (such as those used in anesthesia), with accumulation of drug, or in combination with other CNS depressant medications, respiratory depression may occur.

There is little demonstrable difference in therapeutic outcomes for anxiety among the medications in the benzodiazepine class, although there are considerable differences in half-lives, potency, and ability to cross the blood–brain barrier, which affect therapeutic decisions. Higher potency benzodiazepines (alprazolam, clonazepam, and lorazepam) have greater affinity for $GABA_A$ receptors and exhibit a greater net effect. One exception is alprazolam, which is indicated to be superior for the treatment of panic disorder.

Benzodiazepines can be administered orally, intramuscularly, or intravenously. Administered orally, absorption is rapid and complete. Benzodiazepines are divided into four subclasses; ultra-short acting, short acting with a half-life of 6 hours or less (triazolam), intermediate acting with a half-life of 6 to 24 hours (temazepam), and long acting with a half-life or more than 24 hours (diazepam). Although flurazepam has a short half-life of 2.5 hours, it is metabolized to active metabolites, resulting in a total half-life of 47 to 100 hours. Plasma protein binding differs across the class, ranging from 70% to 99%. Benzodiazepines readily cross the blood–brain and placental barriers and are excreted in breast milk. They are not recommended for pregnant or nursing patients. Older adults have increased sensitivity to benzodiazepines, partially related to decreased clearance; for this reason, benzodiazepines are not recommended due to the risk of cognitive impairment, delirium, falls, fractures, and motor vehicle accidents. Avoidance in older adult patients with delirium, dementia, or a history of falls or fractures is recommended by the Beers panel (American Geriatric Society Beers Criteria Update Expert Panel, 2019). Being lipid soluble, benzodiazepines bind to adipose tissue reservoir and may have prolonged effects in obese patients.

Most benzodiazepines are metabolized in the liver by the cytochrome (CYP) P3A4 system. Erythromycin, clarithromycin, ritonavir, itraconazole, ketoconazole, nefazodone, and grapefruit juice may alter the rate of metabolism of benzodiazepines. Excretion of metabolites is via the kidney. Caution in the use of benzodiazepines on patients with hepatic or renal dysfunction is advised.

Adverse effects of benzodiazepines manifest as an exaggeration of the expected response or a toxic response including sedation, lightheadedness, dizziness, decreased reaction time, impairment of mental and physical function, GI upset, prolonged sedation or drowsiness, vertigo, and antegrade amnesia. Paradoxical CNS stimulation may occur in older adults. Alcohol can intensify all CNS effects. Multiple drug interactions can occur (Table 33.1) and so a careful review of medication history is recommended. When prescribing for anxiety, treatment is highly individualized. Dosing should remain as low as possible, for as short a time as possible, while also implementing alternative therapies to assist patients in self-management of their anxiety. Common doses of anxiety management medications are listed in Table 33.2.

PRACTICE PEARLS

Benzodiazepines

Patients on a benzodiazepine regularly for longer than 2 weeks should be tapered off the medication gradually to avoid uncomfortable withdrawal symptoms.

Diazepam

Diazepam (Valium) is often considered the prototype for the class of benzodiazepines. Diazepam has a rapid onset but long duration of action.

Pharmacokinetics. Oral, intranasal, intramuscular, and rectal forms are available. Diazepam is readily absorbed when administered orally, and the onset of action is rapid. Diazepam is highly protein bound, up to 98%. Although the half-life of the drug is approximately 48 hours, the duration of action is prolonged by active metabolites, which have a half-life of up to 100 hours. Excretion is via the kidney, and drug accumulation can occur with repeated dosing.

Indications. Diazepam is indicated for the treatment of anxiety disorders, alcohol withdrawal, skeletal muscle relaxation, preanesthesia, and status epilepticus.

Adverse Effects. CNS adverse effects tend to be dose dependent, are characteristic of the class, and include dizziness, vertigo, confusion, syncope, depression, ataxia, and headache. Anterograde amnesia can occur at therapeutic doses and can be intensified by alcohol. Tolerance can develop. Physical and psychological dependence can occur with or without misuse or abuse. Risk for falls, especially in older adults, is increased. Elevated liver enzymes have been reported.

Contraindications. It is not recommended that diazepam be used in older adults or in those who are pregnant or nursing. Concomitant use with antiepileptic medications may increase risk of suicide. Caution should be used when the patient has sleep apnea or respiratory insufficiency. Use in patients with renal or hepatic disease should include

TABLE 33.1	Medication Interactions With Benzodiazepines and Serotonergic Anxiolytics	
Medication	**Interacting Medication**	**Possible Effects**
Alprazolam	Cimetidine, omeprazole, macrolides	Increased effects of alprazolam
	Grapefruit juice	Increased effects of alprazolam leading to increased sedation
	Ketoconazole	Increased effects of alprazolam
Diazepam	Phenobarbital	Additive effect – CNS depression
Lorazepam, clonazepam	Valproate	Increased effects of benzodiazepine
Alprazolam, clonazepam	Carbamazepine	Decreased levels of benzodiazepine
Clonazepam, diazepam	Phenytoin	Decreased levels of benzodiazepine, unpredictable effect on phenytoin
All benzodiazepines	Digoxin	Increased half-life of digoxin
	Tricyclic antidepressants	Potentiates CNS effect of both drugs, plasma levels of TCAs may increase
	Sertraline, antihistamines, barbiturates, fluoxetine, alcohol	Additive CNS depression
Serotonergic anxiolytic buspirone (Buspar)	Tricyclic antidepressants, SSRIs, MAOIs	Increases potential for serotonin syndrome
	Ketoconazole, nefazodone, itraconazole, ritonavir, grapefruit juice	May increase serum levels of buspirone
	Rifampin, dexamethasone, phenytoin, phenobarbital, carbamazepine	May decrease serum levels of buspirone
	Cetirizine, antihistamines	Increased CNS depression

CNS, Central nervous system; *MAOIs*, monoamine oxidase inhibitors; *SSRIs*, selective serotonin reuptake inhibitors; *TCAs*, tricyclic antidepressants.

TABLE 33.2 **Dosing for Selected Benzodiazepines and Serotonergic Anxiolytics**

Medication	Indication	Dosage	Comments
Alprazolam (Xanax)	For short-term management of transient symptoms of anxiety or for GAD	*Adults:* Begin with 0.25–0.5 mg orally three times daily. May increase at intervals of 3–4 days up to a maximum of 4 mg/day. *Older or debilitated adults:* Begin with 0.25 mg three times daily; may increase gradually as tolerated to maximum of 4 mg/day.	If discontinuation becomes necessary, daily dose should be decreased by no more than 0.5 mg every 3 days. Some patients may require a more gradual and individualized taper.
	Panic disorder	*Adults:* Begin with 0.5 mg orally three times daily. May be increased gradually as tolerated (no more than 1 mg/day at intervals of 3–4 days). May require more than 4 mg. Mean effective dose in clinical trials was 5–6 mg/day. Maximum dosage: 10 mg/day. *Older or debilitated adults:* Begin with 0.25 mg orally two or three times daily. Dose may be increased gradually as tolerated at intervals of 3–4 days. **Extended-release tablets:** *Adults:* 0.5–1 mg orally once daily, preferably in the morning. Increase by no more than 1 mg/day at intervals of every 3–4 days as needed and as tolerated. Usual dose: 3–6 mg once daily. Maximum dosage: 10 mg/day. *Older or debilitated adults:* Initially, 0.5 mg orally once daily, preferably in the morning. May increase gradually (at least every 3–4 days) as tolerated. Maximum dosage: 10 mg/day.	
Chlordiazepoxide (Librium)	Anxiety disorders or for short-term relief of symptoms of anxiety	*Adults:* 5–10 mg orally three to four times daily for mild to moderate symptoms, or 20–25 mg orally three to four times daily for severe symptoms. Maximum dosage: 100 mg/day. *Older or debilitated adults:* 5 mg orally two to four times daily. *Children and adolescents ≥6 yr:* May begin with 5 mg orally two to four times daily. Dose may be increased in some pediatric patients to 10 mg two to three times daily. Maximum dosage: 30 mg/day.	May be given without regard to food. Paradoxical reactions (e.g., excitabililty, agitation, irritability) have occurred in patients with mental illness.
Clonazepam (Klonopin)	Panic disorder	*Adults:* Begin with 0.25 mg orally twice daily. May increase to 1 mg/day after 3 days according to response and tolerability. Maximum dosage: 4 mg/day orally.	For older adults, begin at low dose range and monitor closely. If discontinuation is necessary, gradually decrease by 0.125 mg twice daily every 3 days.

TABLE 33.2 Dosing for Selected Benzodiazepines and Serotonergic Anxiolytics—cont'd

Medication	Indication	Dosage	Comments
Diazepam (Valium)	Anxiety disorders or for short-term relief of anxiety symptoms	*Adults:* 2–10 mg two to four times daily. Use lower initial doses in debilitated adults. Maximum dosage: 40 mg/day. *Older adults:* 2–2.5 mg orally once or twice daily. May increase gradually according to response and patient tolerability. Maximum dosage: 40 mg/day. *Infants ≥6 months, children, and adolescents:* May begin with 1–2.5 mg orally three or four times daily. Dose may be increased as needed and as tolerated.	If using oral solution forms, use only the calibrated dropper provided and may squeeze the medication into liquid or semisolid foods such as water, juice, soda, applesauce, or pudding.
Lorazepam (Ativan)	Short-term management of anxiety or GAD	**IR formulations:** *Adults, adolescents, and children ≥12 yr:* Begin with 2–3 mg/day orally given in 2–3 divided doses. Usual dosage: 2–6 mg/day. Maximum dosage: 10 mg/day. *Older adults or debilitated patients:* Begin with 1–2 mg/day orally given in 2–3 divided doses. Usual dosage: 2–6 mg/day. Maximum dosage: 10 mg/day. **ER formulations:** *Adults and older adults:* Begin with dosing consistent with the total daily dose of lorazepam given orally once daily in the morning. Usual dosage: 2–6 mg/day. Maximum dosage: 10 mg/day.	Efficacy of use for more than 4 months for anxiety disorders and sleep has not been evaluated. Taper gradually for discontinuation. ER formulations can be used in patients who have been receiving stable, evenly divided, three-times-daily dosing with IR products. Give first dose of ER the morning after the day of discontinuation of a lorazepam IR product.
	Short-term treatment of insomnia due to anxiety or situational stress	**IR formulations:** *Adults, adolescents, and children ≥12 yr:* 2–4 mg orally at bedtime as needed. *Older adults:* Use a lower dose to initiate (1–2 mg orally) and titrate as needed. Usual dosage: 2–4 mg orally at bedtime.	
Oxazepam (Serax)	Treatment of anxiety	*Adults and adolescents:* Mild to moderate symptoms: 10–15 mg orally three to four times daily. Severe anxiety: 15–30 mg orally three to four times daily. Maximum dosage: 120 mg/day. *Older adults:* Begin with 10 mg orally three times daily; may increase with caution up to 15 mg three to four times daily if needed and tolerated. Maximum dosage: 60 mg/day.	Periodically reassess for need of continued treatment.
Serotonergic anxiolytic buspirone (Buspar)	GAD or short-term relief of symptoms of anxiety	*Adults:* Begin with 7.5 mg orally two times daily, then increase as needed by 5 mg/day every 2–3 days. Usual dose: 15–30 mg/day given in 2–3 divided doses. Maximum dosage: 60 mg/day. *Older adults:* Begin with 5 mg orally twice daily, then increase as tolerated by 5 mg every 2–3 days. Usual dosage: 15–30 mg/day. Maximum dosage: 60 mg/day.	Should be taken in a consistent manner with regard to food (with or without food).

ER, Extended release; *GAD,* generalized anxiety disorder; *IR,* immediate release.

monitoring. Diazepam is contraindicated in children younger than 6 months of age, and in patients with closed-angle glaucoma.

Monitoring. During long-term therapy, renal and hepatic function should be monitored. Complete blood count (CBC) should be monitored secondary to reports of neutropenia with long-term use.

Alprazolam

In general, alprazolam is used for temporary, short-term management of anxiety disorders and has high abuse potential. An extended-release form is available for generalized anxiety disorder as an adjunct to selective serotonin reuptake inhibitors (SSRIs), although medications with less addiction potential are advised. Rebound panic attacks and withdrawal can occur even when tapering of the medication is performed.

Pharmacokinetics. When administered orally, alprazolam is readily absorbed, with a rapid onset of action, an intermediate duration of action, and a half-life of 8 to 37 hours, depending on the formula. Approximately 80% is bound to protein. Metabolism in the liver results in little to no active metabolites. Excretion is via the renal system.

Indications. Alprazolam is indicated for the treatment of anxiety disorder and panic disorder (with or without agoraphobia).

Adverse Effects. As with other benzodiazepines, exaggeration of CNS depressant effects is responsible for many adverse effects of alprazolam, such as sedation, drowsiness, and increased risk for falls. Additionally, agitation, abnormal dreams, personality changes, rage, and aggression have been reported. Physiologic and psychologic dependence can occur. Tolerance is possible.

Contraindications. Extreme caution should be exercised in prescribing alprazolam to patients with a history of substance abuse. Withdrawal and rebound of symptoms can occur, even with short-term use. Use of alprazolam in those who are pregnant or nursing is contraindicated.

Monitoring. No laboratory monitoring is recommended.

Temazepam

Used as a hypnotic for insomnia, temazepam is preferred over the older hypnotic, flurazepam, related to temazepam having a shorter half-life and no active metabolites. Abrupt discontinuation of the medication after prolonged use can result in the withdrawal effects of irritability, rebound insomnia, and perceptual disturbances, which can occur after as little as 2 weeks of daily use.

Pharmacokinetics. Temazepam is readily absorbed, with quick onset of action of 30 to 60 minutes and a half-life of approximately 8 to 15 hours. Metabolism is by conjugation in the liver, with excretion of inactive metabolites via the renal system.

Indications. Temazepam can be used for short-term management of insomnia.

Adverse Effects. As with other hypnotic benzodiazepine agents, temazepam can cause abnormal sleep-related behavior, including eating, making phone calls, or driving a car with no memory of the event. Other adverse effects include manifestations of CNS depression such as excess sedation, tolerance, physiologic and psychologic dependence, lethargy, confusion, and a feeling of being hungover.

Contraindications. Temazepam is contraindicated (has a black box warning) in pregnancy and is cautioned in breastfeeding. Caution is also advised in patients with symptoms of or a diagnosis of depression, which may be exacerbated; a history of suicide attempt; or suicide ideation. Caution should be exercised in patients with renal or hepatic impairment and in older adults related to increased risk for falls and reduced clearance.

Monitoring. Routine monitoring is not recommended, except for monitoring of liver function in patients with preexisting hepatic impairment.

Serotonergic Anxiolytics

Buspirone

Used for generalized anxiety disorder without CNS depression or sedation, buspirone has no anticonvulsant action and does not cause muscle relaxation. Considered to be relatively safe, buspirone has few drug–drug interactions and can be given at high doses with minimal risk of dependence. Buspirone can precipitate increased anxiety if used in patients with panic disorders.

Pharmacokinetics. Buspirone is well absorbed when given orally, with extensive first-pass metabolism that can be decreased by administering with food, resulting in higher serum levels. This effect should be maintained with a consistent dosing pattern of with or without food. Buspirone is highly protein bound and lipid soluble, and readily crosses the blood–brain barrier. The half-life is 1 to 10 hours, with a slow onset of action of 1 to 2 weeks and peak action occurring at approximately 6 weeks of continuous use. Metabolism is in the liver. Approximately 30% to 65% is excreted in the urine as metabolites, with the balance excreted via the feces.

Indications. Buspirone is used to treat generalized anxiety disorder. It can also be used for the short-term relief of anxiety symptoms.

Adverse Effects. The side effects reported most frequently are lightheadedness, dizziness, headache, and insomnia. Although drowsiness or sedation is not considered to be a major side effect of buspirone, patients should still observe caution when engaging in activities that require alertness when first starting the medication.

Contraindications. Buspirone is not intended for use in panic disorders and may precipitate increased panic effects. Due to the potential for prolonging half-life with resultant drug accumulation, buspirone is not recommended for patients with hepatic or renal dysfunction. Although animal studies demonstrate no teratogenic effects, well-controlled studies in females are not available. Use in pregnancy should weigh potential risks and benefits. Buspirone is not recommended for patients who are nursing as the extent of excretion via breast milk is not well understood.

Monitoring. Routine laboratory monitoring is not typically recommended.

Nonbenzodiazepine GABA$_A$ Receptor Modulators (Benzodiazepine Receptor Agonists)

Nonbenzodiazepine hypnotics are used to induce sleep. The hallmark of this class is very rapid onset of action. Three medications in this class are available in the United States: zolpidem, zaleplon, and eszopiclone. All are Schedule IV medications and can cause tolerance, physical dependence, and withdrawal symptoms if used chronically. All can also cause abnormal thought processes and behaviors, even at reduced doses. Episodes of patients engaging in activities such as eating, driving, and sex, with total amnesia of the events in the morning, have been reported. In 2018, the U.S. Food and Drug Administration (FDA) recognized these effects as sufficiently urgent to issue a black box warning indicating that drug-induced complex sleep-related behaviors are possible and that people experiencing these behaviors should not take drugs from this class. The FDA recommends use of the nonbenzodiazepine class for no more than 7 to 10 days. Alcohol should be avoided when taking these medications.

Patients may experience somnolence, dizziness, blurred vision, or headache the morning following use, in some cases sufficient to impair reaction time and alertness. When taking the medication to mitigate middle-of-the night awakening, at least four hours should be available before the patient needs to awaken and engage in normal activities. Effects may be exaggerated in older adults and may lead to falls or confusion. Older adults should be started at lower doses to help mitigate these effects. Common dosages for sleep medications are listed in Table 33.3.

Zolpidem

There is little difference among the drugs in the nonbenzodiazepine class, except for individual response. However, females eliminate zolpidem at a slower rate so should be started at lower doses. Zolpidem is available in immediate-release, controlled-release, and sublingual formulas. The controlled-release formula, while useful for maintaining sleep throughout the night, presents increased risk for next-morning impairment.

Pharmacokinetics. Zolpidem is well absorbed in all forms. Onset of action is approximately 30 to 90 minutes. For fastest onset of action, all formulas should be taken on an empty stomach. The half-life varies from 1 to 2 hours, depending on formula. Zolpidem is metabolized in the liver and excreted via the kidneys.

Indications. Zolpidem is used to treat insomnia characterized by difficulty initiating or maintaining sleep. Use should be restricted to 7 to 10 days, after which the patient should be reevaluated for underlying conditions.

Adverse Effects. Zolpidem is subject to the adverse effects of the nonbenzodiazepine benzodiazepine-receptor agonists, with dizziness and headache occurring most frequently. While confusion is relatively frequent, the highest incidence occurs in adults over the age of 70.

Contraindications. Dosage should be adjusted for patients with hepatic impairment. Renal impairment does not appear to result in drug accumulation. Zolpidem readily crosses the placental barrier and may cause fetal depression. Excretion in breast milk may cause sedation in the infant. Avoiding breastfeeding for five half-lives after a dose is recommended. Caution should be used in patients experiencing depression as the medication may worsen or incite suicidal ideation. Patients with a history of drug-induced complex sleep-related behaviors should not take this medication.

Monitoring. Specific laboratory monitoring is not recommended.

Melatonin and Melatonin Receptor Agonists

Melatonin, a hormone produced in the pineal gland, regulates the circadian, or sleep–wake, cycle Melatonin is produced in response to reduced light entering the eye. The melatonin secretion signal is sent to the pineal gland by the optic nerve. Commercially produced melatonin can be taken in the evening, mimicking natural production, to induce sleep. It should be noted that commercially produced melatonin is not FDA regulated. A melatonin receptor agonist, ramelteon (Rozerem), binds selectively to MT1 and MT2 receptors, producing the same stimulation as melatonin produced by the body. Related to the specific receptor stimulation, ramelteon has a low potential for abuse and is not a controlled substance. Physical dependence is unlikely. When administered for 6 months, no tolerance was noted. This medication is most useful for patients having trouble initiating sleep. Alcohol should be avoided when taking ramelteon.

Ramelteon

Pharmacokinetics. Ramelteon is well absorbed when administered orally (although a high-fat meal can

> **BLACK BOX WARNING!**
>
> **Nonbenzodiazepine Benzodiazepine-Receptor Agonists**
>
> Sedative-hypnotic agents can cause complex sleep-related behaviors such as preparing and eating food, driving while not fully awake, conducting phone calls, and engaging in sexual activity. In some cases, patients have no memory of these events. These behaviors are more common in patients taking nonbenzodiazepine benzodiazepine-receptor agonists (NBRAs) than other sedative-hypnotics.
>
> NBRAs are contraindicated in patients with a history of drug-induced complex sleep-related behaviors.

TABLE 33.3   Dosing for Select Medications Used for Insomnia

Class/Medication	Indication	Dosage	Comments
Nonbenzodiazepine GABA_A Receptor Modulators			
Zolpidem (Ambien)	Short-term insomnia characterized by difficulty with sleep initiation	**IR tablets (maximum dose 10 mg/day):** *Adult females:* 5 mg orally at bedtime. *Adult males:* 5–10 mg orally at bedtime. *Older or debilitated adults:* 5 mg orally at bedtime. **SL tablets (e.g., Edluar) (maximum dose 10 mg/day):** *Adult females:* 5 mg SL at bedtime. *Adult males:* 5–10 mg SL at bedtime. *Older or debilitated adults:* 5 mg SL at bedtime. **Lingual spray (Zopimist) (maximum spray 10 mg/day):** *Adult females:* Begin with 5 mg orally (1 spray in mouth over the tongue) immediately before bedtime. *Adult males:* Begin with 5–10 mg orally (1–2 sprays into mouth and over the tongue) immediately before bedtime. *Older adults or debilitated patients:* 5 mg orally (1 spray into mouth and over the tongue) immediately before bedtime.	For IR, ER, lingual spray, and SL (Edluar) formulations, give immediately before bedtime and with at least 7–8 hr remaining before planned time of awakening. For SL dosage (Intermezzo only), use only if the patient has at least 4 hr remaining before the planned time of waking. Always use lowest effective dose.
	Insomnia characterized by difficulties with sleep onset and/or sleep maintenance	**Extended release (maximum dose 12.5 mg/day):** *Adult females:* Begin with 6.25 mg orally immediately before bedtime. *Adult males:* Begin with 6.25–12.5 mg orally immediately before bedtime. *Older and debilitated adults:* Begin with 6.25 mg orally immediately before bedtime.	
	Insomnia characterized by middle-of-the-night awakening that is followed by difficulty returning to sleep	**SL tablets (Intermezzo only):** *Adult females:* 1.75 mg SL taken once per night if needed for a middle-of-the-night awakening followed by difficulty returning to sleep. *Adult males:* 3.5 mg SL once per night if needed for a middle-of-the night awakening followed by difficulty returning to sleep (use 1.75 mg if taking other CNS depressants). *Older adults:* 1.75 mg SL taken once per night if needed for a middle-of-the night awakening followed by difficulty returning to sleep.	

TABLE 33.3 Dosing for Select Medications Used for Insomnia—cont'd

Class/Medication	Indication	Dosage	Comments
Zaleplon (Sonata)	Short-term insomnia	*Adults:* 10 mg orally at bedtime. Maximum dosage: 20 mg/day. *Older, debilitated, low-weight adults or patients with hepatic insufficiency:* 5 mg at bedtime. Maximum dosage: 10 mg/day.	May take either at bedtime or after an attempt to fall asleep without medication. Must have at least 4 or more hr of sleep time remaining. Avoid taking with or immediately after a heavy, high-fat meal as it will reduce absorption and reduce medication effects on sleep latency.
Eszopiclone (Lunesta)	Short-term insomnia	*Adults:* Begin with 1 mg orally at bedtime. May be titrated to 2–3 mg at bedtime. Maximum dose: 3 mg. *Older or debilitated adults:* Begin with 1 mg orally at bedtime. May increase to maximum dose of 2 mg.	Should have at least 7-8 hours before planned time of awakening. Higher doses more likely to cause next-day impairment while performing activities that require full mental alertness (e.g., driving, operating machinery, making major decisions).
Melatonin Receptor Agonist			
Ramelteon (Rozerem)	Short-term or chronic insomnia with delayed sleep onset	*Adults and older adults:* 8 mg taken within 30 min of bedtime.	Do not take with or immediately after a high-fat meal. Efficacy has been shown up to 6 months.

ER, Extended release; *GABA*, gamma-aminobutyric acid; *IR*, immediate release; *SL*, sublingual.

significantly delay absorption) and has significant first-pass effect. Once distributed, ramelteon is approximately 82% protein bound. Onset of action is approximately 30 minutes. Metabolized in the liver, the medication is mainly excreted in the urine, with small quantities in the feces.

Indications. Ramelteon is used for the treatment of acute or chronic insomnia characterized by delayed sleep onset.

Adverse Effects. Ramelteon is generally well tolerated. The most frequently reported events were headache, morning drowsiness, dizziness, and fatigue. Rarely, angioedema has been reported.

Contraindications. Caution should be used for patients with mild to moderate hepatic disease. Ramelteon should be avoided completely in patients with severe hepatic disease. Adequate and well-controlled studies of the use of ramelteon during pregnancy and breastfeeding are not available. The risk-to-benefit ratio should be considered in pregnancy and breastfeeding.

Monitoring. With long-term use, liver function tests (LFTs) should be performed periodically.

BOOKMARK THIS!

Clinical Practice Guidelines

- The American Psychiatric Association provides access to a number of clinical practice guidelines to help ensure evidence-based practice: https://www.psychiatry.org/psychiatrists/practice/clinical-practice-guidelines
- The American Academy of Sleep Medicine™ provides access to a number of clinical practice guidelines that can inform primary care practice: https://aasm.org/clinical-resources/practice-standards/practice-guidelines.
- The U.S. Department of Veterans Affairs provides VA/DoD clinical practice guidelines to inform best practices on a variety of topics, including select mental health and sleep disorders: https://www.healthquality.va.gov/index.asp.
- The American Academy of Child & Adolescent Psychiatry provides resources for primary care providers, including guidelines for the assessment and treatment of children and adolescents with anxiety disorders: https://www.aacap.org/AACAP/Resources_for_Primary_Care/Practice_Parameters_and_Resource_Centers/Practice_Parameters.aspx

Prescriber Considerations for Antianxiety and Insomnia Therapy

Clinical Practice Guidelines

Generalized Anxiety Disorder

Anxiety disorder management includes both pharmacologic and nonpharmacologic intervention. Several classes of medications are approved for the management of generalized anxiety disorder, including antidepressants, benzodiazepines, and nonbenzodiazepine GABA$_A$ receptor modulators. The general consensus among agencies such as the American Psychiatric Association (https://www.psychiatry.org/) and the Anxiety and Depression Association of America (https://adaa.org/) is that pharmacologic therapy is most effective when augmented with psychotherapy and/or psychosocial therapy, although scientific evidence varies in support of this concept (Fig. 33.1).

First-line therapy for generalized anxiety disorder is aimed at helping the patient to understand their condition and to apply various coping mechanisms that address both cognition and behavior. Such interventions as cognitive restructuring, teaching subjective assessment of symptoms, applied relaxation, problem-solving, and interpersonal psychotherapy are used.

Medications may be added as the patient undertakes the work of self-awareness. Antidepressants may be employed. Medications specific to anxiety management, such as benzodiazepines, may be used for short-term management or intermittently to control symptoms.

Generalized Insomnia

Short-term insomnia, which affects 30% to 50% of the population (Sateia et al., 2017), is considered to have a duration of 3 months or less. The condition becomes chronic if it is experienced for more than 3 months, with at least 3 episodes per week. The American Academy of Sleep Medicine provides guidance for primary care providers in diagnosing primary insomnia (Box 33.3).

Treatment of insomnia seeks to accomplish not only improved length and quality of sleep but alleviation of daytime impairment related to insufficient or inadequate sleep and rest. Initial interventions should be aimed at underlying causes such as comorbid conditions, acute or chronic pain, or situational causes. All patients should be educated about good sleep hygiene (see Box 33.2). These are steps patients can take on their own and are part of cognitive-behavioral sleep therapy, which should be instituted for all patients experiencing sleep disturbance. For short-term insomnia, pharmaceutical intervention can be added for periods not to exceed 10 days. Short- or intermediate-acting sedatives such as triazolam; nonbenzodiazepine GABA$_A$ receptor modulators such as zolpidem; or ramelteon, a melatonin receptor agonist, are recommended. Patients should be advised to take the medication only when needed. The sleep diary should be continued to monitor treatment success or identify patterns or relapses. Patients may also benefit from alternative modalities such as relaxation techniques (guided imagery, focused breathing, meditation, visualization of peaceful places or situations), aromatherapy, music therapy, and warm baths.

Clinical Reasoning for Antianxiety and Insomnia Therapy

Consider the individual patient's health problem requiring anxiety or insomnia therapy. Management of anxiety or insomnia should be individualized to the patient. Initial diagnosis must take into account the possibility of medical or mental health comorbidities causing or contributing to the symptoms of anxiety or insomnia. Assessment of the individual's coping and self-management skills will assist in tailoring treatment to be optimally effective. Inquiry should be made into the patient's perception of impairment they experience related to their anxiety or insomnia as patient expectations may alter treatment options.

Determine the desired therapeutic outcome based on the degree of anxiety or sleep management needed for the patient's health problem. Both impairment from anxiety disorders and tolerance of the effects of insomnia are subjective. While one patient may be very alarmed at prolonged time to sleep onset, another may be only mildly concerned. Similarly, one patient's response to anxiety disorders may be severe enough to self-perpetuate an anxiety cycle while another patient may have sufficient coping skills to mitigate all but the most intense anxiety attack. For that reason, it is imperative to include the patient in treatment planning to ensure that expectations are met.

Assess the medication selected for its appropriateness for an individual patient by considering the medication's side effects and the patient's age, race/ethnicity, comorbidities, and genetic factors. Older adult patients should not be prescribed benzodiazepines. If unavoidable, only very low doses should be used for short periods. For all other classes of sedatives and hypnotics, older adults should be started on reduced doses to ascertain patient response. Older adults may be more susceptible to the depressant CNS effects of the medications, which may result in falls or preventable accidents. For zolpidem, female patients should be started at half the normal dose related to gender differences in clearance of the drug. All patients should be made fully aware of black box warnings on nonbenzodiazepine GABA$_A$ receptor modulators, including the potential for drug-induced complex sleep-related behaviors such as eating, making telephone calls, or driving with no memories of those events in the morning.

Initiate the treatment plan with the selected medication by first providing adequate patient education to ensure the patient's understanding and promote full participation in the anxiety or insomnia therapy. Patients should be fully educated on their diagnosis of anxiety or insomnia. Causes of the conditions should be discussed to bring attention to the impact of lifestyle or individual habits on the course and management of the disorder. Nonpharmacologic interventions

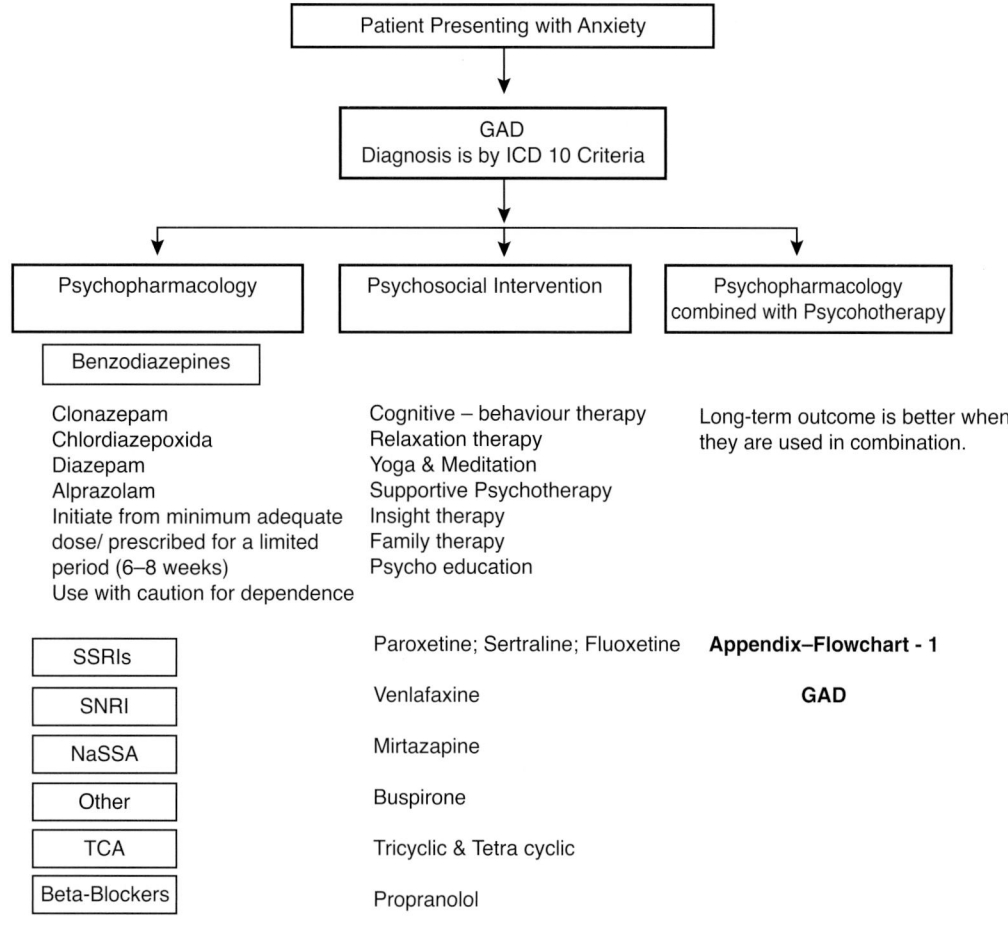

• **Fig. 33.1** Example of algorithmic approach to management of anxiety. (From Gautam, S., Jain, A., Gauram, M., Vahia, V., & Gautam, A. [2016]. Clinical practice guidelines for the management of generalised anxiety disorder [GAD] and panic disorder [PD]. *Indian Journal of Psychiatry, 59*[Suppl 1], 67–73.)

• **BOX 33.3** **Evaluation for Sleep Disorders**

The American Academy of Sleep Medicine guidelines indicate that diagnosing insomnia must include, at a minimum, the following evaluations:

1. Medical and mental health history for comorbid conditions
2. Medication history
3. Family history to identify familial insomnia patterns
4. As part of the social history, careful evaluation for use of substances that may interfere with sleep, such as caffeine, cough and cold medications, substances of abuse, etc.
5. A sleepiness assessment such as the Epworth Sleepiness Scale
6. A sleep diary (minimum of 2-week duration)

Unless a comorbid condition is suspected, laboratory, imaging and other testing is not indicated.

Adapted from Chawla, J., Park, Y., & Passaro, E. 2020. *Insomnia guidelines*. Medscape. https://emedicine.medscape.com/article/1187829-guidelines.

Ensure complete patient and family understanding about the medication prescribed for anxiety or insomnia therapy using a variety of education strategies. For support, patients may wish to include family members in the discussion of management of anxiety disorders. All medication instructions should be provided in written form to assist in recall. Patients and family members should participate in treatment development, with their goals taken into consideration. For insomnia, patients should be encouraged to keep a sleep diary to assist with tracking patterns of sleep. The teach-back method should be employed to ensure understanding of goals and medication directions.

Conduct follow-up and monitoring of patient responses to anxiety or insomnia therapy. Patients being treated for anxiety should be monitored periodically for medication use to be sure tolerance or overuse has not developed. During these follow-up visits, reinforcement of lifestyle and nonpharmacologic management of anxiety should be performed.

Routine monitoring of patients with short-term insomnia is not indicated. Patients being treated for chronic insomnia should periodically monitor the effects of treatment with a sleep journal. Monitoring for appropriate use and encouragement of nonpharmacologic interventions should occur at each follow-up visit.

should always be instituted prior to or in conjunction with pharmacologic agents. Patients should be made aware of the importance of their active participation in treatment, including lifestyle adjustments.

TABLE 33.4 Examples of Herbal/Drug Interactions That May Affect Patients Taking Antianxiety or Antinsomnia Agents

Product	Comments
Ashwagandha	Increased risk for interactions with benzodiazepines and anticonvulsants
Cannabis	Increased risk for sedation with antianxiety medications and hypnotics
Chamomile	Effects may be addictive with CNS depressants; may increase effect of insomnia drugs
Kava kava	Potential interactions with ethanol; may increase effects of CNS depressants (particularly benzodiazepines, antidepressants, and sedative hypnotics)
Lavender	May increase effects of sedative effects and antianxiety agents such as lorazepam, diazepam, and alprazolam
Melatonin	Excessive dosages may cause morning sedation or drowsiness
Passionflower	Potential interactions with antianxiety agents, antidepressants, hypnotics, and sedatives; may increase sedative effects of zolpidem, zaleplon, eszopiclone, and ramelteon
Skullcap	Increases sedative effect of benzodiazepines, drugs used to treat insomnia, and alcohol
St. John's wort	Potential interactions with antidepressants (including SSRIs, tricyclics, MAOIs), narcotics, other CNS depressants, reserpine, and digoxin
Valerian	Increased effects/toxicity with CNS depressants, sedative hypnotics (barbiturates), antidepressants, anxiolytics, antihistamines, benzodiazepines, drugs to treat insomnia, and tricyclics

CNS, Central nervous system; *MAOIs,* monoamine oxidase inhibitors; *SSRIs,* selective serotonin reuptake inhibitors.

Teaching Points for Antianxiety and Insomnia Therapy

Health Promotion Strategies

- Provide patients with information about nonpharmacologic strategies that can be effective in reducing anxiety, such as medication, massage, pet therapy, healthy eating, and increased physical activity.
- Carefully review the patient's medications and lifestyle to address any issues that may be increasing anxiety or affecting sleep, such as use of caffeine, nicotine, alcohol, beta agonists, thyroid medications, or certain OTC medications.
- Assess for underlying substance use disorders that may affect the patient while presenting as concerns about anxiety or sleep problems.
- Refer patients for outside support in mental health if they are experiencing personal stressors such as parent-

ing, relationship or family issues, or financial problems that may require professional help.
- Recommend sleep hygiene to all patients to help promote optimal sleep practices.
- Provide patients with resources about sleep that may inform sleep practices with aging (see https://www.cdc.gov/sleep/about_sleep/how_much_sleep.html).

Patient Education for Medication Safety

- Avoid alcohol while taking any medication that treats anxiety or insomnia due to increased risk of drowsiness/sedation.
- Until you are fully aware of the side effects of the medication you are taking, avoid driving, using heavy machinery, or making major decisions.
- Benzodiazepine medications are for treatment of acute anxiety and should only be used on a short-term basis as recommended by your primary care provider.
- Implement sleep hygiene strategies (see Box 33.2) to promote better, more restful sleep.
- Take medications for sleep right before bedtime as they tend to work very quickly. To avoid daytime drowsiness or feelings of a sleep hangover, do not take sleep medications within 6 to 8 hours of your scheduled wake-up time.
- Tell your provider if you have a history of any unusual sleep-related behaviors (such as sleepwalking, eating, or making phone calls during sleep) after taking sleep-hypnotic agents.
- Avoid taking herbal products for insomnia or anxiety without notifying your primary care providers (Table 33.4).
- Work with your health care providers to determine which stress management techniques work best for you. It may take several attempts to learn the best fit.

Application Questions for Discussion

1. Patients may experience situational anxiety including that related to public speaking. What strategies might a person utilize to mitigate the "fight or flight" effect?
2. Chronic insomnia, lasting longer than 3 months with 3 or more episodes per week, can be very distressing to patients. Discuss the order of interventions, from nonpharmacologic to pharmacologic, that would be used.
3. Discuss age, gender, and comorbidity effects on dosing patients with sedatives or hypnotic agents.

Selected Bibliography

American Alliance for Health Sleep. (2017). *Healthy sleep habits.* Retrieved from http://sleepeducation.org/essentials-in-sleep/healthy-sleep-habits.

American Geriatric Society Beers Criteria Update Expert Panel. (2019). American Geriatrics Society 2019 Updated Beers Criteria for Potentially Inappropriate Medication Use in Older Adults. *Journal of the American Geriatrics Society, 67,* 674–694.

Anxiety and Depression Association of American. (2015). *Clinical practice review for GAD.* Retrieved from https://adaa.org/resources-professionals/practice-guidelines-gad.

Brunton, L. L., Hilal-Dandan, R., & Knollmann, B. C. (2017). *Goodman and Gilman's The Pharmacological Basis of Therapeutics* (*13th ed.*). New York: McGraw Hill Professional.

Chawla, J., Park, Y., & Passaro, E. (2020). *Insomnia guidelines*: Medscape. Retrieved from https://emedicine.medscape.com/article/1187829-guidelines.

Colten, H. R., & Altevogt, B. M. (2006). *Extent and health consequences of chronic sleep loss and sleep disorders*. Retrieved from https://ncbi.nlm.nih.gov/books/nbk19961.

Elsevier. Clinical pharmacology powered by ClinicalKey®. (2019-[cited 2020 August]). Retrieved from http://www.clinicalkey.com.

Gautam, S., Jain, A., Gauram, M., Vahia, V., & Gautam, A. (2016). Clinical practice guidelines for the management of generalised anxiety disorder (GAD) and panic disorder (PD). *Indian Journal of Psychiatry, 59*(Suppl 1), 67–73.

Grossman, S., & Mattson Porth, C. (2013). *Porth's Pathophysiology: Concepts of Altered Health States* (*9th ed.*). New York: Lippincott Williams & Wilkens.

Memorial Sloan Kettering Cancer Center. (2021). *Search about herbs*. Retrieved from https://www.mskcc.org/cancer-care/diagnosis-treatment/symptom-management/integrative-medicine/herbs/search.

Sateia, M., Buysse, D., Krystal, A., Neubauer, D., & Heald, J. (2017). Clinical practice guideline for the pharmacologic treatment of chronic insomnia in adults: An American Academy of Sleep Medicine clinical practice guideline. *Journal of Clinical Sleep Medicine, 13*(2), 307–349.

U.S. National Library of Medicine. (2017). Understanding benzodiazepine and non-benzodiazepine sedative use. Retrieved from https://clinicaltrials.gov/ct2/show/NCT02833272.

34

Mood Disorder Medications

CHERYL ZAMBROSKI AND MELANIE COMBS

Overview

Mood disorder, sometimes called *affective disorder*, is an overarching term covering depressive disorder, bipolar disorder, and their subtypes. Whatever the specific psychiatric diagnosis, the patient experiences a sustained disorder of their emotional state.

Major depression is considered one of the most common mood disorders experienced by adults in the United States. In 2017, approximately 7% of adults and 13% of adolescents 12 to 17 years of age experienced at least one major depressive episode (National Institute of Mental Health [NIMH], 2019). The NIMH (2017) also estimates that approximately 4% of adults in the United States experience bipolar disorder at some time in their lives. In addition, recent evidence suggests that as many as 17% of patients treated for depression in primary care may have unrecognized bipolar disorder (Devaney et al., 2019). The onset of the COVID-19 pandemic exacerbated the mental health challenges, including depression, that are faced by patients who may present to primary care providers for treatment.

A number of risk factors are associated with depression, including a positive family history, history of trauma, substance abuse, major life changes, recent loss, and history of domestic abuse or violence. For some patients, the onset of depression is associated with the adverse effects of certain medications they are taking, such as beta-blockers, proton pump inhibitors, or benzodiazepines. In those cases, changing the medications may relieve the depressive symptoms. For other patients, their depression may be associated with one of a variety of commonly occurring illnesses such as Parkinson's disease, cancer, coronary heart disease, or heart failure. In these cases, treatment may be more complex.

The United States Preventive Services Task Force (USPSTF) recommends screening for depression in the general adult population, including pregnant and postpartum females, as well as adolescents 12 to 18 years of age. Adequate systems are in place to ensure accurate diagnosis, effective treatment, and appropriate follow-up (Sui et al., 2016).

In general, depression is initially treated in the primary care setting. Patients who should be referred to a psychiatrist include those who fail to achieve remission, have symptoms of psychosis or severe symptoms, or have depression as well

as another comorbid psychiatric illness. Life-threatening situations, such as the risk of suicide, must be referred to the emergency department. Children and adolescents often present with complex situations and should be referred to a specialist.

Formal definitions of major depression and bipolar disorder as well as their diagnostic subtypes are included in the *Diagnostic and Statistical Manual of Mental Disorders, Fifth Edition* (*DSM-5*), published by the American Psychiatric Association (Box 34.1 and Box 34.2). Accurate diagnosis is essential in order to choose appropriate pharmacologic treatment and help prevent significant adverse effects. Failure to differentiate major depression from bipolar illness while prescribing any antidepressant to treat depressive symptoms may result in mania or hypomania. While this chapter focuses primarily on the treatment of major depression, primary care providers should recognize key medications used in the treatment of bipolar disorder and their associated risks and benefits. Whatever the disorder, it is imperative to conduct suicide screening for any patient exhibiting signs of depressive illness. All primary care providers should recognize key local and national support systems for patients in crisis, including the National Suicide Prevention Lifeline, the U.S. Department of Veterans Affairs Suicide Prevention website, and the American Foundation for Suicide Prevention.

> ### BOOKMARK THIS!
>
> **Resources for Suicide Prevention**
> - National Suicide Prevention Lifeline: 1-800-273-8255, https://suicidepreventionlifeline.org
> - U.S. Department of Veterans Affairs Suicide Prevention: https://www.mentalhealth.va.gov/suicide_prevention
> - American Foundation for Suicide Prevention: https://afsp.org

Relevant Physiology

Neurotransmitters are endogenous chemical substances synthesized in the neuron and stored in vesicles located in the synaptic knob of the presynaptic neuron. In response to an

---

• BOX 34.1 DSM-5 Criteria for Major Depressive Disorder

DSM-5 Criteria for Major Depressive Disorder

A. Five (or more) of the following symptoms have been present during the same 2-week period and represent a change from previous functioning; at least one of the symptoms is either (1) depressed mood or (2) loss of interest or pleasure.

    Note: Do not include symptoms that are clearly attributable to another medical condition.

  1. Depressed mood most of the day, nearly every day, as indicated by either subjective report (e.g., feels sad, empty, hopeless) or observation made by others (e.g., appears tearful). (Note: In children and adolescents, it can be irritable mood.)

  2. Markedly diminished interest or pleasure in all, or almost all, activities most of the day, nearly every day (as indicated by either subjective account or observation).

  3. Significant weight loss when not dieting, or weight gain (e.g., a change of more than 5% of body weight in a month) or decrease or increase in appetite nearly every day. (Note: In children, consider failure to make expected weight gain.)

  4. Insomnia or hypersomnia nearly every day.

  5. Psychomotor agitation or retardation nearly every day (observable by others, not merely subjective feelings of restlessness or being slowed down).

  6. Fatigue or loss of energy nearly every day.

  7. Feelings of worthlessness or excessive or inappropriate guilt (which may be delusional) nearly every day (not merely self-reproach or guilt about being sick).

  8. Diminished ability to think or concentrate or indecisiveness nearly every day (either by subjective account or as observed by others).

  9. Recurrent thoughts of death (not just fear of dying), recurrent suicidal ideation without a specific plan, or a suicide attempt or a specific plan for committing suicide.

B. The symptoms cause clinically significant distress or impairment in social, occupational, or other important areas of functioning.

C. The episode is not attributable to the physiological effects of a substance or to another medical condition.

    Note: Criteria A through C represent a major depressive episode.

    Note: Responses to a significant loss (bereavement, financial ruin, losses from a natural disaster, a serious medical illness or disability) may include the feelings of intense sadness, rumination about the loss, insomnia, poor appetite, and weight loss as noted in Criterion A, which may resemble a depressive episode. Although such symptoms may be understandable or considered appropriate to the loss, the presence of a major depressive episode in addition to the normal response to a significant loss should also be carefully considered. This decision inevitably requires the exercise of clinical judgment based on the individual's history and the cultural norms for the expression of distress in the context of loss.

D. The occurrence of the major depressive episode is not better explained by schizoaffective disorder, schizophrenia, schizophreniform disorder, delusional disorder, or other specified and unspecified schizophrenia spectrum and other psychotic disorders.

E. There has never been a manic or a hypomanic episode.

    Note: This exclusion does not apply to all of the manic-like or hypomanic-like episodes that are substance-induced or are attributable to the physiological effects of another medical condition.

From American Psychiatric Association. (2013). Diagnostic and statistical manual of mental disorders (5th ed.). Washington, DC: Author.

---

electric impulse, the neurotransmitters are released from the presynaptic neurons by a process of exocytosis into the synaptic cleft. Once in the synaptic cleft, the neurotransmitters bind with their target postsynaptic receptors on the postsynaptic neurons, conveying information to target cells. This may lead to an inhibitory or excitatory action potential. Of note, presynaptic neurons can synthesize more than one neurotransmitter and postsynaptic neurons can have multiple neurotransmitter-specific receptors. Excess neurotransmitters can be broken down into component parts by select enzymes as well as through active removal via reuptake pumps to be recycled. Neurotransmitters widely present in the brain include acetylcholine, norepinephrine, serotonin, dopamine, histamine, gamma-aminobutyric acid (GABA), and glutamate.

Three major types of monoaminergic neurons found in the brain are implicated in regulating mood. They are the serotonergic neurons (also called 5-HT), which use serotonin as their neurotransmitter; noradrenergic neurons, which use norepinephrine as their neurotransmitter; and dopaminergic neurons, which use dopamine as their neurotransmitter. While other neurotransmitters play a role in

mood and mental health, the focus here is on these three major monoaminergic neurons.

Serotonergic neurons are located mainly in the area of the brain stem called the *nucleus raphe*. Pathways originating in the nucleus raphe project across the cerebral cortex, limbic system, hypothalamus, basal ganglia, and brain stem. These pathways contribute to mood, emotion, appetite, sleep, movement, sexual function, responses to stress, and cognition.

Noradrenergic neurons are located in the central and peripheral nervous systems. Central noradrenergic neurons originate in the brain stem; they send projections to various parts of the brain, including the cerebral cortex, hippocampus, cerebellum, amygdala, and hypothalamus, and play a role in attention, memory, information processing, and sleep/wakefulness. Peripheral noradrenergic neurons are involved in the "fight or flight" response, acting on alpha and beta receptors as well as adipose cells.

Dopaminergic neurons are located in the substantia nigra, the medial mesencephalic tegmentum, and the hypothalamus. Dopamine is involved in mood, attention, memory, sleep/

• BOX 34.2   DSM-5 Criteria for Bipolar I Disorder

DSM-5 Criteria for Bipolar I Disorder

For a diagnosis of bipolar I disorder, it is necessary to meet the following criteria for a manic episode. The manic episode may have been preceded by and may be followed by hypomanic or major depressive episodes.

Manic Episode

A. A distinct period of abnormally and persistently elevated, expansive, or irritable mood and abnormally and persistently increased goal-directed activity or energy, lasting at least 1 week and present most of the day, nearly every day (or any duration if hospitalization is necessary).

B. During the period of mood disturbance and increased energy or activity, three (or more) of the following symptoms (four if the mood is only irritable) are present to a significant degree and represent a noticeable change from usual behavior:
1. Inflated self-esteem or grandiosity.
2. Decreased need for sleep (e.g., feels rested after only 3 hours of sleep).
3. More talkative than usual or pressure to keep talking.
4. Flight of ideas or subjective experience that thoughts are racing.
5. Distractibility (i.e., attention too easily drawn to unimportant or irrelevant external stimuli), as reported or observed.
6. Increase in goal-directed activity (either socially, at work or school, or sexually) or psychomotor agitation (i.e., purposeless non–goal-directed activity).
7. Excessive involvement in activities that have a high potential for painful consequences (e.g., engaging in unrestrained buying sprees, sexual indiscretions, or foolish business investments).

C. The mood disturbance is sufficiently severe to cause marked impairment in social or occupational functioning or to necessitate hospitalization to prevent harm to self or others, or there are psychotic features.

D. The episode is not attributable to the physiological effects of a substance (e.g., a drug of abuse, a medication, other treatment) or to another medical condition.

Note: A full manic episode that emerges during antidepressant treatment (e.g., medication, electroconvulsive therapy) but persists at a fully syndromal level beyond the physiological effect of that treatment is sufficient evidence for a manic episode and, therefore, a bipolar I diagnosis.

Note: Criteria A through D constitute a manic episode. At least one lifetime manic episode is required for the diagnosis of bipolar I disorder.

From American Psychiatric Association. (2013). Diagnostic and statistical manual of mental disorders (5th ed.). Washington, DC: Author.

---

wakefulness, and pleasure and reward and also has an effect on movement. The role of dopaminergic pathways is discussed in greater detail in Chapter 36, Thyroid Medications.

Pathophysiology

Multiple factors may contribute to the onset of depressive symptoms and the diagnosis of depression. Genetic, environmental, psychological, socioeconomic, and neurochemical etiologies have been proposed, thereby increasing the complexity of diagnosis and treatment. The vast majority of pharmacologic interventions are directed toward neurochemical etiologies, particularly related to serotonin, norepinephrine, and dopamine. Currently, the role of inflammatory cytokines in depression is being studied and may guide certain therapies.

The most common hypothesis associated with the diagnosis of depression as it relates to pharmacologic treatment is the *monoamine deficiency hypothesis*, which essentially says that depression is a result of an insufficient amount of at least one monoamine: serotonin, norepinephrine, or dopamine. The theory suggests that increasing the availability of these neurotransmitters results in decreased symptoms of depression. The most common antidepressants affect serotonin, norepinephrine, and/or dopamine in varying degrees.

While the monoamine deficiency hypothesis is often used to explain the effects of antidepressants, it does not explain the latency period between the initiation of therapy

and the effects of the medication. Alternate hypotheses are proposed to better explain the pathophysiology of major depressive disorder and responses to antidepressant medications. For example, the *neuroplasticity hypothesis* suggests that chronic stress and increased glucocorticoids may cause atrophy of neurons in the hippocampus, while the *neurogenesis hypothesis* suggests that chronic stress decreases the development of new neurons in the hippocampus. Chronically elevated glucocorticoid levels over time decrease the volume of the hippocampus, whether by atrophy of mature neurons or impairment in the development of new neurons. As the hippocampus is reduced in volume, there is failure of the negative feedback on the hypothalamic-pituitary-adrenal axis (HPAA), further increasing glucocorticoid levels. These hypotheses help explain depression and provide routes for improved pharmacologic intervention.

Bipolar illness is characterized by significant shifts in mood that cycle between symptoms of depression and mania. While the severity of symptoms may vary, bipolar illness can significantly affect mood, energy, and behavior as well as overall quality of life. In addition, patients with bipolar illness are at increased risk for suicidal ideation and suicide.

The pathophysiology of bipolar illness is poorly understood. It is considered to be caused by a variety of complex factors, including genetic, immunologic, neurobiological, and environmental stressors. Abnormalities in the amygdala and prefrontal cortex may also be a factor.

Antidepressant Therapy

Antidepressants are among the most widely prescribed medications in the United States. In fact, they are the third most used drug class behind antihyperlipidemic agents and analgesics (National Center for Health Statistics, 2019). Antidepressants are generally considered effective for moderate to severe depression and are sometimes recommended in cases of mild depression. According to the Centers for Disease Control and Prevention (CDC), from 2011 through 2014, nearly 13% of people age 12 or older reported taking an antidepressant in the previous month, with long-term antidepressant use most common (Pratt et al., 2017). In addition, 25% of those who had taken antidepressants in the previous month had taken them for more than 10 years. More recently, Brody and Gu (2020) reported that slightly over 13% of adults 18 years of age and older had taken antidepressants with the previous 30 days, with use higher among women (17.7%) than men (8.4%). Use of antidepressants was higher in non-Hispanic Whites (16.6%) than in non-Hispanic Blacks (7.8%), Hispanics (6.5%), and non-Hispanic Asians (2.8%).

When prescribing an antidepressant, the primary care provider should consider several factors, including the patient's and their family's history of using specific antidepressants, the side-effect profile of the medication, adverse events associated with the medication, potential drug interactions with the patient's current medications, and the patient's ability to adhere to the plan of care.

Potential Adverse Effects Associated With Antidepressant Therapy

Increased Risk of Suicidal Ideation and Suicide Associated With Antidepressant Therapy

In the early 2000s, the U.S. Food and Drug Administration (FDA) issued a black box warning regarding the increased risk of suicidal ideation and suicide in children, adolescents, and young adults who use antidepressants. The risk is considered greatest within the first few months of therapy. It is important to recognize that there has been significant controversy regarding the continuation of the black box warning. In fact, the warning was modified slightly in 2007 to recognize that depression itself is associated with increased risk of suicide. Also, some fear that, out of an abundance of caution, primary care providers may underprescribe antidepressants to those who may benefit from their use (Fornero et al., 2019). Nevertheless, at the time of this writing, unless otherwise noted, all antidepressants carry a black box warning for suicidal ideation and suicide risk.

Cautious use of antidepressants is not limited to the young. The federal Omnibus Budget Reconciliation Act (OBRA) regulates the use of antidepressants in residents of long-term care facilities and requires that all such residents receiving antidepressants be monitored closely for worsening of depression and suicidal behavior or thinking, especially during initiation of therapy and during dose changes.

BLACK BOX WARNING!

Suicide Risk With Antidepressant Therapy

The FDA issued a black box warning regarding the increased risk of suicidal ideation and suicide in children, adolescents, and young adults who are prescribed antidepressants. The risk is increased early in therapy. The FDA recommends that all patients being treated for depression be monitored for clinical worsening, suicidality, and/or unusual changes in behavior, particularly during the first few months of therapy and at times of dosage change (increase or decrease).

Careful assessment, monitoring, and follow-up is important when prescribing antidepressants.

Serotonin Syndrome and Antidepressant Therapy

Serotonin syndrome is a potentially fatal condition that results from an overabundance of serotonin. Toxic levels of serotonin can result from combinations of serotonergic medications, drug abuse, or additional agents such as St. John's wort (Box 34.3). These substances can induce serotonin syndrome via a number of mechanisms. For example, tryptophan can increase serotonin synthesis, monoamine oxidase inhibitors (MAOIs) can decrease metabolism of serotonin, and drugs such as cocaine and amphetamines can increase the release of serotonin. Lithium and opiates can activate $5HT_1$ receptors, selective serotonin reuptake inhibitors (SSRIs) can inhibit 5HT uptake, and several second-generation antipsychotics can antagonize $5\text{-}HT_{2A}$ receptors. All of these conditions can result in toxic concentrations of serotonin.

The likeliest cause of serotonin syndrome in mood disorder therapy is combination therapy of drugs from differing classes, particularly SSRIs, MAOIs, and serotonin norepinephrine reuptake inhibitors (SNRIs). Furthermore, second-generation antipsychotics, opiates, and St. John's

•BOX 34.3 Medications That Can Increase the Risk for Serotonin Syndrome

- Nonselective and irreversible MAOI A and B (e.g., Isocarboxazid, Isoniazid, Phenelzine)
- Nonselective and reversible MAOI A and B (e.g., Linezolid)
- Selective and irreversible MAOI B (e.g., Selegiline [nonselective at higher doses] Rasagiline)
- Selective and reversible MAOI A (e.g., Moclobemide Methylene blue)
- SSRIs (e.g., paroxetine, escitalopram, fluoxetine)
- SNRIs (e.g., Venlafaxine, desvenlafaxine, duloxetine)
- TCAs (e.g., Clomipramine, imipramine)
- Select opioids and other pain medications (e.g., tramadol, meperidine, methadone, fentanyl)
- Cough, cold and allergy (e.g., Dextromethorphan ["DM"], chlorpheniramine)
- Natural health products (including St. John's wort, L-tryptophan, diet pills)
- Illicit drugs (including Ecstasy [MDMA], amphetamine, cocaine

Adapted from Foong, A. L., Grindrod, K. A., Patel, T., & Kellar, J. (2018). Demystifying serotonin syndrome (or serotonin toxicity). *Can Fam Phys* 64(10), 720–727.

Mild	Moderate	Late
Anxiety	Agitation/restlessness	Confusion/delirium
Insomnia	Hyperreflexia	Fever (>38.5°C)
Mydriasis	Hyperthermia	Rhabdomyolysis
Tremor	Flushing	Muscle rigidity
Nausea/vomiting	Diaphoresis	Seizures
Diarrhea	Hyperthermia (<38.5°C)	
Elevated blood pressure	Myoclonus	
Tachycardia		

Adapted from Foong, A. L., Grindrod, K. A., Patel, T., & Kellar, J. (2018). Demystifying serotonin syndrome (or serotonin toxicity). *Can Fam Phys*, 64(10), 720–727; Bartlett, D. (2017). Drug-induced serotonin syndrome. *Crit Care Nurse*, 37[1], 49–54. http://doi.org/10.4037/ccn2017169; and Scotton, W. J., Hill, L. J., Williams, A. C., & Barnes, N. M. (2019). Serotonin syndrome: Pathophysiology, clinical features, management, and potential future directions. *Int J Tryptophan Res*, 12, 1178646919873925-1178646919873925. http://doi.org/10.1177/1178646919873925.

wort are associated with serotonin syndrome when used in combination with other serotonergic drugs.

Symptoms associated with serotonin syndrome range from mild to deadly. Patients typically present with a mental status change ranging from anxiety to agitation, delirium, or even coma, as well as neuromuscular symptoms ranging from mild tremor to sustained clonus or cogwheel rigidity and autonomic symptoms such as diarrhea, diaphoresis, or hyperthermia that may be severe (Box 34.4) These symptoms typically arise within several hours to one day after increasing the dose of a current medication or adding an additional medication that increases serotonin. A thorough patient history can help the primary care provider differentiate from other disorders such as anticholinergic toxicity, antidepressant withdrawal symptoms, and neuroleptic malignant syndrome. Patients with moderate to severe symptoms should be referred to a hospital immediately for supportive treatment as symptoms can progress rapidly.

QUALITY AND SAFETY

MAOIs and Risk of Serotonin Syndrome

Combining MAOIs with SSRIs, SNRIs, tricyclic antidepressants, St. John's wort, or any other drugs that affect serotonin should be separated by at least 14 days to avoid the risk of serotonin syndrome.

Hyponatremia and Antidepressant Therapy

Although relatively infrequent, hyponatremia may occur in patients taking antidepressants. Older adults are at a higher risk, particularly if they are taking sodium-depleting diuretics or are dehydrated. The risk of hyponatremia is considered higher within the first 2 to 4 weeks of therapy, with the risk decreasing over time (Lien, 2018). Hyponatremia

with sodium levels as low as 110 mmol/L may occur as a result of inappropriate antidiuretic hormone secretion. The risk for hyponatremia is considered higher with the use of SSRIs and SNRIs than with tricyclic antidepressants (TCAs) and noradrenergic and specific serotonergic antidepressants. Signs and symptoms associated with hyponatremia include headache, impaired memory, weakness, restlessness, and confusion. Patients with severe hyponatremia may experience hallucinations, seizures, coma, and even death.

Sexual Dysfunction and Antidepressant Therapy

Sexual dysfunction is a common adverse effect associated with antidepressant therapy that can have a significant effect on quality of life as well as increase nonadherence to therapy. The highest risk for sexual dysfunction is with the serotonergic antidepressants, such as SSRIs and SNRIs. The extent of sexual dysfunction can vary between and within classes of medications, so it is important to provide patients with information regarding the potential for sexual dysfunction and to maintain open communication with patients to ensure the reporting of symptoms. Symptoms can include decreased libido, decreased or diminished orgasm, erectile dysfunction, or ejaculation delay or dysfunction. One drug, bupropion SR, has consistently been shown to be relatively free of sexual side effects, so it may be an option for patients who have been significantly affected by serotonergic antidepressants.

Antidepressants and Underlying Bipolar Illness

The use of antidepressants in patients with underlying bipolar disorder can precipitate mania or hypomania. Because depression may be the presenting symptom of bipolar illness, it is important to carefully screen patients with bipolar disorder prior to beginning antidepressant therapy. Screening should include a detailed patient and family history of any mental illness or suicide. In addition, if after beginning antidepressant therapy, the patient exhibits symptoms of mania or hypomania, discontinue the antidepressant and refer the patient to specialty practitioners for further diagnosis and treatment.

QUALITY AND SAFETY

Antidepressants and Mania or Hypomania

Antidepressants can precipitate hypomania or mania in susceptible individuals. A thorough history is important to determine whether the patient has a history of symptoms associated with hypomania or mania. The Mood Disorder Questionnaire (MDQ) may be useful in evaluating patient symptoms (Hirschfeld et al., 2000).

Major classes of antidepressants include SSRIs, SNRIs, norepinephrine and dopamine reuptake inhibitors, serotonin modulators, and TCAs (Table 34.1). One category, MAOIs, is used far less frequently due to the need for severe dietary restrictions and the potential for serious adverse effects. As such, use of MAOIs should be reserved for treatment-resistant depression in consultation with a specialty practitioner.

TABLE 34.1 Antidepressants

Category/Medication	Indication	Dosage	Considerations and Monitoring
Selective Serotonin Reuptake Inhibitors			
Fluoxetine	Major depression	**Oral dosage (immediate-release capsules, tablets, or oral solution):** *Adults:* Begin with 20 mg/day, may increase by 10–20 mg after several weeks as needed and tolerated. Maximum dosage: 80 mg/day. *Children and adolescents 8–17 yr:* Begin with 10–20 mg orally once daily. Lower-weight children begin with 10 mg/day. Usual effective dosage: 10–20 mg/day. Maximum dosage: 60 mg/day. **Once-weekly maintenance treatment of depression:** *Adults:* 90 mg orally once weekly, beginning 7 days after last 20-mg daily dose.	Ideal for those in whom compliance is an issue. Longest half-life of any antidepressant. Less likely to experience discontinuation syndrome. Full effects may take 4 weeks or longer. Final guidance on length of therapy is available using APA Clinical Practice Guidelines. Monitor for hyponatremia with SSRIs. Use with caution in those with anorexia nervosa or those in which weight loss is undesired.
Paroxetine (Paxil)	Major depressive disorder	**Oral dosage (immediate-release formulations):** *Adults:* 20 mg once daily initially, usually in the morning. Increase as needed in 10-mg increments in, at minimum, once-weekly intervals. Maximum dosage: 50 mg/day. *Older or debilitated adults:* 10 mg once daily initially, may increase if needed by 10 mg in, at minimum, once-weekly intervals. Maximum dosage: 40 mg/day. **Oral dosage (controlled-release formulations):** *Adults:* 25 mg once daily initially, usually in the morning. May increase if needed in 12.5-mg increments in, at minimum, once-weekly intervals. Maximum dosage: 62.5 mg/day. *Older or debilitated adults:* 12.5 mg once daily initially. May increase by 12.5 mg in, at minimum, once-weekly intervals. Maximum dosage: 50 mg/day orally.	Periodically reassess the need for continued treatment. Monitor weight. Paroxetine is not FDA approved for use in children and adolescents younger than 18 years of age.
Sertraline (Zoloft)	Major depressive disorder	**Oral dosage:** *Adults:* 50 mg once daily. Lower initial dose may be used to minimize adverse effects. If necessary, increase at intervals of not less than 1 week. Maximum dosage: 200 mg/day orally.	Periodically reassess the need for continued treatment. Use with caution in those with history of seizure disorder. Dosage adjustments are recommended in patients with hepatic disease. Caution is recommended when prescribing to patients with closed-angle glaucoma.

Continued

TABLE 34.1   Antidepressants—cont'd

Category/Medication	Indication	Dosage	Considerations and Monitoring
Citalopram (Celexa)	Major depressive disorder	**Oral dosage:** *Adults ≤60 yr:* 20 mg once daily initially. Increase in increments of 20 mg at intervals of no less than 1 week based on response and tolerability. Maximum dosage: 40 mg/day in the general population and 20 mg/day in poor metabolizers of CYP 2C19 due to the potential for QT prolongation. *Adults >60 yr:* 20 mg orally once daily is the recommended and maximum dosage.	Periodically reassess the need for continued treatment. Not indicated for any condition in pediatric patients younger than 18 years of age. Higher dosages are not recommended due to an association with QT prolongation.
Escitalopram (Lexapro)	Major depressive disorder	**Oral dosage:** *Adults:* 10 mg once daily is the initial and recommended dose. May be increased to 20 mg once daily after a minimum of 1 week. Maximum dosage: 20 mg/day. *Older adults:* 10 mg once daily is the initial and recommended dose. *Children and adolescents 12–17 yr:* 10 mg once daily is the initial and recommended dose. If clinically indicated, may increase to 20 mg once daily after a minimum of 3 weeks.	Periodically reassess the need for continued treatment. Should be used with caution in patients with a history of seizure disorder.
Serotonin Modulators			
Vilazodone	Major depressive disorder	*Adults:* 10 mg orally once daily with food for 7 days, then 20 mg once daily with food for 7 days. Then may increase after a minimum of 7 days between dosage increases. Target dosage: 20–40 mg once daily with food. Maximum dosage: 40 mg/day.	Use cautiously in patients with hepatic disease due to extensive metabolism.
Serotonin Norepinephrine Reuptake Inhibitors			
Desvenlafaxine	Major depressive disorder	*Adults:* 50 mg orally once daily initially. Dose range: 50–400 mg/day. An additional benefit has not been observed with doses >50 mg/day. Maximum dosage: 400 mg/day. Reduced doses may be advisable in older adults.	False-positive urine drug screen may occur for amphetamine or phencyclidine in patients who have received desvenlafaxine. Monitor blood pressure regularly.
Duloxetine	Major depressive disorder	20 mg orally twice daily. Target maintenance dosage: 60 mg/day.	Contraindicated in patients with uncontrolled closed-angle glaucoma. Avoid use in patients with chronic hepatic disease or cirrhosis. Use caution in older adults; can cause orthostatic hypotension.
Levomilnacipran	Major depression	Initially, 20 mg orally daily for 2 days, then increase to 40 mg daily. Recommended dose range: 40–120 mg once daily, with or without food. Maximum dosage: 120 mg orally once daily.	Monitor for hyponatremia. Dosage adjustments are recommended in patients with moderate (CrCl: 30–59 mL/min) or severe (CrCl: 15–29 mL/min) renal impairment. Not approved for use in those younger than 18 years of age. Not studied in those who are pregnant or breastfeeding.

TABLE 34.1	Antidepressants—cont'd			

Category/Medication	Indication	Dosage	Considerations and Monitoring
Venlafaxine	Major depression	75 mg orally daily in 2 or 3 divided doses initially. Typically started at 37.5 mg to assess tolerability. If needed, may increase by 75 mg orally daily at intervals no less than every 4 days. Maximum dosage: 225 mg/day in divided doses.	May cause false-positive urine drug screen for amphetamine or phencyclidine. Safety and efficacy not established in those younger than 18 years of age. Monitor blood pressure regularly. Dosage reductions are recommended in all stages of renal impairment.
Norepinephrine Dopamine Reuptake Inhibitor			
Buproprion	Major depression	**Immediate-release tablets:** *Adults:* 100 mg orally twice daily. May increase to three times daily with no single dose >150 mg. **Sustained-release tablets:** *Adults:* 150 mg orally in the morning; titrate to 150 mg twice daily after minimum of 4 days. May gradually increase to 150–200 mg twice daily. **Extended-release tablets:** *Adults:* 150 mg once daily in the morning. After a minimum of 4 days, may increase to 300 mg once daily. Maximum dosage: 450 mg once daily.	Antidepressant effect typically occurs within 1–3 weeks, with maximal effects at approximately 4 weeks. Use lowest dose that maintains remission of depressive symptoms. Contraindicated in those with seizure disorder or conditions that increase the risk of seizure. Monitor weight during therapy.
	Prevention of seasonal major depressive disorder episodes	**Extended-release tablets:** Begin treatment in the autumn, with 150 mg orally once daily in the morning. May increase to 300 mg daily through the winter season. Taper during the early spring.	Monitor for worsening tics or Tourette's disorder. Use with caution during pregnancy; use during pregnancy only if the potential benefit justifies the potential risk to the fetus. Useful in smoking cessation and weight loss.
Nonadrenergic and Specific Serotonergic Antidepressants			
Mirtazepine	Major depression	15 mg orally once daily at bedtime initially. If needed, may increase no sooner than every 1–2 weeks. Effective dosage range: 15–45 mg daily. Maximum dosage: 45 mg/day. Older adults may need slower titration schedules.	Sedating effects may be helpful in treating depression-associated insomnia. Regular monitoring of CBC, LFTs, and creatinine/BUN. Appetite stimulant; helpful in those with poor appetite associated with depression. Not FDA approved for use in children or adolescents. Increased plasma concentrations can occur in patients with moderate and severe renal impairment. Use cautiously in patients with hypercholesterolemia or hypertriglyceridemia.

Continued

TABLE 34.1   Antidepressants—cont'd

Category/Medication	Indication	Dosage	Considerations and Monitoring
Serotonin Antagonist and Reuptake Inhibitor			
Trazodone	Major depression	*Adults:* Begin with 150 mg orally daily in divided doses. May increase by 50 mg/day every 3–4 days as tolerated. Maximum dosage: 400 mg/day. Older adults may require lower doses to start.	Monitor blood pressure, heart rate, and thyroid function. Safety and efficacy not established in those younger than 18 years of age. Prolongs the QT/QTc interval.
Tricyclic Antidepressant			
Amitriptyline	Major depression	*Adults:* Begin with 75 mg orally daily in divided doses or 50–100 mg once daily at bedtime. For outpatients, may increase the daily dose 25 mg to 50 mg at weekly intervals, with maximum dosage 150 mg/day. *Older adults:* 10–25 mg orally at bedtime initially. Titrate slowly as tolerated. Maintenance dosage: 50–100 mg daily. In some patients, 40 mg/day orally.	Use lowest effective dose. Avoid in patients with cardiovascular disease. Safety and efficacy not established in those younger than 12 years of age. Can cause significant sedation. Use with extreme caution in those with seizure disorder. Discontinue several days before elective surgery because of the risk of adverse reactions during surgery. May have significant anticholinergic effects, especially in older adults. May be more prone to sunburn.
Nortriptyline	Major depressive disorder	*Adults:* 25–50 mg orally daily in divided doses or once daily at bedtime. May be increased if needed to maximum dosage of 150 mg/day. *Older adults:* 10–25 mg orally at bedtime. May increase to 30–50 mg daily in divided doses or once daily at bedtime.	Contraindicated in those in active recovery phase of MI. Discontinue several days before elective surgery because of the risk of adverse reactions during surgery.

APA, American Psychiatric Association; *BUN,* blood urea nitrogen; *CBC,* complete blood count; *CrCl,* creatinine clearance; *FDA,* U.S. Food and Drug Administration; *LFT,* liver function test; *MI,* myocardial infarction; *SSRIs,* selective serotonin reuptake inhibitors.

Medication Categories

Selective Serotonin Reuptake Inhibitors

Selective serotonin reuptake inhibitors (SSRIs) are the medications most widely used to treat major depression and anxiety disorders. While SSRIs are similar in efficacy to many other antidepressants, they are much safer and more easily tolerated than the first-generation antidepressants, including TCAs and MAOIs.

SSRIs increase the amount of serotonin (also called 5-hydroxytryptamine or 5HT) available in the synaptic space by inhibiting the reuptake of serotonin by the serotonin transporter (SERT) at the presynaptic axon terminal. As a result, increased serotonin is available to stimulate postsynaptic receptors. In addition, serotonin autoreceptors are down regulated and desensitized, resulting in increased serotonin release in the axon terminals. SSRIs have fewer anticholinergic, antihistaminic, and cardiovascular effects than TCAs.

Beyond treatment of depression, select SSRIs have been approved for use in treating generalized anxiety disorder, posttraumatic stress disorder (PTSD), panic disorder, social anxiety disorder, obsessive-compulsive disorder, premenstrual dysphoric disorder, hot flashes, and premature ejaculation. When prescribing an SSRI, primary care providers should base their choice on such factors as drug interactions and the patient's response history to select SSRIs.

The most common adverse effect in patients taking SSRIs is mild to moderate nausea, particularly during the first 2 weeks of therapy. Additional gastrointestinal (GI) effects include dry mouth, dyspepsia, diarrhea or constipation, and loss of appetite. These symptoms often are alleviated by taking the medication with food.

TABLE 34.2	Common Symptoms of Antidepressant Withdrawal	
Somatic	**Psychological**
Dizziness	Anxiety
Light-headedness	Insomnia
Shocklike sensations	Irritability
Paresthesia	Decreased concentration
Fatigue	Hypomania
Headache	Mood swings
Nausea	Suicidal thoughts
Diarrhea	Nervousness
Visual disturbances	Anger outbursts
Tremors	Insomnia
Tachycardia	Nightmares
Hypertension or hypotension	Depression
Flushing	

From Foreman, R. M., Zappas, M., & Whitely, C. (2020). Antidepressant withdrawal: A guide for primary care clinicians. *Journal for Nurse Practitioners, 16*[3], 191–194. http://doi.org/10.1016/j.nurpra.2019.12.013.

Other adverse effects associated with SSRIs include sexual dysfunction, QT prolongation (except for paroxetine), impaired platelet aggregation, hyponatremia, and dermatologic/hypersensitivity reactions. There may be an increased risk of osteoporotic bone fractures. Infants born to mothers taking SSRIs may experience neonatal abstinence syndrome.

SSRIs carry a black box warning regarding the risk of increased suicidal thoughts/suicidal ideation in children and young adults, particularly during the first few months of therapy. Careful screening and monitoring of suicidality is required. Sudden discontinuation of SSRIs may result in withdrawal symptoms such as nausea, dizziness, tremor, fatigue, irritability, and headaches (Table 34.2). The symptoms are more likely in SSRIs with a shorter half-life. Symptoms typically begin within 1 to 3 days of discontinuing and may last for up to 2 weeks. Slow tapering of the dose can minimize these symptoms.

Fluoxetine

Pharmacokinetics. Fluoxetine is administered orally and absorbed by the GI tract, with achievement of steady state in approximately 3 to 4 weeks. While food can slightly delay absorption, it does not affect the degree of absorption. Fluoxetine is highly protein bound (approximately 95%) and well distributed, and is demethylated in the liver to several metabolites that can be excreted by the kidneys. Fluoxetine is a potent inhibitor of cytochrome (CYP) 2D6 and CYP 2C19 and a weak inhibitor of CYP 3A4 and CYP 2C9. The half-life is typically about 4 to 6 days and as long as 7 to 12 days in patients with liver impairment. While older adults metabolize fluoxetine similarly to younger adults, lower or less frequent dosages are recommended.

Indications. Fluoxetine can be used in the treatment of major depression in daily or weekly forms. It can also be used

in combination with olanzapine (a second-generation antipsychotic) in the treatment of treatment-resistant depression or for the acute treatment of depressive episodes of bipolar I depression. Of note, fluoxetine can also be used for the treatment of obsessive-compulsive disorder and panic disorder.

Adverse Effects. The most common adverse effects include nausea, anorexia, dyspepsia, diarrhea, and xerostomia (more than 10% of patients). Other common adverse effects include anxiety, insomnia, asthenia, and headache. Sexual side effects can include decreased libido (1% to 11%), erectile dysfunction (2% to 7%), and ejaculation dysfunction (2% to 7%). Increased appetite and weight gain can occur (1%). Prolongation of the QT interval as well as ventricular dysrhythmias are uncommon. Palpitations, chest pain, and hypertension have occurred in 1% or more of patients. Hypothyroidism was reported in 0.1% to 1.0% of patients during premarketing testing. Increased risk of bleeding may occur due to impaired platelet aggregation in rare cases.

Contraindications. Fluoxetine is contraindicated in patients taking MAOIs due to the risk of serotonin syndrome. It should be used with caution in patients with a history of seizure disorder, hepatic disease, or QT prolongation and ventricular dysrhythmias.

Monitoring. For patients at risk for QT prolongation, baseline and periodic electrocardiogram (ECG) assessments are recommended. Monitor weight and blood pressure regularly. Thyroid function tests may be indicated in some patients.

Sertraline

Pharmacokinetics. Sertraline is administered orally and undergoes extensive first-pass metabolism. Single-dose bioavailability of the tablets is generally equal to an equivalent dose of oral solution. While sertraline is highly protein bound, its presumed binding site is the alpha-1 glycoprotein rather than albumin. As a result, sertraline does not compete with warfarin or propranolol for binding sites. Sertraline is metabolized by several CYP 450 enzymes, and in general, inhibition of one enzyme by another drug is not considered to affect sertraline concentrations. Sertraline does inhibit CYP 2D6 in vivo; therefore it may be necessary to reduce the dosage of concomitant drugs that are metabolized by CYP 2D6. Average half-life is 26 hours.

Indications. Sertraline can be used in the treatment of major depression and premenstrual dysphoric disorder in adults. It can also be used to treat PTSD.

Adverse Effects. The most common adverse effects associated with sertraline are GI related and include diarrhea, nausea, anorexia, and dry mouth. Other common adverse effects are insomnia, drowsiness, and fatigue. Sexual side effects include ejaculation dysfunction, decreased libido, and orgasm dysfunction. Visual side effects including mydriasis, blurred vision, and ocular hypertension have also been reported in patients taking sertraline. Neonatal abstinence syndrome has been reported in infants exposed to sertraline in utero.

Contraindications. Sertraline is contraindicated in patients who are receiving or expect to receive MAOI therapy within a

14-day window to avoid serotonin syndrome. Caution should be used in patients who have a suspected history of mania or hypomania, as use of antidepressants may trigger manic symptoms. Sertraline should be avoided in patients who are taking disulfiram due to the alcohol content of the concentrate formulation. Use caution in patients with a history of seizure disorder and in patients receiving electroconvulsive therapy. Use with caution in older adults who may be at risk for hyponatremia, such as those taking diuretics or who are prone to dehydration.

Sertraline should be used cautiously in patients at risk for cardiovascular dysrhythmias due to the potential for QT prolongation. Avoid in patients with osteoporosis due to increased risk of bone fracture. Dosage adjustments may be needed in patients with liver disease.

Sertraline is not recommended for use during pregnancy. Infants who were exposed to sertraline in utero have been reported to experience neonatal abstinence syndrome. Sertraline has been found in low levels in breast milk. While no adverse effects have been found in small studies, it is important to monitor the infant for adverse effects and for careful evaluation of the risk/benefits to the health of the mother vs. the health of the infant.

PRACTICE PEARLS

Antidepressant Use in Lactation

Use of sertraline, paroxetine, or nortriptyline by patients who are breastfeeding has resulted in undetectable or low concentrations in the serum of the breastfed infants. As a result, these medications may be the best choices after considering risks and benefits to the health of the mother vs. the health of the infant.

Monitoring. As with other SSRIs, patients should be monitored for hyponatremia and increased risk for bleeding. In addition, monitor for symptoms of mania or hypomania in patients who may have undiagnosed bipolar disorder.

Citalopram

Pharmacokinetics. Citalopram is well absorbed after oral administration. Peak plasma concentrations are attained about 4 hours after dosing. Citalopram is metabolized by the liver. A lower maximum daily dosage is recommended in patients who are poor metabolizers of CYP 2C19 or who are receiving a CYP 2C19 inhibitor due to dose-dependent QT prolongation. Steady-state plasma concentrations are achieved within approximately 1 week.

Indications. Citalopram is used to treat major depression.

Adverse Effects. The most common adverse effects are drowsiness, xerostomia, nausea, and insomnia. Approximately 11% of patients experienced hyperhidrosis in clinical trials. Other infrequent adverse effects include anorexia, diarrhea, nausea and vomiting, and anxiety. Sexual side effects include ejaculation dysfunction (about 6%), decreased libido (1.3%), and anorgasmia (1.1%). Although rare, citalopram can cause

cardiovascular adverse effects such as cardiac dysrhythmias (including cardiac arrest), changes in blood pressure (hypotension or hypertension as well as orthostatic hypotension), chest pain, myocardial infarction, and heart failure. Citalopram can cause dose-dependent QT prolongation.

Contraindications. Citalopram is contraindicated in patients who have experienced any hypersensitivity to citalopram or escitalopram. It is contraindicated in patients who have been or will be on MAOI therapy within a 14-day window to avoid serotonin syndrome. Citalopram is not recommended for patients who have or are at increased risk for QT prolongation. Ensure adequate levels of potassium and magnesium prior to and during therapy with citalopram. Use the lowest doses in patients who are 60 years of age or older or who have liver impairment.

PHARMACOGENETICS

Citalopram

Use caution when prescribing citalopram to patients who are poor metabolizers of CYP 2C19 or who are receiving CYP 2C19 inhibitors due to the risk of QT prolongation. Use the lower maximum daily dose and monitor the patient carefully.

Monitoring. Due to the risk of QT prolongation, ECG monitoring is recommended while patients are taking citalopram to treat depression. Citalopram should be discontinued in patients who experience persistent QTc measurements above 500 ms. Ensure adequate potassium and magnesium.

Serotonin Norepinephrine Reuptake Inhibitors

Serotonin norepinephrine reuptake inhibitors (SNRIs) are similar in overall effectiveness to SSRIs in managing depression. The major difference is their effect on inhibiting the reuptake of serotonin and norepinephrine. Various medications within the SNRI class differ in their affinity for serotonin vs. norepinephrine receptors. For example, venlafaxine has a 30 times higher affinity for serotonin reuptake inhibition than norepinephrine, while milnacipran has a three times greater affinity for norepinephrine than serotonin. Their effect on norepinephrine receptors is hypothesized to explain the effectiveness of SNRIs in the treatment of chronic pain.

The most common adverse reaction in SNRIs is nausea, which is typically transient in nature. Other GI effects include dry mouth, constipation, and vomiting. Other common effects associated with this class include headache, dizziness, and insomnia; these rarely result in discontinuation of treatment.

QUALITY AND SAFETY

Drug Interactions: Linezolid

Linezolid, an antibiotic that may be used in community-acquired pneumonia, is also a nonselective MAOI. Use of linezolid with serotonergic drugs such as SSRIs, SNRIs, TCAs, and MAOIs may result in severe serotonin syndrome.

Venlafaxine

Pharmacokinetics. Venlafaxine is given orally and is well absorbed in the GI tract. Food does not affect absorption. Venlafaxine is extensively metabolized in the liver. Medications that potently inhibit both CYP 2D6 and CYP 3A4 may increase the risk of toxicity. Elimination occurs primarily by the kidneys. Dosage adjustments are required in patients with decreased renal function.

Indications. Venlafaxine can be used to treat major depression. In addition, it has been used to treat general anxiety disorder, social phobia, and panic disorder.

Adverse Effects. The most common adverse effects are nausea, headache, and dose-dependent weight loss (up to 47% of patients). Others include insomnia, xerostomia, and dizziness. Sexual side effects include ejaculation dysfunction (up to 19%) and impotence (up to 6%) in males and orgasm dysfunction (2% to 5%) in females. Dose-depended hypertension has occurred in as many as 13% of patients. Cardiovascular abnormalities including QT prolongation, tachycardia, bradycardia, ventricular dysrhythmias, angina pectoris, and myocardial infarction are rare. Rapid withdrawal of venlafaxine has resulted in seizures.

Contraindications. Venlafaxine is contraindicated in patients receiving MAOIs. Use cautiously in patients with a history of seizures. Older patients, patients taking diuretics, and those prone to dehydration may be at greater risk for hyponatremia. Use cautiously in patients with hypertension due to the risk of increased blood pressure. Avoid in patients with a history of or a family history of long QT syndrome and in patients with conditions that may increase the risk of QT prolongation. Dosage reductions are recommended in patients with liver or renal impairment.

Monitoring. Patients who are receiving venlafaxine should be monitored for increased blood pressure and heart rate, especially after beginning therapy and with dosage increases. If elevated levels occur, patients may require a dosage reduction or even discontinuation of venlafaxine. Furthermore, due to the risk of decreased platelet aggregation, monitor for increased bleeding. Avoid abrupt discontinuation of venlafaxine to prevent withdrawal symptoms.

Duloxetine

Pharmacokinetics. Duloxetine is well absorbed, administered orally, and widely distributed throughout the body. It is highly protein bound (over 90%). It is metabolized in the liver by CYP 2D6 and CYP 1A2. The mean half-life is approximately 12 hours. Duloxetine is primarily excreted as metabolites in the urine (70%) and feces (20%).

Indications. Duloxetine can be used to treat major depression and generalized anxiety disorder. It has also been used to effectively treat pain associated with diabetic neuropathy, fibromyalgia, and chronic musculoskeletal pain.

Adverse Effects. The most common adverse effects are nausea, headache, mild weight loss, and dry mouth. Other, less common adverse effects include drowsiness, fatigue, mild abdominal pain, and sexual side effects. Elevated liver enzymes and liver damage are possible, particularly in patients with a history of liver disease or cirrhosis.

Contraindications. Duloxetine is contraindicated in patients requiring MAOI therapy due to the risk of serotonin syndrome. It should not be used within 14 days of discontinuation of MAOIs. Avoid abrupt discontinuation of duloxetine due to the risk of withdrawal syndrome. Duloxetine is contraindicated in patients with uncontrolled closed-angle glaucoma and should be used cautiously in patients with controlled closed-angle glaucoma as it may increase the risk of mydriasis. Use caution in patients with preexisting hypotension as orthostatic hypotension and syncope may occur, particularly during the first week of treatment or after dose increases. Dosages above 60 mg/day and coadministration of antihypertensive medications or CYP 1A2 inhibitors increase the risk of hypotension. Avoid in patients with a history of seizure disorders. Duloxetine should not be prescribed to patients with chronic liver disease or cirrhosis, or to those who are heavy users of alcohol (or have alcoholism). Do not use duloxetine in patients with end-stage renal disease.

PRACTICE PEARLS

Life Span Considerations With SNRIs

SNRIs meet the Beers Criteria as potentially inappropriate medications for older adults. They should be avoided in those with a history of falls or fractures, unless safer alternatives are not available. If used, monitor for orthostatic hypotension and hyponatremia, both of which pose a greater risk to older adults.

There are no well-controlled studies on the use of duloxetine in pregnancy. Infants exposed to duloxetine in the last trimester may experience neonatal abstinence syndrome.

Monitoring. It is important to monitor blood pressure and pulse, especially with initiation of therapy and dosage increases, due to the risk of orthostatic hypotension. Teach caregivers to monitor for increased agitation, irritability, or unusual changes in behavior or signs of suicidality.

Norepinephrine and Dopamine Reuptake Inhibitors

Norepinephrine and dopamine reuptake inhibitors, as the name implies, are thought to act by blocking select norepinephrine and dopamine receptors located in the presynaptic neuron. This allows greater availability of norepinephrine and dopamine in the synaptic cleft for transmission to the postsynaptic neuron. In contrast to SSRIs, bupropion does not cause weight gain or sexual dysfunction, so it may be preferable for some patients. In addition, bupropion can be used to offset sexual side effects associated with SSRIs, and it does not have antihistamine or anticholinergic effects.

Bupropion

Pharmacokinetics. Bupropion is administered orally and may be taken with or without food. It is approximately

85% protein bound. Bupropion is metabolized in the liver into three active metabolites. While the half-life varies for each metabolite, the metabolites are typically excreted in the urine. Onset of action is usually within 1 to 3 weeks.

PHARMACOGENETICS

Bupropion

Bupropion is extensively metabolized by CYP 2B6. As a result, significant interactions are possible with drugs that are metabolized by or are inhibitors or inducers of CYP 2B6.

Indications. Bupropion is used to treat major depression and prevent depression associated with seasonal affective disorder, and has been used as an adjunct to psychosocial interventions for tobacco cessation.

Adverse Effects. Although rare, bupropion is associated with an increased risk of seizures. Seizure risk increases with doses over 450 mg/day. Common adverse effects include headache, insomnia, agitation, nausea, vomiting, and dry mouth. Bupropion has also been associated with anorexia and weight loss. Infrequently, patients may experience cardiovascular effects including hypertension or hypotension, palpitations, syncope, and chest pain.

Contraindications. Bupropion is contraindicated in patients with anorexia and bulimia nervosa, brain tumors or any intracranial mass, seizures, or seizure disorder. It should not be used in patients receiving MAOIs. It should be used cautiously in patients with an increased risk for seizures, such as those with substance use disorders or metabolic disorders or those who are using any medications that may lower the seizure threshold.

Monitoring. Patients may experience weight loss while taking bupropion. Monitor the patient for changes in blood pressure or ECG. To avoid insomnia, recommend that the patient take the medication in the morning.

Serotonin Modulator Antidepressants

Serotonin modulator antidepressants act by inhibiting the reuptake of serotonin as well as acting as partial agonists of postsynaptic $5HT_{1A}$ receptors. They are used as alternatives to SSRIs and SNRIs in the treatment of major depression. While the response rates of serotonin modulators are similar to those of SSRIs and SNRIs in the treatment of depression, they are less likely to be effective in the treatment of anxiety. The two main serotonin modulators are vilazodone and vortioxetine. Drug interactions that may occur are a result of metabolism by the CYP 450 isoenzymes. Vilazodone is metabolized by CYP 3A4 and vortioxetine by CYP 2D6. As a result, dosage adjustments may be required.

Adverse effects are similar to other serotonergic antidepressants and include nausea, dry mouth, diarrhea, and constipation. Central nervous system (CNS) effects include insomnia, restlessness, dizziness, and paresthesia. Rare adverse effects include impaired platelet aggregation and hyponatremia. Sexual dysfunction may occur in males and females. Like other antidepressants, serotonin modulators carry a black box warning regarding an increased risk of suicidal thoughts and behaviors in children, adolescents, and young adults.

Vilazodone

Pharmacokinetics. Vilazodone is administered orally, with peak concentrations occurring within about 4 to 5 hours. Bioavailability is enhanced when administered with food rather than on an empty stomach. Vilazodone is widely distributed, highly protein bound, and extensively metabolized in the liver by CYP 3A4. Concurrent use of strong CYP 3A4 inhibitors may result in a 50% increase in plasma concentrations, while concurrent use of strong CYP 3A4 inducers can decrease systemic exposure of the drug by about 45%. The half-life of vilazodone is approximately 25 hours. Excretion of unchanged vilazodone occurs through the urine and feces.

Indications. Vilazodone is used in the treatment of major depression in adults.

Adverse Effects. The most common adverse effects associated with vilazodone are mild diarrhea (28% of patients), nausea (23%), and headache (up to 15%). Sexual side effects occur in about 6% of patients. Sudden discontinuation of vilazodone can result in withdrawal symptoms. While vilazodone has not been associated with clinically significant effects on blood pressure, heart rate, or ECG, palpitations have occurred at higher dosages.

Contraindications. Vilazodone is contraindicated in patients receiving MAOI therapy. Patients should avoid alcohol while taking vilazodone. There are no adequate studies to determine the impact of vilazodone on pregnancy and breastfeeding; however, neonates exposed to serotonergic drugs in utero may experience neonatal abstinence syndrome. Risks and benefits of the use of antidepressants in pregnant and breastfeeding patients should be carefully evaluated.

Monitoring. Laboratory monitoring is not specifically required in patients taking vilazodone.

Noradrenergic and Specific Serotonergic Antidepressants

Noradrenergic and specific serotonergic antidepressants have chemical structures similar to TCAs. Originally introduced in the 1990s, these drugs are typically reserved for major depressive disorder that is not responsive to other agents. They have similar side effects to TCAs.

Mirtazapine

Pharmacokinetics. Mirtazapine is administered orally and may be given with or without food, with no significant effects on absorption. It is distributed by plasma proteins (approximately 85%) and is extensively metabolized by the liver. Half-life ranges from 20 to 40 hours, with females having significantly longer half-lives than males (37 vs. 26 hours, respectively). Elimination is primarily in the urine (75%), with about 15% via the feces. Dose reductions may be needed in older adults as well as those with liver or renal impairment.

Indications. Mirtazapine is indicated for the treatment of major depression.

Adverse Effects. The most common adverse effects are mild drowsiness (54% of patients) and mild weight gain (up to 49%) relating to histamine blockade associated with mirtazapine's effects. Others include hypercholesterolemia and hypertriglyceridemia. Mild xerostomia occurs in about 25% of patients. Although rare, bone marrow suppression with agranulocytosis was reported in patients during premarketing clinical trials.

Contraindications. Mirtazapine is contraindicated in patients who are taking MAOIs due to the risk of serotonin syndrome. Use with caution in patients with hypercholesterolemia or hypertriglyceridemia as well as in patients with renal or hepatic disease. Avoid abrupt discontinuation of mirtazapine due to the risk of withdrawal symptoms.

Monitoring. Laboratory work indicated for patients taking mirtazapine includes complete blood count (CBC) with differential, liver function tests (LFTs), and serum creatinine/blood urea nitrogen (BUN). Monitor lipid profile in at-risk patients. Advise patients that this medication may cause drowsiness, so they should avoid driving, using heavy machinery, or making major decisions until they are aware of the medication's effects.

Serotonin Antagonist and Reuptake Inhibitors

Serotonin antagonist and reuptake inhibitors (SARIs) block $5-HT_{2A}$ and/or $5-HT_{2C}$ receptors and inhibit reuptake of serotonin. In addition, SARIs typically have mild to moderate alpha and histamine receptor blocking action. Trazodone acts as a serotonin agonist at higher doses and as an antagonist at low doses.

Trazodone

Pharmacokinetics. Trazodone is well absorbed when given orally and may be given with food to decrease nausea. It is distributed highly protein bound. Trazodone is metabolized by the liver, primarily by CYP 3A4. As a result, concurrent use of CYP 3A4 inhibitors may require decreased doses of trazodone while concurrent use of CYP 3A4 inducers may require higher doses. Potent CYP 3A4 inhibitors may increase the risk of trazodone-associated cardiac arrhythmias. Elimination of trazodone is primarily through the urine.

Indications. Trazodone is indicated for adults with major depression.

Adverse Effects. The most common adverse effects are drowsiness, dizziness, and headache. Nausea, vomiting, and blurred vision occur in more than 10% of patients. Additional adverse effects are constipation, diarrhea, and weight gain or loss. Slightly fewer than 10% of patients experience insomnia; these patients may take trazodone during the day. Cardiac dysrhythmias can occur but are less common than with other TCAs.

Contraindications. Trazodone is contraindicated in patients taking MAOIs. It should be used cautiously in patients during the acute recovery phase of myocardial infarction due to increased risk of dysrhythmias. Avoid using trazodone with other CNS depressants due to the risk of oversedation. Trazodone should be used cautiously in patients with hepatic disorders.

Monitoring. Determine the effect of trazodone on depressive symptoms as well as on sleep patterns. Monitor for increases in heart rate and blood pressure. If the increase is significant, the patient may require a dosage adjustment or an alternative antidepressant.

Tricyclic Antidepressants

Tricyclic antidepressants (TCAs) were first used in the late 1950s to treat depression. They are characterized by a core chemical structure with three rings. Like SNRIs, TCAs are believed to inhibit reuptake of serotonin and norepinephrine, leading to increased availability of the neurotransmitters in the synaptic cleft. TCAs with a secondary amine side chain (e.g., nortriptyline, desipramine) have a greater effect on norepinephrine reuptake, while TCAs with a tertiary amine side chain (e.g., amitriptyline, imipramine, doxepin) have a greater effect on serotonin reuptake. In addition, TCAs inhibit cholinergic, histamine, and α1-adrenergic receptors as well as interfere with sodium channels, thus potentially resulting in cardiac dysrhythmias.

TCAs are considered second-line treatment for depression and are typically reserved for patients with severe symptoms who do not respond to first-line medications. While considered as effective as SSRIs in the treatment of mild to moderate depression, TCAs have an increased incidence of uncomfortable side effects and increased risk for adverse events.

Common use of TCAs is hampered by their anticholinergic and antihistaminic effects. Examples of associated anticholinergic effects include dry mouth, urinary retention, constipation, blurred vision, and orthostatic hypotension. Secondary amine TCAs typically are better tolerated than tertiary amines. In general, TCAs with tertiary amine side chains cause more sedation, anticholinergic effects, and cardiac effects.

While they are considered second-line treatment for depression, TCAs are also used in the treatment of neuropathic pain (e.g., diabetic peripheral neuropathy, postherpetic neuropathy), prevention of migraines, and fibromyalgia. In general, dosages for these disorders are approximately 50% less than those required for major depression. The focus in this chapter is on the use of TCAs in depression.

Amitriptyline

Pharmacokinetics. While amitriptyline can be administered intramuscularly, it is typically given orally. It is well absorbed by the GI tract and, as with other TCAs, is highly protein bound and widely distributed in plasma and tissues. Amitriptyline is metabolized in the liver to nortriptyline. The half-life of amitriptyline is 10 to 50 hours, while the half-life of nortriptyline is 20 to 100 hours. Amitriptyline is excreted in the urine and feces. It can be several weeks before the patient experiences an antidepressant effect.

Indications. Amitriptyline is indicated for the treatment of major depression.

Adverse Effects. The most common adverse effects are drowsiness, orthostatic hypotension, and xerostomia. In addition to xerostomia, other anticholinergic effects include blurred vision, constipation, urinary retention, and delirium (particularly in older adults). Headache and hyperhidrosis are also common. Severe adverse effects are rare but include oliguria, seizures, and dysrhythmias.

Contraindications. Amitriptyline is contraindicated in patients who are in the acute phase of recovery from a myocardial infarction due to risk of sudden death. It should not be used in patients receiving MAOI therapy due to the risk of serotonin syndrome. There are no sufficient studies on the use of amitriptyline during pregnancy, so this drug should only be used if the risks outweigh the benefits. Amitriptyline is excreted in breast milk, so it should be avoided in those who are breastfeeding.

Monitoring. Teach patients to report any vision changes that may result with amitriptyline as they may require a thorough ophthalmologic exam. Monitor for blood pressure and heart rate changes. Laboratory work that should be evaluated in patients taking amitriptyline includes thyroid function studies, LFTs, and ECGs. Administration at night may reduce some of the more common adverse effects.

Doxepin

Pharmacokinetics. Doxepin is well absorbed from the GI tract; however, administration with high-fat meals can delay the time to reach maximum concentration. As a result, doxepin should not be taken within 3 hours of meals. Plasma protein binding of doxepin is approximately 80%. Doxepin is extensively metabolized in the liver, primarily by CYP2C19 and CYP2D6. Patients who are poor metabolizers of CYP2D6 and CYP2C19 are at increased risk for adverse reactions. Antidepressant effects can take 2 or more weeks to stabilize, but adverse effects may be seen within a few hours.

Indications. Doxepin can be used in the treatment of major depression and/or anxiety. It can also be effective for the treatment of insomnia characterized by difficulties with sleep maintenance.

Adverse Effects. The most common adverse effect associated with doxepin is drowsiness. This can be advantageous for patients with insomnia as it can be given at night for best effect. Other adverse effects include anticholinergic effects (e.g., dry mouth, vision changes, urinary retention, and constipation), sexual dysfunction, and orthostatic hypotension. Doxepin can cause QT prolongation and other cardiac dysrhythmias, with higher risks at increased doses and in older adults. Weight gain is common for patients taking doxepin.

Contraindications. Doxepin is contraindicated in patients who are in the acute recovery phase of acute myocardial infarction due to the risk of cardiac dysrhythmia and sudden death. It should not be used in patients with urinary retention due to the risk of anticholinergic effects. Doxepin should be avoided in patients with a history of psychosis because it can precipitate psychotic symptoms. Rarely, patients may experience neutrophil depression with

leukopenia, agranulocytosis, neutropenia, thrombocytopenia, anemia, and pancytopenia.

Monitoring. Teach patients to take doses at bedtime to reduce daytime drowsiness. Rarely, patients may experience stimulation from doses at bedtime; if this occurs, the dose should be taken in the morning. Avoid taking doxepin within 3 hours of eating a meal, particularly as it delays absorption and may result in daytime sleepiness. Monitor weight, heart rate, ECG, LFT, and CBC.

Monoamine Oxidase Inhibitors

Monoamine oxidase inhibitors (MAOIs) were introduced in the 1950s as a treatment for depression. While they were an effective treatment at one time, they are rarely used today due to multiple adverse reactions, drug interactions, and the need for dietary restrictions in order to avoid complications. As a result, they are discussed only briefly in this chapter.

MAOIs act by inhibiting the enzyme that breaks down norepinephrine, serotonin, dopamine, and tyramine. Increasing the availability of these neurotransmitters may reduce symptoms of depression; however, unintended consequences of the inhibition of monoamine oxidase in the GI tract and liver can cause absorption of a large amount of tyramine from certain foods. This increase in tyramine can ultimately lead to increased norepinephrine released from adrenergic storage sites, resulting in severe hypertension. In addition, MAOIs interfere with the hepatic metabolism of a variety of drugs. As a result, MAOIs should only be prescribed by specialty providers and not in primary care.

Phenelzine

Pharmacokinetics. Phenelzine is completely absorbed from the GI tract, with peak plasma concentrations reached 2 to 4 hours following administration. It is rapidly metabolized in the liver. Phenelzine is excreted primarily as metabolites in the urine. Onset of action can range anywhere from 7 days to 8 weeks.

Indications. Phenelzine is reserved for treatment-resistant depression, including atypical depression.

Adverse Effects. Common adverse effects include headache, dizziness, drowsiness, and xerostomia. Patients also experience mild to moderate weight gain and peripheral edema. Elevated liver enzymes are common. Phenelzine has been associated with mild to moderate orthostatic hypotension in patients who have a history of hypertension. Less common adverse effects include tremor, rash, insomnia, and hyperhidrosis. Severe CNS effects are rare and may include psychosis, ataxia, delirium, and mania. The most significant adverse reactions associated with phenelzine, as with other MAOIs, is the risk for severe hypertension and hypertensive crisis. This can be triggered by intake of substances high in tyramine or tryptophan, such as aged cheese, beer, red wine, and cured meats, as well as by noradrenergic medications.

Contraindications. MAOIs are contraindicated in patients receiving any other monoamine inhibitor therapy. It is imperative to carefully review all medications to avoid drug–drug interactions. Phenelzine should not be used in patients with alcoholism or heavy alcohol use. To avoid severe drug–drug interactions, at least 14 days should separate prescription of any serotonergic drug and phenelzine. Of note, if the patient is taking fluoxetine, at least 5 weeks should separate discontinuation of fluoxetine and initiation of phenelzine. Phenelzine is not recommended in patients with a history of renal or liver disease. Older adults are at higher risk for drug accumulation and should be monitored carefully.

Monitoring. Monitor blood pressure and heart rate regularly. Laboratory results that should be monitored include LFTs and creatinine/BUN. Dietary restrictions should be carefully reviewed with patients and their families at the start of and during therapy. Dietary restrictions should continue for at least 14 days after cessation of therapy. Phenelzine acts as a pyridoxine antagonist, resulting in vitamin B6 deficiency. Supplementation of vitamin B6 may be warranted.

Bipolar Therapy

In general, pharmacologic management of bipolar illness is directed toward the goal of mood stabilization without significant adverse effects. First-line medications for treatment include lithium as well as or in combination with select antiepileptics (Table 34.3) and second-generation

antipsychotics (Table 34.4). For the purposes of this chapter, lithium will be discussed in greater detail. While dosages for antiepileptics and second-generation antipsychotics are provided in Table 34.3 and Table 34.4, more details about these medications are provided in Chapters 29 and 35.

Lithium was approved for use in the United States in the early 1970s for management of acute mania and long-term stabilization of bipolar illness. The mechanism of action is not well understood; however, lithium may affect the synthesis and release of serotonin, norepinephrine, and dopamine, or potentially reduce the release of the excitatory neurotransmitter glutamate. As a positively charged ion, lithium may affect electrical conductivity in neurons. If overstimulation of neurons is a factor in bipolar illness, lithium may affect sodium and potassium ions at the cell membrane, leading to greater stability of electrical impulses in the neuron. Because of its effect on electrical conductivity, lithium can have a wide range of effects on the body. In fact, a major consideration for lithium therapy is the narrow therapeutic index requiring careful symptom monitoring and regular measurement of serum lithium levels.

Lithium
Pharmacokinetics. Lithium is available as lithium carbonate and lithium citrate. Lithium carbonate is much

TABLE 34.3	Medications for Bipolar Disorder		
Category/Medication	Indication	Dosage	Considerations and Monitoring
Lithium	Bipolar disorder	**Immediate release and capsules:**	Narrow therapeutic window (0.6–1.2 mEq/L).
		Adults: Recommended starting dose: 300 mg orally three times daily. Obtain serum lithium concentrations after 3 days (draw levels 12 hr after last oral dose) and regularly until patient is stabilized. Increase dose by 300 mg every 3 days to the desired effect. When titrating for acute mania, usual dosage range is 600 mg orally two to three times daily with serum lithium 0.8–1.2 mEq/L until patient stabilized. Then, usual maintenance dosage range: 300–600 mg orally two or three times daily. Target titration to serum lithium levels between 0.8 and 1 mEq/L.	Toxic at >1.5 mEq/L.
			Older adults may respond at lower levels of 0.4–0.6 mEq/L.
			Monitor serum lithium levels regularly and adjust the doses accordingly. Typically, lithium levels should be assessed every 1–2 weeks until the patient is stabilized.
			Use cautiously in patients with renal impairment or renal disease.
			Use cautiously in patients with thyroid disease, especially hypothyroidism.
			Can cross placenta and is excreted in breast milk.
			Has been shown to prolong QT interval.
		Older adults typically respond to a lower dosage and may exhibit toxicity at lower serum concentrations than younger adults; consider lower doses and slower titration.	Interacts with many drugs.
			Avoid any situations or medications that may lead to hyponatremia, volume depletion, or dehydration that may cause lithium toxicity.
			Patients should maintain a normal diet, including salt, and adequate fluid intake (e.g., 2500 to 3000 mL).
			Patients with acute mania may require dosage range of 600 mg two or three times daily.

Continued

TABLE
34.3
Medications for Bipolar Disorder—cont'd

Category/Medication	Indication	Dosage	Considerations and Monitoring
Mood Stabilizers			
Carbamazepine	Acute mania and mixed episodes associated with bipolar disorder	*Adults:* 200 mg orally twice daily initially. Increase every 3–4 days to achieve serum carbamazepine concentration of 8–12 mcg/mL. Usual dose range: 600–1600 mg/day in divided doses. Used as monotherapy or as adjunct therapy with lithium. Should be prescribed to children only by specialty prescribers.	Monitor serum levels, LFTs, reticulocyte counts, and creatinine/BUN. Monitor for agranulocytosis and aplastic anemia. Contraindicated in those with bone marrow suppression. Use caution in patients with hepatic disease. Monitor closely in those with cardiac disease. Monitor closely for hyponatremia. Older adults may be more susceptible to confusion or agitation, cardiac side effects, or SIADH. Can cause fetal harm when administered during pregnancy.
Lamotrigine	Long-term maintenance treatment of bipolar disorder to delay the occurrence of mood episodes in patients treated for acute mood episodes with standard therapy	*Adults:* **Note:** Medication errors have been reported with lamotrigine starter kits. There are three different starter kits with titration schedules dependent on concurrent medications. Patients must receive the correct kit to avoid overdosing or underdosing. Follow guidelines carefully. *Maintenance dose:* 100–200 mg once or twice daily. Dosages determined based on concurrent medications. See practice guidelines.	Discontinue immediately if rash occurs at any time during treatment as it may indicate a life-threatening condition such as Stevens-Johnson syndrome or toxic epidermal necrolysis. Acetaminophen can be hepatotoxic. Avoid use in patients who have cardiac conduction disorders, ventricular arrhythmias, or cardiac disease or abnormality. Coadministration of certain drugs may need to be avoided or dosage adjustments may be necessary; review drug interactions. Not recommended for treatment of acute manic or mixed episodes.
Valproic acid, divalproex sodium	Acute mania associated with bipolar disorder with or without psychotic features	**Extended release:** *Adults:* 750 mg/day orally in divided doses initially. Increase dosage as rapidly as possible to lowest effective dose that produces desired clinical effect or desired serum concentrations. Maximum recommended dosage: 60 mg/kg/day.	Therapeutic levels: 50–125 mcg/mL. In the treatment of acute mania, levels up to 125 mcg/mL may be seen. For maintenance therapy, levels <100 mcg/mL are generally desirable. Monitor serum ammonia. Contraindicated in patients with hepatic disease or significant hepatic dysfunction. Advise females of childbearing potential to use effective contraception while taking valproate. Dietary folic acid supplementation is recommended before conception in patients using valproate.

BUN, Blood urea nitrogen; *LFTs*, liver function tests; *SIADH*, syndrome of inappropriate antidiuretic hormone secretion

more widely used due to its longer shelf life. It is completely absorbed through the GI tract and may be given without regard to meals. Half-life is typically between 18 and 36 hours in adults and may be shorter or longer during acute episodes of mania or depression. Lithium does not undergo metabolism and is excreted primarily by the kidneys (approximately 95%). Onset of the acute antimanic effect typically occurs within 5 to 7 days of therapy. Full therapeutic effect may require 10 to 21 days.

Indications. Lithium is used for the treatment of bipolar disorder. It can be used in patients experiencing acute mania and for maintenance therapy.

TABLE 34.4 Second-Generation Antipsychotics for Depression and/or Bipolar Disorder

Category/Medication	Indication	Dosage	Considerations and Monitoring
Aripiprazole	Acute treatment of mania and mixed episodes and maintenance treatment of bipolar disorder (bipolar I disorder)	*Adults:* Initial monotherapy for acute or maintenance therapy: 15 mg orally once daily. If used as adjunct to lithium or valproate, use 10–15 mg. May increase if needed/tolerated. Use lowest effective dose. Maximum dosage: 30 mg/day. **IM dosage (monthly extended-release IM suspension [e.g., Abilify Maintena]):** *Adults:* For maintenance therapy: initial and maintenance dose is 400 mg IM once monthly, with subsequent maintenance doses administered no sooner than 26 days after previous injection. At initiation, oral aripiprazole (10–20 mg/day) or other oral antipsychotic should be continued for 14 consecutive days to maintain therapeutic concentrations during initiation of IM aripiprazole therapy. Once stabilized, may reduce to 300 mg IM once monthly in patients experiencing adverse effects.	Monitor HbA1c, prolactin, lipids, LFTs, and weight. False-positive urine drug screen may occur for amphetamines. May increase compulsive urges, particularly for gambling, and the inability to control these urges. Monitor for metabolic syndrome. Periodic evaluation for movement disorders is recommended. Review drug interactions carefully. In patients classified as poor metabolizers of CYP2D6 or in patients who are taking a CYP3A4 inhibitor, follow practice guidelines carefully for dosage adjustments.
	Adjunctive treatment of major depression	*Adults:* Initially, 2–5 mg orally once daily as an adjunct to previously established antidepressant treatment. Adjust dose in increments of up to 5 mg at intervals of no less than 1 week each. The effective dose range is 2–15 mg orally once daily.	
Asenapine	Bipolar disorder (bipolar I disorder), including mania or mixed episodes	**Adults:** *Acute treatment of manic or mixed episodes (monotherapy):* Initially, 5–10 mg sublingually twice daily. Responding patients should generally continue treatment beyond the acute episode. Maximum dosage: 20 mg/day sublingually. *Adjunct therapy to lithium or valproate for acute treatment of manic or mixed episodes:* 5 mg sublingually twice daily initially. Then may increase to 10 mg sublingually twice daily based upon response and tolerability. Responding patients should generally continue treatment beyond the acute episode. Maximum dosage: 20 mg/day sublingually. *Maintenance treatment as monotherapy:* Initially, continue on dose that patient received during stabilization. If receiving 10 mg sublingually twice daily, may decrease to 5 mg sublingually twice daily as tolerated. Reevaluate to assess need for continued treatment. Maximum dosage: 20 mg/day sublingually. **Children and adolescents ≥10 yr:** *For acute treatment of manic or mixed episodes (monotherapy):* Initially, 2.5 mg sublingually twice daily. Dose may be increased to 5 mg sublingually twice daily after 3 days, then to 10 mg sublingually twice daily after an additional 3 days. Adjust as tolerated within the range of 2.5–10 mg sublingually twice daily. Maximum dosage: 20 mg/day.	Monitor AIMS, weight, lipids, HbA1c, LFTs, and prolactin. Use cautiously in older adults. Should be used with caution in patients with hematological disease. Contraindicated in patients with severe hepatic impairment. Use cautiously in patients with a history of substance abuse. Advise patients to avoid eating or drinking for 10 minutes after administration.

Continued

TABLE
34.4 **Second-Generation Antipsychotics for Depression and/or Bipolar Disorder—cont'd**

Category/Medication	Indication	Dosage	Considerations and Monitoring
Risperidone	Bipolar disorder (bipolar I disorder), including acute mania or mixed episodes and maintenance therapy	*Adults:* Initially, 2–3 mg orally once daily as monotherapy or as adjunct to lithium or valproate. If needed, adjust dose by 1 mg daily at intervals of no less than 24 hr. Maximum dosage: 6 mg/day for bipolar disorder. *Older adults:* Initially, 0.5 mg orally twice daily. If needed, adjust dose by 1 mg daily at intervals of no less than 24 hr. Usual dosage range: 1–6 mg/day. Slower titration or divided doses may be needed in older adults due to potential for impaired renal function and increase in drug toxicity. *Children and adolescents 10–17 yr:* Initially, 0.5 mg orally once daily in the morning or evening as monotherapy. May administer in divided doses to increase tolerability. Adjust dose at intervals of at least 24 hr and in increments of 0.5–1 mg/day as tolerated to recommended target dose range of 1–2.5 mg/day. Doses >2.5 mg/day do not appear to provide additional therapeutic benefits.	Use lowest effective dosage. Monitor AIMS, weight, blood glucose, LFTs, HbA1c, lipids, TFTs, and prolactin. Monitor for drug-induced movement disorders. Monitor for metabolic syndrome. Elevations in prolactin may result in infertility in males and females.
Cariprazine	Mania or mixed episodes associated with bipolar disorder	*Adults:* Initially, 1.5 mg orally once daily with or without food. Dose should be increased to 3 mg orally once daily on day 2. Further dose adjustments can be made in 1.5–3-mg increments based upon response and tolerability. Recommended range: 3–6 mg orally once daily. Maximum dosage: 6 mg/day orally.	Monitor AIMS, weight, LFTs, TFTs, lipids, HbA1c, blood glucose, and prolactin. Use cautiously in patients with a history of seizure disorder. Carefully review drug interactions.
	Bipolar depression	Initially, 1.5 mg orally once daily with or without food. May increase to 3 mg once daily on day 15. Maximum dosage: 3 mg/day.	
Olanzapine	Bipolar disorder (bipolar I disorder), including mania or mixed episodes	*Adults:* For acute treatment of manic or mixed episodes, monotherapy: beginning with 10–15 mg orally once daily is recommended. May increase in increments/decrements of 5 mg, at no less than 24-hr intervals. Maintenance therapy: typically 5–20 mg orally/day. *Debilitated or older adults:* May require lower doses at initiation and management. *Adolescents:* Acute treatment of manic or mixed episodes as monotherapy: begin with 2.5 or 5 mg orally once daily, with target dose of 10 mg/day. Increase in increments/decrements of 2.5 or 5 mg, at no less than 24-hr intervals. Effective dose range: 2.5–20 mg/day. Maximum dosage: 20 mg/day orally.	Monitor AIMS, weight, blood pressure, heart rate, blood glucose, HbA1c, lipids, TFTs, LFTs, and prolactin. Not approved for adolescents as an adjunct to valproate or lithium.
	For use in combination with fluoxetine for treatment-resistant depression	*Adults not at risk for hypotension:* Begin with olanzapine 5 mg orally and fluoxetine 20 mg orally once daily in the evening. Adjust olanzapine to 5–20 mg and fluoxetine to 20–50 mg. Maximum daily dose: 18 mg of olanzapine and 75 mg of fluoxetine. *Older or debilitated adults, or those at risk for hypotension:* Begin with olanzapine 2.5–5 mg and fluoxetine 20 mg orally once daily in the evening. Titrate slowly. Usual effective adult dose range: olanzapine 5–20 mg and fluoxetine 20–50 mg/day. Maximum daily dose: 18 mg of olanzapine and 75 mg of fluoxetine.	

TABLE 34.4	Second-Generation Antipsychotics for Depression and/or Bipolar Disorder—cont'd			
Category/Medication	Indication	Dosage	Considerations and Monitoring
Lurasidone	Depression associated with bipolar I disorder	*Adults:* Initially, 20 mg orally once daily with food (at least 350 calories) as monotherapy or as adjunctive therapy to lithium or valproate. Titrate slowly. Effective range: 20–120 mg/day. Maximum dosage: 120 mg/day. *Children and adolescents ≥10 yr:* Begin with 20 mg orally once daily as monotherapy, taken with food (at least 350 calories). After 1 week, may be increased. Effective dose range is 20–80 mg/day as monotherapy. Maximum dosage: 80 mg/day orally.	Monitor AIMS, weight, blood glucose, LFTs, lipids, HbA1c, and prolactin. Use cautiously in patients with seizures, a history of seizure disorder, or conditions that potentially lower the seizure threshold. Use cautiously in patients with renal disease. Review drug interactions carefully.
Ziprasidone	Bipolar disorder, including monotherapy treatment of mania or mixed episodes and as an adjunct to lithium or valproate in maintenance therapy	*Adults:* Begin with 40 mg orally twice daily with food. On day 2, increase to 60 or 80 mg twice daily. Range: 40–80 mg orally twice daily. Maximum dosage: 160 mg/day orally. As an adjunct to lithium or valproate, continue at the same dose on which the patient was stabilized; range 40–80 mg orally twice daily.	Monitor AIMS, weight, blood glucose, LFTs, lipids, HbA1c, and prolactin. Monitor ECG for QT prolongation. Safety and efficacy of ziprasidone use in children and adolescents < 18 yr have not been established.

AIMS, Abnormal involuntary movement scale; *ECG,* electrocardiogram; *IM,* intramuscular; *LFTs,* liver function tests; *TFTs,* thyroid function tests.

Adverse Effects. The most common adverse effect is mild nausea and vomiting, occurring in more than 50% of patients. If occurring early in therapy, taking the medication with food may reduce this adverse effect. If occurring later in therapy, it may be a sign of lithium toxicity. Mild hand tremor can occur in 25% to 50% of patients; this may be managed by a slight reduction in dose or the addition of a beta-blocker. If the hand tremor is severe, it may be an indicator of lithium toxicity. Weight gain of up to 5 to 10 kg is common, occurring in up to 50% of patients. Other adverse effects include dizziness, fatigue, increased thirst, and polyuria. If the polyuria leads to dehydration, this can lead to toxicity. Rare but severe adverse reactions include glomerulonephritis, nephrotic symptoms, serotonin syndrome, neuroleptic malignant syndrome, and seizures. See Table 34.5 for signs and symptoms of lithium toxicity.

Contraindications. Clearance of lithium is dependent on glomerulofiltration rates. As a result, serum lithium levels should be monitored carefully in patients requiring lithium for symptom management. ECG changes may occur in patients with cardiovascular disease, even with therapeutic doses of lithium. Use cautiously in older adults and those with increased comorbidity due to increased risk for medication interactions. In addition, older adults may experience benefits at lower doses and lower serum lithium levels.

Monitoring. Careful monitoring of lithium is required through serum lithium concentration levels. An initial serum lithium is recommended after 3 days, drawn 8 to 12 hours following the last oral dose. Lithium levels should be checked at least every 1 to 2 weeks until the patient is stabilized. Once stabilized, levels should be monitored every 6 to 12 weeks for 6 months unless the patient's condition warrants more frequent monitoring. Serum lithium levels greater than 1.5 mEq/L are associated with toxicity (see

BLACK BOX WARNING!

Lithium

Prior to prescribing lithium, providers must ensure that facilities are available for prompt and accurate evaluation of lithium concentrations, recognizing that lithium has a narrow therapeutic index. Serum lithium levels greater than 1.5 mEq/L are likely to produce at least some degree of toxicity (see Table 34.5). Serum lithium levels should be monitored consistently throughout therapy.

PRACTICE PEARLS

Lithium and Creatinine Clearance (CrCl)

- CrCl at least 90 mL/min: no dosage adjustments are necessary.
- CrCl 30 mL/min to 89 mL/min: start with a dosage that is less than in patients with normal renal function and titrate slowly with frequent monitoring for lithium toxicity.
- CrCl less than 30 mL/min: avoid use.

TABLE 34.5	Toxicities Associated With Excessive Plasma Levels of Lithium
Plasma Lithium Level (mEq/L)	**Signs of Toxicity**
<1.5	Nausea, vomiting, diarrhea, thirst, polyuria, lethargy, slurred speech, muscle weakness, fine hand tremor
1.5–2	Persistent GI upset, coarse hand tremor, confusion, hyperirritability of muscles, ECG changes, sedation, incoordination
2–2.5	Ataxia, giddiness, high output of dilute urine, serious ECG changes, fasciculations, tinnitus, blurred vision, clonic movements, seizures, stupor, severe hypotension, coma, death (usually secondary to pulmonary complications)
> 2.5	Symptoms may progress rapidly to generalized convulsions, oliguria, and death

ECG, Electrocardiogram; *GI*, gastrointestinal.

To keep lithium levels within the therapeutic range, plasma drug levels should be monitored routinely. Levels should be measured every 2 to 3 days at the beginning of treatment and every 3 to 6 months during maintenance therapy.

Treatment of acute overdose is primarily supportive; there is no specific antidote. The severely intoxicated patient should be hospitalized. Hemodialysis is an effective means of lithium removal and should be considered whenever drug levels exceed 2.5 mEq/L.

From Burchum, J., & Rosenthal, L. [2018]. *Lehne's pharmacotherapeutics for advanced practice providers*. St. Louis: Elsevier.

Table 34.5). Risk for toxicity is increased by a variety of factors including dehydration, hyponatremia, renal insufficiency, and drug interactions.

Additional laboratory monitoring recommended for patients on lithium therapy includes baseline creatinine/BUN, CBC, thyroid function, serum electrolytes, serum calcium, ECG in patients over 40 years of age, and EEG in patients with a history of seizures. Pregnancy tests should be included for all females of childbearing age. These should be repeated at least every 6 to 12 months and as needed.

Because patients with bipolar illness are at risk for suicidal ideation and suicide, instruct patients and their families to report new or worsening changes in mood or behavior. Provide information regarding local and national resources for crisis prevention and intervention.

Prescriber Considerations for Mood Disorder Therapy

Clinical Practice Guidelines

Clinical practice guidelines for treatment of depression and bipolar illness are provided by the American Psychiatric Association. The *Diagnostic and Statistical Manual of Mental Disorders* (*DSM–5*) provides diagnostic criteria for

depression, bipolar, and related disorders to help guide primary care practitioners in differentiating symptoms that may be similar.

Clinical Reasoning for Mood Disorder Therapy

Consider the individual patient's health problem requiring medication for mood disorders. Which specific symptoms are being targeted? For example, is the patient experiencing significant sleep disruption? Changes in appetite? Low mood? Are they experiencing anhedonia or perhaps racing thoughts? Consider specific patient characteristics; are there

---

BOOKMARK THIS!

Clinical Practice Guidelines for Psychiatric Evaluation in Adults

The American Psychiatric Association provides practice guidelines for the psychiatric evaluation of adults. These guidelines include topics such as substance use assessment, and review of psychiatric symptoms, trauma history, and psychiatric treatment history, as well as guidelines for involving patients in treatment decisions. They can be found at https://psychiatryonline.org/doi/full/10.1176/appi.books.9780890426760.pe01.

---

certain side effects that will be more detrimental for this patient (e.g., weight gain or elevation in blood sugar)? Are there underlying medical causes for the mood disorder, such as thyroid disfunction, vitamin B12 deficiency, or sequalae from traumatic brain injury?

Determine the desired therapeutic outcome based on the degree of medication therapy needed for the patient's health problem. Regularly assess symptoms and evaluate therapy goals for each patient. If a patient has achieved their therapy goals, they may consider discontinuing antidepressant therapy. Has the

---

PRACTICE PEARLS

Lithium Use in Pregnancy and Lactation

Maternal exposure to lithium poses significant risk for adverse pregnancy and neonatal complications. All females of childbearing age should be provided information for best contraceptive practices. Breastfeeding is not recommended in patients taking lithium as it is excreted in breast milk. Refer to specialty practitioners should the patient consider becoming pregnant while taking lithium.

patient been on the prescribed therapy for a sufficient length of time? Is this an acute or a chronic illness? How will the patient determine when they "feel better"? Consider both subjective and objective factors. If the decision is made to discontinue antidepressant therapy, carefully taper the medication while educating patients regarding potential withdrawal symptoms and when to contact the provider.

Assess the medication therapy used for its appropriateness for an individual patient by considering the medication's side effects and the patient's age, race/ethnicity, comorbidities, and genetic factors. Always assess the patient's compliance and willingness to adhere to the treatment plan. For example, fluoxetine is useful in those for whom noncompliance is a concern due to its long half-life, which would decrease the incidence of unpleasant withdrawal symptoms. Lithium should be taken consistently due to the need for maintaining consistent blood levels. Also, doses may need to be adjusted, particularly in older adults or in those with renal insufficiency. Be alert to specific side effects that may be most problematic for the patient and whether the side effects improve symptoms. For example, mirtazapine typically causes drowsiness and increased appetite, making it ideal for those with insomnia and poor appetite. Regularly assess for the potential for medication, food, or beverage interactions, including over-the-counter (OTC), herbal, and dietary supplements the patient is currently taking. Are there cultural factors that may affect adherence?

Initiate the treatment plan with the selected medication by first providing adequate patient education to ensure the patient's understanding and promote full participation in the mood disorder medication therapy. Carefully assess for the patient's understanding of the treatment plan (how and when to take the medication), potential side effects, and when to call the provider. Assess for patient willingness or "buy-in" to adhere to the treatment plan. Does the patient believe this medication will be helpful to address their current symptoms? Is additional education needed? Are there support services that may improve monitoring and adherence? If the patient is not fully engaged with the treatment plan, they are at much greater risk for nonadherence and symptom exacerbation.

Ensure complete patient and family understanding about the medication prescribed for antidepressant therapy using a variety of education strategies. Provide patients and families with education regarding onset of action, potential adverse effects, and recommendations for follow-up, including nonpharmacologic strategies to reduce depressive symptoms. Reinforce the need to contact the primary care provider or emergency services should there be an increase in suicidal thoughts.

Conduct follow-up and monitoring of patient responses to medication therapy. Initially, follow-up is recommended within 2 weeks to assess for tolerability and to monitor for emergence of worsening suicidality or activation of underlying mania. In addition, evidence suggests that cognitive behavioral therapy or mindfulness-based cognitive therapy can help patients discontinue antidepressants

without increasing the risk of relapse/recurrence, but they are resource intensive (Maund et al., 2019).

Teaching Points for Mood Disorder Therapy

Health Promotion Strategies

- Discuss nonpharmacologic activities that may help reduce symptoms of depression.
- Refer patients to mental health care providers in the community to assist them in developing cognitive/behavioral or other strategies to manage their symptoms.
- Discuss exercises that patients may be able to incorporate into their activities of daily living.
- Review "rescue" coping skills (call a friend, participate in vigorous physical activity, do a calming activity, etc.). Include discussions of having an "emergency plan" should symptoms increase.
- Discuss the benefit of following a healthy diet and the need to fuel the body with whole foods when possible.
- Review strategies such as mindfulness meditation that may be helpful. Provide written instructions, or information on how to access mindfulness resources online. There are a number of free smartphone apps that may be helpful.
- Discuss healthy coping skills and overall stress management.
- Review sleep hygiene strategies.
- Encourage smoking cessation.
- Address the use of alcohol and illicit substances that may contribute to symptoms, and provide resources as needed.

Patient Education for Medication Safety

- Many patients require at least 6 to 12 months of therapy after achieving a positive response to antidepressant medications. Work closely with your primary care provider before you decide to discontinue your medications.
- Take the medication as prescribed, even though you may no longer be experiencing symptoms. Stopping medications too early can result in relapse/recurrence of symptoms.
- While you may have some improvement in symptoms after about 2 weeks, it typically takes 4 to 8 weeks to achieve an optimal effect.
- Sometimes it takes several dosage adjustments or medication changes to achieve the best overall outcome.
- Contact your primary care provider if you experience serious side effects or adverse effects. These may be minimized by switching to a different medication.
- If you have any suicidal thoughts after beginning or while taking these medications, please don't hesitate to contact the National Suicide Hotline at 1-800-273-8255.
- If you have worsening symptoms of depression, agitation, or irritability, please contact your primary care provider.
- Avoid OTC and herbal medications without discussion with your primary care provider or pharmacist to avoid

dangerous drug interactions.

- If you have any increase in fever, irritability, sweating, or muscle tightness, contact your primary care provider or emergency services as needed.

Application Questions for Discussion

1. As a primary care provider, what patient and safety factors should be considered before prescribing an antidepressant?
2. What should be included in the patient and/or caregiver education plan for a patient who has been prescribed an antidepressant? What should be included in the patient and/or caregiver education plan for a patient who has been prescribed lithium?
3. What local and national resources are available to patients and families in managing depressive or bipolar symptoms? What financial resources are available to support nonpharmacologic interventions such as cognitive behavioral therapy?

Selected Bibliography

Alson, A. R., Robinson, D. M., Ivanova, D., Azer, J., Moreno, M., Turk, M. L., & Blackman, K. S. (2016). Depression in primary care: Strategies for a psychiatry-scarce environment. *International Journal of Psychiatry in Medicine, 51*(2), 182–200. http://doi.org/10.1177/0091217416636580.

Arroll, B., Chin, W. Y., Martis, W., Goodyear-Smith, F., Mount, V., Kingsford, D., & MacGillivray, S. (2016). Antidepressants for treatment of depression in primary care: A systematic review and meta-analysis. *Journal of Primary Health Care, 8*(4), 325–334. http://doi.org/10.1071/hc16008.

Bartlett, D. (2017). Drug-induced serotonin syndrome. *Critical Care Nurse, 37*(1), 49–54. http://doi.org/10.4037/ccn2017169.

Brody, D. J., & Gu, Q (2020)Antidepressant use among adults: United States, 2015–2018377. Hyattsville, MD: National Center for Health Statistics NCHS Data Brief.

Burchum, J., & Rosenthal, L. (2018). *Lehne's Pharmacotherapeutics for Advanced Practice Providers*. St. Louis: Elsevier.

Chu, A., & Wadhwa, R. (2020). Selective serotonin reuptake inhibitors. May 15]. In *StatPearls [Internet]*. Treasure Island (FL): StatPearls Publishing. 2020 Jan-. Available from. https://www.ncbi.nlm.nih.gov/books/NBK554406/.

Daveney, J., Panagioti, M., Waheed, W., & Esmail, A. (2019). Unrecognized bipolar disorder in patients with depression managed in primary care: A systematic review and meta-analysis. *General Hospital Psychiatry, 58*, 71–76. http://doi.org/10.1016/j.genhosppsych.2019.03.006.

Elsevier. Clinical pharmacology powered by ClinicalKey®. (2019). Retrieved from http://www.clinicalkey.com.

Foong, A. L., Grindrod, K. A., Patel, T., & Kellar, J. (2018). Demystifying serotonin syndrome (or serotonin toxicity). *Canadian Family Physician, 64*(10), 720–727.

Foreman, R. M., Zappas, M., & Whitely, C. (2020). Antidepressant withdrawal: A guide for primary care clinicians. *Journal for Nurse Practitioners, 16*(3), 191–194. http://doi.org/10.1016/j.nurpra.2019.12.013.

Fornaro, M., Anastasia, A., Valchera, A., Carano, A., Orsolini, L., Vellante, F., & De Berardis, D. (2019). The FDA "black box" warning on antidepressant suicide risk in young adults: More harm than benefits? *Frontiers in Psychiatry, 10*, 294. http://doi.org/10.3389/fpsyt.2019.00294.

Hillhouse, T. M., & Porter, J. H. (2015). A brief history of the development of antidepressant drugs: From monoamines to glutamate. *Experimental & Clinical Psychopharmacology, 23*(1), 1–21. http://doi.org/10.1037/a0038550.

Hirschfeld, R. M. A., Williams, J. B. W., Spitzer, R. L., Calabrese, J. R., Flynn, L., Keck, P. E., & Zajecka, J. (2000). Development and validation of a screening instrument for bipolar spectrum disorder: The Mood Disorder Questionnaire. *American Journal of Psychiatry, 157*(11), 1873–1875. http://doi.org/10.1176/appi.ajp.157.11.1873.

Hussain, L. S., Reddy, V., & Maani, C. V. (2020). Physiology, Noradrenergic Synapse. May 24]. In *StatPearls [Internet]*. Treasure Island (FL): StatPearls Publishing. 2020 Jan-. Available from. https://www.ncbi.nlm.nih.gov/books/NBK540977/.

InformedHealth.org [Internet]. Cologne, Germany: Institute for Quality and Efficiency in Health Care (IQWiG); 2006-. Depression: How effective are antidepressants? [Updated 2020 Jun 18]. Available from https://www.ncbi.nlm.nih.gov/books/NBK361016/.

Köhler, S., Cierpinsky, K., Kronenberg, G., & Adli, M. (2016). The serotonergic system in the neurobiology of depression: Relevance for novel antidepressants. *Journal of Psychopharmacology, 30*(1), 13–22. http://doi.org/10.1177/0269881115609072.

Lien, Y. H. (2018). Antidepressants and hyponatremia. *The American Journal of Medicine, 131*(1), 7–8. https://doi.org/10.1016/j.amjmed.2017.09.002.

Maund, E., Stuart, B., Moore, M., Dowrick, C., Geraghty, A. W. A., Dawson, S., & Kendrick, T. (2019). Managing antidepressant discontinuation: A systematic review. *Annals of Family Medicine, 17*(1), 52–60. http://doi.org/10.1370/afm.2336.

McCormick, U., Murray, B., & McNew, B. (2015). Diagnosis and treatment of patients with bipolar disorder: A review for advanced practice nurses. *Journal of the American Association of Nurse Practitioners, 27*(9), 530–542. http://doi.org/10.1002/2327-6924.12275.

Miller, T. H. (2016). Bipolar disorder. *Primary Care, 43*(2), 269–284. http://doi.org/10.1016/j.pop.2016.02.003.

Moise, N., Falzon, L., Obi, M., Ye, S., Patel, S., Gonzalez, C., & Kronish, I. M. (2018). Interventions to increase depression treatment initiation in primary care patients: A systematic review. *Journal of General Internal Medicine, 33*(11), 1978–1989. http://doi.org/10.1007/s11606-018-4554-z.

National Center for Health Statistics (2019) *Fast Stats: Therapeutic Drug Use.* Available from https://www.cdc.gov/nchs/fastats/drug-use-therapeutic.htm

National Institute of Mental Health (Updated February 2019). *Statistics: Major depression.* Available at https://www.nimh.nih.gov/health/statistics/major-depression.shtml. National Institute of Mental Health (Updated November 2017) *Statistics: Bipolar disorder.* Available at https://www.nimh.nih.gov/health/statistics/bipolar-disorder.shtml.

Ormel, J., Kessler, R. C., & Schoevers, R. (2019). Depression: More treatment but no drop in prevalence: How effective is treatment? And can we do better? *Current Opinion in Psychiatry, 32*(4), 348–354. http://doi.org/10.1097/YCO.0000000000000505.

Pratt, L. A., Brody, D. J., & Gu, Q. (2017). Antidepressant use among persons aged 12 and over: United States, 2011-2014. *NCHS Data Brief,* (283), 1–8.

Qato, D. M., Ozenberger, K., & Olfson, M. (2018). Prevalence of prescription medications with depression as a potential adverse effect among adults in the United States. *JAMA, 319*(22), 2289–2298. http://doi.org/10.1001/jama.2018.6741.

Riihimäki, K. A., Vuorilehto, M. S., Melartin, T. K., & Isometsä, E. T. (2014). Five-year outcome of major depressive disorder in primary health care. *Psychological Medicine, 44*(7), 1369–1379. http://doi.org/10.1017/S0033291711002303.

Scotton, W. J., Hill, L. J., Williams, A. C., & Barnes, N. M. (2019). Serotonin syndrome: Pathophysiology, clinical features, management, and potential future directions. *International Journal of Tryptophan Research: IJTR, 12,* 1–14. http://doi.org/10.1177/1178646919873925.

Sirey, J. A., Banerjee, S., Marino, P., Bruce, M. L., Halkett, A., Turnwald, M., & Kales, H. C. (2017). Adherence to depression treatment in primary care: A randomized clinical trial. *JAMA Psychiatry, 74*(11), 1129–1135. http://doi.org/10.1001/jamapsychiatry.2017.3047.

Siu, A. L. Force, a. t. U. P. S. T. (2016). Screening for depression in adults: US Preventive Services Task Force recommendation statement. *Jama, 315*(4), 380–387. http://doi.org/10.1001/jama.2015.18392.

Smithson, S., & Pignone, M. P. (2017). Screening adults for depression in primary care. *Medical Clinics of North America, 101*(4), 807–821. http://doi.org/10.1016/j.mcna.2017.03.010.

Sub Laban, T., & Saadabadi, A. (2020). Monoamine Oxidase Inhibitors (MAOI). Aug 22]. In *StatPearls [Internet].* Treasure Island (FL): StatPearls Publishing. 2020 Jan-. Available from. https://www.ncbi.nlm.nih.gov/books/NBK539848/.

VandenBerg, A. M. (2020). Major depressive disorder. In J. T. DiPiro, G. C. Yee, L. M. Posey, S. T. Haines, T. D. Nolin, & V. Ellingrod (Eds.), *Pharmacotherapy: A Pathophysiologic Approach* (11th ed.). New York: McGraw-Hill Education.

Walker, E. P., & Tadi, P. (2020). Neuroanatomy, nucleus raphe. Jul 10]. In StatPearls [Internet]. Treasure Island (FL): StatPearls Publishing. 2020 Jan-. Available from. https://www.ncbi.nlm.nih.gov/books/NBK544359/.

35

Antipsychotic Medications

CHERYL H. ZAMBROSKI

Overview

Psychosis is not a specific disorder. Rather, it is a term used to describe a symptom complex in which the patient experiences gross impairment of reality. It is characterized by dysregulation of normal thought processes which may include hallucinations, delusions, and disorganized thinking and speech. Patients with psychotic disorders experience altered cognition and perception which can significantly impact their quality of life.

Psychosis can result from a variety of conditions, including use of certain medications, alcohol withdrawal, bipolar disorder, traumatic brain injury, Alzheimer's disease, and Parkinson's disease. For patients with acute psychosis, focus should be on identifying the cause and effectively treating the symptoms while ensuring patient safety. For patients with chronic illnesses that include psychotic features, early identification, early intervention, and thorough follow-up can enhance quality of life and minimize risk of morbidity and mortality.

Antipsychotic medications, also known as major tranquilizers or neuroleptics, are typically used to reduce symptoms associated with acute and chronic psychosis as well as several other psychiatric illnesses. Although a number of disorders can cause psychotic symptoms, the primary focus of this chapter is the use of antipsychotics to manage behavioral and psychological symptoms associated with schizophrenia. Use of select antipsychotics in depression and bipolar illness is addressed in Chapter 34.

While primary care providers typically do not initially prescribe antipsychotics for schizophrenia, associated comorbidities are often managed in primary care settings in partnership with specialists in psychiatry. Therefore, a good understanding of the medications used to treat schizophrenia is essential. Furthermore, primary care providers act as members of the overall interdisciplinary team contributing to the patient's plan of care by recognition of symptoms, promotion of adherence, and referral to specialty practice.

Pathophysiology

Schizophrenia is a complex, chronic psychiatric disorder affecting about 1% of the population worldwide. Onset of illness is usually late teens and early 20s, with onset slightly earlier in males than females. Symptoms associated with schizophrenia are typically described as *positive* or *negative* (Fig. 35.1). In addition, patients experience *cognitive* symptoms and *affective* symptoms that must be assessed. These symptoms can impact medication adherence as well as overall quality of life.

Risk factors for schizophrenia include genetic predisposition, brain structural abnormalities (e.g., enlargement of the lateral and third ventricles, reduction in the size of the thalamus), and psychological and environmental factors (e.g., prenatal infection, exposure to extreme stressors) or neurobiological abnormalities, particularly regarding increases or decreases in dopamine, serotonin, and glutamate. Other neurotransmitters that may be involved in the etiology of schizophrenia include acetylcholine and gamma-aminobutyric acid (GABA).

Abnormalities in dopamine transmission are implicated as a major factor in the development of schizophrenia. It is generally considered that dopamine hypersensitivity in the mesolimbic pathway of the brain and hypoactivity of dopamine in the prefrontal cortex (*mesocortical pathway*) lead to the symptoms of schizophrenia. Normally, dopamine is transmitted via four major pathways (Fig. 35.2) that originate primarily from the ventral tegmental area (VTA) and substantia nigra in the midbrain. Two of these pathways, the *mesolimbic* and *mesocortical*, are linked to the development of schizophrenia. A basic understanding of these two pathways helps explain the predominant symptoms associated with schizophrenia. The mesolimbic pathway connects the VTA with the nucleus accumbens in the basal forebrain and is associated with the positive symptoms of schizophrenia including hallucinations and delusions. The mesocortical pathway, also originating from the VTA, projects dopaminergic fibers to the prefrontal cortex. Decreased dopamine in the mesocortical pathway is associated with the cognitive and negative symptoms of schizophrenia such as poverty of speech and flattened affect. An

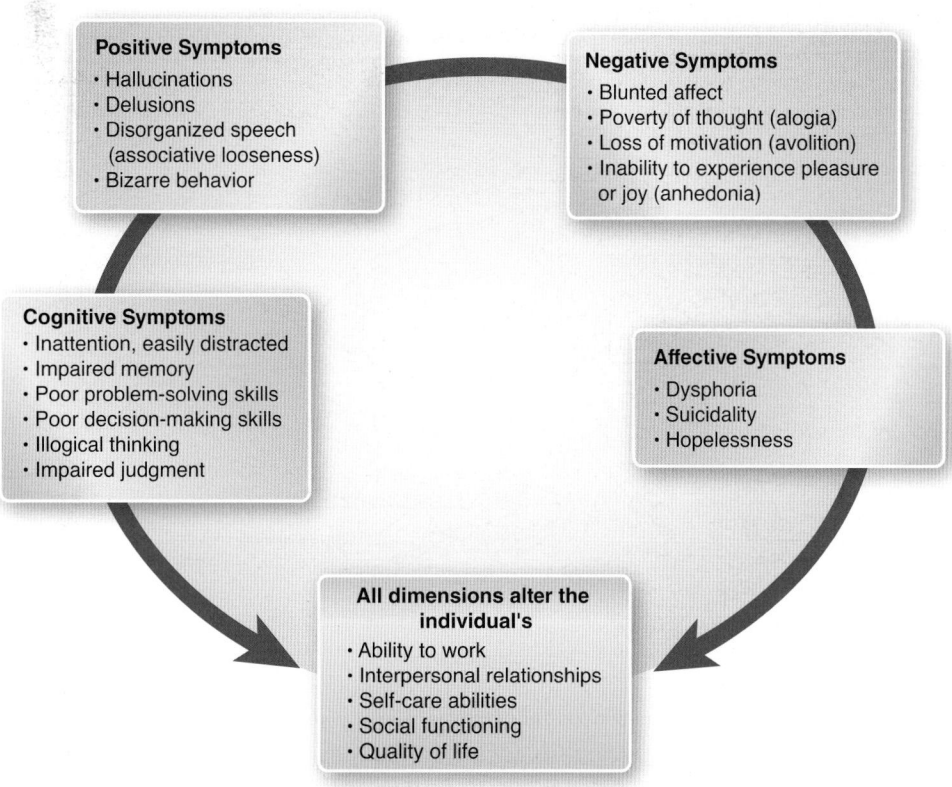

• **Fig. 35.1** Four main symptom groups of schizophrenia. (From Halter, M. [2018]. *Varcarolis' foundations of psychiatric mental health nursing* [8th ed.]. St. Louis: Elsevier.)

understanding of the other two pathways, *nigrostriatal* and *tuberoinfundibular*, helps explain adverse effects commonly associated with the treatment of schizophrenia. The nigrostriatal dopaminergic pathway originates in the substantia nigra of the brain and is primarily associated with purposeful movement. The tuberoinfundibular pathway originates in the hypothalamus and regulates prolactin secretion in the pituitary gland. In other words, blockade of dopamine receptors in the nigrostriatal pathway helps explain disturbances in purposeful movement, and blockade in the tuberoinfundibular pathway helps explain disturbances in prolactin secretion.

The role of serotonin in the etiology of schizophrenia is not well understood; however, it is known that serotonin antagonists can reduce drug-induced movement disorders associated with antipsychotics. In addition, medications that block both serotonin and dopamine, such as risperidone, have improved the symptoms of schizophrenia. It has been theorized that serotonin antagonism in the prefrontal cortex can result in an increase in dopamine, improving negative symptoms and reducing cognitive deficits. Serotonin antagonists alone do not improve symptoms of schizophrenia.

Glutamate has been considered a potentially promising target of therapy for schizophrenia. Glutamate is an excitatory neurotransmitter and the most abundant neurotransmitter in the brain and central nervous system (CNS). It is mediated by the *N*-methyl-*d*-aspartate (NMDA) receptor subtype. The glutamate hypothesis suggests that dysfunction of the NMDA receptor may be part of the etiology of schizophrenia. This was based on clinical findings that patients with exposure to NMDA receptor antagonists such as phencyclidine (PCP) or ketamine resulted in both positive and negative symptoms closely mimicking schizophrenia. Furthermore, an antipsychotic, clozapine, has both weak D_2 receptor blockade and possibly NMDA receptor function enhancement.

Antipsychotic Therapy

Antipsychotic medications are usually categorized as first-generation antipsychotics (FGAs) or second-generation antipsychotics (SGAs). Some of the newer antipsychotic medications are, at times, described as third-generation antipsychotics (TGAs); however, much of the literature classifies these newer antipsychotics as SGAs. FGAs, also called typical or conventional drugs, are primarily used to treat the positive symptoms associated with a psychotic state. SGAs, also called atypical or nonconventional drugs, lead to fewer movement disorders and can be used to treat both positive and negative symptoms of schizophrenia. Still, SGAs are associated with a variety of metabolic effects. The newest group includes aripiprazole, which is a partial dopamine agonist at the D_2 receptors that functions as an agonist when synaptic dopamine levels are low and as an antagonist when they are high. See Table 35.1 for a comparison of select antipsychotics and potential adverse effects.

Neurobiology of Schizophrenia and the Effects of Antipsychotics

The antipsychotics affect a number of neurotransmitters including dopamine, noradrenaline/norepinephrine, serotonin, and GABA. An excess of serotonin may contribute to both the positive and negative symptoms of schizophrenia. GABA regulates dopamine activity and in some people with schizophrenia, there is a loss of GABAergic neurons in the hippocampus, potentially causing hyperactivity of dopamine. Since dopamine is the most studied and most prominent of the neurotransmitters (D_1, D_2, D_3, D_4, and D_5) in schizophrenia, the role of dopamine is presented here.

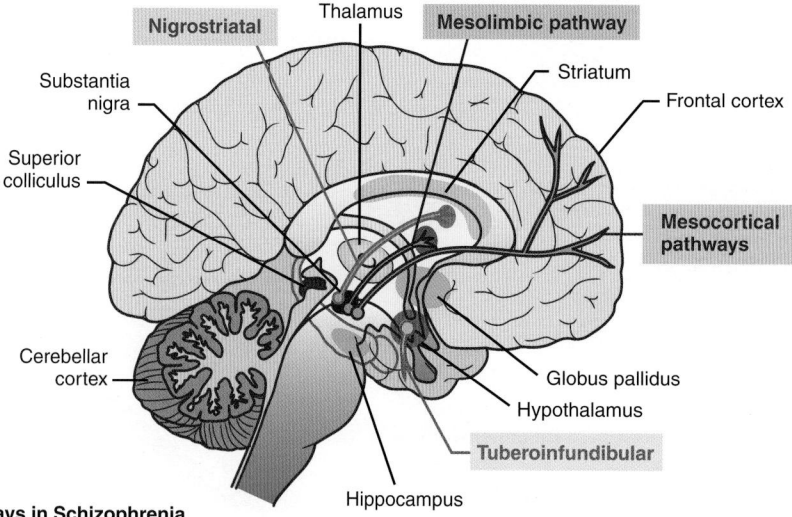

Dopamine Pathways in Schizophrenia

Mesolimbic pathway: reward, motivation, emotions, and positive symptoms of schizophrenia.

Mesocortical pathways: relevant to cognitive function and executive function and negative symptoms of schizophrenia.

Nigrostriatal: normally responsible for purposeful movement.

Tuberoinfundibular: normally responsible for regulation of prolactin.

First-generation antipsychotic (FGA) drugs are potent antagonists/blockers of D_2.

Second-generation antipsychotics (SGA) have less affinity for D_2 receptors, and tend to bind with D_3 and D_4 receptors. Since the expression of D_3 and D_4 is limited to the neurons of the limbic system and cerebral cortex, the action of these drugs is limited to areas involved in the pathology of schizophrenia. Second-generation drugs also inhibit the serotonin (5HT) receptors. Since serotonin inhibits the release of dopamine, the dopaminergic transmission is affected.

The potential serious effects of the SGAs (metabolic effects: weight gain, diabetes, and dyslipidemia) come from the blockade of noradrenaline/norepinephrine (alpha-1), histamine, and acetylcholine.

Dopamine Pathways and Antipsychotic Responses

Dopamine Pathway	Abnormality in Schizophrenia	Responses to Antipsychotic Drugs
Mesolimbic pathway connects the VTA to the nucleus accumbens Associated with reward, motivation, and emotion	Hyperactive in schizophrenia Associated with positive symptoms (hallucinations, delusions, disorganized thought)	**FGA** - D_2 blockage results in reduction in positive symptoms **SGA** - D_3 and D_4 antagonism results in reduction of positive symptoms
Mesocortical pathway made up of dopaminergic neurons that project from the ventral tegmental area to the prefrontal cortex Relevant to cognition, executive function, emotions, and affect	Hypofunction in schizophrenia results in cognitive impairment and negative symptoms (apathy, anhedonia, lack of motivation)	**FGA** - D_2 blockage may result in a worsening of these symptoms **SGA** - Since there are more serotonin (5HT) receptors than D_2 receptors in this area, blockage of 5HT is more profound. Blockage of 5HT may help improve negative symptoms
Tuberoinfundibular pathway consists of dopaminergic projections from the hypothalamus to the pituitary gland Inhibits prolactin release	Unaffected	**FGA** (to a lesser degree SGA) - Blockade of D_2 receptors increases prolactin levels resulting in hyperprolactinemia and lactation
Nigrostriatal pathway - substantial nigra to basal ganglia Responsible for purposeful movement	Unaffected	**FGA** (to a lesser degree SGA) - Long-term blockade of D_2 receptors can cause upregulation (increase response to a stimulus) to those receptors, which may lead to extrapyramidal side effects; e.g., tardive dyskinesia (TD)

• **Fig. 35.2** Neurobiology of schizophrenia and the effects of antipsychotics. (From Halter, M. [2018]. *Varcarolis' foundations of psychiatric mental health nursing* [8th ed.]. St. Louis: Elsevier.)

As noted earlier, antipsychotic therapy is associated with adverse effects relating primarily to the blockade of dopamine receptors. These adverse effects include *drug-induced movement disorders* (DIMDs) such as acute dystonia (also called a dystonic reaction), akathisia, and pseudoparkinsonism (commonly described as *extrapyramidal symptoms* [EPS]). One additional movement disorder, tardive dyskinesia, can develop with long-term use of antipsychotic agents. DIMDs are more common in FGAs, although they still occur in SGAs and TGAs but at lower rates (see Table 35.1). If identified early, many DIMDs can be reversed or treated effectively. Two additional adverse effects, neuroleptic malignant syndrome and metabolic syndrome, will be discussed here.

Acute dystonia usually occurs within the first 24 to 96 hours of treatment but can occur even after a single dose of antipsychotic medication. Symptoms can include torticollis with or without throat tightening, difficulty swallowing, oculogyric crisis, and protrusion of the tongue. It is more likely to occur in young males and in patients using high-potency antipsychotics. Acute dystonia can be frightening, extremely uncomfortable, and life threatening if laryngeal dystonia occurs.

Akathisia is a relatively common and distressing adverse effect associated with antipsychotics, with estimates of prevalence ranging from 18% to 40% (Dilks et al., 2019). Akathisia typically develops within a few weeks of beginning therapy or with dose increases. Symptoms include an intensely unpleasant need to move, with restlessness, pacing, rocking, or an inability to sit or stand still. It may be underdiagnosed or confused with other disorders such as mania, attention deficit hyperactivity disorder (ADHD), or agitated depression. Once it has been identified, treatments may include dose reduction or switching to a different antipsychotic.

Parkinsonism, sometimes called pseudoparkinsonism, mimics Parkinson's disease but occurs in patients taking antipsychotic drugs. Symptoms include tremor, bradykinesia, rigidity, masklike facies, shuffling gait, cogwheeling, and stooped posture. These symptoms are more likely to occur in patients taking FGAs. Symptoms can occur within 5 to 30 days of initiating antipsychotic therapy. Discontinuing the offending drug and switching to another antipsychotic with a decreased risk of EPS may resolve symptoms within weeks to months.

Tardive dyskinesia (TD) is characterized by repetitive involuntary movements of the tongue, face, mouth, and jaw (including protrusion of the tongue), facial grimacing, puffing of cheeks, puckering of mouth, and chewing movements as well as twisting or writhing of the trunk and limbs. These symptoms typically arise months to years after continuous use of antipsychotics. TD may persist even after the antipsychotics are discontinued. Diagnosis may be difficult as TD may coexist with other movement disorders. Careful assessment is vitally important.

Ongoing monitoring of movement disorders can be done using the Abnormal Involuntary Movement Scale (AIMS).

AIMS is designed to measure the presence and severity (from none to severe) of abnormal body movements, including facial and oral movements, extremity movements, and trunk movements (Fig. 35.3). A number of training videos are available online which demonstrate the use of AIMS in evaluating symptoms. Tools such as the Dyskinesia Identification System: Condensed User Scale (DISCUS), Modified Simpson-Angus-Scale (MSAS), and Barnes Akathisia Rating Scale (BARS) are also available (College of Psychiatric and Neurologic Pharmacists [CPNP], 2020).

Neuroleptic malignant syndrome (NMS) is a potentially fatal symptom complex that is associated with an initiation or increase in dose of antipsychotic medications. While the cause of NMS is not completely understood, it is thought to be an idiosyncratic reaction to the initiation of dopamine antagonists or the withdrawal of dopaminergic agents. Symptoms include sudden high fever (as high as 41°C [105.8°F]), autonomic instability (including wide variations in blood pressure), altered mental status, and muscle rigidity (often described as "lead-pipe" rigidity). In addition, patients may have leukocytosis, elevated creatinine kinase secondary to rhabdomyolysis, and acute renal failure. While NMS can occur with FGAs and SGAs, it is more likely with high-potency FGAs such as fluphenazine and haloperidol. NMS is more common in young adults who are at their first exposure to antipsychotic agents.

While SGAs typically have far fewer adverse EPS, they are associated with significant *metabolic effects*. These metabolic effects include weight gain, type 2 diabetes mellitus with insulin resistance, and dyslipidemia (hypercholesterolemia and hypertriglyceridemia), increasing the risk for cardiovascular disease and premature death. The extent of these adverse effects varies among medications, with the greatest risk associated with clozapine and olanzapine (see Table 35.1). Drugs such as quetiapine and risperidone also increase risk for weight gain but at a lesser degree.

Beyond these common adverse effects, the use of antipsychotic therapy includes a risk for potential drug interactions (Table 35.2) and critical black box warnings. For example, use of antipsychotics to treat behavioral problems in patients with dementia is not recommended due to a significant increase in cerebrovascular events. Several SGAs are associated with black box warnings for children and adolescents relating to an increase in suicidal ideation. Knowledge of these warnings is important for primary care providers caring for patients requiring antipsychotic therapy.

Recent clinical practice guidelines suggest that there is no definitive evidence that one generation of antipsychotic (FGA vs. SGA) is superior to another in the treatment of schizophrenia, with the possible exception of clozapine (American Psychiatric Association [APA], 2019). As a result, primary care providers should be aware of adverse and therapeutic effects attributed to both major categories of antipsychotics.

TABLE 35.1   Select Antipsychotics and Incidence of Adverse Effects

Drug	Trade Name	Extrapyramidal Effects[a]	Sedation	Orthostatic Hypotension	Anticholinergic Effects	Metabolic Effects: Weight Gain, Diabetes Risk, Dyslipidemia	Significant QT Prolongation	Prolactin Elevation	Metabolized by CYP3A4
Chlorpromazine	Generic only	Moderate	High	High	Moderate	Moderate	Yes	Low	–
Thioridazine	Generic only	Low	High	High	High	Moderate	Yes	Low	–
Loxapine	Loxitane	Moderate	Moderate	Low	Low	Low	No	Moderate	–
Perphenazine	Generic only	Moderate	Moderate	Low	Low	–	No	Low	–
Fluphenazine	Generic only	Very high	Low	Low	Low	–	No	Moderate	–
Haloperidol	Haldol	Very high	Low	Low	Low	Moderate	Yes	Moderate	–
Pimozide	Orap	High	Moderate	Low	Moderate	–	Yes	Moderate	–
Thiothixene	Navane	High	Low	Moderate	Low	Moderate	No	Moderate	–
Trifluoperazine	Generic only	High	Low	Low	Low	–	No	Moderate	–
Aripiprazole	Abilify	Very low	Low	Low	None	None/low	No	Low	Yes
Asenapine	Saphris	Moderate	Moderate	Moderate	Low	Low	Yes	Low	Slightly
Brexpiprazole	Rexulti	Very low	Very low	Low	None	Low	No	Low	Yes
Cariprazine	Vraylar	Very low	Moderate	Low	Low	Moderate	No	No	Yes
Clozapine	Clozaril, FazaClo, Versacloz	Very low	High	Moderate	High	High	No	Low	Yes
Iloperidone	Fanapt	Very low	Moderate	Moderate	Moderate	Moderate	Yes	Low	Yes
Lurasidone	Latuda	Moderate	Moderate	Low	None	None/low	No	Low	Yes
Olanzapine	Zyprexa	Low	Moderate	Moderate	Moderate	High	No	Low	No
Paliperidone	Invega	Moderate	Low	Low	None	Moderate	Yes	High	Slightly
Quetiapine	Seroquel	Very low	Moderate	Moderate	None	Moderate/high	Yes	Low	Yes
Risperidone	Risperdal	Moderate	Low	Low	None	Moderate	No	High	No
Ziprasidone	Geodon, Zeldox	Low	Moderate	Moderate	None	None/low	Yes	Low	Yes

[a]Incidence here refers to *early* extrapyramidal reactions (acute dystonia, parkinsonism, akathisia). The incidence of *late* reactions (tardive dyskinesia) is the same for all traditional antipsychotics. From Rosenthal, L., & Burchum, J. (2021). *Lehne's pharmacotherapeutics for nurse practitioners and physician assistants* (2nd ed.). St. Louis: Elsevier.

ABNORMAL INVOLUNTARY MOVEMENT SCALE (AIMS)

Public Health Service
Alcohol, Drug Abuse, and Mental Health Administration
National Institute of Mental Health

Name: _____
Date: _____
Prescribing Practitioner: _____

Code: 0 = None
1 = Minimal, may be extreme normal
2 = Mild
3 = Moderate
4 = Severe

Instructions: Complete Examination Procedure before making ratings.

Movement ratings: Rate highest severity observed. Rate movements that occur upon activation one *less* than those observed spontaneously. Circle movement as well as code number that applies.		Rater Date	Rater Date	Rater Date	Rater Date
Facial and Oral Movements	**1. Muscles of facial expression** (e.g., movements of forehead, eyebrows, periorbital area, cheeks, including frowning, blinking, smiling, grimacing)	0 1 2 3 4	0 1 2 3 4	0 1 2 3 4	0 1 2 3 4
	2. Lips and perioral area (e.g., puckering, pouting, smacking)	0 1 2 3 4	0 1 2 3 4	0 1 2 3 4	0 1 2 3 4
	3. Jaw (e.g., biting, clenching, chewing, mouth opening, lateral movement)	0 1 2 3 4	0 1 2 3 4	0 1 2 3 4	0 1 2 3 4
	4. Tongue: Rate only increases in movement both in and out of mouth — *not* inability to sustain movement. Darting in and out of mouth.	0 1 2 3 4	0 1 2 3 4	0 1 2 3 4	0 1 2 3 4
Extremity Movements	**5. Upper (arms, wrists, hands, fingers):** Include choreic movements (i.e., rapid, objectively purposeless, irregular, spontaneous) and athetoid movements (i.e., slow, irregular, complex, serpentine). *Do not include tremor* (i.e., repetitive, regular, rhythmic).	0 1 2 3 4	0 1 2 3 4	0 1 2 3 4	0 1 2 3 4
	6. Lower (legs, knees, ankles, toes) (e.g., lateral knee movement, foot tapping, heel dropping, foot squirming, inversion and eversion of foot)	0 1 2 3 4	0 1 2 3 4	0 1 2 3 4	0 1 2 3 4
Trunk Movements	**7. Neck, shoulder, hips** (e.g., rocking, twisting, squirming, pelvic gyrations)	0 1 2 3 4	0 1 2 3 4	0 1 2 3 4	0 1 2 3 4
Global Judgments	**8. Severity of abnormal movements overall**	0 1 2 3 4	0 1 2 3 4	0 1 2 3 4	0 1 2 3 4
	9. Incapacitation due to abnormal movements	0 1 2 3 4	0 1 2 3 4	0 1 2 3 4	0 1 2 3 4
	10. Patient's awareness of abnormal movements: Rate only patient's report. No awareness 0 Aware, no distress 1 Aware, mild distress 2 Aware, moderate distress 3 Aware, severe distress 4	0 1 2 3 4	0 1 2 3 4	0 1 2 3 4	0 1 2 3 4
Dental Status	**11. Current problems with teeth and/or dentures**	No Yes	No Yes	No Yes	No Yes
	12. Are dentures usually worn?	No Yes	No Yes	No Yes	No Yes
	13. Edentia	No Yes	No Yes	No Yes	No Yes
	14. Do movements disappear in sleep?	No Yes	No Yes	No Yes	No Yes

• **Fig. 35.3** Abnormal Inventory Movement Scale (AIMS). (From Halter, M. [2018]. *Varcarolis' foundations of psychiatric mental health nursing* [8th ed.]. St. Louis: Elsevier.)

BLACK BOX WARNING!

Antipsychotic Medications in Older Adults

Antipsychotics have not received approval from the U.S. Food and Drug Administration (FDA) for the treatment of dementia-related psychosis in older adults, as they are associated with a significantly increased incidence of cerebrovascular events (e.g., stroke, transient ischemic attack), including fatal events.

First-Generation Antipsychotics

FGAs, also known as conventional or typical antipsychotics, were introduced in the early 1950s and revolutionized the treatment of schizophrenia by significantly reducing positive symptoms of psychosis including hallucinations and delusions (Table 35.3). FGAs act primarily by blocking D_2 receptors in the dopamine pathway of the brain. The

AIMS Examination Procedure
Either before or after completing the Examination Procedure, observe the patient unobtrusively, at rest (e.g., in waiting room).

The chair to be used in this examination should be a hard, firm one without arms.

1. Ask patient to remove shoes and socks.
2. Ask patient whether there is anything in his or her mouth (e.g., gum, candy) and, if there is, to remove it.
3. Ask patient about the *current* condition of his or her teeth. Ask patient if he or she wears dentures. Do teeth or dentures bother the patient *now?*
4. Ask patient whether he or she notices any movements in mouth, face, hands, or feet. If yes, ask to describe and to what extent they *currently* bother patient or interfere with his or her activities.
5. Have patient sit in chair with hands on knees, legs slightly apart, and feet flat on floor. Look at entire body movements while in this position.
6. Ask patient to sit with hands hanging unsupported: if male, between legs; if female and wearing a dress, hanging over knees. Observe hands and other body areas.
7. Ask patient to open mouth. Observe tongue at rest within mouth. Do this twice.
8. Ask patient to protrude tongue. Observe abnormalities of tongue movement. Do this twice.
9. Ask patient to tap thumb, with each finger, as rapidly as possible for 10 to 15 seconds, separately with right hand, then with left hand. Observe each facial and leg movement.
10. Flex and extend patient's left and right arms (one at a time). Note any rigidity.
11. Ask patient to stand up. Observe in profile. Observe all body areas again, hips included.
12. Ask patient to extend both arms outstretched in front with palms down. Observe trunk, legs, and mouth.
13. Have patient walk a few paces, turn, and walk back to chair. Observe hands and gait. Do this twice.

• **Fig. 35.3—cont'd**

dopamine blockade results in decreased positive symptoms. FGAs also can block muscarinic cholinergic, H1, and α_1-adrenergic receptors to a lesser degree. As a result, FGAs are associated with a number of uncomfortable side effects and can cause significant DIMDs.

Fluphenazine

Pharmacokinetics. Fluphenazine can be administered via oral, subcutaneous, and intramuscular (IM) routes; this includes the immediate-release and decanoate long-acting oil-based solutions. It is highly plasma protein bound and metabolized in the liver. Oral fluphenazine is rapidly absorbed, but peak plasma concentrations are highly variable due to possible first-pass metabolism in the liver. Immediate-release fluphenazine's onset of action is approximately 1 hour, with a duration of 6 to 8 hours from a single dose. Decanoate injection onset of action is typically within 24 hours. The average interval between injections is 14 days, with a range of 7 to 28 days. Careful adjustment of the oral dose is required before conversion to depot therapy. Plasma concentrations of decanoate preparation approach steady state after 3 months. Excretion is primarily through the kidneys.

Indications. Fluphenazine, a phenothiazine, can be used for the treatment of positive symptoms in patients with schizophrenia. Decanoate forms are used for patients who require long-acting parenteral antipsychotic agents in the management of schizophrenia. IM immediate-acting fluphenazine can be used for acute agitation associated with psychotic disorders.

Adverse Effects. The most common adverse effects are akathisia, weight gain, xerostomia, and pseudoparkinsonism, each occurring in about 10% of patients. Less common effects (1% to 10%) include constipation, dizziness, drowsiness, headache, and dystonic reaction. Hematologic disorders may occur with the use of antipsychotics, with leukopenia, including agranulocytosis, being the most common. Other hematologic abnormalities include eosinophilia, thrombocytopenia, hemolytic anemia, and aplastic anemia. Hyperprolactinemia may occur with effects such as menstrual irregularity, breast enlargement, impotence, and decreased libido. Neuroleptic malignant syndrome is rare but can occur in patients receiving phenothiazine agents.

Contraindications. Fluphenazine is contraindicated in children younger than 12 years of age. It should not be used in any patient with hypersensitivity to phenothiazines. Fluphenazine should not be used in patients with CNS depression, those who use large doses of hypnotic medications, or those who are heavy users of alcohol. Because of potential hematologic effects, it should not be used in patients with hematologic disorders. Due to its anticholinergic effects, fluphenazine should be avoided in patients with benign prostatic hypertrophy (BPH), closed-angle glaucoma, or paralytic ileus. It may increase the risk for QT prolongation.

Monitoring. Patients receiving fluphenazine should be monitored regularly for DIMDs. Monitor complete blood

TABLE 35.2	Examples of Common Drug Interactions With Antipsychotics

Antipsychotic	Drugs Affected
All antipsychotics	↑↓ Phenytoin
Chlorpromazine	↓ Epinephrine, norepinephrine
Clozapine	↑ Risperidone
Olanzapine, quetiapine, risperidone	↓ Dopamine agonists, levodopa
Phenothiazines	↑ Propranolol
	↓ Dexmethylphenidate, bromocriptine
Quetiapine	↑ Lorazepam
Thioridazine	↓ Quetiapine

Drug	Antipsychotic Affected
Aluminum salts	↓ Phenothiazines
Anticholinergics	↓ Phenothiazines
Meperidine, propranolol	↓ Phenothiazines
Carbamazepine	↑ Haloperidol, olanzapine, risperidone
Cimetidine	↑ Quetiapine
Fluoxetine	↑ Haloperidol
Lithium	↑ Phenothiazines, haloperidol
Phenytoin	↓ Quetiapine, thioridazine, haloperidol
3A4, 2D6 inducers	↓ Increase aripiprazole, most second-generation antipsychotics
3A4, 2D6 inhibitors, metoclopramide	↑ Aripiprazole, most second-generation antipsychotics

count (CBC) due to the risk of hematologic complications. Patients should be monitored for hyperprolactinemia. Fluphenazine should not be abruptly discontinued.

Haloperidol

Haloperidol is a non-phenothiazine FGA that was approved by the FDA in the late 1960s as a treatment for psychotic illnesses including schizophrenia. It has also been used as an intervention for agitation in emergent or acute care settings.

Pharmacokinetics. Haloperidol is primarily administered orally and intramuscularly, with intravenous (IV) formulations only used in acute care settings. It is approximately 92% protein bound. Oral doses exhibit extensive first-pass metabolism which occurs in the liver, with cytochrome (CYP) 2D6 and CYP 3A4 as the primary isoenzymes involved. Slow metabolizers of CYP 2D6 appear to be at increased risk of experiencing DIMDs due to delayed clearance of the drug. Approximately 40% of the immediate-release form is excreted renally within 5 days. Half-life

of immediate-release forms is approximately 16 hours in adults. Depot injections typically achieve peak plasma after 5 days, with steady state after the third to fourth dose. Half-life of decanoate form is about 3 weeks.

Indications. Haloperidol can be used in the treatment of patients with schizophrenia. It can also be used in emergent or acute care settings for the treatment of acute agitation in patients with schizophrenia or related psychiatric disorder. Haloperidol can be used in the treatment of severe behavioral disorders in pediatric patients who experience excessive motor activity with conduct disorders.

Adverse Effects. More than 10% of patients can experience DIMDs including akathisia, acute dystonia, and pseudoparkinsonism. Acute dystonia typically appears within the first 24 to 96 hours, pseudoparkinsonism within 1 to 2 weeks, and akathisia within days to several weeks of therapy. TD can occur in patients who have received long-term therapy or after haloperidol therapy is discontinued.

Other common adverse effects include restlessness, tremor, and lethargy. Weight gain can also occur, which may be related to increased prolactin levels or antagonism of histamine-1 receptors, although it is generally less common than with SGAs. Patients receiving injectable medications may have local tissue reactions including injection site pain, swelling, and redness. Haloperidol can cause adverse ocular effects including cataracts, blurred vision, and retinopathy.

Contraindications. Antipsychotics are not FDA approved for use in patients who have dementia-related psychosis. Haloperidol is contraindicated in patients diagnosed with Parkinson's disease, CNS depression, or Lewy body dementia. Abrupt discontinuation of antipsychotics including haloperidol may result in transient dyskinetic movements that resemble TD. Observe patients for symptom exacerbation and dyskinetic movements after the drug is discontinued.

PRACTICE PEARLS

Abrupt Discontinuation of Antipsychotic Medications

Abrupt discontinuation of antipsychotic therapy may result in transient dyskinetic movements that may resemble TD. In addition, abrupt discontinuation can result in nausea, vomiting, diaphoresis, restlessness, anxiety, and agitation. When feasible, drugs should be tapered. Observe for dyskinetic movements as well as return of psychiatric symptoms.

Haloperidol should be used during pregnancy only when the benefits to the mother outweigh the risks to the fetus. Breastfeeding should be avoided in patients who are taking haloperidol.

Monitoring. Patients taking haloperidol should be monitored for movement disorders at 3- to 6-month intervals. Monitor for ocular changes, including cataracts. Teach patients to report any unusual changes in vision. Monitor for any symptoms associated with hyperprolactinemia.

TABLE 35.3	First-Generation Antipsychotic Medications			

Category/ Medication	Indication	Dosage		Considerations and Monitoring
Phenothiazines				
Aliphatics				
Chlorprom-azine[a]	Treatment of schizophrenia	*Adults, mild to moderate symptoms:* Begin with 10 mg orally three to four times daily or 25 mg two to three times daily. *Severe symptoms:* Begin with 25 mg orally three times daily. After 1 or 2 days, daily dosage may be increased by 20–50 mg at semiweekly intervals until patient becomes calm and cooperative.		Recommend use of AIMS assessment to determine presence of adverse effects. Patients on high doses should have regular ophthalmic exams. Older and/or debilitated patients with schizophrenia should begin with lower doses and may require overall lower doses.
Fluphenazine	Treatment of schizophrenia	*Adults:* 2.5–10 mg/day orally every 6–8 hr; may increase gradually as needed and tolerated. Usual maximum dosage: 20 mg/day in divided doses. *Older adults:* 1–2.5 mg orally as single or divided dose; increase as tolerated. Usual maximum dosage: 20 mg/day in divided doses. *Injectable decanoate form:* 6.25–25 mg IM or subcutaneously every 2 weeks.		After response has been obtained, gradual reduction of the dosage to 1–5 mg/day orally for maintenance therapy, often as a single daily dose, is recommended. Adjust to lowest effective and tolerated dose.
Perphenazine	Treatment of schizophrenia	*Adults, adolescents, and children ≥12 yr:* 4–8 mg orally three times daily initially; reduce as soon as possible to minimum effective dosage.		Adjust to maintenance dose at the lowest effective dose. After dosage is stabilized, may be given as a single bedtime dose or in 2 divided doses (one-third in the morning and two-thirds at bedtime) to improve adherence to therapy.
Trifluoperazine	Treatment of schizophrenia	*Adults:* Begin with 2–5 mg orally once to twice daily; may increase gradually as needed and tolerated. Usual doses are 15–20 mg/day in divided doses.		Lower initial doses and slower titration are recommended in older adults or debilitated adults.
Non-Phenothiazines				
Butyrophenone				
Haloperidol	Treatment of schizophrenia	*Adults:* Begin with 0.5–2 mg orally two to three times daily. Severe, chronic, or refractory target symptoms may require 3–5 mg two to three times daily. *Adolescents:* 0.5–5 mg orally daily; may administer in 2 or 3 divided doses. *Children 3–12 yr weighing 15–40 kg:* 0.5 mg orally daily initially; may administer in 2 or 3 divided doses. The usual dosage range is 0.05–0.15 mg/kg/day. **Decanoate depot injection:** *Adults:* Usual IM maintenance dosage range is 50–200 mg every 4 weeks.		Patients should be stabilized on an immediate-release antipsychotic before considering a conversion to haloperidol decanoate for treating schizophrenia in those who require prolonged parenteral therapy. Follow clinical practice guidelines for conversion of oral dosage to depot injection.
Thioxanthenes				
Thiothixene	Treatment of schizophrenia	*Adults, adolescents, and children:* Begin with 2 mg orally three times daily or 5 mg twice daily based on severity of symptoms. Increase dosage gradually based on response and tolerability. Usual dosage is 20–30 mg daily in divided doses.		Use lowest effective dose.

[a]These dosages are associated with treatment in the outpatient setting. *ADHD,* Attention deficit hyperactivity disorder; *AIMS,* Abnormal Involuntary Movement Scale; *IM,* intramuscular.

Second-Generation Antipsychotics

SGAs, sometimes called atypical or conventional antipsychotics, were introduced in the 1990s with the release of clozapine (Table 35.4). In general, SGAs are less likely to cause DIMDs than FGAs, but they are associated with an increased risk of cardiovascular events and premature death secondary to metabolic effects including weight gain, diabetes mellitus, and hyperlipidemia. While FGAs primarily antagonize D_2 receptors, SGAs produce strong blockade of 5-HT3 serotonin receptors and have a lower affinity for D_2 receptors. While the lower affinity for D_2 receptors may be responsible for a lower incidence of movement disorders, the risk is not eliminated completely. As a result, all patients taking antipsychotic medications should be screened regularly for DMIDs.

Risperidone

Pharmacokinetics. Risperidone is available orally in a tablet, disintegrating tablet, or solution and as an injectable for IM or subcutaneous depot routes. Oral forms are completely absorbed and may be given without regard to meals. Peak plasma concentrations occur 1 to 2 hours after administration.

Indications. Risperidone is used for the treatment of schizophrenia in adults and adolescents. It is also used in the treatment of bipolar I disorder, including acute mania or mixed episodes, as well as with maintenance therapy of bipolar I as monotherapy or as an adjunct to lithium or valproate. Steady-state plasma concentrations of IM depot forms are reached after 4 injections and are maintained for 4 to 6 weeks. Steady-state plasma concentrations of the subcutaneous form can be achieved after the second injection, with each injection separated by 28 days. Risperidone is approximately 90% protein bound, with its major active metabolite about 77% protein bound. Risperidone is metabolized to an equally active metabolite, 9-hydroxyrisperidone. Excretion is mainly renal, with a small amount excreted in the feces.

Adverse Effects. As with other SGAs, risperidone can cause weight gain (up to 32% of patients), pseudoparkinsonism ($\leq$28%), akathisia ($\leq$11%), and hyperprolactinemia (>10%). Hyperlipidemia and acute dystonia can occur in up to 6.3% and $\leq$6% of patients, respectively. Movement disorders are more common in patients taking higher doses of risperidone. Other common adverse effects include drowsiness, insomnia, headache, nausea, and constipation. Elevated liver function tests (LFTs) have been reported. Injection site reactions such as pain, swelling, bruising, and induration have occurred in some patients.

Contraindications. Risperidone is contraindicated in the treatment of psychosis in patients with dementia. It should not be used in patients with any significant CNS depression.

Monitoring. As with other antipsychotics, it is important to monitor for DIMDs. Include lab work to detect metabolic abnormalities including changes in blood glucose, HbA1c, serum lipid profile, and serum prolactin. In addition, due to potential adverse effects, monitor LFTs, thyroid function tests, serum creatinine, and serum electrolytes. Fall risk assessments should be completed frequently in at-risk patients. Consistently monitor patients for weight gain, and include weight management strategies as needed.

Clozapine

Clozapine, developed in the late 1980s, was the first of the SGA antipsychotics available. It acts by blocking dopamine receptors with a high affinity for D_4 receptors and a low affinity for D_1 and D_2 receptors. In addition, it blocks serotonin 5-HT2A receptors. With its decreased affinity for select dopamine receptors in the nigrostriatal dopaminergic pathway of the brain, clozapine has a lower incidence of DIMDs. Clozapine also blocks α_1-adrenergic and histamine receptors which can lead to orthostatic hypotension and sedation, respectively. Blockade of muscarinic receptors leads to a range of uncomfortable anticholinergic effects.

Pharmacokinetics. Clozapine is administered orally as tablets, orally disintegrating tablets, and oral suspension. Food does not appear to affect bioavailability. Clozapine is highly protein bound. Metabolism occurs primarily via CYP 1A2, CYP 2D6, and CYP 3A4. Onset of antipsychotic action can take several weeks, with maximum effects typically achieved within several months. Of note, effective dosage is widely variable among individuals. This is due to a weak relationship between the dose of clozapine and serum concentration. Clozapine is almost completely metabolized prior to excretion, with about 50% of the dose excreted in the urine and 30% in the feces primarily as metabolites.

Indications. Clozapine is used for the treatment of schizophrenia in patients whose symptoms have been unresponsive to appropriate courses of other antipsychotics. In addition, clozapine has been used effectively to reduce suicidal behavior in patients with schizophrenia or schizoaffective disorders.

Adverse Effects. The major adverse effect associated with the use of clozapine is a risk of hematologic effects including severe neutropenia with an absolute neutrophil count (ANC) less than 500/microL. Severe neutropenia can lead to severe infection and even death; the risk is greatest during the first 18 weeks and then declines. The most common adverse effects of clozapine include drowsiness (up to 46% of patients), dizziness (15% to 27%), constipation (14% to 25%), increased heart rate (25%), and insomnia (2% to 20%). Nearly 20% of patients experience nausea and vomiting. Hypersalivation can occur in nearly 50% of patients. While usually mild, the hypersalivation and drooling may be severe and troublesome during sleep. Hypersalivation may decrease with reduction of clozapine dosage.

TABLE 35.4 Second-Generation Antipsychotic Medications

Category/ Medication	Indication	Dosage	Considerations and Monitoring
Clozapine	Treatment of refractory schizophrenia that has failed to respond adequately to standard antipsychotic therapies Reduce risk of recurrent suicidal behavior in patients with schizophrenia or schizoaffective disorder	*Adults:* Doses typically begin with 12.5 mg orally once or twice daily on day 1. After day 1, dose may be titrated by 25–50 mg once daily over 2 weeks, up to a dose of 300–450 mg/day in divided doses. Maximum dosage: 900 mg/day.	All patients receiving clozapine must be enrolled in the FDA's Clozapine REMS Program because of the risk of severe neutropenia. All prescribers must be certified in the Clozapine REMS Program. The ANC is the only test result accepted in the Clozapine REMS Program to monitor for neutropenia.
Quetiapine	Treatment of schizophrenia	*Adults and adolescents:* Typically begin with 25 mg orally twice daily, then titrate based on tolerability and response. Usual maintenance dose range is 400–800 mg orally daily. *Extended-release form (SR):* *Adults:* Begin with 300 mg orally once daily, preferably in the evening. Titrate to 400–800 mg once daily, based on response and tolerability. Maximum dosage: 800 mg/day. *Older adults and adolescents:* Typically begin with 50 mg/day, then titrate to usual dose of 400–800 mg/day.	Use AIMS assessment for detection of adverse effects. Inform patient and caregiver to report significant changes in behavior or suicidal ideation. Give extended-release tablets without food or with fewer than 300 calories.
Olanzapine	Treatment of schizophrenia	*Adults not at risk for hypotension:* Usual dose is 5–10 mg orally daily. Doses >10 mg/day not considered more efficacious. Maximum dosage: 20 mg/day. *Older adults:* Begin at 5 mg orally daily. Doses >10 mg/day not considered more efficacious. Maximum dosage: 20 mg/day. *Adolescents:* 2.5–5 mg orally once daily. Target dosage: 10 mg/day. Maximum dosage: 20 mg/day. **IM dosage (extended-release suspension, Zyprexa Relprevv):** *Adults not at risk for hypotension:* 150–300 mg deep IM every 2 weeks or 405 mg IM every 4 weeks.	Debilitated adults or those with factors leading to slower metabolism, including older adults, nonsmokers, and females, are at higher risk for hypotensive reactions. Maintain at lowest effective dosage. Zyprexa Relprevv must be given in a registered health care facility with ready access to emergency response services. Monitor all patients after each injection at the facility for at least 3 hours. Confirm that someone will accompany patient after the 3-hour observation period.

TABLE 35.4 **Second-Generation Antipsychotic Medications—cont'd**

Category/ Medication	Indication	Dosage	Considerations and Monitoring
Asenapine	Treatment of schizophrenia	*Adults, acute treatment:* 5 mg SL twice daily. Maintenance dosage: 5 mg SL twice daily; may increase to 10 mg SL twice daily after 1 week if needed/tolerated. Maximum dosage: 20 mg/day sublingually. *Transdermal patch:* Begin with 3.8 mg/24 hr transdermal; progress to 5.7–7.6 mg/24 hr. Maximum dosage: 7.6 mg/24 hr.	For SL formulation, patient should not eat or drink at least 10 minutes after administration. Instruct patient to avoid applying external heat sources (e.g., heating pad) over the transdermal system since prolonged heat increases asenapine plasma concentrations.
Risperidone	Treatment of schizophrenia	*Adults:* Usually begin at 2 mg orally once daily or 1 mg twice daily. Effective range is 4–16 mg/day. Recommended target dosage is 4–8 mg orally daily. *Older adults:* Typically begin with 0.5 mg orally twice daily. Dose adjustments should be at intervals of at least 24 hr and in increments of 1–2 mg/day as tolerated to the recommended target dose range of 4–8 mg/day orally. Maximum dosage: 16 mg/day. *Adolescents:* Begin with 0.5 mg orally once daily. Effective dosage range is 1–6 mg orally daily. Dosages above 3 mg/day are associated with more adverse events. **Risperidone Consta IM depot dose:** *Adults:* 25 mg IM (deep gluteal or deltoid injection) once every 2 weeks. May supplement with oral dose for 3 weeks after the first injection until adequate plasma concentrations of the depot dose is attained. **Subcutaneous depot dose (Perseris):** *Adults:* Begin with 90–120 mg by abdominal subcutaneous injection once a month. Maximum dosage: 120 mg/ month.	Monitor for EPS with each visit. Titration of response is typically directed toward achieving maximum benefit at lowest safe dose. Monitor for weight gain and refer as needed for nutrition management. Oral disintegrating tablets should not be split or crushed. Before beginning IM or subcutaneous forms of risperidone, tolerability must be established with oral risperidone.
	Treatment of irritability in children and adolescents with autistic disorder	*Children and adolescents 5–17 yr:* If weight is ≥20 kg, begin with 0.5 mg orally daily for at least 4 days, then may increase to recommended dose of 1 mg daily. Maintain this dose for at least 14 days. Thereafter, adjust as clinically necessary at intervals of at least 2 weeks and at increments of 0.5 mg/day. Effective dosage range: 0.5–3 mg orally daily. If weight is 15–19 kg, begin at 0.25 mg orally once daily. May increase to recommended dose by 0.5 mg daily and adjust as necessary at intervals of at least 2 weeks. Effective dosage range: 0.5–3 mg/day.	Once adequate clinical response has been achieved, consider gradually lowering the dose for optimal balance of safety and efficacy. Periodically reassess during long-term therapy.

Continued

TABLE 35.4 Second-Generation Antipsychotic Medications—cont'd

Category/ Medication	Indication	Dosage	Considerations and Monitoring
Iloperidone	Treatment of schizophrenia	*Adults:* Typically begin at 1 mg orally twice daily. May increase in increments of no more than 2 mg twice daily. Target dosage: 6–12 mg twice daily. Maximum dosage: 24 mg/day in divided doses.	Titrate slowly to minimize hypotension. Not recommended for patients with severe liver impairment.
Paliperidone	Treatment of schizophrenia	**Extended-release tablets:** *Adults:* Begin at 3 mg once daily: may increase by 3 mg at intervals of at least 5 days. Maximum dosage: 12 mg/day. *Adolescents and children ≥51 kg:* Initially 3 mg orally once daily. May increase by increments of 3 mg/day at intervals of more than 5 days, if needed. Use lowest effective dose. Maximum dosage: 12 mg/day. *Adolescents and children <51 kg:* Begin with 3 mg orally daily. May increase by 3 mg/day in intervals of at least 5 days. Maximum dosage: 6 mg/day. **IM once-monthly injectable suspension (Invega Sustenna):** *Adults:* Dosage range: 39–234 mg IM every month. **IM 3-month depot injection (Invega Trinza):** *Adults:* Usual dosage range: 273–819 mg IM every 3 months.	Use lowest effective dose. Follow protocols carefully for initiation and missed doses of IM depot injections. Dose adjustment not required in patients with mild to moderate liver impairment. Has not been studied in patients with severe liver impairment. Dose reduction is recommended for patients with CrCl <80 mL/min. Not recommended for patients with severe renal disease.
Lurasidone	Treatment of schizophrenia	*Adults:* 40 mg orally once daily with food (at least 350 calories). Usual dosage: 40–160 mg/day. Maximum dosage: 160 mg/day. *Adolescents:* 40 mg orally once daily with food (at least 350 calories). Usual dosage: 40–80 mg/day. Maximum dosage: 80 mg/day.	Review possible drug interactions carefully as dosage adjustment may be necessary.
Ziprasidone	Treatment of schizophrenia	*Adults:* Begin with 20 mg orally twice daily with food. May be increased up to 80 mg twice daily.	Use cautiously with severe hepatic impairment. Administer with food to increase absorption. Administer at about the same time each day.

AIMS, Abnormal Involuntary Movement Scale (see Fig. 35.3); *ANC*, absolute neutrophil count; *EPS*, extrapyramidal symptoms; *FDA*, U.S. Food and Drug Administration; *IM*, intramuscular; *ODT*, oral disintegrating tablet; *REMS*, Risk Evaluation and Mitigation Strategy; *SL*, sublingual.

Contraindications. Clozapine is contraindicated in patients with agranulocytosis. In addition, there are three black box warnings for clozapine. First, clozapine has been associated with an increased risk of fatal cardiomyopathy or myocarditis, especially during the first month of therapy. The second black box warning concerns the use of clozapine in patients who are taking medications or have conditions that may result in QT prolongation, as bradycardia, severe orthostatic hypotension, syncope, and even cardiac arrest have occurred with clozapine therapy. Finally, as with other antipsychotics, clozapine has a black box warning for use in patients with dementia.

Other precautions include use of anticholinergic medications that can decrease gastrointestinal (GI) motility and result in severe constipation. Use of clozapine may also increase the risk of metabolic syndrome, increasing the risk for cardiovascular events.

QUALITY AND SAFETY

Prescription of Clozapine

Clozapine is available only through the Clozapine Risk Evaluation and Mitigation Strategy (REMS) Program, which restricts prescribers of clozapine. All prescribers, prescriber designees, and dispensing pharmacies must be certified, and all patients must be enrolled in the REMS Program. This is due to the risk of severe neutropenia which can lead to serious infection and even death. More information can be found at https://www.clozapinerems.com.

Monitoring. Follow protocols as recommended by the REMS Program for enrolling, monitoring, and educating patients and evaluating neutropenia. Use the AIMS assessment to monitor for potential movement disorders. Monitor weight, lipid profile, blood glucose, and serum prolactin carefully to reduce the risk of cardiovascular events. Evaluate for any symptoms of dizziness, syncope, or palpitations which may indicate serious adverse events.

Tobacco use increases clearance of clozapine. As a result, patients who smoke should be monitored for decreased response to clozapine and may require increased dosing.

QUALITY AND SAFETY

Discontinuation of Antipsychotics

- Sudden discontinuation of antipsychotic medications can result in withdrawal dyskinesias as well as an increased risk of NMS. In addition, sudden discontinuation of antipsychotics that have strong α-adrenergic receptor blocking effects can result in rebound hypertension, tremor, palpitations, headache, and rebound anxiety.
- Monitor carefully for increased risk of psychiatric symptoms.

Third-Generation Antipsychotics

Aripiprazole

Aripiprazole was the first TGA to be made available; others include brexpiprazole and cariprazine (Table 35.5). These newer drugs typically result in fewer DIMDs due to a slightly different mechanism of action. TGAs affect both dopamine and serotonin receptors, like other antipsychotics. In general, these drugs are partial agonists of the D_2 receptor and the serotonin 5-HT1A receptor. They also act as antagonists at the serotonin 5-HT2A receptors. In addition, they block H1 receptors and α_1-adrenergic receptors.

Pharmacokinetics. Aripiprazole is administered orally or intramuscularly. It is approximately 99% protein bound. Metabolism of aripiprazole occurs mainly through CYP 3A4 and CYP 2D6, with excretion in the urine and feces. Mean half-life is generally 75 to 94 hours for immediate-release formulations. Half-life varies for differing IM depot preparations.

PHARMACOGENETICS

Aripiprazole and CYP 2D6 Poor Metabolizers

Approximately 8% of Caucasians and 3% to 8% of African Americans lack the capacity to metabolize CYP 2D6 substrates. These *poor metabolizers* have a roughly 80% increase in aripiprazole exposure and an approximately 30% decrease in exposure to the active metabolite. As a result, dosage adjustments are recommended in poor metabolizers of CYP 2D6 due to higher aripiprazole concentrations.

Indications. Aripiprazole is used for the treatment of schizophrenia. It can also be used in patients with acute agitation associated with schizophrenia or bipolar I disorder.

Adverse Effects. The most common adverse effects associated with aripiprazole are headache (<27% of patients), weight gain (2.2% to 26.3%), and drowsiness (4% to 23%). Other adverse effects include anxiety, insomnia, nausea, and vomiting. Potential DIMDs include akathisia (2% to 13%), dystonia (2%), pseudoparkinsonism (0.1% to 4%), and TD (unknown). NMS is rare.

Contraindications. There is a black box warning regarding the use of aripiprazole in patients with dementia. Of note, there is also a black box warning regarding the use of aripiprazole in children, adolescents, and young adults who receive it for treatment of major depression, as it may increase suicidal ideation and suicide risk. Use cautiously in patients with risk for QT prolongation as aripiprazole may increase this risk. Use with caution in patients with hematological disease.

Aripiprazole is recommended for use during pregnancy only if the benefits to the mother outweigh the risk to the fetus. It should not be used in patients who are breastfeeding, if possible, as it is excreted in breast milk and may accumulate in the infant due to long elimination half-life.

Monitoring. Evaluate for DIMDs using the AIMS assessment (or a comparable assessment). Monitor for signs

TABLE 35.5	Third-Generation Antipsychotics		
Medication	**Indication**	**Dosage**	**Considerations and Monitoring**
Aripiprazole	Treatment of schizophrenia	**Immediate-release oral dosage forms, tablets, orally disintegrating tablets, oral solution**: *Adults:* 10–15 mg orally once daily as tablets, ODT, or oral solution. *Adolescents:* Begin with 2 mg orally once daily. After 2 days may increase to 5 mg once daily, and after 2 more days may increase to the target dose of 10 mg once daily. **Aripiprazole tablet with sensor to track ingestion (Abilify MyCite)**: *Adults* 10–15 mg once daily. Do not increase the dose before 2 weeks. **IM dose (extended-release injectable suspension [Abilify Maintena]):** *Adults* 400 mg IM once monthly. Once stabilized, may reduce to 300 mg monthly IM based on tolerability.	Do not split/crush the MyCite tablet. The FDA has issued a safety alert to monitor for impulse control disorders (e.g., gambling, binge eating). Review all drug interactions carefully as dosage adjustments may be required. Carefully review all drug inserts and practice guidelines for transition from oral to IM dosages. Brand names vary in terms of dosages and administration. Review carefully.
Brexpiprazole	Treatment of schizophrenia	*Adults:* 1 mg orally once daily, initially. On Day 5, may increase to 2 mg once daily. On Day 8, may increase to 4 mg orally once daily based on response and tolerability. Usual dosage: 2–4 mg once daily. Maximum dosage: 4 mg/day orally. *Older adults:* Begin at low dose range and pwwrogress slowly to response and tolerability. *Adolescents:* Begin with 0.5 mg orally once daily. On Day 5, may increase to 1 mg once daily. On Day 8, may further increase to 2 mg daily. Further titration may be made weekly in 1-mg increments based on response and tolerability. Usual dosage: 2–4 mg once daily. Maximum dosage: 4 mg daily.	May administer without regard to food. In patients who are poor metabolizers of CYP2D6, give one-half of the usual dose. If the patients are receiving another moderate or strong CYP3A4 inhibitor, give one-fourth of the usual dose.
Cariprazine	Treatment of schizophrenia	*Adults:* Begin with 1.5 mg orally. May increase to 3 mg once daily on Day 2. If needed, further dose adjustments can be made in 1.5-mg to 3-mg increments. Usual dosage: 1.5–6 mg once daily. Maximum dosage: 6 mg/day.	May give with or without food. Impact of changes in dose will not be fully reflected in plasma for several weeks. Monitor patient response carefully for several weeks after beginning the drug and after each dosage change.

of metabolic syndrome, including weight gain, lipid profile, and blood glucose as well as serum prolactin. Consider pregnancy testing prior to beginning therapy.

Vesicular Monoamine Transporter Type 2 (VMAT2) Inhibitors

According to recent clinical practice guidelines, VMAT2 inhibitors should be used to treat the severe or disabling symptoms of TD in patients requiring antipsychotic medications (APA, 2019) (Table 35.6). The first available VMAT2 inhibitor, valbenazine, was approved by the FDA in 2017. Normally, VMAT2 acts as a transporter protein found in presynaptic neurons in the CNS. It stores monoamines, including dopamine, for release in the synaptic cleft. These drugs generally decrease dopamine signaling from the presynaptic to the postsynaptic neurons, resulting in reduced motor symptoms.

Valbenazine

Pharmacokinetics. Valbenazine is administered orally. It is metabolized by the liver to form the active metabolite [+]-alpha-dihydrotetrabenazine ([+]-alpha-HTBZ) and by oxidative metabolism, primarily by CYP 3A4/5, to form other minor metabolites. The active metabolite is further metabolized by CYP 2D6. Maximum plasma concentrations of valbenazine are attained in 0.5 to 1 hour. Steady-state plasma concentrations are reached within 1 week. Oral bioavailability of valbenazine is about 49%. The active

PHARMACOGENETICS

Valbenazine

Doses of valbenazine should be adjusted for patients who are poor metabolizers of CYP 2D6. For these patients, the recommended dose is 40 mg/day.

TABLE 35.6	Vesicular Monoamine Transporter Type 2 (VMAT2) Inhibitors			
Medication	**Indication**	**Dosage**	**Considerations and Monitoring**	
Valbenazine	Treatment of tardive dyskinesia	*Adults:* Begin with 40 mg orally once daily. After 1 week, may increase to 80 mg once daily. Dosage of 40–60 mg once daily may be considered. Maximum dosage: 80 mg/day.	May cause an increase in the QTc interval in patients who are poor metabolizers of CYP2D6; therefore recommended dose in these patients is 40 mg/day.	
Deutetrabenazine	Treatment of tardive dyskinesia	*Adults:* Begin with 6 mg orally twice daily. Increase dosage at weekly intervals by increments of 6 mg/day to a maximum total daily dose of 48 mg.	Do not exceed 18 mg/dose or 36 mg/day in patients who are poor CYP2D6 metabolizers. Follow protocols carefully if patient is switching to deutetrabenzine from tetrabenazine. Should be given with food.	

CYP, Cytochrome.

metabolite [+]-alpha-HTBZ reaches maximum concentrations 4 to 8 hours after administration.

Indications. Valbenazine is used for the treatment of TD associated with the use of antipsychotic medications.

Adverse Effects. The most common adverse effect associated with valbenazine is drowsiness (approximately 11% of patients). Infrequently, patients experience anticholinergic effects including xerostomia, constipation, blurred vision, and urinary retention. Patients requiring higher doses may experience hyperprolactinemia and hyperglycemia. Allergic dermatitis, urticaria, pruritis, and reactions consistent with angioedema have occurred.

Contraindications. Valbenazine is contraindicated in patients with hypersensitivity to valbenazine or any components in the formulation. It should be used cautiously in any patient with Parkinson's disease and in those with a history of or risk for prolonged QT interval as it may prolong QT interval in some patients; examples include patients with heart failure, hypertension, coronary artery disease (CAD), hypokalemia, diabetes mellitus, alcoholism, or hepatic dysfunction, or those who use other medications that may worsen QT prolongation. There are insufficient data to provide valbenazine-associated risks in patients who are pregnant or breastfeeding.

Valbenazine may cause parkinsonism in patients with TD secondary to dopamine blockade. These symptoms reportedly occurred within the first 2 weeks after beginning therapy with valbenazine or with increasing the dose. Associated symptoms included tremor, hypokinesia, drooling, gait disturbances, and falls. The symptoms resolved after the dosage was reduced or the drug was discontinued.

Monitoring. Patients taking valbenazine for TD should be screened using the AIMS test or a similar tool for baseline evaluation of TD symptoms. Symptoms should be monitored every 3 to 12 months depending on risk. Also teach patients to report any symptoms that may indicate parkinsonism while taking the medication. Monitor for hyperglycemia or prolactin-related side effects.

Prescriber Considerations for Antipsychotic Therapy

Clinical Practice Guidelines

While antipsychotics are typically prescribed in specialty practices, primary care providers should assess nonadherence to therapy, monitor adverse effects, and provide ongoing patient education. Familiarity with clinical practice guidelines can enhance the provider's contributions to the overall plan of care and help ensure that the patient and family have the resources they need for successful management of the disease and reduction of associated risks.

> **BOOKMARK THIS!**
>
> **APA Clinical Practice Guidelines**
>
> It is important for patients to have access to primary care providers as well as psychiatrists for ongoing monitoring and treatment. Primary care providers may use guidelines in helping to manage overall care for patients with schizophrenia. These include recommendations for patient assessment, pharmacologic management, treatment of select adverse effects, and nonpharmacologic interventions such as cognitive behavioral interventions, psychoeducation, and support for self-care (APA, 2019).
>
> From https://www.psychiatry.org/psychiatrists/practice/clinical-practice-guidelines. Reprinted with permission from the American Journal of Psychiatry, (Copyright © 2020). American Psychiatric Association. All Rights Reserved.

Clinical Reasoning for Antipsychotic Therapy

Consider the individual patient's health problem requiring antipsychotic medication. Patients requiring antipsychotic medications for the treatment of schizophrenia require careful monitoring and evaluation. Primary care providers may recognize changes related to the disease itself, such as positive, negative, and cognitive symptoms, as well as signs and

TABLE 35.7	Assessment Guidelines for Adverse Effects of Medications Used to Treat Schizophrenia	
Assessment	**Baseline**	**Follow-Up**
Diabetes mellitus	Screen for risk factors, FBG	FBG or HbA1c at 4 months after beginning new treatment and at least annually
Hyperlipidemia	Lipid panel	Lipid panel at 4 months after initiating new antipsychotic and at least annually
Metabolic syndrome	Evaluate criteria	Evaluate at 4 months and at least annually
QTc prolongation	ECG at baseline for all medications that may impact QT prolongation or in presence of cardiovascular risk factors	ECG with change in doses or addition of other medications that can prolong QTc intervals particularly in patients with cardiovascular risk factors or elevated baseline QTc intervals
Hyperprolactinemia	Screen for symptoms of hyperprolactinemia Prolactin level if indicated	Screen for symptoms of hyperprolactinemia every visit until stable as indicated for medications known to increase prolactin. Prolactin level if indicated
Drug-induced movement disorders	Assess for symptoms of akathisia, dystonia, parkinsonism, and TD using structured instrument such as the AIMS and DISCUS if needed	Reassess at each visit using structured instrument at a minimum of 6 months with high-risk patients and 12 months for other patients as well as if new symptoms appear

AIMS, Abnormal Involuntary Movement Scale; *DISCUS,* Dyskinesia Identification System: Condensed User Scale; *ECG,* electrocardiogram; *FBG,* fasting blood glucose; *HbA1c,* hemoglobin A1C; *TD,* tardive dyskinesia.

From *The American Psychiatric Association Practice Guideline for the Treatment of Patients with Schizophrenia* (3rd ed.). https://doi.org/10.1176/appi.books.9780890424841. Reprinted with permission from the American Journal of Psychiatry, (Copyright © 2020). American Psychiatric Association. All Rights Reserved.

symptoms associated with the use of antipsychotic medications. For patients who have underlying health issues prior to initiation of antipsychotic medications, such as obesity and substance use, this is particularly important. Maintain strong communication with psychiatry to reinforce treatment plans. Recent clinical practice guidelines from the APA (2019) provide recommendations for baseline and follow-up assessments in patients requiring antipsychotic medications (Table 35.7).

PRACTICE PEARLS

Suicide Risk and Schizophrenia

People with schizophrenia are at increased risk for suicide. Consider implementing suicide screening strategies when caring for patients with schizophrenia.

Determine the desired therapeutic outcome based on the type of antipsychotic medication needed for the patient's health problem. Treatment of schizophrenia is directed toward minimizing positive symptoms and improving negative and cognitive symptoms while decreasing the risk of adverse effects commonly associated with antipsychotic medications. Multiple challenges in treating patients with schizophrenia include uncomfortable adverse effects, lack of resources and follow-up, and comorbid substance use disorder. Knowledge of community resources for patients with chronic mental illness is essential.

Assess the antipsychotic selected for its appropriateness for an individual patient by considering the medication's side effects and the patient's age, race/ethnicity, comorbidities, and genetic

factors. Carefully evaluate all medications for potential drug interactions. Many SGAs are metabolized by the CYP 450 pathway. As a result, it is important to consider other medications that may be inhibitors or inducers of CYP pathways to reduce the risk of an increase or decrease in the medication's effects. Since many SGA antipsychotics prolong the QT interval, carefully evaluate prescribed medications to decrease the risk of cardiac events. Avoid prescribing medications that may increase the risk of sedation or that may block dopamine to reduce adverse effects.

Initiate the treatment plan with the selected medication by first providing adequate patient education to ensure the patient's understanding and promote full participation in the antipsychotic medication therapy. Medication nonadherence is a significant issue for patients requiring antipsychotics. Nonadherence can lead to recurrence of symptoms as well as increased hospitalizations, significant functional decline, and increased mortality. Reasons for nonadherence may include comorbid conditions such as substance use as well as social stigma, lack of access to care coordination, and side effects/adverse effects associated with care.

Improved clinical outcomes are associated with four core interventions: personalized medication management, supported education and employment, family psychoeducation, and resilience-focused individual therapy (Kane et al., 2016). Primary care providers can work closely with specialty practitioners to improve adherence and enhance patient and family outcomes.

Ensure complete patient and family understanding about the medication prescribed for antipsychotic therapy using a variety of education strategies. Patient and family understanding of schizophrenia is essential. The APA (2019) recommends education regarding topics such as diagnosis and symptoms, medications and adverse effects, stress and coping, crisis plans, risks for suicide, and relapse prevention.

The National Alliance on Mental Illness (NAMI) is an excellent resource for patients and families. Provision of local, state, and national resources is important as well. The Substance Abuse and Mental Health Services Administration at www.samhsa.gov includes links for treatment, public information, and information for patients and professionals as well.

> ## BOOKMARK THIS!
> **National Alliance on Mental Illness**
> NAMI is the largest mental health organization dedicated to helping patients and families who are affected by mental illness. Information about mental illness, support groups, and access to links for local chapters is available at www.nami.org.

Conduct follow-up and monitoring of patient responses to antipsychotic medication therapy. Clinical practice guidelines from the APA recommend regular screening for diabetes, hyperlipidemia, metabolic syndrome, QT prolongation, hyperprolactinemia, and DIMDs (APA, 2019). Partnerships with patients, family, and psychiatry can help manage this complex illness and improve patient outcomes.

> ## BOOKMARK THIS!
> **SMI Advisor**
> SMI Advisor (https://smiadviser.org) is a clinical support system recommended by the APA (2019) for clinicians, individuals, and families. It provides access to multiple resources including continuing education opportunities.

Teaching Points for Antipsychotic Therapy

Health Promotion Strategies

- Reinforce the role of medication in reducing symptoms of schizophrenia to help improve adherence to therapy.
- Teach the patient and family about symptoms that may indicate symptom exacerbation.
- Explore community resources that are available to aid the patient and family in managing the illness.
- Maintain strong communication with mental health providers to reduce cardiovascular and metabolic risks associated with schizophrenia.
- If the patient is smoking, refer them to a tobacco cessation program.
- Screen the patient regularly for comorbidities such as cardiovascular disease, obesity, sleep apnea, respiratory illnesses, human immunodeficiency virus (HIV), hepatitis C, and poor oral health.
- Include suicide assessments in primary care visits, and help the patient and family identify resources should the patient experience suicidal thoughts.

- Provide the patient and family with resources to manage stressors that may exacerbate symptoms or reduce adherence to medication therapy.

Patient Education for Medication Safety

- Avoid taking over-the-counter (OTC) medications while taking antipsychotic medications as they may increase the risk of adverse effects.
- To avoid the onset of movement disorders that may resemble TD, do not suddenly stop taking the medication prescribed. Sudden cessation of medication can also result in increased anxiety, agitation, nausea, and vomiting as well as recurrence of schizophrenia symptoms.
- Report the onset of any involuntary movements that are noticed by you or your family.
- Support groups may be available in your community as you learn more about your diagnosis and build strategies to manage your symptoms.
- Make sure to follow up with regular lab work as directed by your providers to help identify adverse effects.
- Participation in cognitive behavioral therapy is recommended by the APA to support you in your recovery.
- If you are using tobacco products, talk to your provider about options for tobacco cessation as tobacco increases the clearance of certain antipsychotics including clozapine.
- If you are taking a VMAT2 inhibitor to treat TD, follow up regularly with your provider and report any symptoms that are similar to Parkinson's disease. These symptoms may indicate the need for an adjustment in dose.
- Good nutrition and physical activity can help decrease the risk of weight gain that occurs with some antipsychotic medications.
- Helpful information on managing your illness can be found through SMI Advisor at https://smiadvisor.org and NAMI at https://www.nami.org/Home.

Application Questions for Discussion

1. A 57-year-old patient diagnosed with schizophrenia has been prescribed clozapine 450 mg/day. You learn that the patient had failed to respond adequately to other antipsychotic agents in the past and has had good results with clozapine in reducing symptoms. You notice that the patient has experienced a 45-pound weight gain in the past 6 months and has an HbA1c of 7.5. What strategies will you use to assist this patient?

2. A 25-year-old male was recently discharged from the hospital following a diagnosis of schizophrenia. Psychiatric services are titrating olanzapine to treat his symptoms. What additional support services will you provide as a primary care provider? What agencies are available to support patients with schizophrenia?

Selected Bibliography

American Psychiatric Association. (2019). *The American Psychiatric Association Practice Guideline for the Treatment of Patients with Schizophrenia* (3rd ed.). Washington, DC: American Psychiatric Association Publishing. https://doi.org/10.1176/appi.books.9780890424841.

Ata, E. E., Bahadir-Yilmaz, E., & Bayrak, N. G. (2020). The impact of side effects on schizophrenia and bipolar disorder patients' adherence to prescribed medical therapy. *Perspectives in Psychiatric Care, 56*(3), 691–696. http://doi.org/10.1111/ppc.12483.

Balu, D. T. (2016). The NMDA receptor and schizophrenia: From pathophysiology to treatment. *Advances in Pharmacology, 76*, 351–382. http://doi.org/10.1016/bs.apha.2016.01.006.

Bozymski, K. M., Whitten, J. A., Blair, M. E., Overley, A. M., & Ott, C. A. (2018). Monitoring and treating metabolic abnormalities in patients with early psychosis initiated on antipsychotic medications. *Community Mental Health Journal, 54*(6), 717–724. http://doi.org/10.1007/s10597-017-0203-y.

College of Psychiatric and Neurologic Pharmacists (2020). *Drug-induced movement disorders: A clinical guide to rating scales.* Available at https://cpnp.org/ed/movement-disorders#includes.

Dilks, S., Xavier, R. M., Kelly, C., & Johnson, J. (2019). Implications of antipsychotic use: Antipsychotic-induced movement disorders, with a focus on tardive dyskinesia. *Nursing Clinics of North America, 54*(4), 595–608. http://doi.org/10.1016/j.cnur.2019.08.004.

Elkins, J. C. (2019). Metabolic effects of antipsychotic medications. *Journal for Nurse Practitioners, 15*(8), 609–610. http://doi.org/10.1016/j.nurpra.2019.03.014.

Elsevier. Clinical pharmacology powered by ClinicalKey®. (2019). Retrieved from http://www.clinicalkey.com.

Kalkan, E., & Kavak Budak, F. (2020). The effect of insights on medication adherence in patients with schizophrenia. *Perspectives in Psychiatric Care, 56*(1), 222–228. http://doi.org/10.1111/ppc.12414.

Kane, J. M., Robinson, D. G., Schooler, N. R., Mueser, K. T., Penn, D. L., Rosenheck, R. A., & Heinssen, R. K. (2016). Comprehensive versus usual community care for first-episode psychosis: 2-year outcomes from the NIMH RAISE Early Treatment Program. *American Journal of Psychiatry, 173*(4), 362–372. http://doi.org/10.1176/appi.ajp.2015.15050632.

Keepers, G. A., Fochtmann, L. J., Anzia, J. M., Benjamin, S., Lyness, J. M., Mojtabai, R., Servis, M., Walaszek, A., Buckley, P., Lenzenweger, M. F., Young, A. S., Degenhardt, A., Hong, S. H., & (Systematic Review) (2020). The American Psychiatric Association Practice Guideline for the Treatment of Patients With Schizophrenia. *The American Journal of Psychiatry, 177*(9), 868–872. https://doi.org/10.1176/appi.ajp.2020.177901.

King, C. A., Horwitz, A., Czyz, E., & Lindsay, R. (2017). Suicide risk screening in healthcare settings: Identifying males and females at risk. *Journal of Clinical Psychology in Medical Settings, 24* (1), 8–20. https://doi.org/10.1007/s10880-017-9486-y.

Levin, J. B., Seifi, N., Cassidy, K. A., Tatsuoka, C., Sams, J., Akagi, K. K., & Sajatovic, M. (2014). Comparing medication attitudes and reasons for medication nonadherence among three disparate groups of individuals with serious mental illness. *Journal of Nervous & Mental Disease, 202*(11), 769–773. http://doi.org/10.1097/NMD.0000000000000201.

Maroney, M. (2020). An update on current treatment strategies and emerging agents for the management of schizophrenia. *American Journal of Managed Care, 26*, S55–S61. Retrieved from http://search.ebscohost.com/login.aspx?direct=true&db=cin20&AN=143796714&site=ehost-live.

McCance, K. L., & Huether, S. E. (2019). *Pathophysiology: The Biologic Basis for Disease in Adults and Children* (8th ed.). St. Louis: Elsevier.

Miller, B. J. (2020). Advances in tardive dyskinesia: A review of recent literature. *Psychiatric Times*(4), 1–6. Retrieved from http://search.ebscohost.com/login.aspx?direct=true&db=cin20&AN=142511179&site=ehost-live.

Palmer, M., Campbell, A. R., Finegan, A., & Nelson, L. A. (2019). Identification, assessment, and clinical management of tardive dyskinesia: An update. *Psychiatric Times, 36*(7), 27–30. Retrieved from http://search.ebscohost.com/login.aspx?direct=true&db=cin20&AN=137440448&site=ehost-live.

Patel, J., Galdikas, F. J., & Marwaha, R. (2020). Akathisia. [Updated 2020 Jun 24]*StatPearls [Internet]*. Treasure Island (FL): StatPearls Publishing. Jan-. Available from. https://www.ncbi.nlm.nih.gov/books/NBK519543.

Pillinger, T., Beck, K., & Howes, O. (2017). First-episode schizophrenia and diabetes risk-reply. *JAMA Psychiatry, 74*(7), 763. http://doi.org/10.1001/jamapsychiatry.2017.0765.

Rosenthal, L. D., & Burchum, J. R. (2018). *Lehne's Pharmacotherapeutics for Advanced Practice Providers.* St. Louis: Elsevier.

Sabella, D. (2017). Antipsychotic medications: An evidence-based review of the mechanisms of action, adverse effects, and contraindications of these commonly used drugs…first in a series. *American Journal of Nursing, 117*(6), 36–45. http://doi.org/10.1097/01.NAJ.0000520229.04987.46.

Shin, H. W., & Chung, S. J. (2012). Drug-induced parkinsonism. *Journal of Clinical Neurology, 8*(1), 15–21. https://doi.org/10.3988/jcn.2012.8.1.15.

Yang, A. C., & Tsai, S. J. (2017). New targets for schizophrenia treatment beyond the dopamine hypothesis. *International Journal of Molecular Sciences, 18*(8), 1689. http://doi.org/10.3390/ijms18081689.

36

Thyroid Medications

ERINI SERAG–BOLOS AND TERESA GORE

Overview

The body's metabolic state is greatly influenced by several hormones secreted by the thyroid gland. The American Thyroid Association (ATA) estimates that 20 million Americans have thyroid disease and 60% are unaware of their disease (ATA, n.d.a). *Hypothyroidism* is the most common disease/disorder of the thyroid and results from a decreased production of thyroid hormone. Hypothyroidism occurs in 2% of females and 0.2% of males, affecting one out of 500 Americans (Dlugasch & Story, 2021). *Hyperthyroidism* is a result of an excess release of thyroid hormones. *Hyperthyroidism* occurs in 1% to 3% of the U.S. population and is more common in females (Garmendia Madariaga et al., 2014). The prevalence of hypo- and hyperthyroidism increases as people age.

Relevant Physiology

Regulation of a basal metabolism is achieved through complex coordination of the hypothalamic-pituitary-thyroid feedback control system (Figure 36.1). T_4 and T_3 hormones are released from the thyroid gland in response to circulating serum levels of thyroid-stimulating hormone (TSH), which is secreted by the pituitary gland. In turn, TSH secretion is influenced by thyroid-releasing hormone (TRH), which is secreted by the hypothalamus. The feedback mechanism creates an inverse relationship between serum levels of T_3-T_4 and TSH-TRH. When T_3 and T_4 serum levels rise, TSH and TRH secretions are suppressed.

TRH and TSH levels can be measured directly (Table 36.1). An elevated TSH, along with low circulating levels of free (unbound) T_3 and T_4, is diagnostic of primary hypothyroidism, which is commonly attributed to destruction of the thyroid gland. Conversely, a low or undetectable TSH with high circulating levels of free T_3 and T_4 (FT_3 and FT_4) is diagnostic of hyperthyroidism.

The thyroid gland releases T_4 (90%), T_3 (10%), and reverse T_3 (rT_3) (<1%). T_3 and T_4 have a high affinity for protein. T_3 is 99.7% protein bound, whereas T_4 is 99.97% protein bound. Only the unbound portion is metabolically active. In the peripheral tissue, T_4 is converted to T_3 through the removal of iodine. In most cases, it is necessary to administer only T_4 because the body will produce T_3 from T_4. The physiologic effects of thyroid hormones are attributed to the peripheral T_3.

Thyroid hormones exert their effect on nearly every system of the body through a variety of mechanisms. Basal metabolic rate is regulated by thyroid hormones. Thyroid hormones also influence oxygen consumption; respiratory rate; body temperature; heart rate; stroke volume; stimulation of bone resorption impacting bone formation; enzyme system activity; the rate of fat, protein, and carbohydrate metabolism; fetal development; central nervous system (CNS) development; growth and maturation; and the rate of metabolism of multiple hormones and medications.

This chapter is divided into two parts: Part I: Hypothyroidism and Part II: Hyperthyroidism. Each part

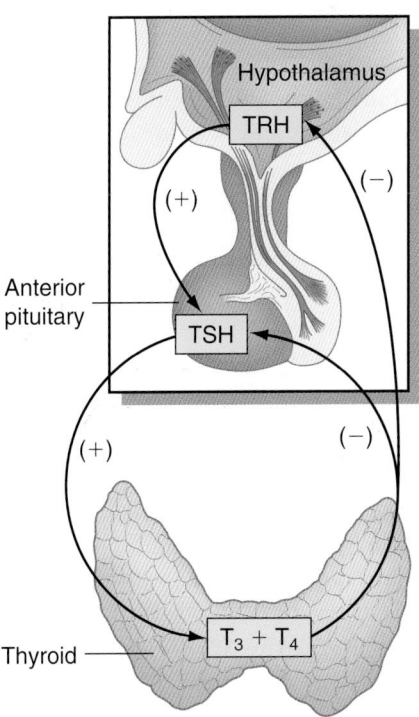

• **Fig. 36.1** Feedback loops for the thyroid gland. (From McCance, K., & Huether, S. [2019]. *Pathophysiology: The biologic basis for disease in adults and children* [8th ed.]. St. Louis: Elsevier.)

TABLE 36.1 Altered Laboratory Findings in Thyroid Dysfunction

Dysfunctional States	TSH	T₄/Free T₄	T₃/Free T₃	Free Thyroxine Index (FTI)	T₃ Uptake	rT₃
Hypothyroid States						
Primary	Increased	Decreased	Decreased	Decreased	Not useful	Normal
Secondary	Normal or decreased	Decreased	Decreased	Decreased	Not useful	Normal
Subclinical hypothyroidism	Increased	Normal	Normal	Normal	Not useful	Normal
Hyperthyroid States						
Primary	Decreased	Increased	Increased	Increased	Increased	Normal
Secondary	Increased	Increased	Increased	Increased	Increased	Normal
Euthyroid						
Sick syndrome	Normal or decreased	Normal or decreased	Decreased	Increased	Not useful	Increased

includes a review of relevant pathophysiology, medications, and an overview of clinical and prescribing guidelines.

HYPOTHYROIDISM

Pathophysiology: Hypothyroidism

Primary hypothyroidism has a variety of causes. Autoimmune disorders, such as Hashimoto's thyroiditis, and iodine deficiencies are the most common causes of hypothyroidism. Another common cause is iatrogenic, which is the result of therapy for thyrotoxicosis or other drugs such as lithium and amiodarone (Surks, 2020). Other causes include idiopathic thyroid atrophy and/or postpartum thyroid disease.

Adults and Older Adults

Adults may develop numerous problems related to a decreased metabolic rate. Cardiovascular, gastrointestinal (GI), musculoskeletal, and neurologic function may be impaired by inadequate thyroid hormones. *Primary hypothyroidism*, the most common form of hypothyroidism, is caused by a failure within the thyroid gland or surgical resection of the gland. *Secondary hypothyroidism* is caused by lack of TSH secretion from the pituitary. *Tertiary hypothyroidism* is caused by lack of TRH secretion from the hypothalamus.

In adults, hypothyroidism is most common in females and is characterized by signs and symptoms consistent with altered energy metabolism, such as fatigue, weight gain, depression, lethargy, constipation, bradycardia, hair thinning, sensitivity to cold, dry skin, peripheral edema, menstrual disturbances, and sometimes a goiter. If severe hypothyroidism is untreated or undertreated, it can progress to life-threatening myxedema and myxedema coma. *Myxedema* is a result of increased permeability of the

capillaries to albumin, producing interstitial edema of the heart, striated muscle, and skin. This leads to a characteristic appearance and physical symptoms, especially of the skin, along with cardiovascular instability. Hypothyroidism is common in older adults. Atypical presentation includes congestive heart failure.

Children

In children, thyroid hormones are essential for overall normal growth and development, especially of the CNS. Without thyroid hormone, development of the CNS is impaired. At-risk neonates should undergo FT₄ and TSH screening as soon as possible after birth. Undetected deficiency of thyroid hormone may begin to affect children shortly after birth (e.g., as cretinism, which is evidenced by intellectual disability, short extremities, enlarged tongue, puffy face, etc.).

Laboratory Testing in Hypothyroidism

Table 36.1 lists altered laboratory findings in thyroid dysfunction. TSH is the most sensitive and useful test in the diagnosis of hypothyroidism. FT₄ and FT₃ are also useful. The amount of circulating and unbound hormones is reduced in patients with this disorder. A thyroid supplement serves to replace inadequate levels of endogenous T₃ and T₄. If an exogenous thyroid hormone is given to a euthyroid patient, endogenous secretion of TSH and TRH will be suppressed, as will the body's production of T₃ and T₄.

Thyroid Hormone Replacement Therapy

Thyroid hormone replacements are available as synthetic preparations or as animal extract preparations. Synthetic formulations are preferred due to standardized bioequivalence and potency. Table 36.2 provides a summary of the pharmacokinetic properties and Table 36.3 provides dosing recommendations of thyroid supplements.

PRACTICE PEARLS

Thyroid Hormone Use in Pregnancy and Lactation

- There is no demonstrated risk to the fetus with the use of hormone replacements during pregnancy. Recommendations are to continue hormone replacement during pregnancy and monitor TSH carefully, as dose adjustments may be required.
- Excretion of thyroid medications in breast milk is minimal. Thyroid hormones are considered compatible with breastfeeding.

Levothyroxine

Pharmacokinetics. As T_4, levothyroxine is a prohormone that becomes deiodinated in peripheral tissues to form T_3. T_4 is poorly absorbed from the GI tract (50% to 80%), but absorption can be increased when it is administered on an empty stomach. Absorption and bioavailability are impacted by food (soybeans, fiber, infant formula). Levothyroxine is highly protein bound and has a half-life of 6 to 7 days; therefore, it takes 4 to 6 weeks to reach full therapeutic effects. Excretion is primarily through the kidneys.

Indications. Oral levothyroxine is the preferred drug of choice for hypothyroidism. (Jonklass et al. 2014) determined that monotherapy with levothyroxine should be considered the standard of care in the treatment of hypothyroidism. The intravenous (IV) form may be used in the treatment of myxedema coma. Of note, the intravenous form is 50% to 75% of the oral dose formulation. Levothyroxine should not be used solely for weight loss.

Adverse Effects. Most common adverse effects include signs and symptoms of overdose (present similarly to hyperthyroidism) such as palpitations, elevated blood pressure, anxiety, headache, diaphoresis, heat intolerance, diarrhea, and insomnia. Also, transient alopecia and reduction in bone mineral density may occur with long-term treatment.

Contraindications. Uncorrected adrenal insufficiency may precipitate adrenal crisis. Other precautions include recent myocardial infarction or hypersensitivity to any of the medication's components. Caution is also warranted in the older adult population, especially in postmenopausal females, as well as in patients with osteoporosis, cardiovascular disease, and diabetes (worsened glycemic control). Numerous drug–drug interactions are present. Noteworthy drug interactions include those that reduce absorption of levothyroxine, such as antacids, iron, proton pump inhibitors (PPIs), and sucralfate, as well as those that affect levothyroxine metabolism, such as rifampin, carbamazepine, phenytoin, and phenobarbital; such drug interactions may necessitate an increase in levothyroxine dosage (Horn & Handsten, 2016).

Monitoring. Lab monitoring of TSH is recommended after about 6 weeks from initiation or dosage adjustment due to a long half-life compared to other agents. Once an appropriate maintenance dose is determined, monitoring should occur after 4 to 6 months, then annually. Additionally, weight, heart rate, blood pressure, and bone mineral density should be evaluated annually. Dosages must be individualized based on clinical response and laboratory parameters.

Liothyronine

Pharmacokinetics. Liothyronine is readily available systemically due to its low affinity to bind to protein. Liothyronine has a rapid onset of action in both oral and IV forms. Following oral administration, the peak response

TABLE 36.2 Pharmacokinetics of Thyroid Supplements

Drug	Absorption	Onset of Action	Time to Peak Concentration	Half–Life	Duration of Action	Protein Bound	Metabolism
Levothyroxine	Variable in GI tract (50%–80%)	3–5 days	2–4 hr	6–7 days	2–3 weeks	99%	Biliary
Liothyronine	Complete in GI tract (95% in 4 hr)	2–4 hr	1–2 hr	2–3 days	3–5 days	99%	Biliary/renal
Liotrix (4 parts T_4, 1 part T_3)	Variable in GI tract but $T_3 < T_4$	T_3: 12–36 hr; T_4: Unknown	T_3: 24–72 hr; T_4: 1–3 weeks	T_3: 2–3 days; T_4: 6–7 days	T_3: 3–5 days; T_4: 1–3 weeks	99%	Biliary/renal
Desiccated thyroid	T_4: 40%–80%; T_3: ~95%	3 hr	T_4: 2–4 hr; T_3: 2–3 days	T_4: 6–7 days; T_3: 0.75 days	1–3 weeks	T_4: >99%	Hepatic/renal

TABLE 36.3	Dosing Recommendations of Thyroid Supplements			
Medication	**Indications**	**Dosage**		**Considerations and Monitoring**
Liothyronine	Hypothyroidism	**Tablet:** *Adults:* 25 mcg/day; increase by 12.5–25 mcg/day every 1–2 weeks. Maximum dosage: 100 mcg/day. *Older adults:* 5 mcg orally once daily; increase 5 mcg/day every 1–2 weeks.		For all thyroid supplements, maintenance dosage is based on thyroid function test results. Reassess treatment option to obtain desired response.

	Congenital hypothyroidism	**Tablet:** *Adolescents and children:*
		
		Initial: 5 mcg/day; increase by 5 mcg every 3–4 days until the desired response is achieved.
		
		Maximum dosage:
		
		    Infants: 20 mcg/day.
		
		    Children 1–3 yr: 50 mcg/day.
		
		    Children >3 yr: adult dose.		

Levothyroxine	Hypothyroidism	**Capsules, tablets, solution:** *Healthy adults <50 yr, children in whom growth and puberty are complete:* Initial dose: 1.6 mcg/kg/day. Increase by 12.5–25 mcg/day every 4–6 weeks. *Older adult or patient with cardiac disease:* Initial dose: 0.25–0.5 mcg/kg/day. Increase by 12.5–25 mcg/day every 4–6 weeks. *Pregnant women:* Initial dose: 1–1.6 mcg/kg/day.		

	Hypothyroidism	*Newborns:* 10–15 mcg/kg; increase dose every 4–6 weeks.
		
		Infants and children:
		
		    0–3 months: 10–15 mcg/kg/day.
		
		    3–6 months: 8–10 mcg/kg/day.
		
		    6–12 months: 6–8 mcg/kg/day.
		
		    1–5 yr: 5–6 mcg/kg/day.
		
		    6–12 yr: 4–5 mcg/kg/day.
		
		    >12 yr: and adolescents in whom growth and puberty are incomplete: 2–3 mcg/kg/day.
				Lower doses of 25 mcg/day should be considered in newborns at risk for cardiac failure.
				
				Adolescents and children >1 yr: Hyperactivity can be minimized if initiated at a dose that is 25% of the recommended replacement dose.

Desiccated thyroid	Hypothyroidism	*Adults:* Initial: 30 or 32.5 mg/day; increase dose in 15- or 16.25-mg increments every 2–3 weeks until adequate replacement dose is determined.		Patients with cardiovascular disease: start at 15 or 16.25 mg/day.

time is 2 to 3 days with a half-life of 2.5 days. Excretion is primarily through the kidneys.

Indications. Liothyronine is approved for use in the adult and pediatric populations. Liothyronine is a synthetic T_3 formulation used for treatment of hypothyroidism. However, due to its short duration of action, liothyronine may not be the best choice for maintenance thyroid replacement. Liothyronine may be an option for patients who remain symptomatic despite T_4 hormone replacement with normal TSH or for preparation of thyroid scan in patients with thyroid cancer. In the event of myxedema coma, injectable liothyronine is approved for use in adults only.

Adverse Effects. Oral administration of liothyronine results in few adverse effects as long as therapeutic levels are maintained. IV liothyronine is associated with a higher incidence of cardiovascular side effects such as tachycardia, cardiac arrhythmia, and myocardial infarction. Older adults or patients with previous cardiovascular disease may be more at risk for adverse cardiac effects. In children, craniosynostosis, premature epiphyseal closure with reduced adult height, and pseudotumor cerebri have been reported.

Contraindications. Contraindications include the use of liothyronine in the presence of uncorrected adrenal cortical insufficiency, untreated thyrotoxicosis, cardiovascular disease including myocardial infarction, and hypersensitivity to any components of the formulation. Caution is warranted in the older adult population, especially in postmenopausal females, as well as in patients with osteoporosis, cardiovascular disease, and diabetes (worsened glycemic control). Allergic reactions may occur in patients with tartrazine (FD & C yellow #5) dye hypersensitivities depending on the formulation or strengths used in therapy; in these cases, increments of the 50-mcg white tablet may be used.

Monitoring. TSH and T_3 may be reevaluated at 1- to 2-week intervals. Once a maintenance dose is determined, monitoring should occur every 4 to 6 months, then annually. Heart rate, blood pressure, and weight should also be checked annually. In pediatric patients, monitor stature at each visit.

Liotrix

Pharmacokinetics. Liotrix has a rapid onset of action of about 3 hours due to the T_3 component. Liotrix binds to protein and is well absorbed. Metabolism occurs in the liver. The half-life of the T_3 component is 2.5 days and the half-life of the T_4 component is 6 to 7 days. Excretion is through the kidneys.

Indications. Liotrix is a synthetic T_4/T_3 (levothyroxine and liothyronine) combination used for treatment of hypothyroidism as an option for patients who remain symptomatic despite use of other preferred formulations. No dose adjustments are required for adults or children with renal or hepatic impairment.

Adverse Effects. Liotrix may be associated with signs and symptoms of hyperthyroidism, although this is rare. Other adverse effects include palpitations, elevated blood pressure, anxiety, headache, diaphoresis, heat intolerance, diarrhea, and insomnia.

Contraindications. The use of liotrix is contraindicated for patients with a history of uncorrected adrenal cortical insufficiency, untreated thyrotoxicosis, cardiovascular disease including myocardial infarction, or hypersensitivity to any components of the formulation. Allergic reactions may occur in patients with tartrazine (FD & C yellow #5) dye hypersensitivities depending on the formulation or strengths used in therapy.

Monitoring. Monitoring of TSH and T_4 should occur every 2 to 3 weeks for necessary dosage adjustments, then every 4 to 6 months after a maintenance dose is determined. Additionally, heart rate and blood pressure should be monitored annually.

Desiccated Thyroid

Pharmacokinetics. Desiccated thyroid has a rapid onset of action of 3 hours and a half-life of 6 to 7 days. Absorption has been shown to vary from 48% to 79% of the administered dose.

Indications. Desiccated thyroid is made from the desiccated thyroid of pigs, sheep, or cows and is standardized by iodine content. Desiccated thyroid is used for the treatment of hypothyroidism as an option for patients who remain symptomatic despite the use of other preferred formulations.

Adverse Effects. Although rare, desiccated thyroid may be associated with signs and symptoms of hyperthyroidism due to overreplacement.

Contraindications. Desiccated thyroid is contraindicated in uncorrected adrenal cortical insufficiency, untreated thyrotoxicosis, and hypersensitivity to any components of the formulation.

Monitoring. Monitoring of TSH and T_4 should occur every 2 to 3 weeks after initiation, then every 4 to 6 months once a maintenance dose is determined. Additionally, heart rate and blood pressure should be monitored annually.

Prescriber Considerations for Hypothyroidism Therapy

Clinical Practice Guidelines

There are several clinical practice guidelines for treating a patient with hypothyroidism. Professional organizations review them periodically and update them as new evidence is produced. One of the most important things to consider when caring for a patient with hypothyroidism is to treat the patient as an individual. When writing the prescription, "dispense as written" should be indicated since not all generic versions are the same. It would be ideal for the patient to stay on the same manufacturer's product. The first medication of choice is levothyroxine and the goal of therapy is to achieve euthyroid state, which usually occurs in 4 to 6 weeks.

> **BOOKMARK THIS!**
>
> **Clinical Practice Guidelines**
> - ATA guidelines: https://www.thyroid.org/professionals/ata-professional-guidelines/
> - 2014 hypothyroidism guidelines: https://www.liebertpub.com/doi/full/10.1089/thy.2014.0028
> - 2017 pregnancy and postpartum guidelines: https://www.liebertpub.com/doi/full/10.1089/thy.2016.0457

Clinical Reasoning for Hypothyroidism Therapy

Consider the individual patient's health problem requiring hypothyroidism therapy. Thorough assessment of the patient's signs and symptoms of presentation, lab values (TSH, T_4, and T_3), and other underlying disease states are necessary to determine initiation of therapy. Concurrent medications that reduce absorption or affect metabolism, such as iron supplementation, antacids, etc., should be considered prior to making dosage adjustments.

Determine the desired therapeutic outcome based on the patient's degree of hypothyroidism. Goals of therapy include symptom relief with normalization of lab values. For newly diagnosed patients, doses should be initiated at the lower range (levothyroxine involves weight-based dosing) and titrated to effect. Follow-up labs should be scheduled based on the specific medication selected according to pharmacokinetic parameters to ensure accuracy.

Assess the selected regimen for its appropriateness for an individual patient by considering the medication's side effects and the patient's age, race/ethnicity, comorbidities, and genetic factors. Once hypothyroidism is determined, levothyroxine is the initial drug of choice and involves weight-based dosing of 1.6 mcg/kg based on ideal body weight. If symptoms remain uncontrolled despite appropriate dose titration, alternative regimens may be considered (see Table 36.3 for age- and weight-appropriate dosages of thyroid supplements).

PRACTICE PEARLS

Life Span Considerations With Thyroid Hormone Supplement

Geriatrics

- Administration of thyroid hormone in supratherapeutic doses may exacerbate cardiovascular disease, particularly angina. It is advisable to start low and gradually increase the dosage.
- Absorption of the medication may increase with aging, so dosage adjustments may be required.
- Consideration must be taken when beginning new medications due to the potential interaction between the medications.

Pediatrics

- Children will require higher doses of medication to meet the metabolic demands of growth and development during the first three years of life.
- In congenital hypothyroidism, therapy may be stopped for 2 to 8 weeks after the patient reaches 3 years of age. If TSH levels remain normal, thyroid supplementation may be discontinued permanently.

Pregnancy

- Adjustment of thyroid hormone supplementation by a 50% increase is common during pregnancy because of increased energy demands. Thus, close monitoring of TSH is indicated.
- Females of child-bearing age with hypothyroidism may experience difficulty conceiving and would benefit from careful evaluation of thyroid hormone levels.

Initiate the treatment plan with the selected medication by first providing adequate patient education to ensure the patient's understanding and promote full participation in the therapy. Patient education is a critical component to empower patients and ensure adherence to the regimen. Information to include within the education plan includes the diagnosis, plan of therapy (medication, dose, frequency, side effects, etc.), and follow-up. Additional key counseling points for levothyroxine include timing the medication dose 1 hour prior to breakfast (to enhance absorption), avoiding missed doses, avoiding timing the dose with other medications that may affect absorption, and staying with one formulation and noting any difference in appearance when picked up at the pharmacy (bioequivalence concerns).

Ensure complete patient and family understanding about the medication prescribed using a variety of education strategies. Use a variety of education strategies, including verbal and written instructions with teach-back to ensure understanding, and provide contact information for follow-up as necessary.

Follow-up and monitor patient responses to hormone therapy. Follow-up and monitoring should include discussions regarding adherence to therapy, effectiveness of treatment with assessment of symptom relief, laboratory monitoring, and patient satisfaction.

Teaching Points for Hypothyroidism Therapy

Health Promotion Strategies

- The most important aspect is to educate the patient about the medications and compliance (skipped or "make-up" dose or changes to dosing regimen).
- Patients should be informed that smoking impacts thyroid hormone secretion and action.
- Treatment with the medication is lifelong.
- Changes in doses should not be initiated with orders based solely on symptoms and lab results.
- Once dose and symptoms are stabilized, annual lab work will be required.
- Offer patient brochures:
  - Adults: https://www.thyroid.org/wp-content/uploads/patients/brochures/Hypo_brochure.pdf
  - Congenital: https://www.thyroid.org/wp-content/uploads/patients/brochures/congenital-hypothyroidism-brochure.pdf
  - Children and adolescents: https://www.thyroid.org/hypothyroidism-children-adolescents/

Patient Education for Medication Safety

- Take the medication daily and as prescribed, 1 hour before breakfast and other medications.
- Stay with one formulation and discuss with the pharmacist if the appearance of supplied tablets is changed.
- Patients with osteoporosis/osteopenia should take recommended amounts of calcium and vitamin D.
- Store medications at room temperature in a dry place and protect from light.
- Keep medications out of reach of children and pets. Tell your provider:
  - About all concurrent prescription and over-the-counter (OTC) medications and supplements.
  - If you are trying to become pregnant, are pregnant, or are breastfeeding.
  - If you are starting any new medications, including amiodarone and lithium, since these are associated with potential medication interactions.

Application Questions for Discussion

1. Which thyroid supplement medication is considered as the first line of therapy?
2. What are key patient counseling points?

3. What are considerations for prescribing hypothyroidism therapy for pregnant patients?

HYPERTHYROIDISM

Overview

Hyperthyroidism is a result of an excess release of thyroid hormone. *Thyrotoxicosis* is the syndrome that develops from an excess of thyroid hormone, regardless of the source. Hyperthyroidism occurs more often in females, and the risk increases with age and smoking. To diagnose the cause of hyperthyroidism, a 24-hour radioiodine uptake scan is completed after oral ingestion of the radioiodine. This test cannot be completed with a pregnant patient (Dlugasch & Story, 2019). Hyperthyroidism usually presents as a hypermetabolic state and requires immediate action to control the symptoms. Undertreated or untreated hyperthyroidism can lead to a thyroid storm, which is life-threatening and requires immediate care in a hospital environment.

Pathophysiology: Hyperthyroidism

Excessive synthesis of thyroid hormone increases the individual's basal metabolism to potentially fatal levels. Cardiovascular and neurologic function may be markedly stimulated, resulting in systemic collapse. Diagnosis is based on symptoms, physical findings, 24-hour radioiodine uptake scan, and laboratory findings. TSH will be suppressed, and T_3 and T_4 will be increased. See Table 36.1 for altered laboratory findings in thyroid dysfunction. The presentation of thyrotoxicosis is highly variable and may include palpitations, tremor, nervousness/anxiety, heat intolerance, increased sweating/moist skin, fatigue, muscle cramps and weakness, diarrhea, hyperreflexia, and sometimes goiter and exophthalmos.

Medications such as lithium and amiodarone can affect the thyroid gland and its function. Amiodarone has a high level of iodine content in the medication. Lithium is concentrated in higher levels in the thyroid than in the plasma. Medication doses may require adjustments to avoid significant drug interactions.

Subclinical hyperthyroidism involves a low TSH level with normal FT_4 and FT_3 levels. These patients present with no or minimal clinical symptoms of thyrotoxicosis. In these cases, hyperthyroidism is often detected by the lab values ordered due to vague complaints from the patient.

Graves' Disease

The most common cause of thyrotoxicosis is primary hyperthyroidism due to *Graves' disease*, an autoimmune process from autoantibodies binding the TSH receptors on the thyroid gland to stimulate hormone production (Braimon & Rieke, 2017; Dlugasch & Story, 2019). If the patient has Graves' eye disease, a referral should be made to a specialized ophthalmologist (Braimon & Rieke, 2017; Dlugasch & Story, 2019). In Graves' disease, the mnemonic for eye changes that can occur is NOSPECS (Braimon & Rieke, 2017, p. 1142):

- No signs or symptoms
- Only signs, no symptoms
- Soft tissue swelling
- Proptosis
- Extraocular muscle paresis
- Corneal involvement
- Sight loss (optic nerve involvement)

Toxic Nodular Goiter

Toxic nodular goiter is due to the hyperfunctioning of a uninodular or multinodular goiter, with autonomous hyperfunctioning thyroid nodules, leading to a hypermetabolic state. Exposure to iodide is iatrogenic and can impact the function of the thyroid gland. Potential sources include dietary excess, administration of high doses of iodine for radiologic diagnostic procedures, and medications such as amiodarone and lithium. This is diagnosed as *iodism* (iodine poisoning or excessive iodine). Other causes of thyrotoxicosis include thyroid inflammatory diseases such as postpartum thyroiditis and subacute thyroiditis, which is typically caused by viral infections. In thyroiditis, thyrotoxicosis is usually transient but may progress to hypothyroidism in some cases.

Thyroiditis

Thyroiditis is inflammation of the thyroid, which may be subacute or painless. Common causes include postpartum thyroiditis, toxic nodule, or toxic multinodular goiter. In subacute thyroiditis, beta-blockers are used to control the heart rate and rhythm, and nonsteroidal antiinflammatory drugs (NSAIDs) are used for pain control. In painless postpartum thyroiditis, beta-blockers are used for symptom control during the hyperthyroid state. Thionamides (antithyroid medications) and beta-blockers are the first-line medical treatments for hyperthyroidism and toxic nodules. Surgery is the definitive treatment for healthy, younger patients with toxic nodule and toxic multinodular goiter. Radioactive iodine ablation may be used instead in older patients or in those in poor health. For the toxic multinodular goiter, another option for treatment is the use of antithyroid medications, followed by a subtotal thyroidectomy. In these cases, lifelong treatment with thyroid replacements will be necessary.

Thyroid Storm

If hyperthyroidism is undertreated or untreated, or if hypothyroidism is treated too aggressively, the patient may experience thyroid storm, especially after trauma or a complex exacerbation of a medical diagnosis (Braimon & Rieke,

2017; Dlugasch & Story, 2019). A thyroid storm is considered a medical emergency and primary care providers should activate the emergency response system. The goal of treatment is to suppress the thyroid hormones and provide alpha-adrenergic blockade. Long-term treatment may also be warranted. Presenting signs and symptoms of thyroid storm include:

- Tachycardia (120–140 beats/minute) and, at times, atrial fibrillation
- Elevated temperature over 102°F and up to 105°F
- Profuse diaphoresis
- Mental status changes including confusion, agitation, and restlessness that can lead to a comatose state
- GI changes including diarrhea, vomiting, and hepatomegaly with jaundice

Thionamides: Thyroid Hormone Suppressants

The goal of treatment for hyperthyroidism is based on the cause of the disease to achieve a euthyroid state. Thyroid suppressants suppress the synthesis of thyroid hormones. Table 36.4 provides a summary of the pharmacokinetic properties and Table 36.5 provides dosing recommendations for thyroid suppressants.

Methimazole

Pharmacokinetics. Included within the drug class of thionamides, methimazole inhibits thyroid hormone synthesis by blocking the oxidation of iodine in the thyroid gland to inhibit T_3 formation. Following oral administration, peak serum concentrations are reached in 1 to 2 hours. The duration of action is 40 hours. The elimination half-life is 5 to 9 hours. These pharmacokinetic characteristics allow for less frequent dosing.

Indications. Methimazole is used to treat hyperthyroidism in adults and children by preventing the thyroid from producing too much thyroid hormone. Methimazole can be prescribed for Graves' disease and toxic multinodular goiter when thyroidectomy and/or radioactive iodine are not appropriate options. It can also be prescribed before a thyroidectomy or radioactive iodine therapy to halt the hyperthyroidism. Methimazole is the drug of choice in nonpregnant females and during the second and third trimesters of pregnancy.

Adverse Effects. Consistent among the drug class, thionamides may cause significant bone marrow depression including leukopenia and hepatitis. Side effects include nausea, vomiting, constipation, arthralgias, drowsiness, neuritis, headache, vertigo, vasculitis, edema, nephrotic syndrome, lupus-like symptoms, hepatotoxicity, lymphadenopathy, sialadenitis, and skin reactions.

Contraindications. Methimazole is contraindicated for use in patients with a history of agranulocytosis (especially in patients older than 40 years of age) and hypersensitivity to any of the medication's components. Additionally, methimazole should be discontinued at least 3 to 4 days before treatment with radioactive iodine and used cautiously in patients with bone marrow suppression and hepatic disease.

Monitoring. Baseline and periodic monitoring of TSH, T_4, T_3, complete blood count (CBC) with differential, liver function tests (LFTs), and prothrombin/partial thromboplastin time (PT/PTT) are recommended. Serum T_4 and T_3 levels should be monitored prior to initiation of therapy, followed by repeat labs every 3 to 6 weeks until euthyroid levels are reached, and then quarterly thereafter.

Propylthiouracil (PTU)

Pharmacokinetics. PTU has a significantly longer onset of action than methimazole and concentrates in the thyroid gland following absorption. Metabolism occurs through the liver with an elimination half-life of 1 to 4 hours. Excretion is through the kidneys.

TABLE 36.4 — Pharmacokinetics of Thyroid Suppressants

Drug	Absorption	Onset of Action	Time to Peak Concentration	Half–Life	Duration of Action	Protein Bound	Metabolism
Methimazole	99%	12–18 hr	1–2 hr	4–6 hr	36–72 hr	None	Hepatic
Propylthiouracil	53%–88%	24–36 hr	1–2 hr	~1 hr	12–24 hr	80%–85%	Hepatic
Potassium iodide–iodine	–	24–48 hr	10–15 days	–	–	–	–

TABLE 36.5 Dosing Recommendations for Thyroid Suppressants

Medication	Indications	Dosage	Considerations and Monitoring
Methimazole	Hyperthyroidism	**Tablet:** *Adults:* Initial: 15–60 mg/day in 3 divided doses. Maintenance dosage: 5–15 mg/day. *Infants, children, and adolescents:* Initial: 0.4 mg/kg/day in 3 divided doses. Maintenance dosage: 0.2 mg/kg/day.	Monitor TSH. Use lowest maintenance dose to maintain status.
Propylthiouracil	Hyperthyroidism	**Tablet:** *Adults:* Initial: 300 mg/day in 3 divided doses. Maintenance dosage: 100–150 mg/day. *Children 6–17 yr* **only if allergic to OR unable to tolerate methimazole AND if no other treatment available:** Initial dosage: 50 mg/day every 8 hr. Titrate to TSH and free T_4 levels. Usual dosage: 5–7 mg/kg/day.	Second-line therapy for adult patients allergic to methimazole. Use caution due to narrow therapeutic window. Titrate dosage to maintain status. *Children 6-17 yr:* Severe liver injury may occur.
Potassium iodide–iodine	Preparation for thyroidectomy in Graves' disease	Lugol's 5% solution: 5–7 drops (0.25–0.35 mL) orally three times daily for 10 days prior to surgery.	
	Thyroid storm	Lugol's 5% solution: 4–8 drops orally every 6–8 hr after methimazole or PTU. Do not start until 1 hr after methimazole or PTU administration.	

PTU, Propylthiouracil.

Indications. As another drug within the drug class of thionamides, propylthiouracil inhibits thyroid hormone synthesis by blocking the oxidation of iodine in the thyroid gland to inhibit the formation of both T_4 and T_3. It is indicated in patients with Graves' disease or toxic multinodular goiter who cannot tolerate methimazole and cannot undergo surgery or radioactive iodine ablation. This is the drug of choice during a thyroid storm since it inhibits the conversion of T_4 to T_3 in the peripheral tissue.

PRACTICE PEARLS

Propylthiouracil Use in Pregnancy and Lactation

- Propylthiouracil is the drug of choice during the first trimester of pregnancy as it inhibits the conversion of T_4 to T_3 in the peripheral tissue.
- Propylthiouracil is considered compatible with breastfeeding.

Adverse Effects Thionamides may cause leukopenia, agranulocytosis, and hepatitis. Side effects include loss of taste, nausea, vomiting, headache, edema, hepatotoxicity, interstitial nephritis, glomerulonephritis, lupus-like symptoms, arthralgias, neuritis, vertigo, and skin reactions.

Contraindications. Avoid propylthiouracil in patients with a history of agranulocytosis and hypersensitivity to any of the medication's components as well as in patients with hepatic disease or bone marrow suppression. PTU is associated with higher risk for hepatotoxicity compared with methimazole, especially among the pediatric population. PTU should be discontinued 3 to 4 days before treatment with radioactive iodine.

Monitoring. Serum T_4 and T_3 levels should be monitored prior to initiation of therapy, then every 3 to 6 weeks until euthyroid levels are reached. Periodic monitoring of TSH, CBC with differential, LFTs, and PT/PTT is recommended.

Iodides

Pharmacokinetics. Hormone secretion is inhibited within 1 to 2 days, with symptomatic improvement within 2 to 7 days. Replacements can include potassium iodide–iodine solution (e.g., Lugol's solution) and potassium iodide solution (SSKI).

Indications. Increased intrathyroidal concentration of iodine in turn prevents the organification of iodine in the thyroid gland to inhibit hormone synthesis (known as the Wolff-Chaikoff effect). Though not approved by the U.S. Food and Drug Administration (FDA), this drug class is commonly used in severe hyperthyroidism as preparation for thyroidectomy, in patients who cannot tolerate thionamides, and in thyroid storm (Calissendorff & Falhammar, 2017).

Adverse Effects. The most common adverse effects include *iodism*, as symptoms of metallic taste, sore teeth and gums, a burning sensation in the mouth and throat, and GI upset. Additionally, hypersensitivity reactions may present as rash or rhinitis and conjunctivitis.

Contraindications. The use of iodides is contraindicated in patients with hypersensitivity to any of the medication's components. Iodides should be used cautiously in patients with adrenal insufficiency, renal impairment, cardiac disease, bronchitis, and tuberculosis.

Monitoring. Thyroid function tests, basic metabolic panel and, especially, potassium levels should be monitored during therapy.

Prescriber Considerations for Hyperthyroidism Therapy

Clinical Practice Guidelines

There are several clinical practice guidelines for the treatment of hyperthyroidism. Professional organizations review them periodically and update them as new evidence is produced. One of the most important things to consider when caring for a patient with hyperthyroidism is to treat the cause. The goal of therapy is to achieve euthyroid state and prevent thyroid storm.

> **BOOKMARK THIS!**
>
> **Clinical Practice Guidelines**
>
> - ATA guidelines: https://www.thyroid.org/professionals/ata-professional-guidelines/
> - ATA guidelines for diagnosis and management of hyperthyroidism and other causes of thyrotoxicosis (2016): https://www.liebertpub.com/doi/full/10.1089/thy.2016.0229
> - ATA guidelines for adults with thyroid nodules and differentiated thyroid cancer (2015): https://www.liebertpub.com/doi/full/10.1089/thy.2015.0020
> - ATA guidelines for children with thyroid nodules and differentiated thyroid cancer (2015): https://www.liebertpub.com/doi/full/10.1089/thy.2014.0460
> - ATA practice recommendations for radiation safety in treatment of patients with thyroid diseases by radioiodine (2011): https://www.liebertpub.com/doi/full/10.1089/thy.2010.0403

Clinical Reasoning for Hyperthyroidism Therapy

Consider the individual patient's health problem requiring therapy for hyperthyroidism. Thorough assessment of the patient's signs and symptoms of presentation, lab values (TSH, T_4, and T_3), and other underlying disease states is necessary to determine initiation of therapy.

Determine the desired therapeutic outcome based on the patient's health problem. Goals of therapy include symptom relief with normalization of lab values, elimination of excess thyroid hormone, and a reduction in the risk of long-term consequences including osteopenia.

Assess the selected regimen for its appropriateness for an individual patient by considering the medication's side effects and the patient's age, race/ethnicity, comorbidities, and genetic factors. A thorough patient history that includes age, comorbidities, specific signs and symptoms, lab values, and concurrent medications is necessary to determine a patient-specific therapeutic plan. Factors such as age and symptom severity guide the plan of care regarding radioactive or surgical ablation or medication treatment with goals for remission.

Initiate the treatment plan with the selected medication by first providing adequate patient education to ensure the patient's understanding and promote full participation in therapy. Similar to the setting of hypothyroidism, information to include within the education plan includes the diagnosis, plan of therapy (medication, dose, frequency, side effects, etc.), and follow-up. Patient education is a critical component to empower patients and ensure adherence to the regimen.

Ensure complete patient and family understanding about the medication prescribed using a variety of education strategies. Education strategies may include verbal and written instructions with teach-back to ensure understanding. Also, follow-up telephone calls may be initiated by health care providers to ensure understanding as well as contact information for follow-up as necessary.

Conduct follow-up and monitoring of patient response to therapy. Follow-up and monitoring should include ensuring adherence to therapy; ensuring effectiveness of treatment; assessing symptom relief; monitoring lab work; ensuring remission; and determining the need for surgery. Furthermore, if the thyroid gland is removed, thyroid hormone supplements will be initiated and should be monitored for maintenance of goals.

For optimum patient outcomes, referrals are often required. There are several indications for referral to an endocrinologist or ophthalmologist or for hospitalization, especially if the patient is pregnant, has multiple comorbidities, or is experiencing significant complications including exophthalmos. If the patient has Graves' eye disease, a referral should be made to a specialized ophthalmologist (Braimon & Rieke, 2017; Dlugasch & Story, 2019).

Life Span Considerations with Thyroid Hormone Supplement

Geriatrics

- Weight loss and anorexia are more common in older patients than younger patients.
- Geriatric patients are at higher risk for atrial fibrillation and osteoporosis, leading to an increased risk of cardiac complications and fractures.
- Smoking increases the risk for Graves' ophthalmopathy.
- Patient education should include weight management, exercise, and smoking cessation.

Pediatrics

- According to the ATA, the cause of hyperthyroidism in the pediatric population is usually Graves' disease (95% of patients). Treatment options include medications, radioactive iodine (RAI), or thyroidectomy. After RAI or surgery, thyroid supplement therapy will be required for life.

Pregnancy

- Pregnant patients treated for hyperthyroidism should begin with propylthiouracil in the first trimester, then transition to methimazole during the second and third trimesters.
- Thionamides should be prescribed in the lowest possible doses. In such cases, subclinical hyperthyroidism is typically well tolerated.
- Pregnant patients with uncontrolled hyperthyroidism or intolerance to thionamides may be treated with a subtotal thyroidectomy during the second trimester (Fitzgerald, 2020).
- Pregnant patients cannot undergo RAI treatment. Females who have received RAI should inform their health care provider of their diagnosis of Graves' disease due to the need for additional monitoring of fetal thyroid and heart rate since TSIs cross the placenta.

Teaching Points for Hyperthyroidism Therapy

Health Promotion Strategies

- Inform patients of the increased risk of atrial fibrillation, heart failure, angina, and osteoporosis resulting in an increased risk of bone fractures.
- Inform patients of the danger signs of thyroid storm, such as tachycardia, fever, sweating, confusion, restlessness, and agitation.
- Advise patients to avoid herbal supplements and excessive sushi containing seaweed.
- Counsel and educate patients regarding smoking cessation.
- Counsel and educate patients regarding weight and nutrition management.

- Offer brochures to patients:
  - Adults: https://www.thyroid.org/wp-content/uploads/patients/brochures/Hyper_brochure.pdf
  - Children and adolescents: https://www.thyroid.org/hyperthyroidism-children-adolescents/

Patient Education for Medication Safety

- Take the medication as prescribed.
- Take a heart rate reading daily and report if the heart rate is less than 50 or more than 120 beats/min.
- Patients with osteoporosis/osteopenia should take recommended amounts of calcium and vitamin D.
- Store medications at room temperature in a dry place and protect from light.
- Keep medications out of reach of children and pets. Tell your provider:
  - If you have a temperature of 101°F as additional laboratory testing may be required.
  - About all concurrent prescription and OTC medications and supplements.
  - If you are trying to become pregnant, are pregnant, or are breastfeeding.

Application Questions for Discussion

1. What are contraindications associated with thionamide therapy?
2. Which thionamide medications are indicated during each trimester of pregnancy?
3. What are typical symptoms of iodism?

Selected Bibliography

American Thyroid Association.(n.d.a). *General information/Press room.* Available at https://www.thyroid.org/media-main/press-room/.

American Thyroid Association. (n.d.b). *Hyperthyroidism in children and adolescents.* Available at https://www.thyroid.org/hyperthyroidism-children-adolescents/.

Braimon, J. C., & Rieke, S. M. (2017). Thyroid disorders. In T. M. Buttaro, J. Trybulski, P. Polgar-Bailey, & J. Sandberg-Cook (Eds.), *Primary Care: A Collaborative Practice* (5th ed., pp. 1135–1151). St. Louis: Elsevier.

Brashers, V. L., & Huether, S. E. (2019). Mechanisms of hormonal regulation. In K. L. Huether, & K. McCance (Eds.), *Pathophysiology: The Biologic Basis for Disease in Adults and Children* (8th ed., pp. 644–668). St. Louis: Elsevier.

Calissendorff, J., & Falhammar, H. (2017). Lugol's solution and other iodide preparations: Perspectives and research directions in Graves' disease. *Endocrine, 58*(3), 467–473. https://doi.org/10.1007/s12020-017-1461-8.

Dlugasch, L., & Story, L. (2021). *Endocrine function Applied Pathophysiology for the Advanced Practice Nurse,* pp. 447–484. Jones & Bartlett Learning; Burlington, MA.

Edmunds, M. W., & Mayhew, M. S. (2014). Thyroid medications. In M. W. Edmunds, & M. S. Mayhew (Eds.), *Pharmacology for the Primary Care Provider* (4th ed., p. 581). St. Louis: Elsevier.

Fitzgerald, P. A. (2020). Hyperthyroidism (Thyrotoxicosis). In M. A. Papadakis, S. J. McPhee, & M. W. Rabow (Eds.), *Current Medical Diagnosis and Treatment 2020*. New York: McGraw-Hill.

Garmendia Madariaga, A., Santos Palacios, S., Guillén-Grima, F., & Galofré, J. C. (2014). The incidence and prevalence of thyroid dysfunction in Europe: A meta-analysis. *The Journal of Clinical Endocrinology and Metabolism, 99*(3), 923–931. https://doi.org/10.1210/jc.2013-2409.

Horn, J. R., & Handsten, P. D. (2016). Drugs affecting levothyroxine absorption. *Pharmacy Times.* Retrieved December 31, 2019, from https://www.pharmacytimes.com/publications/issue/2016/January2016/Drugs-Affecting-Levothyroxine-Absorption.

Jonklaas, J., & Talbert, R. L (2011). Thyroid disorders. In J. T. DiPiro, R. L. Talbert, G. C. Yee, G. R. Matzke, B. G. Wells, & L. M. Posey (Eds.), *Pharmacotherapy: A Pathophysiologic Approach* (8th ed., pp. 1303–1326). McGraw-Hill: New York.

Jonklaas, J., Bianco, A. C., Bauer, A. J., Burman, K. D., Cappola, A. R., Celi, F. S., Cooper, D. S., Kim, B. W., Peeters, R. P., Rosenthal, M. S., & Sawka, A. M. (2014). Guidelines for the treatment of hypothyroidism: Prepared by the American Thyroid Association Task Force on Thyroid Hormone Replacement. *Thyroid, 24*(12), 1670–1751. https://doi.org/10.1089/thy.2014.0028.

Surks, M. I. (29 January 2020). *Lithium and the thyroid.* UpToDate®. Available at https://www.uptodate.com/contents/lithium-and-the-thyroid.

37

Adrenal Gland Medications

ELEANOR RAWSON

Overview

Adrenal gland medications are commonly referred to as *corticosteroids* and are grouped according to which steroid hormone the medication helps regulate. The two main classifications of corticosteroids are glucocorticoids (Table 37.1) and mineralocorticoids (Table 37.2). The primary glucocorticoid is cortisol, and the primary mineralocorticoid is aldosterone; the medications in this class relate to the regulation of these steroid hormones. A diagnosis of adrenal insufficiency requires the administration of glucocorticoids and a tapering off of the medication at the completion of therapy to prevent withdrawal and adrenal crisis. The side effects of these medications can be severe in patients with underlying coexisting disease, such as hypertension or diabetes, so the selection and dosage of these drugs must be highly individualized to the patient.

Relevant Physiology

The body has two adrenal glands, one located at the top of each kidney, that produce endocrine hormones which help regulate blood pressure, metabolism, and the immune system. The adrenal gland is small and triangular-shaped and is divided into two main parts: the *adrenal medulla* (the center of the gland) and the *adrenal cortex* (the outside of the gland). The adrenal medulla secretes the hormones epinephrine and norepinephrine, which help regulate the fight-or-flight stress response. The adrenal cortex is composed of three layers; from the outermost to the innermost layer, they are the zona glomerulosa, zona fasciculata, and zona reticularis (Fig. 37.1). The adrenal cortex, the focus of this chapter, secretes corticosteroids that include glucocorticoids, mineralocorticoids, and sex hormones (androgens), which are derived from the steroid cholesterol. The main glucocorticoid of the body is cortisol, and the main mineralocorticoid of the body is aldosterone.

Plasma levels of the adrenocortical hormones vary throughout the day. The levels are highest from 2 a.m. to 8 a.m. and lowest from 4 p.m. to midnight. For this reason, it is important to time the administration of glucocorticoid medication so that it simulates endogenous hormone function. Therefore, most glucocorticoid medications are given in the morning.

Zona Glomerulosa

The outermost layer of the adrenal cortex is the zona glomerulosa, and it focuses on the production of aldosterone. Aldosterone, a steroid hormone that is usually bound to a protein so that it can travel in the blood, is the main mineralocorticoid in the body. In the distal convoluted tubule of the kidney, aldosterone causes an increase in sodium reabsorption. Since water is also reabsorbed (water follows the sodium), this results in an increase in blood volume and a subsequent increase in blood pressure. This response increases the overall sodium content of the blood, leading to hypernatremia. The production of aldosterone is mediated by three different mechanisms: a decrease in blood pressure, low sodium, and high potassium in the blood.

The first mechanism, a decrease in blood pressure, is sensed in the kidney; the enzyme renin is produced and released, which then converts angiotensinogen in the blood to angiotensin I. The lungs release angiotensin-converting enzyme (ACE) into the blood, which converts angiotensin I to angiotensin II, one of the most potent vasoconstrictors in the body. Angiotensin II then stimulates a G-protein coupled receptor in the zona glomerulosa. The stimulated G-protein coupled receptor is enacted by guanosine triphosphate (GTP) and combines with adenylate cyclase to convert adenosine triphosphate (ATP) to cyclic adenosine monophosphate (cAMP). This activates protein kinase A, which helps stimulate the steps necessary to convert cholesterol to aldosterone.

The second and third mechanisms are the presence of a low blood content of sodium (hyponatremia) and an elevated potassium level (hyperkalemia). The presence of these electrolyte abnormalities is enough to stimulate the conversion of cholesterol to aldosterone. Again, the presence of aldosterone in the kidney will help reabsorb sodium, thereby increasing blood sodium content, and help excrete potassium in the urine, which will decrease blood potassium content.

Zona Fasciculata

The largest zone of the adrenal cortex, the zona fasciculata, secretes glucocorticoids, specifically cortisol. The secretion of cortisol is controlled mainly by the adrenocorticotropic

TABLE 37.1 Glucocorticoid Medications

Category	Medication	Indication	Dosage	Considerations and Monitoring
Short acting	Cortisone	Adrenal insufficiency	*Oral:* 25–300 mg/day in divided doses.	Monitor glucose and weight gain. Use lowest effective dose to relieve symptoms.
	Hydrocortisone	Adrenal crisis, adrenal insufficiency, inflammation	*Adrenal crisis:* 100 mg IM or IV, followed by 200 mg intravenously over 24 hr (may be divided in 4 doses: 50 mg intravenously every 6 hr). *Adrenal insufficiency:* Variable dosing, 15–25 mg orally, 2–4 doses/day. Example: Three times daily: 10 mg in a.m., 5 mg in early afternoon, 2.5 mg in late afternoon.	Try not to take in late evening or at night since normally very little cortisol is secreted at these times. When using a variable dose throughout the day, keep larger doses in the morning.
Intermediate acting	Prednisone	Autoimmune disorders	*Oral:* 5–60 mg/day in divided doses.	Use lowest dose required to relieve symptoms.
	Prednisolone	Autoimmune disorders	*Oral:* 5–60 mg/day in divided doses. *IM or IV:* 40–250 mg every 4–6 hr.	Monitor glucose and weight gain. Use lowest effective dose to relieve symptoms.
	Methylprednisolone	Autoimmune disorders, multiple sclerosis, asthma, spinal injury	*Oral:* 5–60 mg/day in divided doses. *IM or IV:* 40–25 mg every 4–6 hr.	Monitor glucose and weight gain. Use lowest effective dose to relieve symptoms.
Long acting	Dexamethasone	Antiinflammatory, airway edema, cerebral edema, nausea and vomiting (perioperative or chemotherapy-induced)	*Oral, IM, or IV:* 0.75–10 mg every 6–12 hr. **Higher doses:** *Chemotherapy-induced nausea and vomiting:* IV/Oral: 5–20 mg every 12 hr. *Postoperative nausea and vomiting:* IV/Oral: 4–10 mg every 12 hr.	Use lowest dose required to relieve symptoms. Has no mineralocorticoid action. Monitor glucose and weight gain.
	Betamethasone	Adrenal insufficiency, premature labor	*IM:* 0.5–9 mg. Up to 12 mg IM prior to premature delivery.	Has no mineralocorticoid action.

TABLE 37.2	Mineralocorticoid Medication		
Medication	**Indication**	**Dosage**	**Considerations and Monitoring**
Fludrocortisone	Adrenal insufficiency, aldosterone insufficiency, congenital adrenal hyperplasia	50–200 mcg/day or can be given every other day.	Decreases the effects of rifampin and hydantoins. Decreases serum levels of salicylates. Given in combination with hydrocortisone. Monitor blood pressure and weight gain. Hypokalemia may be worsened when given with loop diuretics.

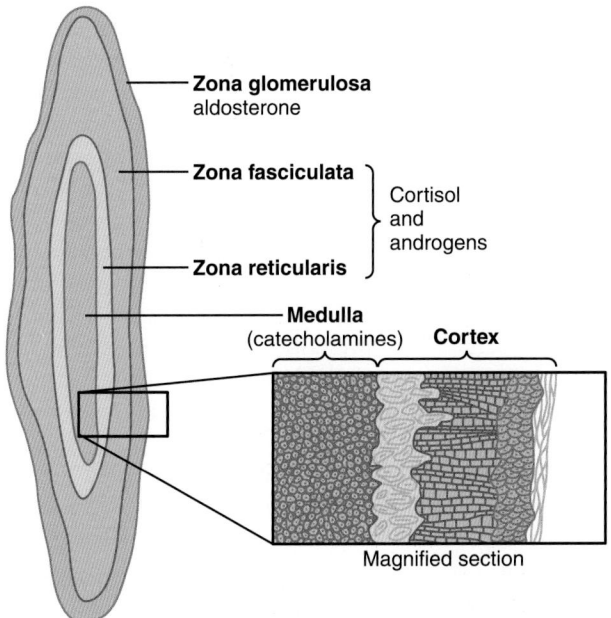

• **Fig. 37.1** Secretion of adrenocortical hormones by the different zones of the adrenal cortex. (From Hall, J. E., & Hall, M. E. [2021]. Adrenocortical hormones. In J. E. Hall & M. E. Hall [Eds.], *Guyton and Hall textbook of medical physiology* [14th ed.], pp. 955-972, Philadelphia: Elsevier.)

hormone (ACTH). ACTH is released by the anterior pituitary after stimulation from the hypothalamus, as part of the hypothalamic-pituitary-adrenal axis (HPAA).

Stressful situations such as injury, infection, and inflammation increase the release of ACTH from the anterior pituitary, leading to an increased release of cortisol. Cortisol has antiinflammatory effects as it blocks many of the inflammatory markers prior to the occurrence of inflammation. Cortisol can even reverse inflammation once it has already begun.

Zona Reticularis

The innermost zone of the adrenal cortex, the zona reticularis, secretes the adrenal androgens (sex hormones) known as dehydroepiandrosterone (DHEA) and androstenedione. Both of these hormones are produced from cholesterol and

released into the blood to travel to the gonads, where they are converted into either estrogen or testosterone.

Pathophysiology

Adrenocortical Insufficiency

There are three types of adrenocortical insufficiency: primary, secondary, and tertiary. *Primary adrenal insufficiency* is usually a result of damage to the adrenal gland and can lead to a decrease in glucocorticoids, mineralocorticoids, and androgens. *Secondary adrenal insufficiency* is the result of decreased hormone production that leads to a decrease in adrenal stimulation, specifically a decrease in ACTH. Administration of glucocorticoids results in an iatrogenic decrease or absent release of ACTH from the pituitary, since there are always high levels of glucocorticoids in the blood. In the absence of ACTH, the adrenal glands do not produce or release endogenous glucocorticoids, which can result in adrenal insufficiency or emergent adrenal crisis. Secondary insufficiency is more common than primary. *Tertiary adrenal insufficiency* is a result of problems with the hypothalamus. Primary insufficiency is associated with both cortisol and aldosterone deficiency, while secondary and tertiary insufficiency are only associated with a deficiency in cortisol.

Symptoms of adrenal insufficiency vary (Box 37.1). Diagnosis of adrenal insufficiency is confirmed with serum cortisol and ACTH laboratory tests, drawn in the morning. Serum cortisol is low in adrenal insufficiency; the type, whether primary or secondary, is determined by the ACTH level.

• Box 37.1	Symptoms of Adrenal Insufficiency

- Fatigue
- Decreased appetite
- Nausea
- Orthostatic hypotension
- Dizziness
- Syncope
- Dyspnea
- Hypoglycemia
- Circulatory collapse

Addison's Disease

Damage to the adrenal glands leads to a primary adrenal insufficiency known as Addison's disease. This disease process decreases or halts release of both cortisol and aldosterone steroid hormones and usually stems from an autoimmune disease that destroys the adrenal gland. Since it is a combined issue, treatment will include both a glucocorticoid and a mineralocorticoid.

Acute Adrenal Insufficiency

Withdrawal from glucocorticoid medications occurs when the steroid is terminated abruptly and can lead to an acute adrenal insufficiency. Administration of steroids leads to an increase in circulating cortisol and aldosterone, which causes the anterior pituitary to stop the release of ACTH. The HPAA is then slowed or stopped, and there is no longer a feedback cycle to keep releasing ACTH, which leads to an adrenal insufficiency. HPAA suppression can be assumed in patients receiving high-dose steroids for more than 3 weeks. It is important to gradually taper off of glucocorticoids to prevent an adrenal crisis. These medications are usually tapered off over many days or weeks, and tapering may be required with as little as 5 to 10 days of taking glucocorticoids. An adrenal crisis is an emergency with symptoms similar to other adrenocortical insufficiency presentations, and it can quickly lead to cardiovascular compromise. Fluid resuscitation is extremely important during an adrenal crisis.

Adrenocortical Excess

Adrenocortical excess can be caused by adrenal disease or iatrogenic interventions. Administration of glucocorticoids can lead to an excess of cortisol with subsequent effects in the body. An excess of aldosterone will present as hypertension without an underlying cause.

Cushing's Syndrome

An increased plasma level of cortisol leads to the signs and symptoms of Cushing's syndrome. These include fatigue or mania, growth retardation in children, weight gain, sleeplessness, glucose intolerance/diabetes, hypertension, striae on the skin, and increased bleeding, as well as increased adipose in the face and upper back, leading to a moon face and buffalo hump appearance. Cushing's syndrome can result from exogenous administration of corticosteroids or a tumor in the adrenal gland or pituitary, leading to the increased cortisol levels.

Conn's Syndrome

Primary aldosteronism is an increase in circulating aldosterone, known as Conn's syndrome, and may be caused by an aldosterone-producing adenoma or bilateral adrenal hyperplasia. Hypertension is the main sign, since the increased aldosterone causes an increase in fluid retention. Another sign may be hypokalemia, indicated by increased excretion of potassium. Although hypokalemia is a common sign of Conn's syndrome, this is not always the case as the patient may have a normal potassium in hyperaldosteronism. Surgical treatment includes an adrenalectomy; alternatively, Conn's syndrome can be pharmacologically managed with a mineralocorticoid antagonist such as spironolactone and antihypertensives.

Adrenal Gland Therapy

Glucocorticoids

Pharmacokinetics. All of the glucocorticoids have similar pharmacologic profiles, specifically with their indications, adverse effects, contraindications, and monitoring during drug treatment. These drugs are often compared to one another based on their glucocorticoid and mineralocorticoid potency and how the potency compares to that of cortisol (Table 37.3). It is also important to recognize the equivalent dosages between the drugs. Glucocorticoid therapy is not a contraindication to live-virus vaccines when the glucocorticoid therapy lasts fewer than 14 days; is given in a low to moderate dose; is prescribed for long-term, alternate-day use with short-acting preparations; is prescribed as replacement therapy; or is administered through topical, inhaled, intraarticular, bursal, or tendon injection (American Academy of Pediatrics, 2009).

Indications. All glucocorticoids can be used in the treatment of adrenal insufficiency. Since they decrease the immune response, they are also used to treat allergies and anaphylactic reactions. In addition, they possess antiinflammatory properties.

Adverse Effects. Adverse effects of glucocorticoids include fluid retention (sodium retention and loss of potassium), impaired wound healing, hypotension or hypertension, syncope, muscle weakness and loss of muscle, thromboembolism, seizures, osteoporosis, and hyperglycemia.

Contraindications. During chronic treatment, all of the glucocorticoids suppress normal adrenal function and HPAA response, so these drugs must be tapered when discontinuing use. These patients are at high risk of impaired wound healing and infection, so glucocorticoids should not be given when a patient is septic. Hyperglycemia is a known side effect of corticosteroids and should be closely monitored in diabetic patients. Osteoporosis may occur due to changes in the bones, as well as decreased muscle mass. Electrolyte abnormalities may be present due to fluid retention, resulting in hypernatremia, hypokalemia, or hypocalcemia. Hypertension may result after glucocorticoid administration.

Monitoring. The lowest effective dose possible should be given to decrease the risk of serious side effects, so the patient should be monitored at the lowest dose for relief of symptoms. The patient should also be monitored for signs of Cushing's syndrome, including weight gain, a

TABLE 37.3	Glucocorticoid Potency (Compared Relative to Cortisol)				
Glucocorticoid	Equivalent Dose (mg)	Glucocorticoid Potency	Mineralocorticoid Potency	Plasma Half-Life (minutes)	Biologic Half-Life (hours)
Short Acting					
Cortisol	20.0	1.0	1.0	90	8–12
Cortisone	25.0	0.8	0.8	80–118	8–12
Intermediate Acting					
Prednisone	5.0	4.0	0.3	60	18–36
Prednisolone	5.0	5.0	0.3	115–200	18–36
Triamcinolone	4.0	5.0	0	30	18–36
Methylprednisolone	4.0	5.0	0	180	18–36
Long Acting					
Dexamethasone	0.75	30	0	200	36–54
Betamethasone	0.6	25–40	0	300	36–54

From Dineen, R., Martin-Grace, J., Thompson, C. J., & Sherlock, M. (2020). The management of glucocorticoid deficiency: Current and future perspectives. *Clinica Chimica Acta, 505*, 148–159.

moon-shaped face, and increased upper-back adipose tissue. Glucose should be checked frequently in diabetic patients due to risk of hyperglycemia.

PRACTICE PEARLS

Quality and Safety: Patients With Diabetes

- Hyperglycemia may result from administration of corticosteroids.
- Monitor blood sugars frequently and routinely.

PRACTICE PEARLS

Life Span Considerations With Corticosteroids in Older Adults

- Per the Beers Criteria, avoid corticosteroids in older adults who have or are at high risk of developing delirium because of the potential of inducing or worsening the delirium.
- Use with caution in older adult patients as corticoid replacement may result in exacerbation of other comorbidities such as hypertension, heart failure, osteoporosis, and arthritis.
- Decrease dosages in older adult patients due to their decreased muscle mass, renal function, and plasma volume.

Types of Glucocorticoids

Cortisone

Cortisone is a short-acting glucocorticoid and is often compared to hydrocortisone, although hydrocortisone is preferred to cortisone. It has the equivalent glucocorticoid and mineralocorticoid potency and is slightly less potent than cortisol.

Pharmacokinetics. Cortisone is metabolized in the liver and converted to hydrocortisone. It has a very short half-life of 30 minutes.

Indications. Cortisone is used in the treatment of adrenal insufficiency, allergies, inflammation, and allergic reactions.

Adverse Effects. In addition to the adverse effects listed for all glucocorticoids, cortisone may result in insomnia, nervousness, increased appetite, and dyspepsia.

Contraindications. Cortisone is contraindicated in patients with hypersensitivity to cortisone or any of its components. Refer to general contraindications for all glucocorticoids.

Monitoring. Laboratory monitoring of glucose and potassium is recommended. Monitor vital signs for increases in blood pressure and heart rate. Monitor body weight in adults and children. In children, also monitor growth rate.

Hydrocortisone

Hydrocortisone has mainly glucocorticoid activity, but also has some minor mineralocorticoid activity and is the most frequently prescribed glucocorticoid. If it is taken concomitantly with fludrocortisone, the dose of fludrocortisone will need to be reduced.

Pharmacokinetics. The oral dose is rapidly absorbed, with peak plasma concentration 1 hour after administration. Hydrocortisone has a relatively short half-life (1.5 to 2 hours), so the dose is usually divided throughout the day in either 2 or 3 doses. Metabolism occurs in the liver as well as by cytochrome (CYP) P450.

Indications. Hydrocortisone is used primarily for the treatment of primary and secondary adrenal insufficiency with low cortisol levels and is also used in the emergency setting in cases of adrenal crisis. In addition, it can be used for its antiinflammatory effects as well as in the treatment of autoimmune disorders such as rheumatoid arthritis. Hydrocortisone is also given to treat acute allergic and anaphylactic reactions.

Adverse Effects. In addition to the adverse effects listed for all glucocorticoids, hydrocortisone may cause alterations in behavior and mood. Refer to Practice Pearls for adverse effects that are common to older adults and to patients with diabetes.

Contraindications. Hydrocortisone is contraindicated in patients with hypersensitivity to hydrocortisone or any of its components. Refer to general contraindications for all glucocorticoids.

Monitoring. Most patients with primary adrenal insufficiency will require mineralocorticoid replacement with fludrocortisone, so patients should be monitored for hyponatremia and hyperkalemia, which indicate the need for supplementation.

Prednisone

Prednisone is used for the treatment of autoimmune diseases as it decreases the immune response, which is overactive in disorders such as rheumatoid arthritis and multiple sclerosis. Prednisone has mostly glucocorticoid activity, but it does have a very small amount of mineralocorticoid activity.

Pharmacokinetics. Prednisone is converted in the liver to prednisolone and then metabolized. The half-life is approximately 3.4 to 3.8 hours.

Indications. Prednisone may be used for the treatment of asthma. It is also indicated for autoimmune disorders and for its antiinflammatory properties.

Adverse Effects. Refer to the list of adverse effects listed for all glucocorticoids.

Contraindications. Prednisone is contraindicated in patients with hypersensitivity to it or any of its components. Refer to general contraindications for all glucocorticoids.

Monitoring. Laboratory monitoring of serum glucose and 2-hour postprandial blood glucose, serum potassium, and urinalysis are recommended. Vital signs should be monitored for increases in blood pressure and heart rate. Pulmonary function tests (PFTs) and changes in mental status should also be monitored. In addition, monitor body weight in adults and children. In children, also monitor growth rate.

Prednisolone

Pharmacokinetics. Prednisolone is metabolized in the liver. The half-life is 2.1 to 3.5 hours.

Indications. Prednisolone is used for its antiinflammatory properties and to decrease immune response in autoimmune disorders. Prednisolone has a very small amount of mineralocorticoid activity; it has mostly glucocorticoid properties and slightly higher glucocorticoid potency than prednisone.

Adverse Effects. Refer to the adverse effects listed for all glucocorticoids. Prednisolone may also cause acne, ecchymosis, headache, euphoria, and psychiatric disorders.

Contraindications. Prednisolone is contraindicated in patients with hypersensitivity to it, to any of its components, or to other glucocorticoids. Avoid in patients with systemic fungal infections. Refer to general contraindications for all glucocorticoids.

Monitoring. Recommendations include monitoring of erythrocyte sedimentation rate (ESR) in patients with rheumatoid arthritis. In patients on extended therapy, monitor 24-hour urine for calcium and creatinine, 2-hour postprandial blood glucose, and serum potassium. Monitor vital signs for increases in blood pressure, heart rate, and PFTs. Monitor body weight in adults and children. In children, also monitor growth rate.

Methylprednisolone

Methylprednisolone can be used in the treatment of many autoimmune disorders, including multiple sclerosis, and is also indicated for inflammation. It has no mineralocorticoid activity, only glucocorticoid activity.

Pharmacokinetics. Methylprednisolone is metabolized in the liver and has a half-life of 3.5 hours. The longer half-life makes this drug a good choice for those who are unable to adhere to frequent dosing with hydrocortisone.

Indications. Methylprednisolone is used for the treatment of asthma. It also may be used in combination with other drugs to prevent rejection of a transplanted organ due to its suppression of the immune system.

Adverse Effects. Refer to the adverse effects listed for all glucocorticoids.

Contraindications. Methylprednisolone is contraindicated in patients with hypersensitivity to it or to any of its components. Avoid use in patients with systemic fungal infections. Refer to general contraindications for all glucocorticoids.

Monitoring. Recommendations include monitoring of blood glucose and serum potassium. Monitor vital signs for increases in blood pressure, heart rate, and PFTs. Monitor body weight in adults and children. In children, also monitor growth rate. In cases of prolonged therapy, monitor ophthalmic exam for changes.

Dexamethasone

Dexamethasone has no mineralocorticoid activity. It is 30 times more potent than cortisol and is used exclusively for its glucocorticoid potency.

Pharmacokinetics. The half-life of dexamethasone is 3.5 to 4 hours. It is metabolized in the liver.

Indications. Dexamethasone is used to test for adrenal disorders by assessing the laboratory values of cortisol before and after administration. It is also used as an immune suppressant for many disorders, including autoimmune disorders and skin conditions. Dexamethasone is also used perioperatively to treat airway edema, nausea, and vomiting. In chemotherapy patients, high doses of dexamethasone are used to prevent or treat nausea and vomiting. Dexamethasone is a very strong antiinflammatory medication and can be used to treat cerebral edema.

Adverse Effects. Refer to the adverse effects listed for all glucocorticoids. In addition, serious ophthalmic effects including blindness, exophthalmos, and increased intraocular pressure have been reported.

Contraindications. Dexamethasone is contraindicated in patients with hypersensitivity to it or to any of its components. Avoid use in patients with systemic fungal infections and ocular or periocular infections. Refer to general contraindications for all glucocorticoids.

Monitoring. Recommendations include monitoring of blood glucose, serum cortisol, and potassium levels. Monitor vital signs for increases in blood pressure, heart rate, and PFTs. Monitor body weight in adults and children. In children, also monitor growth rate. In cases of prolonged therapy, monitor intraocular pressures and ophthalmic exam for changes.

Betamethasone

Pharmacokinetics. The half-life of betamethasone is 3 to 5 hours. This long half-life makes it difficult to titrate when adrenal excess occurs. Betamethasone is metabolized in the liver.

Indications. Betamethasone can be used in patients who are expected to deliver prematurely, to prevent respiratory distress in the newborn. This drug is usually given 2 to 3 days before delivery, or immediately before an emergent delivery.

Adverse Effects. Refer to the adverse effects listed for all glucocorticoids. In addition, dermatologic disorders such as acne, atrophy, and pigment changes have been reported.

Contraindications. Avoid use in patients with hypersensitivity to betamethasone, other corticosteroids, or any component of the product. Also avoid in patients with systemic fungal infections and ocular or periocular infections. Refer to general contraindications for all glucocorticoids.

Monitoring. Recommendations include monitoring of blood glucose and serum potassium levels.

Mineralocorticoids

Fludrocortisone

Fludrocortisone is the only mineralocorticoid medication in use today. When fludrocortisone is used to treat Addison's disease, a glucocorticoid such as hydrocortisone is also administered.

Pharmacokinetics. Although fludrocortisone has both glucocorticoid and mineralocorticoid activity, it is used only for its mineralocorticoid activity since the affinity for glucocorticoid receptors is very low. Fludrocortisone is usually given in conjunction with glucocorticoids.

Indications. Fludrocortisone is used to replace primary and secondary adrenocortical deficiency, specifically in cases of Addison's disease.

Adverse Effects. Adverse effects include edema, hypertension, heart failure, hypertrophy of the heart, increased sweating, hypokalemia, muscle weakness, headache, and hypersensitivity reactions.

Contraindications. Fludrocortisone is contraindicated in patients who are allergic to fludrocortisone. Use cautiously in patients with Addison's disease or infection. Fludrocortisone decreases the effects of rifampin and hydantoins. It also decreases serum levels of salicylates when those agents are administered with fludrocortisone.

Monitoring. Check blood pressure frequently due to risk of hypertension. Hypotension may indicate a suboptimal dosage. Monitor patient's weight to assess for edema, specifically swelling of the hands and feet due to water retention. Adventitious breath sounds such as crackles could indicate fluid overload.

PRACTICE PEARLS

Adrenal Gland Medication Use in Pregnancy and Lactation

- Glucocorticoids are pregnancy category C drugs. Use with caution during pregnancy and lactation.
- No controlled data are available for use in humans, but based on animal data, there is a potential risk to the fetus that should be considered.
- To potentially decrease neonatal mortality and morbidity, corticosteroids may be given to a patient with a viable pregnancy who is between 24 and 34 weeks of gestation if premature labor is expected within the next 7 days.

Prescriber Considerations for Adrenal Gland Therapy

Clinical Practice Guidelines

Corticosteroids have a wide variety of clinical practice uses, with guidelines for each type of occurrence. Doses are variable for autoimmune disorders such as rheumatoid arthritis and systemic lupus erythematosus, and treatment usually begins with the lowest effective dose to minimize risk of adverse side effects. Allergies, inflammation, asthma, and anaphylaxis are also treated with corticosteroids, beginning the course of treatment with a low dose and working up until symptoms are relieved or adverse side effects are present.

For adrenal insufficiency, patients are diagnosed based on symptom presentation and laboratory values. They are usually treated with hydrocortisone and then are continuously monitored for glucocorticoid excess and other side effects. The Endocrine Society provides a clinical practice guideline to address the diagnosis and treatment of primary adrenal insufficiency (Bornstein et al., 2016).

Clinical Reasoning for Adrenal Gland Therapy

Consider the individual patient's health problem requiring adrenal gland therapy. The first step is to assess the condition that is being treated with adrenocortical medications and determine the patient's health history. Adrenal insufficiency is determined by decreased circulating levels of cortisol and is diagnosed through laboratory tests. If the patient's ACTH is high, a primary adrenal insufficiency is likely, whereas a low or normal ACTH may signal a secondary adrenal insufficiency. In addition to lab work, correlation of the diagnosis to the presenting symptoms will help contribute to the diagnosis. If the patient is being treated with corticosteroids for an autoimmune disorder, the patient's health care team should already have investigated the disease process.

It is important to review the chosen medication's adverse effects and correlate them with the rest of the patient's history. Specifically, investigate the cardiovascular and endocrine systems for any disorders. Adverse effects of the heart, including hypertension, fluid retention, and heart failure, occur with both glucocorticoid and mineralocorticoid administration. Diabetes mellitus is an endocrine disorder that must be recognized prior to taking these drugs, as they all increase plasma glucose levels, and insulin requirements may be increased during the treatment period.

Determine the desired therapeutic outcome based on the adrenal gland therapy needed for the patient's health problem. In adrenal insufficiency, the main therapeutic outcome is to increase cortisol levels and alleviate all related symptoms. This should be done using the lowest possible dose to halt symptoms such as fatigue, nausea, hypotension, and circulatory collapse. In autoimmune disorders, the goal of therapy is to stop the disease process or to prevent further damage to the body. Also seen with allergies and anaphylaxis, corticosteroids help reduce inflammation and allergy progression.

Assess the medication therapy selected for its appropriateness for an individual patient by considering the medication's side effects and the patient's age, race/ethnicity, comorbidities, and genetic factors. Adrenal insufficiency is best treated with oral hydrocortisone due to its short half-life and the ability to titrate the dose. Adverse effects that occur with all of the glucocorticoids include nausea, vomiting, hypertension, muscle weakness, and osteoporosis, among others. Mainly the cardiovascular and endocrine systems should be evaluated prior to treatment with hydrocortisone. Patients with autoimmune disorders should be assessed for other comorbidities that may impact the administration of hydrocortisone. The lowest dose possible that relieves symptoms should be given. All patients should be monitored for infection before taking corticosteroids. A current infection could become worse after adrenocortical therapy due to immune suppression and hyperglycemia, which allow the infection to worsen.

Initiate the treatment plan with the selected medication by first providing adequate patient education to ensure the patient's understanding and promote full participation in the adrenal gland therapy. It is best to take the total daily dose of hydrocortisone in divided doses, either two or three times daily. Since normal cortisol levels are highest in the morning, to mimic this, it is best to give the largest divided dose

in the morning, and then smaller doses for the remaining dose or doses, hoping by evening that the patient will be able to fall asleep. A typical medication schedule would be to give hydrocortisone 10 mg in the morning, 5 mg in the early afternoon, and 2.5 mg in the late afternoon.

Ensure complete patient and family understanding about the medication prescribed for adrenal gland therapy using a variety of education strategies. The patient should be educated on the benefits and risks of the drug. Risks include all potential adverse side effects that the patient would need to self-monitor. The patient should pay attention to their weight; weight gain may indicate fluid retention and potentially fluid overload. Additionally, signs and symptoms of Cushing's syndrome should be closely watched for due to the risk of glucocorticoid excess.

Conduct follow-up and monitoring of patient responses to adrenal gland therapy. As previously mentioned, the lowest dose possible should be given that effectively reduces the patient's symptoms. The ideal response to adrenocortical treatment is relief of symptoms, using the lowest dose possible. In adrenal insufficiency, the idea is to temporarily increase the cortisol levels with the goal of stimulating the HPAA and thereby decreasing the presentation of symptoms. In autoimmune disorders, the goal of treatment is to reduce the symptoms or stop the progression of the disease process.

In chronic adrenocortical therapy, dosages must be tapered in anyone taking corticosteroids longer than 5 days. The HPAA is no longer functioning properly, and when the medication is stopped, the body is no longer able to make its own cortisol. The patient should be monitored for adrenal insufficiency and, in the emergency setting, for adrenal crisis.

Teaching Points for Adrenal Gland Therapy

Health Promotion Strategies

It is important for patients to play an active role in their health care decisions by participating in the discussions and plan of care. Patients can discuss the risks and benefits with their provider so that they are aware of what symptoms to monitor that are related to taking corticosteroids. A patient could improve their own health by noticing these symptoms and going to a provider for evaluation as soon as possible.

Patient Education for Medication Safety

When prescribing corticosteroids to patients, the patient and provider should discuss the risks and benefits of administration. The patient should be educated on the difference between acute and chronic therapy and the serious adverse effects associated with both, but especially the need to taper off the medication when used for extended periods of time. The patient should be provided with a list of adverse effects, which includes the risks of glucocorticoid excess that present with Cushing's syndrome.

Application Questions for Discussion

1. What monitoring should be continued for diabetic patients taking corticosteroids?
2. When taking both hydrocortisone and fludrocortisone, why might the dose of fludrocortisone need to be reduced?
3. Why is it required to taper off the dosage of medication when discontinuing glucocorticoids?

Selected Bibliography

American Academy of Pediatrics. Immunization in special clinical circumstances (2009). In L. Pickering, C. Baker, D. Kimberlin, & S. Long (Eds.), *Red book: 2009 report of the committee on infectious diseases*. Elk Grove Village, IL: American Academy of Pediatrics.

American College of Obstetricians and Gynecologists. (2017). ACOG committee opinion No. 713: Antenatal corticosteroid therapy for fetal maturation. *Obstetrics & Gynecology, 130*(2), e102–e109. http://doi.org/10.1097/AOG.0000000000002237.

Bornstein, S. R., Allolio, B., Arlt, W., Barthel, A., Don-Wauchope, A., Hammer, G. D., Husebye, E. S., Merke, D. P., Murad, M. H., Stratakis, C. A., & Torpy, D. J. (2016). Diagnosis and treatment of primary adrenal insufficiency: An Endocrine Society clinical practice guideline. *Journal of Clinical Endocrinology & Metabolism, 101*(2), 364–389. https://doi.org/10.1210/jc.2015-1710.

Dineen, R., Martin-Grace, J., Thompson, C. J., & Sherlock, M. (2020). The management of glucocorticoid deficiency: Current and future perspectives. *Clinica Chimica Acta, 505*, 148–159. http://doi.org/10.1016/j.cca.2020.03.006.

Ford, S. M. (2018). *Roach's introductory clinical pharmacology* (11th ed.). Philadelphia: Wolters Kluwer.

Hall, J. E., & Hall, M. E. (2021). Adrenocortical hormones. In J. E. Hall & M. E. Hall [Eds.], *Guyton and Hall textbook of medical physiology* (14th ed.), pp. 955-972, Philadelphia: Elsevier.

Monticone, S., Burrello, J., Tizzani, D., Bertello, C., Viola, A., Buffolo, F., Gabetti, L., Mengozzi, G., Williams, T. A., Rabbia, F., Veglio, F., & Mulatero, P. (2017). Prevalence and clinical manifestations of primary aldosteronism encountered in primary care practice. *Journal of the American College of Cardiology, 69*(4), 1811–1820. http://doi.org/10.1016/j.jacc.2017.01.052.

Nieman, L. K. (2018). Recent updates on the diagnosis and management of Cushing's syndrome. *Endocrinology and Metabolism, 33*(2), 139–146. http://doi.org/10.3803/EnM.2018.33.2.139.

Vaidya, A., Mulatero, P., Baudrand, R., & Adler, G. K. (2018). The expanding spectrum of primary aldosteronism: Implications for diagnosis, pathogenesis, and treatment. *Endocrine Reviews, 39*(6), 1057–1088. https://doi.org/10.1210/er.2018-00139.

Vallerand, A. H., & Sanoski, C. A. (2020). *Davis's drug guide* (17th ed.). Philadelphia: F.A. Davis Company.

Yeoh, P. (2019). Anatomy and physiology of the adrenal gland. In S. Llahana, C. Follin, C. Yedinak, & A. Grossman (Eds.), *Advanced practice in endocrinology nursing* (1st ed.) (pp. 645–656). Cham, Switzerland: Springer Nature Switzerland AG.

38

Diabetes Mellitus Medications

AIMON C. MIRANDA AND REBECCA M. LUTZ

Overview

Diabetes mellitus (DM) describes a group of metabolic disorders characterized and identified by the presence of hyperglycemia in the absence of treatment (World Health Organization [WHO], 2019). This chapter will review the prevalence, definitions, pathology, and therapeutic interventions for type 1 DM (T1DM) and type 2 DM (T2DM).

Prevalence

DM is a common chronic health condition. The number of people affected by DM in the United States and around the world continues to rise. In 2014, 8.5% of adults (422 million) had diabetes worldwide (WHO, 2016). In the United States, the National Diabetes Statistics Report 2020 (Centers for Disease Control and Prevention [CDC], 2020) provides data based on prevalence estimates among the total population as well as estimates based on age, gender, and race/ethnicity. Diabetes affects more than 34 million adults 18 years of age and older. Diabetes is more prevalent in males (14.0%) than females (12.8%). Race and ethnicity estimates reveal variances in diagnosis. White, non-Hispanic adults 18 years of age and older have 15.4% higher rates than Black, non-Hispanics (4.2%), Hispanics (4.9%), or Asians (1.6%).

The multiyear SEARCH for Diabetes in Youth study tracks the incidence of diabetes in youth (Drivers et al., 2020). Unfortunately, the incidence of T1DM and T2DM continues to rise. The highest rates of T1DM were found in those 10 to 14 years of age, in males, and in Whites. After adjusting for age and gender incidence/year, increases were noted among Blacks (2.7%), Hispanics (4.0%), and Asian and Pacific Islanders (4.4%). Dabelea et al. (2017) identified that diabetic complications such as kidney disease, retinopathy, peripheral neuropathy, and cardiovascular diseases were more prevalent in adolescents and young adults with T2DM than T1DM.

Economic Burden

The cost of diabetes and related consequences is rising globally. It is estimated that the cost will reach more than $1.2 trillion by 2030. This is a 61% increase from 2015 to 2030 (Bommer et al., 2018). In the United States, the economic cost associated with diabetes is $327 billion. People with diagnosed diabetes incur additional annual medical expenditures of approximately $9,600 (American Diabetes Association [ADA], 2018).

Relevant Physiology

The pancreas is composed of *endocrine* and *exocrine glands* and the islets of Langerhans. The *exocrine gland* produces and secretes digestive enzymes to break down the proteins, lipids, and carbohydrates found in food. The *endocrine gland* produces and secretes the hormones insulin and glucagon. The *islets of Langerhans* comprise several types of cells with different functions. Of primary interest are the beta cells (β-cells), which secrete insulin and amylin, and the alpha cells (α-cells), which secrete glucagon. A small number of cells secrete gastrin and somatostatin (delta cells [δ-cells]) as well as pancreatic polypeptide (PP-cells) (Brashers & Huether, 2019; Da Silva Xavier, 2018). The opposing actions of insulin and glucagon hormones maintain stable glucose levels.

Insulin is an anabolic hormone critical to the metabolism of carbohydrates, lipids, and protein. Insulin secretion varies depending on chemical, hormonal, and neural factors. In response to increases in blood glucose, β-cells increase insulin secretion, which stimulates glucose transport in muscle and adipose tissue and reduces glucose production by inhibiting the synthesis of glucose in the liver. As blood glucose decreases, the production of glucose in the liver increases, resulting in leveling of blood glucose (Brashers & Huether, 2019; Mann & Bellin, 2016).

Pathophysiology

The primary characteristic of diabetes is the dysfunction or destruction of pancreatic β-cells, resulting in hyperglycemia. This destruction affects insulin secretion and/or action and progresses along a continuum (Skyler et al., 2017). Dysfunction of or destruction of pancreatic β-cells may result from a genetic predisposition, genetic abnormalities, epigenetic processes, insulin resistance, autoimmunity, concurrent illnesses, inflammation, and/or environmental factors.

Diagnosis

DM diagnosis is based on the results of glycosylated hemoglobin (HbA1c) levels, fasting plasma glucose (FPG) levels, oral glucose tolerance testing (OGTT), and random glucose levels in an individual with symptoms. Based on elevations in HbA1c, FPG, and OGTT, patients are classified as normal, prediabetic, or diabetic. Prediabetic patients have elevated HbA1c, FPG, and OGTT. Table 38.1 outlines the specific criteria for diagnosis (ADA, 2021). Table 38.2 offers an overview of the classifications of DM along with descriptions and characteristic features of each type. This chapter will discuss T1DM and T2DM. The other classifications will not be discussed in this chapter.

Type 1 Diabetes Mellitus (T1DM)

T1DM most commonly involves an autoimmune dysfunction and destruction of insulin-producing pancreatic β-cells in the *islets of Langerhans*. The diagnosis is most often made in childhood or early adulthood but may occur across the life span. Initially, autoantibodies are directed to insulin or glutamic acid decarboxylase. Next, additional autoantibodies act against islet antigen-2 or the ZnT8 transporter. This mechanism involves the following three stages (Table 38.3):

- Stage 1: β-cell autoimmunity, normal plasma glucose levels, and no symptoms
- Stage 2: β-cell autoimmunity, abnormal plasma glucose levels, and no symptoms
- Stage 3: β-cell autoimmunity, abnormal plasma glucose levels, and symptoms of diabetes

Factors attributed to β-cell destruction include genetic, environmental, or an interaction between the two. The primary risk factor is genetic with major histocompatibility complex, or MHC (histocompatibility leukocyte antigen [HLA] class II alleles HLA-DR3-DQ2 or HLA-DR4-DQ8 haplotypes, or both) (Pociot & Lernmark, 2016; Atkinson, 2012). Clinical manifestations of T1DM include polydipsia, polyuria, polyphagia, unexplained weight loss, numbness in extremities, dysesthesias, recurrent infections, fatigue, blurred vision, hyperglycemia, and hypoglycemia (ADA, 2018; Ramachandran, 2014). Maintaining plasma glucose within acceptable levels by administering exogenous insulin is the mainstay of current therapy (ADA, 2021).

Type 2 Diabetes Mellitus (T2DM)

T2DM is the most common classification of DM and includes 90% to 95% of all diabetes cases (ADA, 2020). T2DM does not involve autoimmune β-cell destruction nor is it attributed to other known causes. Insulin deficiency (secretion) and resistance are the hallmark characteristics.

T2DM is a complex disease. Initially considered a disease of adults, children and adolescents are increasingly being diagnosed. There are a variety of causes, and risk factors are multifactorial (Box 38.1).

Diabetes Mellitus Therapy

There are several factors to consider when selecting diabetes mellitus medications, including concomitant diseases, medication efficacy and safety, medication cost, and patient preferences regarding the route of administration (i.e., oral versus subcutaneous injections). Other factors include baseline HbA1c, the compelling need to minimize hypoglycemia, minimizing weight gain, or promoting weight loss. Table 38.4 provides an overview of drug-specific and patient-specific considerations when selecting pharmacologic therapies.

Insulin

Insulins are proteins that bind to cell wall receptors to allow cellular utilization of glucose. Insulin lowers blood glucose levels by stimulating peripheral glucose uptake, particularly in skeletal muscle and fat, and by inhibiting hepatic glucose production. An adequate supply of insulin is needed for transport of glucose across the cell membrane to sustain life.

Most insulin used today is produced by deoxyribonucleic acid (DNA) recombinant technology and is synthesized in a nonpathogenic strain of *Escherichia coli* bacteria or *Saccharomyces cerevisiae* fungus. Advantages of using synthetic human insulin include a decrease in the production of insulin antibodies and a diminished risk for the development of lipodystrophy at the injection site.

Insulin analogs are insulin preparations that are produced by modifying the structure of human insulin. Changing human insulin properties with amino acid substitutions improves the pharmacokinetic profile for optimal

TABLE 38.1	Diagnostic Criteria for Diabetes Mellitus			
	HgA$_{1c}$	Fasting Plasma Glucose (FPG)	Oral Glucose Tolerance Test (OGTT)	Random Plasma Glucose Test
Normal	<5.7%	<100 mg/dL	<140 mg/dL	NA
Prediabetes	5.7–6.4%	100–125 mg/dL	140–199 mg/dL	NA
Diabetes	≥6.5%	≥126 mg/dL	≥200 mg/dL	≥200 mg/dL

NA, Not applicable.
Adapted from American Diabetes Association [2020]. *2. Classification and diagnosis of diabetes: Standards of medical care in diabetes 2020. Diabetes Care* 43[Suppl. 1], S14–S31. https://doi.org/10.2337/dc20-S002.

TABLE 38.2	Classifications and Description/Characteristics of the Different Types of Diabetes

Classification	Description
Type 1 diabetes	β-cell destruction (mostly immune mediated) and absolute insulin deficiency. β-cell destruction may be rapid or slower in progression. Onset most common in childhood and early adulthood but may occur throughout the life span. Little or no insulin secretion. Low or undetectable levels of C-peptide in blood or urine. Insulin dependent. Comorbidities may be present.
Type 2 diabetes	Most common type (90–95% of diabetes cases). Adults, but increasing number of children/adolescents affected. Various degrees of β-cell dysfunction. Insulin resistance. Commonly associated with overweight/obesity, reduced physical activity, unhealthy lifestyle and behavioral patterns, fetal malnutrition, and increasing fetal exposure to hyperglycemia during pregnancy. Additional comorbidities may be present.
Slowly evolving, immune-mediated diabetes of adults	Similar to slowly evolving type 1 diabetes in adults but more often has features of the metabolic syndrome. Criteria: • >35 yr at diagnosis, positivity for GAD autoantibodies. • A single GAD autoantibody and retains greater β-cell function. • No need for insulin therapy in the first 6–12 months after diagnosis.
Ketosis-prone type 2 diabetes	Presents with ketosis and insulin deficiency but later does not require insulin. Common episodes of ketosis. Not immune mediated.
Diabetes mellitus in pregnancy	Type 1 or type 2 diabetes first diagnosed during pregnancy.
Gestational diabetes mellitus	Hyperglycemia below diagnostic thresholds for diabetes in pregnancy.
Monogenic diabetes Monogenic defects of β-cell function Monogenic defects in insulin action	Caused by specific gene mutations. Clinical manifestations require different treatment. Clinical manifestations may occur in the neonatal period, others by early adulthood. Caused by specific gene mutations. Features of severe insulin resistance without obesity. Diabetes develops when β-cells do not compensate for insulin resistance.
Diseases of the exocrine pancreas	Injury to the pancreas, caused by trauma, tumor, inflammation, etc., or, for example, pancreatitis, neoplasia, or cystic fibrosis. Various conditions result in hyperglycemia.
Endocrine disorders	Occurs in diseases with excess secretion of hormones (e.g., growth hormone, cortisol, glucagon, epinephrine) that antagonize insulin action.
Drug or chemical induced	Medicines and chemicals can impair insulin secretion or action and destroy β-cells. Examples include glucocorticoids, thyroid hormone, thiazides, and alpha- and beta-adrenergic agonists.
Infection-related diabetes	Some viruses have been associated with diabetes, including congenital rubella, coxsackie B, cytomegalovirus, adenovirus, and mumps.
Uncommon specific forms of immune-mediated diabetes	Associated with rare immune-mediated diseases.
Other genetic syndromes sometimes associated with diabetes	Many genetic disorders and chromosomal abnormalities increase the risk of diabetes: • Genetic syndromes associated with severe early-onset obesity • Chromosomal abnormalities of Down syndrome, Klinefelter's syndrome, and Turner's syndrome • Neurological disorders, particularly Friedreich's ataxia, Huntington's chorea, and myotonic dystrophy
Unclassified diabetes	Diabetes that does not clearly fit into other categories. Used temporarily when there is not a clear diagnostic category at time of diagnosis.

GAD, Glutamic acid decarboxylase.

Adapted from World Health Organization [2019]. Classification of Diabetes Mellitus 2019. ISBN: 978-92-4-151570-2.

<table>
<tr><td>TABLE 38.3</td><td colspan="4">**Classification and Diagnostic Criteria**</td></tr>
<tr><td></td><td>**Stage 1**</td><td>**Stage 2**</td><td>**Stage 3**</td></tr>
<tr><td>Characteristics</td><td>Autoimmunity
Normoglycemia
Presymptomatic</td><td>Autoimmunity
Dysglycemia
Presymptomatic
Multiple autoantibodies</td><td>New-onset hyperglycemia
Symptomatic
Clinical symptoms</td></tr>
<tr><td>Diagnostic Criteria</td><td>Multiple autoantibodies
No IGT or IFG</td><td>Dysglycemia: IFG and/or IG
FPG 100–125 mg/dL (5.6–6.9 mmol/L)
2-h PG 144–199 mg/dL (7.8–11.0 mmol/L)
HbA1c 5.7–6.4% (39–47 mmol/mol) or ≥10% increase in HbA1c</td><td>Diabetes by standard criteria</td></tr>
</table>

FPC, Fasting plasma glucose; *HbA1c*, hemoglobin A1c; *IFG*, impaired fasting glucose; *IGT*, impaired glucose tolerance; *IG*, impaired glycemia ; *PG*, plasma glucose. From American Diabetes Association (2021). Standards of Medical Care in Diabetes—2021. *Diabetes Care,* 44(Suppl. 1). https://care.diabetesjournals.org/content/44/Supplement_1

• BOX 38.1 Causes and Risk Factors Associated With Type 2 Diabetes Mellitus

- Overweight/obesity
- Increased abdominal body fat
- Illness, infection, or the use of certain drugs
- Increasing age
- Lack of physical activity
- History of gestational diabetes
- Comorbid diseases such as hypertension or dyslipidemia
- Genetic predisposition
- Certain race/ethnicity groups

Data from American Diabetes Association. (n. d.). *Diabetes risk overview.* https://www.diabetes.org/diabetes-risk; and Centers for Disease Control and Prevention (2021, September 20). *Diabetes risk factors.* https://www.cdc.gov/diabetes/basics/risk-factors.html.

---

physiologic insulin replacement. The course of action of the various insulins and insulin analogs varies considerably in different individuals or even within the same individual. The characteristics of activity (time of onset, time to peak, and duration) also vary among the different products available. The rate of insulin absorption or onset of action is known to be affected by the site of injection, exercise, and other variables.

PRACTICE PEARLS

Insulin Formulations

There are several different formulations of insulin with varying durations of action depending on the patient's needs. Insulin comes in rapid-, short- intermediate-, and long-acting formulations. Insulin also comes in vials and prefilled pens. There are also premixed insulin products containing two different formulations of insulin or insulin with a glucagon-like peptide-1 (GLP-1) receptor agonist product. Table 38.5 provides an overview of the characteristics and duration of action of the different formulations.

Insulin Glargine

Pharmacokinetics. Endogenous insulin distributes widely throughout the body. Peripheral tissues inactivate a small portion, but the liver and kidneys metabolize most of the insulin. Insulin glargine is a long-acting insulin that is metabolized at the carboxyl terminus of the β chain with formation of two active metabolites: M1 (21A-Gly-insulin) and M2 (21A-Gly-des-30B-Thr-insulin). Insulin is filtered and reabsorbed by the kidneys. The onset of glucose-lowering activity is 1.5 hours. The duration of action for insulin glargine is 24 hours, with a constant concentration/time profile and no pronounced peak effect.

Indications. Insulin glargine is indicated for the treatment of T1DM and transient neonatal DM. It is also indicated for the treatment of T2DM inadequately managed by diet, exercise, and oral hypoglycemics, and for the treatment of new-onset T2DM in overweight children and adolescents.

Adverse Effects. Hypoglycemia is the most common adverse reaction. The incidence of hypoglycemia varies, with severe hypoglycemia occurring less frequently. Weight gain may occur with insulin therapy, due to the effects of insulin and the decrease in glucosuria. Hypokalemia may be possible, as insulin facilitates the uptake of potassium intracellularly. Long-term use of insulin causes *lipodystrophy*, which is the accumulation of subcutaneous fat around an injection site that has been used repeatedly. *Lipoatrophy*, which is the breakdown of adipose tissue at the injection site, may occur at a site that has repeated injections.

Contraindications. Insulin glargine is contraindicated in patients with hypersensitivity to insulin glargine or its components and during episodes of hypoglycemia.

Monitoring. Patients should have their blood glucose checked regularly and glycosylated hemoglobin A1c (HbA1c) checked routinely. Due to the risk of hypoglycemia, divide into two doses if the daily dose exceeds 100 units.

TABLE
38.4 **Drug-Specific and Patient-Specific Considerations in Pharmacologic Therapies**

Medication	Efficacy	Risk of Hypoglycemia	Weight Change	Formulation	Renal Considerations
Metformin	High	No	Neutral (potential for modest loss)	Oral	Contraindicated with eGFR <30 mL/min/1.73 m²
SGLT2 Inhibitors	Intermediate	No	Loss	Oral	Renal dose adjustment required
GLP-1 RAs	High	No	Loss	Subcutaneous; oral (semaglutide)	Renal dose adjustment required (exenatide, lixisenatide)
DPP-4 Inhibitors	Intermediate	No	Neutral	Oral	Renal dose adjustment required (sitagliptin, saxagliptin, alogliptin); can be used in renal impairment

No dose adjustment required for linagliptin |
Thiazolidinediones	High	No	Gain	Oral	No dose adjustment required
Sulfonylureas (second generation)	High	Yes	Gain	Oral	Glyburide: not recommended
Insulin	Highest	Yes	Gain	Subcutaneous	Lower doses required with a decrease in eGFR; titrate per clinical response

DPP-4, Dipeptidyl peptidase-4; *eGFR*, estimated glomerular filtration rate; *GLP-1 RAs*, glucagon-like-peptide receptor agonists; *SGLT2*, sodium-glucose cotransporter 2.
Adapted from American Diabetes Assocation: 9. Pharmacologic approaches to glycemic treatment: Standards of medical care in diabetes—2020. *Diabetes Care* 43[Suppl. 1], S98–S110. https://doi.org/10.2337/dc20-S009.

TABLE
38.5 **Insulin Product Characteristics and Duration of Action**

Insulins	Compounds	Onset	Peak	Duration
Rapid Acting	Lispro	5–15 min	30–90 min	3–4 hr
	Glulisine	5–15 min	1–3 hr	3–5 hr
	Aspart	5–15 min	30–90 min	3–4 hr
	Inhaled insulin[a]	~12 min	35–55 min	1.5–4.5 hr
Short Acting	Human regular	30–60 min	2–4 hr	6–8 hr
Intermediate Acting	Human NPH	2–4 hr	6–10 hr	10–16 hr
Concentrated Human Regular Insulin	U-500 human regular insulin	15–30 min	4–8 hr	13–24 hr
Long Acting	Glargine	2 hr	No peak	20–24 hr
	Detemir	1 hr	No peak	6–24 hr
	Degludec	1 hr	~12 hr	24–36 hr
Premixed Insulin Products	NPH/regular 70/30	30 min	2–12 hr	Up to 24 hr
	Lispro 50/50	15–30 min	0.8–4.8 hr	12–24 hr
	Lispro 75/25	15–30 min	1–6.5 hr	12–24 hr
	Aspart 70/30	10–20 min	1–4 hr	18–24 hr
Premixed Insulin/GLP-1 RA Products	Glargine/Lixisenatide	Refer to individual agents		
	Degludec/Liraglutide	Refer to individual agents		

[a]Powder formulation.
GLP-1 RA, Glucagon-like-peptide receptor agonist; *NPH*, neutral protamine HEgedorn.

Noninsulin Oral Glucose-Lowering Agents

Noninsulin oral agents offer improved glycemic control for patients with T2DM when lifestyle modifications do not provide optimal control. These agents may be used as monotherapy or in combination. Table 38.6 and Table 38.7 provide an overview of these noninsulin oral glucose-lowering agents.

Biguanides

Biguanides primarily decrease hepatic glucose production. They also have minor effects on insulin sensitivity in both the liver and peripheral tissues. They have no direct effect on the pancreas and therefore do not enhance insulin secretion. Biguanides have been shown to decrease triglycerides and low-density lipoproteins (LDLs) and increase high-density lipoproteins (HDLs). Metformin is an oral biguanide and is a first-line treatment for T2DM. Metformin was chosen as the initial medication therapy due to its efficacy, safety, and cost.

Metformin

Pharmacokinetics. Metformin is administered orally. The medication is distributed rapidly into the peripheral body tissues and fluids. The highest concentrations are found in the gastrointestinal (GI) tract with lower concentrations in the kidneys, liver, and salivary glands. Metformin is not metabolized by the liver and is excreted by the kidneys, largely unchanged, through the active tubular process. The average elimination half-life in the plasma is 6.2 hours in patients with normal renal function. Metformin is distributed and accumulates in red blood cells, which leads to a longer elimination half-life in blood (17.6 hours).

Indications. Metformin is indicated for the treatment of T2DM as monotherapy or in combination with other antidiabetic agents.

Adverse Effects. The most common side effects experienced by patients are GI effects. In clinical trials, diarrhea was experienced by 53.2% of patients receiving immediate-release metformin. Extended-release formulations have been reported to have a lower incidence of diarrhea (roughly 9.6%). Nausea and vomiting have been reported in 6.5% to 25.5% of patients, with lower incidences reported in extended-release products. Other GI effects include flatulence, indigestion or dyspepsia, abdominal pain or discomfort, anorexia, dysgeusia, and change in stool appearance. Frequent side effects tend to decline with continued use and can be minimized by using lower doses or extended-release formulations.

The risk of hypoglycemia is not common and more likely reported when metformin is used with other antidiabetic agents. Metformin has been reported to decrease the absorption of vitamin B_{12}, possibly due to interference of B_{12} absorption from B_{12}-intrinsic factor complex. It has very rarely been associated with anemia and is rapidly reversible with discontinue of metformin and/or vitamin B_{12} supplementation. Mild weight loss occurs with metformin use and can be expected with almost any patient.

Contraindications. Metformin should not be used in patients with known metformin hypersensitivity. It should not be used for T1DM or to treat diabetic ketoacidosis (DKA). Metformin is contraindicated in patients with metabolic acidosis and should not be used in patients with lactic acidosis. Metformin is contraindicated in patients with an eGFR below 30 mL/min/1.73m². Metformin should be discontinued at the time of or before receiving radiographic contrast in patients with an estimated glomerular filtration rate (eGFR) between 30 and 60 mL/min/1.73 m²; in patients with hepatic disease, alcoholism, or heart failure; or in patients who will be receiving intra-arterial iodinated contrast. Mannitol may be given post-procedure, and patients' renal function should be closely monitored prior to restarting metformin.

Monitoring. Blood glucose, complete blood count (CBC), HbA1c, liver function tests (LFTs), and serum creatinine/blood urea nitrogen (BUN) should be monitored while the patient is taking metformin.

SGLT2 Inhibitors

Sodium-glucose cotransporter 2 (SGLT2) inhibitors work by inhibiting the SGLT2 in the proximal renal tubules, reducing reabsorption of filtered glucose from the tubular lumen, and lowering the renal threshold for glucose. SGLT2 is expressed in the proximal renal tubules. SGLT2 is the main site of filtered glucose reabsorption; reduction of filtered glucose reabsorption and lowering of the renal threshold for glucose results in increased urinary excretion of glucose, thereby reducing plasma glucose concentrations. SGLT2 inhibitors are reported to reduce HbA1c by 0.4% to 1.16% from baseline over study durations ranging from 12 to 78 weeks.

SGLT2 inhibitor-induced glycosuria results in a daily caloric deficit of 250 to 450 kcal, resulting in a reported 2- to 3-kg weight loss over 12 weeks of therapy. The weight loss has been shown to plateau around 6 months, with a loss of approximately 3 kg maintained long term. SLGT2 inhibitors also reduce sodium reabsorption and increase sodium delivery to the distal tubules, which may decrease cardiac preload/afterload and down-regulate sympathetic activity as well as reduce both systolic and diastolic blood pressure.

SGLT2 inhibitors are generally recommended as second- and third-line therapy for T2DM. They have minimal risk of hypoglycemia and have been found to have cardiorenal

TABLE 38.6 Noninsulin Oral Glucose-Lowering Agents

Category/Medication	Indication	Dosage	Considerations and Monitoring
Biguanides			
Metformin	Diabetes mellitus, type 2 as monotherapy or in combination	*Immediate release:* 500 mg twice daily or 850 mg once daily. *Extended release:* 500 mg once daily; increase daily dose by 500 mg/week as needed to maximum dosage of 2000 mg once daily.	BBW regarding risk of lactic acidosis.
SGLT2 Inhibitors			
Dapagliflozin	Diabetes mellitus, type 2	5 mg once daily; may increase to 10 mg once daily.	Adjust dose for renal impairment. Contraindicated in ESKD or on dialysis.
Empagliflozin	Diabetes mellitus, type 2	10 mg once daily; may increase to 25 mg once daily.	Adjust dose for renal impairment. Contraindicated in ESKD or on dialysis.
Canagliflozin	Diabetes mellitus, type 2	100 mg once daily; may increase to 300 mg once daily.	Adjust dose for renal impairment. Contraindicated in ESKD or on dialysis. BBW regarding approximately twofold increase in lower limb amputations.
Ertugliflozin	Diabetes mellitus, type 2	5 mg once daily; may increase to 15 mg once daily.	Adjust dose for renal impairment. Contraindicated in ESKD or on dialysis.
DPP-4 Inhibitors			
Alogliptin	Diabetes mellitus, type 2	25 mg once daily.	Requires caution in hepatic impairment, but no dosage adjustments are necessary.
Saxagliptin	Diabetes mellitus, type 2	2.5–5 mg once daily.	
Linagliptin	Diabetes mellitus, type 2	5 mg once daily.	Only agent in this class that does not require renal dosage adjustments.
Sitagliptin	Diabetes mellitus, type 2	100 mg once daily.	
Sulfonylureas (Second Generation)			
Glimepiride	Diabetes mellitus, type 2	1–8 mg once daily.	
Glipizide	Diabetes mellitus, type 2	2.5–40 mg/day.	Preferred sulfonylurea in renal insufficiency.
Glyburide	Diabetes mellitus, type 2	1.25–20 mg/day.	Associated with higher incidence of hypoglycemia. Longer-duration sulfonylurea is not recommended for use in older adults.
Thiazolidinediones			
Pioglitazone	Diabetes mellitus, type 2	15–45 mg once daily.	
Rosiglitazone	Diabetes mellitus, type 2	4–8 mg/day once daily or in 2 divided doses.	

BBW, Black box warning; *CV,* cardiovascular; *DPP-4,* dipeptidyl peptidase-4; *ESKD,* end-stage kidney disease; *GI,* gastrointestinal; *HF,* heart failure; *MACE,* major adverse cardiovascular events; *SGLT2,* sodium-glucose cotransporter 2; *T2DM,* type 2 diabetes mellitus.

TABLE 38.7	Combination Oral Products
Medications	**Brand**
Sitagliptin	Januvia
Sitagliptin and metformin	Janumet, Janumet XR
Sitagliptin and ertugliflozin	Steglujan
Linagliptin	Tradjenta
Linagliptin and empagliflozin	Glyxambi
Linagliptin and metformin	Jentadueto, Jentadueto XR
Dapagliflozin and metformin	Xigduo XR
Dapagliflozin and saxagliptin	QTERN
Glyburide and metformin	Glucovance
Repaglinide and metformin	
Empagliflozin and metformin	Synjardy, Synjardy XR
Saxagliptin and metformin	Kombiglyze XR
Alogliptin and metformin	Kazano
Canagliflozin and metformin	Invokamet, Invokamet XR
Glipizide and metformin	
Pioglitazone and metformin	Actoplus MET
Ertugliflozin and metformin	Segluromet
Dapagliflozin, saxagliptin, and metformin	Qternmet XR
Empagliflozin, linagliptin, and metformin	Trijardy XR

protective effects, such as reduction in cardiovascular death, nonfatal myocardial infarction, nonfatal stroke, cardiovascular mortality, hospitalization for heart failure, need for renal-replacement therapy, renal disease-related death, and albuminuria. All agents in this class require dose adjustment in renal impairment. All agents are contraindicated in patients with end-stage renal disease or on dialysis. No dose adjustments are required for mild to moderate hepatic impairment, but it is worth noting that canagliflozin, dapagliflozin, and ertugliflozin have not been studied in severe hepatic impairment.

Dapagliflozin

Pharmacokinetics. Dapagliflozin is primarily metabolized by UGT1A9 to an inactive metabolite (dapagliflozin 3-O-glucuronide). The half-life of dapagliflozin is approximately 12.9 hours, with a peak plasma time of 2 hours. It is excreted through the urine and feces. Patients with mild, moderate, or severe renal impairment have higher systemic exposure compared to patients with normal renal function. In patients with severe hepatic impairment, mean

maximum serum concentration (Cmax) and area under the curve (AUC) were increased up to 40% and 67%, respectively.

Indications. Dapagliflozin is used primarily as an adjunct to diet and exercise to improve glycemic control in adults with T2DM, and reduce the risk of hospitalization for heart failure in patients with T2DM and established cardiovascular disease or multiple cardiovascular risk factors.

Adverse Effects. The major adverse reaction reported in clinical trials was the incidence of genitourinary fungal infections and urinary tract infections (UTIs), possibly due to the mechanism of the drug. Other adverse reactions included the risk of hypoglycemia when combined with insulin or insulin secretagogue. This was not seen in clinical trials of dapagliflozin monotherapy. Dapagliflozin results in osmotic diuresis, which may lead to reductions in intravascular volume. Adverse reactions related to this include hypotension, orthostatic hypotension, dehydration, and hypovolemia.

Contraindications. Dapagliflozin is contraindicated in patients with a known hypersensitivity reaction to dapagliflozin. Dapagliflozin is not indicated for the treatment of T1DM or for the treatment of DKA. Dapagliflozin is contraindicated in patients with renal failure or severe renal impairment. Estimated glomerular filtration rate should be assessed prior to initiation of treatment and periodically afterward.

Monitoring. Renal function should be assessed prior to initiation of therapy and periodically thereafter. HbA1c should be assessed twice yearly in patients who have stable glycemic control and are meeting treatment goals, or quarterly in patients not meeting treatment goals or with therapy changes. Due to the natriuretic effects of the medication, volume status should be monitored.

Empagliflozin

Pharmacokinetics. Empagliflozin is administered orally. It is approximately 86.2% protein bound. The primary route of metabolism is glucuronidation by the uridine 5'-disphospho-glucuronosyltransferases UGT2B7, UGT1A3, UGT1A8, and UGT1A9. The elimination half-life is estimated at 12.4 hours. The medication is excreted in the feces and urine as mostly unchanged parent drug.

Indications. Empagliflozin is indicated for the treatment of T2DM as an adjunct to diet and exercise to improve glycemic control. It also reduces the risk of cardiovascular mortality in adults with T2DM and established cardiovascular disease.

Adverse Effects. Empagliflozin can increase hematocrit. It can also increase the risk of hypoglycemia when combined with insulin or insulin secretagogue. Hyperlipidemia may occur and has been reported. Arthralgia was reported in clinical trials. Empagliflozin results in osmotic diuresis, which may lead to intravascular volume contraction and volume depletion. There is a risk of UTI, and patients with a history of chronic or recurrent UTI were more likely to experience a UTI. Fatal cases of DKA have been reported in patients receiving empagliflozin. Renal-related adverse reactions may occur, particularly in patients with moderate renal impairment.

Contraindications. Contraindications to empagliflozin are similar to those for dapagliflozin. Empagliflozin is contraindicated in patients with known hypersensitivity to empagliflozin.

Monitoring. Renal function should be assessed prior to initiation of therapy and periodically thereafter. HbA1c should be assessed twice yearly in patients who have stable glycemic control and are meeting treatment goals, or quarterly in patients not meeting treatment goals or with therapy changes. Due to the natriuretic effects of the medication, volume status should be monitored (Box 38.2).

DPP-4 Inhibitors

Dipeptidyl peptidase-4 (DPP-4) inhibitors potentiate the effects of the incretin hormones glucagon-like-peptide (GLP-1) and glucose-dependent insulinotropic peptide (GIP) by inhibiting their breakdown by DPP-4. When blood glucose concentrations are normal or elevated, GLP-1 and GIP increase insulin synthesis and release from pancreatic β-cells. GLP-1 also slows gastric emptying time and lowers glucagon secretion from pancreatic α-cells, leading to reduced hepatic glucose production. By increasing concentrations of GLP-1 and GIP, DPP-4 inhibitors reduce fasting and postprandial glucose concentrations in a glucose-dependent manner.

The first DPP-4 inhibitor, sitagliptin, was approved by the U.S. Food and Drug Administration (FDA) in October 2006 as a once-daily oral medication. It can be used as monotherapy or combined with metformin or a thiazolidinedione. It reduces fasting and postprandial hyperglycemia in patients with T2DM and does not cause weight gain or hypoglycemia. The different DPP-4 inhibitors are distinctive in their metabolism (saxagliptin is metabolized in the liver and sitagliptin is not, linagliptin and alogliptin are not extensively metabolized), excretion, recommended dosage, and daily dosage required for effective treatment. They are similar in efficacy in lowering HbA1c levels, safety profile, and patient tolerance (Dicker, 2011). DPP-4 inhibitors have been shown to reduce HbA1c at 24 weeks by 0.5% to 0.7% when compared to placebo. They are, in general, recommended as second- or third-line therapy. Because of their favorable efficacy/safety profile, they are well suited for

---

• BOX 38.2   Cardiac Benefits and Adverse Effects of SGLT2 Inhibitors

SGLT2 inhibitors carry additional beneficial cardiorenal effects for patients with T2DM. Although the exact mechanism is unknown, it is believed to be related to glycosuria and natriuresis. These effects lead to uricosuria and a reduction in plasma uric acid and plasma volume, lowering of cardiac preload, and reduced arterial pressure and stiffness, possibly resulting in afterload reduction. Despite these benefits, SGLT2 inhibitors carry risks not seen with other antidiabetic agents, such as increased risk for severe urinary tract infections, intravascular volume contraction, risk of diabetic ketoacidosis, and association with Fournier's gangrene.

---

older adults, patients with renal or hepatic impairment, and those at risk for hypoglycemia.

Sitagliptin

Pharmacokinetics. Sitagliptin is administered orally and is not highly protein bound (38%). Metabolism is a minor pathway of elimination, with approximately 16% of the dose excreted as metabolites that do not contribute significantly to its activity. It is metabolized by cytochrome (CYP) 3A4 and CYP 2C8. Elimination occurs primarily through renal excretion and involves active tubular secretion, with approximately 79% of the dose excreted unchanged in the urine. Sitagliptin is a substrate for human organic anion transporter-3 (hOAT-3) and P-glycoprotein (P-gp) but does not inhibit P-gp mediated transport. Based on this, it is unlikely to cause interaction with other drugs that utilize these pathways. Clinical data also suggest that it is not susceptible to clinically meaningful pharmacokinetic interaction by co-administered medications. Due to its renal excretion, the dose does need to be adjusted for renal impairment.

Indications. Sitagliptin is indicated for the treatment of T2DM in combination with diet and exercise.

Adverse Effects. In clinical trials, the overall incidence of adverse reaction in patients taking sitagliptin was similar to that reported with placebo. Discontinuation rates were also similar between both groups. The most commonly reported adverse reaction was nasopharyngitis. During postmarketing surveillance, serious allergic reactions have been reported and have typically occurred within 3 months of initiation.

Contraindications. Sitagliptin is contraindicated in patients with known sitagliptin hypersensitivity. A severe hypersensitivity risk has been reported during the first 3 months of therapy. Sitagliptin should not be used in patients with T1DM or for the treatment of DKA.

Monitoring. During the use of sitagliptin, blood glucose, HbA1c, and serum creatinine and BUN should be monitored.

Linagliptin

Pharmacokinetics. Linagliptin is administered orally. Protein binding is concentration dependent. The effective half-life is 12 hours. Metabolism is a minor pathway of elimination and a small fraction is metabolized to an inactive metabolite, with more than 90% of the drug excreted unchanged. Eighty-five percent (85%) of the dose is excreted via the enterohepatic system (80%) or urine (5%) within 4 days of dosing. Due to its pharmacokinetics, it is the only medication in the class that does not require dose adjustment for renal impairment.

Indications. Linagliptin is indicated for the treatment of T2DM in combination with diet and exercise.

Adverse Effects. Adverse effects are similar to sitagliptin. In clinical trials, myalgia was reported but the incidence was not noted. During postmarketing surveillance, rhabdomyolysis has also been reported.

Contraindications. Linagliptin carries the same contraindications as the other agents in this medication class.

Monitoring. During the use of sitagliptin, blood glucose, HbA1c, serum creatinine, and BUN should be monitored.

Sulfonylureas (Second Generation)

Sulfonylureas enhance insulin secretion primarily by binding to sulfonylurea receptor 1 (SUR 1) on β-cells. This causes a decrease in potassium permeability and membrane depolarization. The subsequent increase in intracellular calcium ions causes exocytosis of insulin from secretory granules. Other results include suppression of hepatic glucose production through entry of insulin into the portal vein and increased muscle glucose uptake via elevated insulin levels.

The efficacy of sulfonylurea is dependent on β-cell functionality, which decreases with the progression of T2DM. The second-generation agents are more potent and have a better safety profile than first-generation sulfonylureas. The sulfonylureas have equivalent efficacy and lower HbA1c by 1% to 2%, but they may differ in their duration of action, potency, and propensity to cause hypoglycemia. Glyburide has a higher incidence of hypoglycemia compared to other sulfonylureas, especially in older adults and in patients with renal impairment. Sulfonylureas can cause minor weight gain.

Glipizide

Pharmacokinetics. Glipizide is administered orally and is rapidly and completely absorbed from the GI tract. First-pass metabolism is not significant. Glipizide is extensively metabolized to inactive metabolites in the liver. Approximately 90% of the dose is excreted as biotransformation products and less than 10% is excreted in the urine and feces. The half-life ranges from 2 to 5 hours. Glipizide is a CYP 2C9 substrate; therefore CYP 2C9 inhibitors or inducers may affect medication exposure.

Indications. Glipizide is indicated for the treatment of T2DM as an adjunct to diet and exercise to improve glycemic control.

Adverse Effects. Sulfonylureas are generally well tolerated. Hypoglycemia is the most common side effect. Although not frequently observed in clinical trials, the incidence is much higher in clinical practice. Hypoglycemia may be a result of excessive dosing but can also be aggravated by other factors such as alcohol use or interfering medications (e.g., β-blockers). Many of the GI adverse effects to glipizide are dose related and transient. The most frequently reported GI-related effects with immediate-release glipizide include nausea, diarrhea, constipation, and dyspepsia. Common GI side effects with glipizide XL include nausea, dyspepsia, constipation, and vomiting. These GI symptoms may subside by reducing the dose or dividing the daily dose.

Sulfonylureas may cause allergic and nonallergic dermatologic reactions. Allergic skin reactions include erythema, rash eruptions, urticaria, and eczema. Dizziness, drowsiness, and headache have been reported in about 2% of patients treated with glipizide immediate-release formulations. In patients taking glipizide XL, there have been reports of headache, dizziness, nervousness, and tremor. Some of these more common neurologic effects may be related to

low blood sugar, are usually transient, and seldom require discontinuation of the medication.

Contraindications. Glipizide is contraindicated in patients with a hypersensitivity to glipizide, sulfonamide derivatives, or any component of the formulation, patients with T1DM, and for the treatment of DKA.

Monitoring. Patients taking glipizide should have their blood glucose, glucose-6-phosphate dehydrogenase (G6PD) activity, and HbA1c monitored. Hemolytic reactions are possible with sulfonylureas but are not common. Treatment of patients with G6PD deficiency with sulfonylureas can lead to hemolysis and hemolytic anemia.

Thiazolidinediones

Thiazolidinediones (TZDs) increase sensitivity in the adipose tissue, skeletal muscle, and liver by improving control of glycemic utilization. This in turn reduces circulating insulin levels. Functioning β-cells are required for these medications to work. Specifically, these drugs are agonists for peroxisome proliferator-activated receptors-γ (PPAR-γ), which are found in adipose tissue, skeletal muscle, and the liver. Activation of PPAR-γ receptors regulates the insulin-responsive genes involved in the control of glucose production, transport, and utilization and facilitates the regulation of fatty acid metabolism.

TZDs produce similar glycemic control. Pioglitazone is a TZD associated with fewer negative changes in cholesterol profile as well as lower triglyceride and LDL levels when compared to rosiglitazone. When used as monotherapy, TZDs have shown a 0.5% to 1.4% reduction in HbA1c. The onset of glycemic reduction is delayed. In patients without high-risk or established cardiovascular disease, heart failure, or chronic kidney disease, TZDs are a therapeutic option that needs to be considered with the risk of medication-related side effects such as heart failure, edema, decreased bone mineral density, and weight gain. Weight gain can be dose related and is due to increased adipose tissue mass and fluid retention.

Rosiglitazone

Pharmacokinetics. Rosiglitazone is administered orally. Protein binding to albumin occurs at a rate of approximately 99.8%. The major route of metabolism includes N-demethylation and hydroxylation, followed by conjugation with sulfate and glucuronic acid. Metabolism is extensive, with no unchanged drug detected in the urine. Metabolites are active, but they have less activity than the parent compound and do not contribute to insulin-sensitizing activity. The half-life is about 3 to 4 hours.

Indications. Rosiglitazone is indicated for the treatment of T2DM as an adjunct to diet and exercise to improve glycemic control.

Adverse Effects. Adverse effects of the GI system have been reported and include abdominal pain, diarrhea, nausea, and vomiting. In clinical trials, peripheral edema was reported. Postmarketing reports include volume expansion. Rosiglitazone has been associated with new-onset or exacerbation of heart failure. It has also been reported to affect lipid panels and is associated with increases in total, LDL, and HDL cholesterol, and decreases in free fatty acids.

Contraindications. Rosiglitazone is contraindicated in patients with known rosiglitazone hypersensitivity. It is active only in the presence of insulin and should not be used for T1DM or for the treatment of DKA. Initiation of therapy is contraindicated in patients with New York Heart Association (NYHA) Class III or IV heart failure.

Monitoring. Patients on rosiglitazone should have their blood glucose and HbA1c monitored. In addition, LFTs and weight should be monitored. Although not observed in clinical trials, postmarketing experience has reported hepatitis, with elevated liver enzymes.

BLACK BOX WARNING!

Thiazolidinediones

Thiazolidinediones may cause or exacerbate congestive heart failure. Patients on these agents should be closely monitored for signs and symptoms of congestive heart failure (e.g., rapid weight gain, edema, dyspnea), particularly after initiation or dose increases. If heart failure develops, treat accordingly and consider dose reduction or discontinuation of thiazolidinediones. Thiazolidinediones are not recommended for use in any patients with symptomatic heart failure. Initiation of therapy is contraindicated in patients with NYHA Class III or IV heart failure.

Noninsulin Injectable Glucose Lowering Agents

Noninsulin injectable agents are a treatment option for T2DM patients who have not achieved glycemic control with noninsulin oral agents or for those who are unable to take the noninsulin oral agents. Noninsulin injectable agents may be used as monotherapy or in combination with noninsulin oral agents. Table 38.8 provides an overview of noninsulin injectable agents.

GLP-1 Receptor Agonists

Incretins are hormones that are released from the gut after ingestion of carbohydrates or fat; they often are found in low concentrations in persons with T2DM. The incretin that has received the most attention is GLP-1. Incretins stimulate insulin secretion in pancreatic β-cells that have been shown to restore both phases of insulin release. GLP-1 regulates glucose homeostasis via multiple complementary actions and along with other incretins is known to do the following:

- Stimulate glucose-dependent endogenous insulin secretion
- Inhibit endogenous glucagon secretion
- Suppress appetite and induce satiety
- Reduce rate of gastric emptying
- Protect β-cells from cytokine- and free fatty acid-mediated injury

GLP-1 receptor agonists bind and activate the GLP-1 receptor, enhancing insulin secretion, slowing gastric emptying, suppressing glucagon secretion, reducing food intake

by reducing appetite, and promoting β-cell proliferation. GLP-1 receptor agonists are generally recommended as second- or third-line therapy for T2DM. For patients with HbA1c levels above target despite dual/triple therapy with metformin and other antidiabetic medication, GLP-1 receptor agonists are the preferred injectable medication compared to insulin due to similar or even better efficacy in HbA1c reduction, reduced risk of hypoglycemia, and promotion of weight loss. The efficacy and safety of the medications in this class are similar, and medications differ by their frequency in administration. Some of the agents in this class do carry indications for proven cardiac benefits, with the strongest evidence for liraglutide, semaglutide, and dulaglutide.

GLP-1 receptor agonists are injectable agents; except for semaglutide, which is available as an injectable and oral agent. Exenatide and lixisenatide require dosage adjustments based on renal impairment, but none of the agents in this class requires any dosage adjustments for hepatic impairment.

Exenatide

Pharmacokinetics. Exenatide is given via subcutaneous administration. Exenatide is predominately eliminated by glomerular filtration. The half-life is 2.4 hours. Renal impairment can lead to accumulation of the medication due to reduced clearance.

Indications. Exenatide is indicated for the treatment of T2DM in combination with diet and exercise.

Adverse Effects. Adverse effects on the GI system are the most common. Nausea and vomiting are the most common reason for discontinuation. The effect is dose dependent and appears to decrease in frequency and severity over time. Other GI effects include diarrhea, gastroesophageal reflux, dyspepsia, anorexia, abdominal distention, constipation, and flatulence. Hypoglycemia has been reported in patients taking exenatide as monotherapy and also in patients on concomitant antidiabetic medications.

Contraindications. Exenatide is contraindicated in patients who have experienced exenatide hypersensitivity or hypersensitivity to any of its inactive ingredients. It is not to be used in patients with T1DM or for the treatment of DKA. Extended-release exenatide suspension is contraindicated in patients with a personal or family history of certain types of thyroid cancer.

Monitoring. Lab studies include serum glucose, HbA1c, renal function, and triglycerides. HbA1c should be checked two to four times yearly based on glycemic control and treatment goals. If the patient is not meeting treatment goals or maintaining stable glycemic levels, or if the treatment plan is modified, consider more frequent checks. Office visits should include monitoring body weight and signs and/or symptoms of pancreatitis or gallbladder disease.

Semaglutide
Pharmacokinetics. Semaglutide is the only GLP-1 receptor agonist that is administered subcutaneously or

TABLE 38.8	Noninsulin Injectable Glucose-Lowering Agents		
Category/Medication	Frequency	Duration	Considerations and Monitoring
GLP-1 Receptor Agonists			
Albiglutide	Once weekly	Long acting	
Exenatide	Twice daily	Short acting	Renal impairment.
Exenatide (extended release)	Once weekly	Long acting	Renal impairment.
Dulaglutide	Once weekly	Long acting	Indicated for treatment of T2DM and CV risk reduction. Indicated for reduction of CV mortality in T2DM patients with multiple CV disease risk factors.
Semaglutide	Once weekly	Long acting	Only agent in this class that is also available as a once-daily tablet. Indicated for treatment of T2DM and CV risk reduction. Renal impairment.
Liraglutide	Once daily	Short acting	Also carries FDA-approved indication for weight loss in patients with obesity. Indicated for treatment of T2DM and CV risk reduction.
Lixisenatide	Once daily	Short acting	
Amylin Mimetic			
Pramlintide	Prior to meals	Short acting	Requires careful selection of patient due to medication properties.

CV, Cardiovascular; *FDA,* U.S. Food and Drug Administration; *GLP-1,* glucagon-like-peptide; *T2DM,* type 2 diabetes mellitus.

orally. Following oral administration, the maximum concentration is reached within 1 hour. Following subcutaneous administration, the maximum concentration is reached in 3 to 5 days. Semaglutide is more than 99% bound to plasma albumin and undergoes proteolytic cleavage of the peptide backbone and sequential β-oxidation of the fatty acid side-chain. Excretion is through urine and feces. The elimination half-life is approximately 1 week. For subcutaneous administration, similar medication exposure is achieved regardless of administration in the abdomen, thigh, or upper arm. The absolute bioavailability for subcutaneous administration is 89%.

Indications. Semaglutide is indicated for the treatment of T2DM in combination with diet and exercise. It is also indicated for the reduction of cardiovascular mortality and cardiovascular events in T2DM patients who also have established cardiovascular disease.

Adverse Effects. Adverse events of the GI system are the most commonly reported adverse effects. In monotherapy trials with subcutaneous injection, severe hypoglycemia was not reported but symptomatic hypoglycemia did occur. Cholelithiasis was reported in placebo-controlled trials.

Contraindications. Semaglutide is contraindicated in patients who have experienced semaglutide hypersensitivity. It is not to be used in patients with T1DM or for the treatment of DKA. Semaglutide is contraindicated in patients with a personal or family history of certain types of thyroid cancer.

Monitoring. Blood glucose and HbA1c should be monitored while on semaglutide.

Amylin Mimetics

Pramlintide is an analog of amylin; it is an endogenous peptide that is secreted in conjunction with insulin by pancreatic β-cells. Pramlintide produces the same physiologic effects as are caused by amylin, but it is stable enough to be used as a medication. Amylin is known to do the following:
- Suppress glucagon production, especially in the postprandial state
- Reduce postprandial hepatic glucose production
- Delay gastric emptying time
- Centrally mediate induction of satiety
- Reduce postprandial glucose levels

Pramlintide

Pharmacokinetics. Pramlintide is administered via subcutaneous injection, with an absolute bioavailability of 30% to 40%. Pramlintide is not extensively bound to blood cells or albumin; approximately 40% of the medication is bound in plasma. The half-life is approximately 48 minutes and the therapeutic effects last approximately 3 hours. Pramlintide is extensively metabolized by the kidneys, with a biologically active metabolite that has a similar half-life to the parent compound.

Indications. Pramlintide is indicated for the treatment of T1DM and T2DM.

Adverse Effects. Nausea is the most commonly reported adverse effect, with a higher frequency reported in patients with T1DM. It is reported as mild to moderate, dose dependent, and decreasing in incidence over time. Other GI effects include vomiting, abdominal pain, and anorexia. Headache, fatigue, and dizziness have been reported but may be more related to hypoglycemia. Pramlintide does not cause hypoglycemia, but when used with insulin, the risk is increased.

Injection-site reactions have been reported postmarketing. These reactions are mild and typically resolve within a few days to 1 week. Pramlintide needs to be at room temperature before administration, and injection sites should be rotated to reduce potential injection-site reactions. Other adverse effects reported include cough, pharyngitis, arthralgia, and pancreatitis.

Contraindications. Pramlintide is contraindicated in patients with gastroparesis, as it slows down the rate of gastric emptying. It is also contraindicated in patients with hypoglycemia unawareness. Pramlintide is contraindicated in patients with a known pramlintide hypersensitivity or any of its components. The formulation contains metacresol, and there have been reports of localized reactions and general myalgias with its use.

Monitoring. Prior to initiation of therapy, current and most recent glucose monitoring data, history of insulin-induced hypoglycemia, current insulin regimen, and weight should be reviewed. During therapy, blood glucose and HbA1c should be monitored.

Prescriber Considerations for Diabetes Mellitus Medication Therapy

Clinical Practice Guidelines

PRACTICE PEARL

Clinical Practice Guidelines

- Standards of Medical Care in Diabetes—2021. American Diabetes Association. Available at https://doi.org/10.2337/dc21-Sint.
- Consensus Statement by the American Association of Clinical Endocrinologists and American College of Endocrinology (AACE/ACE) on the Comprehensive Type 2 Diabetes Management Algorithm – 2020 Executive Summary. Available at https://doi.org/10.4158/CS-2019-0472.
- 2019 Update to Management of Hyperglycaemia in Type 2 Diabetes, 2018. A Consensus Report by the American Diabetes Association (ADA) and the European Association for the Study of Diabetes (EASD). Available at https://doi.org/10.1007/s00125-019-05039-w.
- Recommendations for Managing Type 2 Diabetes in Primary Care, 2017. International Diabetes Federation. Available at https://www.idf.org/e-library/guidelines/128-idf-clinical-practice-recommendations-for-managing-type-2-diabetes-in-primary-care.html.

Note: This is not an exhaustive list of guidelines or practice statements. Please refer to additional resources for organizations of interest.

Every year, the ADA updates the clinical guidelines for glycemic management (ADA, 2021). Recommendations from the ADA's 2020 updates include implementation of the Chronic Care Model to improve the quality of diabetic care. The six core elements comprising this model are a proactive, team-based approach; self-management; decision support based on evidence and current guidelines; the use of clinical information systems; the development of community resources and policies; and quality-oriented health care systems. Baptista et al. (2016) recommend using an approach combining all six core elements for improved health outcomes.

Clinical Reasoning for Diabetes Mellitus Therapy

Consider the individual patient's health problem requiring diabetes mellitus therapy. It is important to correctly diagnose the type of diabetes and identify any comorbid conditions. Patients with indicators of high-risk or established cardiovascular disease, chronic kidney disease, or heart failure may require selective medication classes based on these characteristics. For patients without those indicators or comorbidities, considerations should be individualized based on compelling needs such as the need to minimize hypoglycemia, minimize weight loss or promote weight gain, and medication cost.

Determine the desired therapeutic outcome based on the degree of glycemic control needed for the patient. Control of blood glucose levels is important to prevent progression and further complications. Selection of a medication is based on previously mentioned factors and the results of periodic HbA1c levels. If the patient's HbA1c is above the goal, intensification of the medication regimen is needed.

Assess the selected agent for its appropriateness for an individual patient by considering the medication's side effects and the patient's age, race/ethnicity, comorbidities, and genetic factors. Primary care providers should consider a variety of factors prior to initiating therapy. Adults 65 years of age or older may benefit from less stringent HbA1c parameters, as well as frequent evaluations of HbA1c and fasting blood glucose levels to monitor glycemic control dependent on comorbidities or multimorbidities and side effects (ADA, 2020). HbA1c levels are higher in racial minorities than in non-Hispanic White patients with T2DM (Smalls et al., 2020). Mexican Americans had higher levels of HbA1c than those identifying as unspecified/mixed-race or non-Hispanic Black. Genetic variants related to T2DM are linked with metformin, TZDs, sulphonylureas, and DPP-4 inhibitors. A review of the literature suggests that although multiple genetic variants have been identified, the full impact of these variants on individualized therapy has not been fully established (Mannino et al., 2019).

Initiate the treatment plan with the selected medication by first providing adequate patient education to ensure the patient's understanding and promote full participation in the diabetes mellitus therapy. Promoting patient understanding begins with a clear, concise explanation of the diagnosis of hyperglycemia/diabetes. Patients must understand that management of their diabetes is a lifelong commitment. Managing diabetes requires learning new skills to manage medications, diet, and exercise. Health care providers should evaluate the patient's confidence and abilities in comparison to the level of care required (Chaudhury et al., 2017).

Ensure complete patient and family understanding about the medication prescribed for diabetes mellitus therapy using a variety of education strategies. Medication education should include the name, dose, and frequency; instruction on self-administration (oral or subcutaneous); potential side effects; and treatment goals. It is also important to include education on avoiding and managing hypoglycemia and hyperglycemia.

In addition to providing education on the medication regimen, health care providers should encourage diabetes education. Diabetes self-management education and support (DSMES) that is skills based, patient centered, and longitudinal may increase the likelihood of successful health outcomes. Topics covered in DSMES programs include understanding diabetes and diabetes treatment, healthy eating, physical activity, medication regimens, checking blood sugar, reducing risk from other health problems, and mental health concerns (CDC, 2018).

Conduct follow-up and monitoring of patient responses to diabetes mellitus therapy. Follow-up visits should begin with a review of the patient's understanding of diabetes and an interval medical history. Each visit should also include a review of medication-taking behaviors including a discussion of medication cost and access, medication side effects, an assessment of risk for complications including the incidence and severity of hypoglycemic events, laboratory evaluation of HbA1c and metabolic targets, diabetes self-management behaviors, nutrition, psychosocial health, and the need for referrals, immunizations, or other routine health maintenance screening (ADA, 2020).

Teaching Points for Diabetes Mellitus Therapy

Health Promotion Strategies

- Wear medical alert identification.
- Be alert for signs and symptoms of low blood sugar (hypoglycemia) or high blood sugar (hyperglycemia). See Box 38.3.
- Call your primary care provider or 9-1-1 or ask someone to call for you if you experience episodes of low or high blood sugar that do not respond to treatment.
- Check your blood sugar and keep a record to bring to your primary care provider. Follow instructions for managing low or high blood sugar levels.
- Always have 15 Gm of carbohydrates on hand in case your blood sugar drops. Examples include glucose tablets or oral glucose gel (follow the instructions on the package), hard candy, and 4 ounces of juice or soda (regular, not sugar free).
- Keep a record of when episodes of low or high blood sugar occur. Be sure to tell your primary care provider about the episodes.

• Box 38.3   Signs and Symptoms of Hypoglycemia and Hyperglycemia

Hypoglycemia

- Feeling shaky
- Being nervous or anxious
- Sweating, chills, and clamminess
- Irritability or impatience
- Confusion
- Fast heartbeat
- Feeling lightheaded or dizzy
- Hunger
- Nausea
- Color draining from the skin (pallor)
- Feeling sleepy
- Feeling weak or having no energy
- Blurred/impaired vision
- Tingling or numbness in the lips, tongue, or cheeks
- Headaches
- Coordination problems, clumsiness
- Nightmares or crying out during sleep
- Seizures

Hyperglycemia

- High blood sugar
- High levels of sugar in the urine
- Frequent urination
- Increased thirst

- Avoid driving or operating machinery until you know how you react to the medications or if you experience signs and symptoms of low or high blood sugar.
- Notify your primary care provider of changes in vision, signs of infection (fever, chills, pain), dizziness, seizures, pain or infection at injection sites, or a change in mood or behavior.
- If you can't afford your medications, tell your primary care provider immediately. Do not skip medications.
- Foot care is important. Check your feet daily for redness, pain, ingrown toenails, rash, or irritations. Notify your primary care provider of any changes to your feet.
- Complete all laboratory work and attend all appointments as instructed.

Patient Education for Medication Safety

- Tell your primary care provider of any allergies to drugs or components of any drug and report any side effects at drug injection sites.
- Use medications exactly as prescribed. If you miss a dose, call your primary care provider or follow previous instructions.
- Store medications as instructed and keep them away from children.
- Do not share your medications with others.

Application Questions for Discussion

1. What is the most common adverse effect of insulin glargine?
2. Which medication would be a poor choice for a 54-year-old male with diabetes and heart failure?
3. Which medications improve control of glycemic utilization by increasing sensitivity in the adipose tissue, skeletal muscle, and liver?

Selected Bibliography

American Diabetes Association (2018). Economic costs of diabetes in the U.S. in 2017. *Diabetes Care, 41*, 917–928. https://doi.org/10.2337/dci18-0007.

American Diabetes Association (2021). Standards of Medical Care in Diabetes—2021. *Diabetes Care, 44*(Suppl. 1). https://care.diabetesjournals.org/content/44/Supplement_1.

American Diabetes Association (2020). Standards of Medical Care in Diabetes—2020. *Diabetes Care, 43*(Suppl. 1), S1–S212. https://professional.diabetes.org/content-page/practice-guidelines-resources.

American Diabetes Association. (n. d.). *Diabetes risk overview.* https://www.diabetes.org/diabetes-risk.

Atkinson, M. A. (2012). The pathogenesis and natural history of type 1 diabetes. *Cold Spring Harbor Perspectives in Medicine, 2*(11), a007641. http://doi.org/10.1101/cshperspect.a007641.

Baptista, D. R., Wiens, A., Pontarolo, R., Regis, L., Reis, W. C. T., & Correr, C. J. (2016). The chronic care model for type 2 diabetes: A systematic review. *Diabetology & Metabolic Syndrome, 8*(7). https://doi.org/10.1186/s13098-015-0119-z.

Bommer, C., Sagalova, V., Heesemann, E., Manne-Goehler, J., Atun, R., Barnighausen, T., Davies, J., & Vollmer, S. (2018). Global economic burden of diabetes in adults: Projections from 2015 to 2030. *Diabetes Care, 41*, 963–970. https://doi.org/10.2337/dc17-1962.

Brashers, V. L., & Huether, S. E. (2019). Mechanisms of hormonal regulation. In K. L. McCance, & S. E. Huether (Eds.), *Pathophysiology. The Biologic Basis for Disease in Adults and Children* (8th ed.) (pp. 644–667). St. Louis: Elsevier.

Centers for Disease Control and Prevention. (CDC). (2018). *Self-management education: Learn more. Feel better.* Centers for Disease Control and Prevention, U.S. Department of Health & Human Services. Available at https://www.cdc.gov/learnmorefeelbetter/programs/diabetes.htm.

Centers for Disease Control and Prevention. (CDC). (2020). *National Diabetes Statistics Report, 2020.* Centers for Disease Control and Prevention, U.S. Department of Health & Human Services. Available at https://www.cdc.gov/diabetes/pdfs/data/statistics/national-diabetes-statistics-report.pdf.

Centers for Disease Control and Prevention (CDC). (2021). *Diabetes risk factors.* Centers for Disease Control and Prevention, U.S. Department of Health & Human Services. https://www.cdc.gov/diabetes/basics/risk-factors.html.

Chaudhury, A., Duvoor, C., Dendi, V. S. R., Kraleti, S., Chada, A., Ravilla, R., Marco, A., Shekhawat, N. S., Montales, M. T., Kuriakose, K., Sasapu, A., Beebe, A., Patil, N., Musham, C. K., Lohani, G. P., & Mirza, W. (2017). Clinical review of antidiabetic drugs: Implications for type 2 diabetes mellitus management. *Frontiers in Endocrinology, 8*(6). http://doi.org/10.3389/fendo.2017.00006.

Da Silva Xavier, G. (2018). The cells of the islets of Langerhans. *Journal of Clinical Medicine, 7*(3), 54. http://doi.org/10.3390/jcm7030054.

Dabelea, D., Stafford, J. M., Mayer-Davis, E. J., D'Agostino, R., Dolan, L., Imperatore, G., Linder, B., Lawrence, J. M., Marcovina, S. M., Mottl, A. K., Black, M. H., Pop-Busui, R., Saydah, S., Hamman, R. F., & Pihoker, C. (2017). Association of type 1 diabetes vs type 2 diabetes diagnosed during childhood and adolescence with complications during teenage years and young adulthood. *Journal of the American Medical Association, 317*(8), 825–835. https://doi.org/10.1001/jama.2017.0686.

Dicker, D. (2011). DDP-4 inhibitors: Impact on glycemic control and cardiovascular risk factors. *Diabetes Care, 34*(Suppl. 2), S276–S278.

Drivers, J., Mayer-Davis, E. J., Lawrence, J. M., Isom, S., Dabela, D., Dolan, L., Imperatore, G., Marcovina, S., Pettitt, D. J., Pihoker, C., Hamman, R. F., Saydah, S., & Wagenknecht, L. E. (2020). Trends in incidence of type 1 and type 2 diabetes among youths – selected counties and Indian reservations, United States, 2002–2015. *MMWR Morbidity and Mortality Weekly Report, 69*, 161–165. http://dx.doi.org/10.15585/mmwr.mm6906a3.

Garber, A. J., Handlesman, Y., Grunberger, G., Einhorn, D., Abrahamson, M. J., Barzilay, J. I., Blonde, L., Bush, M. A., DeFronzo, R. A., Garber, J. R., Garvey, W. T., Hirsch, I. B., Jellinger, P. S., McGill, J. B., Mechanick, J. I., Perreault, L., Rosenblit, P. D., Samson, S., & Umpierrez, G. E. (2020). Consensus statement by the American Association of Clinical Endocrinologists and American College of Endocrinology on the comprehensive type 2 diabetes management algorithm –2020 executive summary. *Endocrine Practice, 26*(1), 107–139. http://doi.org/10.4158/CS-2019-0472.

International Diabetes Federation (2017). *Recommendations for Managing Type 2 Diabetes in Primary Care, 2017.* Available at www.idf.org/managing-type2-diabetes.

Kochanek, K. D., Murphy, S. L., Xu, J. Q., & Arias, E. (2019). Deaths: Final data for 2017. *National Vital Statistics Reports, 68*(9), 1–77. Available at https://www.cdc.gov/nchs/data/nvsr/nvsr68/nvsr68_09-508.pdf.

Mann, E., & Bellin, MD. (2016). Secretion of insulin in response to diet and hormones. *Pancreapedia: Exocrine Pancreas Knowledge Base, 1.0. March 30, 2016.* American Pancreatic Association. http://doi.org/10.3998/panc.2016.3.

Mannino, G. C., Andreozzi, F., & Sesti, G. (2019). Pharmacogenetics of type 2 diabetes mellitus, the route toward tailored medicine. *Diabetes Metabolism Research and Reviews, 35*, e3109. https://doi.org/10.1002/dmrr.3109.

Pociot, F., & Lernmark, A. (2016). Genetic risk factors for type 1 diabetes. *The Lancet, 387*(10035), 2331–2339. http://doi.org/10.1016/S0140-6736(16)30582-7.

Ramachandran, A. (2014). Know the signs and symptoms of diabetes. *The Indian Journal of Medical Research, 140*(5), 579–581. Available at https://www.ncbi.nlm.nih.gov/pmc/articles/PMC4311308/.

Skyler, J. S., Bakris, G. L., Bonifacio, E., Darsow, T., Eckel, R. H., Groop, L., Groop, P-H., Handelsman, Y., Insel, R. A., Mathiew, C., McElvaine, A. T., Palmer, J. P., Puliese, A., Schatz, D. A., Sosenko, J. M., Wilding, J. P. H., & Ratner, R. E. (2017). Differentiation of diabetes by pathophysiology, natural history, and prognosis. *Diabetes, 66*, 241–255. http://doi.org/10.2337/db16-0806.

Smalls, B. L., Ritchwood, T. D., Bishu, K. G., & Egede, L. E. (2020). Racial/ethnic differences in glycemic control in older adults with type 2 diabetes: United States 2003–2014. *International Journal of Environmental Research and Public Health, 17*(3), 950. http://doi.org/10.3390/ijerph17030950.

World Health Organization (2016). *World Health Organization Global Report on Diabetes.* World Health Organization. Available at http://apps.who.int/iris/bitstream/10665/204871/1/9789241565257_eng.pdf?ua=1.

World Health Organization (2019). *Classification of diabetes mellitus.* World Health Organization. Available at https://apps.who.int/iris/handle/10665/325182.

39

Principles for Prescribing Antiinfective Medications in Primary Care

CONSTANCE G. VISOVSKY

Overview

In general, the prescribing of antiinfective medication, particularly antibacterial medication, has undergone great scrutiny over the past decade. Antibiotic resistance patterns are of particular concern as organism resistance rises and infections become untreatable because the pipeline for new antibiotics is slim (Centers for Disease Control and Prevention [CDC], 2018). It is important for the primary care practitioner to access the most recent clinical practice guidelines for the treatment of specific infections. Although there are prescribing guidelines, the primary care practitioner must consider the individual patient's disease and current illness, medical history, allergies, and risk factors, as well as consider the pharmacokinetics and pharmacodynamics of the medication, before creating a treatment plan. Selecting an antibiotic that will provide optimal treatment for infections, minimize adverse effects, and reduce the development of resistance is a critical first step. The emphasis in this unit is on the use of oral medications in treating conditions commonly seen in the primary care setting.

Relevant Physiology

The taxonomy of bacteria has changed with the advent of genome sequencing of organisms that contributes to new information about the genetics of bacteria. Currently, 40% of the strains of validly published species and subspecies have been sequenced (Garrity, 2016). Table 39.1 provides information on bacterial pathogens. Bacteria are small, single-celled organisms with a simple internal structure that lacks a nucleus but contains deoxyribonucleic acid (DNA) that floats freely or is in a twisted, thread-like mass. Bacterial cells are generally surrounded by two protective coverings: an outer cell wall and an inner cell membrane. Bacteria contain extensions that often cover the surface of the cell, known as *flagella* or *pili,* which help the bacteria move and attach to a host. The human body contains many bacteria, most of which are harmless and some of which are even helpful. A relatively small number of species cause disease. Fig. 39.1 shows an image of *Escherichia coli.*

Classification of Antiinfective Medications

Antiinfectives, especially antibiotics, vary widely in their ability to control or kill bacteria and other microbes. Broad-spectrum antibiotics are effective against a wide variety of bacteria, while narrow-spectrum antibiotics are effective against only a few types of bacteria.

Antiinfectives can be used to suppress the growth of or kill bacteria and other microbes. For example, some antiinfectives, such as the penicillins and cephalosporins, work to promote cell lysis of the bacteria by disrupting the bacterial cell wall. Sulfonamides work by inhibiting an enzyme needed to make folic acid. For bacteria to survive, a folic acid precursor known as para-aminobenzoic acid (PABA) must be taken up and converted into folic acid. If this process is disrupted, the bacteria die.

PRACTICE PEARLS

Mechanisms of Antiinfectives

- Inhibit cell wall synthesis
- Inhibit enzymes and metabolites
- Increase cell permeability
- Inhibit protein synthesis
- Inhibit synthesis of DNA and ribonucleic acid (RNA)
- Suppress viral replication

TABLE
39.1 **Important Pathogens**

Morphology	Aerobe vs. Anaerobe	Organism	Most Important Pathogen	Disease Caused
BACTERIA				
Gram Positive				
Cocci	Aerobe	Staphylococcus	S. aureus	Skin and soft tissue infective endocarditis Osteomyelitis, bacteremia, toxic shock syndrome
	Anaerobe	Streptococcus	S. pyogenes group A β-hemolytic (GABH)	Pharyngitis/rheumatic fever Impetigo Endocarditis
	Anaerobe	Enterococcus	E. faecalis	Wound, UTI, endocarditis
	Anaerobe	Pneumococcus	S. pneumoniae	Pneumonia Meningitis
Rods	Anaerobe	Bacillus	B. anthracis	Anthrax
		Actinomyces	A. israelii	Cervicofacial
			A. haemolyticum	Pharyngitis
	Aerobe	Corynebacterium	C. diphtheriae	Diphtheria
		Listeria		Listeriosis
	Anaerobe	Clostridium	L. monocytogenes	Gas gangrene
			C. perfringens	Enteritis
			C. difficile	Severe diarrhea, colitis
			C. tetani	Tetanus
			C. botulinum, Clostridium butyricum, Clostridium baratii	Botulism
Gram Negative				
Cocci	Aerobe	Neisseria	N. gonorrhoeae	Gonorrhea
			N. meningitidis	Meningitis
	Aerobe	Moraxella	M. catarrhalis	Otitis media, sinusitis, pneumonia
Bacilli	Aerobe	Pseudomonas	P. aeruginosa	Bacteremia
ENTEROBACTERIA				
Rod-shaped bacilli	Anaerobe	Escherichia	E. coli	Gastroenteritis
		Shigella	S. dysenteriae	Shigellosis dysentery
		Salmonella	S. typhi	Typhoid fever
			S. enteritidis	Gastroenteritis
	Anaerobe	Klebsiella	K. pneumoniae	UTI, various
		Proteus	P. mirabilis	UTI, various
			P. vulgaris	UTI, various
	Aerobe	Yersinia	Y. pestis	Plague
	Anaerobe	Enterobacter	E. cloacae	Nosocomial infections such as pneumonia, septicemia, UTI, wound infection, meningitis in newborns
		Serratia	S. marcescens	Pneumonia, UTI, bacteremia, biliary tract infection, wound infection, meningitis, endocarditis
		Citrobacter	C. freundii	UTI, wound infection, respiratory infection, meningitis, sepsis
		Morganella	M. morganii	Sepsis, abscess, chorioamnionitis, cellulitis
	Anaerobe	Vibrio	V. cholerae	Cholera
	Microaerophilic	Helicobacter	H. pylori	Gastritis, PUD

TABLE 39.1 **Important Pathogens—cont'd**

Morphology	Aerobe vs. Anaerobe	Organism	Most Important Pathogen	Disease Caused
Small bacilli	Aerobe	Haemophilus	H. influenzae	Sinusitis, otitis, bronchitis, pneumonia
	Aerobe	Bordetella	B. pertussis	Whooping cough
	Anaerobe	Pasteurella	P. tularensis	Tularemia
			P. multocida	Animal bite infections
	Microaerophilic	Campylobacter	C. jejuni	Gastroenteritis
	Aerobe	Gardnerella	G. vaginalis	Vaginitis
		Legionella	L. pneumophila	Legionnaire's pneumonia
	Aerobe	Nocardia	N. asteroides	Pulmonary endocarditis, systemic infection
	Anaerobe	Bacteroides	B. fragilis	Anaerobic peritoneal infection, intraabdominal infection, peritonitis, abscess
	Aerobe	Prevotella (formerly Bacteroides)	P. melaninogenica	URIs
Acid fast	Aerobe	Mycobacterium	M. tuberculosis	Tuberculosis
			M. avium	Bronchitis, etc
			M. leprae	Leprosy
Mycoplasma	Aerobe	Mycoplasma	M. pneumoniae	Atypical pneumonia
			M. hominis	Wound infection, abscess, arthritis, osteitis, peritonitis, pneumonia, meningitis, sepsis
		Ureaplasma	U. urealyticum	Infection of urinary tract and vagina; can be passed from mother to infant during birth
Spirochetes	Anaerobe	Treponema	T. pallidum	Syphilis
			T. pallidum sub	Yaws
	Anaerobe	Borrelia	B. burgdorferi	Lyme disease
Rickettsia	Aerobe	Rickettsia	R. rickettsii	Rocky Mountain spotted fever, typhus
PROTOZOA				
Flagellates, ciliates, sarcodina, and sporozoans	Anaerobe	Chlamydia	C. trachomatis	Lymphogranuloma venereum, urethritis, and cervicitis
	Aerobe		C. psittaci	Psittacosis
			C. pneumoniae	Pneumonia
	Anaerobe	Trichomonas	T. vaginalis	Trichomonas vaginitis
		Entamoeba	E. histolytica	Amebiasis colitis
		Cryptosporidium	C. parvum	Diarrhea
		Giardia	G. lamblia	Diarrhea
		Leishmania	Many species	Skin lesions
		Plasmodium	P. falciparum	Malaria
	Aerobe	Plasmodium	P. vivax	Malaria
			P. malariae	Malaria
	Anaerobe		P. ovale	Malaria
Intestinal coccidian	Anaerobe and aerobe	Toxoplasma	T. gondii	Toxoplasmosis

Continued

TABLE 39.1	Important Pathogens—cont'd			
Morphology	Aerobe vs. Anaerobe	Organism	Most Important Pathogen	Disease Caused
HELMINTHIC				
Invertebrates with elongated, flat or round worm bodies	Aerobe	Tapeworms, round-worms, and fluke infections	Trematode Cestode	Schistosomiasis
			Nematode	Anisakiasis
	Anaerobe	*Ascaris*	*A. lumbricoides*	Ascariasis Enterobiasis
	Aerobe	*Trichinella*	*T. spiralis*	Trichinosis

UTI, Urinary tract infection; *URI*, upper respiratory infection; *PUD*, peptic ulcer disease.

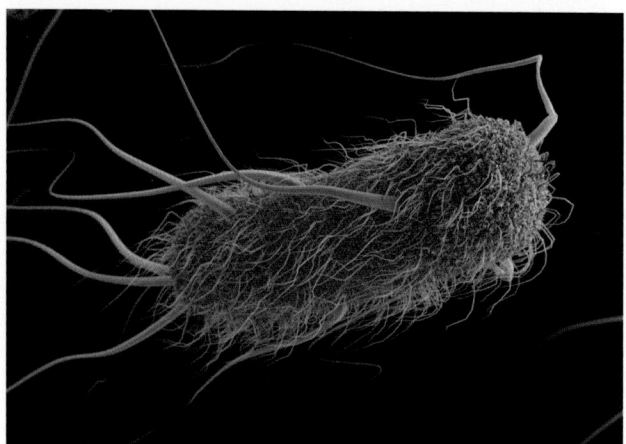

• **FIG. 39.1** A computer-generated image of *E. coli*. (Image credit: Alissa Eckert and Jennifer Oosthuizen, CDC)

Antiinfective Medication Prescribing Practices

Infections are among the most common reasons for primary care visits. Respiratory tract infections include acute upper respiratory infections (URIs), bronchitis, pneumonia, chronic sinusitis, acute pharyngitis, and otitis media. Other infections commonly seen in the primary care setting are urinary tract infections (UTIs), eye infections such as conjunctivitis, ear infections such as otitis media and externa, and skin infections such as cellulitis and impetigo.

Over the course of a year, approximately 4 million individuals receive care and services in a nursing home. Antibiotics are among the most prescribed medications in nursing homes, with 50% to 70% of residents receiving an antibiotic over the course of a year. Overall, antibiotic prescription rates for children have declined, from 75 million prescriptions in 2011 to about 64 million prescriptions in 2014. However, antibiotic prescription rates for adults have risen slightly, from about 192 million in 2011 to 198 million in 2014. Children younger than 2 years of age and adults age 65 or older receive the most antibiotic prescriptions.

In 2016 alone, more than 269 million prescriptions for oral antiinfective medications were written in the United States. Although the efficacy of antiinfectives in decreasing mortality and morbidity is unquestioned, the overuse and abuse of these products have led to drug resistance.

More difficult or detailed clinical problems will require the clinician to review additional anatomic, physiologic, or microbiologic texts before making treatment decisions.

Accurate identification of the causative organism is the most critical clinical decision. This is possible through simple laboratory tests, such as a Gram stain. Some organisms require more extensive testing that must be done in a commercial laboratory. Knowledge of which organisms are endemic in the community during a specific season and which organisms seem to have developed resistance to different drugs is also important for the primary care provider.

Patient Assessment

To prescribe an antiinfective, the first step is to take a thorough history of the patient's present illness, past medical and surgical history as appropriate, allergies, smoking habits, all medications the patient is taking, and previous antibiotic treatment. If the patient reports a previous allergic reaction, determining the type of reaction is necessary to distinguish a true hypersensitivity reaction from expected side effects. Inquire about recent travel, work history, and exposure to high-risk environments (e.g., college and military dormitories, child care centers, patient care facilities, ill family members).

The best practice is to confirm a diagnosis of bacterial infection before placing a patient on an antibiotic. It is important for patients and family members to understand and distinguish the differences between bacterial and viral infections, the latter which do not need treatment with an antibiotic.

At least 90% of URIs are caused by viruses. When treating infections, assess for the expected symptoms or signs that indicate a bacterial infection. Consider obtaining an appropriate culture and sensitivity test. If the patient has signs and symptoms that indicate *probable* bacterial infection, consider empirical treatment until culture results are available. The signs and symptoms that indicate bacterial infection are not always clear. Generally, signs and symptoms include fever (often higher than 101°F), lymphadenopathy, swelling, redness, and pain. The primary care provider must have a high index of suspicion for bacterial infection, order appropriate testing, and recognize the severity of a patient's illness when determining a treatment plan.

Some cardinal signs that indicate a serious bacterial infection include the following:

- *Loss of appetite:* When accompanied by fever, loss of appetite can signal the presence of a significant infection. Maintenance of appetite with fever is a reliable indicator of localized or limited infection.
- *Symptoms of dehydration:* Ask the patient to describe their fluid intake. Consider the potential for dehydration even in cases of minor illness. Inquire whether the patient reports dizziness when standing, an unsteady walk, orthostatic changes in blood pressure, urine concentration of 1.025 to 1.030, or dry mucous membranes. Pronounced changes in behavior or mental status may be observed in children or in older adults with serious infections.
- *Absence of fever:* Patients with diabetes or with immature or aging immune systems may have a serious infection but fail to mount a febrile response to infection, as the immune system may not release pyrogens. High or persistent fever in children or adults is often a sign of serious illness.

Although minor infections account for most visits to primary care practices, consider referral to a specialist for unusual symptoms or unusual responses to treatment. Infectious disease and pulmonary specialists are highly attuned to knowledge of community-acquired infections and their treatment, as well as to the more exotic presentations. Simple localized infection may progress to septic shock within hours, and the primary care provider must not discount the ominous symptoms of shaking chills and soaring temperatures or decreased temperature with changes in mental status that require emergency attention.

Identification of Gram-Positive vs. Gram-Negative Organisms

Identification of a bacterial organism as gram positive or gram negative helps the primary care provider make the critical decision of choosing an appropriate antiinfective that will be effective against the specific organism. A test called a *Gram stain* is used to identify bacteria by the composition of their cell walls, and was named for Hans Christian Gram, who developed the technique in 1884. Gram-positive bacteria do not have an outer membrane and thus can pick up the stain, while gram-negative bacteria cannot. Another variable that is important in decision-making is whether bacteria are aerobic or anaerobic, which determines where in the body the organism will grow and potentially cause infection.

The Gram stain is a laboratory test that is used to determine whether the infection is resulting from a gram-positive or gram-negative organism. Gram-positive bacteria appear purple in color and gram-negative bacteria appear pink. The shape, arrangement, and size of the organism can provide further information to help in identify it. Common shapes seen on the Gram stain include *cocci*, which are sphere shaped; *bacilli*, which resemble rods; and *coccobacilli*, which are a combination of the two. To perform a Gram stain, the technician applies bacteria to a slide. Next, crystal violet dye is applied, which stains the bacteria purple. Iodine is then applied, which helps the dye bind to the peptidoglycan layer of the cell wall, and this is followed by acetone, which washes away the dye. The purple dye remains on gram-positive bacteria as a result of the strong bond between the bacteria and a thick peptidoglycan layer, but it washes away from gram-negative bacteria, which has a thin peptidoglycan layer. As stated earlier, gram-positive bacteria retain the staining dye and appear deep violet on the microscopic slide. Gram-negative bacteria do not retain the dye and appear a pink-red color on the slide.

Anaerobes are organisms that can grow in the absence of oxygen. This characteristic allows them to grow in necrotic tissue and poorly aerated portions of the respiratory tract. Mycobacteria such as the tuberculosis organism do not uptake Gram stain; they have very tough cell walls and are difficult to kill. Yeasts are gram positive; rickettsia are gram negative.

Sensitivity Testing

Sensitivity testing or *susceptibility testing* determines an organism's response to antimicrobial medications by exposing a standardized concentration of the organism to specific concentrations of antimicrobial medication. Sensitivity testing can be done for bacteria, fungi, and viruses. Sensitivity testing occurs in vitro and may not account for many other patient-related factors, such as pharmacodynamics and pharmacokinetics, the patient's immune status, or other factors that influence treatment success. Throat, blood, urine, or other specimens should be sent to hospital-based or commercial laboratories for culture and sensitivity testing. Antibiotic effectiveness against an organism is determined by exposing the organism to various antibiotics. This piece of critical information is needed by the clinician to make an effective treatment decision in cases where drug resistance is likely.

Resistance to Antiinfective Medications

Antimicrobial resistance is recognized as a serious threat to health. New resistance mechanisms are emerging and spreading globally, threatening therapeutic options for infectious diseases. The CDC estimates that each year in the

United States alone, antibiotic-resistant bacteria cause more than 2 million illnesses and about 23,000 deaths. Resistance to antibiotics can be a natural progression or, more concerning, acquired over time. When organisms become less susceptible to treatment with antiinfectives over time, acquired resistance develops and the need for newer, more effective antiinfectives becomes urgent.

In 2017, the World Health Organization (WHO) conducted an analysis of the pipeline for antibacterial development and warned of a substantial lack of new antibiotics under development to treat an increasing number of resistant infections. Inappropriate and excessive antimicrobial prescribing is linked to the emergence of antimicrobial-resistant bacteria such as extended spectrum β-lactamase (ESBL)-producing gram-negative bacteria, as well as the specific acquisition of methicillin-resistant *Staphylococcus aureus* (MRSA). Since 80% of antimicrobial prescribing occurs in primary care, advanced practitioners in primary care have a key role in antibiotic stewardship. The safe use of antibiotics lies also in restricting the prescription to the minimum duration required for efficacy. The notion that ceasing antibiotic treatment early would result in antibiotic resistance is no longer supported by evidence, while taking antibiotics for longer durations than necessary is known to increase the risk of resistance (Llewelyn et al., 2017). Lastly, there is a decided lack of treatment options, especially for multidrug-resistant and gram-negative pathogens, some of which are implicated in the development of common infections such as pneumonia and UTIs. Antibiotic resistance can directly contribute to severe or untreatable infections in the future if antibiotic stewardship is lacking.

BOOKMARK THIS!

Antibiotic Stewardship

Centers for Disease Control and Prevention. (2017). *Antibiotic Use in the United States, Progress and Opportunities*. U.S. Department of Health and Human Services. Available at https://www.cdc.gov/antibiotic-use/stewardship-report/pdf/stewardship-report.pdf.

Mechanisms of Antimicrobial Resistance

Organisms have several mechanisms for developing drug resistance. It is important to note that the use of antibiotics can lead to the promotion of drug-resistant organisms. Under normal conditions, organisms have the means to keep one another in check. However, if some organisms develop resistance to an antibiotic, the resistant organism kills off sensitive microbes only, allowing the resistant organisms to continue to grow. Antibiotics that are broader in spectrum tend to kill off more organisms. These medications are the most likely to promote resistance.

The use of any antiinfective agent in primary care is associated with the emergence of resistant organisms. Overuse

and inappropriate use can exacerbate conditions in terms of the selection of resistant bacterial strains. Regardless of appropriate or inappropriate antiinfective use, bacteria exposed to antimicrobial agents can develop resistance through the following mechanisms:

- Acquisition of genes that can produce enzymes that inactivate the antimicrobial agent. Common drug resistance–producing enzymes are collectively known as *penicillinases*, and the most prevalent of these is β-lactamase.
- Acquisition of efflux pumps capable of draining the antimicrobial agent from the bacterial cell prior to any bactericidal or bacteriostatic effects. Such efflux pumps can confer multidrug resistance, such as MRSA or resistance to tetracycline, due to active efflux.
- Acquisition of several genes capable of eliminating the antimicrobial binding site during synthesis of the bacterial wall.
- Mutations occurring in the gene that encode the target protein so that it no longer binds the drug. Examples of bacteria that are resistant to antibiotics through mutation include *Mycobacterium tuberculosis*, *Escherichia coli*, and *Staphylococcus aureus*.
- Bacterial mutations that occur via transduction, transformation, and/or conjugation, with the resultant mutated form resistant to one or more classes of antimicrobials.
  - *Transduction* occurs when a virus that contains DNA infects the bacteria. The virus that infects the bacteria contains plasmids of bacterial DNA that contain genes for various functions, including one that provides drug resistance. Incorporation of these plasmids makes the newly infected bacterial cell resistant and capable of passing on the trait of resistance. One plasmid carries the code for penicillinase. An example is *S. aureus*. Others contain codes for resistance to erythromycin, tetracycline, or chloramphenicol.
  - *Transformation* involves transfer of DNA that is free in the environment into the bacteria. Examples include penicillin resistance in pneumococci and *Neisseria*.
  - *Conjugation* is the transfer of DNA from one organism to another during mating. This occurs predominantly among gram-negative bacilli such as Enterobacteriaceae and *Shigella flexneri*.

These factors, together over time, cause decreased penetration to the target site, alteration of the target site, and inactivation of the antibiotic by a bacterial enzyme that causes bacterial resistance. Antimicrobials are becoming less effective because of the exchange of genetic material, selection pressure, and mutations over time among pathogens. Concurrently, the total number of new antimicrobial agents under development is decreasing. Consequences that clinicians and patients face in the current antimicrobial therapy environment range from initial therapy failure, to increased medical care costs associated with the management of drug-resistant infections, to the ultimate crisis: patient mortality. Primary care providers should educate patients regarding the potential dangers of antibiotics killing sensitive bacteria but leaving resistant organisms to grow and multiply.

Mechanism of Action of Antiinfective Medications

Antiinfectives are classified as bacteriostatic or bactericidal in action. *Bacteriostatic agents* inhibit growth; *bactericidal agents* kill bacteria. Antiinfectives provide these effects through different mechanisms of action, including the following:

- Inhibition of cell wall synthesis, such as that seen with β-lactam antiinfectives (e.g., penicillins, cephalosporins, cephamycins, carbapenems, monobactams), vancomycin, antifungal agents, and bacitracin
- Direct action on the cell membrane to alter permeability and cause leakage of intracellular compounds; for example, the bactericidal action of polymyxin and nystatin
- Effects on the function of ribosomal subunits that inhibit protein synthesis; examples include the bacteriostatic actions of tetracycline, erythromycin, clindamycin, and chloramphenicol
- Binding of ribosome subunits to alter protein synthesis and cause cell death; for example, the bactericidal action of aminoglycosides
- Changes in nucleic acid metabolism, as seen in the bactericidal actions of rifampin, quinolones, and metronidazole
- Blockage of specific essential metabolic steps by antimetabolites; for example, the bactericidal actions of sulfonamides and trimethoprim
- Inhibition of viral enzymes essential for DNA synthesis by nucleic acid analogs that produce bacteriostatic activity

Principles of Treatment With Antiinfective Medications

> **BOOKMARK THIS!**
>
> **Clinical Guidelines**
> - Guidelines from the Infectious Diseases Society of America: www.idsociety.org
> - Agency for Healthcare Research and Quality National Clearinghouse for Guidelines: www.guidelines.gov

Antiinfective Treatment Criteria

Treatment with antiinfectives requires the primary care provider to select an antiinfective medication that meets the following criteria:
- Most effective
- Narrowest spectrum

- Lowest toxicity
- Lowest potential for allergy
- Most cost effective

Prophylaxis With Antiinfective Medications

The emergence of antibiotic resistance requires the primary care provider to carefully consider antibiotic prophylaxis. Occasionally, prophylaxis with an antiinfective agent is indicated. If a single effective nontoxic drug can be used to prevent or eradicate an infection after it has been introduced, then prophylaxis may be successful. Prophylaxis often is not successful in preventing colonization or infection by microorganisms present in the environment. An example of traditional use of a prophylaxis is that used for prevention of bacterial endocarditis by group A streptococcus, but this procedure has been challenged in some studies. Treatment for a sexually transmitted disease after exposure is often effective. Attempts are being made to provide prophylaxis for human immunodeficiency virus (HIV) postexposure.

Prophylaxis is sometimes attempted for patients at increased risk of bacterial infection, such as those undergoing organ transplantation, cancer chemotherapy, and HIV treatment, where the immune response may be diminished or lacking. However, prophylactic treatment may negatively impact normal flora and allow infection to occur with drug-resistant strains, thus defeating the purpose of the prophylaxis.

Antibiotic Selection

Choose the most cost-effective antibiotic with the narrowest spectrum, lowest toxicity, and lowest potential for allergy to decrease the risk of resistance. Table 39.1 lists common problems seen in the primary care setting and the antiinfectives to which each organism is usually susceptible. Consider both drug characteristics and patient characteristics when choosing an antibiotic.

Characteristics of Antiinfective Medications

Antibacterial medications tend to alter normal flora. Normal flora help prevent overgrowth and infection by pathogenic bacteria. Change in this flora places the patient at risk for superinfection, typically by yeast. The wider the spectrum of the antibacterial, the greater the alteration in normal flora, and the greater the risk of a superinfection. Choose the antibiotic with the narrowest spectrum that is effective against the organism causing the infection.

Certain antiinfectives are more likely than others to produce allergic reactions. Patients with a history of atopic allergy are particularly susceptible to the development of allergic reactions to antiinfectives. The penicillins and sulfonamides are the most frequent causes of allergic reaction. Certain viral infections increase the frequency of rash in response to penicillin. This reaction often happens when amoxicillin is given to a patient with mononucleosis and is not necessarily an allergic reaction. Antiinfectives also can potentially cause a *drug fever*, which is a fever that develops and coincides with administration of a drug and disappears after the discontinuation of the drug, when no other cause for the fever can be found after a physical examination and laboratory investigation.

The side effects and potential adverse effects resulting from the use of antiinfectives vary and need to be considered when contemplating an antiinfective regimen. Antiinfectives differ in terms of the frequency and severity of adverse reactions. Gastrointestinal (GI) problems such as nausea, vomiting, diarrhea, and GI distress are often caused by the administration of antiinfectives. One of the common side effects of taking antibiotics is loose bowel movements (diarrhea), as the antibiotic disrupts the normal, healthy bacteria in the gut that promote regular bowel function. The primary care provider might recommend the use of probiotics following antibiotic treatment to help repopulate healthy strains of bacteria. Patients must be prepared for the expected side effects and potential adverse effects of the prescribed antiinfective to achieve compliance with the treatment regimen. The appropriate strategies for self-management of side effects, which adverse effects to report, and when to report them are crucial aspects of patient education.

Once an oral antiinfective is taken, the medication dissolves in the GI tract and the dissolved medication passes through the intestinal wall into the bloodstream. This is followed by *medication distribution* follows, which is the movement of medication to and from the blood and various tissues of the body (fat, muscle, and brain tissue) and the relative proportions of the drug in the tissues. Some antiinfectives penetrate specific sites better than others. Thus, the location of the infection plays an important role in antiinfective prescribing. For example, rifampin is highly fat soluble and rapidly enters the brain, but penicillin, a water-soluble antibiotic, does not.

The liver is involved in the metabolism of some antiinfectives. The macrolides clarithromycin, erythromycin, and troleandomycin are inhibitors of the cytochrome (CYP) P450 3A4 system. Clindamycin and erythromycin are substrates of the 3A4 system. Before antiinfectives are prescribed, it is important to check for drug interactions. For patients with hepatic dysfunction, alterations in dosage and the monitoring of liver enzymes often are required.

The kidney is involved in the elimination of most antiinfective medications. Monitor renal function and decrease the dose if renal impairment is present. This is critically important when prescribing aminoglycosides. The primary care provider must know how to calculate creatinine clearance (CrCl) and how to reduce dosages in patients with renal impairment. It is important to follow the appropriate dosing schedule to maintain serum and tissue concentrations of the antibiotic. The medication must be taken at regular intervals, and the primary care provider is responsible for writing a prescription that describes precisely how the patient is to take the medication. For example, an antibiotic to be taken three times daily should be taken every 8 hours, not at each of the patient's three meals, so the clinician must be precise in writing the prescription.

Factors That Affect Antibiotic Selection

Patient factors that traditionally influence antibiotic decisions include the severity of the illness, the age of the patient, the presence of comorbid illness, laboratory results (i.e., cultures), the presence of organ dysfunction, and allergy history. The severity of illness is the most important factor that must be considered when deciding how aggressively to treat the infection, as well as the length of treatment. If the patient is experiencing mental confusion, has low oxygen saturation or unstable vital signs, and is unable to take the medication orally or maintain adequate hydration, admission to the hospital is most likely required. Comorbid conditions can affect the patient's response to antiinfective therapy. Older patients tend to have more chronic illnesses, are more susceptible to infection, and generally require a longer duration of treatment. The presence of organ dysfunction will require the primary care provider to consider whether dose reductions or monitoring of laboratory tests is needed. Conditions that reduce circulation, such as diabetes and heart failure, may limit delivery of an antibiotic to an infected site. Knowledge of laboratory results such as cultures and white blood cell counts can be used in the selection of an appropriate antiinfective. A thorough medication allergy history will also factor into the selection of an antiinfective.

Prescriber Considerations for Antiinfective Therapy

Clinical guidelines for prescribing antiinfective medications have been developed for the treatment of many common infections. These guidelines have been developed as the result of analysis of valid research and scientific studies and have been issued by federal agencies and professional groups. Be aware that clinical practice guidelines are revised and are updated regularly. To practice in accordance with accepted standards, the primary care provider is expected to follow accepted clinical practice guidelines regarding antiinfectives. For example, when the CDC issues a guideline for the treatment of strep infection of the throat that includes 10 days of antibiotic therapy, clinicians are expected to adhere to this standard of practice.

BOOKMARK THIS!

Clinical Practice Guidelines for Prescribing Antiinfectives

- CDC:
  - Adults: https://www.cdc.gov/antibiotic-use/community/for-hcp/outpatient-hcp/adult-treatment-rec.html
  - Children: https://www.cdc.gov/antibiotic-use/clinicians/pediatric-treatment-rec.html?CDC_AA_refVal=https%3A%2F%2Fwww.cdc.gov%2Fantibiotic-use%2Fcommunity%2Ffor-hcp%2Foutpatient-hcp%2Fpediatric-treatment-rec.html
- Infectious Diseases Society of America: https://www.idsociety.org/practice-guideline/alphabetical-guidelines/

Treatment Site

Determination of the infectious site to be treated is an important consideration. Skin, eye, and vaginal infections can be treated via local application of medication. In some cases, drainage of the site is necessary, such as in empyema and abscesses. Antiinfectives alone do not replace the necessary local treatment of incision and drainage. If foreign objects are associated with an infection, they must be removed to achieve infection clearance.

Treatment Length

Always establish a definite duration of treatment; do not begin an open-ended course. If necessary, a course of therapy can be extended if the patient evaluation reveals the need for continuation beyond the originally defined period.

Whether to discontinue a course of antiinfectives once started can be a difficult choice. If the culture shows that bacteria are resistant to the agent currently in use, it is clear that the provider must discontinue the medication originally prescribed and substitute one to which the bacteria are susceptible, if the patient is still ill. In general, primary care providers should emphasize to patients that it is important to complete the prescribed course of antiinfectives, even if the symptoms are gone. This is necessary to completely eradicate the offending organism, not just the ones most susceptible to the antibiotic, while leaving resistant bacteria alive. On the other hand, the primary care provider should discontinue an antibiotic that was started based on empirical evidence if the culture is negative.

Selected Bibliography

Centers for Disease Control and Prevention. (2017). Antibiotic Use in the United States, Progress and Opportunities. Atlanta, GA: U.S. Department of Health and Human Services, CDC; 2017.

Centers for Disease Control and Prevention. (2018). *About antibiotic resistance*. Available at https://www.cdc.gov/drugresistance/about.html.

Eyler, R. F., & Shvets, K. (2019). Clinical pharmacology of antibiotics. *Clinical Journal of the American Society of Nephrology, 14*, 1080–1090.

Garrity, G. M. (2016). A new genomics-driven taxonomy of bacteria and archaea: Are we there yet? *Journal of Clinical Microbiology, 54*(8), 1956–1963. http://doi.org/10.1128/JCM.00200-16.

Kmietowicz, Z. (2017). Few novel antibiotics in the pipeline, WHO warns. *The BMJ, 358*, j4339. http://doi.org/10.1136/bmj.j4339.

Llewelyn, M. J., Fitzpatrick, J. M., Darwin, E., et al. (2017). The antibiotic course has had its day. *The BMJ, 358*, j4339. j3418.017;358.

Mack, I., & Bielicki, J. (2019). What can we do about antimicrobial resistance? *The Pediatric Infectious Disease Journal, 38*(6S Suppl 1), S33–S38. http://doi.org/10.1097/INF.0000000000002321.

McCullough, A. R., Pollack, A. J., Plejdrup Hansen, M., Glasziou, P., Looke, D., Britt, H. C., & Del Mar, C. B (2017). Antibiotics for acute respiratory infections in general practice: Comparison of prescribing rates with guideline recommendations. *The Medical Journal of Australia, 207*(2), 65–69. http://doi.org/10.5694/mja16.01042.

Ness, V., Price, L., Currie, K., & Reilly, J. (2016). Influences on independent nurse prescribers' antimicrobial prescribing behavior: A systematic review. *Journal of Clinical Nursing, 25*, 1206–1217. http://doi.org/10.1111/jocn.13249.

Tarrant, C., Colman, A. M., Chattoe-Brown, E., Jenkins, D. R., Mehtar, S., Perera, N., & Krockow, E. M. (2019). Optimizing antibiotic prescribing: Collective approaches to managing a common-pool resource. *Clinical Microbiology and Infection, 25*, 1356–1363.

40

Penicillins

KRISTY M. SHAEER

Overview

The discovery of penicillin in 1928 by Alexander Fleming led to a decrease in morbidity and mortality rates from communicable diseases. Fleming observed the bactericidal effect of *Penicillium notatum* and this led to the discovery and isolation of the first beta-lactam antibiotic, penicillin. Many organisms that were initially highly susceptible to penicillin have developed resistance. However, penicillins are still effective against many gram-positive bacteria and a few gram-negative bacteria. Penicillins are relatively inexpensive and widely used to treat mild to moderately severe infections of the skin, ear, sinus, and upper respiratory tract. Penicillins are naturally occurring or synthetic with differing antimicrobial activity. Table 40.1 provides an overview of penicillins.

Classification

Penicillins are considered beta-lactam antibiotics, with the basic structure including a four-membered beta-lactam (cyclic amide), a five-membered thiazolidine ring (6-aminopenicillanic acid), and a side chain. The spectrum of activity for each penicillin varies based on the side chain of each derivative and may afford some unique pharmacokinetic properties. Penicillins are bactericidal, which means they cause bacterial destruction and cell death by binding to penicillin-binding proteins (PBPs) and ultimately inhibiting cell wall synthesis. PBPs (e.g., transpeptidases) are essential enzymes for catalyzing the formation and maintenance of the peptidoglycan cell wall structure. The binding of the penicillin molecules causes the bacterial cell wall to weaken, which ultimately leads to cell lysis and death. Penicillins are used to treat a variety of infections caused by susceptible bacteria, including those in the *Streptococcus*, *Staphylococcus*, *Clostridium*, *Neisseria*, and *Listeria* genera.

Antibiotic Resistance

The development of resistance by gram-positive and gram-negative bacteria leads to treatment challenges. The effectiveness of the penicillins' antimicrobial activity against

bacteria depends on three factors: the ability of the penicillins to reach the PBPs, the inactivation of penicillins by bacterial enzymes, and the low affinity some of the PBPs have to penicillins.

The ability of penicillins to reach the PBPs depends on the structure of the bacterial cell wall. The cell wall of gram-positive bacteria consists of two layers: the cytoplasmic membrane and a thick cell wall. Despite the thickness, the cell wall can be easily penetrated by penicillins. The cell wall of gram-negative bacteria consists of three layers: the cytoplasmic membrane, a thin cell wall, and an outer membrane that is difficult for penicillins to penetrate. Only certain penicillins (e.g., ampicillin, amoxicillin, and piperacillin) can cross the cell wall and reach PBPs on the cytoplasmic membrane.

In some instances, bacterial enzymes inactivate penicillins, rendering them ineffective against an organism. Bacterial enzymes called *beta-lactamases* are enzymes that hydrolyze the beta-lactam ring. Beta-lactamases that act exclusively on penicillins are known as *penicillinases*. *Penicillinases* are produced by gram-positive bacteria in larger quantities and gram-negative bacteria in smaller quantities to confer resistance. For example, *Staphylococcus aureus*, a gram-positive cocci bacterium, developed resistance to penicillins due to the production of penicillinases. In general, penicillinase-producing strains of bacteria are resistant to benzylpenicillin; phenoxymethylpenicillin; and amino-, carboxy-, and ureidopenicillins.

The third mechanism of resistance is associated with the genetically altered PBP response of some bacteria to penicillins. Methicillin-resistant *Staphylococcus aureus* (MRSA) are bacteria that produce PBPs with a low affinity for penicillins, making them resistant not only to methicillin but also to all penicillins.

Pharmacokinetics

In the presence of inflammation, penicillins readily penetrate most tissues and body fluids, including cerebrospinal fluid, the joints, and the eyes. All penicillins are readily and actively (30% to more than 90%) excreted by the renal tubules and most are eliminated unchanged in the urine. Table 40.2 provides a summary of dose adjustments based

TABLE 40.1 Overview of Penicillins

Drug Classification	Generic Name	Usual Routes	Possible Spectrum of Activity
Natural Penicillins	Penicillin G Penicillin V	IM, IV, oral	*Streptococcus* spp., *Neisseria* spp., *Pasteurella multocida*, many oropharynx anaerobes, spirochetes (e.g., T. *pallidum*), others
Aminopenicillins	Ampicillin Ampicillin/Sulbactam Amoxicillin Amoxicillin/Clavulanate	IM, IV, oral IV Oral Oral	*Staphylococcus aureus* (methicillin-susceptible strains and use only ampicillin/sulbactam and amoxicillin/clavulanate), coagulase-negative staphylococci (methicillin susceptible), *Streptococcus* spp., L. monocytogenes, *influenzae*, E. coli, *Proteus mirabilis*, *Enterococci* spp., *Neisseria meningitidis* (penicillin sensitive), *Moraxella cataharralis*, *Acinetobacter baumannii* (ampicillin/sulbactam only), *Pasteurella multocida*, many oropharynx anaerobes and gut anaerobes (including B. *fragilis*)
Penicillinase-resistant penicillins	Dicloxacillin Oxacillin Nafcillin	Oral, IV	*Staphylococcus aureus* (methicillin susceptible), viridans group streptococci, coagulase-negative staphylococci (methicillin susceptible); lesser activity against S. *pneumoniae* and S. *pyogenes* compared to natural penicillins
Ureidopenicillins	Piperacillin/Tazobactam	IV	*Enterococcus faecalis* (ampicillin or amoxicillin sensitive), *Staphylococcus aureus* (methicillin-susceptible strains), coagulase-negative staphylococci (methicillin-susceptible strains), *Haemophilus influenzae*, *Moraxella cataharralis*, *Enterobacteriaceae* (e.g., E. coli, *Klebsiella* spp., *Serratia* spp., *Citrobacter* spp., *Enterobacter* spp.), *Pseudomonas aeruginosa*, many anaerobes including B. *fragilis*

IM, Intramuscular; IV, intravenous.

TABLE 40.2 Dosing Based on Renal Impairment

Medication	Age	CrCl or GFR	Dose Adjustment
Penicillin G	Adults: CrCl	>50 mL/min	No dosage adjustment needed.
		10–50 mL/min	Reduce dose by 25% and keep the same interval.
		<10 mL/min/1.73 m² in patients with uremia	Manufacturer recommendation: 1 full loading dose, then 50% of usual dose every 4–5 hr.
		<10 mL/min	Consider extending dosing interval to every 12 hr depending on severity of infection. Manufacturer recommendation: 1 full loading dose, then 50% of usual dose every 8–10 hr.
Penicillin V	Adults and pediatrics	No dosage adjustment is necessary in adult patients. No recommendations for pediatric patients.	Consider <10 mL/min, extending dosing interval to every 8 hr.
Dicloxacillin	Adults and pediatrics	No dosage adjustment needed.	
Oxacillin		No dosage adjustment needed.	
Ampicillin	Adults: CrCl	>50 mL/min	1–2 g IV every 4–6 hr.
		10–50 mL/min	1–2 g IV every 6–8 hr.
		<10 mL/min	1–2 g IV every 8–12 hr.

Continued

TABLE 40.2   Dosing Based on Renal Impairment—cont'd

Medication	Age	CrCl or GFR	Dose Adjustment
Ampicillin/ sulbactam	Adults: CrCl	≥30 mL/min	1.5–3 g IV every 6 hr.
		15–29 mL/min	1.5–3 g IV every 12 hr.
		<15 mL/min	1.5–3 g IV every 24 hr.
Ampicillin	Pediatrics: CrCl	>50 mL/min	No adjustment needed.
		30–50 mL/min	Same mg/kg/dose and extend interval to every 6 hr.
		10–29 mL/min/1.73 m²	Same mg/kg/dose and extend to every 8–12 hr.
		<10 mL/min/1.73 m²	Same mg/kg/dose and extend to every 12 hr.
Ampicillin/ sulbactam	Pediatrics: CrCl and based on ampicillin component	≥30 mL/min	No adjustment needed.
		15–29 mL/min	Usual mg/kg/day IV every 12 hr.
		<15 mL/min	Usual mg/kg/day IV every 24 hr.
Amoxicillin	Adults: CrCl	>30 mL/min	No dosage adjustment needed.
		10–30 mL/min	Consider decreasing dose by 50% in patients who require higher dose (e.g., 1 g orally every 8–12 hr). 250–500 mg orally every 12 hr depending on severity of infection. Do not use 875-mg tablet strength or extended-release tablet for dosing.
		<10 mL/min	250–500 mg orally every 24 hr, depending on severity of infection. Do not use 875-mg tablet strength or extended-release tablet for dosing.
	Pediatrics: CrCl	10–30 mL/min	Same dose every 12 hr.
		<10 mL/min	Same dose every 24 hr.
Piperacillin/ tazobactam	Adults: CrCl	≥40 mL/min	No dosage adjustment needed.
		20–40 mL/min	For suspected or confirmed infection with *P. aeruginosa,* reduce dose to 3.375 Gm (3 Gm piperacillin and 0.375 Gm tazobactam) IV every 6 hr. For all other indications, reduce dose to 2.25 Gm (2 Gm piperacillin and 0.25 Gm tazobactam) IV every 6 hr.
		≤20 mL/min	For suspected or confirmed infection with *P. aeruginosa,* reduce dose to 2.25 Gm (2 Gm piperacillin and 0.25 Gm tazobactam) IV every 6 hr. For all other indications, reduce dose to 2.25 Gm (2 Gm piperacillin and 0.25 Gm tazobactam) IV every 8 hr.
	Pediatrics: CrCl	>40 mL/min	No dosage adjustment needed.
		20–40 mL/min	Same mg/kg/dose every 8 hr.
		<20 mL/min	Same mg/kg/dose every 12 hr.

CrCl, Creatinine clearance; *GFR,* glomerular filtration rate; *IV,* intravenous.

on creatinine clearance (CrCl) and glomerular filtration rates (GFRs). Penicillins exhibit minimal liver excretion (Baietto et al., 2014).

Allergic Reactions to Penicillins

Since 1980, studies have demonstrated that 2% or less of the population report allergies to other penicillin derivatives (Joint Task Force on Practice Parameters, 2010). Almost 10% of patients report an allergy to penicillin, but the majority (90%) of patients who undergo testing will demonstrate tolerance to these agents (Joint Task Force on Practice Parameters, 2010). Although some patients may have true IgE-mediated penicillin allergies, this is rare and occurs in approximately 1% of the population (Joint Task Force on Practice Parameters, 2010). IgE-mediated penicillin reactions occur within minutes to 1 to 2 hours and include sudden anaphylaxis with hypotension, wheezing, bronchospasm, angioedema itching, and urticaria (Bhattacharya, 2010). Approximately 50% of patients with IgE-mediated penicillin allergy lose their sensitivity after 5 years; this rises to 80% after 10 years. Board-certified allergists can utilize skin sensitivity testing to assess current risk status. Caution is advised in patients who previously experienced severe hypersensitivity syndromes such as Stevens-Johnson syndrome, toxic epidermal necrolysis, serum sickness, acute interstitial nephritis, hemolytic anemia, and drug rash with eosinophilia and systemic symptoms (DRESS). Positive penicillin skin sensitivity testing indicates the presence of IgE antibodies to penicillin. In addition to the hypersensitivity type reactions, Table 40.3 provides an overview of the systemic adverse reactions most associated with penicillin.

Contraindications and Precautions for Penicillins

Any patient reporting an IgE-mediated hypersensitivity reaction to one type of penicillin may have cross-sensitivity reactions with other agents with similar side chains (Joint Task Force on Practice Parameters, 2010). However, patients often may tolerate another penicillin or can undergo a desensitization to receive the preferred agent. Common drug–drug interactions associated with concomitant penicillin use can be found in Table 40.4.

A false-positive reaction for glucose in the urine has been observed in patients receiving penicillin and using Benedict's solution, Fehling's solution, or Clinitest tablets for urine glucose testing. However, this reaction has not been observed with Tes-tape (glucose Enzymatic Test Strip, USP, Lilly) or Clinistix. Patients with diabetes mellitus who test their urine for glucose should use glucose tests based on enzymatic glucose oxidase reactions.

TABLE 40.3 Overview of Systemic Adverse Reactions to Penicillins

Body System Affected	Adverse Reaction
Central Nervous System	Encephalopathy
	Headache
	Neurotoxicity
	Seizures
Gastrointestinal	Antibiotic-associated pseudomembranous colitis
	Constipation
	Diarrhea
	Epigastric distress
	Nausea
	Vomiting
Skin	Contact dermatitis
	Pruritus
	Rash
	Urticaria
Musculoskeletal	Arthralgia
	Myalgia
Liver	Elevated liver enzymes
Renal Effects	Elevated creatinine/BUN
Metabolic Effects	Hypernatremia
	Hypokalemia
Hematologic Effects	Agranulocytosis
	Bone marrow depression
	Granulocytopenia
	Hemolytic anemia
	Neutropenia
	Thrombocytopenia

BUN, Blood urea nitrogen.

TABLE 40.4 Drug–Drug Interactions

- Aminoglycosides and ureidopenicillin (if higher concentrations of both agents)
- Hormonal contraceptives
- Probenecid: increase penicillin serum concentrations
- Anticoagulants and antiplatelets: may cause prolonged bleeding
- Methotrexate: monitored for methotrexate toxicity
- High doses parenteral penicillin may cause hyperkalemia with concomitant use of:
  - Potassium-sparing diuretics
  - Angiotensin-converting inhibitors
  - Potassium-containing medications
  - Potassium salts

PRACTICE PEARLS

Penicillin Use in Pregnancy and Lactation

- Penicillins are generally safe in pregnancy. Animal studies failed to reveal evidence of fetal harm and no adverse effects have been reported during human use.
- Penicillins are excreted in breast milk. Unless the infant is allergic to penicillins, breastfeeding is generally safe during maternal penicillin therapy.
- Penicillins may cause diarrhea, candidiasis, and skin rash in breastfeeding babies. The infant should be observed for potential effects.

Penicillin Therapy

Natural Penicillins

Penicillin G (Benzylpenicillin)

The natural penicillins are also known as *narrow-spectrum* penicillins. This group includes penicillin G (benzyl penicillin) and penicillin V (also known as penicillin VK). Table 40.5 provides a summary of the natural penicillins.

Pharmacokinetics. Penicillin G is available in intravenous (IV) or intramuscular (IM) preparations as potassium penicillin G, procaine penicillin G, benzathine penicillin G,

TABLE 40.5   Natural Penicillins

Medication	Indication	Dosage	Considerations and Monitoring
Penicillin G benzathine	Pharyngitis (*Group A beta-hemolytic streptococcal*) Rheumatic fever prophylaxis	*Adults:* 1.2 million units IM as a single injection. *Children and adolescents ≥27 kg:* 1.2 million units IM as a single injection. *Infants and children <27 kg:* 600,000 units IM as a single injection.	Black box warning: avoid IV administration Monitor: serum creatinine/BUN
	Syphilis (*T. pallidum*) Primary, secondary, or early latent (<1-year duration)	*Adults:* 2.4 million units IM as a single injection. *Infants, children, and adolescents:* 50,000 units/kg IM, up to adult dose of 2.4 million units as a single injection.	
	Syphilis (*T. pallidum*) Syphilis (>1-year duration) Syphilis of unknown duration	*Adults:* 2.4 million units IM once weekly for 3 successive weeks. The total dose is 7.2 million units. *Infants, children, and adolescents:* 50,000 units/kg IM, up to adult dose of 2.4 million units, once weekly for 3 successive weeks. The total dose is 150,000 units/kg up to a maximum dose of 7.2 million units.	
	Neurosyphilis and congenital syphilis (*T. pallidum*)	Consult current CDC guidelines.	
Penicillin G procaine	Pharyngitis (Group A beta-hemolytic streptococcal)	*Adults:* 600,000–1 million units IM daily × 10 days. *Infants, children, and adolescents:* ≥60 lb: 600,000 units IM <60 lb: 300,000 units IM	
	Neurosyphilis, ocular syphilis, or otosyphilis (alternative)	Adults: penicillin procaine 2.4 million units IM daily every 24 hr plus probenecid 500 mg orally every 6 hr for 10–14 days.	Considered if compliance ensured.
Penicillin VK	Pharyngitis (Group A beta-hemolytic streptococcal)	*Adults:* 125–250 mg orally every 6–8 hr for 10 days. *Children and adolescents 12–17 yr:* 125–250 mg orally every 6–8 hr for 10 days. *Children ≤27 kg:* : 250 mg orally every 8–12 hr for 10 days. *Children >27 kg:* 500 mg orally every 8–12 hr for 10 days. Maximum dosage: *Adults, older adults, adolescents, and children ≥12 yr:* 2 Gm/day orally.	*All ages:* Current practice guidelines may differ from FDA-approved dosage. Oral penicillin should not be used in patients at high risk for endocarditis.
	Skin and skin structure infections	*Adults, adolescents, and children 12–17 yr:* Streptococcal infection: 125–250 mg orally every 6–8 hr for 5–10 days. Staphylococcal infections: 250–500 mg orally every 6–8 hr for 10 days.	

BUN, Blood urea nitrogen; *CDC,* Centers for Disease Control and Prevention; *FDA,* U.S. Food and Drug Administration; *IM,* intramuscular; *IV,* intravenous.

and sodium penicillin G. The potassium and sodium penicillin G IV preparations are rapidly absorbed, with peak blood levels reached in about 5 to 15 minutes depending on the rate of infusion. The absorption of procaine and benzathine penicillins occurs more slowly. Procaine penicillin has a peak concentration within 2 to 3 hours in adults and 3 to 6 hours in children. Benzathine penicillin has a peak concentration within 48 hours in adults and 24 hours in children. This slow absorption provides continuously sustained blood levels, which makes it the recommended preparation for the treatment of *Treponema pallidum*. In older children and adults, the half-life is very short (about 30 minutes). Approximately 75% to 89% of the circulating drug is protein bound. Excretion occurs within the kidneys but may be delayed in neonates, young infants, and patients with impaired renal function.

Indications. The natural penicillins are effective against aerobic gram-positive organisms (*Streptococcus pneumoniae*, *Streptococcus pyogenes*, *Streptococcus agalactiae*, viridans group streptococci, and possibly *Corynebacterium* spp. and *Enterococcus faecalis*); aerobic gram-negative organisms (*Neisseria meningitidis*); the anaerobes that reside in the oropharynx (e.g., *Bacteroides* spp. [excludes *B. fragilis*]); *Peptostreptococcus* sp.; *Clostridium* sp. (excludes *Clostridioides difficile*); *Prevotella* spp.; and spirochetes (including *T. pallidum*) (Geddes et al., 2018a). IM penicillin G benzathine or aqueous penicillin G is the recommended first-line treatment of choice for *T. pallidum* infections (Shatsky, 2009). Additional indications for natural penicillin use include *S. pyogenes*-associated pharyngitis, scarlet fever, cellulitis, necrotizing fasciitis, bone and joint infections, bacteremia, *S. agalactiae*-associated skin and soft tissue infections, bacteremia and meningitis, meningococcal meningitis, and streptococci-associated endocarditis (may use in combination with an aminoglycoside for a shorter duration of therapy in some patients).

Adverse Effects. The severity of adverse effects can range from a minor rash to life-threatening anaphylaxis. There is no direct relationship between the size of the penicillin dose and the intensity of the adverse effect. Acute generalized exanthematous pustulosis (AGEP) may present 2 to 3 weeks after the first dose. AGEP presents as a nonfollicular, pustular, erythematous rash with an associated fever above 100.4°F. In children, AGEP may also include laryngeal stridor and high fever. Penicillin procaine formulation has been associated with dizziness, heart palpitations, auditory or visual disturbances, and fear of impending death that typically resolves within about 15 to 30 minutes.

Contraindications. Penicillin in contraindicated in the presence of a viral infection unless a coinfection with a susceptible bacterium is identified. A history of a true IgE-mediated penicillin allergic (hypersensitivity/anaphylactic) reaction to any penicillin is an absolute contraindication. Use with caution in patients with cephalosporin hypersensitivity or carbapenem hypersensitivity. Dose reductions may be necessary in patients with renal impairment or renal failure.

BLACK BOX WARNING!

Penicillin G Benzathine

- Inadvertent IV administration of penicillin G benzathine has been associated with cardiorespiratory arrest and death.
- Administer by deep IM injection only.

Monitoring. Monitor renal function (serum creatinine/blood urea nitrogen or BUN). Large doses of penicillin administered to patients with renal impairment have been associated with seizures. Monitor kidney function in patients with renal impairment, neonates, young infants, older adults, and those who are acutely ill. Penicillin G blood concentrations may be decreased following hemodialysis.

Penicillin V (Penicillin VK)

Penicillin V (also known as phenoxymethylpenicillin potassium and penicillin VK) is an acid-stable derivative of penicillin G and is available in an oral preparation.

Pharmacokinetics. Penicillin V is available in an oral preparation that is absorbed from the upper part of the small bowel. Serum levels peak within 30 to 60 minutes after dosing. Only about 25% of the dose is absorbed. Penicillin V is primarily excreted by the kidneys through glomerular filtration and tubular secretion. Excretion may be delayed in neonates, young infants, and patients with impaired renal function. Like penicillin G, penicillin V distributes into pleural, pericardial, ascitic, peritoneal, and synovial fluids, as well as the lung, urine, middle ear, and inflamed meninges. It distributes poorly in the maxillary sinuses and inflamed tonsils (Geddes et al., 2018b).

Indications. Penicillin V is recommended for the treatment of streptococcal pharyngitis/tonsillitis, scarlet fever, mild to moderately severe skin and skin structure infections, *S. pneumoniae* infections, and necrotizing ulcerative gingivitis, and is recommended as the primary prevention of rheumatic fever. The preferred oral preparation due to its stability in stomach acid, penicillin V may be taken with meals. Oral penicillin V should not be used to treat *T. pallidum* infections.

Adverse Effects. Approximately 10% of the population may report allergies to penicillins. Fortunately, patients with true IgE-mediated penicillin allergies are rare, though severity can range from a minor rash to life-threatening anaphylaxis. There is no direct relationship between the size of the penicillin dose and the intensity of the adverse effect.

Contraindications. Penicillin V in contraindicated in the presence of a viral infection unless a concomitant bacterial infection has been identified. The use of penicillin V in a patient with a history of a true IgE-mediated penicillin allergic (hypersensitivity/anaphylactic) reaction to any penicillin is an absolute contraindication. Use with caution in patients with cephalosporin hypersensitivity or carbapenem hypersensitivity. Consider the presence of pseudomembranous colitis in patients with a history of ulcerative colitis or other inflammatory bowel disease or who present with diarrhea (for more than 1 week) as this may reduce the absorption of penicillin V (Geddes et al., 2018b). Dose reductions may be necessary in patients with renal impairment or renal failure. Penicillin V should not be used in patients at high risk for endocarditis (e.g., prosthetic heart valve). Patients with phenylketonuria or those who require restriction of phenylalanine intake should be warned that some penicillin V powders contain phenylalanine and some contain aspartame. Aspartame is metabolized to phenylalanine in the GI tract after oral administration.

Monitoring. Limited data are available in patients with a CrCl less than 10 mL/min, but providers should consider adjusting medication dosages. Monitor renal function (serum creatinine/BUN). Monitor for seizure activity when utilizing large doses of penicillin. Monitor kidney function

in patients with renal impairment, neonates, young infants, older adults, and those who are acutely ill.

Narrow-Spectrum Penicillins: Beta-Lactamase (Penicillinase)–Resistant Penicillins

Penicillins in this category include nafcillin, oxacillin, and dicloxacillin. These second-generation penicillins are semi-synthetic modifications of natural penicillins that are resistant to inactivation by beta-lactamases (e.g., penicillinases). These drugs have a narrow spectrum of gram-positive antimicrobial activity against methicillin-susceptible *Staphylococcus aureus* (MSSA) and methicillin-susceptible coagulase-negative staphylococci. Though beta-lactamase–resistant penicillins show activity against penicillin-susceptible *Streptococcus pneumoniae*, *Streptococcus pyogenes*, and viridans group streptococci, the natural penicillins are preferred due to increased potency. These agents have no activity against enterococci and gram-negative organisms and limited to no activity against anaerobic organisms. They are the drugs of choice for most staphylococcal infections but are ineffective against MRSA. Nafcillin is administered primarily by the IV route but can be given intramuscularly. Oxacillin may be given via an IV or IM route. Dicloxacillin is available as an oral preparation. Table 40.6 provides a summary of the beta-lactamase–resistant penicillins.

Oxacillin, Dicloxacillin, and Nafcillin

Oxacillin, dicloxacillin, and nafcillin are similar in chemical structure and pharmacokinetic properties.

Pharmacokinetics. Oxacillin achieves peak concentration within 5 minutes when administered intravenously and within 30 minutes when administered intramuscularly. Approximately 92% to 93% is protein bound (Smith, 2018). Between 45% and 50% of an oxacillin dose is metabolized by the liver to active and inactive metabolites and is cleared

TABLE 40.6	Narrow-Spectrum Penicillins: Beta-Lactamase–Resistant Penicillins		
Medication	**Indication**	**Dosage**	**Considerations and Monitoring**
Dicloxacillin	Bacteremia, skin and skin structure infections, bone and joint infections, pneumonia, or endocarditis due to infections due to *Staphylococcus* sp.	*Adults, adolescents, and children ≥40 kg*: 125 mg orally every 6 hr for mild infections, 250–500 mg orally every 6 hr for moderate infections, and 1000 mg orally every 6 hr for severe infections. *Infants, children, and adolescents <40 kg*: 12.5–25 mg/kg/day orally in equally divided doses every 6 hr (maximum: 500 mg/dose) for mild to moderate infections and 25–50 mg/kg/day orally in equally divided doses every 6 hr (maximum: 500 mg/dose) for severe infections. *Neonates*: safety and efficacy have not been established.	No dosage adjustments for renal impairment. Maximum daily dose for adults, older adults, and adolescents: 4 Gm orally. Maximum daily dose for children: Not available.
	Mastitis	*Adults*: 125–500 mg orally every 6 hr for 10–14 days.	

TABLE 40.6 Narrow-Spectrum Penicillins: Beta-Lactamase–Resistant Penicillins—cont'd

Medication	Indication	Dosage	Considerations and Monitoring
Oxacillin	Bacteremia, skin and skin structure infections, bone and joint infections, pneumonia, or endocarditis due to infections due to *Staphylococcus* sp.	*Adults*: 0.25–0.5 Gm IV or IM every 4–6 hr for mild to moderate infections and 1–2 Gm IV or IM every 4–6 hr for severe infections. *Children and adolescents ≥40 kg*: 0.25–0.5 Gm IV or IM every 4–6 hr for mild to moderate infections and 1 Gm IV or IM every 4–6 hr for severe infections. *Children and adolescents <40 kg*: 50 mg/kg/day IV or IM divided every 6 hr for mild to moderate infections and 100 mg/kg/day IV or IM divided every 4–6 hr for severe infections. *All neonates*: 25 mg/kg/day IV or IM.	No dosage adjustments for renal impairment. Maximum dosage limits: *Adults, older adults, and children ≥40 kg:* 6 Gm/day IV or IM. *Infants and children <40 kg*: 100 mg/kg/day IV or IM. *Neonates*: 25 mg/kg/day IV or IM.
	Bacterial meningitis	*Adults*: 2 Gm IV every 4 hr. *Children and adolescents ≥40 kg*: severe infections: 1 Gm IV every 4–6 hr. *Children and adolescents <40 kg*: severe infections: 100 mg/kg/day IV divided every 4–6 hr. *All neonates*: Age birth–7 days: 75 mg/kg/day IV divided every 8–12 hr (guideline dosing). Age 8–28 days: 150–200 mg/kg/day IV divided every 6–8 hr (guideline dosing). Age >28 days: 200 mg/kg/day IV divided every 6 hr (guideline dosing).	
	Pneumonia, community-acquired pneumonia	*Adults*: 0.25–0.5 Gm IV or IM every 4–6 hr for mild to moderate infections and 1 Gm IV or IM every 4–6 hr for severe infections. *Children and adolescents ≥40 kg*: 1 Gm IV or IM every 4–6 hr. *Infants 4–11 months, children, and adolescents <40 kg*: severe infections:100 mg/kg/day IV or IM divided every 4–6 hr. *Infants 1–3 months*: 100 mg/kg/day IV or IM divided every 4–6 hr for severe infections. *All neonates*: 25 mg/kg/day IV or IM.	
	Mastitis	*Adults*: 1–2 Gm IV every 4 hr for 10–14 days. *Infants 1–2 months*: 100–200 mg/kg/day IV divided every 4–6 hr. *Neonates*: refer to resources for alternate treatment recommendations.	
	Infective endocarditis	*Adults*: severe infections: 2 Gm IV every 6 hr. *Children and adolescents ≥40 kg*: severe infections: 1–2 Gm IV every 4–6 hr. *Children and adolescents <40 kg*: severe infections: 100 mg/kg/day IV divided every 4–6 hr. *All neonates*: 25 mg/kg/day IV.	

IM, Intramuscular; *IV*, intravenous.

by the biliary tract. Oxacillin distributes into bone, bile, the biliary tract, pleural and synovial fluids, inflamed meninges, and most organs of the body. It also crosses the placenta. Oxacillin and its metabolites are excreted primarily in the urine via tubular secretion and glomerular filtration. Approximately 30% of an oral oxacillin dose is absorbed, with peak serum levels occurring within 30 to 120 minutes. Oxacillin is classified as generally safe in pregnancy as animal studies have failed to reveal evidence of fetal harm and no adverse effects have been reported during human use.

Dicloxacillin is formulated for oral dosing only. Approximately 30% of a dose is metabolized by the liver. About 95% to 99% of the circulating drug is protein bound. Dicloxacillin is distributed into bone, bile, pleural and synovial fluids, and most organs in the body, and reaches minimal levels within the cerebrospinal fluid if uninflamed. It also crosses the placenta. Dicloxacillin is well absorbed from the gastrointestinal (GI) tract. Oral bioavailability is 35% to 76%, but generally less than 50%. Peak serum levels of dicloxacillin occur within 30 to 120 minutes following an oral dose. Food in the stomach inhibits the rate and extent of absorption, thus dicloxacillin should be taken on an empty stomach, preferably 1 hour prior to or 2 hours following a meal. Dicloxacillin and its metabolites are excreted into the urine primarily via tubular secretion and glomerular filtration. Dicloxacillin is classified as generally safe in pregnancy as animal studies have failed to reveal evidence of fetal harm and no adverse effects have been reported during human use.

Nafcillin achieves peak concentration within 5 minutes when administered intravenously and within 60 minutes when administered intramuscularly. Approximately 90% is protein bound. Between 60% and 70% of a nafcillin dose is metabolized by the liver to active and inactive metabolites; clearance is via the biliary tract (Avdic, 2018). Nafcillin distributes into bone, bile, the biliary tract, pleural and synovial fluids, inflamed meninges, and most organs of the body. It also crosses the placenta. Nafcillin is excreted primarily in the urine via tubular secretion and glomerular filtration. Approximately 30% of an oral dose is absorbed, with peak serum levels occurring within 30 to 120 minutes.

Indications. Oxacillin and nafcillin are indicated for bacteremia, skin and skin structure infections, bone and joint infections, pneumonia, and endocarditis due to staphylococcus (mostly *S. aureus*) infection, bacterial meningitis, pneumonia, community-acquired pneumonia, mastitis, and infective endocarditis. Dicloxacillin is indicated for the treatment of infections involving *S. aureus* (e.g., skin and soft tissue, bone and joint, and respiratory tract).

Adverse Effects. Interstitial nephritis (eosinophilia, hematuria, proteinuria, and renal insufficiency) infrequently occurs with oxacillin. Hepatotoxicity (e.g., fever, nausea, vomiting, and elevated liver function tests or LFTs), rash, and reversible neutropenia have been seen with oxacillin. Injection-site reaction following IM injections have occurred. Phlebitis may occur with IV administration. Nafcillin has been associated with hypokalemia and altered kidney function (Viehman et al., 2016).

Contraindications. Do not use narrow-spectrum penicillin in patients with hypersensitivity to penicillins. Prescribe with caution in patients with inflammatory bowel disease or other GI illnesses due to the potential for pseudomembranous colitis. As with other penicillin therapy, use with caution in patients with suspected cross-sensitivities to cephalosporin or carbapenem. Use with caution in patients

with preexisting hepatic dysfunction in patients who have tested positive for human immunodeficiency virus (HIV) as hepatotoxicity has been shown to be more common in this population. Use oxacillin cautiously in patients with fluid and electrolyte imbalance and those with heart failure or hypertension due to high sodium content.

Monitoring. Monitor complete blood count (CBC) with differential, LFTs, and renal function (serum creatinine/BUN and urinalysis). Decreased renal function may increase half-life with a subsequent increase in serum levels. Dose adjustments may be necessary in cases of severely decreased renal function for dicloxacillin.

Broad-Spectrum Penicillins: Aminopenicillins

With the addition of an amino group side chain, this group of penicillins has a broader spectrum of activity compared to the natural penicillins. Amoxicillin and ampicillin are the two aminopenicillins used in clinical practice today. They can be effective against infections caused by *Streptococci* spp., *Listeria monocytogenes*, *Enterococcus faecalis*, *Proteus mirabilis*, *E. coli*, *Salmonella* and *Shigella* species, *H. pylori*, *H. parainfluenzae*, and *H. influenzae*. The aminopenicillins are not effective against beta-lactamase–producing gram-positive and gram-negative bacteria. *Salmonella* and *Shigella* have rising rates of resistance and their use is often avoided for these infections.

The addition of beta-lactamase inhibitors such as sulbactam (ampicillin) and clavulanic acid (amoxicillin) extends the antimicrobial activity of ampicillin and amoxicillin to include some organisms that produce beta-lactamases (methicillin-susceptible *S. aureus* and coagulase-negative staphylococci, *H. influenzae*, *Enterobacteriaceae*, anaerobes, etc.). This combination makes them additionally effective against susceptible *Haemophilus influenzae*, *E. coli*, *Proteus mirabilis*, enterococci, and *Neisseria meningitidis* (penicillin sensitive). Over the past 40 years, *N. gonorrhoeae* strains have developed resistance to penicillin G, ampicillin, and amoxicillin (Geddes et al., 2018c). The spectrum is further broadened to have activity against anaerobic organisms such as *Clostridium* spp. (excluding *C. difficile*), *Peptococcus* spp., *Peptostreptococcus* spp., and *Bacteroides* spp. (including *B. fragilis*). Table 40.7 provides a summary of the broad-spectrum penicillins.

Ampicillin and Ampicillin/Sulbactam

Ampicillin was discovered in 1958 and became the first broad-spectrum semisynthetic penicillin in clinical use. When it is combined with a beta-lactamase inhibitor (e.g., sulbactam), antimicrobial activity is extended against some organisms that produce beta-lactamases. Sulbactam is only available in fixed-dose combinations with IV ampicillin. Sulbactam is a derivative of the penicillin that irreversibly binds to a beta-lactamase to prevent degradation of ampicillin. Sulbactam lacks significant antibacterial activity, except for cases of *Neisseria* spp. and *Acinetobacter baumannii*.

TABLE 40.7 Broad-Spectrum Penicillins: Aminopenicillins

Medication	Indication	Dosage	Considerations and Monitoring
Ampicillin	Respiratory tract infection (upper and lower)	*Adults:* 250 mg orally every 6 hr. *Children and adolescents:* 50–100 mg/kg/day orally divided every 6–8 hr. Maximum dosage: 1000 mg/day recommended by FDA. Maximum dosage: 2 Gm/day recommended by AAP.	FDA and AAP guideline dosing varies. Adults and pediatrics: renal impairment; see Table 40.2.
	Gonorrhea	*Adults:* 3.5 Gm orally as a single dose in conjunction with 1 Gm probenecid. *Children <20 kg:* 100 mg/kg/day orally divided every 6 hr. *Children >20 kg:* 3.5 Gm orally as a single dose in conjunction with 1 Gm probenecid.	
	Infections of digestive tract and genitourinary tract	*Adults:* 500 mg orally every 6 hr. *Infants, children, and adolescents:* 100 mg/kg/day orally every 6 hr. IV or IM dosages are based on weight. Refer to current guidelines.	
Ampicillin/ Sulbactam	Skin and skin structure infections	*Adults:* 1.5 Gm (1 Gm ampicillin and 0.5 Gm sulbactam) or 3 Gm (2 Gm ampicillin and 1 Gm sulbactam) IV or IM every 6 hr for 2–4 weeks. *Children and adolescents:* 100–200 mg/kg/day ampicillin component (300 mg/kg/day ampicillin; sulbactam) IV or IM divided every 6 hr for up to 14 days. *Adults, adolescents, and children:* Maximum dose: 2000 mg ampicillin/dose.	Renal impairment: see Table 40.2.
	Severe infection (e.g., meningitis, resistant streptococcus pneumonia)	*Children and adolescents:* 200–400 mg ampicillin/kg/day IV or IM divided every 6 hr. Maximum dose: 2000 mg ampicillin/dose.	
	Moderate to severe gynecologic infections or intraabdominal infections	*Adults:* 1.5 Gm (1 Gm ampicillin and 0.5 Gm sulbactam) or 3 Gm (2 Gm ampicillin and 1 Gm sulbactam) IV or IM every 6 hr. *Adolescents:* 3 Gm ampicillin/sulbactam IV every 6 hr with doxycycline.	
Amoxicillin	Upper respiratory tract infections, skin and/or subcutaneous tissue, general ear/nose/throat infections	**Oral immediate release:** *Adults: mild/moderate infections:* 500 mg orally every 12 hr or 250 mg orally every 8 hr. *Adults: severe infections:* 875 mg orally every 12 hr or 500 mg orally every 8 hr. *Infants and children >3 months (>40 kg): mild/moderate infections:* 250 mg orally every 8 hr or 500 mg orally every 12 hr. *Infants and children >3 months (<40 kg): mild/moderate infections:* 20 mg/kg/day orally in divided doses every 8 hr (maximum dose: 250 mg/dose) or 25 mg/kg/day orally in divided doses every 12 hr (maximum dose: 500 mg/dose). *Infants and children >3 months (>40 kg): severe infections:* 500 mg orally every 8 hr or 875 mg orally every 12 hr. *Neonates and infants ≤3 months:* 30 mg/kg/day orally given in divided doses every 12 hr.	Renal impairment: see Table 40.2.

Continued

Broad-Spectrum Penicillins: Aminopenicillins—cont'd

Medication	Indication	Dosage	Considerations and Monitoring
	Acute otitis media, uncomplicated	*Adults:* 500 mg orally every 12 hr or 250 mg orally every 8 hr for mild/moderate infections and 875 mg orally every 12 hr or 500 mg orally every 8 hr for severe infections.	
		Children 6 months–12 yr with mild/moderate infection: 80–90 mg/kg/day orally in 2 divided doses; duration of therapy is based on age of child; <2 yr, 10 days; 2–5 yr, 7 days; 6–12 yr, 5–7 days (guideline dosage).	
		Children 6 months–12 yr with severe infection: 80–90 mg/kg/day orally in 2 divided doses for 10 days (guideline dosage).	
	Pharyngitis, tonsillitis	**Oral extended release:**	
		Adults and adolescents ≥12 yr: 775 mg orally once daily, taken within 1 hr of finishing a meal, for 10 days.	
Amoxicillin/ Clavulanic acid	Acute otitis media, skin and/or subcutaneous tissue, sinusitis, UTI, lower respiratory tract infection	**Immediate-release tablet, suspension:**	Renal impairment: see Table 40.2.
		Adults and children >40 kg: mild/moderate infection: 250 mg (amoxicillin component) orally every 8 hr or 500 mg (amoxicillin component) orally every 12 hr for 5–7 days.	
		Immediate-release tablet, suspension:	
		Adults and children >40 kg: severe infection: 500 mg (amoxicillin component) orally every 8 hr or 875 mg (amoxicillin component) orally every 12 hr for 5–7 days.	
		Children <3 months: 125 mg/5 mL suspension: 30 mg/kg/day (amoxicillin component) orally divided every 12 hr.	
		Children >3 months and <40 kg: 125 mg/5 mL suspension or 250 mg/5 mL suspension, 125 mg or 250 mg chewable tablet: 20–40 mg/kg/day (amoxicillin component) orally divided every 8 hr for 10 days, depending on severity of infection.	
		Children >3 months and < 40 kg: 200 mg/5 mL or 400 mg/5 mL suspension, 200 mg or 400 mg chewable tablet: 25–45 mg/kg/day (amoxicillin component) orally divided every 12 hr for 10 days, depending on severity of infection.	
		Children >3 months: 600 mg/5 mL suspension, recurrent or persistent infection: 90 mg/kg/day (amoxicillin component) orally divided every 12 hr for 10 days.	
	Community acquired pneumonia, sinusitis	**Extended-release tablet containing 1000 mg amoxicillin and 62.5 mg clavulanate per tablet:**	
		Adults and adolescents >40 kg: 2 tablets (2000 mg amoxicillin component) orally every 12 hr for 5–10 days.	
		Children >3 months: 90 mg/kg/day (amoxicillin component) orally in 2 divided doses; for children ≥5 yr, maximum dosage is 4000 mg/day.	

AAP, American Academy of Pediatrics; *FDA,* U.S. Food and Drug Administration; *IM,* intramuscular; *IV,* intravenous; *UTI,* urinary tract infection.

Pharmacokinetics. Ampicillin is distributed into the lungs, liver, gallbladder, appendix, maxillary sinus, prostate, other tissues, and body fluids such as skin blisters, middle ear effusions, bronchial secretions, urine, and pleural, peritoneal, and synovial fluids. Ampicillin crosses to inflamed meninges, intestinal mucosa, the placenta, and breast milk. Renal excretion is primarily through tubular secretion and glomerular filtration. In patients with normal renal function, the elimination half-life of ampicillin is 60 to 90 minutes. Absorption varies depending on the route of administration.

When given orally, approximately 30% to 55% is absorbed. IV and IM routes depend on the milligram (mg) of dosing, with absorption rates of 40–150 mcg/mL. Peak serum concentrations of ampicillin occur almost immediately after a 15-minute IV infusion, within 1 hour after an IM dose, and within 1 to 2 hours after oral dosing.

Indications. Ampicillin is used primarily to treat infections caused by susceptible organisms. Infections include bacteremia, meningitis, upper and lower respiratory tract infections, skin and skin structure infections, GI infections, genitourinary tract infections, and infective endocarditis. Ampicillin/sulbactam is considered a drug of choice in patients with animal (e.g., dog and cat) bite wound infections. When indicated, oral ampicillin should be administered 1 hour before or 2 hours after a meal for maximal absorption.

Adverse Effects. Systemic effects have been noted within the central nervous system (CNS), GI system, skin, musculoskeletal system, liver and kidneys, and hematological system. The most common side effects associated with ampicillin are rash and diarrhea. The concern for cross-sensitivity is likely associated with similarities in side chains. For example, ampicillin's side chain is identical to the cephalosporins cephalexin and cefaclor and amoxicillin's to cefadroxil and cefprozil, respectively (Geddes et al., 2018c). Patients who are allergic to penicillin may be allergic to aminopenicillins, but that is not always the case, and allergic reactions can wane with time (Geddes et al., 2018c). Consult an allergist for consideration of an oral-graded challenge or desensitization if use is warranted in patients with high suspicion for an allergic reaction. In 40% to 100% of patients with susceptible infections and concurrent mononucleosis, nonallergic rashes (generalized, maculopapular, and pruritic) similar to an IgE-mediated allergic reaction have been reported. This rash, due to administration of ampicillin in patients with mononucleosis, appears to be temporary and does not recur if these same patients receive the antibiotic after recovery from their viral illness (Geddes et al., 2018c). Oral ampicillin is more likely to cause adverse GI effects such as diarrhea. Sulbactam has minimal toxicity concerns, and any adverse effects occurring with the combination formula are due to the penicillin classification.

Contraindications. Avoid in all patients with a hypersensitivity to penicillin or a beta-lactamase. Ampicillin should not be used in patients in which susceptibility has not been determined or in those with viral infection. Use with caution in patients at risk for *C. diff*-associated diarrhea and pseudomembranous colitis.

Monitoring. Monitor renal status (serum creatinine and BUN) as well as hepatic (LFTs) and hematologic function. Table 40.2 details the ampicillin and ampicillin/sulbactam monitoring and dose adjustments required for adult and pediatric patients based on CrCl levels and GFRs. Observe signs and symptoms of anaphylaxis during administration of the first dose. Monitor patients for adverse reactions that may occur during ampicillin therapy. Monitor for AGEP that may occur 2 to 3 weeks after the initial dose.

Amoxicillin and Amoxicillin/Clavulanic Acid

Amoxicillin is the second most used medication within the broad-spectrum semisynthetic beta-lactam antibiotics. Oral amoxicillin is more stable to gastric acid than oral ampicillin, which makes amoxicillin the drug of choice. This enhanced gastric stability increases the bioavailability of the drug and lowers the incidence of diarrhea. When oral therapy is indicated, amoxicillin is preferred. Amoxicillin is also available in combination with a fixed-dose of clavulanic acid, an inhibitor of bacterial beta-lactamases. The addition of clavulanic acid increases the incidence of GI adverse effects compared with amoxicillin alone (Gordon, 2018). Amoxicillin and amoxicillin/clavulanic acid are the drugs of choice for initial treatment of acute otitis media and acute bacterial sinusitis.

Pharmacokinetics. Amoxicillin is widely distributed into most body mucosa, tissues, bones, organs, and fluids, including inflamed meninges. Bioavailability ranges from 74% to 92% due to enhanced gastric stability. Excretion occurs through tubular secretion and glomerular filtration, with approximately 60% of the drug excreted within 6 to 8 hours. With normal renal function, the half-life is approximately 60 to 90 minutes. Peak concentrations of amoxicillin and amoxicillin/clavulanic acid are reached approximately 1 hour and approximately 3 hours after administration, respectively.

Indications. Amoxicillin and amoxicillin/clavulanic acid are available in immediate- and extended-release formulations with similar spectrum activity as ampicillin and ampicillin/sulbactam (excluding *A. baumannii*). Treatment indications include upper and lower respiratory tract infections (community-acquired pneumonia, pharyngitis, tonsillitis), skin and skin structure infections, urinary tract infections or UTIs (e.g., cystitis), and *H. pylori*. Amoxicillin is not recommended for empiric use for UTIs due to high rates of resistance to *E. coli* and poor efficacy. Amoxicillin is not recommended for treatment of gonorrhea due to high rates of resistance. Amoxicillin/clavulanic acid is considered a drug of choice in patients with animal (dog and cat) bite wound infections. Infants younger than 3 months of age require modified dosages because of incompletely developed renal function.

Adverse Effects. The concern for cross-sensitivity is likely associated with similarities in side chains. For example, amoxicillin's side chain is identical to cefadroxil and cefprozil (Geddes et al., 2018c). Patients who are allergic to penicillin may be allergic to aminopenicillins, but that is not always the case, and allergic reactions can wane with time. Episodes of oral candidiasis or vaginal candidiasis may occur. Amoxicillin use during early childhood has been associated with developmental defects (tooth discoloration) affecting permanent teeth (Hong et al., 2011). Discoloration was eliminated or improved with brushing or dental cleaning in the majority of cases.

Contraindications. Amoxicillin and amoxicillin/clavulanic acid are contraindicated in patients with an IgE-mediated penicillin hypersensitivity. Consult an allergist for consideration of an oral-graded challenge or desensitization if use is warranted in patients with high suspicion for an allergic reaction. Exercise caution when prescribing to patients with hypersensitivities to cephalosporin or carbapenem or who have allergies or atopic conditions including asthma, eczema, hives, or hay fever. Avoid use in patients with mononucleosis as a high incidence of skin rashes has been reported in these patients. Amoxicillin/clavulanic acid is contraindicated for use in any patient with a previous history of drug-induced cholestasis, jaundice, or preexisting hepatic disease. Do not use the extended-release tablet in patients with CrCl levels of 30 mL/min or less. The use of amoxicillin may lead to false-negative diagnostic testing for *H. pylori*, so it is recommended to avoid the use of amoxicillin in the 4 weeks prior to diagnostic testing. In patients with phenylketonuria, the use of chewable tablets is contraindicated because this preparation contains phenylalanine. Primary care providers should consider an alternate route of administration.

Monitoring. Monitor renal and liver function during therapy. Monitor for adverse effects, particularly hypersensitivity reactions during the first dose. Dosage adjustments are recommended in patients with CrCl levels of 30 mL/min or less and in patients who are receiving dialysis.

Extended-Spectrum Penicillins: Ureidopenicillins

Piperacillin/Tazobactam

Piperacillin is a broad-spectrum, semisynthetic beta-lactam antibiotic available with a fixed-dose combination of tazobactam, a beta-lactamase inhibitor. Combining piperacillin with tazobactam extends the antimicrobial spectrum to include some organisms that produce beta-lactamases (*S. aureus, H. influenzae, Enterobacteriaceae*, etc.). Similar to some other beta-lactamase inhibitors, tazobactam has minimal toxicity concerns. Adverse effects that occur with the

combination products are due to the penicillin component. Table 40.8 provides a summary of the extended-spectrum penicillins.

Pharmacokinetics. Piperacillin/tazobactam used to be available only as a 30-minute IV infusion. However, 3-hour extended-infusion piperacillin-tazobactam therapy has gained traction over the past decade to maximize the pharmacokinetics compared to intermittent-infusion administration (Lodise et al., 2007), particularly in critically ill patients with gram-negative infections (Chen et al., 2019). Widespread drug distribution into tissues and body fluids (blisters, urine, peritoneal, pleural, middle ear) includes inflamed meninges, intestinal mucosa, lung, female reproductive tissues (uterus, ovary, and fallopian tube), interstitial fluid, and bile (Teng & Thursky, 2018). Excretion occurs primarily through tubular secretion and glomerular filtration. Peak serum concentrations are immediate. In patients with hepatic or renal failure, the half-life of piperacillin/tazobactam increases as organ function decreases. Pediatric patients with renal impairment require dose adjustments, and these are outlined in Table 40.2.

Indications. Piperacillin/tazobactam is indicated for the treatment of serious hospital-acquired infections, intraabdominal infections, polymicrobial skin and soft-tissue infections, and febrile neutropenia. Piperacillin/tazobactam is often considered a first-line treatment option for infections involving *Pseudomonas aeruginosa*. The spectrum is further broadened to have activity against more gram-negative organisms (e.g., *Enterobacteriaceae*), anaerobic organisms such as *Clostridium* spp. (excluding *C. difficile*), *Peptococcus* spp., *Peptostreptococcus* spp., and *Bacteroides* spp. (including *B. fragilis*).

Adverse Effects. Piperacillin/tazobactam is generally well tolerated, but the most common adverse effects are GI and dermatologic in nature. These may induce *C. difficile* colitis, but this is less common compared to aminopenicillins and third-generation cephalosporins (Teng & Thursky, 2018). The piperacillin/tazobactam combination product contains a total of 2.79 mEq (64 mg) of sodium per gram of

TABLE 40.8	**Extended-Spectrum Penicillins: Ureidopenicillins**		
Medication	**Indication**	**Dosage**	**Considerations and Monitoring**
Piperacillin/ tazobactam	Intra-abdominal infections, community acquired pneumonia, hospital acquired pneumonia, skin and/ or subcutaneous tissue infections, gynecological infections	*Adults and children >40 kg*: 3.375 Gm IV every 6 hr (total daily dose: 12 Gm piperacillin/1.5 Gm tazobactam) for 7–10 days. *Children ≥9 months and <40 kg*: piperacillin 100 mg/tazobactam 12.5 mg/kg IV every 8 hr for 7–10 days. *Children 2–9 months*: piperacillin 80 mg/tazobactam 10 mg/kg IV every 8 hr for 7–10 days.	Renal impairment: see Table 40.2.

IV, Intravenous.

piperacillin, which may lead to hypernatremia in patients receiving high doses of the drug and may subsequently cause further electrolyte disturbances such as hypokalemia. Platelet dysfunction and prolonged bleeding time may occur because piperacillin can bind to platelets to prevent aggregation. In a small number of patients (1% or less), reports of adverse effects also include hepatitis, jaundice, and elevated hepatic enzymes.

Contraindications. Piperacillin/tazobactam is contraindicated in patients with penicillin or beta-lactamase hypersensitivity. Consult an allergist for consideration for graded-challenge or desensitization if use is warranted in patients with high suspicion for an allergic reaction. Use with caution in patients with restricted salt intake and renal impairment or renal failure, because the drug is eliminated via renal mechanisms.

Monitoring. Dosage adjustments are required in patients with renal impairment or in those who are receiving dialysis. Monitor creatinine, BUN, CBC with differential, prothrombin time, partial thromboplastin time, serum electrolytes, LFTs, and urinalysis. Also monitor for signs of bleeding, and for signs of anaphylaxis during first dose.

PRACTICE PEARLS

Life Span Considerations With Penicillin Therapy

- Infants: Penicillins are generally considered safe, though transmission through breastfeeding does occur. Be alert for hypersensitivity reactions.
- Children and adolescents: Penicillins are considered safe and are commonly used for bacterial infections.
- Pregnancy and breastfeeding: Penicillins are generally safe in pregnancy as animal studies have failed to reveal evidence of fetal harm and no adverse effects have been reported during human use. Penicillins do enter breast milk. Recommendations are to use only if clearly needed.
- Older adults: Dose adjustments may be required due to changes in drug metabolism and excretion (e.g., renal function).

Prescriber Considerations for Penicillin Therapy

Clinical Practice Guidelines

The ability of the health care provider to access and utilize treatment guidelines improves patient outcomes. Treatment guidelines for the use of penicillins are available from several national organizations, including the Infectious Diseases Society of America, the Pediatric Infectious Disease Society, the American Academy of Pediatrics, the American Academy of Family Practice Physicians, the American Heart Association, and the American Thoracic Society.

BOOKMARK THIS!

Clinical Guidelines for Penicillin Therapy[a]

- Infectious Diseases Society of America: Updated Guideline on Group A Streptococcal Pharyngitis (http://news.idsociety.org/idsa/issues/2012-09-27/13.html)
- 2021 Sexually Transmitted Diseases Treatment Guidelines (https://www.cdc.gov/std/treatment-guidelines/syphilis.htm)
- Antibiotic Use for Community Acquired Pneumonia (CAP) in Neonates and Children: 2016 Evidence Update (https://www.who.int/selection_medicines/committees/expert/21/applications/s6_paed_antibiotics_appendix3_cap.pdf)
- Diagnosis and Treatment of Adults with Community-Acquired Pneumonia. An Official Clinical Practice Guideline of the American Thoracic Society and Infectious Diseases Society of America (https://www.idsociety.org/practice-guideline/community-acquired-pneumonia-cap-in-adults/)

[a] **NOTE:** This is not an exhaustive list of practice guidelines.

Clinical Reasoning for Penicillin Therapy

Consider the individual patient's health problem requiring penicillin therapy. Identification of the infecting organism, sensitivity of the organism to the penicillin, and the patient's clinical status should be considered prior to prescribing these agents.

Determine the desired therapeutic outcome based on the patient's health problem. Antibiotic therapy is primarily used to treat active infectious diseases. In some cases, the use of prophylaxis therapy is recommended. Guidelines recommend the use of prophylactic penicillin therapy for the following:

- A subset of select patients undergoing dental procedures
- The prevention of bacterial infections in children with sickle cell disease (Nishimura, 2017; Witherspoon & Drotar, 2006)
- Patients at increased risk of developing infective endocarditis and at high risk of experiencing adverse outcomes from infective endocarditis (Matiasz & Rigolin, 2018)
- Individuals with complement deficiencies who are on agents that may increase their risk for meningococcal disease (e.g., eculizumab)

Assess the selected penicillin for its appropriateness for an individual patient by considering the medication's side effects and the patient's age, race/ethnicity, comorbidities, and genetic factors. Before initiating penicillin therapy, a clinical evaluation of the patient is suggested. Parameters include allergies to the selected penicillin, susceptibility of the organism, comorbidities such as renal impairment/failure, and the risk of other adverse effects.

Initiate the treatment plan with the selected medication by first providing adequate patient education to ensure the patient's understanding and promote full participation in the penicillin therapy. Patient education regarding the use of penicillin therapies includes the need to complete the full course of antibiotics even when the patient begins to feel better.

Ensure complete patient and family understanding about the medication prescribed using a variety of education strategies. The CDC provides a variety of patient handouts and electronic messaging related to antibiotic use and stewardship. Written instructions should include the name, dose, length of time (number of days or doses), route (if oral, whether to take with or without food), and adverse effects that should be reported to the health-care provider.

Conduct follow-up and monitoring of patient responses to penicillin therapy. The effectiveness of penicillin therapy is monitored by clinical reassessment (e.g., improvement in or resolution of signs and symptoms of an infectious disease). Monitor patient status for adverse and/or early signs of toxic effects.

Teaching Points for Penicillin Therapy

Health Promotion Strategies

Improving health outcomes while decreasing antibiotic resistance is a key point in antibiotic stewardship. Health-care providers and patients play a role in antibiotic stewardship.

Provider strategies include the following:
- Prescribe antibiotics only when indicated.
- Educate patients on the public health risks associated with inappropriate antibiotic use.

Patient strategies include the following:
- Complete the entire course of antibiotics.
- Do not take medications prescribed to others.
- Follow up with your health-care provider as directed.

Patient Education for Medication Safety

Medication safety begins with patient education that includes how, when, and why to take the prescribed medication, what information the provider needs, and when to contact the provider. The following points should be addressed when prescribing penicillin antibiotics:
- Amoxicillin, amoxicillin/clavulanic acid: oral preparations may be taken with meals, milk, formula, or juice, or on an empty stomach. Taking with meals may decrease GI upset.
- Take all of the doses of your medicine as directed. Do not skip doses or stop your medicine early.
- Have your blood or urine checked as requested by your provider.
- Store all drugs at room temperature in a dry place unless otherwise instructed.
- Protect medications from light.
- Keep all drugs out of the reach of children and pets.
- Tell your provider:
  - If you have an allergic reaction to amoxicillin, other penicillins, cephalosporin antibiotics, other

medicines, foods, dyes, or preservatives; if you have asthma; and if you have kidney disease
- If you develop any signs of an adverse reaction such as breathing problems; change in urine color or trouble urinating; watery diarrhea or black, tarry stool; bleeding or bruising; change in color of the eyes; or peeling, redness, or blistering of the mouth or skin
- If you have a history of phenylketonuria, as some chewable tablets contain phenylalanine
- If you are pregnant, are trying to get pregnant, or are breastfeeding
- If your symptoms do not improve in 2 or 3 days or if they become worse.
- If you are diabetic; certain brands of urine glucose test strips may read as a false positive
- About all of the prescription drugs, OTC drugs, natural products, and/or vitamins you are currently taking
- Birth control pills may not work properly while on this medication. Concomitant use of antibiotics and combination contraceptives may result in decreased contraceptive efficacy; however, significant differences in contraceptive failure rates were not demonstrated during a study of oral contraceptives with or without antibiotics and no significant difference in exposure was observed with the use of the vaginal ring. If a typical failure rate of 1% to 3% is a concern, consider additional forms of birth control.
- Do not treat diarrhea with OTC products. Contact your doctor if you have diarrhea that lasts more than 2 days or if the diarrhea is severe and watery.

Application Questions for Discussion

1. Are penicillins safe and effective for the treatment of viral infections?
2. What are the considerations for prescribing penicillins to patients with a previously documented allergy to this class of drug?
3. What factors should be considered when educating the patient on prophylactic penicillin therapy?

Selected Bibliography

Avdic, E. (2018). Nafcillin. In M. L. Grayson, S. E. Cosgrove, S. M. Crowe, W. Hope, J. S. McCarthy, J. Mills, J. W. Mouton, & D. L. Patterson (Eds.), *Kucers' the Use of Antibiotics (e-book): A Clinical Review of Antibacterial, Antifungal, Antiparasitic and Antiviral Drugs* (7th ed.). Boca Raton, FL: CRC Press, Taylor & Francis Group.

Baietto, L., Corcione, S., Pacini, G., Di Perri, G., D'Avolio, A., & De Rosa, F. G. (2014). A 30-years review on pharmacokinetics of antibiotics: Is the right time for pharmacogenetics? *Current Drug Metabolism, 15*(6), 581–598. https://doi.org/10.2174/1389200215666140605130935.

Bhattacharya, S. (2010). The facts about penicillin allergy: A review. *Journal of Advanced Pharmaceutical Technology and Research, 1*(1), 11–17. Retrieved from https://www.ncbi.nlm.nih.gov/pmc/articles/PMC3255391/.

Centers for Disease Control and Prevention. (2021, July 22). *Sexually transmitted infections treatment guidelines, 2021: Syphilis during pregnancy.* https://www.cdc.gov/std/treatment-guidelines/syphilis-pregnancy.htm.

Chen, M., Buurma, V., Shah, M., & Fahim, G. (2019). Evaluation of studies on extended versus standard infusion of beta-lactam antibiotics. *American Journal of Health-System Pharmacy, 76*(18), 1383–1394. https://doi.org/10.1093/ajhp/zxz154.

Geddes, A. M., Gould, I. M., Roberts, J. A., Trubiano, J. A., & Grayson, M. L (2018a). Benzylpenicillin (Penicillin G). In M. L. Grayson, S. E. Cosgrove, S. M. Crowe, W. Hope, J. S. McCarthy, J. Mills, J. W. Mouton, & D. L. Patterson (Eds.), *Kucers' the Use of Antibiotics (e-book): A Clinical Review of Antibacterial, Antifungal, Antiparasitic and Antiviral Drugs* (7th ed.). Boca Raton, FL: CRC Press, Taylor & Francis Group.

Geddes, A. M., Gould, I. M., Roberts, J. A., Grayson, A. L., & Cosgrove, S. E (2018b). Ampicillin and amoxicillin. In M. L. Grayson, S. E. Cosgrove, S. M. Crowe, W. Hope, J. S. McCarthy, J. Mills, J. W. Mouton, & D. L. Patterson (Eds.), *Kucers' the Use of Antibiotics (e-book): A Clinical Review of Antibacterial, Antifungal, Antiparasitic and Antiviral Drugs* (7th ed.). Boca Raton, FL: CRC Press, Taylor & Francis Group.

Geddes, A. M., Gould, I. M., & Roberts, J. A. (2018c). Phenoxypenicillins. In M. L. Grayson, S. E. Cosgrove, S. M. Crowe, W. Hope, J. S. McCarthy, J. Mills, J. W. Mouton, & D. L. Patterson (Eds.), *Kucers' the Use of Antibiotics (e-book): A Clinical Review of Antibacterial, Antifungal, Antiparasitic and Antiviral Drugs* (7th ed.). Boca Raton, FL: CRC Press, Taylor & Francis Group.

Gordon, D (2018). Amoxicillin-clavulanic acid. In M. L. Grayson, S. E. Cosgrove, S. M. Crowe, W. Hope, J. S. McCarthy, J. Mills, J. W. Mouton, & D. L. Patterson (Eds.), *Kucers' the Use of Antibiotics (e-book): A Clinical Review of Antibacterial, Antifungal, Antiparasitic and Antiviral Drugs* (7th ed.). Boca Raton, FL: CRC Press, Taylor & Francis Group.

Hong, L., Levy, S. M., Warren, J. J., & Broffitt, B. (2011). Amoxicillin use during early childhood and fluorosis of later developing tooth zones. *Journal of Public Health Dentistry, 71*(3), 229–235. https://doi.org/10.1111/j.1752-7325.2011.00254.x.

Joint Task Force on Practice Parameters. American Academy of Allergy, Asthma and Immunology; American College of Allergy, Asthma and Immunology; Joint Council of Allergy, Asthma and Immunology. (2010). Drug allergy: An updated practice parameter. *Annals of Allergy, Asthma, & Immunology, 105*(4), 259-273. Retrieved from https://www.aaaai.org/Aaaai/media/MediaLibrary/PDF%20Documents/Practice%20and%20Parameters/drug-allergy-updated-practice-param.pdf.

Lodise, Jr. T. P., Lomaestrod, B., & Drusano, G. L (2007). Piperacillin-tazobactam for pseudomonas aeruginosa infection: Clinical implications of an extended-infusion dosing strategy. *Clinical Infectious Diseases, 44*(3), 357–363. https://doi.org/10.1086/510590.

Matiasz, R., & Rigolin, V. H. (2018). 2017 focused update for management of patients with valvular heart disease: Summary of new recommendations. *Journal of the American Heart Association, 7*(1), Article e007596. http://doi.org/10.1161/JAHA.117.007596.

Nishimura, R. A., Otto, C. M., Bonow, R. O., Carabello, B. A., Erwin, J. P.3rd, Fleisher, L. A., Jneid, H., Mack, M. J., McLeod, C. J., O'Gara, P. T., Rigolin, V. H., Sundt, T. M.3rd, & Thompson, A. (2017). AHA/ACC focused update of the 2014 AHA/ACC guideline for the management of patients with valvular heart disease. *Journal of the American College of Cardiology, 70*(2), 252–289. Retrieved from http://dx.doi.org/10.1016/j.jacc.2017.03.011.

Shatsky, M. (2009). Evidence for the use of intramuscular injections in outpatient practice. *American Family Physician, 79*(4), 297–300. Retrieved from https://www.aafp.org/afp/2009/0215/p297.pdf.

Shulman, S. T., Bisno, A. L., Clegg, H. W., Gerber, M. A., Kaplan, E. L., Lee, G., Martin, J. M., & Van Beneden, C. (2012). Clinical practice guideline for the diagnosis and management of group A streptococcal pharyngitis: 2012 Update by the Infectious Diseases Society of America. *Clinical Infectious Diseases, 55*(10), 1279–1282. https://doi.org/10.1093/cid/cis629.

Smith, J. M. (2018). Isoxazolyl penicillins: oxacillin, cloxacillin, dicloxacillin, and flucloxacillin. In M. L. Grayson, S. E. Cosgrove, S. M. Crowe, W. Hope, J. S. McCarthy, J. Mills, J. W. Mouton, & D. L. Patterson (Eds.), *Kucers' the Use of Antibiotics (e-book): A Clinical Review of Antibacterial, Antifungal, Antiparasitic and Antiviral Drugs* (7th ed.). Boca Raton, FL: CRC Press, Taylor & Francis Group.

Teng, J., & Thursky, K (2018). Piperacillin-tazobactam. In M. L. Grayson, S. E. Cosgrove, S. M. Crowe, W. Hope, J. S. McCarthy, J. Mills, J. W. Mouton, & D. L. Patterson (Eds.), *Kucers' the Use of Antibiotics (e-book): A Clinical Review of Antibacterial, Antifungal, Antiparasitic and Antiviral Drugs* (7th ed.). Boca Raton, FL: CRC Press, Taylor & Francis Group.

Viehman, J. A., Oleksiuk, L, M., Sheridan, K., R., Byers, K. E., He, P., Falcione, B. A., & Shields, R. K (2016). Adverse events lead to drug discontinuation more commonly among patients who receive nafcillin than among those who receive oxacillin. *Antimicrobial Agents and Chemotherapy, 60*(5), 3090–3095. https://doi.org/10.1128/AAC.03122-15.

Witherspoon, D., & Drotar, D. (2006). Correlates of adherence to prophylactic penicillin therapy in children with sickle cell disease. *Journal of Children's Health Care, 35*(4), 281–296. https://doi.org/10.1207/s15326888chc3504_1.

41

Cephalosporins

REBECCA M. LUTZ

Overview

In 1945, Giuseppe Brotzu isolated the fungus *Cephalosporium acremonium* (now known as *Acremonium chrysogenum*). This fungus was effective against the gram-negative *Salmonella typhi*, which caused typhoid fever. Over the next two decades, new cephalosporin antibiotics were derived from the original fungal sample. The first cephalosporin was brought to market in the 1960s.

Cephalosporins are semisynthetic, broad-spectrum bactericidal antibiotics. They are beta-lactam antibiotics with the ability to resist beta-lactamase. The nucleus is a beta-lactam ring attached to a six-member sulfur-containing dihydrodaidzein ring (Fig. 41.1). Cephalosporin antibiotics bind to penicillin-binding proteins (PBPs). Their actions inhibit bacterial cell wall synthesis and activate autolysins, which causes lysis, leading to cell death. Their low toxicity makes them well tolerated. Unfortunately, this tolerance has led to their widespread use. Table 41.1 provides a list of indications and susceptible bacteria.

Pharmacokinetics

Drug distribution occurs in the urine and the pleural, peritoneal, synovial, and pericardial fluids. Variability in half-life, absorption, elimination, and central nervous system (CNS) penetration exists among the drugs. Cephalosporins are primarily excreted by the kidneys. Dose adjustment is required depending on the creatinine clearance (CrCl). Table 41.2 provides the parameters for dose adjustments.

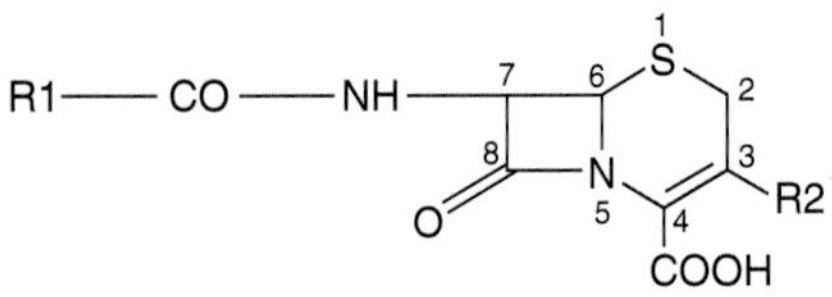

• **Fig. 41.1** Structure of cephalosporin. (From Kalman, D., & Barriere, S. L. [1990]. Review of the pharmacology, pharmacokinetics, and clinical use of cephalosporins. *Texas Heart Institute Journal, 17*[3], 203–215. Available at https://europepmc.org/backend/ptpmcrender.fcgi?accid=PMC324918&blobtype=pdf.)

Commonalities exist primarily in the areas of adverse effects and cross-reactivity, contraindications, and monitoring parameters. Drug–drug interactions are noted in Table 41.3.

Allergic Reactions and Cross-Reactivity

Cephalosporins can cause IgE-mediated reactions. Severe type-1 anaphylactic reactions are rare. Symptoms include urticaria, angioedema, and anaphylactic shock. This type of reaction happens within minutes of administration.

More common adverse reactions in both adult and pediatric patients include a maculopapular rash, nausea, vomiting, diarrhea, and itching (Miller et al., 2011;

TABLE 41.1	Therapeutic Indications and Susceptible Bacteria	
Indications	**Susceptible Bacteria**
Mild to moderate respiratory tract infections: Acute maxillary sinusitis Acute bacterial exacerbations of chronic bronchitis and secondary infections of acute bronchitis Community-acquired pneumonia	*Streptococcus pneumoniae, Haemophilus influenzae, H. parainfluenzae, Moraxella catarrhalis*
Acute bacterial otitis media	*S. pneumoniae, H. influenzae, M. catarrhalis*
Pharyngitis and tonsillitis	*Streptococcus pyogenes* (group A beta-hemolytic streptococci)
Mild to moderate skin and skin structure infections	Susceptible staphylococci or streptococci
Mild to moderate urinary tract infections	*E. coli, Klebsiella, Proteus mirabilis*
Uncomplicated gonorrhea	*Neisseria gonorrhoeae*

TABLE 41.2   Recommended Dose Adjustments Based on Creatinine Clearance

Cephalosporin Generation	Medication	Creatinine Clearance	Dose Adjustment
First Generation	**Cephalexin**	≥60 mL/min	None
		30–59 mL/min	None; do not exceed 1 Gm/day
		15–29 mL/min	250 mg every 8 to 12 hr
		5–14 mL/min and not yet on dialysis	250 mg every 24 hr
		1–4 mL/min and not yet on dialysis	250 mg every 48 to 60 hr
	Cefadroxil	≥50 mL/min	No dose adjustment necessary
		25–50 mL/min	Administer every 12 hr
		10–24 mL/min	Administer every 24 hr
		0–9 mL/min	Administer every 36 hr
Second Generation	**Cefprozil**	<30 mL/min	50% of standard dose at the usual interval
Third Generation	**Cefdinir**	*Adults:* <30 mL/min	300 mg daily
		Children: <30 mL/min/1.73 m^2	7 mg/kg once daily (up to 300 mg/day)
	Cefixime	>60 mL/min	None
		21–59 mL/min	*Adults and pediatrics:* Do not use tablet or chewable tablet *Adults: Oral suspension:* Reduce recommended dose by approximately 35%. *Pediatrics:* No specific recommendations. Consider using adult recommendations to reduce recommended dose by approximately 35%.
		≤20 mL/min	*Adults: Reduce recommended dose by approximately 50%.* *Pediatrics:* No specific recommendations. Consider using adult recommendations to reduce recommended dose by approximately 50%.
	Ceftibuten	>50 mL/min	None
		30–49 mL/min	200 mg every 24 hr or 4.5 mg/kg every 24 hr
		5–29 mL/min	100 mg every 24 hr or 2.25 mg/kg every 24 hr
	Ceftriaxone	Renal impairment	None
		Renal and hepatic impairment	Do not exceed 2 Gm/day

Bhattacharya, 2010). Adverse effects common to all cephalosporins are found in Table 41.4.

Cross-reactions between individual cephalosporins may occur. Cross-reactions between cephalosporins, penicillins, and aminopenicillins also occur. These types of reactions are related to similarities between the R1 side chains (Chaudhry et al., 2019; Bhattacharya, 2010). Prior to prescribing a cephalosporin to a penicillin-allergic patient, the health care provider should review the reported penicillin reaction and consider skin testing (Joint Task Force on Practice Parameters et al., 2010). The American Academy of Pediatrics endorsed the use of cephalosporins for the treatment of acute bacterial sinusitis and acute otitis media in patients with allergies to penicillin (Pichichero, 2005). The patient should be observed for signs and symptoms of anaphylaxis during the first dose.

TABLE 41.3 Drug–Drug Interactions With Cephalosporins

Medication	Effects
Antacids containing magnesium or aluminum Iron supplements	Decreased absorption of cephalosporin
Carbamazepine	Elevated levels with concomitant administration
Diuretics	Concomitant administration adversely affects renal function
Probenecid	Increasesd half-life and excretion of cephalosporin
Live vaccines	Decreased immunologic response to vaccine
Warfarin and anticoagulants	Increased risk of bleeding

TABLE 41.4 Common Adverse Effects of Cephalosporins

Body System Affected	Common Adverse Effects
Hypersensitivity	Anaphylaxis, angioedema, erythema multiforme or erythema nodosum, exfoliative dermatitis, fever, maculopapular rash Stevens-Johnson syndrome, toxic epidermal necrolysis
Dermatologic	Cutaneous moniliasis, diaphoresis, flushing, urticaria
Cardiovascular	Chest pain, hypotension, palpitations, syncope, tachycardia, vasodilation
Gastrointestinal	Abdominal cramps and pain, anorexia, *C. difficile*–associated diarrhea, colitis including pseudomembranous colitis, constipation, diarrhea, dyspepsia, flatulence, glossitis, ileus, melena, nausea, peptic ulcer, thirst, upper GI bleeding, vomiting
Genitourinary	Dysuria, hematuria, interstitial nephritis
Hemic and lymphatic	Agranulocytosis, aplastic anemia, eosinophilia, hemolytic anemia, neutropenia, pancytopenia, thrombocytopenia
Hepatic	Cholestasis; elevations in SGPT, SGOT, alkaline phosphatase; hepatomegaly; hepatitis; jaundice
Metabolic and nutritional	Glucosuria
Musculoskeletal	Arthralgia, muscle cramps, myalgia, stiffness or spasms, rhabdomyolysis
Nervous system	Anxiety, confusion, dizziness, fatigue, headache, hyperactivity, hypertonia, insomnia, lethargy, nervousness, paresthesia, somnolence, vertigo
Renal	Elevations in BUN and creatinine, renal failure, toxic nephropathy
Respiratory	Asthma, bronchospasm, dyspnea, interstitial pneumonitis, pneumonia, rhinitis

BUN, Blood urea nitrogen; *SGOT*, serum glutamic oxaloacetic transaminase; *SGPT*, serum glutamic pyruvic transaminase.

Contraindications and Precautions to Cephalosporins

Cephalosporins in general are considered safe and do not require drug-level monitoring.

Alterations in gastrointestinal (GI) flora may lead to an overgrowth of *Clostridium (C.) difficile*, which may lead to a wide range of adverse outcomes including increased morbidity and mortality. Health care providers are encouraged to monitor all patients with known GI diseases, particularly colitis.

PRACTICE PEARLS

Cephalosporin Use in Pregnancy and Lactation

- Evidence is inconclusive or is inadequate for determining fetal risk when used in patients who are pregnant or of childbearing potential. Weigh the potential benefits of drug treatment against the potential risks before prescribing this drug during pregnancy.
- Cephalosporins cross the placenta and are excreted in breast milk.
- Maternal medication is usually compatible with breastfeeding.

Cephalosporin Therapy

Each successive group of cephalosporins is called a *generation*. The oral preparations of the first-, second-, and third-generation cephalosporins are the most commonly used in the primary care setting. Ceftriaxone sodium, a third-generation cephalosporin, is also used in a parenteral formulation in primary care settings. Table 41.5 provides dosing recommendations for the first-, second-, and third-generation cephalosporins.

First Generation

First-generation cephalosporins (e.g., oral: cephalexin, cefadroxil) are highly effective against gram-positive bacteria. The efficacy of first-generation cephalosporins against gram-negative bacteria and their resistance to beta-lactamases is low compared to the future generations. There is no CNS penetration. Therapeutic use includes the treatment of infections of the skin and soft tissue, urinary tract, throat, ear, and lower respiratory system.

TABLE 41.5 Recommended Dosing of First-, Second-, and Third-Generation Cephalosporins

Cephalosporin Generation	Medication	Indications	Dosage	Considerations and Monitoring
First Generation	Cephalexin	Upper and lower respiratory tract infections	*Adults:* 250 mg every 6 hr or 500 mg every 12 hr orally for 7–14 days. Maximum dosage: 4 Gm/day. *Adolescents and children:* 25–100 mg/kg orally in divided doses for 7–14 days. Maximum dosage: 2 Gm/day.	Renal impairment: see Table 41.2. Not FDA approved for use in infants.
		Community-acquired pneumonia, otitis media	*Adolescents and children:* 75–100 mg/kg/day orally in divided doses for 10 days. Maximum dosage: 4 Gm/day.	
		Bone and joint infections	*Adults:* 250 mg every 6 hr or 500 mg every 12 hr orally for 7–14 days. Maximum dosage: 4 Gm/day. *Adolescents and children:* 50–100 mg/kg/day orally in divided doses for 10 days. Maximum dosage: 4 Gm/day.	
		Skin and skin structure infections, genitourinary infection	*Adults:* 250 mg every 6 hr or 500 mg to 4 Gm every 12 hr orally in divided doses for 7–14 days. Maximum dosage: 4 Gm/day. *Adolescents and children:* 25–50 mg/kg/day orally in divided doses for 7–14 days. Maximum dosage: Impetigo: 1 Gm/day; other skin and skin structure infections: 2 Gm/day.	
	Cefadroxil	Uncomplicated UTI	*Adults:* 1–2 Gm/day orally in divided doses. Maximum dosage: 2 Gm/day. *Adolescents, children, infants:* 30 mg/kg/day orally in divided doses every 12 hr. Maximum dosage: 2 Gm/day.	See Table 41.2.

Continued

TABLE 41.5 **Recommended Dosing of First-, Second-, and Third-Generation Cephalosporins—cont'd**

Cephalosporin Generation	Medication	Indications	Dosage	Considerations and Monitoring
		Skin and skin structure infections	*Adults:* 1 Gm/day orally in divided doses. Maximum dosage: 2 Gm/day. *Adolescents, children, infants:* 30 mg/kg/day orally every 12 hr. Impetigo in adolescents and children: May dose at 30 mg/kg/day once or twice daily. Maximum dosage: 1 Gm/day.	
		Streptococcal pharyngitis, tonsilitis	*Adults:* 1 Gm/day orally in 1–2 divided doses for 10 days. Maximum dosage: 2 Gm/day. *Adolescents and children:* 30 mg/kg/day orally in 1–2 divided doses for 10 days. Maximum dosage: 1 Gm/day.	
Second Generation	Cefaclor	Pharyngitis, tonsillitis	**Extended release:** *Adults and adolescents ≥16 yr:* 375 mg orally every 12 hr for 7–10 days. **Immediate release:** *Adults:* 250–500 mg orally every 8 hr *Adolescents, children, infants:* 20–40 mg/kg/day orally in 3 divided doses every 8 hr or in 2 divided doses every 12 hr	Guidelines do not recommend cefaclor for Group A streptococcal pharyngitis to prevent rheumatic fever. Maximum dosage: *Adults immediate release:* 1.5 Gm/day; *adults extended release:* 1 Gm/day. Maximum dosage: *Adolescents ≥16 yr immediate and extended release:* 1 Gm/day.
		Otitis media, lower respiratory tract infections, skin and skin structure infections, UTI	**Immediate release:** *Adults:* 250–500 mg orally every 8 hr *Adolescents, children, infants:* 20-40 mg/kg/day orally in divided doses every 8 hr. **Extended release:** *Adults and adolescents ≥16 yr:* 375 mg orally every 12 hr for 7–10 days.	Maximum dosage: *Adolescents ≤15 yr and children immediate release:* 1 Gm/day. Maximum dosage: *Infants oral suspension:* 40 mg/kg/day orally. No dose adjustment for moderate to severe renal impairment.
		Acute bacterial exacerbations of chronic bronchitis	**Extended release:** *Adults:* 500 mg orally every 12 hr for 5–7 days. *Adolescents ≥16 yr:* 500 mg orally every 12 hr for 7 days.	
		Secondary bacterial infections of acute bronchitis	**Extended release:** *Adults and adolescents ≥16 yr:* 500 mg orally every 12 hr for 7 days.	

TABLE 41.5	Recommended Dosing of First-, Second-, and Third-Generation Cephalosporins—cont'd			
Cephalosporin Generation	**Medication**	**Indications**	**Dosage**	**Considerations and Monitoring**
	Cefprozil	Pharyngitis, tonsilitis	*Adults and adolescents ≥13 yr*: 500 mg orally every 24 hr for 10 days. *Children 2–12 yr*: 7.5 mg/kg/dose orally every 12 hr for 10 days. Maximum dosage: 250 mg/dose.	Renal impairment: see Table 41.2. Maximum dose (unless otherwise specified for specific indications): *Adults and adolescents:* 1000 mg/day *Children 6 month–12 yr:* 30 mg/kg/day.
		Acute bacterial exacerbation of chronic bronchitis	*Adults:* 500 mg orally every 12 hr for 5–7 days. *Adolescents:* 500 mg orally every 12 hr for 10 days.	FDA treatment recommendation is 10 days.
		Otitis media	*Infants and children 6 months–12 yr:* 15 mg/kg/dose orally every 12 hr for 10 days. Maximum dosage: 500 mg/dose.	
		Skin and skin structure infections	*Adults and adolescents ≥13 yr:* 250–500 mg orally every 12 hr or 500 mg every 24 hr for 10 days. *Children 2–12 yr:* 20 mg/kg/dose orally every 24 hr for 10 days. Maximum dosage: 500 mg/dose.	
		Acute sinusitis	*Adults and adolescents ≥13 yr:* 250–500 mg orally every 12 hr for 10 days. *Children 6 months–12 yr:* 7.5–15 mg/kg/dose orally every 12 hr for 10 days. Maximum dosage: 500 mg/dose.	*All ages:* Use higher dosage for moderate to severe infections
Third Generation	Cefdinir	Acute bacterial exacerbation of chronic bronchitis, pharyngitis, tonsillitis	*Adults and adolescents ≥13 yr*: 300 mg orally every 12 hr for 5–10 days or 600 mg orally once daily for 10 days. Maximum dosage: 600 mg/day.	Renal impairment: see Table 41.2. Guidelines do not recommend cefaclor for Group A streptococcal pharyngitis to prevent rheumatic fever.
		Acute bacterial otitis media, pharyngitis, tonsillitis	*Infants and children ≥6 months*: 7 mg/kg/dose orally every 12 hr (Maximum dosage: 300 mg/dose) orally for 5–10 days, or 14 mg/kg/dose (Maximum dosage: 600 mg/dose) orally once daily for 10 days.	

Continued

TABLE 41.5 Recommended Dosing of First-, Second-, and Third-Generation Cephalosporins—cont'd

Cephalosporin Generation	Medication	Indications	Dosage	Considerations and Monitoring
		Acute maxillary sinusitis	*Adults and adolescents ≥13 yr:* 300 mg orally every 12 hr or 600 mg once daily for 10 days. Maximum dosage: 600 mg/day. *Infants and children ≥6 months:* 7 mg/kg/dose orally every 12 hr (Maximum dosage: 300 mg/dose) orally for 10 days or 14 mg/kg/dose (Maximum dosage: 600 mg/dose) orally once daily for 10 days.	Not recommended by the Infectious Disease Society of America (IDSA) for empiric monotherapy of acute bacterial sinusitis due to variable rates of *S. pneumoniae* resistance.
		Community-acquired pneumonia	*Adults and adolescents ≥13 yr:* 300 mg orally every 12 hr for 10 days. Maximum dosage: 600 mg/day.	
		Skin and skin structure infections	*Adults and adolescents ≥13 yr:* 300 mg orally every 12 hr for 10 days. Maximum dosage: 600 mg/day. *Children ≥6 months:* 7 mg/kg orally every 12 hr. Maximum dosage: 300 mg/day.	
	Cefixime	Pharyngitis, tonsillitis (*S. pyogenes* infections)	*Adults and adolescents >12 yr or ≥45 kg:* 400 mg orally divided every 12–24 hr for at least 10 days. Maximum dosage: 400 mg/day. *Children 6 months–12 yr or ≤45 kg:* 8 mg/kg orally divided every 12–24 hr for at least 10 days. Maximum dosage: 8 mg/kg/day.	Renal impairment: see Table 42.2. Guidelines do not recommend cefixime for Group A streptococcal pharyngitis to prevent rheumatic fever.
		Otitis media	**Chewable tablet, suspension:** *Adults:* 400 mg orally divided every 12–24 hr. Maximum dosage: 400 mg/day. *Adolescents >12 yr or ≥45 kg with severe disease:* 400 mg orally divided every 12–24 hr for 10 days. Maximum dosage: 400 mg/day. *Children 6 months–12 yr or ≤45 kg with severe disease:* 8 mg/kg/day orally divided every 12–24 hr. Maximum dosage: 8 mg/kg/day.	**Alternate dose:** Children 6 years and older with mild to moderate disease, a 5- to 7-day course. Children 2 to 5 years with mild to moderate disease, a 7-day course is acceptable.

TABLE 41.5 Recommended Dosing of First-, Second-, and Third-Generation Cephalosporins—cont'd

Cephalosporin Generation	Medication	Indications	Dosage	Considerations and Monitoring
		Acute exacerbation of chronic bronchitis	*Adults and adolescents >12 yr or ≥45 kg:* 400 mg orally divided every 12–24 hours for 5–7 days. Maximum dosage: 400 mg/day. *Children 6 months–12 yr or ≤45 kg:* 8 mg/kg/dose orally divided every 12–24 hours for 5–7 days. Maximum dosage: 8 mg/kg/day.	
		Uncomplicated UTI	*Adults and adolescents >12 yr or ≥45 kg:* 400 mg orally divided every 12–24 hr. *Children 6 months–12 yr or ≤45 kg:* 8 mg/kg/day orally divided every 12–24 hr for 7–14 days.	
	Ceftibuten	Acute exacerbation of chronic bronchitis	*Adults and adolescents ≥12 yr:* 400 mg orally once daily for 10 days.	Renal impairment: see Table 41.2. Maximum dosage:
		Pharyngitis, tonsilitis, otitis media	*Adults and adolescents ≥12 yr:* 400 mg orally once daily for 10 days. *Infants and children 6 months–12 yr:* 9 mg/kg/day orally once daily for 10 days.	*Adults, adolescents, and children to ≥6 months:* 400 mg/day *Infants ≤6 months:* Safety and efficacy not established
	Ceftriaxone	Bacteremia and sepsis, UTI	**Intravenous or Intramuscular:** *Adults:* 1–2 Gm every 12–24 hr. Maximum dosage: 4 Gm/day. *Adolescents, children, and full-term infants:* 50–75 mg/kg/day every 12–24 hr. Maximum dosage: 2 Gm/day.	
		Uncomplicated gonorrhea (excluding pharyngitis)	*Adults:* 250 mg dose IM one time.	Guideline dosing varies.
		Lower respiratory tract infections, community-aquired pneumonia	*Adults:* 1–2 Gm every 12–24 hr. Maximum dosage: 4 Gm/day. *Adolescents, children, and infants:* 50–100 mg/kg/day every 12–24 hr. Maximum dosage: 4 Gm/day.	

UTI, Urinary tract infection.

Cephalexin

Pharmacokinetics. Cephalexin is available in capsule and tablet forms and as a powder for suspension. Cephalexin is well absorbed in the GI tract and may be given with or without meals. The majority of the drug is excreted unchanged by the renal system. The half-life is approximately 1 hour in patients with normal renal function.

Indications. Cephalexin is indicated for the treatment of impetigo, infections of the skin and/or subcutaneous tissue, osteomyelitis, otitis media, respiratory tract infections, streptococcal pharyngitis, and urinary tract infections (UTIs). Cephalexin is ineffective against most strains of *Enterobacter*, *Morganella morganii*, *Proteus vulgaris*, *Pseudomonas*, and *Acinetobacter calcoaceticus*.

Adverse Effects. Common adverse effects include diarrhea and nausea. More serious effects include Stevens-Johnson syndrome, toxic epidermal necrolysis, *C. difficile* colitis, increased prothrombin time, thrombocytopenia, allergic reactions, seizures, interstitial nephritis, and angioedema.

Contraindications. Avoid in patients with known hypersensitivity to cephalexin or other members of the cephalosporin class. Use with probenecid is not recommended. Use caution in patients with a history of renal impairment and with GI diseases such as colitis. Cephalexin may cause increased plasma concentrations and renal clearance of metformin.

Monitoring. Monitor electrolytes, complete blood count (CBC) including platelets, and liver and kidney function in all patients. Dose adjustments are required in patients with renal impairment and are based on age and CrCl levels. Monitor for increased prothrombin time in at-risk patients (e.g., in cases of liver or renal impairment, anticoagulant or prolonged antibiotic therapy, malnutrition). Monitoring and dose adjustment of metformin are recommended in patients concomitantly taking cephalexin and metformin. Observe for signs of hypersensitivity reactions, antibiotic-associated diarrhea, and other superinfections.

Cefadroxil

Pharmacokinetics. Cefadroxil is available in capsules, tablets, and suspension form. The drug may be administered with or without food. Cefadroxil is rapidly absorbed after oral administration. Approximately 90% of the drug is excreted unchanged in the urine within 24 hours.

Indications. Cefadroxil is approved for use in adults and pediatrics and as alternative treatment in penicillin-allergic patients. Indications include the treatment of skin and skin structure infections caused by susceptible staphylococci and/or streptococci; pharyngitis and/or tonsillitis caused by *Streptococcus pyogenes* (group A beta-hemolytic streptococci); and UTIs caused by the *E. coli*, *P. mirabilis*, or *Klebsiella* species.

Adverse Effects. Cefadroxil may result in a false-positive direct Coombs' test, though the causative mechanism is unknown. Commonly occurring side effects include nausea, diarrhea, stomatitis, vaginal itching or discharge, and joint aches and pains. Serious adverse effects including erythema multiforme, Stevens-Johnson syndrome, *C. difficile* diarrhea, thrombocytopenia, and liver failure have been reported. Patients should be advised to report the new onset of a rash, urticaria, arthralgia, fever, malaise, and/or enlarged lymph nodes.

Contraindications. Cefadroxil is contraindicated in patients with hypersensitivity to cephalosporins or penicillins. Use with caution in patients with renal impairment or with a history of colitis.

Monitoring. Monitor electrolytes, CBC including platelets, and liver and kidney function in all patients. Observe for signs of hypersensitivity reactions and signs of antibiotic-associated diarrhea and other superinfections. A false-positive reaction for ketones in the urine may occur with tests using nitroprusside. Cephalosporins occasionally cause a positive direct Coombs' test.

Second Generation

Second-generation cephalosporins and the cephamycins (e.g., oral: cefaclor, cefprozil, cepuroxime) are generally effective against *E. coli*, *Proteus mirabilis*, *Klebsiella* species, *Haemophilus influenzae*, *Moraxella catarrhalis*, *Streptococcus pneumoniae*, *Staphylococcus aureus*, *Streptococcus pyogenes*, and coagulase-negative staphylococci, though there are some individual drug differences. *Pseudomonas*, *Campylobacter*, *Acinetobacter calcoaceticus*, *Legionella*, and most strains of *Serratia* and *Proteus vulgaris* are resistant to second-generation cephalosporins. Some strains of *Morganella morganii*, *Enterobacter cloacae*, and *Citrobacter* spp. are also resistant. CNS penetration remains poor. Indications include the treatment of infections of the ear, upper and lower respiratory systems, and urinary tract, as well as gonorrhea, meningitis, and sepsis.

Cefaclor

Pharmacokinetics. Cefaclor may be administered without regard to food, though peak concentrations are reached more quickly when the drug is taken on an empty stomach. Half-life is approximately 1 hour in patients with normal renal function. Half-life is prolonged in patients with impaired renal function. Excretion occurs in the urine, with 60% to 85% of the drug excreted unchanged.

Indications. Cefaclor is approved for the treatment of acute bacterial exacerbation of chronic bronchitis, acute otitis media, acute bronchitis – secondary bacterial infection, skin and skin structure infections, lower respiratory infections, pharyngitis, tonsillitis, and UTIs. Individual indicators may require a specific formula for administration.

Adverse Effects. Cefaclor has a significant number of adverse effects. The most frequent are those of the GI system. Diarrhea is more common than nausea or vomiting. Other adverse effects include eosinophilia, genital pruritus, moniliasis, and vaginitis. A serum-sickness–like reaction is a rare (fewer than 0.5%) hypersensitivity reaction seen more frequently in pediatric patients than in adults. In rare instances, anaphylaxis, Stevens-Johnson syndrome, and toxic epidermal necrolysis have been reported.

Contraindications. Use with caution in patients with renal impairment, though dose adjustment is not usually recommended. Cefaclor is contraindicated in those with hypersensitivity to cefaclor and other cephalosporins. Use with caution in patients with known colitis or other GI diseases.

Monitoring. Monitor liver and renal function during therapy. Evaluate effectiveness of therapy by resolution of infective symptoms.

Cefprozil

Pharmacokinetics. The capsule, solution, tablet, and suspension formulations are bioequivalent. Fasting does not impact absorption from the GI tract, which is approximately 95%. The time to peak concentration is 1 to 2 hours. The half-life is 90 minutes in infants older than 6 months and in children. In adults with normal renal function, the half-life is about 1 hour, and extends up to 6 hours depending on the degree of impairment. Hepatic impairment affects half-life (about 2 hours). Renal excretion is approximately 60%.

Indications. Indications include secondary bacterial infection resulting in acute bronchitis, acute bacterial exacerbation of chronic bronchitis, acute otitis media, uncomplicated infections of skin and/or subcutaneous tissue, pharyngitis, acute sinusitis, and tonsillitis. Cefprozil is recommended as an alternative treatment for sinusitis and otitis media in patients unresponsive to amoxicillin. Cefprozil is not effective against methicillin-resistant staphylococci, *Enterococcus faecium*, or most strains of *Acinetobacter*, *Enterobacter*, *Morganella morganii*, *Proteus vulgaris*, *Providencia*, *Pseudomonas*, *Serratia*, or *Bacteroides fragilis*.

Adverse Effects. Cefprozil is well tolerated. Only about 2% of patients stop therapy due to adverse effects. The most common adverse effects are from GI complaints such as nausea, diarrhea, vomiting, and abdominal pain. Elevations in liver values occur in 2% or less of patients.

Contraindications. Cefprozil is contraindicated in patients with known allergy to the cephalosporin class of antibiotics. Consider alternate formulas in patients with phenylketonuria since cefprozil oral suspension contains phenylalanine 28 mg/5 mL.

Monitoring. Monitor renal studies prior to and during therapy. Observe for signs of superinfection and response to therapy.

Third Generation

Third-generation cephalosporins (e.g., oral: cefdinir, cefixime, ceftibuten; parenteral: ceftriaxone) provide therapy for gram-negative and gram-positive organisms. They are most effective against the following:

- Gram-negative bacteria (gram-negative meningitis, Lyme disease, *Pseudomonas pneumonia*, gram-negative sepsis,

streptococcal endocarditis, melioidosis, penicillinase-producing *Neisseria gonorrhea*, chancroid, and gram-negative osteomyelitis)
- Bacteria resistant to the first- and second-generation cephalosporins (*Klebsiella*, *Haemophilus influenzae*, and *E. coli*)

They are less effective against gram-positive bacteria (*Streptococcus* and *Staphylococcus* species).

Commonalities exist regarding adverse effects, contraindications, and recommendations for monitoring. Common adverse effects include stomach discomfort, nausea or vomiting, diarrhea, fungal infection, rash or itching, injection-site reactions, coagulation disorders and bleeding, seizures, neurotoxicity, and disulfiram-like reactions. Known contraindications to third-generation cephalosporins include patients with known cephalosporin allergy and severe anaphylactic reaction to other drugs. Monitor patients for severe anaphylactic reactions. Obtain culture for sensitivity reports prior to therapy.

Cefdinir

Pharmacokinetics. Peak onset occurs within 2 to 4 hours. Excretion occurs primarily through the renal system. The half-life is approximately 2 hours. Cefdinir may be taken with or without meals.

Indications. Cefdinir has been approved by the U.S. Food and Drug Administration (FDA) for the treatment of exacerbation of chronic obstructive pulmonary disease (COPD), acute otitis media, community-acquired pneumonia, acute sinusitis, uncomplicated skin and skin structure infections, and *Streptococcus pyogenes* pharyngitis (group A).

Adverse Effects. Stevens-Johnson syndrome and toxic epidermal necrolysis have been reported (Arumugham & Cascella, 2020). The most common adverse effect is diarrhea, reported in adult and pediatric patients.

Contraindications. Cefdinir is contraindicated in patients with known allergy to the cephalosporin class of antibiotics. Cefdinir is ineffective against methicillin-resistant staphylococci, *Pseudomonas*, and *Enterobacter* species. The oral suspension form contains sucrose and should be avoided in patients with diabetes. Safety and efficacy in children younger than 6 months of age have not been established.

Monitoring. Monitor serum creatinine and blood urea nitrogen (BUN) in patients with renal impairment. Adjust dosing depending on CrCl levels. Monitor prothrombin time. Observe for signs of superinfection.

Cefixime

Pharmacokinetics. Cefixime is widely distributed and well absorbed. Peak serum concentration occurs within 2 to 8 hours. The half-life is 3 to 4 hours in patients with normal renal function. Primary excretion occurs in the urine, followed by secondary excretion in the bile.

Indications. FDA-approved indications include the treatment of uncomplicated UTIs, otitis media, pharyngitis, and tonsillitis; acute exacerbations of chronic bronchitis;

and uncomplicated gonorrhea (cervical/urethral) caused by susceptible bacteria. The suspension form results in higher peak blood levels than the tablet when administered at the same dose in pediatric patients with otitis media.

Adverse Effects. Diarrhea was the most frequently reported adverse effect. Patient reports also included abdominal pain, dyspepsia, loose stools, nausea, and vomiting. Additional adverse effects include those common to all cephalosporins.

Contraindications. Cefixime is contraindicated in patients with known allergy to cefixime or other cephalosporins. Safety and efficacy in pediatric patients younger than 6 months of age have not been established. Discontinue use in nursing mothers.

Monitoring. Dose adjustment is required when CrCl levels are less than 60 mL/min. Obtain CBC, renal function tests, and liver function tests (LFTs) periodically with prolonged therapy. Monitor for improvement, and consider retesting after 14 days in patients treated for pharyngeal gonorrhea.

Ceftibuten

Pharmacokinetics. Ceftibuten oral capsules and suspension are rapidly absorbed with proportional plasma concentrations. Peak action occurs within 2 to 6 hours. In adults and children without renal impairment, half-life is approximately 2 hours. Plasma half-life increases and total clearance decreases in patients with renal impairment. Excretion occurs within 24 hours and is primarily via the kidneys and feces.

Indications. Ceftibuten is indicated for the treatment of acute bacterial exacerbations of chronic bronchitis, acute bacterial otitis media, pharyngitis and tonsillitis caused by gram-positive *Streptococcus pneumoniae* (penicillin-susceptible strains only) and *Streptococcus pyogenes*, and gram-negative *Haemophilus influenzae* and *Moraxella catarrhalis*.

Adverse Effects. Adults reported nausea as the most common adverse effect. Less common adverse effects include headache, diarrhea, dyspepsia, dizziness, abdominal pain, and vomiting. In the pediatric population, diarrhea was more commonly reported in children younger than 2 years of age.

Contraindications. The oral suspension form contains sucrose and should be avoided in the diabetic patient. Safety and efficacy in infants younger than 6 months of age have not been established.

Monitoring. Monitor CBC and hepatic and renal functions. Observe for signs of superinfection or serum-sickness–like reactions. Monitor for signs of improvement. Dose adjustments are required for patients with renal impairment.

Ceftriaxone

Pharmacokinetics. After intramuscular (IM) injection, ceftriaxone is almost completely absorbed within 2 to 3 hours. The half-life is approximately 5 to 8 hours in adults. In neonates and children, the half-life is 4 to

6 hours. Ceftriaxone is excreted in the urine. The remainder is excreted in the bile and feces. Comparisons of older adults and patients with renal or hepatic impairment to healthy adults revealed little change in pharmacokinetic properties.

Indications. Ceftriaxone is approved for the treatment of lower respiratory tract infections, acute bacterial otitis media, skin and skin structure infections, UTIs, uncomplicated gonorrhea, pelvic inflammatory disease, bacterial septicemia, bone and joint infections, intraabdominal infections, and meningitis caused by susceptible organisms. Organisms resistant to ceftriaxone include methicillin-resistant staphylococci, most strains of group D streptococci and enterococci (*Enterococcus [Streptococcus] faecalis*), and *C. difficile*.

Adverse Effects. The most common adverse effects include injection-site warmth, tightness, and induration; eosinophilia; thrombocytosis; elevations of serum glutamic oxaloacetic transaminase (SGOT) or serum glutamic pyruvic transaminase (SGPT); diarrhea; hypersensitivity reaction; and leukopenia. In 3-day-old neonates with extremely low birth weights, there is an increased risk of candidiasis compared with other antibiotics.

Contraindications. Ceftriaxone is contraindicated in patients with known allergy to the cephalosporin class of antibiotics. Do not prescribe to hyperbilirubinemic neonates younger than 28 days of age at risk for bilirubin encephalopathy. Alcohol should be avoided to decrease disulfiram-like reactions that lead to nausea, vomiting, flushing, dizziness, headache, and generalized hangover-like symptoms (Arumugham & Cascella, 2020). Use with caution in patients with known GI disease, impaired vitamin K synthesis or storage, or hepatic or renal impairment.

Monitoring. Monitor CBC and hepatic and renal function. Monitor coagulation studies in patients with a known risk of bleeding (Arumugham & Cascella, 2020). Monitor signs of adverse reactions and antibiotic-associated diarrhea. Adjust dosages in patients with combined significant hepatic and renal disease.

Fourth and Fifth Generations

The fourth- and fifth-generation cephalosporins offer the highest efficacy against gram-negative bacteria. Available only in parenteral form, they are not frequently used in the primary care setting. These classifications will not be reviewed in detail in this chapter.

Fourth-generation drugs are indicated for moderate to severe, complicated infections. They are effective against gram-positive cocci including methicillin-susceptible *Staphylococcus aureus* (MSSA), *Streptococcus* spp., *P. aeruginosa*, and enteric gram-negative *bacilli* (Chaudhry et al., 2019).

Fifth-generation drugs are effective against gram-positive cocci including MSSA, methicillin-resistant *Staphylococcus aureus* (MRSA), and *Streptococcus* spp. as well as many enteric gram-negative rods. Ceftobiprole offers additional antimicrobial coverage against *Enterococcus faecalis* and

Pseudomonas aeruginosa (Chaudhry et al., 2019). Fifth-generation cephalosporins are not effective against extended-spectrum beta-lactamase producers, *Acinetobacter baumannii*, or *Stenotrophomonas maltophilia*.

Prescriber Considerations for Cephalosporin Therapy

Clinical Practice Guidelines

Numerous organizations offer practice guidelines. These guidelines are commonly listed by diagnosis rather than by classification of medication.

BOOKMARK THIS!

Clinical Guidelines

- American Academy of Dermatology (AAD): https://www.aad.org/
- American Academy of Neurology (AAN): https://www.aan.com/
- American Academy of Pediatrics (AAP): https://www.aap.org/
- American Thoracic Society (ATS): https://www.thoracic.org/professionals/
- Infectious Disease Society of America (IDSA): https://www.idsociety.org/practice-guideline/practice-guidelines/#/+/0/date_na_dt/desc/
- Pediatric Infectious Diseases Society (PIDS): https://pids.org/

Clinical Reasoning for Cephalosporin Therapy

Consider the individual patient's health problem requiring the use of a cephalosporin. Health care providers should carefully assess the patient's clinical status to differentiate between a viral and a bacterial infection. If a bacterial infection is identified, the next step is to determine the appropriate cephalosporin based on culture and sensitivity reports.

Determine the desired therapeutic outcome based on the patient's health problem. Cephalosporin therapy is prescribed to treat active bacterial infections as well as for prophylaxis in specific situations. Health care providers should be familiar with the current clinical guidelines.

Assess the cephalosporin selected for its appropriateness for an individual patient by considering the medication's side effects and the patient's age, race/ethnicity, comorbidities, and genetic factors. Prior to initiating cephalosporin therapy, the health care provider should conduct a thorough review of the patient history, including current and past medical history, clinical status, previous allergic reactions, and current medication therapy. Review the side-effect profile, contraindications, and monitoring parameters of the selected drug.

Initiate the treatment plan with the selected medication by first providing adequate patient education to ensure the patient's understanding and promote full participation in cephalosporin therapy. Prior to beginning cephalosporin therapy, the health care provider should educate the patient on the diagnosis, suspected causative factor, and treatment recommendations. Patient education should include the name of the antibiotic, dosage instructions, and common adverse effects. The patient should be advised of the duration of therapy and expected results.

Ensure complete patient and family understanding about the medication prescribed for cephalosporin therapy using a variety of education strategies. Strategies to improve patient education include verbal and written instructions, electronic messaging/reminders, and follow-up calls. Prior to leaving the office, the patient should be asked to repeat back the instructions. If electronic patient portals are used in the practice, the provider should consider a demonstration of the portal.

Conduct follow-up and monitoring of patient responses to cephalosporin therapy. Advise the patient to seek emergent care if adverse effects occur. Advise the patient of follow-up laboratory and medical appointments. Monitor laboratory results and adjust medication therapy as required.

Teaching Points for Cephalosporin Therapy

Health Promotion Strategies

The health care provider should be aware of appropriate antibiotic prescribing principles. Shared decision-making concepts should be used to guide discussions. All patients should be educated on the appropriate use of antibiotics and the need to complete the entire course of therapy.

Counsel patients to consider alternative contraceptive measures during antibiotic therapy. Instruct patients to notify their provider of any response that would suggest an allergic reaction.

Patient Education for Medication Safety

Tell your provider if you:
- Are allergic to cephalosporin, penicillin, or any other drugs, foods, dyes, or preservatives
- Develop any response that would suggest an allergic reaction
- Are pregnant or thinking of becoming pregnant and/or breastfeeding
- Develop diarrhea that becomes severe, does not stop, or is bloody. Do not take any medicine to stop diarrhea until you have talked to your doctor.
- Are diagnosed with:
  - Phenylketonuria
  - Kidney disease
  - Liver disease
  - Digestive problems such as colitis
- Are taking any other medications, including prescription and nonprescription medicines, vitamins, and herbal supplements. Examples:
  - Birth control pills
  - Blood thinners such as warfarin

- Diuretics such as furosemide or hydrochlorothiazide
- Other antibiotic medicine, such as streptomycin or neomycin
- Probenecid

Application Questions for Discussion

1. Cross-reactions between cephalosporins, penicillins, and aminopenicillins are due to similarities in which side chain?
2. Cephalosporins are primarily excreted by which system?
3. Which cephalosporin is commonly used in the parenteral formula in the primary care setting?

Selected Bibliography

American Academy of Pediatrics. (2001). The transfer of drugs and other chemicals into human milk. *Pediatrics, 108*, 776–1030. Available at http://www.e-lactancia.org/media/papers/DrugsBF-Pediatrics-2001.pdf.

Arumugham, V. B., & Cascella, M. (2020). *Third Generation Cephalosporins*. In StatPearls [Internet]. Treasure Island (FL): StatPearls Publishing. 2020 Jan-. Available at https://www.ncbi.nlm.nih.gov/books/NBK549881/.

Bhattacharya, S. (2010). The facts about penicillin allergy: A review. *Journal of Advanced Pharmaceutical Technology & Research, 1*(1), 11–17. Available at https://www.ncbi.nlm.nih.gov/pubmed/22247826.

Chaudhry, S. B., Veve, M. P., & Wagner, J. L. (2019). Cephalosporins: A focus on side chains and ß-lactam cross-reactivity. *Pharmacy, 7*(3), 103. Available at https://doi.org/10.3390/pharmacy7030103.

Joint Task Force on Practice Parameters; American Academy of Allergy, Asthma and Immunology; American College of Allergy, Asthma and Immunology; Joint Council of Allergy, Asthma and Immunology. (2010). Drug allergy: An updated practice parameter. *Annals of Allergy, Asthma & Immunology, 105*(4), 259–273. https://doi.org/10.1016/j.anai.2010.08.002.

Kalman, D., & Barriere, S. L. (1990). Review of the pharmacology, pharmacokinetics, and clinical use of cephalosporins. *Texas Heart Institute Journal, 17*(3), 203–215. Available at https://europepmc.org/backend/ptpmcrender.fcgi?accid=PMC324918&blobtype=pdf.

Miller, L. E., Knoderer, C. A., Cox, E. G., & Kleiman, M. B. (2011). Assessment of the validity of reported antibiotic allergic reactions in pediatric patients. *Pharmacotherapy, 31*(8), 736–741. https://doi.org/10.1592/phco.31.8.736.

Pichichero, M. E. (2005). A review of evidence supporting the American Academy of Pediatrics recommendation for prescribing cephalosporin antibiotics for penicillin-allergic patients. *Pediatrics, 115*(4), 1048–1457. https://doi.org/10.1542/peds.2004-1276.

42
Tetracyclines

REBECCA M. LUTZ

Overview

Tetracyclines were discovered in the 1950s. Current tetracyclines are broad-spectrum, semisynthetic, bacteriostatic antibiotics. These drugs work by inhibiting protein synthesis, which suppresses bacterial growth and replication. All of the tetracyclines have similar structure, antimicrobial actions, and adverse effects. The differences exist primarily within their pharmacokinetic principles.

Primary care providers most commonly use tetracycline and doxycycline. Doxycycline is used more often than tetracycline. The use of tetracyclines as a treatment for skin disorders is discussed in this chapter as well as in Chapter 3. The use of tetracyclines to manage periodontal diseases will not be discussed in this chapter. Tetracycline therapy used in the treatment of the syndrome of inappropriate antidiuretic hormone secretion (SIADH) will not be discussed in this chapter.

Tetracyclines are labeled for use against a wide variety of gram-positive and gram-negative bacteria, spirochetes, obligate intracellular bacteria, and protozoan parasites. They cover infections caused by *Escherichia coli*, *Enterobacter aerogenes*, *Shigella* spp., *Acinetobacter* spp., *Bacteroides* spp., *Haemophilus influenzae* (upper respiratory tract only), *Klebsiella* spp. (lower respiratory tract only), *Mycoplasma pneumoniae* (lower respiratory tract only), *Streptococcus pneumoniae*, *Streptococcus pyogenes*, *Chlamydia trachomatis*, *Haemophilus ducreyi*, and *Klebsiella granulomatis*. Tetracycline is an effective treatment for skin and skin structure infections caused by *Staphylococcus aureus* or *S. pyogenes*, *Rickettsiae*, *Borrelia* spp., and *Vibrio cholera*. Tetracyclines are labeled for use as adjunctive therapy in situations where the primary drug of choice is contraindicated, such as in diseases caused by *Actinomyces* species, *Bacillus anthracis*, *Clostridium* spp., *Treponema pallidum*, *Chlamydophila psittaci*, *Yersinia pestis*, *Francisella tularensis*, *Brucella* spp., *Bartonella bacilliformis*, and *Fusobacterium fusiforme*.

Antibiotic Resistance

All tetracyclines exhibit similar antimicrobial activity. Cross-resistance is common and thus decreases the usefulness of tetracyclines. Resistance occurs on local levels due to prescribing practices and frequency of use within communities (World Health Organization, n.d.). Tetracycline resistance occurs through efflux, ribosomal protection, and enzymatic inactivation. Efflux occurs when the unchanged drug is pumped out of the bacteria. Ribosomal protection allows the ribosome to continue to function. During enzymatic inactivation, degradation occurs within the cell.

Pharmacokinetics

Since the discovery of tetracyclines in the 1950s, additional generations have been developed. The second-generation semisynthetic compounds, doxycycline and minocycline, were developed via modification of the tetracycline core in the 1960s and 1970s. In the early 2000s, minocycline was structurally modified to derive tigecycline, an intravenous (IV) preparation. In 2018, omadacycline (IV and oral) and eravacycline (IV) were approved by the U.S. Food and Drug Administration (FDA). Like tigecycline, these agents were designed to be active against tetracycline-resistant organisms specifically.

The tetracyclines suppress bacterial growth by inhibiting protein synthesis by binding to the 30S ribosomal subunit and possibly the 50S ribosomal subunit(s). They may also cause alterations in the cytoplasmic membrane. The tetracyclines distribute well into most body fluids and tissues except cerebrospinal fluid (CSF). They cross the placenta and are distributed into breast milk (see Practice Pearls: Tetracycline Use in Pregnancy and Lactation).

Classification

The tetracyclines are divided into three groups: short acting (tetracycline), intermediate acting (demeclocycline), and long acting (doxycycline, minocycline). The groupings also depend on lipid solubility. Tetracycline has relatively low lipid solubility. Doxycycline and minocycline have relatively high lipid solubility. Tetracycline and doxycycline are available in oral and IV formulations. Oral absorption occurs in the stomach, duodenum, and small intestine. Oral absorption of tetracycline, demeclocycline, and doxycycline is reduced by food. Minocycline absorption is not affected by food.

Adverse Effects

All tetracyclines may cause adverse effects, and the most common is a fixed drug reaction (Hamilton & Guarascio, 2019). In general, severe adverse effects such as IgE-mediated immediate-type anaphylactic hypersensitivity reactions are rare and nonfatal with treatment (Hamilton & Guarascio, 2019). The most common adverse effects include those to the central nervous, dermatologic, gastrointestinal (GI), hematologic, hepatic, and renal systems. Table 42.1 provides a summary

TABLE 42.1 Adverse Effects of Tetracyclines

Body System Affected	Adverse Reaction	Body System Affected	Adverse Reaction
Cardiovascular	Abnormal color	Hematologic Effects	Eosinophilia
	Autoimmune vasculitis		Hemolytic anemia
	Pericardial effusion		Leukemoid reaction
	Pericarditis		Neutropenia
Central Nervous System	Headache		Thrombocytopenia
	Blurred vision, diplopia, vision loss	Hepatic	Hepatitis
	Dizziness, light-headedness, vertigo		Hepatotoxicity
	Myopathy		Increased liver enzymes
Dermatologic	Dry skin and itching		Steatosis of liver
	Erythema multiforme	Immunologic Effects	Anaphylaxis
	Fixed drug eruptions		Drug-induced systemic lupus erythematosus
	Hyperpigmentation		Hypersensitivity reaction
	Onycholysis		Jarisch Herxheimer reaction
	Phototoxicity		Sweet's syndrome
	Stevens-Johnson syndrome		Lupus erythematosus
	Toxic epidermal necrolysis	Musculoskeletal Effects	Disorder of bone development
	Verruca vulgaris		Drug-induced myopathy
Endocrine/ Metabolic	Acidosis	Neurologic Effects	Antibiotic-induced neuromuscular blocking
	Azotemia		Bulging fontanelle
	Hyperphosphatemia		Dizziness
	Hypoglycemia		Headache
	Increased body temperature		Inflammatory neuropathy
	Increased serum blood urea nitrogen		Lightheadedness
	Thyroid cancer		Pseudotumor cerebri
	Thyroid dysfunction		Raised intracranial pressure
Gastrointestinal	Black hairy tongue		Vertigo
	Clostridium difficile colitis	Ophthalmic Effects	Abnormal color vision
	Diarrhea		Scleral discoloration
	Dysphagia		Visual field scotoma
	Enterocolitis	Renal	Acute renal failure
	Esophagitis		Azotemia
	Gastrointestinal ulcer		Increased blood urea nitrogen
	Generalized enamel hypoplasia associated with ingestion of drugs		Fanconi syndrome
	Glossitis		Nephrotoxicity
	Loss of appetite	Respiratory	Nasopharyngitis
	Nausea		
	Pancreatitis		
	Soft tissue lesion of pelvic region		
	Tongue discoloration		
	Tooth discoloration		
	Ulcer of esophagus		
	Upset stomach		
	Vomiting		

of adverse effects. Patients with acne who are treated concomitantly with tetracycline antibiotics and isotretinoin risk development of pseudotumor cerebri. Concomitant therapy is rare to the well-known risk of pseudotumor cerebri, increasing antibiotic resistance of Propionibacterium acnes, and the burden associated with navigating the iPLEDGE® program (Reserva et al., 2019).

Contraindications

Absolute contraindications to the tetracyclines include patients with known tetracycline hypersensitivity. Patients with hepatic and renal disease should be monitored closely for evidence of toxicity. In children 4 months to 8 years of age, tetracyclines should be avoided due to the disruption of enamel formation resulting in discoloration of permanent teeth, except when other drugs are ineffective or contraindicated.

Box 42.1 provides a summary of drug–drug interactions. These interactions are seen in prescriptions and over-the-counter (OTC) medications, including common antacids. The health care provider should check all drug interactions among the patient's medications before

PRACTICE PEARLS

Tetracycline Use During Pregnancy and Lactation

- Tetracycline readily crosses the placenta and may result in delays and/or alterations in skeletal development and bone growth of the fetus.
- Do not use tetracycline in the second half of pregnancy unless the potential benefits from treatment outweigh the potential risks to the fetus.
- Avoid use in those who are breastfeeding and those who are taking oral contraceptives.

• Box 42.1 Tetracyclines: Common Drug and Food Interactions

- Avoid concomitant administration with these drugs:
  - Aminolevulinic acid (systemic)
  - Intravesical bacillus Calmette–Guérin (BCG)
  - Cholera vaccine
  - Mecamylamine
  - Methoxyflurane
  - Retinoic acid derivatives
  - Strontium ranelate
- Monitor and/or consider alternative therapy due to impaired absorption of tetracycline with antibiotics (including beta-lactams), minerals and antacids (including calcium, magnesium, and iron), and dairy products (including milk).
- Refer to resources for a complete listing of the food and drug interactions with tetracycline.

Data from May, D. B. (2020). Tetracyclines. UpToDate. Retrieved February 16, 2022 from https://www.uptodate-com.ezproxy.hsc.usf.edu/contents/tetracyclines?search=Tetracyclines&source=search_result&selectedTitle=2~142&usage_type=default&display_rank=1#H20.

prescribing tetracyclines. Table 42.2 provides a summary of common tetracyclines.

Tetracycline Therapy

Tetracycline Hydrochloride

Tetracycline is the least expensive and most widely used member of the tetracycline family. When employed systemically, the drug has the indications, pharmacokinetics, adverse effects, and drug interactions that describe the tetracyclines as a group. Like most tetracyclines, tetracycline hydrochloride should not be administered with food and is contraindicated for patients with renal impairment.

Pharmacokinetics. Tetracycline hydrochloride is classified as a short-acting tetracycline. Tetracycline has poor penetration into CSF but is readily distributed to other body tissues and fluids. Absorption takes place mainly in the stomach and upper intestine, with absorption rates between 77% and 88% when administered orally. Peak concentrations occur in 2 to 5 hours, depending on the dosage. Excretion occurs in the urine and feces (Agwuh & MacGowan, 2006).

Indications. Tetracycline is indicated in the treatment of mild to moderate upper and lower respiratory tract infections, sexually transmitted infections, and skin and skin structure infections, and as adjunctive therapy when the drug of choice is contraindicated.

Adverse Effects. Though uncommon, adverse effects include those similar to all tetracycline preparations. The risk of adverse effects in children younger than 8 years of age and in females who are pregnant, breastfeeding, or using oral contraceptives is significant. Photosensitivity is common, and patients should be advised to avoid ultraviolet exposure.

Contraindications. Avoid tetracycline hydrochloride in patients with hypersensitivity to tetracycline, tetracycline-class antibacterial drugs, or any component of the formulation. Avoid in patients with significant renal impairment (see monitoring and alternate dosing) due to decreased absorption rates. Avoid the use of tetracycline in conjunction with iron and antacid products or any other products that contain aluminum, magnesium, calcium, zinc, and milk. Alternate therapies should be considered in pregnant or breastfeeding patients, children younger than 8 years of age, and females taking oral contraceptives.

Monitoring. Monitor for adverse side effects. GI effects may signal *Clostridium difficile* infection or hepatotoxicity. Recommendations include baseline kidney and liver function studies, thyroid profile, and a complete blood count (CBC), with follow-up monitoring every 3 months if the patient is under long-term treatment. As renal function decreases, the serum half-life of tetracycline increases. Table 42.3 provides dosing guidelines based on creatinine clearance (CrCl) (Munar & Singh, 2007). Assess for *C. difficile* if the patient develops diarrhea.

Doxycycline

Doxycycline is a long-acting, second-generation tetracycline. Doxycycline is usually well tolerated by patients, and in patients with renal failure it is the drug of choice. Adverse

TABLE 42.2 **Tetracyclines**

Medication	Indication	Dosage	Considerations and Monitoring
Tetracycline	Upper/lower respiratory system, skin and skin structure infections, bacterial UTI	*Adults and older adults:* 250–500 mg orally every 6–12 hr. Maximum dosage: 2 Gm/day. *Children ≥9 yr and adolescents:* 25–50 mg/kg/day orally in divided doses every 6 hr. Maximum dosage: 50 mg/kg/day orally up to 2 Gm/day orally.	Take on an empty stomach. Tetracycline is approved for a wide variety of disease processes when penicillin is contraindicated.
Doxycycline	Upper and lower respiratory tract infection, UTI, adjunctive therapy to acne vulgaris	**Formulations excluding Doryx MPC delayed release** *Adults, adolescents, and children ≥8 yr weighing ≥45 kg:* 100 mg/day every 12 hr orally on day 1, then once daily. For severe infection, including chronic UTI: 100 mg orally every 12 hr. *Adolescents and children ≥8 yr weighing <45 kg:* 2.2 mg/kg/dose every 12 hr orally on day 1, then 2.2 mg/kg/dose orally once daily. For severe infection, including chronic UTI: 2.2 mg/kg/dose every 12 hr. Maximum dosage: 100 mg/dose. **Doryx MPC delayed-release** *Adults, adolescents, and children ≥8 yr weighing ≥45 kg:* 120 mg orally every 12 hr on day 1, then 60 mg orally every 12 hr or 120 mg orally once daily. For severe infections, including chronic UTI, continue 120 mg orally every 12 hr. *Adolescents and children ≥8 yr weighing <45 kg:* 2.65 mg/kg/dose orally every 12 hr on day 1, then 1.3 mg/kg/dose orally every 12 hr or 2.6 mg/kg/dose orally once daily. For severe infections, 2.6 mg/kg/dose orally every 12 hr. Maximum dosage: 120 mg/dose.	Sinusitis treatment in patients with beta-lactam allergy: 200 mg orally once daily for 5–7 days.
	Community-acquired pneumonia	**Formulations excluding Doryx MPC delayed release** *Adults:* 100 mg orally every 12 hours for at least 5 days. *Adolescents and children ≥8 yr:* 2–4 mg/kg/day orally in 1–2 divided doses for 5–10 days. Maximum dose: 200 mg/day.	As monotherapy for outpatients without comorbidities or risk factors for MRSA or *P. aeruginosa.*
	Acne rosacea	**Delayed release:** *Adults:* 40 mg orally once daily in the morning.	Efficacy beyond 16 weeks and safety beyond 9 months have not been established.
	Early Lyme disease (erythema migrans)	**Formulations excluding Doryx MPC delayed release** *Adults:* 100 mg orally every 12 hr or 200 mg orally once daily for 10–14 days. *Adolescents and children >8 yr and ≥45 kg:* 100 mg orally every 12 hr for 10–14 days.	
	Sexually transmitted infections		Treatment of sexually transmitted infections depends on pathogen, infection status, and pregnancy status. Refer to FDA and current practice guidelines.

TABLE 42.2 Tetracyclines—cont'd

Medication	Indication	Dosage	Considerations and Monitoring
Omadacycline	CAP	*Adults:* 300 mg orally twice on day 1, then 300 mg orally once daily for 7–14 days.	*Neonates, infants, children, and adolescents:* Safety and efficacy have not been established.
	ABSSSI	*Adults:* 450 mg orally once daily for 2 days, then 300 mg once daily for 7–14 days.	
Sarecycline	Non-nodular moderate to severe acne vulgaris	*Adults, adolescents, and children ≥9 yr:* Based on weight: • 33–54 kg: 60 mg once daily. • 55–84 kg: 100 mg once daily. • 85–136 kg: 150 mg orally once daily.	If no improvement after 12 weeks, reassess treatment.
Demeclocycline	Skin and skin structure infections due to *Staphylococcus aureus* or *Streptococcus pneumoniae,* upper and lower respiratory tract infections, UTI caused by *Klebsiella* spp.	*Adults:* 150 mg orally four times daily or 300 mg orally twice daily. Maximum dosage: 600 mg/day. *Children ≥8 yr and adolescents:* 7–13 mg/kg/day orally in divided doses every 6–12 hr. Maximum dosage: 600 mg/day.	Although FDA approved, pediatric dosing is uncommon and rarely used.

ABSSSI, Acute bacterial skin and skin structure infection; *CAP,* community-acquired pneumonia; *FDA,* U.S. Food and Drug Administration; *MRSA,* methicillin-resistant *Staphylococcus aureus; UTI,* urinary tract infection.

TABLE 42.3 Tetracycline Dose Based on Creatinine Clearance (CrCl)

	Creatinine Clearance (CrCl)	Administer Indicated/Recommended Dose
Adults, adolescents, and children ≥9 yr	>90 mL/min	No dosage adjustment needed.
	51–90 mL/min	Extend dosing interval to every 8–12 hr.
	10–50 mL/min	Extend dosing interval to every 12–24 hr.
	<10 mL/min	Extend dosing interval to every 24 hr.

effects are few compared to other tetracyclines (Hamilton & Guarascio, 2019).

Pharmacokinetics. Doxycycline is distributed into most body tissues and fluids. There is poor distribution to saliva, aqueous humor, and CSF. Oral absorption of doxycycline from immediate- and delayed-release products is 90% to 100%. Peak serum concentrations are reached between 1.5 and 4 hours depending on the formulation. Serum half-life ranges from 12 to 25 hours. Peak absorption occurs 2 to 4 hours after oral dosing (Agwuh & MacGowan, 2006). Because of its extended half-life, doxycycline can be administered once daily on an empty stomach to increase absorption.

Indications. Labeled indications include *Bartonella* spp., *Brucellosis,* acute exacerbations of chronic obstructive pulmonary disease, malaria, rosacea, periodontitis, Q fever, Rocky Mountain spotted fever, and sexually transmitted infections caused by *Chlamydia trachomatis* or lymphogranuloma venereum. The primary care provider should refer to current treatment guidelines as doxycycline

has numerous indications for prophylactic or adjunctive therapy or when the drug of choice is contraindicated. Preparations are available in immediate-release and extended-release formulas. In some instances, the once- or twice-daily dosing regimens make doxycycline the preferred drug of choice.

Adverse Effects. The most common adverse effects are those affecting the respiratory system and the cardiovascular system. Nephrotoxicity may occur, though it is less common with doxycycline than with the other tetracyclines. Renal failure is rarely reported after the administration of doxycycline.

Contraindications. Doxycycline is contraindicated in patients with known hypersensitivity to tetracyclines, during pregnancy, and in infants and children up to 8 years of age. Use with caution in patients with a known sulfite hypersensitivity. This reaction is more common in patients with asthma than in nonasthmatic patients. Delayed excretion may be observed in patients with a creatinine clearance (CrCl) less than 10 mL/minute.

Monitoring. Monitor liver function tests (LFTs), creatinine, and blood urea nitrogen (BUN). Monitor effectiveness in patients using proton pump inhibitor therapy or with decreased levels of hydrochloric acid resulting from gastrectomy or gastric bypass surgery.

Omadacycline

Omadacycline is a relatively new aminomethylcycline antibiotic in the tetracycline class of drugs. Omadacycline is active against vancomycin-resistant *Enterococcus* (VRE) and methicillin-resistant *Staphylococcus aureus* (MRSA), gram-negative organisms, and anaerobes (Barber et al., 2018). Prescribing guidelines from Paratek Pharmaceuticals (2018) include information for the treatment of:

- Community-acquired pneumonia (CAP) caused by *Streptococcus pneumoniae*, *Staphylococcus aureus* (methicillin-susceptible isolates), *Haemophilus influenzae*, *Haemophilus parainfluenzae*, *Klebsiella pneumoniae*, *Legionella pneumophila*, *Mycoplasma pneumoniae*, and *Chlamydophila pneumoniae*
- Acute bacterial skin and skin structure infections (ABSSSIs) caused by *Staphylococcus aureus* (methicillin-susceptible and methicillin-resistant isolates), *S. lugdunensis*, *S. pyogenes*, *S. anginosus* group, *Enterococcus faecalis*, *Enterobacter cloacae*, and *K. pneumoniae*

Pharmacokinetics. Omadacycline does not require dosing adjustments in patients with renal or hepatic disease. Food decreases the rate and extent of absorption; therefore, recommendations are to administer with water on an empty stomach. Half-life elimination after oral dosing is 13.45 to 16.83 hours. The time to peak after oral dosing is 2.5 hours. Excretion after oral dosing occurs primarily in the feces (77.5% to 84.0%) with the remainder excreted in urine. No dosage adjustments are recommended for patients with renal or liver impairment.

Indications. Omadacycline is available in oral and IV formulations. Treatment recommendations for CAP include an IV loading dose followed by oral dosing for 7 to 14 days. Treatment recommendations for ABSSSI call for the administration of 450 mg orally once daily for 2 days (or IV loading dose), then 300 mg orally once daily for 7 to 14 days.

Adverse Effects. In addition to the adverse effects common to other drugs in the tetracyclines classification, hypertension, insomnia, headache, increased gamma-glutamyl transferase, increased serum alanine aminotransferase, and increased serum aspartate aminotransferase (2% to 4% of patients) may occur. GI effects are common, with more than 10% of patients reporting nausea, vomiting, constipation, or diarrhea.

Contraindications. Similarities exist with other tetracyclines. Avoid in patients with hypersensitivity to omadacycline, tetracycline-class antibacterial drugs, or any component of the formulation, and during pregnancy/infancy/childhood up to 8 years of age. Omadacycline is not recommended in patients who are pregnant. Omadacycline is not recommended when breastfeeding. Breastfeeding may resume 4 days after the final dose of omadacycline.

Monitoring. Monitor response to therapy, particularly in patients with CAP and those who are at higher risk for mortality. Monitor renal and liver function. Monitor patients for effectiveness of treatment. Evaluate the patient's history and all medications. Consider alternative therapy or dosage adjustments.

Minocycline

Minocycline is a long-acting, second-generation tetracycline. Minocycline was approved for use in the United States in 1971. Disadvantages to minocycline are its expense and its adverse effects on the vestibular system. It is available in an extended-release formulation for acne and a topical formulation for periodontal disease.

Pharmacokinetics. Minocycline is well absorbed orally, even when taken with food. The distribution includes most body fluids and tissues except for poor central nervous system (CNS) penetration. Minocycline is metabolized by the liver. Half-life with oral dosing is approximately 16 hours, with peak action times between 1 and 4 hours depending on the preparation.

Indications. Minocycline is most frequently used for the treatment of acne. Other uses include the treatment of infections caused by *Vibrio cholerae*, gram-negative infections caused by *Acinetobacter* spp., *Escherichia coli*, *Enterobacter aerogenes*, *Shigella* spp., and *Chlamydia trachomatis*. It can treat respiratory infections caused by *Haemophilus influenzae*, *Klebsiella* spp., *Mycoplasma pneumonia*, *Streptococcus pneumoniae*, and urinary tract infections (UTIs) caused by *Klebsiella*. Minocycline is used as second-line therapy in a variety of infections when the primary therapy is contraindicated.

Adverse Effects. Minocycline is unique among the tetracyclines in that it can damage the vestibular system, causing unsteadiness, lightheadedness, and dizziness. Ophthalmic effects include abnormal color vision, scleral discoloration, and visual field scotoma (partial loss of vision or blind spot). Ototoxicity manifests as dizziness, vertigo, nausea/vomiting, and ataxia.

Contraindications. Minocycline is contraindicated in patients with hypersensitivity to minocycline or other tetracyclines, and during pregnancy/infancy/childhood up to 8 years of age. Extended-release preparations are not approved for use in children younger than 12 years of age. Use with caution in patients with hepatic impairment or those taking other hepatotoxic drugs. Use with caution in patients with a CrCl less than 80 mL/minute.

Monitoring. Monitor antinuclear antibodies (ANAs), CBC, and LFTs. In patients with impaired renal function, monitor serum creatinine, BUN, and magnesium. Monitor visual disturbances. Advise patients experiencing vestibular dysfunction to avoid performing tasks that require mental alertness, such as operating machinery or driving. During long-term treatment, monitor thyroid studies and for signs of cancer (Pollock et al., 2016). Monitor for adverse effects common to all tetracyclines.

Prescriber Considerations for Tetracycline Therapy

Clinical Practice Guidelines

Multiple professional organizations offer guidelines for the effective use of tetracyclines:

- American College of Clinical Pharmacy
- American Thoracic Society with the Infectious Diseases Society of America (ATS/IDSA)
- Centers for Disease Control and Prevention (CDC)
- Infectious Diseases Society of America (IDSA)
- The Infectious Diseases Society of America with the Pediatric Infectious Diseases Society (IDSA/PIDS)
- U.S. Department of Health & Human Services (HHS)
- World Health Organization (WHO)

Clinical Reasoning for Tetracycline Therapy

Consider the individual patient's health problem requiring tetracycline therapy. The first consideration is whether the organism will respond therapeutically to this class of antibiotics. The use of culture and sensitivities is recommended. Surveillance conducted by the local health department provides regional guidance on bacterial resistance levels.

Determine the desired therapeutic outcome based on the patient's health problem. Tetracycline therapy is primarily used in the treatment of active infections. The goal of therapy is the complete resolution of the infection with limited to no adverse effects. In patients with recurrent infections, the goal is to return to baseline or better.

Assess the tetracycline selected for its appropriateness for an individual patient by considering the medication's side effects and the patient's age, race/ethnicity, comorbidities, and genetic factors. Prior to the initiation of treatment, the health care provider must determine whether treatment can effectively be monitored in the outpatient or inpatient setting. Dosing should be based on age considerations; comorbidities such as decreased hepatic, renal, or cardiac function; and the presence of concomitant disease or other drug therapies.

Initiate the treatment plan with the selected medication by first providing adequate patient education to ensure the patient's understanding and promote full participation. Patient education prior to initiating treatment includes:

- The diagnosis and implications of no treatment
- The selected tetracycline as the preferred option
- Alternative treatment options available
- The therapeutic goal

Ensure complete patient and family understanding about the medication prescribed for antibiotic therapy using a variety of education strategies. There are a variety of strategies to increase patient and family understanding:

- Assess patient and family understanding by asking them to repeat their diagnosis and treatment plan.
- Offer demonstrations, videos, or video links.
- Provide printed material.

Conduct follow-up and monitoring of patient responses to antibiotic therapy. Effective tetracycline therapy results in the resolution of signs and symptoms of infection. In some cases, effectiveness is measured by the prevention of disease (e.g., malaria). Monitor patient status for adverse and/or early signs of toxic effects.

Teaching Points for Tetracycline Therapy

Health Promotion Strategies

- Be sure to tell your primary care provider about allergies to tetracycline or any other part of this drug, any other drugs, foods, or substances.
- Tell your provider if you are pregnant, suspect you may be pregnant, are on oral contraceptives, are breastfeeding, or plan to breastfeed.
- Tell your provider about all of your drugs (prescription, OTC, natural products, vitamins) and health problems, particularly kidney or liver disease.
- Do not take tetracyclines with:
  - Multivitamins, calcium, or iron supplements
  - Laxatives that contain magnesium
  - Milk products (because they contain calcium)
  - Antacids containing magnesium, aluminum, or both
- Sunburn occurs easily with tetracyclines. Avoid sun, sunlamps, and tanning beds. Use sunscreen and wear protective clothing and eyewear.
- Complete the full course of treatment, even if you begin to feel better earlier.

Patient Education for Medication Safety

- Omadacycline should be taken with water on an empty stomach (after fasting more than 4 hours); avoid food and drink (except water) for 2 hours after taking.
- To reduce the risk of esophageal irritation or ulceration, do not take at bedtime.
- Have your bloodwork checked as ordered by your primary care provider.
- Avoid sun, sunlamps, and tanning beds. Use sunscreen and wear clothing and eyewear that protects you from the sun.
- Tetracyclines may decrease the effects of oral contraceptives, resulting in recommendations of alternative forms of contraception. In addition to using oral contraceptives, use an alternate form of birth control when taking this medication.
- It is important to keep follow-up and laboratory appointments for blood work. Reschedule missed follow-up or laboratory appointments as soon as possible.
- If you get pregnant while taking this drug, call your provider right away.

Application Questions for Discussion

1. Are tetracyclines safe and effective for the treatment of all bacterial infections?
2. What are the considerations for prescribing tetracyclines to patients younger than 8 years of age?

3. What factors should be considered when educating the patient about ultraviolet exposures while on tetracyclines?

Selected Bibliography

Agwuh, K. N., & MacGowan, A. (2006). Pharmacokinetics and pharmacodynamics of the tetracyclines including glycylcyclines. *Journal of Antimicrobial Chemotherapy, 58*(2), 256–265. https://doi.org/10.1093/jac/dkl224.

Barber, K. E., Bell, A. M., Wingler, M. J. B., Wagner, J. L., & Stover, K. R. (2018). Omadacycline enters the ring: A new antimicrobial contender. *Pharmacotherapy, 38*(12), 1194–1204. https://doi.org/10.1002/phar.2185.

Hamilton, L. A., & Guarascio, A. J. (2019). Tetracycline allergy. *Pharmacy, 7*(3), 104. https://doi.org/10.3390/pharmacy7030104.

May, D. B. (2020). Tetracyclines. *UpToDate.* Retrieved February 16, 2022 from https://www-uptodate-com.ezproxy.hsc.usf.edu/contents/tetracyclines?

Munar, M. Y., & Singh, H. (2007). Drug dosing adjustments in patients with chronic kidney disease. *American Family Physician, 75*(10), 1487–1496. Retrieved from https://www.aafp.org/afp/2007/0515/p1487.html.

Paratek Pharmaceuticals (2018). NUZYRA. Highlights of prescribing information. Retrieved from https://www.accessdata.fda.gov/drugsatfda_docs/label/2018/209816_209817lbl.pdf.

Pollock, A. J., Seibert, T., & Allen, D. B. (2016). Severe and persistent thyroid dysfunction associated with tetracycline-antibiotic treatment in youth. *The Journal of Pediatrics, 173*, 232–234. https://doi.org/10.1016/j.jpeds.2016.03.034.

Reserva, J., Adams, W., Perlman, D., Vasicek, B., Joyce, C., Tung, R., & Swan, J. (2019). Coprescription of isotretinoin and tetracyclines for acne is rare: An analysis of the national ambulatory medical care survey. *The Journal of Clinical and Aesthetic Dermatology, 12*(10), 45–48. Epub 2019 Oct 1. PMID: 32038749; PMCID: PMC6937145.

World Health Organization. (n.d.). Antimicrobial resistance. Retrieved August 14, 2019, from https://www.who.int/antimicrobial-resistance/en/.

43

Macrolides

CHERYL H. ZAMBROSKI

Overview

Macrolides are considered to be among the most widely prescribed antibiotics worldwide (Hansen et al., 2019). The most common macrolides are erythromycin, clarithromycin, and azithromycin. They are used for a variety of infections, including acute upper and lower respiratory disorders, skin infections, and sexually transmitted infections, and to eradicate *H. pylori* infections. Macrolides are frequently used as the drug of choice for patients who are allergic to penicillin.

Macrolides are effective in treating a variety of gram-positive and gram-negative aerobes. They work by binding to bacterial 50S ribosomal subunits in sensitive bacteria, thus inhibiting protein synthesis. While macrolides are generally considered bacteriostatic, they can be bactericidal in certain specific bacteria or in high doses. Macrolides have extensive tissue penetration and can achieve high intracellular concentration. This results in an increased likelihood of eradication of intracellular pathogens.

Acquired bacterial resistance to macrolides can occur and must be considered in choosing appropriate antibiotic therapy. Resistance to macrolides occurs through two primary mechanisms. First, a specific gene called the *erythromycin ribosome methylation gene* (or *erm gene*) alters the 50S ribosomal subunit binding site. This gene is transported from one bacterium to another, thus reducing the sensitivity of the bacteria to macrolides. The second mechanism of increased resistance is the increased action of macrolide efflux pumps, thereby pumping out macrolides before they have a chance to reach the 50S ribosomal subunit. These mechanisms have led to increased resistance of many gram-positive bacteria. To illustrate the impact of acquired antibiotic resistance, macrolides were considered first-line therapy for outpatient adults with community-acquired pneumonia (CAP) in the

---

BOOKMARK THIS!

Antibiotic Resistance

Resistance to macrolides is increasing and varies across the United States and globally. The Center for Disease Dynamics, Economics & Policy provides antibiotic resistance and antibiotic consumption data from countries across the globe at https://resistancemap.cddep.org/.

2007 American Thoracic Society/Infectious Diseases Society of America (ATS/IDSA) Guidelines. Slightly more than one decade later, the updated guidelines include macrolides as "conditionally recommended" for CAP based on macrolide resistance levels in the community (Metlay et al., 2019).

Macrolide Therapy

Macrolides are a class of broad-spectrum antibiotics used in primary care for a number of infections, including CAP, sexually transmitted infections (STIs), and upper respiratory infections. Three macrolides—erythromycin, azithromycin, and clarithromycin—are systemically active and can have bacteriostatic or bactericidal activity depending on certain conditions or specific microorganisms. One additional macrolide, fidaxomicin, has minimal systemic absorption and is indicated for the treatment of pseudomembranous colitis secondary to *Clostridium difficile*.

The most common side effects are gastrointestinal (GI) disturbances, including mild abdominal pain, nausea, vomiting, and diarrhea. These may be decreased by taking the drugs with food. Severe adverse effects are less likely. While cardiac toxicity is very commonly referred to as an adverse effect of macrolides, a systematic review by Hansen and colleagues (2019) showed that in clinical studies there was no difference in the incidence of cardiac problems between the macrolide group and the placebo group. Also, they did not find significant liver, blood, skin, soft tissue, or respiratory symptoms with macrolides compared to placebo. The primary issue regarding the use of macrolides is the growing global concern of antibiotic resistance.

The significant differences between erythromycin and the newer macrolides include GI tolerability, a broader spectrum of activity, and dosing frequency. Macrolides are active primarily against gram-positive organisms, including *S. pyogenes* and *Streptococcus pneumoniae*. The newer macrolides have added effectiveness against gram-negative bacteria and anaerobes. Azithromycin and clarithromycin have significantly increased potency against gram-negative bacteria and anaerobes. They generally are reserved for more complicated infections such as CAP, exacerbation of chronic obstructive pulmonary disease (COPD), and sinusitis. See Table 43.1 for indications and dosing recommendations of common macrolides.

TABLE 43.1   Macrolides

Category/ Medication	Indication	Dosage	Considerations and Monitoring
Erythromycin	Mild to moderately severe lower respiratory tract infections	*Adults*: Erythromycin base: 250 mg orally every 6 hr or 333 mg orally every 8 hr or 500 mg orally every 12 hr. Doses up to 4 Gm/day may be used for severe infections. Twice-daily dosing is not recommended for doses more than 1 Gm/day. *Adults*: Erythromycin ethylsuccinate: 1.6 Gm/day orally divided every 6–12 hr. Doses up to 4 Gm/day may be used for severe infections. *Adults*: Erythromycin stearate 250 mg orally every 6 hr or 500 mg orally every 12 hr. Doses up to 4 Gm/day may be used for severe infections. Twice-daily dosing is not recommended with doses more than 1 Gm/day. *Infants, children, and adolescents*: 30–50 mg/kg/day (maximum dosage: 1–2 Gm/day) orally in 3–4 divided doses of erythromycin base, estolate, ethylsuccinate, or stearate.	Frequent dosing schedule may affect adherence. GI side effects are more common with erythromycin than with other macrolides, although erythromycin estolate has a lower rate of GI side effects than erythromycin ethylsuccinate.
	Legionnaire's disease	500 mg to 1 Gm orally (of erythromycin base, estolate, or stearate) every 6 hr or 400 mg to 1 Gm orally (of erythromycin ethylsuccinate) every 6 hr.	
	Mild to moderately severe upper respiratory tract infections, including group A beta-hemolytic streptococcal pharyngitis	*Adults*: 250–500 mg (of erythromycin base, estolate, or stearate) orally every 6 hr or 400–800 mg (of erythromycin ethylsuccinate) orally every 6 hr for 10 days. *Infants, children, and adolescents*: 30–50 mg/kg/day orally in 3–4 divided doses for 10 days. Maximum dosage: 1–2 Gm/day.	
	Prevent recurrent attacks of rheumatic fever	*Adults, adolescents, and children*: 250 mg orally (of erythromycin base, estolate, or stearate) twice daily or 400 mg orally (of erythromycin ethylsuccinate) twice daily. Follow clinical practice guidelines for precise duration of therapy.	
	Listeriosis	*Adults*: 250–500 mg (of erythromycin base, estolate, or stearate) orally every 6 hr or 400–800 mg (of ethylsuccinate) orally every 6 hr. Up to 4 Gm/day may be used in severe infections. *Infants, children, and adolescents*: 30–50 mg/kg/day orally in 3–4 divided doses. Usual maximum dosage: 2 Gm/day.	
	Nongonococcal urethritis or chlamydial infections, including urogenital infections	As an alternative to azithromycin or doxycycline, erythromycin base 500 mg orally or erythromycin ethylsuccinate 800 mg orally four times daily for 7 days.	
	Intestinal amebiasis in patients unable to receive metronidazole	*Adults*: 250 mg orally every 6 hr for 10–14 days. *Infants, children, and adolescents*: 30–50 mg/kg/day (maximum dosage: 1 Gm/day) orally in 3–4 divided doses for 10–14 days.	
Azithromycin	CAP	*Adults*: Immediate-release forms 500 mg orally on day 1, followed by 250 mg orally once daily for at least 5 days as monotherapy for patients without comorbidities or risk factors for MRSA or *P. aeruginosa* and as part of combination therapy for patients with comorbidities. *Adolescents, children, and infants 6 months to 12 yr*: 10 mg/kg/dose (maximum: 500 mg/dose) orally for 1 day, followed by 5 mg/kg/dose (maximum: 250 mg/dose) orally once daily for 4 days.	Dosage adjustment recommendations for patients with liver or renal impairment; however, caution should be used in patients with CrCl <10 mL/min. Always make sure to follow the most current clinical practice guidelines available.

TABLE 43.1	Macrolides—cont'd		
Category/ Medication	**Indication**	**Dosage**	**Considerations and Monitoring**
	Mild to moderate acute bacterial exacerbations of chronic bronchitis	Recommended dose is either 500 mg orally once daily for 3 days (e.g., Zithromax Tri-Pak) or 500 mg orally on first day of therapy, followed by 250 mg orally once daily for 4 days (e.g., Z-Pak).	
	Uncomplicated skin and skin structure infections	*Adults*: Recommended dose is 500 mg orally on first day of therapy, followed by 250 mg orally once daily for 4 days.	
Clarithromycin	Acute exacerbations of chronic bronchitis	**Regular-release tablets or oral suspension:** *Adults*: 250–500 mg orally every 12 hr for 7–14 days; dose and duration are dependent on organism. For *M. catarrhalis* and *S. pneumoniae*, 250 mg orally every 12 hr for 7–14 days. For *H. influenzae*, 500 mg orally every 12 hr for 7–14 days. For *H. parainfluenzae*, 500 mg orally every 12 hr for 7 days. **Extended release:** *Adults*: 1000 mg orally every 24 hr for 7 days.	Regular-release tablets and oral suspension may be given with or without food. Extended-release tablets should be given with food.
	CAP	**Regular-release tablets or oral suspension:** *Adults*: 500 mg orally every 12 hr for at least 5 days as monotherapy for outpatients without comorbidities or risk factors for MRSA or *P. aeruginosa* and as part of combination therapy. FDA-approved labeling recommends 250 mg orally every 12 hr for 7–14 days. *Adolescents*: 7.5 mg/kg/dose (maximum: 250 mg/dose) orally every 12 hr for 5–10 days. *Infants and children 6 months–12 yr*: 7.5 mg/kg/dose (maximum: 250 mg/dose) orally every 12 hr for 10 days. **Extended release:** *Adults*: 1000 mg orally once daily for at least 5 days as monotherapy for outpatients without comorbidities or risk factors for MRSA or *P. aeruginosa* and as part of combination therapy for outpatients with comorbidities. FDA-approved labeling recommends 7-day treatment.	
Fidaxomicin	Pseudomembranous colitis or *C. difficile*–associated diarrhea	*Adults, adolescents, and children weighing ≥12.5 kg*: 200 mg orally twice daily for 10 days. *Infants and children ≥6 months weighing 9–12.4 kg*: 160 mg orally twice daily for 10 days. *Infants and children ≥6 months weighing 7–8 kg*: 120 mg orally twice daily for 10 days. *Infants ≥6 months and older weighing 4–6 kg*: 80 mg orally twice daily for 10 days.	May be given with or without food. Available as tablets or in granules for suspension. Follow packaging instructions carefully for reconstitution of suspension. Can be used as initial treatment in severe/nonsevere cases or in recurrence for patients previously treated with vancomycin. Fidaxomicin does not require renal or hepatic dose adjustments because of its minimal systemic absorption.

CAP, Community-acquired pneumonia; *CDC*, Centers for Disease Control and Prevention; *COPD*, chronic obstructive pulmonary disease; *CrCl*, creatinine clearance; *FDA*, U.S. Food and Drug Administration; *GI*, gastrointestinal; *MRSA*, methicillin-resistant *Staphylococcus aureus*.

Erythromycin

Pharmacokinetics. Erythromycin can be delivered via a variety of routes, including oral, topical, and ophthalmic (for discussion of the ophthalmic route, see Chapter 4). Erythromycin is highly protein bound and distributed widely into most body tissues, except for the brain and cerebrospinal fluid (CSF). Excretion is predominantly via bile, with only small amounts found in the urine.

Because erythromycin is inactivated by stomach acid, different formulations have been developed to prevent this effect, leading to the greatest absorption taking place in the duodenum. Oral erythromycin is available in ethylsuccinate, stearate, and estolate preparations and as erythromycin base. More recently, oral erythromycin has become available in encapsulated pellets. All forms are similarly effective. Peak serum levels of free erythromycin are typically achieved in 1 to 4 hours and range from 0.1 to 2 mcg/mL. The normal half-life of erythromycin in healthy adults is approximately 1.5 hours. Renal impairment can prolong half-life up to 6 hours.

PHARMACOGENETICS

Drug Interactions With Erythromycin

Erythromycin and clarithromycin are cytochrome (CYP) 3A4 enzyme system inhibitors, as well as substrates and inhibitors of P-glycoprotein. Administration of erythromycin or clarithromycin with drugs primarily metabolized via CYP 3A4 can result in significant drug interactions. Because azithromycin does not affect CYP 3A4, it is associated with fewer drug interactions.

Indications. Erythromycin can be used to treat a variety of illnesses commonly addressed in primary care, including upper and lower respiratory tract disorders, various skin infections, and a number of sexually transmitted and urogenital infections. It can also be used in the treatment of pelvic inflammatory disease, prevention of rheumatic fever, and treatment of intestinal amebiasis in patients unable to receive metronidazole. Of note, erythromycin may be used as a prokinetic agent for patients with gastroparesis.

Erythromycin is active against a variety of gram-positive and gram-negative bacteria. Examples of sensitive gram-positive bacteria include *Streptococcus pneumoniae*, *Streptococcus pyogenes* (group A beta-hemolytic streptococci), *Listeria monocytogenes*, and *Staphylococcus aureus*. Gram-negative bacteria sensitive to erythromycin include *Haemophilus influenzae*, *Legionella pneumophila*, *Helicobacter pylori*, *Chlamydia trachomatis*, and *Neisseria gonorrhoeae*. Erythromycin can be used to treat primary syphilis caused by *Treponema pallidum* in nonpregnant patients who are allergic to penicillin.

Adverse Effects. The most common adverse effects associated with erythromycin are GI related. They include nausea, vomiting, diarrhea, and anorexia. These effects are often dose related. Rarely, patients who are taking tablets or capsule forms of erythromycin may experience symptoms of esophagitis. Approximately 5% of patients may experience symptoms of hepatotoxicity that can persist for several weeks after the medication is discontinued. Rare cases of serious cardiovascular adverse effects have been associated with erythromycin, including prolonged QT interval, torsade de pointes, other ventricular arrhythmias, and even cardiac arrest. Severe diarrhea, abdominal tenderness, and abdominal cramping may be symptoms of pseudomembranous colitis, although this is rare. Topical application of erythromycin can result in pruritis, xerosis, peeling of skin, skin tenderness, and redness.

Contraindications. Erythromycin is contraindicated in patients with a history of macrolide hypersensitivity. It should be used cautiously in patients with impaired liver or biliary function or who regularly use alcohol. It should be used cautiously in patients with inflammatory bowel disorders or other GI disorders. Erythromycin should be avoided in patients with known QT prolongation or with a history of proarrhythmic conditions. It should be used cautiously in patients with a seizure disorder. Erythromycin is considered pregnancy category B and should be used with caution in patients who are breastfeeding.

Monitoring. Liver function should be monitored in patients who are taking erythromycin for extended periods. Evaluate for changes in the electrocardiogram (ECG), particularly in patients with cardiovascular risk factors. All patients with STIs who are sensitive to erythromycin should be screened for other STIs at the time of diagnosis and then evaluated for follow-up strategies to reduce the risk of reinfection.

Azithromycin

Pharmacokinetics. Absorption of azithromycin is rapid following oral administration. Both tablets and immediate-release oral suspension may be taken with or without food. The extended-release oral suspension should be taken on an empty stomach. Elimination is in the feces, with less than 10% excreted in the urine. While no dosage adjustment is required, use with caution in patients with a creatinine clearance (CrCl) less than 10 mL/min.

PRACTICE PEARLS

Macrolides and Sexually Transmitted Infections

Erythromycin and azithromycin are commonly recommended treatment options for a variety of STIs. Always refer to the most recent clinical practice guidelines for a specific medication regimen.

Indications. Azithromycin is effective against a wide variety of infections due to aerobic gram-positive organisms and gram-negative infections. Gram-positive organisms sensitive to azithromycin include methicillin-susceptible *Staphylococcus aureus*, *Streptococcus pneumoniae*, *Streptococcus pyogenes* (group A beta-hemolytic streptococci), *Streptococcus sp.*, viridans group, and *Mycobacterium avium*. Aerobic gram-negative organisms include *Haemophilus influenzae*, *Moraxella catarrhalis*, *Neisseria gonorrhoeae*, *Heliobacter* *pylori*, and *Legionella pneumophila*. Other organisms include *Chlamydia trachomatis*, *Chlamydophila pneumoniae*, and *Mycoplasma pneumoniae*. Azithromycin can be used to treat CAP, bronchitis, uncomplicated skin infections, pelvic inflammatory disease, and uncomplicated gonorrhea of the cervix, urethra, rectum, and pharynx. Azithromycin may be used in human immunodeficiency virus (HIV)-infected patients with mycobacterium avium complex infection who are intolerant to clarithromycin. It can be used for the treatment of nongonococcal urethritis and other urogenital infections.

Adverse Effects. The most common adverse effects associated with azithromycin are typically GI related and include diarrhea, nausea, vomiting, abdominal pain, and anorexia. GI-related symptoms are frequent in adults receiving single oral-dose regimens and in pediatric patients receiving higher doses. Patients may experience photosensitivity, rash, or itching of the skin. Rarely, serious skin reactions such as Stevens-Johnson syndrome and toxic epidermal necrolysis have occurred. Elevations of liver enzymes may occur in a small percentage (1% to 2%) of patients. Azithromycin has been associated with pseudomembranous colitis and other superinfections such as oral candidiasis, vaginitis, and fungal superinfection; however, these are rare. Cardiovascular adverse reactions including chest pain and palpitations are rare (fewer than 1%).

Contraindications. Azithromycin is contraindicated in patients with hepatic disease or who have known azithromycin or macrolide hypersensitivity. It should be used cautiously in patients with a history of cardiovascular disease and dysrhythmias. It may be associated with prolonged QT intervals; however, the risk is less with azithromycin than with clarithromycin or erythromycin.

QUALITY AND SAFETY

Macrolides and Prolonged QT Intervals

Use macrolides cautiously in patients with cardiac disease or other conditions or medications that increase the risk of QT prolongation. Remember that females, older patients, and patients with diabetes mellitus, thyroid disease, malnutrition, alcoholism, or hepatic impairment may be at increased risk for QT prolongation.

Monitoring. Patients receiving systemic azithromycin should be monitored for signs and symptoms of liver dysfunction, and therapy should be discontinued if signs or symptoms occur. Azithromycin may mask or delay symptoms of incubating syphilis, so monitoring for all STIs should occur using the most recent practice guidelines. Monitor for signs of superinfection.

Clarithromycin

Pharmacokinetics. Clarithromycin is available in several oral preparations including immediate- and extended-release tablets and as an oral suspension. Immediate-release tablets and the oral suspension may be given without regard to food, while the extended-release tablets should be given with food. Clarithromycin is well absorbed from the GI tract, with bioavailability slightly reduced via first-pass metabolism. Protein binding varies between approximately 42% and 70%. Clarithromycin is well distributed through the body, achieving higher concentrations in the tissues than in serum. It is excreted through the kidneys in urine as well as in bile.

Indications. Clarithromycin is used to treat a variety of infections that result from gram-positive and gram-negative aerobes. Gram-positive organisms sensitive to clarithromycin include methicillin-susceptible *Staphylococcus aureus*, *Streptococcus pneumoniae*, *Streptococcus pyogenes* (group A beta-hemolytic streptococci), and *Mycobacterium avium*. Aerobic gram-negative organisms include *Haemophilus influenzae*, *Moraxella catarrhalis*, *Neisseria gonorrhoeae*, *Heliobacter pylori*, and *Legionella pneumophila*. Other susceptible organisms include *Chlamydophila pneumoniae* and *Mycoplasma pneumoniae*. Unlike erythromycin and azithromycin, clarithromycin is not effective against *Chlamydia trachomatis*. It can be used to treat CAP, bronchitis, pharyngitis, sinusitis, acute otitis media, and uncomplicated skin and skin structure infections. Clarithromycin is effective for the treatment of *Mycobacterium avium* complex (MAC) infection in HIV-infected patients and nongonococcal urethritis.

Adverse Effects. The most common adverse effects are nausea and vomiting (approximately 25% of patients) and dysgeusia (approximately 19%). Slightly fewer than 10% of patients experience mild diarrhea, headache, flatulence, mild abdominal pain, and mild rash. Fewer than 5% of patients have elevated liver function tests (LFTs). Rarely, patients may experience cardiac dysrhythmias, including QT prolongation and atrial fibrillation.

Contraindications. Clarithromycin is contraindicated in all patients with a history of hypersensitivity to macrolides and those with a history of jaundice and/or liver dysfunction. It should be used cautiously in patients with a history of cardiac dysrhythmias and in patients taking medications that may prolong the QT interval. Clarithromycin is considered pregnancy risk category C and is not recommended for use during pregnancy unless there is no alternative. It has not been thoroughly evaluated for use in breastfeeding patients.

Monitoring. Monitor for any signs of superinfection, particularly *Candida*, as overgrowth can occur with clarithromycin therapy. Monitoring of LFTs should also be considered. To reduce GI effects, patients may take the medication with food.

PRACTICE PEARLS

Macrolide Use in Pregnancy and Lactation

Erythromycin and azithromycin are considered pregnancy risk category B; clarithromycin is considered pregnancy category C. Erythromycin is generally considered safe during breastfeeding.

Prescriber Considerations for Macrolide Therapy

Clinical Practice Guidelines

In October 2019, the ATS and the IDSA updated the 2007 guidelines for the diagnosis and treatment of CAP (Metlay et al., 2019). For healthy individuals with CAP and no comorbidities or risk factors for methicillin-resistant *Staphylococcus aureus* (MRSA) or *Pseudomonas aeruginosa*, macrolides are an option for therapy (if local pneumococcal resistance is less than 25%). For patients with comorbidities, combination therapy with a beta-lactam antibiotic plus a macrolide or doxycycline is recommended.

Clinical practice guidelines for STIs were updated in 2021 and can be found on the Centers for Disease Control and Prevention (CDC) website: https://www.cdc.gov/std/. Macrolides are considered as options for the treatment of a variety of STIs, including chlamydia, nongonococcal urethritis and other urogenital infections, and gonorrhea.

BOOKMARK THIS!

Clinical Guidelines for Diagnosis and Treatment of Adults With CAP

- The ATS and the IDSA have updated the 2007 guidelines: https://www.atsjournals.org/doi/10.1164/rccm.201908-1581ST.

Clinical Reasoning for Macrolide Therapy

Consider the individual patient's health problem requiring macrolide therapy. Be sure to carefully determine the need for macrolide therapy given the increasing incidence of antibiotic resistance. For patients who are candidates for macrolide therapy, caution should be taken with dosing in the presence of severe renal or hepatic impairment or when potential drug interactions with the patient's current drug regimen are identified. For cases in which antibiotics may not be indicated, such as in suspected otitis media, follow practice guidelines to determine whether treatment with antibiotics is appropriate.

Determine the desired therapeutic outcome based on the macrolide therapy needed for the patient's health problem. The goal of macrolide therapy is to eradicate the infection without significant adverse effects, particularly superinfection. Considering the possible risk of QT prolongation, use caution in prescribing these drugs to patients with known cardiovascular disease who are taking other medications that may impact the QT interval.

Assess the macrolide selected for its appropriateness for an individual patient by considering the medication's side effects and the patient's age, race/ethnicity, comorbidities, and genetic factors. Doses for children should be carefully determined to minimize the risk of under- or overdosage. Age, weight, and severity of illness are essential factors in determining dosage for children when prescribing macrolides and are reflected in dosage recommendations. Lower doses of macrolides generally are not necessary for older adults, provided they do not have severe renal or hepatic impairment. It is essential to carefully consider drug interactions as erythromycin and clarithromycin are metabolized by the CYP 450 3A4 system and interact with a wide variety of drugs that are also metabolized by that system.

Initiate the treatment plan with the selected macrolide by first providing adequate patient education to ensure the patient's understanding and promote full participation in the therapy. It is vital to help patients understand the need to complete the full course of medication, even if they feel better, to reduce the risk of antibiotic resistance. These medications may cause GI distress, but these symptoms may be reduced by taking the medication with a full glass of water or food. It is also important to determine whether the patient is pregnant or planning to become pregnant while on macrolides, particularly when choosing which medication to prescribe.

Ensure complete patient and family understanding about the medication prescribed for macrolide therapy using a variety of education strategies. Teach-back strategies can be helpful in ensuring patient and family understanding. Also, patients and families may find smartphone medication reminder apps to be useful to ensure adherence to the full course of medication. Instruct the patient to notify their provider if their symptoms do not improve in 48 to 72 hours or if they worsen. Because of potential drug interactions, teach the patient to avoid adding any new herbal or over-the-counter (OTC) medications while taking macrolides. Always provide and reinforce information about safe sex practices to reduce STIs.

Conduct follow-up and monitoring of patient responses to macrolide therapy. Follow-up varies based on the specific condition and clinical practice guidelines. The patient should be instructed to follow up should they experience severe diarrhea or any significant adverse effects.

Teaching Points for Macrolide Therapy

Health Promotion Strategies

- Consider the cost of erythromycin compared to newer macrolides. Erythromycin is less expensive but may have more GI effects and require more frequent dosing, which may affect patient adherence. Azithromycin and clarithromycin typically have greater absorption, longer half-lives, and a broader spectrum of activity than erythromycin.
- All patients who are diagnosed with or have a suspected STI such as HIV, syphilis, chlamydia, or gonorrhea should undergo broad testing for other STIs. Perform follow-up testing as recommended by current clinical practice guidelines.
- Consider using the Center for Disease Dynamics, Economics & Policy antibiotic resistance maps and, if available, local antibiograms, to guide prescribing practices.
- Provide patients with information to reduce infection including hand hygiene, safe sex practices, and obtaining recommended vaccines to prevent pneumonia and other infectious diseases.

Patient Education for Medication Safety

- Take medications with a full glass of water.
- Do not chew, cut, or crush the tablets unless specifically indicated on the medication packaging.
- Stop taking the medication and notify your primary care provider if you develop a skin rash, redness, blistering, or itchiness.
- Report severe, watery diarrhea to your primary care provider as this may be an indication of a more serious infection.
- Avoid direct sunlight exposure while taking macrolides due to the risk of photosensitivity, particularly with azithromycin.
- Clarithromycin may be taken with or without food. It should not be refrigerated. It should be shaken well before each use.
- Azithromycin tablets can be taken without regard to food. The oral suspension should be given on an empty stomach.
- Make sure to take the prescription as prescribed to decrease the risk of antibiotic resistance.

Application Questions for Discussion

1. Discuss safe sex practices for patients who present with symptoms associated with an STI. What community and public health resources are available beyond primary care?
2. How would you determine which infections or adverse medication effects would merit primary care follow-up versus specialty care follow-up?
3. What do the resistance maps indicate for appropriate antibiotic use in your region of the country?

Selected Bibliography

Beauduy, C. E., & Winston, L. G. (2017). Tetracyclines, macrolides, clindamycin, chloramphenicol, streptogramins, & oxazolidinones. In B. G. Katzung (Ed.), *Basic & Clinical Pharmacology* (14th ed.). New York: McGraw-Hill Education.

Burcham, J., & Rosenthal, L. (2016). *Lehne's Pharmacology for Nursing Care* (10th ed.). St. Louis: Elsevier.

Cheng, Y.-J., Nie, X.-Y., Chen, X.-M., Lin, X.-X., Tang, K., Zeng, W.-T., & Wu, S.-H. (2015). The role of macrolide antibiotics in increasing cardiovascular risk. *Journal of the American College of Cardiology, 66*(20), 2173–2184. http://doi.org/10.1016/j.jacc.2015.09.029.

Elsevier. Clinical pharmacology powered by ClinicalKey®. (2019). Retrieved from http://www.clinicalkey.com.

Gruenberg, K., & Guglielmo, B. J. (2020). Erythromycin group (macrolides). In M. A. Papadakis, S. J. McPhee, & M. W. Rabow (Eds.), *Current Medical Diagnosis and Treatment 2020*. New York: McGraw-Hill Education.

Hansen, M. P., Scott, A. M., McCullough, A., Thorning, S., Aronson, J. K., Beller, E. M., & Del Mar, C. B. (2019). Adverse events in people taking macrolide antibiotics versus placebo for any indication. *Cochrane Database of Systematic Reviews* (1). http://doi.org/10.1002/14651858.CD011825.pub2.

Haran, J. P., & Volturo, G. A. (2018). Macrolide resistance in cases of community-acquired bacterial pneumonia in the emergency department. *The Journal of Emergency Medicine, 55*(3), 347–353. http://doi.org/10.1016/j.jemermed.2018.04.031.

Workowski, K. A., & Bolan, G. A. (2015). Sexually transmitted diseases treatment guidelines, 2015. *Morbidity and Mortality Weekly Report (MMWR) Recommendations and Reports, 64*(3), 1–137.

Metlay, J. P., Waterer, G. W., Long, A. C., Anzueto, A., Brozek, J., Crothers, K., & Whitney, C. G. (2019). Diagnosis and treatment of adults with community-acquired pneumonia. An official clinical practice guideline of the American Thoracic Society and Infectious Diseases Society of America. *American Journal of Respiratory and Critical Care Medicine, 200*(7), e45–e67. http://doi.org/10.1164/rccm.201908-1581ST.

44

Fluoroquinolones

CHERYL H. ZAMBROSKI

Overview

Quinolones, represented by the drug *nalidixic acid*, were discovered in the early 1960s as a byproduct of chloroquine synthesis. Nalidixic acid was a narrow spectrum antibiotic used to treat urinary tract infections (UTIs). Unfortunately, nalidixic acid was associated with a very high adverse effect profile. By adding a fluorine radical to the chemical structure of the nalidixic acid, scientists developed the next generation of quinolone medications, called *fluoroquinolones*. At this time, the quinolone nalidixic acid is off the market in favor of the newer, broad-spectrum fluoroquinolones. Still, many references use the terms *quinolone* and *fluoroquinolone* interchangeably. For the purposes of this discussion, the term *fluoroquinolone* will be used.

Fluoroquinolones are effective in treating a variety of conditions caused by select gram-positive or gram-negative bacteria, including infections of the gastrointestinal (GI) tract, bone and joint infections, skin and skin structure infections (e.g., bite wounds, diabetic foot ulcers, and surgical incision site infections), and select cases of community-acquired pneumonia (CAP). One medication, ciprofloxacin, is recommended as a preferred therapy for postexposure prophylaxis to *Bacillus anthracis* (anthrax). Ophthalmic and otic forms of fluoroquinolones are discussed in Chapter 4.

Fluoroquinolones act by disrupting the process of bacterial synthesis and are considered bactericidal. They can do this through two mechanisms. First, fluoroquinolones inhibit deoxyribonucleic acid (DNA) gyrase (also known as topoisomerase II). Normally, DNA gyrase helps unwind/relax the supercoiled DNA, a step critical to the process of transcription and replication. Fluoroquinolones can bind to DNA gyrase, preventing the smooth unwinding of the supercoiled DNA strand, leading to breaks in DNA and cell death. The second mechanism is through inhibition of topoisomerase IV. Topoisomerase IV normally helps to separate linked daughter chromosomes at the end of DNA replication. By binding to topoisomerase IV, fluoroquinolones stop the separation, ultimately leading to cell death.

The primary target of action for fluoroquinolones differs for gram-negative and gram-positive bacteria. In general, medications that primarily target DNA gyrase are effective against gram-negative bacteria. Medications that primarily inhibit topoisomerase IV are effective against gram-positive bacteria. A newer fluoroquinolone, delafloxacin, is considered dual targeting because it is equally potent against DNA gyrase and topoisomerase IV.

Bacterial resistance to fluoroquinolones typically develops by mutations in chromosomal genes. These mutations usually affect the target enzymes DNA gyrase and/or topoisomerase IV. The mutation then reduces the affinity of the antibiotic to the target enzyme. Other mechanisms of resistance are through *intracellular plasmids* that reduce sensitivity to the fluoroquinolone, and *efflux pumps* that limit intracellular accumulation of medication.

> ### BOOKMARK THIS!
>
> **FDA Medication Guides**
>
> The U.S. Food and Drug Administration (FDA) provides access to guides containing information on a wide variety of medications and medication classes at https://www.fda.gov/drugs/drug-safety-and-availability/medication-guides. The guides are updated with the newest drug labeling and provide information for primary care providers as well as patients.

While the side effects of fluoroquinolones are generally mild, such as mild diarrhea or headache, fluoroquinolones must be used cautiously due to the potential for serious adverse effects. The FDA enhanced the black box warning on fluoroquinolone labels for systemic use due to the risk for disabling and potentially permanent adverse effects on tendons, muscles, joints, nerves, and the central nervous system (CNS) that may occur even in healthy patients taking this class of medication (FDA, 2016). Examples of these effects include tendonitis, tendon rupture, peripheral neuropathy, and seizures. Potential psychiatric adverse reactions include anxiety, restlessness, delirium, hallucinations, nightmares, and memory impairment.

> ### QUALITY AND SAFETY
>
> **FDA Warning for Fluoroquinolone Antibiotics**
>
> In December 2018, the FDA announced that fluoroquinolones can increase the risk of aortic dissection or aortic tear. Therefore, fluoroquinolones should be avoided in patients with a history of aortic aneurysm and in those who are at risk for aortic aneurysm. This includes older adults and those with genetic risk such as Marfan or Ehlers-Danlos syndrome.

Attempted or completed suicides have been reported, particularly in patients with a history of depression (Box 44.1). More recently, the FDA (2018) announced that fluoroquinolones may increase the risk of aortic dissection or aortic tear.

Because of the risk of adverse effects, the FDA recommends fluoroquinolones be used only when other options are not available for treating uncomplicated conditions (such as acute bacterial sinusitis, acute bronchitis, and UTIs) because of the risk of adverse effects. For treatment of more complicated infections such as bone or joint infections, pneumonia, or intraabdominal infections, the benefits of fluoroquinolones may outweigh the risks.

Fluroquinolone Therapy

Fluoroquinolones are available for use in patients with select gram-positive and gram-negative infections. Older available fluoroquinolones include ciprofloxacin and ofloxacin. Newer ones include levofloxacin, gemifloxacin, delafloxacin, and moxifloxacin. Of the newer fluoroquinolones, gemifloxacin and moxifloxacin have greater activity in treating anaerobes. Gemifloxacin, levofloxacin, and moxifloxacin are commonly considered the *respiratory fluoroquinolones* as they are active against a variety of bacterial pathogens such as *H. influenzae*, *S. pneumoniae*, *Legionella*, *Mycoplasma*, and *Chlamydophila pneumoniae*.

BOOKMARK THIS!

Antibiotic Resistance Map

As it does for many antibiotics, the Center for Disease Dynamics, Economics & Policy offers a resistance map that can help guide primary care providers in selecting the most effective medications for their patients. See https://resistancemap.cddep.org/index.php.

Caution must be used in prescribing any fluoroquinolones related to the risk of food–drug interactions (Box 44.2). For example, bioavailability of oral fluoroquinolones is significantly decreased when given with cations found in calcium and iron supplements, antacids including aluminum and magnesium, zinc salts, multivitamins, and milk and milk-containing products. As a result, it is important to separate the timing of these substances by at least 2 hours. If possible,

• **BOX 44.2** Examples of Common Drug–Food Interactions with Fluoroquinolones[a]

Drug	Reaction
Theophylline/ Aminophylline	Increased risk of seizures if taking with ciprofloxacin
Warfarin	Increased anticoagulant activity
Antacids	Can decrease absorption by up to 90%
Clozapine	Ciprofloxacin increases plasma level of clozapine as much as 80%
Dairy products or other foods high in calcium or iron	Can decrease absorption by up to 90%
Orange juice and calcium-fortified orange juice	Can decrease clinical efficacy and potentially increase resistance to fluoroquinolones
Antidiabetic agents	May cause severe hypoglycemia
NSAIDs	Increased risk of CNS stimulation and seizures
Corticosteroids	Increased risk of tendon rupture, particularly in older adults
Drugs that prolong the QT interval	Ciprofloxacin, ofloxacin, gemifloxacin, levofloxacin, and moxifloxacin may increase the risk for QT prolongation. Only delafloxacin does not affect the QT interval.

[a]There are many other drug–drug and drug–food interactions with fluoroquinolones. The primary care provider should check all drug interactions among the patient's medications before prescribing any fluoroquinolone.

CNS, Central nervous system; *NSAIDs*, nonsteroidal antiinflammatory drugs.

---

it is best for patients to avoid them altogether while taking fluoroquinolones. Nonsteroidal antiinflammatory drugs (NSAIDs) can increase the risk of CNS stimulation and seizures if taken with fluoroquinolones. Patients taking corticosteroids while taking fluoroquinolones are at increased risk of tendon rupture. See Table 44.1 for indications and dosing recommendations of common fluoroquinolones.

Ciprofloxacin

Pharmacokinetics. Oral ciprofloxacin can be prescribed in immediate- or extended-release tablets or as a suspension. In general, ciprofloxacin is rapidly absorbed; however, food may delay absorption of the immediate-release tablets. There is no delay in absorption with extended-release tablets or suspension. Ciprofloxacin undergoes minimal first-pass metabolism and is well distributed in most tissues. It is predominantly excreted via urine or fecal routes. Normal half-life is approximately 4 hours but may be delayed up to 6 to 9 hours for patients with renal impairment. Older adults may have higher plasma concentrations related to decreased renal clearance.

Indications. Ciprofloxacin is effective in treating a variety of infections of the bone, joints, and skin (including animal bites). It can be used for infections of the GI tract including gastroenteritis and infectious diarrhea. When combined with metronidazole, ciprofloxacin is used in cases

TABLE
44.1   **Fluoroquinolones**

Medication	Indication	Dosage	Considerations and Monitoring
Levofloxacin	Mild to moderate complicated UTI or acute pyelonephritis	750 mg orally every 24 hr for 5 days or 250 mg orally every 24 hr for 10 days.	Due to the serious and potentially permanent adverse effects associated with them, fluoroquinolone antibiotics should be used only where alternatives cannot be used.
	Mild to moderate uncomplicated UTI	250 mg orally every 24 hours for 3 days.	
	Acute bacterial exacerbations of chronic bronchitis	500 mg orally every 24 hours for 5–7 days.	
	CAP	750 mg orally every 24 hr for at least 5 days or 500 mg orally every 24 hr for 7–14 days.	Duration of antibiotic therapy should be continued until the patient achieves clinical stability for at least the recommended duration.
Moxifloxacin	Mild to moderate CAP Acute bacterial exacerbation of chronic bronchitis	400 mg orally once daily for at least 5 days.	Avoid use in pregnant and breastfeeding patients unless the benefit outweighs the risk.
	Acute bacterial sinusitis	400 mg orally once daily for 10 days.	Moxifloxacin and levofloxacin offer increased gram-positive activity compared with ciprofloxacin, particularly with *S. pneumoniae*.
	Uncomplicated skin and skin structure infections due to *S. aureus* (MSSA) and *S. pyogenes*	400 mg orally once daily for 7 days.	
Ciprofloxacin	Acute, uncomplicated UTI (acute cystitis) in females	**Immediate-release tablets:** 250 mg orally every 12 hours for 3 days. **Extended-release tablets:** 500 mg orally once daily for 3 days.	For older patients and patients with renal impairment, calculate creatinine clearance to guide dose requirements.
	Mild to moderate UTIs and for the treatment of severe and/or complicated UTIs, including pyelonephritis	**Immediate-release tablets:** 250–500 mg orally every 12 hr for 7–14 days. **Extended-release tablets:** 1000 mg orally once daily for 7-14 days.	Levofloxacin, moxifloxacin, ciprofloxacin, ofloxacin, gemifloxacin, and norfloxacin have the potential to prolong the QT interval.
	CAP **Note:** Not a drug of first choice in the treatment of presumed or confirmed pneumonia secondary to *S. pneumoniae*	500–750 mg orally every 12 hr for 7–14 days.	Delafloxacin has not shown clinically relevant effect on cardiac repolarization.
	Skin and skin structure infections, including diabetic foot ulcers, surgical incision site infections, and animal bite wounds	500–750 mg orally every 12 hr for 7–14 days.	Delafloxacin has shown increased activity against *S. aureus* and may maintain activity for organisms showing resistance to other fluroquinolones.
	Enteric infections, including acute gastroenteritis and infectious diarrhea	500 mg orally every 12 hr for 5–7 days.	
	Chronic bacterial prostatitis	500 mg orally every 12 hr for 28 days.	
Ofloxacin	Bacterial prostatitis due to *E. coli*	300 mg orally every 12 hr for 6 weeks.	
	Uncomplicated UTI due to *E.coli* or *K. pneumoniae*	200 mg orally every 12 hours for 3 days.	
	Uncomplicated UTI due to other pathogens	200 mg orally every 12 hours for 7 days.	
	Complicated UTIs	200 mg every 12 hours for 10 days.	
	Infections of skin and skin structure due to susceptible organisms	400 mg orally every 12 hr for 10 days.	
	CAP	400 mg orally every 12 hr for 10 days.	

TABLE 44.1	Fluoroquinolones—cont'd		
Medication	Indication	Dosage	Considerations and Monitoring
Gemifloxacin	Acute bacterial exacerbation of chronic bronchitis	320 mg orally once daily for at least 5 days.	
	CAP as monotherapy for outpatients with comorbidities		
Delafloxacin	Acute bacterial skin and skin structure infections	450 mg orally every 12 hr for 5–14 days.	
	CAP	450 mg orally every 12 hr for 5–10 days.	

CAP, Community-acquired pneumonia; *MSSA*, methicillin-susceptible *Staphylococcus aureus*; *UTI*, urinary tract infection.

PHARMACOGENETICS

Ciprofloxacin

Ciprofloxacin inhibits the cytochrome (CYP) 1A2 isoenzyme. Administration of ciprofloxacin with other drugs that are metabolized by CYP 1A2 may result in increased plasma concentrations and therefore may cause clinically significant pharmacodynamic side effects. In addition, some data suggest that ciprofloxacin is an inhibitor of the CYP 3A4 isoenzyme.

of community-acquired intra-abdominal infections such as acute diverticulitis and acute cholecystitis. It may be combined with clindamycin as an option for moderate to severe diabetic wound infections.

Ciprofloxacin is generally more effective against gram-negative than gram-positive organisms. Gram-negative bacteria that may be sensitive to ciprofloxacin include various species of *Campylobacter*, *Klebsiella*, *Salmonella*, *Shigella*, and *Vibrio*. Unfortunately, many strains of *E. faecalis* are only moderately susceptible to ciprofloxacin due to increasing resistance patterns.

Gram-positive organisms that may be sensitive to ciprofloxacin include *Staphylococcus sp*. and *Streptococcus sp*. However, it is important to consider growing resistance patterns. For example, ciprofloxacin should be used cautiously in treatment of infections related to pneumococcus and *Staphylococcus aureus* due to increased rates of resistance.

Adverse Effects. See Box 44.1 for black box warnings. Other adverse effects associated with systemic ciprofloxacin include nausea, diarrhea, and pharyngitis. Although relatively infrequent, adverse reactions affecting special senses, such as dysgeusia, hearing loss, nystagmus, tinnitus, or visual impairment, may occur in fewer than 1% of patients. Agranulocytosis, severe allergic reactions, and angioedema are rare. Up to 1.3% of patients may have abnormal liver function tests (LFTs). Cases of severe hepatotoxicity have been reported (fewer than 1%). Blood glucose disturbances, including hyperglycemia and

hypoglycemia, have been reported in fewer than 1% of adult patients receiving systemic ciprofloxacin.

Contraindications. Ciprofloxacin is contraindicated for anyone with known sensitivity to quinolones or fluoroquinolones. It should be used cautiously in patients with cardiac dysrhythmias or other cardiovascular conditions that may predispose to dysrhythmias. It should be avoided in patients with a history of peripheral neuropathy or with any other known or suspected CNS disorder. Use of ciprofloxacin during pregnancy and breastfeeding should be avoided due to lack of well-controlled studies unless the potential benefits justify the potential risks.

Monitoring. Patients taking ciprofloxacin should be monitored for onset of musculoskeletal symptoms. If any emerge, the patient should hold their medication and contact their provider. Diabetic patients should monitor their blood sugar frequently. Educate the patient to notify the provider for any rash, dizziness, or changes in vision.

Moxifloxacin

Pharmacokinetics. Oral moxifloxacin is widely distributed in the body, with good penetration in respiratory tissues and fluids. It is approximately 30% to 50% protein bound and has been detected in abdominal tissues and fluids, mucosa of the sinuses, nasal and bronchial secretions, saliva, skeletal muscle, skin blister fluid, and subcutaneous tissue. Moxifloxacin metabolism does not involve CYP 450 enzymes. Elimination is typically via the urine and feces. Half-life is approximately 12 hours.

QUALITY AND SAFETY

Dosing Requirements for Fluoroquinolones

When compared to other fluoroquinolones, moxifloxacin is the only drug in this class that does not require renal impairment dosing. In general, other fluoroquinolones require dosing adjustments for creatinine clearances (CrCl) less than 50 mL/min.

Indications. Moxifloxacin can be used as monotherapy for patients with mild to moderate CAP who have comorbidities. It can be used for treatment of uncomplicated skin and skin structure infections due to *Staphylococcus aureus* and *Streptococcus pyogenes* or for complicated skin and skin structure infections due to *Enterobacter cloacae*, *Escherichia coli*, *Klebsiella pneumoniae*, or *Staphylococcus aureus*. Moxifloxacin may be used in cases of acute bacterial exacerbation of chronic bronchitis or acute bacterial sinusitis, but only when alternatives are not available, due to the potential for adverse effects.

Adverse Effects. See Box 44.1 for black box warnings. The most common adverse effects are mild and include nausea, diarrhea, and headache. Candidiasis, vaginal infection, fungal infection, and gastroenteritis are rare, occurring in fewer than 1% of patients. Abnormal liver function and elevated liver enzymes are also rare. Blood dyscrasias are uncommon but may include coagulopathy, thrombocytopenia, neutropenia, and agranulocytosis. Moxifloxacin may affect blood glucose in patients with diabetes who are receiving insulin or oral hypoglycemic agents.

Contraindications. Moxifloxacin is contraindicated in patients with quinolone/fluoroquinolone hypersensitivity. It should be avoided in patients with myasthenia gravis, a history of peripheral neuropathy, cardiovascular illnesses (including cardiac dysrhythmias), or any disorder that would increase the risk of adverse effects. It should not be used in patients who are pregnant or breastfeeding unless the potential benefits outweigh the risks.

Monitoring. Moxifloxacin may be given without regard to food, including milk and dietary supplements containing calcium. Give at least 4 hours before or 8 hours after giving ferrous sulfate, sucralfate, or dietary supplements containing iron, magnesium, or zinc. These substances interfere with medication absorption.

Remind patients to avoid excessive sunlight exposure due to photosensitivity. If they must be exposed to sunlight, patients should wear protective clothing.

Monitor liver and renal function studies for patients requiring moxifloxacin. Discontinue if any signs or symptoms indicating serious adverse effects occur.

PRACTICE PEARLS

Fluoroquinolone Use in Pediatrics

While fluoroquinolones are typically not recommended in pediatric patients due to the potential for musculoskeletal adverse effects, current recommendations from the American Academy of Pediatrics (AAP) Committee on Infectious Diseases include reserving the use of systemic quinolones for multidrug-resistant infections when other alternatives are not feasible, safe, or effective (Jackson & Schutze, 2016).

Levofloxacin

Pharmacokinetics. Oral levofloxacin is rapidly absorbed and has a bioavailability of 99%. It is 24% to 28% bound to serum protein and is widely distributed into body tissues.

In fact, lung tissue concentrations are approximately 2 to 5 times higher than plasma concentrations. Peak plasma concentrations occur approximately 1 to 2 hours after dosing. Food increases time to peak concentration by approximately 1 hour. In addition, food decreases peak concentration by approximately 14% after tablet administration and 25% after oral solution administration. Levofloxacin undergoes limited metabolism and approximately 87% is excreted unchanged in the urine. Mean half-life in adults is 6 to 8 hours.

Indications. Levofloxacin can be effective against a variety of organisms, including *Streptococcus pneumoniae*, *Staphylococcus aureus*, *Haemophilus influenzae*, *Enterococcus faecalis*, *Streptococcus pyogenes*, *Moraxella catarrhalis*, and *Proteus mirabilis*. Levofloxacin can be used for the treatment of mild to moderate complicated UTIs or acute pyelonephritis, as monotherapy for CAP outpatients with comorbidities, and for the treatment of chronic bacterial prostatitis.

Adverse Effects. See Box 44.1 for black box warnings. The most common adverse effect associated with levofloxacin is dysgeusia, occurring in at least 10% of patients. GI adverse effects are relatively infrequent, occurring in fewer than 10% of patients, and include nausea, vomiting, diarrhea or constipation, abdominal pain, and dyspepsia. Other infrequent adverse effects include mild headache, insomnia, or dizziness. Rarely, severe reactions including renal failure, seizures, pancreatitis, hyperkalemia, ventricular tachycardia, and cardiac arrest may occur.

Contraindications. Levofloxacin is contraindicated in patients with known quinolone/fluoroquinolone hypersensitivity. It should be used cautiously in patients with known psychiatric history, cardiovascular disease, or history of tendinopathy or tendonitis. Use cautiously for patients with renal insufficiency or dehydration. Older adults, females, and patients with diabetes, alcoholism, thyroid disease, or liver disease may be at greater risk for QT prolongation.

Monitoring. For patients with a history of renal impairment, monitor serum creatinine/blood urea nitrogen (BUN). Teach patients to report any new-onset chest pain, joint pain, or significant diarrhea. Also, educate patients to notify the primary care provider if they experience any increase in psychiatric symptoms.

Prescriber Considerations for Fluroquinolone Therapy

Clinical Practice Guidelines

In 2019, the American Thoracic Society (ATS) and the Infectious Diseases Society of America (IDSA) updated their clinical guidelines for CAP (Metlay et al., 2019). Highlights from the 2019 update include consideration of antibiotic resistance levels prior to antibiotic selection as well as the risk-benefit profiles of each medication. In 2007, β-lactam/macrolide and β-lactam/fluoroquinolone combinations were given equal weighting for standard empiric therapy of CAP. In the current guidelines, although both are accepted, evidence is in favor of the β-lactam/macrolide combination over the β-lactam/fluoroquinolone combination. The respiratory fluoroquinolones may be given as monotherapy for CAP patients with comorbidities.

> ### BOOKMARK THIS!
>
> **Infectious Diseases Society of America**
>
> The IDSA provides access to current clinical practice guidelines to help primary care providers and patients make decisions regarding the best way to treat select clinical issues. See https://www.idsociety.org/practice-guideline/practice-guidelines#/name_na_str/ASC/0/+.

Clinical Reasoning for Fluoroquinolone Therapy

Consider the individual patient's health problem requiring fluoroquinolone therapy. The most important question to ask is: are there alternative antibiotics with lower adverse effect profiles than fluoroquinolones? Next, it is important to learn the antibiotic resistance pattern in the practice area and to use this information to help guide the appropriateness of the use of the fluoroquinolone.

Determine the desired therapeutic outcome based on the fluoroquinolone needed for the patient's health problem. The goal is eradication of the infection without significant adverse effects. Adherence to treatment can reduce the risk of antibiotic resistance, so consider the dosing schedule as well as cost and patient self-care ability.

Assess the fluoroquinolone selected for its appropriateness for an individual patient by considering the medication's side effects and the patient's age, race/ethnicity, comorbidities, and genetic factors. Older patients are more likely than others to have reduced renal function, which increases the half-life of the fluoroquinolone. Dosages should be adjusted in patients with impaired renal function. Also, older adults are more prone to develop tendon rupture and adverse CNS reactions. Systemic quinolones, including ciprofloxacin, should be used with caution in patients with CNS disorders (such as seizures) or cerebrovascular disease (such as cerebral arteriosclerosis), or other risk factors that may predispose them to seizures or lower the seizure threshold. Patients with cardiovascular conditions are at greater risk for QT prolongation, aortic dissection, or aortic tear. Avoid use in patients with genetic disorders affecting the aorta.

Initiate the treatment plan with the selected fluoroquinolone by first providing adequate patient education to ensure the patient's understanding and promote full participation in the medication therapy. All patient education efforts must include the importance of adherence to the full course of antibiotic therapy. In addition, recognition of potential adverse effects associated with use of the fluoroquinolones is imperative. Advise patients of diet and medication timing to avoid interactions (e.g., calcium products and zinc and iron supplements).

Ensure complete patient and family understanding about the fluoroquinolone prescribed for therapy using a variety of education strategies. Use of verbal and written patient education materials on the importance of medication compliance as well as reminder applications available for use with smartphones may be helpful in reminding patients when to take their medication. Assess the patient's ability to adhere to the treatment plan and involve family members as needed.

Conduct follow-up and monitoring of patient responses to fluoroquinolone therapy. Consider black box warnings to help determine treatment plans and the need for patient education. For patients with a history of renal or liver impairment, monitor serum creatinine/BUN and LFTs. Teach patients to report any new-onset chest pain, joint pain, or significant diarrhea. Let patients know to notify their primary care provider if they experience any increase in psychiatric symptoms.

Teaching Points for Fluoroquinolone Therapy

Health Promotion Strategies

- Reinforce that it is critically important to avoid missing doses and to take the full course of medication to help combat antibiotic resistance.
- Teach the patient signs and symptoms that may indicate adverse reactions to fluoroquinolone therapy.
- Instruct diabetic or prediabetic patients that fluoroquinolones may impact blood sugar, so their use requires careful monitoring.
- Remind patients to contact their primary care provider or pharmacist before taking any over-the-counter (OTC) medications.
- Only use antibiotics when it is clear that the origin of the infection is bacterial rather than viral. Antibiotic stewardship is imperative.

Patient Education for Medication Safety

- Seek medical attention immediately if you experience sudden, severe, or constant pain in the stomach, chest, or back. This may indicate severe vascular adverse effects from the fluoroquinolones.
- Notify your primary care provider before you start taking a fluoroquinolone if you have a history of cardiovascular disease including aneurysm, high blood pressure, or hardening of the arteries, or if you have genetic conditions such as Marfan syndrome.
- Although rare, these medications may cause neurological problems such as confusion, anxiety, mood changes, and tremor. Notify your provider immediately if you have any new or worsening mental health problems or thoughts of suicide.
- This medication may cause tendon problems or injuries. Notify your provider if you have muscle weakness, pain, joint swelling, or tenderness.
- Follow medication directions carefully to reduce drug–food interactions with fluoroquinolones. Avoid taking products containing iron, calcium, or zinc within 2 to 4 hours of taking fluoroquinolones.
- Notify your provider if you have prediabetes or diabetes as these medications may affect your blood sugar.

- Avoid taking this medication if you are pregnant or trying to become pregnant or if you are breastfeeding.
- Notify your provider if you have a history of mental illness or are taking any medications for mental illness.
- Do not take OTC medications, particularly NSAIDs, without talking to your primary care provider or your pharmacist due to increased risk of adverse effects.
- Notify your provider if you have any severe diarrhea or if your diarrhea lasts more than 2 days.
- This medication increases your sensitivity to sunlight. Avoid exposure to direct sunlight or tanning beds. If you are out in the sun, use protective clothing.

Application Questions for Discussion

1. An older adult patient is convinced that the only treatment for an infection is antibiotics. You recognize that the current symptoms the patient is experiencing indicate a viral etiology. What is your strategy to improve the patient's understanding about viral vs. bacterial etiology of infection while maintaining or increasing patient satisfaction?
2. Using the antibiotic resistance map at https://resistance-map.cddep.org/index.php, what are the antibiotic resistance patterns in your region? How will you address this issue with other providers in your practice? In your region?
3. Discuss risks and benefits when choosing between β-lactam/macrolide combination and β-lactam/fluoroquinolones for select patients with CAP. When would you choose the fluoroquinolone combination over the macrolide combination?

Selected Bibliography

Bennett, A. C., Bennett, C. L., Witherspoon, B. J., & Knopf, K. B. (2019). An evaluation of reports of ciprofloxacin, levofloxacin, and moxifloxacin-associated neuropsychiatric toxicities, long-term disability, and aortic aneurysms/dissections disseminated by the Food and Drug Administration and the European Medicines Agency. *Expert Opinion on Drug Safety, 18*(11), 1055–1063. http://doi.org/10.1080/14740338.2019.1665022.

Burchum, J. R., & Rosenthal, L. D. (2018). *Lehne's Pharmacotherapeutics for Advanced Practice Providers.* St. Louis: Elsevier.

Elsevier. Clinical pharmacology powered by ClinicalKey®. (2019). Retrieved from http://www.clinicalkey.com.

Jackson, M. A., & Schutze, G. E. (2016). The use of systemic and topical fluoroquinolones. *Pediatrics, 138*(5), Article e20162706. http://doi.org/10.1542/peds.2016-2706.

Jacoby, G. A. (2005). Mechanisms of resistance to quinolones. *Clinical Infectious Diseases, 41*(Suppl. 2), S120–S126. http://doi.org/10.1086/428052.

Kennedy, W. K., Jann, M. W., & Kutscher, E. C. (2013). Clinically significant drug interactions with atypical antipsychotics. *CNS Drugs, 27*(12), 1021–1048. http://doi.org/10.1007/s40263-013-0114-6.

Meng, C., Shu-yi, Z., Fabriaga, E., Pian-hong, Z., & Quan, Z. (2018). Food–drug interactions precipitated by fruit juices other than grapefruit juice: An update review. *Journal of Food & Drug Analysis, 26*(2), 1–11. http://doi.org/10.1016/j.jfda.2018.01.009.

Merel, S. E., & Paauw, D. S. (2017). Common drug side effects and drug–drug interactions in elderly adults in primary care. *Journal of the American Geriatrics Society, 65*(7), 1578–1585. http://doi.org/10.1111/jgs.14870.

Metlay, J. P., Waterer, G. W., Long, A. C., Anzueto, A., Brozek, J., Crothers, K., & Whitney, C. G. (2019). Diagnosis and treatment of adults with community-acquired pneumonia. An official clinical practice guideline of the American Thoracic Society and Infectious Diseases Society of America. *American Journal of Respiratory and Critical Care Medicine, 200*(7), e45–e67. http://doi.org/10.1164/rccm.201908-1581.

U.S. Food and Drug Administration (2018). *Drug safety communication: FDA warns about increased risk of ruptures or tears in the aorta blood vessel with fluoroquinolone antibiotics in certain patients* [Press release]. Retrieved from https://www.fda.gov/drugs/drug-safety-and-availability/fda-warns-about-increased-risk-ruptures-or-tears-aorta-blood-vessel-fluoroquinolone-antibiotics.

U.S. Food and Drug Administration. (2016). *FDA drug safety communication: FDA updates warnings for oral and injectable fluoroquinolone antibiotics due to disabling side effects* [Press release] https://www.fda.gov/drugs/drug-safety-and-availability/fda-drug-safety-communication-fda-updates-warnings-oral-and-injectable-fluoroquinolone-antibiotics

45

Sulfonamides

KRISTY M. SHAEER

Overview

Sulfonamides were the first class of effective synthetic, broad-spectrum antimicrobial medications introduced in the 1930s, offering multiple clinical uses. This chapter reviews the sulfonamides and the combination drug of sulfamethoxazole with trimethoprim (SMZ/TMP or SMX/TMP). SMZ/TMP is the most used sulfonamide for respiratory, urinary, and gastrointestinal (GI) infections.

Relevant Physiology

Sulfonamides are *bacteriostatic*, which means they prevent cell growth or replication without killing the organism and require the aid of host defenses to clear tissues of the infecting microorganism. However, when SMZ is combined with TMP, this results in bactericidal action when synergy is achieved (Trubiano & Grayson, 2018). Sulfonamides inhibit folic acid synthesis within bacteria. P-aminobenzoic acid (PABA) combines with pteridine. Biosynthesis leads to the formation of tetrahydrofolic acid, which is an essential component required by deoxyribonucleic acid (DNA), ribonucleic acid (RNA), and proteins. Sulfonamides have a structure similar to PABA and competitively inhibit dihydropteroate synthetase and, ultimately, dihydrofolic acid synthesis. This prevents the occurrence of the necessary conversion of PABA to folic acid and ultimately disrupts the ability of bacteria to complete the biosynthetic formation of tetrahydrofolic acid (Beauduy & Winston, 2021). Fig. 45.1 represents the actions of sulfonamides and trimethoprim.

Classification

Sulfonamides act against gram-positive and gram-negative organisms, protozoa, and fungi. Therapeutic uses of a sulfonamide as monotherapy or as a combination (SMZ/TMP) include the treatment of genitourinary tract infections, otitis media, acute bronchitis, community-acquired pneumonia (CAP), skin and soft tissue infections, prostatitis, and sexually transmitted diseases. In the primary care setting, silver sulfadiazine, prescribed in the treatment of burns, is available as a topical preparation. Ophthalmic preparations are also readily available. Sulfonamides are useful for prophylaxis against some specific organisms (e.g., *Pneumocystis jirovecii*, *Toxoplasma gondii*, *Bordetella pertussis*, and *Plasmodium falciparum*) and recurrence of some infections (e.g., spontaneous bacterial peritonitis, particularly in the immunocompromised and high-risk populations). Susceptible bacteria, depending on community rates of resistance, include *Escherichia coli* and *Staphylococcus aureus* (community-acquired methicillin-resistant *Staphylococcus aureus* [MRSA]). Other organisms that are typically susceptible to SMZ/TMP include *B. pertussis*, *P. jirovecii*, *Bartonella henselae*, *Chlamydia trachomatis* (not a current guideline recommendation), *Nocardia* spp., *Listeria monocytogenes*, *Mycobacterium marinum* and *fortuitum*, *Cyclospora* spp., and *Isospora* spp.

Antibiotic Resistance

Bacterial resistance varies within communities and is often associated with usage rates. As with other classifications of antibiotics, health care providers should refer to current guidelines and local reporting of antibiotic resistance for appropriate drug selection. SMZ/TMP resistance is generally plasmid or chromosome mediated. Chromosomally mediated mechanisms of resistance include mutations in dihydrofolate reductase, alterations in the pathway for bacterial DNA synthesis, and modification in bacterial cell wall permeability to SMZ/TMP, which typically result in low-level resistance. However, plasma-mediated resistance typically results in high-level resistance to the TMP component and is readily transferred among *Enterobacteriaceae* and *S. aureus* (Trubiano & Grayson, 2018). Examples of acquired resistance are diarrheal illnesses caused by *E. coli*, *Salmonella* spp., *Shigella* spp., and *Cholera* spp. in countries where these organisms are endemic. There is no clinical role for SMZ/TMP in the treatment of *P. falciparum*-associated malaria due to the development of resistance (Trubiano & Grayson, 2018).

Historically, sulfonamides were avoided for the treatment of group A beta-hemolytic streptococcal (*S. pyogenes*) infections due to resistance leading to clinical failure. However, Bowen et al. (2012) reevaluated this and demonstrated success with using SMZ/TMP with *S. pyogenes* infections and found resistance rates were falsely elevated due to

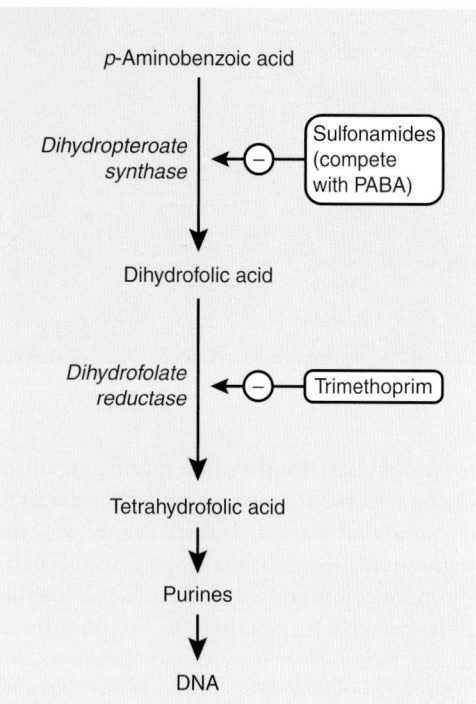

• **Fig. 45.1** Actions of sulfonamides and trimethoprim. (From Katzung, B. G. (2018). *Basic & clinical pharmacology* [14th ed.] New York: Mc-Graw-Hill Education.)

TABLE 45.1	Sulfonamide Dosing Based on Level of Renal Impairment	
Level of Renal Impairment	**Dosage Adjustment**
Creatinine clearance >50 mL/min	No dosage adjustment needed.
Creatinine clearance 10–50 mL/min	Decrease dosage by 50%. Consider extending dosing interval to every 12–24 hr.
Creatinine clearance <10 mL/min	Discontinue use. Consider extending dosing interval to every 24 hr.

the presence of thymidine in the culture media. Still, two patient case series by Gelfand et al. (2013) include cautionary points for clinical practice, as good clinical trial data to support the use of sulfonamides for the treatment of *S. pyogenes* skin and soft tissue infections are greatly lacking and usage may lead to poor outcomes.

> **PRACTICE PEARLS**
>
> **Clinical Indications for SMZ/TMP**
>
> • SMZ/TMP is not a first-line treatment for infections involving the upper respiratory tract (e.g., otitis media and sinusitis) that are often caused by *S. pneumoniae* or *H. influenzae* due to increased rates of resistance leading to treatment failures. However, another culprit of these infections, *M. catarrhalis*, is rarely associated with SMZ/TMP resistance.
> • SMZ/TMP is commonly used to treat skin and soft tissue infections and urinary tract infections (UTIs). However, local resistance and patient culture and sensitivity should be considered.

Pharmacokinetics

Systemic sulfonamides (oral and intravenous [IV] preparations) suitable for treating bacterial infections are classified as short or intermediate acting and are well absorbed by the GI tract. Oral sulfonamides are 70% to 100% bioavailable. They readily distribute to and penetrate all fluids and tissues

in the body, including the central nervous system (CNS). Sulfonamides are metabolized within the liver. Excretion is by glomerular filtration within the kidneys. Table 45.1 outlines recommended dose adjustments based on estimated creatinine clearance (CrCl).

Topical sulfonamides treat infections of the skin and mucous membranes, as well as infections due to burns. When applied topically to the skin or mucous membranes, these drugs are rarely absorbed, and thus rarely cause systemic effects.

Allergic Reactions to Sulfonamides

Approximately 1.6% to 8% of the general population and 50% to 60% of those with human immunodeficiency virus (HIV) report sulfa allergies (Trubiano & Grayson, 2018). A chart review by Geller et al. (2018) identified SMZ/TMP administration in 19% to 25% of allergic reactions. Hypersensitivity reactions are especially frequent with topical sulfonamides. The most common reaction (90%) is a benign maculopapular exanthem. These maculopapular rashes are often accompanied by fever. This reaction tends to occur after 7 to 12 days of therapy (Abrams et al., 2019). Table 45.2 provides an overview of common systemic adverse reactions and Table 45.3 provides an overview of cross-sensitivity and hypersensitivity reactions to sulfonamides.

Sulfonamides are associated with a variety of hypersensitivity (allergic) reactions ranging from mild to severe. Reactions to sulfonamide metabolites occur at the N1 and N4 amino nitrogens on the heterocyclic ring and contribute to their higher incidence of allergic-type reactions. Reactions include Type I–IV (Blumenthal et al., 2019). Rarely occurring with the use of sulfonamide antibiotics, Type I (IgE-mediated) reactions include urticaria, angioedema, and anaphylaxis with cardiovascular collapse. These reactions typically occur within minutes to hours after drug administration. Type II (cytotoxic) reactions lead to cytopenia and nephritis and occur in fewer than 3 to 15 days after drug administration. Type III (immune complex) reactions include serum sickness and vasculitis and typically

TABLE 45.2	Overview of Systemic Adverse Reactions to Sulfonamides	
	Adverse Reaction	
Newborn	Jaundice	
	Hemolytic anemia	
	Kernicterus	
Body System Affected	**Adverse Reaction**	
Central nervous system	Drug-induced aseptic meningitis	
	Delirium tremor	
	Gait disturbances	
	Ataxia, depression, hallucinations, headache, insomnia, peripheral neuropathy/neuritis, seizures, tinnitus, and vertigo	
Cardiovascular	Drug-induced long QT syndrome	
	Congenital long QT syndrome	
	Hyperkalemia	
Gastrointestinal	Nausea, vomiting, and diarrhea	
	Pseudomembranous colitis (antibiotic-associated colitis)	
	Hepatotoxicity, including jaundice	
	Diffuse hepatocellular necrosis	
	Hypersensitivity hepatitis	
	Hepatic failure	
Acute intermittent porphyria	Precipitate an acute attack of porphyria	
Renal impairment	Crystalluria	
	Urolithiasis and nephrolithiasis	
	Interstitial nephritis	
	Nephrotoxicity	
	Elevated BUN and creatinine	
Skin	Erythema, urticaria, angioedema, and photosensitivity	
	Rash: maculopapular, exanthematous, purpuric, and petechial	
Hematologic effects	Agranulocytosis	
	Aplastic anemia	
	Eosinophilia	
	Hyperfibrinogenemia	
	Hypoprothrombinemia	
	Thrombocytopenia	
	Leukopenia	
	Hemolytic anemia in patients with G6PD	
	Methemoglobinemia	

BUN, Blood urea nitrogen; *G6PD*, glucose-6-phosphate dehydrogenase

TABLE 45.3	Hypersensitivity with Sulfonamides	
Hypersensitivity	**Sulfadiazine Sulfamethoxazole**	
Immunologic	Anaphylaxis	
	Serum sickness, arthralgia, drug fever, and chills	
	Generalized exanthem (eruptive skin rash that may be associated with fever or other systemic symptoms)	
	Drug reaction with eosinophilia and systemic symptoms (DRESS)	
	Drug-induced hypersensitivity reaction (DIHS)	
	Stevens–Johnson syndrome (SJS)	
	Toxic epidermal necrolysis (TEN)	
	Hepatitis, pneumonitis, and interstitial nephritis	
	Henoch-Schönlein purpura	

PRACTICE PEARLS

Allergic Reaction and Cross-Reactivity

- Stop sulfonamide therapy immediately if a rash develops. Note, however, that most rashes do not present until 7 to 14 days after therapy initiation. The agent may be continued if the rash is mild and nonprogressive.
- The chemical structure of SMZ differs from other sulfa-containing drugs (e.g., thiazide diuretics, furosemide, dapsone, and darunavir). These other agents can be prescribed even if the patient has an allergy to SMZ.

Contraindications to Sulfonamides

The injectable preparation of SMZ/TMP contains sodium metabisulfite, so it should not be used in patients with sulfite hypersensitivity. This hypersensitivity occurs in patients with a diagnosis of asthma more frequently than in nonasthmatic patients. Cross-reactivity with nonantimicrobial sulfonamides (e.g., thiazide diuretics, loop diuretics, protease inhibitors, sulfonylureas, celecoxib, acetazolamide, sumatriptan, sotalol, and probenecid) is a theoretical consideration for patients with a reported sulfa allergy (Trubiano & Grayson, 2018). Clinically significant cross-reactivity between antimicrobial and nonantimicrobial sulfonamides has not been appreciably demonstrated (Hemstreet & Page, 2006). In 2010, the Joint Task Force on Practice Parameters; the American Academy of Allergy, Asthma & Immunology (AAAAI); the American College of Allergy, Asthma and Immunology (ACAAI); and the Joint Council of Allergy, Asthma and Immunology (JCAAI) concluded that there currently is no evidence to support cross-reactivity with nonantimicrobial sulfonamides in patients with reported allergy to antimicrobial sulfonamides.

occur 2 weeks after administration. Type IV reactions result in acute generalized exanthematous pustulosis (AGEP), Stevens-Johnson syndrome, toxic epidermal necrolysis, and drug rash with eosinophilia and systemic symptoms (DRESS) days to weeks after administration.

Controversy exists concerning the use of sulfonamide therapy in patients with a G6PD deficiency. Drug references vary depending on source. Health care providers should base therapy decisions on diagnosis, prior use of sulfa-containing medications without adverse effects, and potential for future safe use (Glader, 2021).

Sulfonamide Therapy

Oral Sulfonamides

Oral sulfonamides available in the United States include sulfadiazine (generic only) and sulfamethoxazole/trimethoprim (SMZ/TMP, available as Bactrim, Bactrim DS, Septra, Septra DS, Sulfatrim, Sulfatrim Pediatric, and Sultrex Pediatric). Table 45.4 provides a summary of the oral sulfonamides.

Sulfamethoxazole/Trimethoprim (SMZ/TMP)

Sulfamethoxazole/trimethoprim is a fixed-dose combination of a sulfonamide antibiotic (sulfamethoxazole) and a second antibiotic (trimethoprim) used for mild to moderate bacterial infections and as prophylaxis against opportunistic infections. Sulfamethoxazole competitively inhibits dihydropteroate synthetase, preventing the production of dihydrofolate from paraaminobenzoic acid. Trimethoprim inhibits dihydrofolate reductase, preventing reduction of dihydrofolate into tetrahydrofolate, as shown in Fig. 45.1.

Due to the combination effect, antibiotic resistance to SMZ/TMP is less compared to either drug alone. SMZ/TMP was approved for use as a combination antibiotic in the United States in 1973.

SMZ/TMP is available in a fixed 5:1 ratio. Tablet formulations contain 200, 400, or 800 mg of sulfamethoxazole and 80 or 160 mg of trimethoprim. The dosing considerations are based on the trimethoprim component. SMZ/TMP is approved by the U.S. Food and Drug Administration (FDA) for use in adults and children to treat acute infective exacerbation of chronic obstructive pulmonary disease (COPD), UTIs, acute otitis media, traveler's diarrhea, and shigellosis as well as for treatment and prophylaxis of *Pneumocystis jirovecii*.

Pharmacokinetics. SMZ/TMP is rapidly and well absorbed (90% to 100%) from the GI tract and excreted through the kidneys. SMZ/TMP is widely distributed and absorbed throughout all body tissues and fluids, including the CNS (with high doses). Tissue and fluid concentration levels vary. SMZ/TMP crosses the placenta and enters breast milk. Protein binding capacity is 70% for sulfamethoxazole and 44% to 62% for trimethoprim. Excretion of 85% sulfamethoxazole and 67% trimethoprim occurs with normal kidney function. The half-life of sulfamethoxazole ranges from 6 to 12 hours. The half-life of trimethoprim ranges from 6 to 17 hours in patients with normal renal function. Renal insufficiency increases the half-lives of both sulfamethoxazole and trimethoprim.

TABLE 45.4	Oral Sulfonamides			
Medication	**Indication**	**Dose**		**Considerations and Monitoring**
Sulfamethoxazole/ trimethoprim (SMZ/TMP)	Urinary tract infection, including pyelonephritis and cystitis	*Adults ≥18 yr:* 800 mg sulfamethoxazole/160 mg trimethoprim orally every 12 hr for 10–14 days.		Maximum dosing recommendations.
		Females with acute, uncomplicated cystitis: 800 mg sulfamethoxazole/160 mg trimethoprim orally every 12 hr for 3 days.		Monitor creatinine clearance.
		Females with pyelonephritis: 800 mg sulfamethoxazole/160 mg trimethoprim orally every 12 hr for 14 days.		
		Children and adolescents 3–17 yr: 8 mg/kg/day (trimethoprim component) orally divided every 12 hr for 10 days. (Max: 160 mg trimethoprim/800 mg sulfamethoxazole per dose)		
		Infants and children ≥2 months to 2 yr: 8 mg/kg/day (trimethoprim component) orally divided every 12 hr for 10 days (Max: 160 mg trimethoprim/800 mg sulfamethoxazole per dose).		
Sulfadiazine	Urinary tract infection including pyelonephritis and cystitis	*Adults:* Initially: 2–4 Gm orally as a loading dose. Maintenance: 2–4 Gm orally daily in 3–6 divided doses.		Monitor creatinine clearance.
		Infants ≥2 months and children: Initially: 75 mg/kg orally or 2 Gm/m² orally as a loading dose. Maintenance: 150 mg/kg/day orally or 4 Gm/m²/day orally, in 4–6 divided doses (Maximum dosage: 6 Gm/day).		
		Infants ≤2 months: Contraindicated.		

Indications. SMZ/TMP is active against a wide range of gram-positive and gram-negative bacteria, fungi, and parasites. Therapeutic uses include the treatment of UTIs (including pyelonephritis and cystitis), otitis media, shigellosis, and pneumocystis pneumonia caused by *P. jiroveci*, pneumocystis pneumonia prophylaxis in HIV-infected patients, otitis media, acute exacerbations of COPD, gastroenteritis, infectious diarrhea, GI infections, traveler's diarrhea (e.g., *Salmonella*, *Shigella*, *E. coli*, and *Cyclospora*), and nocardiosis. In addition, SMZ/TMP can be used for treatment of infections involving *L. monocytogenes*, *Nocardia* spp., and *Staphylococci.*

Adverse Effects. The most common adverse effects are photosensitivity, pseudo elevation in serum creatinine, abdominal upset, nausea, vomiting, and rash and pruritus. Published case reports showed that SMZ/TMP has been associated with an increased risk of sudden cardiac death due to drug-induced long QT syndrome and congenital long QT syndrome (Fazio et al., 2013). At higher doses, reversible hyperkalemia may occur due to TMP's action as a potassium-sparing diuretic; this effect is potentiated if TMP is used in combination with potassium-sparing diuretics, especially in patients with risk factors such as renal disease. However, high doses of SMZ/TMP may cause hyperkalemia independent of renal status.

Contraindications. Despite the frequent use of SMZ/TMP in the primary care setting, there is an extensive list of potential contraindications. Contraindications to SMZ/TMP include any patient with cross-sensitivities or hypersensitivities to SMZ/TMP. SMZ/TMP should be avoided in patients with G6PD deficiency, long QT syndrome, congenital long QT syndrome, folate deficiency, megaloblastic anemia, hyperkalemia, sulfadiazine hypersensitivity, trimethoprim hypersensitivity, severe renal impairment (CrCl less than 15 mL/minute), renal disease, renal failure, marked hepatic damage, or hepatic disease. SMZ/TMP should be avoided in infants younger than 2 months of age. Avoidance of SMZ/TMP while breastfeeding is recommended if the infant is jaundiced, premature, or has known or suspected G6PD deficits.

Monitoring. Monitor complete blood counts (CBCs) with differential, liver functions tests (LFTs), platelet counts, and serum creatinine/blood urea nitrogen (BUN). In patients taking high doses of trimethoprim, those with renal impairment, or those taking angiotensin-converting enzyme (ACE) inhibitors, angiotensin receptor blockers (ARBs), potassium-sparing diuretics, aldosterone antagonists, and potassium supplements, it is recommended that the serum potassium be monitored on days 7 to 10 upon commencing treatment (Trubiano & Grayson, 2018).

Sulfadiazine (Generic)

Pharmacokinetics. Sulfadiazine is a short-acting sulfonamide antibiotic available in the United States only as a generic preparation (Holmes & Grayson, 2018).

PRACTICE PEARLS

SMZ/TMP Use in Pregnancy and Lactation

- Oral sulfonamides cross the placental barrier during all stages of gestation. Fetal blood levels average 70% to 90% of maternal levels.
- Oral sulfonamides show evidence of fetal risk when used near term due to the potential for jaundice, hemolytic anemia, and kernicterus in the newborn. Manufacturers do not recommend use during pregnancy, but the Centers for Disease Control and Prevention (CDC) Opportunistic Infections guidelines recommend SMZ/TMP for treatment and prophylaxis of *P. jirovecii* pneumonia (Kaplan et al., 2009).
- SMZ/TMP is excreted in breast milk, but the American Academy of Pediatrics (AAP) considers it to be compatible with breastfeeding.

Sulfadiazine is easily absorbed from the GI tract and binds to protein. Excretion of approximately 60% to 85% occurs within 48 to 72 hours. Half-life in patients with normal renal function is roughly 17 hours. In patients with a CrCl of less than 10 ml/minute, the elimination half-life is approximately 34 hours. Sulfadiazine distributes well throughout the body and tissues, including the CNS.

Indications. FDA-approved indications include UTIs; acute otitis media due to *H. influenzae* in combination with penicillin; chancroid; treatment and prophylaxis for toxoplasmic encephalitis; *H. influenzae* meningitis with parenteral streptomycin; adjunctive therapy for malaria for chloroquine-resistant *P. falciparum*; adjunctive therapy for meningococcal meningitis; treatment of nocardiosis; recurrent rheumatic fever; rheumatic fever prophylaxis; trachoma; and trachomatous follicular conjunctivitis. Prescribing information differs between the manufacturer resources and the CDC clinical guidelines. Providers are advised to consult references for current prescriptive information for diseases not listed here.

Adverse Effects. The most common side effects are photosensitivity, diarrhea, nausea, vomiting, GI upset, rash, and fever. Sulfadiazine is less soluble and more likely to crystallize in urine, especially in patients with impaired renal function or dehydration that may result in concentrated acidic urine. Crystalluria may be avoided by adequate hydration (more than 2 to 3 liters daily), alkalinizing the urine to a pH greater than 7.15, and monitoring the urine for crystalluria or hematuria (Trubiano & Grayson, 2018).

Contraindications. Contraindications to sulfadiazine include any patient with an allergy to sulfamethoxazole, given the similarity in chemical structures. Contraindications also include neonates and infants younger than 2 months of age, except as adjunctive therapy with pyrimethamine for the treatment of congenital toxoplasmosis, pregnancy at term, and mothers who are breastfeeding infants younger than 2 months of age. Precautions include patients with G6PD deficiency and hepatic and renal impairment. Sulfadiazine may decrease cyclosporine concentrations, increase phenytoin concentrations, increase the international normalized ratio (INR) in patients on warfarin therapy, and increase the risk of hypoglycemia if taken concomitantly with sulfonylureas.

Monitoring. Assess CBC with differential, platelet counts, and urinalysis before, during, and after therapy. Monitor renal function tests and adjust dosages dependent on renal status. If a patient develops rash and pruritus, the drug may be continued and managed supportively, but it can be discontinued if symptoms are progressive. Monitor for adequate hydration and urinary output.

Topical Sulfonamides

Topical sulfonamides treat infections of the skin and mucous membranes, as well as infections due to second- and third-degree burns. When applied topically to the nonskin or mucous membranes, these drugs are minimally systemically absorbed unless there are severe burns and no detrimental systemic effects have been documented (Trubiano & Grayson, 2018). The preparations have a low incidence of hypersensitivity and are suitable for use in the primary

care setting. Table 45.5 provides a summary of the topical sulfonamides.

Silver Sulfadiazine

Silver sulfadiazine is not absorbed through intact skin. It is formed by combining the weak acid, sulfadiazine, with silver nitrate to form a white, slightly soluble complex silver salt. Silver sulfadiazine employs antibacterial effects by binding to bacterial cell membranes and, to a lesser extent, the cell wall. When silver sulfadiazine encounters skin, sulfadiazine is slowly released and then absorbed to various extents. This reaction is dependent on the presence of chlorides and other anions in the exudate and is greater during eschar separation than in the early postburn period when renal function may be altered (Fox & Modak, 1974). The free silver may react with both the sulfhydryl groups of bacterial enzymes and DNA, combining its bactericidal action with the bacteriostatic action of the sulfonamide against many organisms (Fox & Modak, 1974).

Pharmacokinetics. Once absorbed into body tissue, silver sulfadiazine crosses cell membranes. Silver sulfadiazine is metabolized by the liver and excreted by the kidneys. Elimination half-life is 10 hours. Systemic concentrations of sulfadiazine may reach therapeutic levels.

TABLE 45.5	Topical Sulfonamides			
Medication	**Indication**	**Dose**		**Considerations and Monitoring**
Silver sulfadiazine (1% cream)	Urinary tract infection, including pyelonephritis and cystitis	*Adults, adolescents, and children:* Apply topically to a thickness of approximately 1.6 mm (1/16th of an inch) twice daily (Max dose: 2 applications/day). *Infants ≥2 months:* Apply topically to a thickness of about 1.6 mm (1/16th of an inch) twice daily. Maximum dosage: 2 applications/day.		Maximum dosing recommendations.
Sulfacetamide	Acne, bacterial infection of the eye, conjunctivitis, bacterial infection of the skin, seborrhea	**Lotion and suspension:** *Adults and adolescents ≥12 yr:* Apply a thin film of 10% lotion topically to affected areas twice daily. **Ophthalmic ointment (gel) and solution:** *Adults and infants/children ≥2 months:* apply approximately {1/2}-inch ribbon of 10% gel OR instill 1–2 drops of 10% solution into conjunctival sacs(s) of affected eye(s) every 3–4 hr and at bedtime; taper by increasing time intervals as condition responds; usual duration 7–10 days. *Adults and adolescents ≥12 yr:* • Topical cream: apply 10% cream topically to affected area twice daily for 8–10 days. • Topical foam: massage 10% foam topically into affected area one to three times daily; rinse thoroughly with plain water. • Topical gel: wash affected areas with 10% gel twice daily for 8–10 days; rinse thoroughly with plain water. • Topical liquid wash: wash affected areas with 10% liquid twice daily for 8–10 days; rinse thoroughly with plain water. • Topical shampoo: apply 10% shampoo to wet hair and massage into scalp at least twice weekly; rinse thoroughly.		

Indications. Silver sulfadiazine does not inhibit folic acid synthesis like other sulfonamides. Silver sulfadiazine does suppress bacterial colonization in patients with second- and third-degree burns. Silver sulfadiazine possesses activity against gram-positive and gram-negative bacteria and against yeast. Organisms that may be susceptible to topical silver sulfadiazine include *Staphylococcus aureus, S. epidermidis, beta-hemolytic streptococci, Enterococci* spp., *Corynebacterium diphtheriae, Clostridium perfringens, Klebsiella* spp., *E. coli, Enterobacter* spp., *Citrobacter* spp., *Proteus* spp., *P. aeruginosa, Stenotrophomonas maltophilia, Morganella morganii, Providencia* spp., *Serratia* spp., *Acinetobacter* spp., and *Candida albicans.*

Adverse Effects. Transient leukopenia characterized by decreased neutrophil count occurs within 2 to 4 days after initiating therapy and rebounds to normal within 2 to 3 days. Recovery is not influenced by continuation of silver sulfadiazine therapy. An increased incidence of leukopenia has been reported in patients treated concurrently with the rarely used H2RA, cimetidine. Photosensitivity can occur when large areas of burns are treated. Additional rare adverse effects may include skin necrosis, erythema multiforme, skin discoloration, burning sensation, rashes, and interstitial nephritis.

Contraindications. Contraindications to sulfadiazine include any patient with cross-sensitivities or hypersensitivities to the drug or its components. Avoid silver sulfadiazine in patients who are hypersensitive to the drug or any of the other ingredients in the formulation. Because sulfonamide therapy is known to increase the possibility of kernicterus, silver sulfadiazine should not be used in pregnant patients approaching or at term, in premature infants, or in newborn infants during the first 2 months of life. Topical sulfonamides are incompatible with preparations containing silver. Providers should weigh the risks and benefits in the event of severe maternal burns. Preparations are not recommended during breastfeeding.

PRACTICE PEARLS

Silver Sulfadiazine Use in Pregnancy and Lactation

- **Pregnancy:** There are no data on the use of silver sulfadiazine in pregnant females. Kernicterus in a newborn infant is possible if significant amounts of maternally applied silver sulfadiazine cream are absorbed systemically. Topical silver sulfadiazine should only be used during pregnancy if the maternal benefit outweighs the potential risk to the fetus. However, near- or at-term use is contraindicated. Silver is not substantially absorbed systemically, but sulfadiazine may be absorbed systemically if applied to large areas or over prolonged periods of time.
- **Breastfeeding:** It is unknown whether silver sulfadiazine is excreted in human milk. Consider the benefits of breastfeeding to the infant versus the health of the mother. Manufacturers recommend avoiding breastfeeding if maternal use is required.

PRACTICE PEARLS

Silver Sulfadiazine and G6PD Deficiency

- Sulfonamides are rarely systemically absorbed when applied to the skin, eye, or mucosal membranes if the skin is intact. In cases of severe breaches, absorption may occur but rarely is associated with systemic adverse effects.
- Use cautiously in patients with G6PD deficiency and hepatic or renal impairment.

Monitoring. During extended periods of use, monitor for a reduction in wound or ulcer size and signs of closure. Laboratory examinations include CBC with differential, LFTs, platelet count, and serum creatinine/BUN. If required, administer intramuscular (IM) injections cautiously to patients receiving silver sulfadiazine. Monitor patients receiving concomitant IM injections as there may be bleeding, bruising, or hematomas at the injection site due to platelet effects secondary to silver sulfadiazine therapy.

Sulfacetamide

Sulfacetamide is a synthetic antibiotic used for treating certain infections of the eye and a variety of dermatologic disorders (e.g., acne). Sulfacetamide sodium ophthalmic is available as a 10% water-soluble solution or ointment. For dermatologic disorders, the drug is available as a 10% solution in lotions, gels, washes, and shampoos.

Pharmacokinetics. Sulfacetamide sodium is bacteriostatic and the pharmacokinetic activity is similar to other sulfonamides. Sulfacetamide sodium ophthalmic solution penetrates ocular fluid and tissues. No pharmacokinetic data are available regarding systemic absorption for topical sulfacetamide (lotions, gels, washes, and shampoos).

Indications. Susceptible organisms are streptococci, staphylococci, *E. coli, Klebsiella pneumoniae, Pseudomonas pyocyanea, Salmonella* species, *Proteus vulgaris, Nocardia,* and *Actinomyces.* Topical sulfonamides do not provide adequate coverage against *Neisseria* species, *Serratia marcescens,* or *Pseudomonas aeruginosa.*

Sulfacetamide sodium ophthalmic solution is used in the treatment of conjunctivitis, corneal ulcers, and other superficial ophthalmic infections caused by susceptible organisms. Topical sulfacetamide is available as lotions, gels, washes, and shampoos. Therapeutic usage includes the treatment of susceptible organisms resulting in acne vulgaris, seborrheic dermatitis, and secondary bacterial skin infections.

Adverse Effects. In addition to the previously mentioned adverse effects associated with this classification, bacterial and fungal corneal ulcers have developed during treatment with sulfonamide ophthalmic solutions. Product manufacturers warn that sulfacetamide sodium ophthalmic ointment may retard corneal wound healing resulting from trauma or surgery. Ophthalmic solutions and ointment may cause blurred vision, sensitivity to bright light, and headache. Topical sulfacetamide may cause local irritation.

Contraindications. Avoid in patients with hypersensitivity to sulfonamides, sulfonylureas, thiazide or loop diuretics, or any ingredient of the preparation. Topical sulfonamides are incompatible with preparations containing silver. Advise patients not to wear contact lenses while using this medicine.

Monitoring. Laboratory monitoring is not necessary. Monitor and offer advice against continuous use as this may result in overgrowth of nonsusceptible organisms.

PRACTICE PEARLS

Sulfacetamide Use in Pregnancy and Lactation

- There are limited studies on the teratogenic effects of ophthalmic and topical preparations of sulfacetamide.
- Consider the use of ophthalmic and topical preparations of sulfacetamide in pregnancy only if the potential benefit justifies the potential risk to the fetus.

Prescriber Considerations for Sulfonamide Therapy

Clinical Practice Guidelines

When considering antibiotic therapy, concepts of antibiotic stewardship are important to keep in mind. The provider should consider the etiology of the disease, the likelihood of bacterial susceptibility to sulfonamide drugs, and levels of antimicrobial resistance within the community. Providers should also refer to published guidelines from national organizations. By following these recommendations, there is the potential to decrease the risk of adverse effects, the risk of superinfections, antimicrobial and antibiotic resistance, and health care costs to treat unintended consequences (Klugman, 2003).

Clinical Reasoning for Sulfonamide Therapy

Consider the individual patient's health problem requiring sulfonamide therapy. Appropriate assessment of the patient is an essential component of the diagnostic process. Consider the patient presentation and whether the symptomatology and clinical findings are consistent with an infectious process suitable for treatment with sulfonamides. Community antimicrobial resistance to sulfonamides is also important to consider.

Determine the desired therapeutic outcome based on the patient's health problem. For patients with a new onset of infection, the desired outcome is complete resolution of the infection with limited to no adverse effects. In patients with recurrent infections, the goal is to return to baseline or better. In patients requiring prophylaxis with sulfonamides, the goal is to prevent infection.

BOOKMARK THIS!

Clinical Practice Guidelines

- American Academy of Pediatrics
  - Group A streptococcal pharyngitis: https://doi.org/10.1093/cid/cis629
  - Acute bacterial sinusitis: https://doi.org/10.1542/peds.2013-1071
- American Heart Association: https://www.ahajournals.org/doi/10.1161/cir.0b013e31829e8776
- American Thoracic Society: https://www.atsjournals.org/doi/full/10.1164/rccm.201908-1581ST
- Infectious Diseases Society of America
  - Vertebral osteomyelitis: https://doi.org/10.1093/cid/civ482
  - Uncomplicated cystitis and pyelonephritis: https://doi.org/10.1093/cid/ciq257
  - Skin and soft tissue infection: https://doi.org/10.1093/cid/ciu296
  - Group A streptococcal pharyngitis: https://doi.org/10.1093/cid/cis629
  - Acute bacterial sinusitis: https://doi.org/10.1093/cid/cis370
- Pediatric Infectious Diseases Society: https://www.aafp.org/afp/2012/0715/p196.html

---

Assess the selected medication for its appropriateness for an individual patient by considering the medication's side effects and the patient's age, race/ethnicity, comorbidities, and genetic factors. A thorough patient history and exam is the first step to making the diagnosis. Consideration of past medical history, comorbidities, and genetics affects the prescribing of sulfonamide therapy. Once a diagnosis is determined, providers should review current prescribing guidelines and local antibiotic and antimicrobial resistance patterns.

Initiate the treatment plan with the selected medication by first providing adequate patient education to ensure the patient's understanding and promote full participation in antibiotic therapy. Concepts of shared decision-making include a thorough review of the diagnosis, treatment goal, and plan of care. This empowers the patient as a full partner in the plan of care and provides an avenue for improved health outcomes.

Ensure complete patient and family understanding about the medication prescribed using a variety of education strategies. Information to include in educational plans comprises the diagnosis; plan of care, including the use of any medication, side effects, food and drug interactions; and method of administration. A variety of education modes such as verbal and written instruction, referrals to electronic resources, and having the patient explain the process to the provider ensure increased levels of understanding of the goal of therapy.

Conduct follow-up and monitoring of patient responses to therapy. Follow-up evaluation depends on the diagnosis and length of treatment. For the treatment of acute, episodic, nonrecurrent conditions such as an uncomplicated cystitis, follow-up may not be required or may consist of an electronic contact by phone, text, or email. In cases that are more complicated or where long-term therapy is required, more intense follow-up is expected. Follow-up includes evaluation of treatment effectiveness, adherence to therapy, laboratory monitoring, and patient satisfaction and willingness to continue therapy.

Teaching Points for Sulfonamide Therapy

Health Promotion Strategies

Health promotion strategies associated with the use of antibiotic therapy include improving individual health outcomes and limiting the risk of antibiotic and antimicrobial resistance. The use of antimicrobial drugs when not indicated (e.g., wrong medication or no infection) increases the patient's risk of experiencing adverse effects from the drug, delays patient healing, and risks spreading the infection. Specific strategies include the following:

- Patients should complete the entire course of antibiotics.
- Patients should not share their medications with others.
- Patients should follow up with their health care provider for questions regarding health status.

Patient Education for Medication Safety

Decreasing the risk associated with medication administration is the key to patient education. Health care providers should stress the following points with patients:

- Oral medications should be taken with a full glass (8 ounces) of water. Drink several additional noncaffeinated beverages during the day, unless otherwise directed by your doctor.
- Complete the prescribed course of treatment, even though symptoms may abate before the full course is over.
- Avoid vitamin C or acidifying drinks such as cranberry juice as these may increase the risk for crystals to form in urine.
- Do not use silver sulfadiazine on the face as the medication can cause skin discoloration.
- Avoid or limit sunlight (UV) exposure and use sunscreens since the skin will be photosensitive and reactions may occur.
- Have blood or urine checked as requested by your provider.
- Store all drugs at room temperature in a dry place unless otherwise instructed.
- Protect medications from light.
- Keep all drugs out of the reach of children and pets. Tell your provider:
- If your symptoms or health problems do not get better or if they become worse

- About all of your prescription drugs, over-the-counter (OTC) drugs, or any natural products or vitamins you currently take
- If you have an allergy to sulfadiazine or any other part of this drug or an allergy to any other drugs, foods, or other substances
- If you have any previous health diagnoses such as kidney or liver disease, HIV or AIDS, G6PD deficiency, anemias, thyroid disease, diabetes, or any other conditions
- If you are pregnant and near term or breastfeeding

Application Questions for Discussion

1. Are sulfonamides safe and effective for the treatment of group A beta-hemolytic streptococcal infections?
2. What are the considerations for prescribing sulfonamides to pregnant or lactating patients?
3. What factors should be considered when educating the patient on sulfonamide therapy?

Selected Bibliography

Abrams, E., Netchiporouk, E., Miedzybrodzki, B., & Ben-Shoshan, M. (2019). Antibiotic allergy in children: More than just a label. *International Archives of Allergy and Immunology, 180,* 103–112. https://doi.org/10.1159/000501518.

Beauduy, C.E., Winston, L.G. (2021). Sulfonamides, trimethoprim, & quinolones. In B. G. Katzung & T. W. Vanderah (Eds.). Basic & clinical pharmacology (15th ed.). New York: McGraw Hill.

Blumenthal, K. G., Peter, J. G., Trubiano, J. A., & Phillips, E. J. (2019). Antibiotic allergy. *Lancet, 393*(10167), 183–198. https://doi.org/10.1016/S0140-6736(18)32218-9.

Bowen, A. C., Lilliebridge, R. A., Tong, S. Y. C., Baird, R. W., Ward, P., McDonald, M. I., Currie, B. J., & Carapetis, J. R. (2012). Is *Streptococcus pyogenes* resistant or susceptible to trimethoprim-sulfamethoxazole? *Journal of Clinical Microbiology, 50*(12), 4067–4072. https://doi.org/10.1128/JCM.02195-12.

Fazio, G., Vernuccio, F., Grutta, G., & Re, G. L. (2013). Drugs to be avoided in patients with long QT syndrome: Focus on the anaesthesiological management. *World Journal of Cardiology, 5*(4), 87–93. https://doi.org/10.4330/wjc.v5.i4.87.

Fox, Jr., C. L., & Modak, S. M (1974). Mechanism of silver sulfadiazine action on burn wound infections. *Antimicrobial Agents Chemotherapy, 5*(6), 582–588. https://doi.org/10.1128/aac.5.6.582.

Gelfand, M. S., Cleveland, K. O., & Ketterer, D. C. (2013). Susceptibility of *Streptococcus pyogenes* to trimethoprim-sulfamethoxazole. *Journal of Clinical Microbiology, 51*(4), 1350. https://doi.org/10.1128/jcm.03329-12.

Geller, A. I., Lovegrove, M. C., Shehab, N., Hicks, L. A., Sapiano, M. R. P., & Budnitz, D. S. (2018). National estimates of emergency department visits for antibiotic adverse events among adults—United States, 2011–2015. *Journal of General Internal Medicine, 33*(7), 1060–1068. https://doi.org/10.1007/s11606-018-4430-x.

Glader, B. (2021). Genetics and pathophysiology of glucose-6-phosphate dehydrogenase (G6PD) deficiency. https://www-uptodate-com.ezproxy.hsc.usf.edu/contents/genetics-and-pathophysiology-of-glucose-6-phosphate-dehydrogenase-g6pd-deficiency?search=sulfonamide%20and%20G6PD&source=search_result&selectedTitle=1~150&usage_type=default&display_rank=1. Accessed February 25, 2021.

Hemstreet, B. A., & Page, R. L.2nd. (2006). Sulfonamide allergies and outcomes related to use of potentially cross-reactive drugs in hospitalized patients. *Pharmacotherapy, 26*(4), 551–557. https://doi.org/10.1592/phco.26.4.551.

Holmes, N. E., & Grayson, M. L (2018). Sulfonamides. In M. L. Grayson, S. E. Cosgrove, S. M. Crowe, W. Hope, J. S. McCarthy, J. Mills, J. W. Mouton, & D. L. Patterson (Eds.), *Kucers' the Use of Antibiotics (e-book): A Clinical Review of Antibacterial, Antifungal, Antiparasitic and Antiviral Drugs* (7th ed.). Boca Raton, FL: CRC Press.

Joint Task Force on Practice Parameters, American Academy of Allergy, Asthma and Immunology, the American College of Allergy, Asthma and Immunology, & Joint Council of Allergy, Asthma and Immunology. (2010). Drug allergy: An updated practice parameter. *Annals of Allergy, Asthma, & Immunology, 105*(4), 259–273. https://doi.org/10.1016/j.anai.2010.08.002.

Kaplan, J. E., Benson, C., Holmes, K. K., Brooks, J. T., Pau, A., & Masur, H. Centers for Disease Control and Prevention (CDC), National Institutes of Health, & HIV Medicine Association of the Infectious Diseases Society of America. (2009). Guidelines for prevention and treatment of opportunistic infections in HIV-infected adults and adolescents: Recommendations from CDC, the National Institutes of Health, and the HIV Medicine Association of the Infectious Diseases Society of America. *Morbidity and Mortality Weekly Report, Recommendations and Reports, 8*(RR-4). 1-CE4. https://pubmed.ncbi.nlm.nih.gov/19357635.

Klugman, K. P. (2003). Implications for antimicrobial prescribing of strategies based on bacterial eradication. *International Journal of Infectious Diseases, 7*(1), S27–S31. https://doi.org/10.1016/S1201-9712(03)90068-3.

Trubiano, J. A., & Grayson, M. L (2018). Trimethoprim and trimethoprim–sulfamethoxazole (Cotrimoxazole). In M. L. Grayson, S. E. Cosgrove, S. M. Crowe, W. Hope, J. S. McCarthy, J. Mills, J. W. Mouton, & D. L. Patterson (Eds.), *Kucers' the Use of Antibiotics (e-book): A Clinical Review of Antibacterial, Antifungal, Antiparasitic and Antiviral Drugs* (7th ed.). Boa Raton, FL: CRC Press.

46

Antitubercular Medications

CHERYL H. ZAMBROSKI

Overview

Tuberculosis (TB) is the 13th leading cause of death worldwide and the leading cause of death by a single infectious agent (World Health Organization [WHO], 2021). While cases of TB in the United States have decreased significantly over the past five decades, roughly 7000 cases were identified in 2020 (Centers for Disease Control and Prevention [CDC], 2021). Cases were reported in all 50 states and the District of Columbia. Any health care provider, including those in primary care, is required to report suspected cases of TB within 24 hours to notify the local board of health in the community where the cases reside (CDC, 2012).

Treatment of TB is typically initiated and followed by infectious disease specialists and public health officials. Nevertheless, primary care providers may care for patients who require screening for TB, have been diagnosed with latent TB, or are undergoing treatment for TB. Also, primary care providers should be attentive to the possibility that patients may present with symptoms of active TB, especially if they come from an at-risk population.

According to the CDC (2016), two main categories of people are at high risk for developing TB (Box 46.1). The first category includes those who have been recently infected with TB bacteria, such as people who have been in close contact with infected persons or exposed to groups with high rates of TB transmission. The second category includes those with medical conditions that weaken the immune system, such as HIV/AIDS and diabetes, or who are taking certain medications. Up to 13 million people in the United States are living with latent TB infection (CDC, 2021), so it is critically important that the primary care provider

recognizes those patients with weakened immune systems who are most vulnerable to contracting TB and/or progressing to active disease.

Pathophysiology

TB is caused by the organism *Mycobacterium tuberculosis*. The organism is transmitted person to person through aerosolized droplets (also called *droplet nuclei*). These droplets are expelled from the infected person, usually to those within close contact, through coughing, sneezing, speaking, or singing. The droplets can remain in the air for up to several hours. Following inhalation, the droplets carrying the TB bacilli can travel through the bronchi and bronchioles, ultimately reaching the alveolar sacs and resulting in *primary infection*.

Once the patient is infected, the TB bacteria begin to multiply. Typically, the immune and inflammatory systems are able to contain the bacilli. Neutrophils and macrophages in the lung phagocytize the bacilli to help prevent the spread of the infection. Unfortunately, *Mycobacterium tuberculosis* is resistant to phagocytosis through the inhibition of lysosomes. This leads to the multiplication of the TB bacilli within the cell and localized infection. Also, the TB infection can spread through the bloodstream or to the lymphatic system, initiating an immune response. Over time, macrophages, neutrophils, and lymphocytes fight to wall off colonies of bacilli, resulting in a *tubercle*, a granulomatous lesion containing the bacteria. Scar tissue grows around the tubercle, and in most cases the bacteria are killed by the immune system. In other cases, however, the TB bacteria remain alive and become dormant, resulting in *latent tuberculosis infection* (LTBI). In many cases, the dormant TB remain dormant for life. For patients who are immunocompromised, the bacilli continue to replicate and spread through the blood and lymphatics to other parts of the body, such as the kidneys, bone, or liver.

TB disease (often referred to as *active TB*) results when the patient's immune and inflammatory responses cannot adequately contain the TB bacteria. This may occur initially following the primary infection with TB or through reactivation of the LTBI. Reactivation is more likely to occur in patients with illnesses such as human immunodeficiency virus (HIV), cancer, diabetes, or renal failure, as well as in patients with poor nutritional status or those who are taking

• BOX 46.1 Patients at Risk for Developing TB

Persons Who Have Been Recently Infected With TB Bacteria

- Close contacts of a person with infectious TB disease
- Persons who have emigrated from areas of the world with high rates of TB
- Children younger than 5 years of age who have a positive TB test
- Groups with high rates of TB transmission, such as homeless persons, illicit injectable drug users, and persons with HIV infection
- Persons who work or reside with people who are at high risk for TB in facilities or institutions such as hospitals, homeless shelters, correctional facilities, nursing homes, and residential homes for those with HIV

Persons With Medical Conditions That Weaken the Immune System

Infants and young children often have weak immune systems. Other people can also have weak immune systems, especially people with any of these conditions:

- HIV infection
- Substance abuse
- Silicosis
- Diabetes mellitus
- Severe kidney disease
- Low body weight
- Organ transplants
- Head and neck cancer
- Medical treatments such as corticosteroids or organ transplant
- Specialized treatment for rheumatoid arthritis or Crohn's disease

From Centers for Disease Control and Prevention (2016). *TB risk factors*. https://www.cdc.gov/tb/topic/basics/risk.htm.

immunosuppressant medications such as those who have received organ transplants. TB disease ultimately is characterized by progressive necrosis and cavitation of lung tissue as well as spread of the organism. Without treatment, death from TB disease may result.

LTBI is typically asymptomatic. Active disease, however, is characterized by symptoms of fatigue, unintentional weight loss, loss of appetite, low-grade fever, and night sweats. As the disease progresses, patients typically develop a productive cough that becomes more frequent over time. Chest pain, dyspnea, and hemoptysis may occur. For those who experience extrapulmonary TB disease, additional symptoms of pyelonephritis, meningitis, peritonitis, or bone marrow suppression may occur. See Box 46.2 for a comparison of LTBI and TB disease.

The CDC works closely with public health officials to find and treat cases of TB to eventually eliminate TB in the United States (CDC, 2021). Cases are identified using two main testing methods: the Mantoux tuberculin skin test (TST) and interferon-gamma release assays (IGRAs). The CDC recommends that people with recent exposure, who work in high-risk settings, and who are from areas with a high incidence of TB be screened for TB. Other risk groups include people who inject illicit drugs, people with HIV infection, babies, young children, and older adults.

Tuberculin skin testing strategy varies with the likelihood of exposure to TB and the risk of disease progression (Lewinson et al., 2017). In general, the Mantoux TST is an acceptable test for determining exposure to TB (Table 46.1). Intradermal injection of 0.1 mL of purified protein derivative (PPD) tuberculin typically produces a discrete, pale elevation of skin 6 to 10 mm in diameter. PPD interpretation criteria are listed in Box 46.3. The TST should be read 48 to 72 hours after the injection is given. The patient should be taught to wait 48 hours at a minimum. If the patient returns after more than 3 days and the results appear

• BOX 46.2 Differences Between Latent Tuberculosis Infection and Active TB Disease

Latent Tuberculosis Infection	Active TB Disease
No symptoms or physical findings suggestive of TB disease.	Symptoms may include one or more of the following: fever, cough, chest pain, weight loss, night sweats, hemoptysis, fatigue, and decreased appetite.
TST or IGRA result is usually positive.	TST or IGRA result is usually positive.
Chest radiograph is typically normal.	Chest radiograph is usually abnormal. However, it may be normal in persons with advanced immunosuppression or extrapulmonary disease.
If done, respiratory specimens are smear and culture negative.	Respiratory specimens are usually smear and culture positive. However, they may be negative in persons with extrapulmonary disease or minimal or early pulmonary disease.
Cannot spread TB bacteria to others.	May spread TB bacteria to others.
Should consider treatment for LTBI to prevent TB disease.	Needs treatment for TB disease.

IGRA, Interferon-gamma release assay; *TST*, tuberculin skin test.
From Centers for Disease Control and Prevention National Center for HIV/AIDS, Viral Hepatitis, STD, and TB Prevention. (2013). *Latent tuberculosis infection: a guide for primary health care providers*. U.S. Department of Health and Human Services Centers for Disease Control and Prevention.

TABLE 46.1 Medications Used for TB Prevention and Screening

Category/Medication	Indication	Dosage	Considerations and Monitoring
PPD			
Tuberculin PPD	TB diagnosis (latent TB or active TB disease)	Inject 0.1 mL (5 TU) intradermally into volar or dorsal surface of forearm. After 48–72 hr, inspect injection site for induration; erythema at the injection site has no diagnostic value. Measure and record diameter of induration in mm; lack of induration should be recorded as 0 mm. Positive reaction is determined by induration size and patient's medical history. **Two-step method:** Inject 0.1 mL (5 tuberculin units [TU]) intradermally into the volar or dorsal surface of the forearm. After a period of 48–72 hr, observe the injection site for induration. If the first skin test is negative, a second 0.1-mL intradermal test is given 1–4 weeks later. The injection site is again inspected after 48–72 hr. A positive reaction (≥10 mm) to the second test indicates a past or old infection. If the second test was negative, any future positive skin test should indicate a skin test conversion.	Certain patient populations (such as older adults, neonates, and infants <6 weeks of age, immunosuppressed persons, and persons with active infection) may have a decreased response to the PPD. The two-step method is preferred for the initial screening in adults who will undergo routine tuberculin skin testing. Use of the two-step method helps distinguish between a boosted reaction and a skin test conversion.
Vaccine			
BCG vaccine	TB prophylaxis in patients who have not been previously infected with *Mycobacterium tuberculosis* but who are at high risk of exposure NOTE: BCG vaccination is recommended for infants and children with negative TST who are at high risk of intimate and prolonged exposure to persistently untreated or ineffectively treated persons with infectious pulmonary TB or who are continuously exposed to persons with TB who are resistant to INH and RIF and cannot be separated from the infectious person(s)	0.2–0.3 mL should be dropped on the skin and administered using a multiple puncture disc. Additional vaccine may be dropped on the skin after initial application to ensure a "wet" vaccine site, and revaccination may be necessary.	Tuberculin skin testing should be performed prior to vaccination. Vaccination is recommended only for certain health care workers, infants, and children who are tuberculin-negative to a recent skin test with 5 tuberculin units. Epinephrine (1:1000) injection and other agents used in the treatment of anaphylaxis should be available in the event of a serious allergic reaction. Providers must give the patient or guardian the Vaccine Information Statements from the manufacturer before each immunization. Record the manufacturer and lot number of the vaccine; date of administration; and name, address, and phone number of the person who administered the vaccine in the recipient's permanent medical record. Provider should wear gloves, gown, and mask while giving the vaccine.

BCG, Bacillus Calmette–Guérin vaccine; *INH*, Isoniazid; *mm*, millimeters; *PPD*, purified protein derivative; *RIF*, rifampin; *TB*, tuberculosis; *TU*, tuberculin units.

• **BOX 46.3**   **Reading TB Skin Tests**

The reaction to the skin test should be read by a health care provider 48–72 hours after the injection. The reading should be based on a measurement of induration (swelling), not erythema. The diameter of the induration should be measured transversely to the long axis of the forearm.
An induration of ≥5 mm is considered positive for:

- HIV-positive persons
- Persons who have had recent contact with TB patients
- Persons with fibrotic changes on chest X-ray consistent with old healed TB
- Patients with organ transplants and other immunosuppressed individuals (e.g., receiving equivalent of prednisone ≥15 mg/day for ≥1 month)

An induration of ≥10 mm is considered positive for:

- Recent arrivals to the U.S. (<5 years) from high-prevalence countries
- Illicit users of injectable drugs
- Residents and employees of high-risk congregate settings (e.g., prisons, jails, nursing homes, long-term care facilities, hospitals and other health care facilities, residential facilities for AIDS patients, and homeless shelters)
- Mycobacteriology laboratory personnel
- Persons with high-risk clinical conditions (e.g., diabetes mellitus, silicosis, high-dose corticosteroid therapy, other immunosuppressive therapy, cancer, hematologic diseases [e.g., leukemia and Hodgkin's disease], end-stage renal disease, intestinal bypass or gastrectomy, low body weight [≤10% ideal body weight])
- Children <4 years of age or children and adolescents exposed to adults in high-risk categories

An induration of ≥15 mm is considered positive for:

- Persons with no known risk factors for TB

From Clinical Pharmacology powered by ClinicalKey®. (2019). Elsevier. http://www.clinicalkey.com.

negative, the test must be repeated. Only the induration, not the erythema, is measured in millimeters. A positive TST does not differentiate between past exposure to TB, latent TB, or active TB. If the skin test is positive, a chest X-ray is indicated. If the chest X-ray shows signs of active or latent TB, microscopic examination of sputum smears as well as sputum culture are recommended.

When feasible, an IGRA rather than a TST is preferred in certain conditions (Lewinson et al., 2017). These include patients older than 5 years of age who are unlikely to return for reading their TST, who have received the Bacillus Calmette–Guérin (BCG) vaccination, or who are likely to be infected and have a low or intermediate risk of disease progression. The feasibility of IGRA testing varies due to cost, availability, and burden.

Acid-fast bacilli smear microscopy is recommended for all patients suspected of having pulmonary TB. Because the organism grows slowly, a definitive diagnosis via a sputum culture takes up to 6 weeks. A diagnostic nucleic acid amplification test (NAAT) on the initial respiratory specimen from patients suspected of having pulmonary TB can be used as evidence of extrapulmonary TB.

TB treatment is focused on curing the patient and minimizing the risk of transmission (Nahid et al., 2016). All suspected and confirmed cases of TB should be reported to the local public health department for recommendations and case management. Primary care providers may work closely with public health authorities and case managers to facilitate treatment and adherence of patients to medication therapy.

Antitubercular Therapy

Antitubercular medication therapies vary based on whether the patient is experiencing LTBI or active disease. In general, four treatment regimens are effective for the treatment of LTBI (Table 46.2). The shortest duration of therapy is a 3-month course of Isoniazid (INH). Rifapentine (RPT) is recommended for its convenient, once-weekly dosing schedule. For drug-susceptible TB disease, first-line treatment regimens require a combination of four primary medications, including INH, Rifampin (RIF), Pyrazinamide (PZA), and Ethambutol (EMB) (Table 46.3). Second-line medications may be required; however, these are typically less effective and more toxic than the first-line medications, so they are generally reserved for disseminated TB and/or cases of drug-resistant TB (Table 46.4). Medications used for TB screening and the primary first-line treatment agents will be discussed here.

Mantoux Tuberculin Skin Test

The purpose of the Mantoux TST is to screen for individuals with LTBI and to screen for those who are infected with *Mycobacterium tuberculosis* and have active TB. To perform the test, PPD tuberculin, isolated from culture media filtrates of a human strain of *Mycobacterium tuberculosis,* is injected intradermally. Once an individual has become sensitized to the mycobacterial antigens, the skin test appears to stimulate or activate previously sensitized T-cells to evoke a delayed hypersensitivity reaction at the site of the PPD administration. The patient's response to the test determines whether they might be infected with *Mycobacterium tuberculosis* (Box 46.3).

Pharmacokinetics. PPD skin tests are administered intradermally. The hypersensitivity reaction results in a measurable induration at the injection site. This reaction typically begins within 5 to 6 hours of administration, with maximal reaction occurring after 48 to 72 hours.

PRACTICE PEARLS

Reading TB Skin Tests in Older Adults

Older adults may have decreased sensitivity to the tuberculin PPD. As a result, reaction to the TST may develop more slowly; maximal induration may not be achieved until after 72 hours.

Indications. The PPD skin test is used to screen for latent and active TB. In general, the two-step method is preferred for the initial screening in adults who are undergoing a routine TST. Use of this method helps to distinguish between a boosted reaction and skin test conversion.

TABLE 46.2 Drug Regimens for Microbiologically Confirmed Pulmonary Tuberculosis Caused by Drug-Susceptible Organisms

Regimen	Intensive Phase		Continuation Phase			Regimen Effectiveness
	Drug[a]	Interval and Dose[b] (Minimum Duration)	Drugs	Interval and Dose[b,c] (Minimum Duration)	Range of Total Doses	Comments[c,d]
1	INH RIF PZA EMB	Daily for 56 doses (8 weeks), or 5 days weekly for 40 doses (8 weeks)	INH RIF	Daily for 126 doses (18 weeks), or 5 days weekly for 90 doses (18 weeks)	182–130	This is the preferred regimen for patients with newly diagnosed pulmonary tuberculosis.
2	INH RIF PZA EMB	Daily for 56 doses (8 weeks), or 5 days weekly for 40 doses (8 weeks)	INH RIF	Three times weekly for 54 doses (18 weeks)	110–94	Preferred alternative regimen in situations in which more frequent DOT during continuation phase is difficult to achieve.
3	INH RIF PZA EMB	Three times weekly for 24 doses (8 weeks)	INH RIF	Three times weekly for 54 doses (18 weeks)	78	Use regimen with caution in patients with HIV and/or cavitary disease. Missed doses can lead to treatment failure, relapse, and acquired drug resistance.
4	INH RIF PZA EMB	Daily for 14 doses, then twice weekly for 12 doses	INH RIF	Twice weekly for 36 doses (18 weeks)	62	Do not use twice-weekly regimens in HIV-infected patients or patients with smear-positive and/or cavitary disease. If doses are missed, then therapy is equivalent to once weekly, which is inferior.

Regimen Effectiveness: Greater → Lesser

[a]DOT, Directly observed therapy; EMB, ethambutol; HIV, human immunodeficiency virus; INH, isoniazid; PZA, pyrazinamide; RIF, rifampin. Other combinations may be appropriate in certain circumstances; additional details are provided in the section "Recommended Treatment Regimens."

[b]When DOT is used, drugs may be given 5 days/week and the necessary number of doses adjusted accordingly. Although there are no studies that compare 5 with 7 daily doses, extensive experience indicates this would be an effective practice. DOT should be used when drugs are administered <7 days/week.

[c]Based on expert opinion, patients with cavitation on initial chest radiograph and positive cultures at completion of 2 months of therapy should receive a 7-month (31-week) continuation phase.

[d]Pyridoxine (vitamin B₆), 25–50 mg/day, is given with INH to all persons at risk of neuropathy (e.g., pregnant patients; breastfeeding infants; persons with HIV; patients with diabetes, alcoholism, malnutrition, or chronic renal failure; or patients with advanced age). For patients with peripheral neuropathy, experts recommend increasing pyridoxine dose to 100 mg/day."See [426]. Alternatively, some U.S. tuberculosis control programs have administered intensive-phase regimens 5 days/week for 15 doses (3 weeks), then twice weekly for 12 doses.

From Nahid, P., Dorman, S. E., Alipanah, N., Barry, P. M., Brozek, J. L., Cattamanchi, A., ... Peloquin, C. A. (2016). Official American Thoracic Society/Centers for Disease Control and Prevention/Infectious Diseases Society of America clinical practice guidelines: Treatment of drug-susceptible tuberculosis. *Clinical Infectious Diseases, 63*(7), e147–e195. https://doi.org/10.1093/cid/ciw376.

| TABLE 46.3 | First-Line Antitubercular Medications | | |

Medication	Indication	Dosage[a]	Considerations and Monitoring
Isoniazid	TB prophylaxis or latent TB infection in nonimmunocompromised patients; treatment of TB infection in combination with other antitubercular agents; TB prophylaxis in HIV-infected patients when a newly positive skin test (5 mm or more) is confirmed or when the patient has been in contact with someone with active INH-sensitive TB regardless of skin test result	*TB prophylaxis or latent TB:* 300 mg orally once daily or 900 mg/dose orally twice weekly for 9 months. *TB in nonimmunocompromised patients:* 5 mg/kg (maximum dose: 300 mg) orally administered daily or 5 days/week OR 15 mg/kg (maximum dose: 900 mg) orally administered once, twice, or three times weekly. The usual initial treatment regimen is INH plus PZA, EMB, and RIF administered daily or 5 days/week DOT for 2 months; daily or 5 days/week DOT for 2 weeks, then twice weekly for 6 weeks; or three times/week DOT for 2 months.	Always check most recent clinical practice guidelines prior to recommendation of any medication for TB. Active TB must be excluded prior to beginning TB prophylaxis. Food may decrease absorption of INH; take 1 hr before or 2 hr after meals. Administer with 25–50 mg pyridoxine (vitamin B_6) each day to decrease the risk of peripheral neuropathy. For patients with peripheral neuropathy, may increase to 100 mg/day. For pregnant patients whose risk for active TB is low, some experts recommend waiting until after delivery to start therapy.
Ethambutol	Treatment of TB infection in combination with other antitubercular agents	15 mg/kg/dose (maximum dose: 1.5 Gm) orally once daily in treatment-naïve patients and 25 mg/kg/dose (maximum dose: 2.5 Gm) orally once daily in patients who have previously received therapy. After 60 days, decrease to 15 mg/kg orally once daily. The usual initial treatment regimen is INH plus PZA, EMB, and RIF once daily or five times weekly DOT for 2 months; once daily or five times weekly DOT for 2 weeks then twice weekly for 6 weeks; or three times weekly DOT for 2 months.	Should be given with food to decrease gastric irritation. Visual acuity and color discrimination tests should be administered prior to beginning EMB and monthly after starting therapy.
Rifampin	Treatment of TB infection in combination with other antitubercular agents	10 mg/kg/dose (maximum dosage: 600 mg/dose) orally once daily or two, three, or five times weekly. The usual initial treatment regimen is INH plus PZA, EMB, and RIF administered once daily or five times weekly DOT for 2 months; once daily or five times weekly DOT for 2 weeks, then twice weekly for 6 weeks; or three times weekly DOT for 2 months.	Take at least 1 hr before or 2 hr after a meal to increase absorption of the drug. Antacids may decrease absorption of RIF; give at least 1 hr before taking any antacids. Contents of capsules may be mixed with applesauce or jelly to ease swallowing.
PZA	Treatment of TB infection in combination with other antitubercular agents	15–30 mg/kg/dose orally once daily (maximum dosage: 3 Gm/day) or 50–70 mg/kg/dose (based on lean body weight) orally twice weekly. The usual initial treatment regimen is INH plus PZA, EMB, and RIF given once daily or five times weekly DOT for 2 months; once daily or five times weekly DOT for 2 weeks then twice weekly for 6 weeks; or three times weekly DOT for 2 months.	May be administered without regard to meals.
Rifabutin	Treatment of TB as an alternative to RIF in combination with other antitubercular agents	5 mg/kg (usual dose: 300 mg) orally once daily or two, three, or five times weekly. Initial treatment phase is rifabutin plus PZA, EMB, and INH once daily OR three or five times weekly. See guidelines for treatment of patients with HIV.	Rifabutin is used in patients who are taking protease inhibitors or nonnucleoside reverse transcriptase inhibitors or in patients who have experienced intolerance to RIF.

TABLE 46.3 First-Line Antitubercular Medications—cont'd

Medication	Indication	Dosage[a]	Considerations and Monitoring
Rifapentine	Active TB in conjunction with at least one other antituberculosis agent; TB prophylaxis or the treatment of latent tuberculosis infection in patients at high risk for progression to active TB	For active TB, once weekly dosage is 10–20 mg/kg. For latent TB or TB prophylaxis, rifapentine is given in combination with INH. For adults weighing ≥50 kg, 900 mg orally once weekly for 3 months. For adults weighing 32.1–49.9 kg, 750 mg orally once weekly for 3 months.	Rule out active TB disease before initiating therapy for latent tuberculosis.

[a]*DOT,* Directly observed therapy; *EMB,* ethambutol; *HIV,* human immunodeficiency virus; *INH,* Isoniazid; *PZA,* pyrazinamide; *RIF,* rifampin; *TB,* tuberculosis.
See clinical practice guidelines for treatment of specialty populations such as HIV, adolescents, children, and infants.

TABLE 46.4 Examples of Second-Line Agents for Patients Resistant to or Unable to Tolerate Usual Agents[a]

Medication	Indication	Dosage	Considerations and Monitoring
Cycloserine	Treatment of active pulmonary and extrapulmonary TB infection (in combination with other antitubercular agents) as second-line therapy	*Adults:* 10–15 mg/kg total (usually 250–500 mg orally once or twice daily). *Children:* 15–20 mg/kg total (orally, in 1–2 divided doses).	To relieve or prevent neurotoxic effects of cycloserine, add pyridoxine to regimen. Contraindicated in severe renal impairment. May use "no sugar added" chocolate pudding or fruit jelly to aid in giving drugs to children. Monitor CBC, renal function, and cycloserine levels as needed.
Streptomycin	Treatment of TB infection in combination with other antituberculosis agents as second-line therapy	*Adults:* IM route only, 15 mg/kg/ dose daily or 5 days/week. Some clinicians prefer 25 mg/kg three times weekly. Patients with decreased renal function may require the 15 mg/kg dose be given only three times weekly to allow for drug clearance. *Infants, children, and adolescents:* 15–40 mg/kg total once daily or 5 days/week or 25–30 mg/kg two or three times weekly. See guidelines for length of treatment.	Watch for symptoms of ototoxicity and nephrotoxicity. Inject deeply into a large muscle mass. May use muscles of the mid-lateral thigh. In children, the preferable site is the mid-lateral thigh.
Ethionamide	Treatment of drug-resistant TB infection as part of combination therapy	*Adults:* 15–20 mg/kg total orally divided once or twice daily. Start with 250 mg orally once daily and increase as tolerated (usually 250–500 mg once or twice daily). *Children:* 15–20 mg/kg total (divided 1–2 times daily). See guidelines for length of treatment.	May cause GI upset, metallic taste, or loss of appetite. Take with food to minimize GI upset.
Levofloxacin	Treatment of TB in combination with other antituberculosis agents as second-line therapy	*Adults:* 500–1000 mg daily. Inadequate dosage information for children.	Administer 1 hr before or 2 hr after eating and at least 2 hr before or 2 hr after any antacid, multivitamin, or other medication that contains divalent or trivalent cations.
Moxifloxacin	Treatment of drug-susceptible TB infection as part of combination therapy; considered second-line agent	*Adults:* 400 mg daily or 5 days a week. Inadequate dosage information for children. See guidelines for length of treatment.	Separate the administration of products containing magnesium, aluminum, iron, or zinc, including antacids and multivitamins, by at least 4 hr before or 8 hr after administration. May be given with or without food.

[a]Work in concert with state and local public health officials for adequate treatment of drug-resistant TB.
CBC, Complete blood count; *GI,* gastrointestinal; *IM,* intramuscular; *TB,* tuberculosis.

Adverse Effects. Patients may experience localized erythema at the injection site. Infrequently, patients may experience mild discomfort, itching, or rash. Allergic reactions are rare.

PRACTICE PEARLS

TB Skin Test Boosted Reaction

According to the CDC (2016), a two-step TST is used to detect past TB infection in individuals who may have decreased skin reactivity to tuberculin. These individuals, when given a TST years after TB infection, may have a false-negative result at the first test. With the second test, these individuals may have a positive skin test or "boosted reaction." This would be interpreted as TB infection.

Contraindications. Use of PPD is contraindicated in anyone who has been diagnosed with TB or has had a previous allergic reaction to PPD. The primary care provider should have access to epinephrine should the patient experience a severe allergic reaction. Patients with chronic renal failure may have a decreased response to the PPD.

Monitoring. See Box 46.3 for PPD interpretation criteria. It is essential to recognize that infected neonates and infants younger than 6 weeks of age may not develop a delayed hypersensitivity reaction because their immune system is not fully developed. PPD sensitivity develops anywhere from 3 weeks to 3 months after initial TB infection in older infants and children.

Isoniazid (INH)

Pharmacokinetics. Following oral administration, INH is absorbed from the gastrointestinal (GI) tract, with peak serum levels attained within 1 to 2 hours. Food decreases the rate and extent of absorption. INH is widely distributed into all body tissues and fluids, including cerebrospinal fluid (CSF). It crosses the placenta and is distributed into breast milk. Metabolism occurs in the liver. INH has been associated with several drug interactions relating to affected cytochrome (CYP) P450 isoenzymes. It is a potent inhibitor of CYP 2C19 and an inhibitor of CYP 3A4 in vitro. INH weakly inhibits CYP 2A6, CYP 2C9, and CYP 2D6. Approximately 75% of the drug is excreted in the urine, with the remainder in the feces, saliva, and sputum.

Indications. INH is effective against *Mycobacterium tuberculosis*. It is used for the treatment of TB infection in combination with other antitubercular medications, for TB prophylaxis, and for the treatment of LTBI. INH can also be used in the treatment of patients with HIV infection who have a newly positive TB skin test (5 mm or more), or who have been in contact with someone with active INH-sensitive tuberculosis regardless of skin test result.

Adverse Effects. The two most common adverse effects are peripheral neuropathy (more than 40% of patients) and elevated liver enzymes (10% to 20%). Peripheral neuropathy symptoms typically occur with doses of at least 16 to 24 mg/kg/day. It is also more likely in patients with diabetes or alcoholism and those who are malnourished. The risk of

peripheral neuropathy may be reduced through coadministration of pyridoxine (vitamin B_6). The risk of hepatitis is highest in patients between 35 and 64 years of age. Additional neurotoxic effects are rare but may include seizures, encephalopathy, memory impairment, psychosis, and optic neuritis.

Contraindications. Hepatitis is an absolute contraindication for INH (black box warning). The risk of hepatitis is increased in Black and Hispanic females. INH is contraindicated in patients who develop severe hypersensitivity reactions, including drug-induced hepatitis, previous INH-associated hepatic injury, or any severe adverse reactions. It should be used very cautiously in older adults and in any patient with a chronic hepatic disease such as alcoholism, cirrhosis. or chronic hepatitis C. Because INH is excreted in the kidneys, it should be used cautiously in patients with severe renal impairment.

BLACK BOX WARNING!

Isoniazid

Isoniazid is associated with risk for serious hepatotoxicity. Severe and possibly fatal hepatitis can occur with isoniazid therapy.

The use of INH in pregnancy should be avoided unless the benefits outweigh the risk. All females should be monitored carefully for hepatic dysfunction. While INH is excreted in breast milk, it has not been shown to produce toxic effects in infants. Oral pyridoxine is recommended to decrease the risk of peripheral neuropathy for the pregnant or breastfeeding patient and the infant.

Monitoring. All patients taking INH should have baseline liver function tests (LFTs) and monthly assessment for symptoms of liver injury (Fig. 46.1). If the LFTs are abnormal, it is imperative to monitor them periodically. Patients should be taught to immediately report any signs or symptoms consistent with liver damage: examples include anorexia, nausea, dark urine, fatigue, persistent fever, and right upper-quadrant tenderness. If signs are indicative of liver damage, INH should be discontinued and alternative treatments initiated.

Rifampin (RIF)

Rifampin is the most commonly used member of the rifamycin class; other members include rifapentine and rifabutin. While rifamycins (including rifampin) have multiple drug interactions (see Box 46.4), they are still considered a vital part of TB treatment.

Pharmacokinetics. The pharmacokinetics of RIF in infants and children are similar to those seen in adults. In general, RIF is absorbed rapidly from the GI tract after oral administration. Peak serum levels are typically attained within 2 to 4 hours. Because food decreases RIF absorption by about 30%, it should be given about 1 hour before or 2 hours after meals. RIF is approximately 80% protein bound and is widely distributed into most body tissues and fluids. It is metabolized in the liver to an active metabolite and is primarily excreted in the feces and urine. Elimination half-life in adults is 3 to 5 hours and decreases with prolonged use.

Activity	Baseline	Month of Treatment Completed 1	2	3	4	5	6	7	8	End of Treatment Visit
MICROBIOLOGY										
Sputum smears and culture[1]	☐	☐	☐	☐	☐					☐
Drug susceptibility testing[2]	☐			☐						
IMAGING										
Chest radiograph or other imaging[3]	☐		☐							☐
CLINICAL ASSESSMENT										
Weight[4]	☐	☐	☐	☐	☐	☐	☐	☐	☐	
Symptom and adherence review[5]	☐	☐	☐	☐	☐	☐	☐	☐	☐	
Vision assessment[6]	☐	☐	☐	☐	☐	☐	☐	☐	☐	
LABORATORY TESTING										
AST, ALT, bilirubin, alkaline phosphate[7]	☐	☐	☐	☐	☐	☐	☐	☐	☐	
Platelet count[8]	☐	☐	☐	☐	☐	☐	☐	☐	☐	
Creatinine[8]	☐	☐	☐	☐	☐	☐	☐	☐	☐	
HIV[9]	☐									
Hepatitis B and C screen[10]	☐									
Diabetes Screen[11]	☐									

• **Fig. 46.1** Baseline and follow-up evaluations for patients treated with first-line tuberculosis medications. Shading around boxes indicates activities that are optional or contingent on other information. Footnote: [1]Obtain sputa for smear and culture at baseline, then monthly until 2 consecutive specimens are negative. Collecting sputa more often early in treatment for assessment of treatment response and at end of treatment is optional. At least one baseline specimen should be tested using a rapid molecular test. [2]Drug susceptibility for isoniazid, rifampin, ethambutol (EMB), and pyrazinamide should be obtained. Repeat drug susceptibility testing if patient remains culture positive after completing 3 months of treatment. Molecular resistance testing should be performed for patients with risk for drug resistance. [3]Obtain chest radiograph at baseline for all patients, and also at month 2 if baseline cultures are negative. End-of-treatment chest radiograph is optional. Other imaging for monitoring of extrapulmonary disease. [4]Monitor weight monthly to assess response to treatment; adjust medication dose if needed. [5]Assess adherence and monitor improvement in tuberculosis symptoms (e.g., cough, fever, fatigue, night sweats) as well as development of medication adverse effects (e.g., jaundice, dark urine, nausea, vomiting, abdominal pain, fever, rash, anorexia, malaise, neuropathy, arthralgias). [6]Patients on EMB: baseline visual acuity (Snellen test) and color discrimination tests, followed by monthly inquiry about visual disturbance and monthly color discrimination tests. [7]Liver function tests only at baseline unless there were abnormalities at baseline, symptoms consistent with hepatotoxicity develop, or for patients who chronically consume alcohol, take other potentially hepatotoxic medications, or have viral hepatitis or history of liver disease, human immunodeficiency virus (HIV) infection, or prior drug-induced liver injury. [8]Baseline for all patients. Further monitoring if there are baseline abnormalities or as clinically indicated. [9]HIV testing in all patients. CD4 lymphocyte count and HIV RNA load if positive. [10]Patients with hepatitis B or C risk factor (e.g., injection drug use, birth in Asia or Africa, or HIV infection) should have screening tests for these viruses. [11]Fasting glucose or hemoglobin A1c for patients with risk factors for diabetes according to the American Diabetes Association including: age >45 years, body mass index >25 kg/m^2, first-degree relative with diabetes, and race/ethnicity of African American, Asian, Hispanic, American Indian/Alaska Native, or Hawaiian Native/Pacific Islander. Abbreviations: ALT, alanine aminotransferase; AST, aspartate aminotransferase. (From Nahid, P., Dorman, S. E., Alipanah, N., Barry, P. M., Brozek, J. L., Cattamanchi, A., … Peloquin, C. A. [2016]. Official American Thoracic Society/Centers for Disease Control and Prevention/Infectious Diseases Society of America clinical practice guidelines: Treatment of drug-susceptible tuberculosis. *Clinical Infectious Diseases*, *637*], e147–e195. https://doi.org/10.1093/cid/ciw376)

PHARMACOGENETICS

Rifampin

Rifampin is a significant inducer of many CYP P450 isoenzymes and drug transporters, including CYP 3A4, CYP 1A2, CYP 2B6, CYP 2C8, CYP 2C9, CYP 2C19, CYP 2D6, and P-glycoprotein. Drug–drug interactions are common with the use of rifampin.

Indications. RIF is used for treatment of all forms of active TB infection in combination with other antitubercular agents. Of note, it is also recommended as antimicrobial chemoprophylaxis for close contacts of a person with invasive meningococcal disease to eliminate meningococci from the nasopharynx. It is not used for the treatment of active meningococcal infection.

Adverse Effects. Common GI disturbances have been reported in patients taking RIF and include nausea, vomiting, flatulence, abdominal cramps, diarrhea, and pyrosis. These occur more frequently in patients taking RIF more than twice weekly. In general, the GI disturbances are relatively mild and do not require discontinuation of the therapy.

RIF can cause yellow-orange discoloration of urine, sweat, saliva, tears, sputum, and even teeth. It is important to advise patients who wear soft contact lenses that discoloration of the lens from tears may be permanent.

Although rare, patients may experience systemic hypersensitivity and cutaneous reactions including Stevens-Johnson syndrome and toxic epidermal necrolysis.

• BOX 46.4   Examples of Common Drug Interactions with Rifamycins[a]

Drug	Comments
Warfarin	Monitor PT/INR; may require increase in warfarin dose while taking rifamycin agent
Corticosteroids	Monitor patient carefully; may require increase in dose of corticosteroids while taking rifamycin agent
Lamotrigine	Therapeutic drug monitoring required; may require dosage increase to manage symptoms
Calcium channel blockers including verapamil, nifedipine, and diltiazem	Monitor patient's cardiovascular status; may require a change in medication to a different category while taking rifamycin agent
Sulfonylurea hypoglycemic agents	Monitor blood glucose; may require changing to another agent
Simvastatin, Fluvastatin	Monitor hypolipemic effect; may require another antihyperlipidemic agent
Levothyroxine	Monitor TSH; may require increase dose while taking rifamycin agent
Corticosteroids	May need to increase dose of corticosteroid while taking any rifamycin agent
Enalapril	May require a dose increase or change to another agent
NNRTIs	RIF decreases exposure to all NNRTIs
Benzodiazepines	Monitor patient response; may require dose increase or an alternative psychiatric medication

[a]There are many other drug–drug interactions with rifamycins. The healthcare provider should check all drug interactions among the patient's medications before prescribing any medication while the patient is on antitubercular therapy.

INR, International normalized ratio; NNRTI, nonnucleoside reverse transcriptase inhibitor; PT, prothrombin time; TSH, thyroid-stimulating hormone.

Adapted from Nahid, P., Dorman, S. E., Alipanah, N., Barry, P. M., Brozek, J. L., Cattamanchi, A., . . . Vernon, A. (2016). Official American Thoracic Society/Centers for Disease Control and Prevention/Infectious Diseases Society of America clinical practice guidelines: Treatment of drug-susceptible tuberculosis. Clinical Infectious Diseases, 63(7), e147–e195. http://doi.org/10.1093/cid/ciw376.

Anaphylaxis is rare. The incidence of these reactions is more common in patients who take RIF more than twice weekly.

Hepatotoxicity may occur in patients taking RIF. Severity may range from transient, asymptomatic elevations in LFTs to symptomatic hepatitis to fulminant hepatic failure. Severe hepatic abnormalities are more common in patients taking RIF in combination with other hepatotoxic medications.

Other adverse effects include elevations in blood urea nitrogen (BUN) and uric acid; central nervous system (CNS) effects such as headache, ataxia, decreased ability to concentrate, and mental confusion; thrombocytopenia; and vitamin K-deficient coagulation abnormalities. Deficiencies in vitamin B_6 and vitamin D have occurred. Females may experience menstrual irregularities.

Contraindications. RIF is contraindicated in patients with known RIF or rifamycin hypersensitivity. Patients with impaired liver function should receive RIF only if essential and then with careful follow-up. It should be used cautiously in patients with a history of coagulation disorders or who have chronic hepatic disease as it may increase the risk of vitamin K-dependent coagulation abnormalities. Patients who wear soft contact lenses should avoid using them while on RIF therapy. RIF should be used cautiously in patients with diabetes mellitus who are being treated with medications that are potentially hepatotoxic.

Monitoring. LFTs should be monitored before initiating RIF therapy and every 2 to 4 weeks during treatment. Also, monitor for signs and symptoms of liver dysfunction, particularly during prolonged treatment and if given with other hepatotoxic drugs. Discontinue RIF if signs or symptoms of hepatic damage occur or worsen.

Because vitamin D deficiency has been reported in patients taking long-term RIF, it is essential to monitor vitamin D levels. Monitor prothrombin time/international normalized ratio (INR) and platelet count, particularly in patients at risk for vitamin K-dependent coagulopathy. Supplementation of these important vitamins may be necessary.

QUALITY AND SAFETY

Directly Observed Therapy

Clinical practice guidelines (Nahid et al., 2016) recommend that directly observed therapy (DOT) be used as opposed to self-administered therapy (SAT) for treatment of patients with all forms of tuberculosis.

Ethambutol (EMB)

Pharmacokinetics. EMB is administered orally, with peak levels achieved within 2 to 4 hours. It is widely distributed, with high concentrations in the lungs, kidneys, and saliva. EMB is partly metabolized in the liver and excreted primarily in the urine (about 65%), with 20% to 25% excreted in the feces. Half-life is typically 3.5 hours; half-life is prolonged in patients with renal disease.

Indications. EMB is active against *Mycobacterium sp.* and *Mycobacterium tuberculosis* infection. It is primarily used in combination with other antitubercular medications for the treatment of TB infection.

Adverse Effects. Optic neuritis is one of the most significant adverse effects associated with EMB therapy. Symptoms include diminished visual acuity, loss of color discrimination, reduction of visual fields, and the presence of scotomata. Visual changes are typically dose related (25 mg/kg/day) and are reversible. Nevertheless, blindness has occurred.

Other adverse effects associated with EMB therapy include hypersensitivity reactions, hepatitis, hepatotoxicity, GI complaints, joint pain, and peripheral neuropathy. Fever, malaise, headache, and dizziness have occurred. Hyperuricemia and blood dyscrasias, including leukopenia, neutropenia, and thrombocytopenia, have occurred.

Contraindications. EMB is contraindicated in patients with optic neuritis and in neonates, infants, and children younger than 13 years of age who are unable to report visual changes. Consideration should be given to patients with visual defects such as cataracts or diabetic retinopathy, so ensure that an accurate visual assessment is conducted before beginning and while on EMB therapy. It should be used cautiously in patients with renal or hepatic impairment. EMB is pregnancy category B and is considered safe in breastfeeding.

Monitoring. Ophthalmologic exams including visual acuity and color discrimination tests should be conducted before the initiation of EMB therapy; these exams should be repeated monthly during EMB use (Nahid et al., 2016). In addition, patients with cataracts, diabetic retinopathy, and inflammatory eye conditions as well as those receiving more than 15mg/kg/day of EMB should be carefully monitored for visual changes related to the medication rather than to their primary visual condition. Monitor liver function studies, platelet count, serum creatinine/BUN, and serum uric acid.

Pyrazinamide (PZA)

Pharmacokinetics. PZA is administered orally and is rapidly absorbed from the GI tract. The plasma half-life is 9 to 10 hours and it is primarily excreted in the urine (70%) via glomerular filtration. Half-life may be increased up to 26 hours in patients with renal impairment.

Indications. PZA is effective against *Mycobacterium tuberculosis*. It is used in combination with other drugs to treat TB.

Adverse Effects. The most common adverse effects associated with PZA administration are mild arthralgia and myopathy. GI effects such as nausea, vomiting, and anorexia have been reported. Although rare, hematologic complications, angioedema, and hepatotoxicity are possible with PZA therapy.

Contraindications. PZA is contraindicated in patients with a history of severe or chronic hepatic disease and should be used cautiously in patients with alcoholism. It should not be given to patients with gout and should be used cautiously in patients with hyperuricemia. PZA is classified as pregnancy category C and is generally not recommended in patients during pregnancy. In females with HIV, PZA has been given after the first trimester. PZA is distributed in breast milk. Consideration should be given for the risks and benefits of giving PZA to breastfeeding females with TB.

Monitoring. Baseline LFTs should be performed initially and then every 2 to 4 weeks as indicated during treatment. Discontinue PZA if the patient experiences signs or symptoms of liver damage. Serum uric acid levels should be evaluated at baseline and throughout treatment in patients with a history of gout.

> **PRACTICE PEARLS**
>
> **Rifampin Therapy**
>
> Remember to tell patients taking rifampin that their urine, sweat, saliva, and tears may turn orange-yellow. Patients who wear contact lenses should avoid wearing them while taking rifampin.

> **PRACTICE PEARLS**
>
> **Isoniazid Use in Pregnancy and Lactation**
>
> Pyridoxine supplementation is recommended in pregnant and breastfeeding patients taking isoniazid to reduce the risk for drug-induced neuropathy.

Prescriber Considerations for Antitubercular Therapy

Clinical Practice Guidelines

The American Thoracic Society (ATS), Infectious Diseases Society of America (IDSA), and the CDC published clinical practice guidelines for the diagnosis of TB in adults and children (Lewinsohn et al., 2017) as well as clinical practice guidelines for the treatment of drug-susceptible TB (Nahid et al., 2016). Both can be accessed through the CDC TB Professional Tools link at https://www.cdc.gov/tb/education/professionaltools.htm.

> **BOOKMARK THIS!**
>
> **CDC TB Products and Publications**
>
> The CDC provides links to up-to-date information and clinical practice guidelines on TB-related topics such as drug-resistant TB, testing and diagnosis, TB in special populations, and TB and HIV. See https://www.cdc.gov/tb/publications/guidelines/default.htm.

Clinical Reasoning for Antitubercular Therapy

Consider the individual patient's health problem requiring antitubercular medication therapy. It is important to gather an accurate history in determining the patient's likelihood of exposure to TB. Is the primary care provider testing for latent TB or is the patient exhibiting symptoms of active TB? Treatment of latent TB reduces the risk of progression to active TB in the future. About 10% of patients become sick with TB in the future as a result of having LTBI. Treatment should begin after determining that the patient does not have active TB. If the patient is exhibiting signs and symptoms of active TB, it is imperative to work closely with the local public health department to decrease the risk of spread and increase the likelihood of completion of treatment. The public health department will help to identify individuals who have been in contact with the patient and may also be at risk.

Determine the desired therapeutic outcome for the patient with latent or active TB. For patients with latent TB, the desired outcome is eradication of the TB organism through medication therapy using a short course of combination therapy with once-weekly INH plus rifapentine for 12 weeks using DOT or SAT (Borisov et al., 2018). Patients with active TB will require a combination of intensive medication therapy followed by a continuation phase of medication for up to 6 to 9 months (or longer if the patient is drug resistant or there are any interruptions in treatment) to eradicate the TB organism.

Assess the antitubercular medication selected for its appropriateness for an individual patient by considering the medication's side effects and the patient's age, race/ethnicity, comorbidities, and genetic factors. Consider first-line recommended treatments for cases of latent TB vs. active TB disease as supported by the CDC's clinical practice guidelines. Because the majority of TB medications are hepatotoxic, it is critical to evaluate the patient for a history of liver disease and/or alcohol use. If the patient has a history of alcohol use disorder, work closely with mental health resources to determine support systems available to help the patient reduce or abstain from alcohol. In addition, monitoring liver function will be critical. Baseline visual acuity and color discrimination tests will be important for patients beginning INH and/or EMB.

Initiate the treatment plan with the selected medication by first providing adequate patient education to ensure the patient's understanding and promote full participation in the antitubercular medication therapy. According to Jeffries and colleagues from the CDC (2017), the ultimate responsibility for ensuring quality and completeness of TB-related services rests with state and local public health agencies. Nevertheless, the primary care provider should work closely with public health agencies to reinforce the treatment plan and educate the patient and family regarding the need for adherence to the prescribed medication regimen. TB treatment requires anywhere from 12 weeks for patients diagnosed with latent TB to 6 to 9 months for patients with drug-sensitive TB. Patients with drug-resistant TB may require up to 2 years of treatment. Continue to support patient follow-up for usual primary care including acute and chronic illness management.

Ensure complete patient and family understanding about the medication prescribed for antitubercular therapy using a variety of education strategies. Use the multiple resources available from the CDC to support patient and family understanding of the illness. Follow up with state agencies to garner additional resources. For example, the Florida Department of Public Health provides access to a wide variety of resources for patients and families at www.floridahealth.gov/diseases-and-conditions/tuberculosis/tb-resources.html.

Conduct follow-up and monitoring of patient responses to antitubercular medication therapy. Clinical practice guidelines

(Nahid et al., 2016) provide recommendations for baseline and follow-up testing for patients taking first-line TB medications (Fig. 46.1). Evidence indicates that DOT is the preferred method for TB medication administration. This can reduce interruptions in therapy as well as increase the likelihood of identification of adverse effects. Mild GI symptoms may be treated with the addition of antacids which have less effect on absorption than food. Because INH, RIF, and PZA can cause drug-induced hepatotoxicity, it is important to monitor LFTs carefully. If there are signs of hepatotoxicity, discontinue the medication and notify the public health department and/or physician specialist in your area for referral. The ATS provides detailed recommendations for management of drug-induced hepatotoxicity at https://www.thoracic.org/statements/resources/mtpi/hepatotoxicity-of-antituberculosis-therapy.pdf.

Teaching Points for Antitubercular Medications

Health Promotion Strategies

- It is essential that the primary care provider work closely with local public health agencies to reduce the risk of TB transmission and ensure adequate treatment and follow-up.
- Explain to the patient the need to remain at home for the first several weeks of therapy to reduce the risk of spread of infection. When this is not possible, or if there are others in the home, patients may need to wear a respiratory mask. Sputum should be expelled into a tissue and the tissue placed in a closed bag until ready to discard.
- Provide the patient with information about TB diagnosis, transmission, treatment, and adverse effects to enhance medication adherence and outcomes.
- For patients who are non-English–speaking or have limited understanding of English, use a medical interpreter rather than family and friends to enhance patient teaching.
- Follow up on any missed appointments to help decrease the risk of interruption in therapy.
- Reinforce the need to cover the mouth/nose when coughing, sneezing, or speaking loudly.
- Emphasize the need for proper nutrition, avoidance of smoking, and abstinence from alcohol.
- Remind the patient of the need to avoid over-the-counter (OTC) medications that may interact with therapy.
- Teach the patient the risks of nonadherence to treatment, including increased drug resistance, the spread of TB to others, and the risk of significant disease progression that can result in death.

Patient Education for Medication Safety

- Multiple medications are required to treat TB to eradicate the infection and prevent its spread to others.
- Proper nutrition, hydration, and physical activity will be important as you treat and recover from TB.

- Excellent patient information is available from the CDC at https://www.cdc.gov/tb/topic/basics/default.htm. You can find information about signs and symptoms, treatment, and prevention of TB as well as a variety of personal stories from patients with TB and public health officials who work with them.
- It is vitally important to adhere to your medication regimen to treat the infection and reduce the risk of antibiotic resistance to TB medications.
- For those who are participating in programs that include direct observation therapy (DOT), this is to help you adhere to the rigorous medication therapy and to ensure that any adverse effects are discovered early in therapy.
- Notify your primary care provider should you experience any signs or symptoms of liver problems, including loss of appetite, nausea, vomiting, or a yellowing of the skin or eyes. These can indicate severe complications of antitubercular therapy.
- Make sure to cover your mouth when coughing, sneezing, or speaking to reduce the risk of airborne droplets during the early stages of your treatment.
- PZA may cause achiness in your joints. Notify your primary care provider to determine the best actions to treat the discomfort.
- If you are taking INH and/or EMB, make sure to notify your primary care provider if you experience any changes in vision, such as blurred vision or changes in color vision, as these may be signs of a condition called optic neuritis.
- Depending on your medication regimen, you may be asked to take vitamin B_6, vitamin D, and/or vitamin K supplements to help prevent adverse effects associated with antitubercular therapy.
- Because you are taking medications that may affect your liver, it is imperative to avoid alcohol. If avoiding alcohol is a significant issue for you, do not hesitate to contact your primary care provider for referrals to programs in your area that may be helpful.

Application Questions for Discussion

1. You suspect that one of your patients may have been exposed to someone with active TB. Develop an assessment and treatment plan for the patient and their close contacts.
2. What are the requirements in your state or region for reporting suspected TB? Who are the primary contacts?
3. You are responsible for the provision of health care in a local correctional facility. A patient in the facility is now being treated for active TB. What are the practices and policies that will reduce the spread of TB within the facility?

Selected Bibliography

Borisov, A. S., Bamrah Morris, S., Njie, G. J., Winston, C. A., Burton, D., Goldberg, S., & Vernon, A. (2018). Update of recommendations for use of once-weekly Isoniazid-Rifapentine regimen to treat latent *Mycobacterium tuberculosis* infection. *Morbidity and Mortality Weekly Report, 67*(25), 723–726. http://doi.org/10.15585/mmwr.mm6725a5.

Centers for Disease Control and Prevention (CDC). (2013). *Latent Tuberculosis Infection: A Guide for Primary Health Care Providers*: U.S. Department of Health and Human Services, Centers for Disease Control and Prevention. Available at. https://www.cdc.gov/tb/publications/ltbi/default.htm.

Centers for Disease Control and Prevention (CDC). (2012). Menu of suggested provisions for state tuberculosis prevention and control laws: Case identification. Retrieved from https://www.cdc.gov/tb/programs/laws/menu/caseid.htm.

Centers for Disease Control and Prevention (CDC). (2016, March 18). *TB risk factors.* https://www.cdc.gov/tb/topic/basics/risk.htm.

Centers for Disease Control and Prevention (CDC). (2018). *Questions and answers about tuberculosis.* Retrieved from https://www.cdc.gov/tb/default.htm.

Centers for Disease Control and Prevention (CDC). (October 5, 2021) TB incidence in the United States, 1953-2020 *TB cases and case rates per 100,000 population.* https://www.cdc.gov/tb/statistics/tbcases.htm.

Chesnutt, A. N., Chesnutt, M. S., Prendergast, N. T., & Prendergast, T. J. (2020). Pulmonary tuberculosis. In M. A. Papadakis, S. J. McPhee, & M. W. Rabow (Eds.), *Current Medical Diagnosis and Treatment 2020.* New York: McGraw-Hill Education.

Elsevier. Clinical pharmacology powered by ClinicalKey®. (2019). Retrieved from http://www.clinicalkey.com.

Jeffries, C., Lobue, P., Chorba, T., Metchock, B., & Kashef, I. (2017). Role of the health department in tuberculosis prevention and control—Legal and public health considerations. *Microbiology Spectrum, 5*(2). http://doi.org/10.1128/microbiolspec.TNMI7-0034-2016.

Lewinsohn, D. M., Leonard, M. K., LoBue, P. A., Cohn, D. L., Daley, C. L., Desmond, E., & Woods, G. L. (2017). Official American Thoracic Society/Infectious Diseases Society of America/Centers for Disease Control and Prevention clinical practice guidelines: Diagnosis of tuberculosis in adults and children. *Clinical Infectious Diseases, 64*(2), 111–115. http://doi.org/10.1093/cid/ciw778.

McCance, K. L., & Huether, S. E. (2019). *Pathophysiology: The Biologic Basis for Disease in Adults and Children* (8th ed.). St. Louis: Elsevier.

Nahid, P., Dorman, S. E., Alipanah, N., Barry, P. M., Brozek, J. L., Cattamanchi, A., & Vernon, A. (2016). Official American Thoracic Society/Centers for Disease Control and Prevention/Infectious Diseases Society of America clinical practice guidelines: Treatment of drug-susceptible tuberculosis. *Clinical Infectious Diseases, 63*(7), e147–e195. http://doi.org/10.1093/cid/ciw376.

Namdar, R., & Peloquin, C. A. (2020). Tuberculosis. In J. T. DiPiro, G. C. Yee, L. M. Posey, S. T. Haines, T. D. Nolin, & V. Ellingrod (Eds.), *Pharmacotherapy: A Pathophysiologic Approach* (11th ed.). New York: McGraw-Hill Education.

Rosenthal, L. D., & Burchum, J. R. (2018). *Lehne's Pharmacotherapeutics for Advanced Practice Providers.* St. Louis: Elsevier.

World Health Organization (WHO). (2021, October 14). *Tuberculosis: key facts.* Retrieved from https://www.who.int/news-room/fact-sheets/detail/tuberculosis.

47

Antifungal Medications

CHERYL H. ZAMBROSKI

Overview

Fungal infections are widespread and a major public health issue, particularly as the number of immunocompromised patients has grown and the use of broad-spectrum antibiotics has increased. According to Bongomin et al. (2017), nearly 1 billion people worldwide are estimated to have skin, nail, and hair fungal infections. In addition, millions of people are affected by mucosal candidiasis and more than 150 million have serious and possibly fatal fungal infections. Severity may range from mild or asymptomatic, as in many mucocutaneous infections, to life-threatening systemic infections.

Currently the most common fungal diseases include onychomycosis, oral and vaginal candidiasis, and tinea corporis (Centers for Disease Control and Prevention [CDC], 2019). The most common organism responsible for mucosal disease is *Candida albicans*; for skin infections, the *Trichophyton* spp.; and for allergic fungal disease, *Aspergillus fumigatus* (Bongomin et al., 2017).

Fungal diseases that typically affect people who live or travel to certain areas include blastomycosis (U.S. and Canada), coccidiomycosis (southwestern U.S. and parts of Mexico and Central and South America), *Cryptococcus gattii* infection (Pacific Northwest U.S. and British Columbia), and histoplasmosis (associated with bird and bat droppings). A wide variety of infections are opportunistic, affecting those with suppressed immune systems such as those receiving immunosuppressant medications, as well as with those with human immunodeficiency virus (HIV), with cancer, or who have received organ transplants.

An increased incidence of fungal infection can be attributed to a variety of causes, including use of broad-spectrum antibiotics, immunosuppression associated with organ transplants and chemotherapy, treatment of autoimmune disorders, and HIV/AIDS. Fungal infections in transplant patients and those with HIV tend to be severe and usually require treatment for a prolonged period.

A growing number of antifungals are now available for topical or oral use. This chapter discusses the topical and oral antifungals most commonly used in primary care to treat two types of fungal infection: *endemic fungal infection*, such as blastomycosis, histoplasmosis, and sporotrichosis; and *superficial fungal infection*, including those infections not responsive to topical therapy. Fungal infections are typically difficult to treat and require long-term therapy for best results. In addition, systemic antifungals are associated with a significant risk of serious adverse reactions and should be used with caution. Several antifungals are administered parenterally and are used in specialty practices rather than primary care; these are not discussed here.

Relevant Physiology

Fungi can be divided into two broad categories based on morphology: *yeasts* and *molds*. Yeasts are unicellular fungi that are typically round or oval and reproduce by budding. When buds do not separate, they form long chains of yeast cells known as *pseudohyphae*. Molds are multicellular colonies that are composed of tubular structures called *hyphae* which grow by branching and longitudinal extension. Some fungi are dimorphic and can grow as either yeast or molds, depending on environmental conditions.

Fungal and mammalian cells are eukaryocytes. In contrast to bacteria, which are prokaryotes, eukaryocytes have a distinct nucleus, specialized organelles, and a protective cell membrane. Due to the similarity between mammalian cells and fungal cells, antifungal medications may have increased toxic effects on mammalian cells; therefore, antifungal medications must be used cautiously. A key difference between fungal and mammalian cells is the sterol used in the synthesis of their respective cell membranes—ergosterol in fungi and cholesterol in mammals.

Pathophysiology

Mycosis is the presence of parasitic fungi in or on the body. Most fungi that are pathogenic in humans grow as yeast, are nonmotile, and with rare exceptions are not transmissible. Fungal infections can be superficial (i.e., confined to the keratinous layers), subcutaneous, or deeply invasive.

Topical Fungi

Fungal infections of the skin, hair, and nails remain prevalent, and the demand for treatment has increased as safer drugs have been developed. Tinea infections are discussed more thoroughly in Chapter 3 of this text. Some tinea infections require systemic treatment. For example, tinea capitis (most commonly caused by *Trichophyton tonsurans*) usually requires systemic treatment. Tinea corporis (usually caused by *T. rubrum*) frequently responds to topical therapy but may require systemic treatment. Tinea versicolor is caused by *Malassezia furfur* (also known as *Pityrosporum orbiculare*) and frequently requires systemic treatment.

Candida species can normally live on the skin and in the mouth, gut, or vagina of healthy individuals. Yet these organisms can be opportunistic under a variety of conditions. Overgrowth of *Candida* organisms can cause mucosal candidiasis affecting the mouth, throat, esophagus, and vulvovagina. It can also be found on the skin, especially in skin folds in patients with obesity. Risk factors for candidiasis of the mouth, throat, or esophagus can be found in Box 47.1. Vulvovaginal candida is the second most common type of vaginal infection reported in the United States (CDC, 2019). While over-the-counter (OTC) antifungal agents are commonly used to treat vaginal candidiasis, patients who experience infections more than four times yearly or who are diabetic or immunosuppressed may require antifungals by prescription. Risk factors for vulvovaginal candidiasis (VVC) are found in Box 47.2.

Invasive candidiasis is far less common than topical candidiasis. Risk factors for invasive candidiasis (i.e., fungemia and endocarditis) include neutropenia, recent surgery, broad-spectrum antibiotic therapy, indwelling catheters (intravenous [IV] or bladder), and immunodeficiency. HIV infection should be suspected if the patient has invasive candidiasis. Patients with invasive candidiasis typically are hospitalized and require IV medications.

Endemic Mycoses

The primary care provider should be aware of endemic fungal infections in rural and regional populations. Some types of diagnostic cytology, such as skin scraping smears, are inexpensive and are easily done in the outpatient setting. Most of these fungi do not result in systemic infection in immunocompetent persons. However, individuals who are immunocompromised, young children, and older adults may be at higher risk. Although many fungal species have been identified, only the most common are discussed here.

> ### BOOKMARK THIS!
>
> #### CDC Resources on Fungal Diseases
>
> The CDC provides up-to-date information about fungal diseases in the United States and around the world at https://www.cdc.gov/fungal/index.html. Here you will also find information on a specific branch of the CDC, the Mycotic Diseases Branch, which is dedicated to determining the burden of fungal infections and responding to outbreaks worldwide.

Endemic mycoses are infections by fungi commonly found in distinct geographical regions. These fungi can cause disease even in healthy hosts. Infection is caused by inhalation of the organism from the environment during the mold phase. The clinical presentation is generally a nonspecific or atypical pulmonary infection. Many fungi are associated with geographic regions, and these patterns assist primary care providers in making a clinical diagnosis. However, because of opportunities for regional, national, and global travel, careful history in combination with symptom assessment and diagnostic testing is essential. The severity of disease depends on the amount inhaled and the immune response of the patient.

Blastomycosis is caused by the fungus *Blastomyces dermatitidis*. It is endemic to the midwestern, south central, and southeastern states that border the Mississippi and Ohio River basins, the Great Lakes, and Canada. Infection occurs primarily in healthy individuals during occupational or recreational contact with soil from streams and rivers. Although many patients may be asymptomatic, they may present with flulike symptoms including fever, shortness of breath, cough, muscle aches, fatigue, and night sweats. Disseminated infection can cause lesions on the lungs, skin, bones, and reproductive and urinary systems. Skin lesions are typically verrucous or ulcerative and can lead to abscesses with scarring and loss of skin pigment.

Coccidioidomycosis (also called Valley fever) is caused by *Coccidioides immitis*, a mold that grows in soil in arid regions of the southwestern United States, Mexico, and Central and South America. Typically, people who are exposed to the infection recover without medications within several weeks to 1 month. In fact, many patients are asymptomatic, while others experience flulike symptoms with fatigue, cough, fever, night sweats, arthralgia, periarticular swelling, and rash (erythema nodosum). Persistent and severe symptoms require treatment to prevent chronic pulmonary infection with pneumonia, osteomyelitis, meningitis, and multiple organ involvement, even septic shock. Like other fungal diseases, immunosuppressed individuals are most at risk. Other at-risk groups include pregnant females, African Americans, and Filipinos.

• BOX 47.1 Risk Factors for *Candida* Infection of the Mouth, Throat, or Esophagus

- Infants <1 month of age
- People who wear poorly fitted dentures
- People using inhaled corticosteroids for asthma
- People with chronic illnesses including cancer, anemia, diabetes, HIV/AIDS
- People on antibiotic therapy
- People who smoke
- People with xerostomia secondary to medications or other conditions

---

• BOX 47.2 Risk Factors for Vulvovaginal Candidiasis

- Diabetes mellitus
- Use of hormonal contraceptives
- Females who are immunosuppressed
- Current or recent antibiotic therapy
- Pregnancy

Histoplasmosis is caused by *Histoplasma capsulatum*, which is prevalent in the eastern and central parts of United States. It can be found in bird droppings and bat exposure along river valleys, especially the Ohio and Mississippi River valleys. Locations with large bat and/or bird populations are more likely to be affected. Most cases are asymptomatic or involve mild, influenza-like illnesses, go unrecognized, and resolve without medication. More severe infections may present as atypical pneumonia or can present with neurological symptoms such as headache, confusion, neck stiffness, and ataxia. Progressive disseminated infections can be severe and may be fatal. Severe symptoms include marked prostration, fever, dyspnea, and weight loss.

Pneumocystosis is caused by *Pneumocystis jiroveci* (formerly called *Pneumocystis carinii*). This fungus is found in the lungs of many domesticated and wild mammals and is distributed worldwide in humans. It seldom causes illness in immunocompetent people. It causes acute pneumonia in premature or debilitated infants in hospitals and underdeveloped countries, as well as in older children and adults who have weakened cellular immune systems, most commonly due to HIV. Symptoms usually develop over several weeks and include fever, dry cough, shortness of breath, chest pain, and fatigue. Without treatment, it can be fatal in immunosuppressed individuals.

Cryptococcosis is caused by inhalation of *Cryptococcus neoformans*, a yeast that is found worldwide in soil and in bird droppings. It is the most common cause of fungal meningitis.

Cryptococcosis typically infects the lungs or central nervous system (CNS) with symptoms including cough, dyspnea, chest pain, fever, headache, photophobia, nuchal rigidity, confusion, and changes in behavior. Immunocompetent people rarely develop clinically apparent pneumonia. Progressive lung disease and dissemination can occur in patients with immunodeficiency, including HIV.

Aspergillosis is caused by *Aspergillus fumigatus*. The fungus can be found in soil and decaying vegetation as well as in household dust, ornamental plants, and even food and water. Symptoms vary depending on the site of infection but typically include dyspnea, cough, fever, and hemoptysis. Aspergillosis is most common in patients who are immunocompromised such as those with organ or bone marrow transplants and those with HIV.

Antifungal Therapy

Antifungal medications are available to combat both superficial and systemic fungal infections. Superficial fungal infections are far more common; systemic infections are far more serious and may require hospitalization for IV antifungals. This chapter covers antifungal medications that may be used in primary care including the azoles, allylamines, polyenes, and several others (Table 47.1). These medications are available in a variety of forms including topical (e.g., creams, foams, shampoos, and gels) and oral forms. Antifungal medications, particularly oral, should be used

TABLE 47.1	**Antifungal Medications**			
Category/ Medication	**Indication**	**Dosage**		**Considerations and Monitoring**
Azoles				
Clotrimazole	Oropharyngeal, cutaneous, and vulvovaginal candidiasis (VVC); treatment of tinea corporis, tinea cruris, tinea pedis, and tinea versicolor	*For cutaneous candidiasis:* Apply topically to affected skin and surrounding areas twice daily for 2–4 weeks. *For oropharyngeal candidiasis:* Apply transmucosal doses: 10 mg five times daily for 7–14 days for adults and children ≥3 yr. *For tinea pedis, cruris, corporis, and versicolor:* Apply twice daily for 2 weeks (tinea cruris) or 4 weeks (tinea corporis, pedis). *For VVC in adults and adolescents 12–17 yr:* 1 applicatorful of 1% cream (50 mg) vaginally at bedtime for 7 days or 1 applicatorful of 2% cream (100 mg) vaginally at bedtime for 3 days. Cream may be applied externally if extravaginal symptoms.		Troches should be dissolved slowly in the mouth; do not chew. Vaginal application should be used 7 days for pregnant patients and 7–14 days for immunocompromised patients or severe or recurrent VVC. For HIV-infected patients, treat for 3–7 days for uncomplicated cases or at least 7 days for severe or recurrent cases of VVC.

TABLE 47.1 Antifungal Medications—cont'd

Category/ Medication	Indication	Dosage	Considerations and Monitoring
Miconazole	Tinea pedis, tinea corporis, tinea cruris, tinea versicolor, VVC, cutaneous candidiasis, and oropharyngeal candidiasis	*Adults, adolescents, and children ≥2 yr:* Apply topical cream twice daily for 2–4 weeks. *Transmucosal dosage for adults and adolescents ≥16 yr:* Apply one 50-mg buccal tablet to the upper gum region, just above the incisor tooth, once daily for 14 days. For uncomplicated VVC, there are 1-, 3-, and 7-day regimens in which the suppository or applicator is inserted vaginally daily at bedtime. For complicated or recurrent cases, use one 100-mg suppository inserted intravaginally once daily at bedtime for 7–14 consecutive days or one applicatorful (5 Gm) of the 2% cream intravaginally once daily at bedtime for 7–14 consecutive days. The vulvar cream may be used topically externally twice daily for up to 7 days, regardless of the intravaginal regimen utilized.	Apply 2% preparation to the cleansed, dry, infected area as directed. Pregnant patients should not use self-directed OTC preparations of miconazole for VVC.
Econazole	Tinea cruris, tinea corporis, tinea pedis, and tinea versicolor caused by susceptible fungi; cutaneous candidiasis	*Adults:* Apply a sufficient amount of cream to the affected areas once daily for 2 weeks. Cream may be used for tinea pedis for 1 month. For cutaneous candidiasis, the recommended length of therapy is 2 weeks.	Tinea pedis may require treatment for 1 month to reduce possibility of recurrence. Topical foam dosage may be used by adolescents and children >12 yr for tinea pedis for a duration of 4 weeks.
Oxiconazole	Tinea corporis, tinea cruris, and tinea pedis due to *Epidermophyton floccosum, Trichophyton mentagrophytes,* or *Trichophyton rubrum*; tinea versicolor due to *Malassezia furfur*	*Adults, adolescents and children:* Apply 1% cream or lotion to affected and surrounding areas once or twice daily for 2 weeks (tinea cruris, corporis) or 1 month (pedis). Use 1% cream for tinea versicolor once daily for 2 weeks.	If the patient shows no clinical improvement after the treatment period, the diagnosis should be reviewed. Return to normal pigmentation in tinea versicolor may take weeks to months depending on skin type and exposure to sun.
Ketoconazole	Topical treatment: Mucocutaneous candidiasis, seborrheic dermatitis, tinea corporis, tinea cruris, tinea pedis, and tinea versicolor Oral treatment: Chromomycosis, blastomycosis, coccidioidomycosis, histoplasmosis, and paracoccidioidomycosis in patients who have failed or who are intolerant to other therapies	**Oral:** *Adults:* 200 mg orally once daily. Serious infection may require 400 mg orally once daily. *Children ≥2 yr and adolescents:* 3.3 mg/kg orally once daily. Do not exceed 400 mg/day. **Topical:** For mucocutaneous candidiasis, apply to area once daily for 2 weeks. For seborrheic dermatitis on scalp, use 1% shampoo every 3–4 days for up to 8 weeks; use 2% shampoo once on affected area. For cream and foam, apply to affected area twice daily for 4 weeks; for gel, apply once daily for 2 weeks. For tinea corporis, cruris, pedis, and versicolor, apply cream once daily for 2 weeks (corporis, cruris, versicolor) or 6 weeks (pedis).	Oral doses should be used only for treatment of chromomycosis, blastomycosis, coccidioidomycosis, histoplasmosis, and paracoccidioidomycosis in patients who have failed or who are intolerant to other therapies due to risk of adverse effects. For topical forms, teach patient to read package labeling very carefully to apply using proper techniques. For example, shampoos may require user to leave in place for 5 minutes before rinsing.

Continued

TABLE 47.1   Antifungal Medications—cont'd

Category/ Medication	Indication	Dosage	Considerations and Monitoring
Itraconazole	Mild to moderate pulmonary or disseminated extrapulmonary blastomycosis	*Adults:* Sporanox capsule or equivalent: 200 mg orally three times daily for 3 days followed by 200 mg orally once or twice daily for 6–12 months. Maximum dosage: 400 mg/day.	Capsules/tablets and oral solution should not be used interchangeably due to the higher oral bioavailability seen with the oral solution.
	Mild to moderate acute pulmonary histoplasmosis	*Adults:* 200 mg orally once or twice daily for 6 weeks.	Monitor serum itraconazole trough concentration after at least 2 weeks to ensure adequate drug exposure.
	Onychomycosis due to dermatophytes (tinea unguium) in immunocompetent patients	*Adults:* Sporanox capsule or equivalent: for fingernail involvement only, 200 mg twice daily for 1 week, followed by no drug for 3 weeks, then 200 mg twice daily for 1 week. For fingernail and/or toenail involvement, 200 mg orally once daily for 12 weeks.	Itraconazole is recommended for patients with histoplasmosis who have symptoms for more than 1 month. Confirm diagnosis with lab testing prior to initiating therapy.
Fluconazole	Treatment of oropharyngeal candidiasis	*Adults:* 200 mg orally once, then 100 mg orally once daily for 7–14 days. For moderate to severe disease, may prescribe 100–200 mg once daily. *Adolescents:* May prescribe 6 mg/kg/dose (maximum: 200 mg/dose) orally once, then 3 mg/kg/dose (maximum: 100 mg/dose) orally once daily. May give 100–200 mg orally once daily for moderate to severe disease. Treat for 7–14 days. *For infants and children:* 6 mg/kg/dose orally once, then 3 mg/kg/dose orally once daily. A maximum of 400 mg/dose has been recommended. Treat for 7–14 days; a course of at least 14 days may decrease the likelihood of relapse.	Refer to current clinical practice guidelines for HIV-infected patients with oropharyngeal or esophageal candidiasis. May be given without regard to meals.
	Treatment of esophageal candidiasis	*Adults:* 200 mg orally once, then 100 mg orally once daily. Alternatively, 200–400 mg (3–6 mg/kg/dose) orally once daily. Treat for 14–21 days and for at least 2 weeks after resolution of symptoms. *Adolescents:* 6 mg/kg/dose (maximum: 200 mg/dose) orally once, then 3 mg/kg/dose (maximum: 100 mg/dose) orally once daily. Treat for 14–21 days and for at least 2 weeks after resolution of symptoms.	
	For VVC	*Adults:* 150 mg orally as a single dose as an alternative to topical antifungal therapy is recommended by guidelines for uncomplicated VVC. For complicated or severe acute VVC, 150 mg orally every 72 hours for 2–3 doses. For recurrent VVC, 100 mg, 150 mg, or 200 mg orally every 3 days for 3 doses, or alternatively, daily therapy with a topical agent or oral fluconazole for 10–14 days.	
Posaconazole	Oropharyngeal candidiasis	**Immediate-release oral suspension form:** *Adults and adolescents:* 100 mg orally twice daily for 1 day, then 100 mg orally once daily for 13 days. *Adults and adolescents living with HIV:* 400 mg orally twice daily for 1 day, then 400 mg once daily for 7–14 days.	Delayed-release tablets and oral suspension forms are NOT interchangeable due to differences in dosing. Administer suspension form during or within 20 minutes of a full meal to decrease nausea. Use calibrated measuring device to ensure accurate dosing.

TABLE 47.1 **Antifungal Medications—cont'd**

Category/ Medication	Indication	Dosage	Considerations and Monitoring
Allylamines			
Terbinafine	Tinea pedis	*Adults, adolescents, and children ≥12 yr:* Topical 1% OTC spray, apply between the toes twice daily for 1 week; 1% gel, apply between the toes once daily for 1 week; 1% cream, apply between the toes twice daily for 1 week, bottom or sides of feet may be treated for 2 weeks.	For tinea pedis, remind patient to change shoes and socks at least once daily. Improvement of dermal tinea infection is gradual. Improvements in the treated condition may continue for 2–6 weeks after therapy is completed. Wash hands before and after application except when treating hand or fingernail infections. Rub cream, topical solution, or topical gel gently into the affected area(s). Apply an amount sufficient to cover the affected area and the immediate surrounding skin. Avoid getting in the eyes, nose, mouth, or other mucous membranes.
	Tinea cruris, tinea corporis	*Adults, adolescents, and children ≥12 yr:* Topical 1% spray, solution, gel, or cream, apply to affected area once daily for 1 week. Topical 1% prescription gel, apply to affected area and surrounding skin once daily for 1 week.	
	Tinea versicolor due to *Malassezia furfur*	*Adults:* Topical 1% prescription gel, apply to affected area and surrounding skin once daily for 1 week. Topical 1% prescription solution, apply to affected area twice daily for 1 week.	
	Onychomycosis (tinea unguium)	*Adults:* Oral tablets, 250 mg orally once daily. Administer for 6 weeks for fingernails, 12 weeks for toenails.	
Naftifine	Tinea cruris	*Adults:* 1% gel, apply twice daily for 4 weeks; 1% cream, apply once daily for 4 weeks. *Adults, adolescents, and children >12 yr:* 2% cream, apply once daily for 2 weeks.	Creams and gels should be gently massaged into affected area and surrounding skin as directed. 1% cream and 2% gel are effective for *Trichophyton rubrum, Trichophyton mentagrophytes,* and *Epidermophyton floccosum.* 1% gel is effective for *Trichophyton rubrum, Trichophyton mentagrophytes, Trichophyton tonsurans,* and *Epidermophyton floccosum.* 2% cream is effective for *Trichophyton rubrum.* Therapeutic response may be delayed; reevaluate if no clinical improvement is observed after 4 weeks of treatment. Instruct patient to discontinue treatment if irritation or sensitivity develops.
	Tinea pedis	*Adults:* 1% gel, apply twice daily for 4 weeks; 1% cream, apply once daily for 4 weeks. *Adults, adolescents, and children >12 yr:* 2% gel or 2% cream, apply once daily for 2 weeks.	
	Tinea corporis	*Adults:* 1% gel, apply twice daily for 4 weeks; 1% cream, apply once daily for 4 weeks. *Adults, adolescents, and children >12 yr:* 2% cream, apply approximately 0.5 inches once daily for 2 weeks.	
Butenafine	Topical treatment of tinea corporis, tinea cruris, tinea pedis, and tinea versicolor due to susceptible organisms such as *Epidermophyton floccosum, Trichophyton mentagrophytes, Trichophyton rubrum, Trichophyton tonsurans,* and *Malassezia furfur*	*Adults, adolescents, and children ≥12 yr:* For tinea corporis, tinea cruris, and tinea versicolor, apply topical cream to the affected area(s) and to the immediately surrounding skin once daily for 2 weeks. For tinea pedis, apply topical cream to affected area(s) and the immediately surrounding skin once daily for 4 weeks.	

Continued

Antifungal Medications—cont'd

Category/ Medication	Indication	Dosage	Considerations and Monitoring
Polyene			
Nystatin	Cutaneous and mucocutaneous candidiasis, including candidal diaper dermatitis	*Adults, adolescents, children, infants:* Cream or ointment, apply twice daily until healing is complete. Topical powder, apply two or three times daily until healing is complete.	Topical powder is recommended over creams and ointments for moist lesions, particularly in the intertriginous areas of the skin.
	For oropharyngeal candidiasis	*Adults, adolescents, and children:* Oral suspension, 400,000–600,000 units (4–6 mL) orally swished in the mouth four times daily for 7–14 days. *Infants:* 200,000 units (2 mL) orally four times daily; each dose is divided so that one-half of each dose is placed in each side of the mouth. Avoid feeding for 5–10 minutes. Treat for 7–14 days, at least 2 days after symptoms resolve.	Oral suspension should be swished in the mouth so that one-half of each dose is placed in each side of the mouth. Retain in the mouth as long as possible before swallowing. Avoid eating for 5–10 minutes after using the oral suspension.
Other			
Ciclopirox	Mild to moderate onychomycosis of fingernails and toenails without lunula involvement, due to *Trichophyton rubrum* in immunocompetent patients	*Adults, adolescents, and children >12 yr:* Apply topical nail solution (8% nail lacquer) once daily at bedtime to affected nails.	Apply the nail lacquer over the entire nail and 5 mm surrounding skin, over the previous coat for 7 days before removing with alcohol. Use nail file to trim loose nails as needed every 7 days. May require up to 48 weeks of treatment.
	For seborrheic dermatitis of the scalp	1% shampoo can be used in adults and adolescents ≥16 yr. 0.77% gel can be applied to affected scalp areas twice daily for 4 weeks in adults and adolescents ≥16 yr.	For shampoo, wet hair and apply roughly 1 tsp. (5 mL) to the scalp. Up to 10 mL may be used for long hair. Lather and leave on hair and scalp for 3 minutes. Rinse off. Repeat treatment twice weekly for 4 weeks, with a minimum of 3 days between applications.
	Treatment of tinea corporis, tinea cruris, and tinea pedis due to *Candida albicans*	*Adults, adolescents, and children ≥10 yr:* Apply topical dosage (0.77% cream or lotion; and topical suspension) sparingly to affected skin and surrounding areas twice daily, morning and evening; can be used for 4 weeks.	If there is no improvement after 4 weeks of treatment using shampoo, cream, lotion, or suspension, the diagnosis should be reviewed.
Griseofulvin	Tinea corporis, tinea cruris, tinea capitis, tinea barbae	*Adults:* Ultramicrosize tablets, 300–375 mg orally either once daily or in 2–4 divided doses daily. Microsize tablets, 500 mg orally either once daily or in 2–4 divided doses daily. Duration of therapy is variable and should continue until organism is completely eradicated. *Adolescents and children >2 yr:* Ultramicrosize tablets, 5–15 mg/kg/dose orally once daily (maximum: 750 mg/dose) is recommended by the AAP. Microsize tablets, 10–20 mg/kg/day orally in 2 divided doses (maximum dosage: 1 Gm/day) is recommended by the AAP.	Give tablets with a fatty meal to increase absorption Suggested periods of therapy are 2 to 4 weeks for tinea corporis and 4 to 6 weeks for tinea capitis. May be difficult for children to adhere to the therapy Suggested duration of therapy for tinea pedis 4-8 weeks, for onychomycosis of the fingernails 4 months, for toenails 6 months.

TABLE 47.1	Antifungal Medications—cont'd		
Category/ Medication	Indication	Dosage	Considerations and Monitoring
	For tinea pedis, and onychomycosis	*Adults:* Dosage varies based on formulation. Ultramicrosize tablets, 660–750 mg orally either once daily or in 2–4 divided doses. Microsize tablets, 750–1000 mg orally either once daily or in 2–4 divided doses. *Adolescents and children >2 yr:* dosage varies based on formulation. Ultramicrosize tablets, 5–15 mg/kg/dose orally once daily (maximum: 750 mg/dose) is recommended by the AAP. Microsize tablets, 10–20 mg/kg/day orally in 2 divided doses (maximum dosage: 1 Gm/day) is recommended by the AAP.	

AAP, American Academy of Pediatrics; *HIV,* human immunodeficiency virus; *OTC,* over-the-counter; *VVC,* vulvovaginal candidiasis.

cautiously in patients who are experiencing cardiac, renal, or liver disorder due to risk of adverse effects. In addition, drug interactions are common in patients taking select antifungal medications (Table 47.2). More specific details regarding antifungal medications used for integumentary infections can be found in Chapter 3.

Azoles

Azoles are a class of antifungals that are effective against a wide range of yeasts and molds. They act by blocking the biosynthesis of ergosterol, an essential component of fungal cell membranes. This results in inhibition of cell growth and subsequent cell death. All antifungals interact with P450 enzymes, so it is important to consider the potential of drug interactions. Cardiac dysrhythmias and hepatotoxicity are an adverse effect associated with all azole antifungals. These drugs have the *-azole* suffix, with the exception of isavuconazonium.

Clotrimazole

Pharmacokinetics. Clotrimazole is minimally systemically absorbed. Concentrations of oral clotrimazole in saliva may be due to its binding to the oral mucosa. Fungicidal concentrations of vaginal clotrimazole persist for up to 3 days after application.

Indications. Topical preparations of clotrimazole are used for a variety of fungal infections including those secondary to *Epidermophyton floccosum, Trichophyton mentagrophytes, Trichophyton rubrum, Malassezia furfur,* and *Candida albicans.* Oral troche preparations are used as lozenges for oropharyngeal candidiasis. Vaginal cream can be used for VVC.

Adverse Effects. The most common adverse effect, mild to moderate elevation of liver enzymes, is associated with about 15% of patients taking oral lozenges for oropharyngeal candidiasis. In addition, the lozenges may cause mild nausea and an unpleasant mouth sensation. Topical clotrimazole may cause mild skin irritation. Vaginal products may cause mild vaginal burning and itching; however,

this should not be severe. If severe, the patient should notify their primary care provider.

Contraindications. Clotrimazole should be used with caution in patients with azole antifungal hypersensitivity. If there is no improvement in symptoms following initiation of clotrimazole therapy, instruct the patient to report to the primary care provider.

Monitoring. While laboratory monitoring is typically not necessary, patients with underlying conditions using oral lozenges may require monitoring of liver enzymes. If patients who are using the vaginal products experience abdominal pain, fever, or foul-smelling discharge, they should seek follow-up care with a primary care provider.

Ketoconazole

Pharmacokinetics. Topical forms of ketoconazole are not associated with significant systemic absorption. Oral ketoconazole is dissolved in gastric secretions and rapidly absorbed from the stomach. Food can lead to increased absorption. Once absorbed, it is widely distributed and metabolized, with excretion through the feces (approximately 65%) and the urine.

PHARMACOGENETICS

Ketoconazole

Ketoconazole is a substrate and potent inhibitor of the cytochrome (CYP) 3A4 isoenzyme. It also can inhibit CYP 2C19, P-glycoprotein (P-gp), UGT1A1, and UGT2B7. Oral ketoconazole may cause elevated plasma levels of a variety of medications that may prolong the QT interval. The risk may be greater in older patients.

Indications. Topical forms of ketoconazole, including creams, gels, foam, and shampoo, can be used to treat a variety of mucocutaneous conditions. For example, creams can be used to treat mucocutaneous candidiasis, seborrheic dermatitis, tinea corporis, tinea cruris, tinea pedis, and tinea

TABLE 47.2	Examples of Drug Interactions with Antifungal Agents
Antifungal	**Action on Other Drugs**
Ketoconazole	↑Benzodiazepines, buspirone, carbamazepine, corticosteroids, cyclosporine, donepezil, nisoldipine, protease inhibitors, quinidine, sulfonylureas, tacrolimus, TCAs, warfarin, zolpidem
	↓↑ Oral contraceptives
	↓ Theophylline
Fluconazole	↑ Alfentanil, zolpidem, benzodiazepines, buspirone, corticosteroids, cyclosporine, losartan, nisoldipine, phenytoin, sulfonylureas, tacrolimus, theophylline, tricyclic antidepressants, warfarin, zidovudine
	↓↑ Oral contraceptives
Itraconazole	↑ Alfentanil, benzodiazepines, buspirone, calcium channel blockers, carbamazepine, cisapride, corticosteroids, cyclosporine, digoxin, haloperidol, HMG-CoA reductase inhibitors, hydantoins, oral hypoglycemic agents, pimozide, protease inhibitors, quinidine, rifampin, tacrolimus, tolterodine, warfarin, zolpidem
Terbinafine	↑ Caffeine, dextromethorphan
	↓ Cyclosporine
Griseofulvin	↑ Anticoagulants, oral contraceptives, cyclosporine, salicylates
Drugs	**Action on Antifungals**
Antacids, didanosine, sucralfate, proton pump inhibitors, H$_2$-antagonists, isoniazid, rifampin	↑ Ketoconazole
	↓ Ketoconazole
Hydrochlorothiazide	↑ Fluconazole
Cimetidine, rifampin	↓ Fluconazole
Hydantoins, antacids, proton pump inhibitors, H$_2$-antagonists	↓ Itraconazole
Rifampin	↓ Terbinafine

Note: ↑ means increase serum concentration; ↓ means decreased serum concentration.

versicolor. Ketoconazole shampoo may be used to treat seborrheic dermatitis and tinea versicolor. Due to serious adverse infections, oral forms of ketoconazole are reserved for patients who have serious fungal infections that are not sensitive to other antifungals.

Adverse Effects. Adverse effects are generally rare with topical forms of ketoconazole but can include mild pruritus, skin dryness, and erythema; topical ketoconazole may also be associated with site reactions such as burning and photosensitivity. Oral forms of ketoconazole may cause severe hepatotoxicity and are not recommended unless essential in treatment of systemic fungal infections.

Contraindications. Oral or topical ketoconazole should not be used if the patient has a history of azole antifungal hypersensitivity. Ketoconazole is contraindicated in patients with acute or chronic hepatic disease. Avoid accidental ocular exposure of topical ketoconazole products. Foams or gel formulations of topical ketoconazole products are flammable due to alcohol content. Do not use topical forms on the scalp or on any areas of broken or inflamed skin.

BLACK BOX WARNING!

Ketoconazole

The U.S. Food and Drug Administration (FDA) recommends against using oral ketoconazole to treat skin and nail fungal infections due to risk of hepatic injury and potential for adrenal problems. Topical versions have not been linked to liver damage, adrenal problems, or drug interactions.

Monitoring. Ensure that the patient understands the importance of proper topical administration of these products. For example, to be effective, foam applications must be applied directly to the skin rather than over the hair.

Fluconazole

Pharmacokinetics. Fluconazole is well absorbed orally and does not undergo first-pass metabolism. It is widely distributed into body tissues and fluids. Peak concentrations are typically achieved 1 to 2 hours after oral administration. Fluconazole inhibits the CYP 2C19 enzyme as well as the CYP 2C9 and CYP 3A4. It is primarily eliminated unchanged in the urine.

Indications. Oral fluconazole can be used to treat oropharyngeal, esophageal, and VVC. It can also be used to treat urinary tract infections (UTIs) caused by *Candida sp.*

Adverse Effects. Adverse effects can occur in up to 26% of patients. The most common adverse effect is headache (up to 13%). Other adverse effects include mild to moderate nausea, diarrhea, abdominal pain, dizziness, and skin rash. About 1% of patients experience dysgeusia. Although rare, patients may have elevated liver enzymes with possible symptoms of hepatotoxicity.

Contraindications. Fluconazole should be used cautiously in patients with preexisting hepatic disease due to risk of hepatotoxicity, and dysrhythmias such as torsade de pointes. Fluconazole has been associated with QT prolongation. Dosage adjustment is indicated in patients with renal insufficiency or renal failure. Fluconazole should be avoided during pregnancy except in severe fungal infections when benefits outweigh risks. It should be avoided in those who are breastfeeding.

Monitoring. Due to the risk of hepatotoxicity, monitor liver function studies. Monitor renal function tests and serum potassium. In patients who have cardiac risk and/or take medications that may prolong the QTc, monitor for ECG changes. Discontinue fluconazole if any signs and symptoms of hepatotoxicity develop. Advise patients to use caution when driving, operating machinery, or making major decisions until they are aware of the effects of fluconazole. Fluconazole may be given without regard to meals.

Allylamines

Terbinafine

Pharmacokinetics. Terbinafine can be given orally or topically. Oral forms are well absorbed from the gastrointestinal (GI) tract and are widely distributed, including to the CNS, hair, and nail beds. Terbinafine can be detected within the stratum corneum as soon as 24 hours after therapy, and after 2 weeks of therapy it can remain in the skin for up to 3 months. Metabolism is via the liver by at least seven CYP isoenzymes including CYP 1A2, CYP 2C8, CYP 2C9, CYP 2C19, and CYP 3A. Nearly 80% is excreted unchanged in the urine. Topical forms are not extensively absorbed and do not generally result in drug interactions.

Indications. Terbinafine can be used for the treatment of tinea pedis, cruris, capitus, and corporis. It can also be used to treat tinea versicolor due to *Malassezia furfur*. Oral terbinafine can be used in the treatment of onychomycosis as well as tinea capitis.

Adverse Effects. The most common adverse effects associated with oral terbinafine are mild headache (7% to 12.9% of patients) and sore throat (10%). GI side effects are infrequent and include mild abdominal pain, dyspepsia, nausea, and vomiting. Taste and smell disturbances are rare but may result in loss of appetite and weight loss. Approximately 3% of patients may demonstrate elevated hepatic enzymes with symptoms of hepatotoxicity. Blood dyscrasias including anemia, neutropenia, lymphopenia, thrombocytopenia, agranulocytosis, and pancytopenia have been reported in rare cases. Vision changes may occur in up to 5% of patients. Topical terbinafine may result in skin irritation as well as symptoms of itching, burning, and xerosis.

Contraindications. Terbinafine is contraindicated in patients with hepatitis or hepatic disease. It should be used cautiously in patients who are immunosuppressed or who have any immunodeficiency syndromes. Terbinafine should be used cautiously in patients who are pregnant or breastfeeding. Children may be at risk of anxiety, depression, or an increase in suicidal thoughts while taking oral terbinafine; monitor carefully.

Monitoring. Discontinue terbinafine if the patient reports any disturbances in smell or taste. Monitor complete blood count (CBC) with differentials as well as liver function tests (LFTs) during therapy. Monitor for signs of infection, particularly in patients who are immunosuppressed. Make sure to monitor mental status (including risk for suicide) carefully in children who require oral terbinafine.

Polyenes

Polyenes were the first antifungal drugs used clinically. Polyenes have an affinity for ergosterol, which is found in fungal cell membranes. This results in impaired integrity of the cell membrane with loss of intracellular potassium and other cytoplasmic contents, ultimately resulting in cell death. In addition to nystatin, amphotericin is an example of a polyene; however, it is not typically used in primary care.

Nystatin

Pharmacokinetics. Nystatin administered orally is poorly absorbed from the GI tract and excreted almost entirely unchanged in the feces. Topical forms are not absorbed from intact skin or mucous membranes.

Indications. Nystatin is effective in treating a variety of *Candida* species, including *Candida albicans*. It is available for treating oropharyngeal candidiasis, cutaneous and mucocutaneous candidiasis, and candida diaper dermatitis. Nystatin may also be used in patients with intestinal candidiasis.

Adverse Effects. Nystatin is generally well tolerated. Oral forms may result in mild GI disturbances such as nausea, vomiting, and diarrhea. Topical and vaginal forms may cause some skin irritation. Rarely, patients may have an allergic response to nystatin as well as burning, itching, and rash.

Contraindications. Caution should be used in prescribing oral nystatin to pregnant or breastfeeding patients. Topical nystatin is considered safe during breastfeeding. Nystatin suspension may contain sucrose, so it should be used cautiously in patients with diabetes mellitus.

Monitoring. Laboratory monitoring is not needed in patients taking oral or topical forms of nystatin.

Other

Other commonly used antifungals work through slightly different mechanisms. Ciclopirox inhibits essential enzymes by creating large polyvalent cations through chelation. This results in interference in the mitochondrial electron transport processes and energy production. It has both fungicidal and fungistatic properties. Griseofulvin inhibits fungal cell mitosis and nucleic acid synthesis. In addition, it interferes with the function of spindles and cytoplasmic microtubules by binding to α- and β-tubulin in select fungi. It is fungistatic.

Ciclopirox

Pharmacokinetics. Ciclopirox is available only as a topical agent in lotion, gel, cream, and shampoo forms. In addition, it is available as a nail lacquer to treat onychomycosis. As a topical agent, it is distributed in the stratum corneum, epidermis, hair follicles, sebaceous glands, and dermis. The nail lacquer can penetrate the nail plate. Systemic absorption is minimal.

Indications. Ciclopirox is used to treat mild to moderate onychomycosis of the fingernails or toenails without lunula involvement due to *Trichophyton rubrum*. In addition, ciclopirox can be used for topical treatment of tinea corporis, tinea cruris, and tinea pedis. It can be effective in treating cutaneous candidiasis due to *Candida albicans*. Gel and shampoo formulations can be used to treat seborrheic dermatitis of the scalp.

Adverse Effects. The most common adverse effect is mild erythema. This occurred in nearly half of patients using the nail lacquer form. A small percentage (1% to 2%) of patients using nail lacquer experienced side effects including ingrown toenail and change in nail shape. Other topical forms can cause localized reactions including itching, burning, or rash at the application site. In patients using the shampoo formulation, ciclopirox may cause worsening of seborrhea. Other adverse effects associated with the shampoo are headache and ventricular tachycardia. Hair discoloration (particularly with lighter hair) has been reported, albeit rarely, for patients using ciclopirox shampoo. Eye pain and facial swelling were reported in fewer than 1% of patients receiving the topical gel.

Contraindications. Avoid using ciclopirox in patients with evidence of skin irritation or abrasion. Ciclopirox is not recommended for patients with a history of seizure disorder or any patient who is immunosuppressed (including patients taking any form of corticosteroid). While ciclopirox is classified as pregnancy category B, it should be used only if the benefits to the mother outweigh the risk to the fetus. Breastfeeding while on ciclopirox should be avoided. Safety has not been established in those younger than 10 years of age.

Monitoring. Laboratory monitoring is not required in patients taking ciclopirox.

Griseofulvin

Pharmacokinetics. Griseofulvin is only available in oral forms in two tablet sizes: microsize and ultramicrosize. Both forms are mainly absorbed from the duodenum, although the ultramicrosize form is almost completely absorbed while the microsize form has unpredictable oral absorption. Absorption may be enhanced by taking the medication with a high-fat meal. Peak concentrations are typically obtained within 4 to 8 hours after administration. Griseofulvin may induce the CYP 3A4 isoenzyme.

Indications. Griseofulvin can be used to treat tinea corporis, tinea capitis, and tinea barbae caused by organisms including *Trichophyton sp.*, *Microsporum sp.*, and *Epidermophyton sp.* It can also be used to treat tinea pedis and onychomycosis.

Adverse Effects. Patients may experience headaches early in therapy, which tend to dissipate with time. Griseofulvin has been associated with CNS effects including confusion, dizziness, peripheral neuropathy, and paresthesias of the hands and feet with extended therapy. Patients may experience fatigue and insomnia. Other adverse effects include those affecting the GI system such as nausea, vomiting, and diarrhea as well as hematologic adverse effects such as leukopenia and coagulopathy. Patients may experience skin rash that may become severe. Griseofulvin can be hepatotoxic.

Contraindications. Patients should not take griseofulvin if they are hypersensitive to the drug or its components. Of note, griseofulvin is produced by a species of *Penicillium*. As a result, patients with penicillin hypersensitivity might exhibit a cross-sensitivity to griseofulvin. Although this may be theoretical in nature, caution should be used in patients with penicillin, cephalosporin, or carbapenem hypersensitivity.

Griseofulvin is contraindicated in patients with hepatocellular failure and should be used cautiously in patients with hepatic disease. It may exacerbate symptoms of systemic lupus erythematosus. Griseofulvin is contraindicated in patients with porphyria and in those who are pregnant. There are insufficient data to recommend breastfeeding while taking griseofulvin.

Monitoring. Serious adverse effects are more likely with high doses of griseofulvin and/or in patients taking griseofulvin for extensive periods. Monitor patients for hepatic dysfunction and blood abnormalities. If they occur, consider discontinuing therapy. Renal function studies and CBC should be monitored regularly during long-term use.

Griseofulvin Therapy

Griseofulvin tablets should be taken with a fatty meal to enhance absorption.

Prescriber Considerations for Antifungal Therapy

Clinical Practice Guidelines

The Infectious Diseases Society of America (IDSA) is a resource for current clinical practice guidelines for a variety of fungal infections (see https://www.idsociety.org). Fungal infections are challenging to treat, whether systemic or superficial in nature. Treatment is often lengthy and the risk for toxicity from oral doses is high. It is important to determine the particular infectious agent, treat based on current practice guidelines, and follow up. For superficial fungal infections, length of therapy may be extensive with marginal results and risk of reoccurrence.

BOOKMARK THIS!

Clinical Guidelines for Infectious Diseases

Clinical practice guidelines for a variety of fungal infections can be found at the IDSA's website, https://www.idsociety.org. The IDSA is committed to improving the health of individuals, communities, and society through patient care, education, research, and public health relating to infectious diseases.

Clinical Reasoning for Antifungal Medications

Consider the individual patient's health problem requiring antifungal medications. Have you completed thorough diagnostic testing to ensure the best therapies based on the organism involved? Does the patient require oral or topical therapy? Use the least toxic drug possible for the particular infection. It is clear that these drugs have the potential for serious adverse reactions, and drug interactions are a problem.

Determine the desired therapeutic outcome based on the degree of treatment needed for the patient's health problem. Identify the risk factors for specific endemic infections and provide patients with information to minimize risk. Then, consider risks vs. benefits of eradication of the infection. For example, coccidioidomycosis may not require treatment for the primary infection. If it becomes progressive, patients may require hospital admission for IV antifungal agents, followed by oral therapy for up to 6 months. For patients with compromised immune systems, antifungals may be prescribed indefinitely.

Assess the antifungal medication selected for its appropriateness for an individual patient by considering the medication's side effects and the patient's age, race/ethnicity, comorbidities, and genetic factors. Identify common fungi such as *Histoplasma*, *Blastomyces*, and *Coccidioides* which may affect

the community. For example, if the primary care provider practices in an area where *Histoplasma* is common, any patients who are immunosuppressed should avoid high-risk behaviors such as cleaning or remodeling old buildings or working in areas with bird or bat droppings.

Does the patient have a history of liver disorders which may preclude prescription of the antifungal? What other medications is the patient currently taking for other acute or chronic illnesses? Does the patient require lab work prior to taking the medication or during the therapy?

Initiate the treatment plan with the selected antifungal medication by first providing adequate patient education to ensure the patient's understanding and promote full participation in the antifungal medication therapy. Reinforce the need for adherence to treatment plans, as treatments often take weeks. For example, ciclopirox nail lacquer may require months of treatment to eradicate onychomycosis. Teach patients using antifungal agents for vulvovaginal infections to report to their provider abdominal pain, fever, or the presence of foul-smelling discharge, as these may be signs of more serious infection. Provide patients with information to prevent recurrence of the fungal infection.

Ensure complete patient and family understanding about the antifungal medication prescribed for therapy using a variety of education strategies. Teach patients the proper application of the selected medication. Reinforce the importance of adherence to treatment plans to decrease the risk of recurrence.

Conduct follow-up and monitoring of patient responses to antifungal medication therapy. Follow up with patients to ensure effectiveness of treatment. Due to the risk of hepatotoxicity, monitor liver function studies in patients taking antifungal medications. For patients taking terbinafine or griseofulvin, monitor LFTs and CBC and consider discontinuing the medication as soon as the infection is treated.

Teaching Points for Antifungal Therapy

Health Promotion Strategies

- Perform initial cultures. Assess response to therapy with repeat cultures as necessary.
- Assess for signs or symptoms of hepatitis, such as fatigue, anorexia, nausea, vomiting, jaundice, dark urine, and pale stools.
- Perform LFTs before initiating therapy and periodically thereafter for patients requiring oral antifungal agents. In healthy individuals, testing should be done every 4 to 6 weeks. Patients at risk must be monitored carefully and may require biweekly testing.
- Older adults tend to be susceptible to hepatotoxicity and are likely to be on other medications that may interact with these drugs. Lower dosages of these products are required in patients with reduced renal function.
- Itraconazole oral solution is formulated with hydroxypropyl-β-cyclodextrin, which is eliminated by the kidneys. It should not be used in patients with a creatinine clearance (CrCl) lower than 30 ml/minute.
- Patients with endemic infection should observe the following guidelines:

- Continue taking the medication until the prescription is completed. For some illnesses, therapy may require months of treatment.
- Notify the primary care provider if symptoms worsen or if chest pain, increased dyspnea, headache or stiff neck, or any confusion occurs.
- Teach patients with tinea infections to do the following:
  - Keep nails short.
  - Avoid artificial fingernails.
  - If using nail salons, make sure that the salons practice thorough cleaning between clients.
  - Wash clothing regularly.
  - Avoid touching people who have skin infections.
  - Thoroughly clean and dry skin, particularly in areas with skin folds.
  - Avoid sharing clothing if possible.

Patient Education for Medication Safety

All Antifungals

- Take as prescribed. Inadequate treatment periods may result in a poor response or early recurrence of symptoms.
- Immediately report any signs or symptoms of hepatitis such as fatigue, anorexia, nausea, vomiting, jaundice, dark urine, or pale stools.
- Griseofulvin and ketoconazole may cause photosensitivity.
- During treatment, avoid alcohol consumption and medications that contain acetaminophen.

Azoles

- Do not take ketoconazole or itraconazole within 2 hours of taking antacids.
- Take fluconazole without regard for food or gastric acidity restrictions.
- Females of childbearing age should use contraception or abstain from sexual intercourse while on azole therapy.
- Females using intravaginal clotrimazole should abstain from sexual intercourse during treatment. Intravaginal clotrimazole can damage contraceptive barrier devices leading to device failure.
- If the patient is self-administering clotrimazole, do not use for longer than 7 days. If there is no improvement after 3 days, or if the condition persists after 7 days, discontinue the medication and contact provider.

Griseofulvin

- Bioavailability improves when given with food.
- Headaches, if they occur, usually disappear with continued therapy or when griseofulvin is taken with food.
- Notify provider if skin rash or sore throat appears.
- May potentiate effects of alcohol.

Nystatin

- For nystatin oral solution, swish the solution in the mouth to ensure coverage of all surfaces, then swallow the solution to treat the affected mucosa.
- Carefully measure the prescribed dose with the measuring device included in the packaging. Avoid using household measures.

Application Questions for Discussion

1. A 26-year-old female patient presents with complaints of infected toenails and would like to get rid of the infection because it is unsightly. As you conduct your examination and assessment, you learn that the patient describes herself as a social drinker. How would you proceed?
2. You suspect that your patient is experiencing symptoms associated with Valley fever (coccidioidomycosis). Using the most recent clinical practice guidelines for treating newly diagnosed, uncomplicated coccidioidal pneumonia, discuss how you would proceed in treatment. How would your treatment vary if the patient was immunosuppressed?
3. Describe strategies to enhance adherence to topical antifungal therapy, even when length of therapy may be prolonged without evidence of improvement early in therapy.

Selected Bibliography

Alter, S. J., McDonald, M. B., Schloemer, J., Simon, R., & Trevino, J. (2018). Common child and adolescent cutaneous infestations and fungal infections. *Current Problems in Pediatric and Adolescent Health Care, 48*(1), 3–25. http://doi.org/10.1016/j.cppeds.2017.11.001.

Bongomin, F., Gago, S., Oladele, R. O., & Denning, D. W. (2017). Global and multi-national prevalence of fungal diseases—Estimate precision. *Journal of Fungi (Basel, Switzerland), 3*(4), 57. http://doi.org/10.3390/jof3040057.

Campoy, S., & Adrio, J. L. (2017). Antifungals. *Biochemical Pharmacology, 133*, 86–96. https://doi.org/10.1016/j.bcp.2016.11.019.

Centers for Disease Control and Prevention (2019). *Types of fungal diseases.* Available at https://www.cdc.gov/fungal/diseases/index.html.

Clebak, K. T., & Malone, M. A. (2018). Skin infections. *Primary Care, 45*(3), 433–454. http://doi.org/10.1016/j.pop.2018.05.004.

Elsevier. Clinical pharmacology powered by ClinicalKey®. (2019). Retrieved from http://www.clinicalkey.com.

Ely, J. W., Rosenfeld, S., & Seabury Stone, M. (2014). Diagnosis and management of tinea infections. *American Family Physician, 90*(10), 702–710.

Kaushik, N., Pujalte, G. G. A., & Reese, S. T. (2015). Superficial fungal infections. *Primary Care, 42*(4), 501–516. http://doi.org/10.1016/j.pop.2015.08.004.

Kreijkamp-Kaspers, S., Hawke, K., Guo, L., Kerin, G., Bell-Syer, S. E., Magin, P., & van Driel, M. L. (2017). Oral antifungal medication for toenail onychomycosis. *The Cochrane Database of Systematic Reviews, 7*(7). CD010031–CD010031. http://doi.org/10.1002/14651858.CD010031.pub2.

Pappas, P. G., Kauffman, C. A., Andes, D. R., Clancy, C. J., Marr, K. A., Ostrosky-Zeichner, L., & Sobel, J. D. (2015). Clinical practice guideline for the management of candidiasis: 2016 update by the Infectious Diseases Society of America. *Clinical Infectious Diseases, 62*(4), e1–e50. http://doi.org/10.1093/cid/civ933.

Rosenthal, L. D., & Burchum, J. R. (2018). *Lehne's Pharmacotherapeutics for Advanced Practice Providers.* St. Louis: Elsevier.

Saccente, M., & Woods, G. L. (2010). Clinical and laboratory update on blastomycosis. *Clinical Microbiology Reviews, 23*(2), 367–381. https://doi.org/10.1128/CMR.00056-09.

Woo, T. E., Somayaji, R., Haber, R. M., & Parsons, L. (2019). Diagnosis and management of cutaneous tinea infections. *Advances in Skin & Wound Care, 32*(8), 350–357. http://doi.org/10.1097/01.Asw.0000569128.44287.67.

48

Antiviral and Antiretroviral Medications

TRACEY L. TAYLOR AND TERESA GORE

Overview

The human immunodeficiency virus (HIV) pandemic has claimed millions of lives worldwide. The recommended use of antiretroviral agents in clinical practice will continue to evolve as new information from clinical trials and research becomes available. Infectious disease specialists generally provide treatment for patients with HIV infection because of the difficulty involved in keeping current with the latest treatment protocols, and primary care providers generally are concerned with preventing transmission of the virus. Nonetheless, primary care providers must have knowledge of current medication therapies and their side effects because HIV-infected patients rely on them to help evaluate their complaints and, for some, to provide treatment to a limited extent. This chapter will discuss medications most commonly used in the antiretroviral treatment of HIV/AIDS.

Relevant Physiology

HIV is a retrovirus from the family of viruses referred to as *lentiviruses*. Retroviruses are viruses that replicate through the reverse transcriptase enzyme, which allows the virus to incorporate its genome into that of certain host cells. This key enzyme transcripts the ribonucleic acid (RNA) into double-stranded deoxyribonucleic acid (DNA), resulting in insertion of the viruses' genomes into CD4 receptor–containing cells. The primary CD4 receptor–containing cells are tissue-based macrophages and helper T-cells. Three primary categories of human retroviruses have been identified: T-cell leukemia retroviruses, endogenous viruses, and human immunodeficiency viruses (HIV-1 and HIV-2). This chapter discusses only HIV-1 in detail.

The HIV virus attaches to the CD4 protein with the help of coreceptors (CXCR4 or CCR5) found on T-helper lymphocytes and other cells such as macrophages and dendritic cells. The HIV virus then fuses its membrane with that of the host cell and inserts its genetic material into the cytoplasm. The viral genetic material then is transcribed into double-stranded DNA called *proviral DNA* (Fig. 48.1). The

HIV enzyme, reverse transcriptase, is responsible for creating double-stranded DNA from viral RNA. Once produced, this DNA often becomes integrated into the chromosomal DNA of the host cell. The HIV DNA is expressed by the host cell's genetic machinery, which creates new HIV RNA genetic material and messenger RNA. The messenger RNA codes for the development of HIV polyproteins must be cleaved, or separated, into individual proteins by the HIV enzyme protease if infectious virions are to be produced. Once this occurs, new virions are assembled and bud from the host cells' membrane, and then they continue to infect new cells.

According to HIV.gov, one in seven people in the United States is living with HIV and is unaware of their infection. The incidence rate has declined by more than two-thirds since the epidemic of the mid–1980s, and has remained stable from 2014 to 2018 at 13.3 infections per 100,000 people. HIV is not evenly distributed in the United States: the highest rate of new diagnosis continues to occur in the South, and there is a higher occurrence among Blacks/African Americans, in males than in females, and in male-to-male sexual contact. The incidence rate among those 25 to 34 years of age has remained stable, and it has decreased for all other age groups. Current strategies for testing at early ages and treating patients as soon as possible have shown to be effective overall for decreasing the number of new cases.

Pathophysiology: HIV

The defining stages of HIV infection through progression to AIDS have changed over the years as medication treatments have become extremely effective in preventing the opportunistic infections that once led to severe debilitation and death. Generally, the disease starts with a primary infection (primary phase) and then progresses to early, middle, and advanced or late-stage HIV infection or AIDS (advanced or late phase).

The primary phase includes initial acute infection that almost always presents with a mild to moderate viral syndrome which often mimics conditions such as infectious mononucleosis. This stage includes the development of

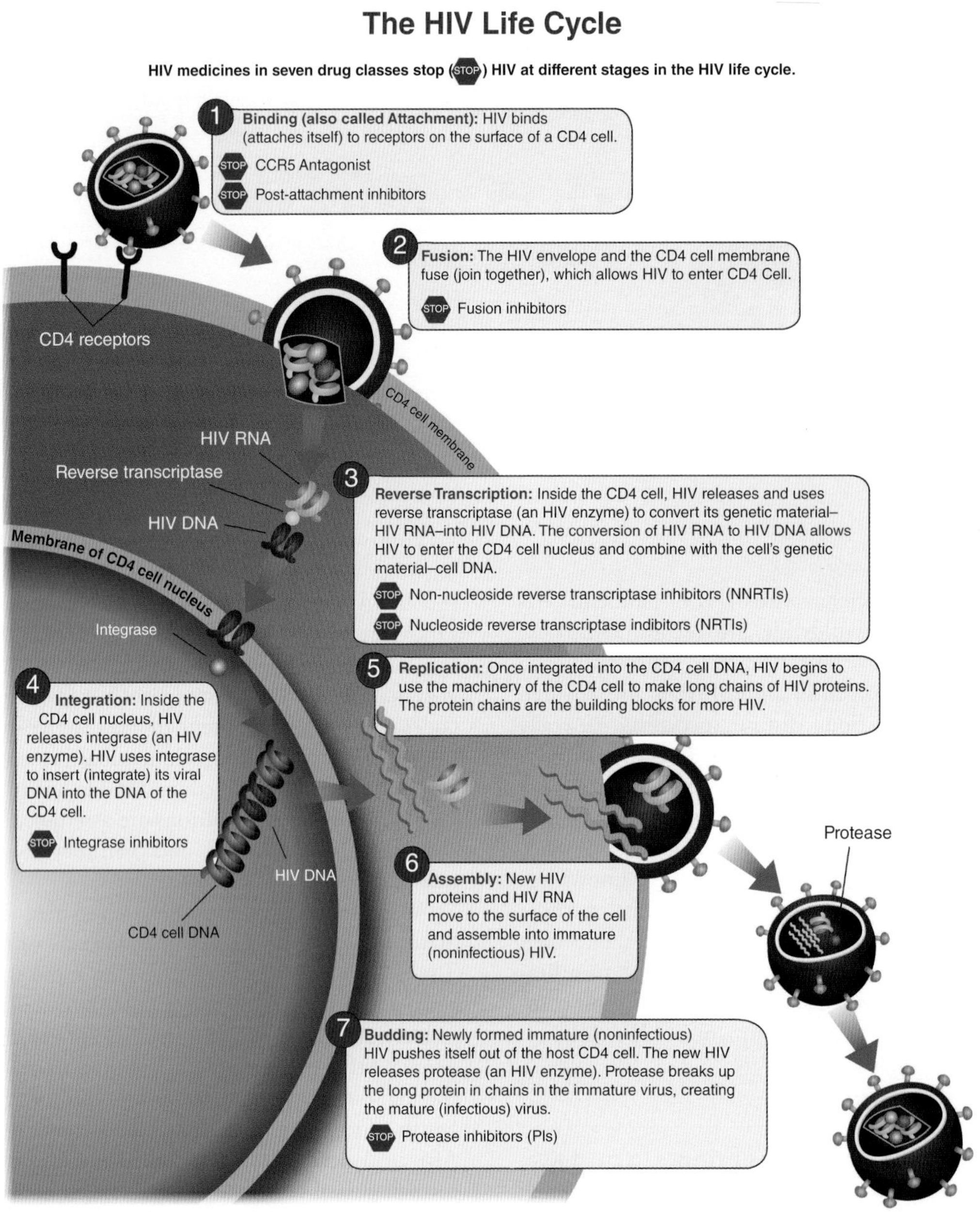

The HIV Life Cycle

HIV medicines in seven drug classes stop (STOP) HIV at different stages in the HIV life cycle.

1 **Binding (also called Attachment):** HIV binds (attaches itself) to receptors on the surface of a CD4 cell.
STOP CCR5 Antagonist
STOP Post-attachment inhibitors

2 **Fusion:** The HIV envelope and the CD4 cell membrane fuse (join together), which allows HIV to enter CD4 Cell.
STOP Fusion inhibitors

CD4 receptors
CD4 cell membrane

HIV RNA
Reverse transcriptase
HIV DNA
Membrane of CD4 cell nucleus

3 **Reverse Transcription:** Inside the CD4 cell, HIV releases and uses reverse transcriptase (an HIV enzyme) to convert its genetic material–HIV RNA–into HIV DNA. The conversion of HIV RNA to HIV DNA allows HIV to enter the CD4 cell nucleus and combine with the cell's genetic material–cell DNA.
STOP Non-nucleoside reverse transcriptase inhibitors (NNRTIs)
STOP Nucleoside reverse transcriptase indibitors (NRTIs)

Integrase

4 **Integration:** Inside the CD4 cell nucleus, HIV releases integrase (an HIV enzyme). HIV uses integrase to insert (integrate) its viral DNA into the DNA of the CD4 cell.
STOP Integrase inhibitors

5 **Replication:** Once integrated into the CD4 cell DNA, HIV begins to use the machinery of the CD4 cell to make long chains of HIV proteins. The protein chains are the building blocks for more HIV.

Protease

HIV DNA

6 **Assembly:** New HIV proteins and HIV RNA move to the surface of the cell and assemble into immature (noninfectious) HIV.

CD4 cell DNA

7 **Budding:** Newly formed immature (noninfectious) HIV pushes itself out of the host CD4 cell. The new HIV releases protease (an HIV enzyme). Protease breaks up the long protein in chains in the immature virus, creating the mature (infectious) virus.
STOP Protease inhibitors (PIs)

• **Fig. 48.1** HIV life cycle. (From HIV Life Cycle. [2021]. Retrieved October 27, 2021, from https://hivinfo.nih.gov/understanding-hiv/infographics/hiv-life-cycle.)

antibodies and the stabilization of viral load levels. This is when the patient is most infectious. Early and middle stages of HIV infection can be asymptomatic and represent the time when the virus entrenches itself into the architecture of the host's immune system. The virus during this time destroys normal lymphoid architecture and creates reservoirs that are difficult to eradicate despite the best medication treatments. CD4 and CD8 cells undergo immunologic changes that render them useless in effectively killing and/or controlling HIV infection, leading to rapid HIV replication and mutation. It is during this stage that CD4 counts decrease dangerously to 200 to 300 cells/mm^3.

The advanced or late phase of HIV infection is characterized by a continued decrease in CD4 counts, with drops to 50 cells/mm^3. The patient experiences neurologic changes that are heralded by dementia, peripheral neuropathy, and myelopathy. Further immune system collapse occurs with the onset of opportunistic infections such as pneumocystis jiroveci pneumonia, toxoplasmosis, mycobacterium avium complex, and multiple viral primary or reactivated infections such as herpes simplex or varicella zoster. Chronic illness leads to constitutional disease with muscle wasting, weight loss, fevers, and severe fatigue. Malignancy with Kaposi's sarcoma is also seen. The compilation of AIDS and the sequelae of opportunistic infections finally result in death.

Antiretroviral Medication Classifications

Genotypic or phenotypic testing is available as an in vitro tool to examine resistance of HIV to antiretroviral agents. Genotypic assays detect drug resistance mutations that are present in reverse transcriptase, protease, and integrase genes. Phenotypic assays measure the ability of the virus to replicate within concentrations of the antiretrovirals. These assays facilitate selection of antiretroviral agents when medication regimens are changed. It is best to consult with an expert who can assist with interpretation of these results.

New guidelines reflect patients with HIV gain more benefit from early diagnosis and immediate treatment. Key benefits of early treatment are an increase in the uptake of antiretroviral therapy (ART) and a decrease in the time required to achieve linkage to care and virologic suppression

for patients. Early treatment results in a reduced risk of HIV transmission and an improved rate of virologic suppression among persons with HIV. Initial ART should begin as soon as possible for most people with HIV.

Currently seven classes of HIV antiretroviral agents have been approved by the U.S. Food and Drug Administration (FDA): nucleoside analog reverse transcriptase inhibitors (NRTIs); non-nucleoside reverse transcriptase inhibitors (NNRTIs); protease inhibitors (PIs); fusion (or entry) inhibitors; integrase inhibitors (or integrase strand transfer inhibitors); CCR5 antagonists; and CD4 and post-attachment inhibitors. Pharmacokinetic enhancers and combination medications are also available. Potent combination therapy has become a worldwide standard of care; morbidity and mortality in the developed world have been substantially reduced where major antiretroviral regimens have been initiated. Balanced against this progress is the identification of a surprising number of major toxic effects, and recognition of medication class cross-resistance and restrictions placed on alternate treatment regimens in the setting of treatment failure. Table 48.1 lists the HIV antiretroviral medications currently approved by the FDA.

TABLE 48.1 FDA-Approved HIV Medicines

Drug Class	Generic Name (Other Names and Acronyms)	Brand Name	FDA Approval Date
Nucleoside Analog Reverse Transcriptase Inhibitors (NRTIs)			
NRTIs block reverse transcriptase, an enzyme that HIV needs to make copies of itself.	Abacavir (abacavir sulfate, ABC)	Ziagen	December 17, 1998
	Emtricitabine (FTC)	Emtriva	July 2, 2003
	Lamivudine (3TC)	Epivir	November 17, 1995
	Tenofovir disoproxil fumarate (tenofovir DF, TDF)	Viread	October 26, 2001
	Zidovudine (azidothymidine, AZT, ZDV)	Retrovir	March 19, 1987
Non-Nucleoside Reverse Transcriptase Inhibitors (NNRTIs)			
NNRTIs bind to and later alter reverse transcriptase, an enzyme that HIV needs to make copies of itself.	Doravirine (DOR)	Pifeltro	August 30, 2018
	Efavirenz (EFV)	Sustiva	September 17, 1998
	Etravirine (ETR)	Intelence	January 18, 2008
	Nevirapine (extended-release nevirapine, NVP)	Viramune	June 21, 1996
		Viramune XR (extended release)	March 25, 2011
	Rilpivirine (rilpivirine hydrochloride, RPV)	Edurant	May 20, 2011

Continued

TABLE 48.1	FDA-Approved HIV Medicines—cont'd		
Drug Class	**Generic Name (Other Names and Acronyms)**	**Brand Name**	**FDA Approval Date**
Protease Inhibitors (PIs)			
PIs block HIV protease, an enzyme that HIV needs to make copies of itself.	Atazanavir (atazanavir sulfate, ATV)	Reyataz	June 20, 2003
	Darunavir (darunavir ethanolate, DRV)	Prezista	June 23, 2006
	Fosamprenavir (fosamprenavir calcium, FOS-APV, FPV)	Lexiva	October 20, 2003
	Ritonavir[a] (RTV)	Norvir	March 1, 1996
	Saquinavir (saquinavir mesylate, SQV)	Invirase	December 6, 1995
	Tipranavir (TPV)	Aptivus	June 22, 2005
Fusion Inhibitors			
Fusion inhibitors block HIV from entering the CD4 T lymphocyte (CD4) cells of the immune system.	Enfuvirtide (T-20)	Fuzeon	March 13, 2003
CCR5 Antagonists			
CCR5 antagonists block CCR5 coreceptors on the surface of certain immune cells that HIV needs to enter the cells.	Maraviroc (MVC)	Selzentry	August 6, 2007
Integrase Strand Transfer Inhibitors (INSTIs)			
Integrase inhibitors block HIV integrase, an enzyme that HIV needs to make copies of itself.	Cabotegravir (cabotegravir sodium, CAB)	Vocabria	January 22, 2021
	Dolutegravir (dolutegravir sodium, DTG)	Tivicay	August 13, 2013
	Raltegravir (raltegravir potassium, RAL)	Isentress	October 12, 2007
		Isentress HD	May 26, 2017
Attachment Inhibitors			
Attachment inhibitors bind to the gp120 protein on the outer surface of HIV, preventing HIV from entering CD4 cells.	Fostemsavir (fostemsavir tromethamine, FTR)	Rukobia	July 2, 2020
Post-Attachment Inhibitors			
Post-attachment inhibitors block CD4 receptors on the surface of certain immune cells that HIV needs to enter the cells.	Ibalizumab-uiyk (Hu5A8, IBA, Ibalizumab, TMB-355, TNX-355)	Trogarzo	March 6, 2018
Pharmacokinetic Enhancers			
Pharmacokinetic enhancers are used in HIV treatment to increase the effectiveness of an HIV medicine included in an HIV treatment regimen.	Cobicistat (COBI, c)	Tybost	September 24, 2014

TABLE 48.1 FDA-Approved HIV Medicines—cont'd

Drug Class	Generic Name (Other Names and Acronyms)	Brand Name	FDA Approval Date
Combination HIV Medicines			
Combination HIV medicines contain two or more HIV medicines from one or more drug classes.	Abacavir and lamivudine (abacavir sulfate/lamivudine, ABC/3TC)	Epzicom	August 2, 2004
	Abacavir, dolutegravir, and lamivudine (abacavir sulfate/dolutegravir sodium/lamivudine, ABC/DTG/3TC)	Triumeq	August 22, 2014
	Abacavir, lamivudine, and zidovudine (abacavir sulfate/lamivudine/zidovudine, ABC/3TC/ZDV)	Trizivir	November 14, 2000
	Atazanavir and cobicistat (atazanavir sulfate/cobicistat, ATV/COBI)	Evotaz	January 29, 2015
	Bictegravir, emtricitabine, and tenofovir alafenamide (bictegravir sodium/emtricitabine/tenofovir alafenamide fumarate, BIC/FTC/TAF)	Biktarvy	February 7, 2018
	Cabotegravir and rilpivirine (CAB and RPV, CAB plus RPV, Cabenuva kit, cabotegravir extended-release injectable suspension and rilpivirine extended-release injectable suspension)	Cabenuva	January 22, 2021
	Darunavir and cobicistat (darunavir ethanolate/cobicistat, DRV/COBI)	Prezcobix	January 29, 2015
	Darunavir, cobicistat, emtricitabine, and tenofovir alafenamide (darunavir ethanolate/cobicistat/emtricitabine/tenofovir AF, darunavir ethanolate/cobicistat/emtricitabine/tenofovir alafenamide, darunavir/cobicistat/emtricitabine/tenofovir AF, darunavir/cobicistat/emtricitabine/tenofovir alafenamide fumarate, DRV/COBI/FTC/TAF)	Symtuza	July 17, 2018
	Dolutegravir and lamivudine (dolutegravir sodium/lamivudine, DTG/3TC)	Dovato	April 8, 2019
	Dolutegravir and rilpivirine (dolutegravir sodium/rilpivirine hydrochloride, DTG/RPV)	Juluca	November 21, 2017
	Doravirine, lamivudine, and tenofovir disoproxil fumarate (doravirine/lamivudine/TDF, doravirine/lamivudine/tenofovir DF, DOR/3TC/TDF)	Delstrigo	August 30, 2018

Continued

TABLE 48.1	FDA-Approved HIV Medicines—cont'd		
Drug Class	**Generic Name (Other Names and Acronyms)**	**Brand Name**	**FDA Approval Date**
	Efavirenz, emtricitabine, and tenofovir disoproxil fumarate (efavirenz/emtricitabine/tenofovir DF, EFV/FTC/TDF)	Atripla	July 12, 2006
	Efavirenz, lamivudine, and tenofovir disoproxil fumarate (EFV/3TC/TDF)	Symfi	March 22, 2018
	Efavirenz, lamivudine, and tenofovir disoproxil fumarate (EFV/3TC/TDF)	Symfi Lo	February 5, 2018
	Elvitegravir, cobicistat, emtricitabine, and tenofovir alafenamide (elvitegravir/cobicistat/emtricitabine/ tenofovir alafenamide fumarate, EVG/COBI/FTC/TAF)	Genvoya	November 5, 2015
	Elvitegravir, cobicistat, emtricitabine, and tenofovir disoproxil fumarate (QUAD, EVG/COBI/FTC/TDF)	Stribild	August 27, 2012
	Emtricitabine, rilpivirine, and tenofovir alafenamide (emtricitabine/rilpivirine/tenofovir AF, emtricitabine/rilpivirine/tenofovir alafenamide fumarate, emtricitabine/rilpivirine hydrochloride/ tenofovir AF, emtricitabine/ rilpivirine hydrochloride/tenofovir alafenamide, emtricitabine/ rilpivirine hydrochloride/tenofovir alafenamide fumarate, FTC/RPV/ TAF)	Odefsey	March 1, 2016
	Emtricitabine, rilpivirine, and tenofovir disoproxil fumarate (emtricitabine/rilpivirine hydrochloride/tenofovir disoproxil fumarate, emtricitabine/rilpivirine/ tenofovir, FTC/RPV/TDF)	Complera	August 10, 2011
	Emtricitabine and tenofovir alafenamide (emtricitabine/tenofovir AF, emtricitabine/tenofovir alafenamide fumarate, FTC/TAF)	Descovy	April 4, 2016
	Emtricitabine and tenofovir disoproxil fumarate (emtricitabine/tenofovir DF, FTC/TDF)	Truvada	August 2, 2004
	Lamivudine and tenofovir disoproxil fumarate (Temixys, 3TC/TDF)	Cimduo	February 28, 2018
	Lamivudine and zidovudine (3TC/ZDV)	Combivir	September 27, 1997
	Lopinavir and ritonavir (ritonavir-boosted lopinavir, LPV/r, LPV/RTV)	Kaletra	September 15, 2000

^aAlthough ritonavir is a PI, it is generally used as a pharmacokinetic enhancer as recommended in the Guidelines for the Use of Antiretroviral Agents in Adults and Adolescents Living with HIV and the Guidelines for the Use of Antiretroviral Agents in Pediatric HIV Infection
From National Institutes of Health. (2021). *FDA-approved HIV medicines.* https://aidsinfo.nih.gov/understanding-hiv-aids/fact-sheets/21/58/fda-approved-hiv-medicines.

Nucleoside Reverse Transcriptase Inhibitors (NRTIs)

NRTIs were the first medication class approved for the treatment of HIV infections (Table 48.2). These are the least potent of the antiretroviral medication classes. NRTIs remain the current standard of care and are effective in the treatment of HIV-1 and HIV-2.

NRTIs interrupt the HIV replication cycle via competitive inhibition of HIV reverse transcriptase and termination of the DNA chain. Reverse transcriptase is an HIV-specific DNA polymerase that allows HIV RNA to be transcribed into single-strand, and ultimately double-strand, proviral DNA and incorporated into the host-cell genome. Proviral DNA chain elongation is necessary before genome incorporation can occur and is accomplished by the addition of purine and pyrimidine nucleosides to the 3′ end of the growing chain. NRTIs are structurally like the DNA nucleoside bases and become incorporated into the proviral DNA chain, resulting in termination of proviral DNA formation.

Abacavir (ABC)

Abacavir (ABC) is a nucleoside analogue human immunodeficiency virus (HIV-1) reverse transcriptase inhibitor. NRTIs interrupt the HIV replication cycle via competitive inhibition of HIV reverse transcriptase and termination of the DNA chain. Reverse transcriptase is an HIV-specific DNA polymerase that allows HIV RNA to be transcribed into single-strand, and

ultimately, double-strand proviral DNA and incorporated into the host-cell genome. Proviral DNA chain elongation is necessary before genome incorporation can occur and is accomplished by the addition of purine and pyrimidine nucleosides to the 3′ end of the growing chain. NRTIs are structurally like the DNA nucleoside bases and become incorporated into the proviral DNA chain, resulting in termination of proviral DNA formation. NRTIs are indicated for patients alone, or in combination with other antiretroviral agents for the treatment of HIV-1 infection in negative HLA-B*5701 allele patients. Abacavir works by decreasing the amount of HIV in the blood. It is not a cure. However, it will decrease the patient's likelihood of developing AIDS and HIV-related illnesses.

Pharmacokinetics. Abacavir is well absorbed and is unaffected by food; plasma half-life is 1.5 hours. It is metabolized by alcohol dehydrogenase and glucuronosyltransferase to inactive metabolites that are eliminated in the urine.

PHARMACOGENETICS

Abacavir Therapy

- Due to potential mitochondrial dysfunction and oxidative stress, NRTIs can uncover predisposed genetic susceptibility to a toxicity phenotype.
- Positive HLB-B*5701 allele patients have a high risk of developing hypersensitivity reaction. Treatment with abacavir is not recommended for these individuals.

PRACTICE PEARLS

Life Span Considerations With NRTIs

Children and Adolescents

- Diagnosis and early treatment are more effective for decreasing HIV-associated illnesses and AIDS. The new guidelines recommend rapid initiation of ART within days of diagnosis with HIV, and no longer recommend initiating ART based on a child's age.
- The guidelines acknowledge the need to postpone initiating therapy based on a patient's clinical or psychosocial factors.

Pregnancy

- Guidelines for individuals of childbearing potential have been updated with revised recommendations on the use of dolutegravir sodium.
- NRTIs are pregnancy category C, meaning risks cannot be ruled out. Limited data are available regarding the safety of administration during pregnancy.
- Pregnancy changes the role of the single nucleotide polymorphisms (SNPs) of ABCC2 and ABCC4 transporters on emtricitabine during pregnancy. Emtricitabine concentration in patients with a specific TT genotype is one- to twofold higher.
- Encourage applicable patients to register by calling the Antiretroviral Pregnancy Registry (APR) at 1-800-258-4263.

Breastfeeding

- ARTs are present in breast milk. Breastfeeding should be avoided while on ARTs due to potential complications.

Older Adult and Geriatric Considerations

- NRTIs are associated with peripheral neuropathy, typically symmetric, distal sensory polyneuropathy. Neuropathy is characterized by painful dysesthesia and/or sensory loss. The range of symptomatic neuropathy is 10% to 25% after 1 year of treatment and increases to more than 50% after 2 years of more neurotoxic NRTIs. The highest incidence of peripheral neuropathy from NRTIs occurs in females, older adults, and those with increased HIV RNA loads.
- Caution should be exercised in the administration of lamivudine in older adults, reflecting the greater frequency of decreased hepatic, renal, or cardiac function and concomitant disease and/or another drug therapy.
- Guidelines have been updated with recommendations for HIV and the older person.
- HIV disease progression is impacted by age and comorbidities.
- The primary care provider must be cognizant of the complexities of management of older persons with HIV due to polypharmacy and the potential for drug–drug interactions.
- New recommendations emphasize the importance of HIV-associated neurocognitive disorder (HAND) recognition and management. HAND can cause poor medication adherence, leading to poor patient outcomes. The older patient will need to be screened for depression, along with management of depression, for better outcomes.

TABLE 48.2 **Characteristics of Nucleoside Reverse Transcriptase Inhibitors**

Generic Name (Abbreviation) Trade Name	Formulations	Dosing Recommendations[a]	Elimination/Metabolic Pathway	Serum/Intracellular Half-Lives	Adverse Events[b]
Abacavir (ABC) Ziagen **NOTE:** Generic tablet formulation is available.	**Ziagen:** • 300-mg tablet • 20-mg/mL oral solution **Generic:** • 300-mg tablet • Also available as FDC with 3TC and ZDV/3TC **FDC Tablets That Contain ABC:[c]** • Epzicom (ABC/3TC) **STRs That Contain ABC:[d]** • Triumeq (DTG/ABC/3TC)	**Ziagen:** • ABC 600 mg orally once daily, or • ABC 300 mg orally twice daily	Metabolized by alcohol dehydrogenase and glucuronyl transferase 82% of ABC dose is excreted in the urine as metabolites of ABC. Dose adjustment is recommended in patients with hepatic insufficiency (see Appendix B, Table 11).	1.5 hr/12–26 hr	Patients who test positive for HLA-B*5701 are at the highest risk of experiencing HSRs. HLA screening should be done before initiating ABC. For patients with a history of HSRs, rechallenge is not recommended. Symptoms of HSRs may include fever, rash, nausea, vomiting, diarrhea, abdominal pain, malaise, fatigue, or respiratory symptoms (e.g., sore throat, cough, or shortness of breath). Some cohort studies suggest an increased risk of MI with recent or current use of ABC, but this risk is not substantiated in other studies.
Emtricitabine (FTC) Emtriva	**Emtriva:** • 200-mg hard gelatin capsule • 10-mg/mL oral solution **FDC Tablets That Contain FTC:[c]** • Descovy (TAF/FTC) • Truvada (TDF/FTC) **STRs That Contain FTC:[d]** • Atripla (EFV/TDF/FTC) • Biktarvy (BIC/TAF/FTC) • Complera (RPV/TDF/FTC) • Genvoya (EVG/c/TAF/FTC) • Odefsey (RPV/TAF/FTC) • Stribild (EVG/c/TDF/FTC) • Symtuza (DRV/c/TAF/FTC)	**Emtriva:** *Capsule:* • FTC 200 mg orally once daily *Oral Solution:* • FTC 240 mg (24 mL) orally once daily See Appendix B, Tables 1 and 2, for dosing information for FDC tablets that contain FTC.	86% of FTC dose is excreted renally. See Appendix B, Table 11, for dosing recommendations in patients with renal insufficiency.	10 hr/>20 hr	Minimal toxicity. Hyperpigmentation/skin discoloration. Severe acute exacerbation of hepatitis may occur in patients with HBV/HIV coinfection who discontinue FTC.

Lamivudine (3TC) Epivir **NOTE:** Generic products are available.	**Epivir:** • 150- and 300-mg tablets • 10-mg/mL oral solution **Generic:** • 150- and 300-mg tablets • Also available as FDC with ABC and ZDV **FDC Tablets That Contain 3TC:**[c] • Cimduo (TDF/3TC) • Epzicom (ABC/3TC) • Temixys (TDF/3TC) **STRs That Contain 3TC:**[d] • Delstrigo (DOR/TDF/3TC) • Dovato (DTG/3TC) • Symfi (EFV 600 mg/TDF/3TC) • Symfi Lo (EFV 400 mg/ TDF/3TC) • Triumeq (DTG/ABC/3TC)	**Epivir:** • 3TC 300 mg orally once daily, or • 3TC 150 mg orally twice daily See Appendix B, Tables 1 and 2, for dosing information for FDC tablets that contain 3TC.	5–7 hr/18–22 hr	Minimal toxicity. Severe acute exacerbation of hepatitis may occur in patients with HBV/HIV coinfection who discontinue 3TC.
		70% of 3TC dose is excreted renally. See Appendix B, Table 11, for dose recommendations in patients with renal insufficiency.		
Tenofovir Alafenamide (TAF) Vemlidy **NOTE:** Vemlidy is available as a 25-mg tablet for the treatment of HBV.	**FDC Tablets That Contain TAF:**[c] • Descovy (TAF/FTC) **STRs That Contain TAF:**[d] • Biktarvy (BIC/TAF/FTC) • Genvoya (EVG/c/TAF/FTC) • Odefsey (RPV/TAF/FTC) • Symtuza (DRV/c/TAF/FTC)	See Appendix B, Tables 1 and 2, for dosing information for FDC tablets that contain TAF.	0.5 hr/150–180 hr	Renal insufficiency, Fanconi syndrome, and proximal renal tubulopathy are less likely to occur with TAF than with TDF. Osteomalacia and decreases in BMD are less likely to occur with TAF than with TDF. Severe acute exacerbation of hepatitis may occur in patients with HBV/HIV coinfection who discontinue TAF. Diarrhea, nausea, headache. Greater weight increase has been reported with TAF than with TDF.
		Metabolized by cathepsin A. See Appendix B, Table 11, for dosing recommendations in patients with renal insufficiency.		

Continued

TABLE 48.2 Characteristics of Nucleoside Reverse Transcriptase Inhibitors—cont'd

Generic Name (Abbreviation) Trade Name	Formulations	Dosing Recommendations[a]	Elimination/Metabolic Pathway	Serum/Intracellular Half-Lives	Adverse Events[b]
Tenofovir diso-proxil fumarate (TDF) Viread **NOTE:** Generic product is available.	**Viread:** • 150-, 200-, 250-, and 300-mg tablets • 40-mg/Gm oral powder **Generic:** • 300-mg tablet **FDC Tablets That Contain TDF:[c]** • Cimduo (TDF/3TC) • Temixys (TDF/3TC) • Truvada (TDF/FTC) **STRs That Contain TDF:[d]** • Atripla (EFV/TDF/FTC) • Complera (RPV/TDF/FTC) • Delstrigo (DOR/TDF/3TC) • Stribild (EVG/c/TDF/FTC) • Symfi (EFV 600 mg/TDF/3TC) • Symfi Lo (EFV 400 mg/TDF/3TC)	**Viread:** • TDF 300 mg orally once daily, or • 7.5 level scoops of oral powder orally once daily (dosing scoop dispensed with each bottle; 1 level scoop contains 1 Gm of oral powder). • Mix oral powder with 2–4 ounces of a soft food that does not require chewing (e.g., applesauce, yogurt). Do not mix oral powder with liquid. See Appendix B, Tables 1 and 2, for dosing information for FDC tablets that contain TDF.	Renal excretion is the primary route of elimi-nation. See Appendix B, Table 11, for dose recommendations in patients with renal insufficiency.	17 hr/>60 hr	Renal insufficiency, Fanconi syndrome, proximal renal tubulopathy. Osteomalacia, decrease in BMD. Severe acute exacerbation of hepatitis may occur in patients with HBV/HIV coinfection who discontinue TDF. Asthenia, headache, diarrhea, nausea, vomiting, flatulence.

NOTE: See original source for Appendix B.

[a]For dose adjustments in patients with renal or hepatic insufficiency, see Appendix B, Table 11. When no food restriction is listed, the ARV drug can be taken with or without food.

[b]Also see Table 17.

[c]See Appendix B, Table 2, for information about these formulations.

[d]See Appendix B, Table 1, for information about these formulations.

3TC, Lamivudine; *ABC,* abacavir; *BIC,* bictegravir; *BMD,* bone mineral density; *DOR,* doravirine; *DRV/c,* darunavir/cobicistat; *DTG,* dolutegravir; *EVG/c,* elvitegravir/cobicistat; *EFV,* efavirenz; *FDC,* fixed-dose combination; *FTC,* emtricitabine; *HBV,* hepatitis B virus; *HLA,* human leukocyte antigen; *HSR,* hypersensitivity reaction; *MI,* myocardial infarction; *RPV,* rilpivirine; *STR,* single-tablet regimen; *TAF* tenofovir alafenamide; *TDF,* tenofovir disoproxil fumarate.

From National Institutes of Health (NIH). (2021). *Characteristics of nucleoside reverse transcriptase inhibitors.* Retrieved October 27, 2021, from https://clinicalinfo.hiv.gov/en/table/appendix-b-table-3-characteristics-nucleoside-reverse-transcriptase-inhibitors.

Indications. Abacavir is used with negative HLA-B*5701 allele HIV patients. It is recommended in combination with other antiretroviral medications.

Adverse Effects. The most common adverse effects (more than 10% of patients) are headache, malaise/fatigue, and nausea/vomiting. Less common side effects (10%) are depression, anxiety, hypersensitivity, diarrhea, muscle pain, hypertriglyceridemia, fever/chills, viral upper respiratory infections, rash, and thrombocytopenia.

Some serious side effects which can occur in less than 1% of patients are Stevens-Johnson syndrome, pancreatitis, hepatic diseases, lactic acidosis, irregular heartbeat, renal disease, and anaphylactoid reaction.

There are 41 medications that have known medication interactions with abacavir: five with major interactions, 28 with moderate interactions, and seven with minor interactions. A full list and details of interactions are available at https://www.drugs.com/drug-interactions/abacavir.html.

There are two disease interactions with abacavir: hepatotoxicity and cardiovascular disease (major interaction) and ethanol (minor interaction).

Contraindications. Abacavir is contraindicated in patients with prior hypersensitivity or allergic reaction to abacavir, in HLA-B*5701-positive patients, and in those with moderate to severe hepatic impairment. It is contraindicated if the patient is taking elvitegravir/cobicistat/emtricitabine/tenofovir disoproxil fumarate.

Monitoring. The primary care provider should monitor closely for potential medication or organ dysfunction interactions for patients receiving abacavir. Monitor liver and renal functions for impairment. Always monitor for over-the-counter (OTC) medications and herbal supplements for potential interactions.

Emtricitabine

Emtricitabine is an NRTI and a cytosine analog phosphorylated to emtricitabine 5′-triphosphate, causing inhibition of HIV- and RNA-dependent DNA polymerase.

Pharmacokinetics. Emtricitabine's oral bioavailability exceeds 93% and is not food dependent. The plasma elimination half-life is 10 hours and the intracellular half-life is more than 24 hours. The majority of emtricitabine is eliminated unchanged in the urine. The dose should be reduced in patients with renal insufficiency.

Indications. For HIV-1 infection, emtricitabine is given alone or in combination with other medications as a component of combination therapy. It is recommended in combination with other antiretroviral medications.

Adverse Effects. Emtricitabine has several adverse effects, and they increase in occurrence and severity when used in conjunction with combination therapies. The most common adverse effects (more than 10% of patients) include diarrhea, dizziness, headache, insomnia, rash, asthenia, nausea, rhinitis, abdominal pain, abnormal dreams, increased creatinine kinase (CK), increased cough, neuritis, and paresthesia. Less common adverse effects (less than 10%) include depression, dyspepsia, vomiting, increased triglycerides, and myalgia. Severe adverse effects (less than 1%) include moderate to severe lactic acidosis.

There are 34 medications that have known medication interactions with emtricitabine: seven with major interactions, 26 with moderate interactions, and one with minor interactions. A full list and details of interactions are available at https://www.drugs.com/drug-interactions/emtricitabine.html.

There are three disease interactions with emtricitabine: hepatitis B disease (major interaction, and hemodialysis and renal dysfunction (minor interaction).

Contraindications. Emtricitabine is contraindicated in patients receiving elvitegravir/cobicistat/emtricitabine/tenofovir disoproxil fumarate and/or lamivudine and dolutegravir sodium, as well as in patients with hypersensitivity

---

BLACK BOX WARNING!

Hypersensitivity Reactions with Abacavir Therapy

- Severe to fatal multiple organ involvement can occur.
- Positive HLA-B*5701 allele patients are at higher risk of hypersensitivity reactions. These reactions have also occurred in negative HLA-B*5701 allele patients.
- All patients should be screened for HLA-B*5701 allele prior to beginning therapy.
- Abacavir therapy is contraindicated in patients with prior hypersensitivity reactions to abacavir and in positive HLA-B*5701 allele patients.
- If hypersensitivity is suspected, discontinue immediately.

PRACTICE PEARLS

Abacavir Therapy

- Prior to beginning therapy, assess for underlying infectious processes: pneumonia, tuberculosis (TB), herpes virus, hepatitis, or fungal infection.
- Prior to beginning therapy, know the patient's HLA-B* allele status.
- Strict adherence to prescribed therapy is essential because nonadherence allows virus(es) to replicate to resistant strains.
- Always monitor for OTC medications and herbal supplements for potential interactions.

BLACK BOX WARNING!

Emtricitabine Therapy

- Nucleoside analogues can cause lactic acidosis as well as severe hepatomegaly with steatosis and the potential for fatality when used alone or in combination with other antiretroviral medications.
- Emtricitabine is not FDA approved for treatment of chronic hepatitis B virus (HBV) infection.
- Emtricitabine can cause severe acute exacerbation of HBV in patients coinfected with HIV-1 and HBV. Discontinue therapy and monitor hepatic function with assessment and laboratory findings for several months. HBV therapy may be initiated if required.

to emtricitabine. Patients taking rifampin should not be receiving emtricitabine.

Monitoring. The primary care provider should monitor closely for potential medication or organ dysfunction interactions for patients receiving emtricitabine. If emtricitabine is used with other antivirals, there is a risk of immune

---

PRACTICE PEARLS

Emtricitabine Therapy

- Remind patients that emtricitabine is not a cure for HIV. It improves their life and decreases complications from HIV.
- The medication can be taken with or without food.
- Monitor liver and renal function routinely.
- Instruct patients about the increased risk for complications if they contract HBV.
- Always monitor for OTC medications and herbal supplements for potential interactions.

---

reconstitution syndrome, including Graves' disease, polymyositis, and Guillain-Barré syndrome.

Non-Nucleoside Reverse Transcriptase Inhibitors (NNRTIs)

NNRTIs resemble false nucleotides by binding within a mechanism to inhibit reverse transcriptase enzyme activity (Table 48.3). NNRTIs must be phosphorylated within target cells to their active triphosphate form. It is important to note that the nucleotide analog reverse transcriptase inhibitor, tenofovir, is included in the same category as a nucleoside subclass. However, the structural difference between nucleotides and nucleosides is that nucleotides already have a phosphate group, so only two steps of phosphorylation are required instead of three. Once these medications are in the active triphosphate form, they work through at least two mechanisms: chain termination and competitive inhibition.

NNRTIs do not require phosphorylation or intracellular processing to be activated. They are noncompetitive,

---

PRACTICE PEARLS

Life Span Considerations With NNRTIs

Children and Adolescents

- Diagnosis and early treatment are more effective for decreasing HIV-associated illnesses and AIDS. The new guidelines recommend rapid initiation of ART within days of diagnosis with HIV, and no longer recommend initiating ART based on a child's age.
- The guidelines acknowledge the need to postpone initiating therapy based on a patient's clinical or psychosocial factors.
- The safety and effectiveness of efavirenz, lamivudine, and tenofovir disoproxil fumarate as a fixed-dose tablet in pediatric patients infected with HIV-1 and weighing at least 35 kg have been established based on clinical studies using the individual components (efavirenz, lamivudine, and tenofovir disoproxil fumarate).
- Doravirine is not FDA approved for HIV patients younger than 18 years of age.
- A patient's stage of puberty directly affects how efavirenz is metabolized and affects its pharmacokinetic properties; therefore, dosage for HIV infection should be based on the Tanner Staging of puberty and not just on age alone.
- Adolescents in early puberty are treated based on the Tanner Staging of puberty, not just age. Patients in Tanner Stages 1 through 3 should follow pediatric dosing schedules found in the pediatric treatment guidelines, whereas those in Tanner Stages 4 and 5 should follow adult dosing schedules.
- Adolescents who are undergoing their growth-spurt period (Tanner Stage 3 for females and Tanner Stage 4 for males) should follow the adult dosing guidelines.

Pregnancy

- The guidelines for individuals of childbearing potential have been updated with revised recommendations on the use of dolutegravir sodium.

- NNRTIs are pregnancy category C, meaning risks cannot be ruled out. Limited data are available regarding the safety of administration during pregnancy.
- Pregnancy changes the role of the SNPs of ABCC2 and ABCC4 transporters on emtricitabine during pregnancy. Emtricitabine concentration in patients with a specific TT genotype is one- to twofold higher.
- Females can take elvitegravir during pregnancy and when trying to become pregnant.
- Encourage patients to register by calling the Antiretroviral Pregnancy Registry (APR) at 1-800-258-4263.

Breastfeeding

- ARTs are present in breast milk. Breastfeeding should be avoided while on ARTs due to potential complications.

Older Adult and Geriatric Considerations

- Caution should be exercised in the administration of lamivudine and doravirine in older adults, reflecting the greater frequency of decreased hepatic, renal, or cardiac function and of concomitant disease and/or another drug therapy.
- Guidelines have been updated with recommendations for HIV and the older person.
- HIV disease progression is impacted by age and comorbidities.
- The primary care provider must be cognizant of the complexities of management of older persons with HIV due to polypharmacy and the potential for drug–drug interactions.
- The geriatric patient will need to be screened for depression, along with management of depression, for better outcomes.

TABLE 48.3 Characteristics of Non-Nucleoside Reverse Transcriptase Inhibitors

Generic Name (Abbreviations) Trade Name	Formulations	Dosing Recommendations	Elimination/ Metabolic Pathway	Serum Half-Life	Adverse Events
Doravirine (DOR) Pifeltro	**Pifeltro:** • 100-mg tablet Also available as part of the STR Delstrigo (DOR/ TDF/3TC)	**Pifeltro:** • DOR 100 mg orally once daily See Appendix B, Table 1, for dosing information for Delstrigo.	CYP 3A4/5 substrate	15 hr	Nausea Dizziness Abnormal dreams
Efavirenz (EFV) Sustiva **NOTE:** Generic product is available.	**Sustiva:** • 50- and 200-mg capsules • 600-mg tablet **Generic:** • 600-mg tablet **STRs That Contain EFV:** • Atripla (EFV/TDF/ FTC) • Symfi (EFV 600 mg/TDF/3TC) • Symfi Lo (EFV 400 mg/TDF/3TC)	**Sustiva:** • EFV 600 mg orally once daily, at or before bedtime Take on an empty stomach to reduce side effects. See Appendix B, Table 1, for dosing information for STRs that contain EFV.	Metabolized by CYP 2B6 (primary), 3A4, and 2A6 CYP 3A4 mixed inducer/inhibitor (more an inducer than an inhibitor) CYP 2B6 and 2C19 inducer	40–55 hr	Rash[a] Neuropsychiatric symptoms[b] Serum transaminase elevations Hyperlipidemia Use of EFV may lead to false-positive results with some cannabinoid and benzodiazepine screening assays QT interval prolongation
Etravirine (ETR) Intelence	**Intelence:** • 25-, 100-, and 200-mg tablets	**Intelence:** ETR 200 mg orally twice daily Take following a meal.	CYP 3A4, 2C9, and 2C19 substrate CYP 3A4 inducer CYP 2C9 and 2C19 inhibitor	41 hr	Rash, including Stevens-Johnson syndrome[d] HSRs, characterized by rash, constitutional findings, and sometimes organ dysfunction (including hepatic failure) Nausea
Nevirapine (NVP) Viramune or Viramune XR **NOTE:** Generic products are available.	**Viramune:** • 200-mg tablet • 50-mg/5-mL oral suspension **Viramune XR:** • 400-mg tablet **Generic:** • 200-mg tablet • 400-mg extended-release tablet, 50-mg/5-mL oral suspension	**Viramune:** • NVP 200 mg orally once daily for 14 days (lead-in period); thereafter, NVP 200 mg orally twice daily, or • NVP 400 mg (Viramune XR tablet) orally once daily Take without regard to meals. Repeat lead-in period if therapy is discontinued for >7 days. In patients who develop mild to moderate rash without constitutional symptoms, continue lead-in dose until rash resolves, but do not extend lead-in period beyond 28 days.	CYP 450 substrate CYP 3A4 and 2B6 inducer Contraindicated in patients with moderate to severe hepatic impairment. Dose adjustment is recommended in patients on hemodialysis.	25–30 hr	Rash, including Stevens-Johnson syndrome[a] Symptomatic hepatitis: • Symptomatic hepatitis, including fatal hepatic necrosis, has been reported • Rash has been reported in approximately 50% of cases. • Symptomatic hepatitis occurs at a significantly higher frequency in ARV-naïve female patients with pre-NVP CD4 counts >250 cells/ mm[3] and in ARV-naïve male patients with pre-NVP CD4 counts >400 cells/mm[3] • NVP should not be initiated in these patients unless the benefit clearly outweighs the risk

Continued

TABLE 48.3	Characteristics of Non-Nucleoside Reverse Transcriptase Inhibitors—cont'd				
Generic Name (Abbreviations) Trade Name	Formulations	Dosing Recommendations	Elimination/ Metabolic Pathway	Serum Half-Life	Adverse Events
Rilpivirine (RPV) Edurant	**Edurant:** • 25-mg tablet **Coformulated STRs That Contain RPV:** • Complera (RPV/TDF/FTC) • Juluca (DTG/RPV) • Odefsey (RPV/TAF/FTC) **Copackaged Intramuscular Regimen:** • Cabenuva (CAB plus RPV)	**Edurant:** • RPV 25 mg orally once daily Take with a meal.	CYP 3A4 substrate	Oral: 50 hr IM: 13–28 weeks	Rash[a] Depression, insomnia, headache Hepatotoxicity QT interval prolongation IM formulation only: • Injection-site reactions (pain, induration, swelling, nodules) • Rare post-injection reaction (dyspnea, agitation, abdominal cramps, flushing) occurring within a few minutes after RPV IM injection; possibly associated with inadvertent IV administration

[a]Rare cases of Stevens-Johnson syndrome have been reported with the use of most NNRTIs; the highest incidence of rash was seen among patients who were receiving NVP.
[b]Adverse events can include dizziness, somnolence, insomnia, abnormal dreams, depression, suicidality (e.g., suicide, suicide attempt, or ideation), confusion, abnormal thinking, impaired concentration, amnesia, agitation, depersonalization, hallucinations, and euphoria. Approximately 50% of patients who are receiving EFV may experience any of these symptoms. Symptoms usually subside spontaneously after 2–4 weeks, but discontinuation of EFV may be necessary in a small percentage of patients. Late-onset neurotoxicities, including ataxia and encephalopathy, have been reported. *3TC*, lamivudine; *ARV*, antiretroviral; *CAB*, cabotegravir; *CD4*, CD4 T lymphocyte; *CYP*, cytochrome P; *DOR*, doravirine; *DTG*, dolutegravir; *EFV*, efavirenz; *ETR*, etravirine; *FTC*, emtricitabine; *HSR*, hypersensitivity reaction; *IM*, intramuscular; *IV*, intravenous; *NNRTI*, non-nucleoside reverse transcriptase inhibitor; *NVP*, nevirapine; *RPV*, rilpivirine; *STR*, single-tablet regimen; *TAF*, tenofovir alafenamide; *TDF*, tenofovir disoproxil fumarate; *XR*, extended release.
Modified from National Institutes of Health (NIH). (2021, June 3). Characteristics of non-nucleoside reverse transcriptase inhibitors (NNRTIs). Retrieved October 27, 2021, from https://clinicalinfo.hiv.gov/en/guidelines/adult-and-adolescent-arv/characteristics-non-nucleoside-reverse-transcriptase-inhibitors.)

binding to reverse transcriptase and inhibiting the function of this enzyme by binding at sites distinct from nucleoside binding sites.

Doravirine

Doravirine is an NNRTI that can be used by adult HIV patients who have not received prior antiretroviral treatment, or to replace the current antiretroviral regimen in those who are virologically suppressed on a stable antiretroviral regimen with no history of treatment failure and no known substitutions associated with resistance to doravirine.

Pharmacokinetics. The peak plasma time for doravirine is 2 hours, and the plasma concentration is 0.962 mcg/mL. Absolute bioavailability is 64%. The half-life is 15 hours, with a median time to maximum plasma concentration of 1 to 4 hours. The concentration rate to reach a steady state is 7 days. Doravirine is metabolized by cytochrome (CYP) 3A4 and eliminated through urine.

Indications. Doravirine is used to treat HIV-1 infection alone or is given in combination with other medications as a component of combination therapy.

Adverse Effects. When doravirine is coadministered with strong CYP 3A inducers, a significant decrease in doravirine plasma concentrations may occur, decreasing the efficacy of the drug. Common side effects are nausea, headache, diarrhea, abdominal pain, and abnormal dreams. Severe side effects are less common and include neuropsychiatric conditions such as insomnia, somnolence, dizziness, and altered sensorium. Immune reconstitution inflammatory syndrome may occur.

There are 165 medications that have known medication interactions with doravirine: 30 with major interactions, 50 with moderate interactions, and 85 with minor interactions. A full list and details of interactions are available at https://www.drugs.com/drug-interactions/doravirine.html.

Contraindications. Doravirine is contraindicated in patients taking strong CYP 3A inducers. Examples of strong CYP 3A inducers include anticonvulsants (carbamazepine, oxcarbazepine, phenobarbital, phenytoin), enzalutamide, rifampin, rifapentine, mitotane, and St. John's wort.

Monitoring. Monitor for hepatic and renal dysfunction. Monitor (and treat, if necessary) for posttreatment acute exacerbation of hepatitis B, if coinfected concurrently.

Efavirenz

Efavirenz is an NNRTI prescribed for the treatment of HIV in adults and pediatric patients. Nervous system side effects occur frequently within the first few days of treatment and usually recede within 2 to 4 weeks. Efavirenz must be avoided in the first trimester of pregnancy. Efavirenz is not to be used as a single HIV treatment or as a single medication added to a failing therapy treatment.

Pharmacokinetics. Time-to-peak plasma concentrations were approximately 3 to 5 hours and steady-state plasma concentrations were reached in 6 to 10 days. Efavirenz is metabolized by the CYP P450 system to hydroxylated metabolites with subsequent glucuronidation of these hydroxylated metabolites. Efavirenz has a half-life of 40 to 55 hours after multiple doses.

Indications. Efavirenz is an ART for treating HIV infection in adults and pediatric patients at least 3 months old and weighing at least 3.5 kg.

Adverse Effects. The most common adverse reactions are impaired concentration, abnormal dreams, rash, dizziness, nausea, headaches, fatigue, insomnia, and vomiting. Some patients may experience lipodystrophy syndrome. Serious psychiatric adverse events have been reported, including depression (up to 19%), anxiety (up to 13%), and nervousness (up to 7%). Dermatologic effects, including skin rash (unspecified), occurred in 26% of adult patients and in 32% of pediatric patients who received

efavirenz during clinical trials. Children tend to have more frequent and severe rashes, with Stevens-Johnson syndrome occurring in 0.1% of adults and in 2.2% of children. Elevated hepatic enzymes can occur. Patients seropositive for hepatitis B and/or hepatitis C had elevations in AST, ALT and serum amylase greater than five times the normal values.

There are 698 medications that have known medication interactions with efavirenz: 216 with major interactions, 437 with moderate interactions, and 13 with minor interactions. A full list and details of interactions are available at https://www.drugs.com/drug-interactions/efavirenz.html.

There are five disease interactions with efavirenz: cholesterol, liver disease, mental symptoms, seizures, and QT prolongation (all are moderate interactions).

Contraindications. Efavirenz, lamivudine, and tenofovir alafenamide tablet combination therapy is contraindicated in those with previous hypersensitivity reaction (Stevens-Johnson syndrome, erythema multiforme, or toxic skin eruptions) and in pregnancy (teratogenesis).

Monitoring. Monitor hepatic function prior to and during treatment with efavirenz, lamivudine, and tenofovir alafenamide tablet combination therapy. Lipids and cholesterol levels need to be monitored in case the levels increase. Liver function tests (LFTs) should be monitored for patients with a history of hepatitis B and C virus infections. Monitor for signs and symptoms of depression, suicide, aggressive behaviors, delusions, and/or paranoia.

Protease Inhibitors (PIs)

One of the final stages of the HIV life cycle is the production of HIV polyproteins, for which coding is provided by the viral messenger RNA. These polyproteins must be cleaved or separated into individual proteins by the HIV enzyme known as *protease* if infectious virions are to be produced.

PIs prevent the protease enzyme from cleaving or separating the essential proteins necessary for production of new infectious virions. (Table 48.4). Drug resistance is common, thus contraindicating monotherapy.

All antiretroviral PIs are substrates of CYP 3A4. Some PIs are also inhibitors of CYP 3A4 (amprenavir, indinavir, lopinavir, ritonavir) and can cause decreased clearance of other drugs. In general, these later drugs should not be given at the same time as other drugs that are heavily metabolized by CYP 3A4.

Atazanavir

Atazanavir (ATV) is a protease inhibitor for the treatment of HIV infection in adults and in pediatric patients at least 3 months of age. Atazanavir is always given in combination with another ART. Atazanavir is used to treat and prevent HIV/AIDS. Atazanavir is used after an accidental needle-stick injury.

Pharmacokinetics. Atazanavir has a half-life of 6.5 hours. It is metabolized by the liver and excreted in the feces and urine. Atazanavir has a bioavailability of 60% to 68% and is 86% protein bound. It is one of the preferred HIV medications for pregnant women new to ART.

PHARMACOGENETICS

Atazanavir Therapy

- PIs are mostly metabolized by CYP 3A4 in the liver.
- Atazanavir increases unconjugated bilirubin in most patients. This is caused by a competitive inhibition of UGT1A1. The presence of allele UGT1A1*28 is strongly related to jaundice. Other alleles of the UGT1A1 are probably involved.

Indications. Atazanavir is indicated for pregnant women, adults, and children at least 6 years of age who are HIV positive. Atazanavir is different from other PIs because it has a lesser effect on the lipid profile and is less likely to cause lipodystrophy. Atazanavir is a part of combination medication therapy.

Adverse Effects. The most common side effects are nausea, headache, yellowish skin, abdominal pain, trouble sleeping, and fever. Severe side effects include rashes (erythema multiforme) and high blood sugar.

PRACTICE PEARLS

Life Span Considerations With PI Therapy

Children and Adolescents

- Diagnosis and early treatment are more effective for decreasing HIV-associated illnesses and AIDS. The new guidelines recommend rapid initiation of ART within days of diagnosis with HIV, and no longer recommend initiating ART based on a child's age.
- The guidelines acknowledge the need to postpone initiating therapy based on a patient's clinical or psychosocial factors.
- The safety and effectiveness of efavirenz, lamivudine, and tenofovir disoproxil fumarate as a fixed-dose tablet in pediatric patients infected with HIV-1 and weighing at least 35 kg have been established based on clinical studies using the individual components (efavirenz, lamivudine, and tenofovir disoproxil fumarate).
- Doravirine is not FDA approved for pediatric HIV patients younger than 18 years of age.
- A patient's stage of puberty directly affects how efavirenz is metabolized and affects its pharmacokinetic properties; therefore, dosage for HIV infection should be based on the Tanner Staging of puberty and not just on age alone.
- Adolescents in early puberty are treated based on the Tanner Staging of puberty, not just age. Patients in Tanner Stages 1 through 3 should follow pediatric dosing schedules found in the pediatric treatment guidelines, whereas those in Tanner Stages 4 and 5 should follow adult dosing schedules.
- Adolescents who are undergoing their growth-spurt period (Tanner Stage 3 for females and Tanner Stage 4 for males) should follow the adult dosing guidelines.

Pregnancy

- Guidelines for individuals of childbearing potential have been updated with revised recommendations on the use of dolutegravir sodium.
- PIs are pregnancy category C, meaning risks cannot be ruled out. Limited data are available regarding the safety of administration during pregnancy.
- Females should use contraceptives during treatment and for 12 weeks after discontinuing due to the long half-life of etravirine.
- Females can take efavirenz during pregnancy or while trying to become pregnant.
- Atazanavir is pregnancy category B, meaning there is no evidence of harm to mother or baby.
- Encourage patients to register by calling the Antiretroviral Pregnancy Registry (APR) at 1-800-258-4263.

Breastfeeding

- ARTs are present in breast milk. Breastfeeding should be avoided while on ARTs due to potential complications.

Older Adult and Geriatric Considerations

- Caution should be exercised in the administration of lamivudine and doravirine in older adults, reflecting the greater frequency of decreased hepatic, renal, or cardiac function and of concomitant disease and/or additional drug therapy.
- Guidelines have been updated with recommendations for HIV and the older person.
- HIV disease progression is impacted by age and comorbidities.
- The primary care provider must be cognizant of the complexities of management of older persons with HIV due to polypharmacy and the potential for drug–drug interactions.

TABLE 48.4	Characteristics of Protease Inhibitors				
Generic Name (Abbreviations) Trade Name	**Formulations**	**Dosing Recommendations**[a]	**Elimination/ Metabolic Pathway**	**Serum Half-Life**	**Adverse Events**[b]
Atazanavir (ATV) Reyataz (ATV/c) Evotaz **NOTE:** Generic products of ATV are available.	**Reyataz:** • 150-, 200-, and 300-mg capsules • 50-mg oral powder/packet **Generic:** • 100-, 150-, 200-, and 300-mg capsules **Evotaz:** • ATV 300-mg/ COBI 150-mg tablet	**Reyataz:** *In ARV-Naïve Patients:* • (ATV 300 mg plus RTV 100 mg) orally once daily; or • ATV 400 mg orally once daily • Take with food. *With TDF or in ARV-Experienced Patients:* • (ATV 300 mg plus RTV 100 mg) orally once daily • Unboosted ATV is not recommended. • Take with food. *With EFV in ARV-Naïve Patients:* • (ATV 400 mg plus RTV 100 mg) orally once daily • Take with food. **Evotaz:** • One tablet orally once daily • Take with food. • The use of ATV/c **is not recommended** for patients who are taking TDF and who have baseline CrCl <70 mL/min (see Appendix B, Table 11, for the equation for calculating CrCl). For dosing recommendations for patients who also are receiving H2 antagonists and PPIs, refer to Table 21a.	**ATV:** • CYP 3A4 inhibitor and substrate • Weak CYP 2C8 inhibitor • UGT1A1 inhibitor **COBI:** • CYP 3A inhibitor and substrate • CYP 2D6 inhibitor Dose adjustment is recommended in patients with hepatic insufficiency (see Appendix B, Table 11).	7 hr	Indirect hyperbilirubinemia PR interval prolongation. First-degree symptomatic AV block has been reported. Use with caution in patients who have underlying conduction defects or who are on concomitant medications that can cause PR prolongation Cholelithiasis Nephrolithiasis Renal insufficiency Serum transaminase elevations Hyperlipidemia (especially with RTV boosting) Skin rash Hyperglycemia Fat maldistribution An increase in serum creatinine may occur when ATV is administered with COBI

Continued

TABLE 48.4 **Characteristics of Protease Inhibitors—cont'd**

Generic Name (Abbreviations) Trade Name	Formulations	Dosing Recommendations[a]	Elimination/Metabolic Pathway	Serum Half-Life	Adverse Events[b]
Darunavir (DRV) Prezista (DRV/c) Prezcobix	**Prezista:** • 75-, 150-, 600-, and 800-mg tablets • 100-mg/mL oral suspension **Prezcobix:** • DRV 800-mg/ COBI 150-mg tablet Also available as part of the STR Symtuza (DRV/c/TAF/FTC)	**Prezista:** *In ARV-Naïve Patients or ARV-Experienced Patients with No DRV Mutations:* • (DRV 800 mg plus RTV 100 mg) orally once daily • Take with food. *In ARV-Experienced Patients with One or More DRV Resistance Mutations:* • (DRV 600 mg plus RTV 100 mg) orally twice daily • Take with food. Unboosted DRV **is not recommended.** Prezcobix: • One tablet orally once daily • Take with food. • Not recommended for patients with one or more DRV resistance-associated mutations. • Coadministering Prezcobix and *TDF is not recommended* for patients with baseline CrCl <70 mL/min (see Appendix B, Table 11, for the equation for calculating CrCl). See Appendix B, Table 1, for dosing information for Symtuza.	**DRV:** • CYP 3A4 inhibitor and substrate • CYP 2C9 inducer **COBI:** • CYP 3A inhibitor and substrate • CYP 2D6 inhibitor	15 hr when combined with RTV 7 hr when combined with COBI	Skin rash: DRV has a sulfonamide moiety; however, incidence and severity of rash are similar in those with or without a sulfonamide allergy; Stevens-Johnson syndrome, toxic epidermal necrolysis, acute generalized exanthematous pustulosis, and erythema multiforme have been reported Hepatotoxicity Diarrhea, nausea Headache Hyperlipidemia Serum transaminase elevation Hyperglycemia Fat maldistribution An increase in serum creatinine may occur when DRV is administered with COBI
Lopinavir/ Ritonavir (LPV/r) Kaletra **NOTE:** LPV is only available as a component of an FDC tablet that also contains RTV.	**Kaletra:** • LPV/r 200-mg/50-mg tablets • LPV/r 100-mg/25-mg tablets • LPV/r 400-mg/100-mg per 5 mL of oral solution. Oral solution contains 42% alcohol.	**Kaletra:** • LPV/r 400 mg/100 mg orally twice daily, or • LPV/r 800 mg/200 mg orally once daily. However, once-daily dosing is not recommended for patients with three or more LPV-associated mutations, pregnant women, or patients receiving EFV, NVP, carbamazepine, phenytoin, or phenobarbital. *With EFV or NVP in PI-Naïve or PI-Experienced Patients:* • LPV/r 500-mg/125-mg tablets orally twice daily (use a combination of 2 LPV/r 200-mg/50-mg tablets plus 1 LPV/r 100-mg/25-mg tablet to make a total dose of LPV/r 500 mg/125 mg), or • LPV/r 533 mg/133 mg oral solution twice daily **Food Restrictions** *Tablet:* • Take without regard to meals. *Oral Solution:* • Take with food.	CYP 3A4 inhibitor and substrate	5–6 hr	GI intolerance, nausea, vomiting, diarrhea Pancreatitis Asthenia Hyperlipidemia (especially hypertriglyceridemia) Serum transaminase elevation Hyperglycemia Insulin resistance/diabetes mellitus Fat maldistribution Possible increase in the frequency of bleeding episodes in patients with hemophilia PR interval prolongation QT interval prolongation and torsades de pointes have been reported; however, causality has not been established

| Ritonavir (RTV)
Norvir

NOTE: Generic is available.

Although RTV was initially developed as a PI for HIV treatment, RTV is currently used at a lower dose of 100–200 mg once or twice daily as a PK enhancer to increase the concentrations of other PIs. | **Norvir:**
• 100-mg tablet
• 100-mg soft gel capsule
• 80-mg/mL oral solution. Oral solution contains 43% alcohol.
• 100-mg single packet oral powder

Also available as part of the FDC tablet Kaletra (LPV/r) | **As a PK Booster (or Enhancer) for Other PIs:**
• RTV 100–400 mg orally daily in 1 or 2 divided doses (refer to other PIs for specific dosing recommendations).

Food Restrictions:
Tablet:
• Take with food.
Capsule and Oral Solution:
• To improve tolerability, take with food if possible. | CYP 3A4 > 2D6 substrate
Potent CYP 3A4 and 2D6 inhibitor

Inducer of UGT1A1 and CYPs 1A2, 2C8, 2C9, and 2C19 | 3–5 hr | GI intolerance, nausea, vomiting, diarrhea
Paresthesia (circumoral and extremities)
Hyperlipidemia (especially hypertriglyceridemia)
Hepatitis
Asthenia
Taste perversion
Hyperglycemia
Fat maldistribution
Possible increase in the frequency of bleeding episodes in patients with hemophilia |

NOTE: See original source for Appendix B.

[a]For dose adjustments in patients with hepatic insufficiency, see Appendix B, Table 11.

[b]Also see Table 20.

ARV, antiretroviral; *ATV,* atazanavir; *ATV/c,* atazanavir/cobicistat; *AV,* atrioventricular; *COBI,* cobicistat; *CrCl,* creatinine clearance; *CYP,* cytochrome P; *DRV,* darunavir; *DRV/c,* darunavir/cobicistat; *EFV,* efavirenz; *FDC,* fixed-dose combination; *FTC,* emtricitabine; *GI,* gastrointestinal; *H2,* histamine H2 receptor; *LPV,* lopinavir; *LPV/r,* lopinavir/ritonavir; *NVP,* nevirapine; *PI,* protease inhibitor; *PK,* pharmacokinetic; *PPI,* proton pump inhibitor; *RTV,* ritonavir; *STR,* single-tablet regimen; *TAF,* tenofovir alafenamide; *TDF,* tenofovir disoproxil fumarate; *UGT1,* uridine diphosphate glucuronyl transferase 1 family.
From National Institutes of Health (NIH). (2021). *Characteristics of protease inhibitors.* Retrieved October 27, 2021, from https://clinicalinfo.hiv.gov/en/table/appendix-b-table-5-characteristics-protease-inhibitors.)

There are 472 medications that have known medication interactions with atazanavir: 199 with major interactions, 242 with moderate interactions, and 31 with minor interactions. A full list and details of interactions are available at https://www.drugs.com/drug-interactions/atazanavir.html.

There are eight disease interactions with atazanavir: heart block, nephrolithiasis, renal impairment, and hemophilia (major interaction); and liver disease, phenylketonuria (PKU), hyperglycemia, and hyperlipidemia (moderate interaction).

Contraindications. Patients with previous episodes of hypersensitivity (Stevens-Johnson symptoms, erythema multiforme, or toxic skin eruptions) should not take atazanavir.

Monitoring. Monitor hepatic and renal functions. Monitor for jaundice.

PRACTICE PEARLS

Atazanavir Therapy

- Atazanavir must be given with other antiretroviral agents.
- Atazanavir can be used in pregnant patients with HIV.
- Atazanavir can be used in patients at least 6 years of age.
- Give atazanavir cautiously to patients with hepatic and renal dysfunction.

Darunavir

Darunavir (DRV) is a PI administered in combination with other ARTs for the treatment of HIV infection in adult and pediatric patients 3 years of age and older to slow the disease progression and prolong life. Darunavir can be co-administered with ritonavir and in combination with other antiretroviral agents.

Pharmacokinetics. Darunavir is rapidly absorbed after oral administration and reaches peak concentrations after 2 to 4 hours. Darunavir has a fast distribution/elimination phase. It has a slower elimination phase, with terminal half-life of 15 hours, when given with ritonavir.

Indications. Darunavir is used to treat and/or prevent HIV infection. It can be given to pregnant women and can prevent the baby from contracting HIV. Patients 18 years of age and older can be administered darunavir. Darunavir can be administered but should *not* be used as initial therapy in children younger than 12 years of age. Darunavir with ritonavir is FDA approved as a component of ART treatment-naïve patients and treatment-experienced children at least 3 years of age.

Adverse Effects. Some of the common side effects of darunavir are diarrhea, nausea, vomiting, heartburn, stomach pain, weakness, headache, skin rash, and fat redistribution. Darunavir can cause elevated blood sugar and liver or pancreas problems.

There are 417 medications that have known medication interactions with darunavir: 84 with major interactions, 315 with moderate interactions, and 18 with minor interactions. A full list and details of interactions are available at https://www.drugs.com/drug-interactions/darunavir.html.

There are three disease interactions with darunavir: hepatotoxicity and hemophilia (major interaction), and hyperglycemia (moderate interaction).

Contraindications. Patients with previous episodes of hypersensitivity (Stevens-Johnson syndrome, erythema multiforme, or toxic skin eruptions) should not take darunavir.

Monitoring. Monitor blood sugar, and liver and renal function.

PRACTICE PEARLS

Darunavir Therapy

- Assess the patient for hyperglycemia.
- Assess the patient's renal and liver function.
- Monitor for jaundice.
- All pediatric patients are dosed based on their weight.

Ritonavir

Subtherapeutic doses of ritonavir (RTV) can cause marked inhibition of CYP 3A4. Therefore, it is used in combination formulations with other PIs to increase efficacy and reduce the number of doses required daily. With decreased daily doses, patient compliance increases.

Pharmacokinetics. Ritonavir is a PI. However, its ability to block CYP 3A–mediated metabolism of atazanavir causes it to become a booster or enhancer. With ritonavir, other drugs such as atazanavir can be given to a larger population of patients.

PHARMACOGENETICS

Ritonavir Therapy

- Dyslipidemia is related to several genetic and environmental determinates.
- Ritonavir-related hypertriglyceridemia is increased in patients with ABCA1, APOA5, APOC1, APOE, and CETP genes.

Indications. Ritonavir is indicated as a component of combination therapy to treat HIV-infected patients. Ritonavir can be given to pediatric and adult patients.

Adverse Effects. Ritonavir can cause life-threatening side effects (especially when given alone due to toxicity) such as pancreatitis, cardiac dysrhythmias, severe allergic reactions, and liver damage. It can also cause redistribution and accumulation of body fat, including buffalo hump, central obesity, peripheral and facial wasting, and breast enlargement. Some common side effects are increased levels of triglycerides and cholesterol, hyperglycemia, immune reconstitution inflammatory syndrome, and increased spontaneous bleeding in hemophilia patients.

There are 582 medications that have known medication interactions with ritonavir: 193 with major interactions, 348 with moderate interactions, and 41 with minor interactions. A full list and details of interactions are available at https://www.drugs.com/drug-interactions/ritonavir.html.

There are five disease interactions with ritonavir: hepatotoxicity and hemophilia (major interaction), and hyperglycemia, hyperlipidemia, and heart block (moderate interaction).

Contraindications. Do not give nonsedating antihistamines, sedative hypnotics, or ergot alkaloids to patients taking ritonavir.

Monitoring. Monitor hepatic, renal, cholesterol, and triglyceride levels. Monitor for increased bleeding in hemophilia patients.

BLACK BOX WARNING!

Ritonavir Therapy

- Ritonavir has potentially serious drug interactions with nonsedating antihistamines, sedative hypnotics, antiarrhythmics, and ergot alkaloids.

PRACTICE PEARLS

Ritonavir Therapy

- Ritonavir is mainly used as a pharmacokinetic enhancer of other PIs; the recommended dose of ritonavir varies with the different PIs.
- Ritonavir oral solution contains a large amount of alcohol. Children may become sick after drinking ritonavir.
- Patients should swallow tablets whole. Do not crush, break, or chew the tablets.
- Ritonavir powder can be mixed in liquids or applesauce/pudding to lessen its bitter aftertaste. The medicine should be ingested within 2 hours of mixing.
- Oral contraceptives are less effective for patients on ritonavir.
- Monitor for increased spontaneous bleeding in hemophilia patients.
- Monitor renal, liver, and pancreatic laboratory values.
- Give with food to decrease the gastrointestinal (GI) side effects.

CD4 Fusion/Entry Inhibitors

The class of medications called *fusion inhibitors* work by preventing the HIV virus from invading the white blood cells, which are the primary targets of the virus. Fusion inhibitors attach themselves to proteins on the surfaces of T-cells or HIV cells (Table 48.5). For HIV to bind to and enter T-cells, the proteins on the outer coat of the HIV cell must bind to the surface receptors on the T-cells. Fusion inhibitors prevent this from happening. Some fusion inhibitors target the gp120 or gp41 on the CD4 protein or, in the case of maraviroc, the CCR5 coreceptor. A profile test should be performed prior to using maraviroc. If entry inhibitors are successful, HIV cannot bind to the surfaces of T-cells or enter them.

PRACTICE PEARLS

Life Span Considerations With Fusion/ Entry Inhibitor Therapy

Children and Adolescents

- Fusion/entry inhibitors can be used in children weighing at least 11 kg.

Pregnancy

- Fusion/entry inhibitors are pregnancy category is C, meaning risks cannot be ruled out. Limited data are available regarding the safety of administration during pregnancy.
- Encourage patients to register by calling the Antiretroviral Pregnancy Registry (APR) at 1-800-258-4263.

Breastfeeding

- Breastfeeding should be avoided while on ARTs due to potential complications.

Older Adult and Geriatric Considerations

- No dose adjustments are required for renal or hepatic impairment.
- Guidelines have been updated with recommendations for HIV and the older person.
- HIV disease progression is impacted by age and comorbidities.
- The primary care provider must be cognizant of the complexities of management of older persons with HIV due to polypharmacy and the potential for drug–drug interactions.

Enfuvirtide (T-20)

Enfuvirtide (T-20) is the only CD4 fusion or entry inhibitor. Enfuvirtide blocks the HIV from entering the CD4 cells of the immune system.

Pharmacokinetics. Enfuvirtide is administered subcutaneously in combination with other antiretroviral agents. It must be administered via subcutaneous injection twice daily; half-life is 3.8 hours and bioavailability is 84.3%. It is metabolized by the hepatic system. The mechanism for excretion is unknown.

TABLE 48.5	Characteristics of the Fusion Inhibitor					
Generic Name (Abbreviation) Trade Name	**Formulation**	**Dosing Recommendation**	**Serum Half-Life**	**Elimination**	**Adverse Events**	
Enfuvirtide (T-20) Fuzeon	**Fuzeon:** • Injectable; supplied as lyophilized powder. • Each vial contains 108 mg of T-20; reconstitute with 1.1 mL of sterile water for injection for delivery of approximately 90 mg/1 mL. • Refer to prescribing information for storage instruction.	**Fuzeon:** • T-20 90 mg/1 mL SQ twice daily	3.8 hr	Expected to undergo catabolism to its constituent amino acids, with subsequent recycling of the amino acids in the body pool	Local injection site reactions (e.g., pain, erythema, induration, nodules and cysts, pruritus, ecchymosis) in almost 100% of patients Increased incidence of bacterial pneumonia HSR occurs in <1% of patients. Symptoms may include rash, fever, nausea, vomiting, chills, rigors, hypotension, or elevated serum transaminases. Re-challenge is not recommended.	

HSR, hypersensitivity reaction; *SQ*, subcutaneous; *T-20*, enfuvirtide
From National Institutes of Health (NIH). (2021). *Characteristics of the fusion inhibitor.* Retrieved October 27, 2021, from https://clinicalinfo.hiv.gov/en/guidelines/adult-and-adolescent-arv/characteristics-fusion-inhibitor.

Indications. Enfuvirtide is indicated for patients with persistent HIV-1 replication despite ongoing ART. Enfuvirtide can be prescribed to adults and children weighing at least 11 kg.

Adverse Effects. The most common side effects are injection site pain, hardening of the skin, erythema, nodules, cysts, and itch. Pneumonia is a serious side effect that can occur. Risks for pneumonia include low initial CD4 count, high initial viral load, intravenous (IV) drug use, smoking, and a history of lung disease. Immune reconstitution syndrome can occur. Other adverse effects include peripheral neuropathy, insomnia, depression, cough, anorexia, flulike symptoms, pneumonia, and dry mouth. Hypersensitivity reactions can occur.

The medications that have known minor to moderate medication interactions with enfuvirtide include cobicistat, rifampin, ritonavir, saquinavir, and tipranavir. These interactions increase or decrease blood level concentrations of HIV medications.

Contraindications. Exercise caution with patients with known lung disease. The only contraindication is known hypersensitivity to enfuvirtide components.

Monitoring. Monitor for injection site side effects. Assess for signs and symptoms of pneumonia.

PRACTICE PEARLS

Enfuvirtide Therapy

• Local injection site reactions have occurred.
• Never administer enfuvirtide near the navel, or over/near skin irregularities (moles, scar tissue, bruises, surgical scars, tattoos, or burn sites).
• Enfuvirtide requires twice-daily injections. This may cause decreased adherence to the medication regimen.
• Teach the patient and/or family how to administer enfuvirtide.
• Monitor for immune reconstitution syndrome.
• Enfuvirtide must be used in combination with other antiretroviral agents.

CCR5 Antagonist

The CCR5 coreceptor antagonist prevents HIV-1 from entering and infecting immune cells by blocking CCR5 cell-surface receptors (Table 48.6). The molecules bind to the hydrophobic pocket to form transmembrane helices blocking the entry of the virus. Approximately 50% or more treatment-experienced patients are infected with CXCR4-tropic virus.

TABLE 48.6   Characteristics of the CCR5 Antagonist

Generic Name (Abbreviation) Trade Name	Formulation	Dosing Recommendations[a]	Serum Half-Life	Elimination/ Metabolic Pathway	Adverse Events[b]
Maraviroc (MVC) Selzentry	**Selzentry:** • 150- and 300-mg tablets	**Selzentry:** • MVC 150 mg orally twice daily when given with drugs that are strong CYP 3A inhibitors (with or without CYP 3A inducers), including PIs (except TPV/r) • MVC 300 mg orally twice daily when given with NRTIs, T-20, TPV/r, NVP, RAL, and other drugs that are not strong CYP 3A inhibitors or inducers • MVC 600 mg orally twice daily when given with drugs that are CYP 3A inducers, including EFV, ETR, etc. (without a CYP3A inhibitor) Take MVC without regard to meals.	14–18 hr	CYP 3A4 substrate	Abdominal pain Cough Dizziness Musculoskeletal symptoms Pyrexia Rash Upper respiratory tract infections Hepatotoxicity, which may be preceded by severe rash or other signs of systemic allergic reactions Orthostatic hypotension, especially in patients with severe renal insufficiency

NOTE: See original source for Appendix B.
[a]For dose adjustment in patients with hepatic insufficiency, see Appendix B, Table 11.
[b]Also see Table 20.
CYP, Cytochrome P; EFV, efavirenz; ETR, etravirine; MVC, maraviroc; NRTI, nucleoside reverse transcriptase inhibitor; NVP, nevirapine; PI, protease inhibitor; RAL, raltegravir; T-20, enfuvirtide; TPV/r, tipranavir/ritonavir.
From National Institutes of Health (NIH). (2021). Characteristics of the CCR5 antagonist. Retrieved October 27, 2021, from https://clinicalinfo.hiv.gov/en/guidelines/adult-and-adolescent-arv/characteristics-ccr5-antagonist.

PRACTICE PEARLS

Life Span Considerations With CCR5 Antagonist Therapy

Children and Adolescents

• CCR5 antagonists can be used in children who are at least 2 years of age.

Pregnancy

• CCR5 antagonists are pregnancy category C, meaning risks cannot be ruled out. Limited data are available regarding the safety of administration during pregnancy.
• Encourage patients to register by calling the Antiretroviral Pregnancy Registry (APR) at 1-800-258-4263.

Breastfeeding

• Breastfeeding should be avoided while on ARTs due to potential complications.

Older Adult and Geriatric Considerations

• No dose adjustments are required for renal or hepatic impairment.
• Guidelines have been updated with recommendations for HIV and the older person.
• HIV disease progression is impacted by age and comorbidities.
• The primary care provider must be cognizant of the complexities of management of older persons with HIV due to polypharmacy and the potential for drug–drug interactions.

Maraviroc

Maraviroc (MVC) is the first CCR5 coreceptor antagonist to receive FDA approval for treating HIV-1 infected patients to optimize their treatment.

Pharmacokinetics. Maraviroc is a CYP 3A4 substrate and requires dosage adjustment when taken with drugs that interact with this P450 isozyme. Maraviroc is excreted in urine and feces. Terminal half-life is 14 to 18 hours. Maraviroc concentrations are higher when administered without a CYP 3A inhibitor.

Indications. Maraviroc is indicated in combination with other antiretroviral agents for use with treatment-experienced

Maraviroc Therapy

- Maraviroc is only effective in the subpopulation of HIV-1 patients with selective tropism for the mutation of the CCR5 receptor virus form.
- A tropism assay should be performed prior to starting maraviroc to determine whether it binds selectively to the CCR5 coreceptor necessary for HIV entrance into CD4 cells.

adult patients infected with CCR5-tropic HIV-1 to optimize therapy. Maraviroc can be administered to pediatric patients age 2 and older weighing 10 kg or more. Noninteracting drugs include tipranavir/ritonavir, nevirapine, raltegravir, all NRTIs, and enfuvirtide. Potent CYP 3A inhibitors include PIs (except tipranavir/ritonavir), delavirdine, elvitegravir/ritonavir, ketoconazole, itraconazole, clarithromycin, and other potent CYP 3A inhibitors (nefazodone, telithromycin).

Adverse Effects. Cough, upper respiratory tract infections, fever, rash, dizziness, muscle and joint pain, diarrhea, nausea, increased hepatic transaminase activity, and sleep or appetite disorders can occur. Immune reconstitution inflammatory syndrome can occur when the immune system begins to recover after treatment with antiretroviral medicine(s). Severe skin and hypersensitivity reactions have occurred prior to hepatotoxicity.

There are 297 medications that have known medication interactions with maraviroc: 39 with major interactions, 256 with moderate interactions, and two with minor interactions. A full list and details of interactions are available at https://www.drugs.com/drug-interactions/maraviroc.html.

There are four disease interactions with maraviroc: hepatotoxicity/liver impairment and renal impairment (major interaction), and cardiovascular disease and hypotension (moderate interaction).

Contraindications. Maraviroc is not indicated in patients with CXCR4-tropic HIV-1 due to apparent lack of efficacy. Maraviroc should be used cautiously in patients with decreased creatinine clearance (CrCl). Maraviroc should not be taken with St. John's wort. Maraviroc is not recommended for children taking potent CYP 3A inducers. Potent CYP 3A inducers include efavirenz, rifampin, etravirine, carbamazepine, phenobarbital, and phenytoin.

Monitoring. Monitor for hepatic function and the presence of a rash/skin abnormalities with fever and flulike symptoms.

BLACK BOX WARNING!

Maraviroc Therapy

CCR5 Antagonist: Hepatotoxicity may be preceded by systemic allergic symptoms, including itchy rash or increased eosinophils.

Maraviroc Therapy

- Monitor patients taking maraviroc without a CYP 3A inhibitor for adverse effects.
- No dose adjustments are required based on race or gender.
- Expect dose adjustments with CYP 3A inhibitors.

Integrase Inhibitors or Integrase Strand Transfer Inhibitors

Integrase inhibitors, also known as integrase strand transfer inhibitors, are used in combination with other antiretroviral medications (Table 48.7). Integrase inhibitors must be given with elvitegravir and ritonavir. Some brand-name products combine these medications into one pill.

Life Span Considerations With Integrase Inhibitor Therapy

Children and Adolescents

- Integrase inhibitors can be used in children who are 2 years of age and older.
- Tablets cannot be chewed, cut, or crushed.
- The use of dolutegravir sodium in neonates, infants, and children weighing less than 30 kg is not FDA approved.

Pregnancy

- There is a risk for embryo-fetal toxicity with neural tube defects if integrase inhibitors are taken at the time of conception through the first trimester.
- Encourage patients to register by calling the Antiretroviral Pregnancy Registry (APR) at 1-800-258-4263.

Breastfeeding

- Breastfeeding should be avoided while on ARTs due to potential complications.

Older Adult and Geriatric Considerations

- Guidelines have been updated with recommendations for HIV and the older person.
- HIV disease progression is impacted by age and comorbidities.
- The primary care provider must be cognizant of the complexities of management of older persons with HIV due to polypharmacy and the potential for drug–drug interactions.
- There is an increased risk for renal failure and decreased hepatic and/or cardiac function with dolutegravir sodium use in patients 65 years of age and older.

Dolutegravir Sodium

Dolutegravir sodium (DTG) can be administered once daily. However, it is not safe to give to females of childbearing age who are not on an effective form of birth control.

TABLE 48.7 Characteristics of Integrase Strand Transfer Inhibitors

Generic Name (Abbreviation) Trade Name	Formulations	Dosing Recommendations[a]	Elimination/Metabolic Pathways	Serum Half-Life	Adverse Events[b]
Bictegravir (BIC)	BIC is available only as a component of the STR Biktarvy (BIC/TAF/FTC).[c]	**Biktarvy:** • 1 tablet orally once daily	CYP 3A4 substrate UGT1A1-mediated glucuronidation	~17 hr	Diarrhea Nausea Headache Weight gain
Cabotegravir (CAB)	Available as part of the copackaged IM long-acting regimen **Cabenuva (CAB IM and RPV IM):** • 400-mg/2-mL vial • 600-mg/3-mL vial *Also available in oral tablet formulation.* **Vocabria (CAB PO):** • 30-mg tablet • Must be obtained from manufacturer for oral lead-in and oral bridging during administration of Cabenuva (CAB IM/RPV IM)	See Appendix B, Table 1, for dosing information for coformulated and co-packaged regimens that contain CAB.	UGT1A1 and UGT1A9-mediated glucuronidation	Oral: 41 hr IM: 6–12 weeks	Headache Nausea Abnormal dreams Anxiety Insomnia Depressive disorders Hepatotoxicity IM formulation only: injection-site reactions (e.g., pain, induration, swelling, nodules)
Dolutegravir (DTG) Tivicay	**Tivicay:** • 10-, 25-, and 50-mg tablets • 5-mg soluble tablet **STRs That Contain DTG:c** • Dovato (DTG/3TC) • Juluca (DTG/RPV) • Triumeq (DTG/ABC/3TC)	*In ARV-Naïve or ARV-Experienced, INSTI-Naïve Patients:* • DTG 50 mg orally once daily *In ARV-Naïve or ARV-Experienced, INSTI-Naïve Patients when Coadministered with EFV, FPV/r, TPV/r, or Rifampin:* • DTG 50 mg orally twice daily *INSTI-Experienced Patients with Certain INSTI Mutations (See Product Label) or with Clinically Suspected INSTI Resistance:* • DTG 50 mg orally twice daily See Appendix B, Table 1, for dosing information for STRs that contain DTG.	UGT1A1-mediated glucuronidation Minor substrate of CYP 3A4	~14 hr	Insomnia Headache Depression and suicidal ideation (rare; usually occurs in patients with preexisting psychiatric conditions) Weight gain Hepatotoxicity Potential for increased risk of NTDs in infants born to individuals who received DTG around the time of conception is lower than previously reported. Refer to INSTI section for more information. HSRs, including rash, constitutional symptoms, and organ dysfunction (including liver injury), have been reported.

Continued

TABLE 48.7

TABLE 48.7 Characteristics of Integrase Strand Transfer Inhibitors—cont'd

Generic Name (Abbreviation) Trade Name	Formulations	Dosing Recommendations[a]	Elimination/Metabolic Pathways	Serum Half-Life	Adverse Events[b]
Elvitegravir (EVG)	EVG is only available as a component of an STR tablet that also contains COBI, FTC, and either TDF or TAF. **STRs That Contain EVG:[c]** • Genvoya (EVG/c/TAF/FTC) • Stribild (EVG/c/TDF/FTC)	**Genvoya:** • 1 tablet orally once daily with food • See Appendix B, Table 11, for recommendations on dosing in persons with renal insufficiency. **Stribild:** • 1 tablet orally once daily with food • **Not recommended** for patients with baseline CrCl <70 mL/min (see Appendix B, Table 11, for the CrCl calculation equation).	**EVG:** • CYP 3A and UGT1A1/3 substrate **COBI:** • CYP 3A inhibitor and substrate • CYP 2D6 inhibitor	EVG/c: ~13 hr	Nausea Diarrhea Depression and suicidal ideation (rare; usually occurs in patients with preexisting psychiatric conditions)
Raltegravir (RAL) Isentress Isentress HD	**Isentress:** • 400-mg tablet • 25- and 10-mg chewable tablets • 100-mg single-use packet for oral suspension **Isentress HD:** • 600-mg tablet	**Isentress** *In ARV-Naïve Patients or ARV-Experienced Patients:* • 400 mg orally twice daily *With Rifampin:* • 800 mg orally twice daily **Isentress HD:** *In ARV-Naïve or ARV-Experienced Patients with Virologic Suppression on a Regimen Containing RAL 400 mg Twice Daily:* • 1200 mg (2 600-mg tablets) orally once daily *With Rifampin:* • Not recommended	UGT1A1-mediated glucuronidation	~9 hr	Rash, including Stevens-Johnson syndrome, HSR, and toxic epidermal necrolysis Nausea Headache Diarrhea Pyrexia CPK elevation, muscle weakness, and rhabdomyolysis Weight gain Insomnia Depression and suicidal ideation (rare; usually occurs in patients with preexisting psychiatric conditions)

NOTE: See original source for Appendix B.

[a]For dose adjustments in patients with hepatic insufficiency, see Appendix B, Table 11. When no food restriction is listed, the ARV drug can be taken with or without food.

[b]Also see Table 20.

[c]See Appendix B, Table 1, for information about these formulations.

3TC, lamivudine; *ABC,* abacavir; *ARV,* antiretroviral; *BIC,* bictegravir; *CAB,* cabotegravir; *COBI,* cobicistat; *CPK,* creatine phosphokinase; *CrCl,* creatinine clearance; *CYP,* cytochrome P; *DTG,* dolutegravir; *EFV,* efavirenz; *EVG,* elvitegravir; *EVG/c,* elvitegravir/cobicistat; *FPV/r,* fosamprenavir/ritonavir; *FTC,* emtricitabine; *HSR,* hypersensitivity reaction; *IM,* intramuscular; *INSTI,* integrase strand transfer inhibitor; *NTD,* neural tube defect; *RAL,* raltegravir; *RPV,* rilpivirine; *STR,* single-tablet regimen; *TAF,* tenofovir alafenamide; *TDF,* tenofovir disoproxil fumarate; *TPV/r,* tipranavir/ritonavir; *UGT1,* uridine diphosphate glucuronyl transferase 1 family. From National Institutes of Health (NIH). (2021). *Characteristics of integrase inhibitors.* Retrieved October 27, 2021, from https://clinicalinfo.hiv.gov/en/guidelines/adult-and-adolescent-arv/characteristics-integrase-inhibitors.

Pharmacokinetics. Dolutegravir sodium has a half-life of approximately 14 hours. This allows for once-daily dosing. Peak plasma concentrations are 2 to 3 hours after oral administration.

PHARMACOGENETICS

Dolutegravir Sodium Therapy

When administering dolutegravir to carriers of UGT1A1 reduced function polymorphisms, a medication dose adjustment is not required.

Indications. Dolutegravir sodium is indicated for the treatment of adult patients infected with strains of HIV that are resistant to multiple other drugs. Dosing occurs in ranges of 50 mg orally daily for adolescents 12 years of age and older; for those weighing 30 to 39 kg, the dose is 35 mg daily, and for those weighing more than 40 kg, the dose is 50 mg daily. Dolutegravir sodium can be used with other HIV medicines in children who are at least 4 weeks of age, weigh at least 3 kg, and have never received an integrase inhibitor.

Adverse Effects. Common side effects include diarrhea, nausea, fatigue, headache, insomnia, and dizziness. Serious side effects can occur and include allergic reactions and hepatic impairment. Immune reconstitution inflammatory syndrome can occur. If signs or symptoms of hypersensitivity reactions develop (severe rash or rash accompanied by fever, general malaise, fatigue, muscle or joint aches, blisters or peeling of the skin, oral blisters or lesions, conjunctivitis, facial edema, hepatitis, eosinophilia, angioedema, or difficulty breathing), discontinue immediately. Use cautiously in patients with hepatitis B or C due to potential for hepatotoxicity. Severe adverse reactions include suicidal ideation, hepatic failure, and teratogenesis. Mild adverse reactions include insomnia, headache, fatigue, weight gain, anxiety, and abdominal symptoms (abdominal pain, nausea, vomiting, diarrhea, and flatulence).

There are 144 medications that have known medication interactions with dolutegravir sodium: 56 with major interactions, seven with moderate interactions, and 81 with minor interactions. A full list and details of interactions are available at https://www.drugs.com/drug-interactions/dolutegravir.html.

Multivitamins with minerals should not be taken at the same time as dolutegravir sodium.

Contraindications. Dolutegravir sodium is contraindicated in pregnancy due to potential increased risk for neural tube birth defects. Dolutegravir sodium should not be prescribed to any person of childbearing potential who is sexually active and is not on effective birth control. Raltegravir is a safer alternative if pregnancy is desired, or if the female patient is not on effective birth control. Patients taking the antiarrhythmic dofetilide should not take dolutegravir sodium.

Monitoring. Monitor hepatic and renal function. Screen frequently for depression and suicidal ideation.

PRACTICE PEARLS

Dolutegravir Sodium Therapy

- Dolutegravir sodium is always used with other antiretroviral medications.
- Dolutegravir sodium should always be taken whole or dispersed in drinking water. It should never be chewed, cut, or crushed.
- Dolutegravir sodium should be taken at least 2 hours before or 6 hours after cation antacids, laxatives, sucralfate, or supplements with iron or calcium.
- Dolutegravir sodium can be taken with or without food.
- The patient's mental status should be screened for depression and suicidal ideation.

Raltegravir

Raltegravir (RAL) was the first integrase inhibitor to receive FDA approval. Combination therapy containing raltegravir has potent antiretroviral activity and is well tolerated.

Pharmacokinetics. Raltegravir has a half-life of 9 hours. It is eliminated in feces and urine.

PHARMACOGENETICS

Raltegravir Therapy

- Increased raltegravir exposure in carriers of UGT1A1 reduced function polymorphisms requires no dose adjustment.

Indications. Raltegravir is a safer alternative if pregnancy is desired, or if the female patient is not on effective birth control. Raltegravir can be prescribed to HIV-1 positive patients weighing at least 25 kg.

Adverse Effects. If signs or symptoms of hypersensitivity reactions develop (including, but not limited to, severe rash or rash accompanied by fever, general malaise, fatigue, muscle or joint aches, blisters or peeling of the skin, oral blisters or lesions, conjunctivitis, facial edema, hepatitis, eosinophilia, angioedema, or difficulty breathing), discontinue use. Raltegravir should be prescribed cautiously in patients with hepatic disease and hepatitis B and C coinfections. Mild adverse effects include headache, insomnia, depression, fatigue, diarrhea, anxiety, and rash. More serious effects include hepatic impairment, neutropenia, nephrolithiasis, myopathy, anemia, hyperglycemia, and rhabdomyolysis.

There are 63 medications that have known medication interactions with raltegravir: 12 with major interactions, 19 with moderate interactions, and 32 with minor interactions. A full list of interactions and details are available at https://www.drugs.com/drug-interactions/raltegravir.html.

There are four disease interactions with raltegravir: hemodialysis, liver disease, myopathy/rhabdomyolysis, and PKU (all moderate interaction).

Contraindications. Patients with PKU should not be administered the chewable tablets because they contain phenylalanine. Do not prescribe for patients with a history of Stevens-Johnson syndrome or toxic epidermal necrolysis.

Monitoring. Monitor for hepatic and renal impairment, immune reconstitution syndrome, autoimmune disease, Graves' disease, Guillain-Barré syndrome, and serious rashes.

PRACTICE PEARLS

Raltegravir Therapy

- Raltegravir is available in chewable tablets for pediatric patients and in powder suspension for neonates and older.
- Dosage considerations may be implemented for hepatic and renal impairment.
- Monitor for renal, hepatic, and red blood cell (RBC) function.

CD4 Post-Attachment Inhibitors

Post-attachment inhibitors block CD4 receptors on the surface of certain immune cells that HIV needs to enter the cells (Table 48.8). By binding to the CD4 receptors, HIV is blocked from attaching to CCR5 and CXCR4 coreceptors and is thereby denied entry into the cell.

PRACTICE PEARLS

Life Span Considerations With CD4 Post-Attachment Inhibitor Therapy

Children and Adolescents

- No guidance related to safety and efficacy in the pediatric and adolescent populations has been described.

Pregnancy

- This drug class has not been studied in pregnancy. However, the drug may traverse the placenta, resulting in transfer to the developing fetus.
- Encourage patients to register by calling the Antiretroviral Pregnancy Registry (APR) at 1-800-258-4263.

Breastfeeding

- Breastfeeding should be avoided while on ARTs due to potential complications.

Older Adult and Geriatric Considerations

- No guidance related to the safety and efficacy in the older adult or geriatric population has been described.

Ibalizumab

Ibalizumab-uiyk received FDA approval in March 2018 and is the first medication approved for this class. It is indicated for heavily treated adults with multidrug-resistant infection who are failing their current ART regimen. It is used in combination with the patient's current ART regimen. Ibalizumab is a humanized monoclonal antibody (mAb) that binds to extracellular domain 2 of the CD4 receptor. The ibalizumab binding epitope is located at the interface between domains 1 and 2, opposite from the binding site, for major

---

TABLE 48.8 Characteristics of the CD4 Post-Attachment Inhibitor

Generic Name (Abbreviation) Trade Name	Formulation	Dosing Recommendations	Serum Half-Life	Elimination/ Metabolic Pathway	Adverse Events
Ibalizumab (IBA) *Trogarzo*	Trogarzo: • Single-dose 2-mL vial containing 200 mg/ 1.33 mL (150 mg/mL) of ibalizumab	Trogarzo: • Administer a single loading dose of IBA 2000 mg IV infusion over 30 minutes, followed by a maintenance dose of IBA 800 mg IV infusion over 15 minutes every 2 weeks. • See prescribing information for additional instructions for preparing, storing, and administering IBA, and for monitoring patients who are receiving IBA.	~64 hr	Not well defined	Diarrhea Dizziness Nausea Rash Hypersensitivity, including anaphylaxis and infusion-related reactions

IBA, Ibalizumab; *IV*, intravenous
From National Institutes of Health (NIH). (2021). *Characteristics of CD4 post-attachment inhibitor.* Retrieved October 27, 2021, from https://clinicalinfo.hiv.gov/en/guidelines/hiv-clinical-guidelines-adult-and-adolescent-arv/characteristics-cd4-post-attachment.

histocompatibility complex class II molecules and gp120 attachment. Ibalizumab does not inhibit HIV gp120 attachment to CD4; however, its post-binding conformational effects block the gp120-CD4 complex from interacting with CCR5 or CXCR4, thus preventing viral entry and fusion.

Pharmacokinetics. Ibalizumab maintenance therapy requires IV infusions every 2 weeks. The elimination half-life is approximately 3 days. It has not been shown to have any interactions. Dose modifications of ibalizumab are not required when administered with any other ARTs or any other drugs.

PHARMACOGENETICS

Ibalizumab Therapy

Genotype changes in the HIV-1 cells could lead to decreased susceptibility to ibalizumab-uiyk; however, the clinical significance has not been established.

Indications. This drug is used to treat adults with HIV-1 infection who have been treated with multiple ARTs and are experiencing drug resistance or regimen failure. It is given in combination with other ARTs.

Adverse Effects. Diarrhea, dizziness, nausea, and rash have been reported in 5% to 8% of patients. Immune reconstitution syndrome is rare. Infusion-related reactions and anaphylaxis have also been reported.

Contraindications. Ibalizumab is contraindicated for any person who experiences hypersensitivity to ibalizumab or any of its components. There are no known significant drug interactions.

Monitoring. Monitor CD4 count and HIV RNA plasma levels. Monitor for infusion-related reactions and anaphylaxis.

PRACTICE PEARLS

Ibalizumab Therapy

- Ibalizumab is given intravenously every 2 weeks as maintenance therapy after an initial loading dose.
- Do not administer as an IV push or bolus.
- Administration is preferred in the cephalic vein, if accessible. Otherwise, another appropriate accessible vein may be used.
- Loading dose should be administered over 30 minutes followed by a 1-hour observation period. If no adverse reactions occur, subsequent maintenance doses may be infused over 15 minutes followed by a 15-minute observation period.
- Flush with 30 mL normal saline (NS) once the infusion is complete.
- Monitor for infusion-related reactions including dyspnea, angioedema, wheezing, chest pain, chest tightness, cough, hot flush, nausea, and vomiting.
- Monitor for anaphylaxis during and after infusion.
- Specific laboratory values that should be monitored include CD4 count and HIV RNA plasma levels.

Pharmacokinetic Enhancers

Pharmacokinetic enhancers (PEs) are not prescribed as monotherapy and are not considered stand-alone treatment for HIV infection. They increase the effectiveness of an HIV medication and are prescribed concomitantly with another ART to boost the effectiveness of that drug. The PE interrupts the absorption of the prime ART, causing the prime ART to remain bioavailable for a longer period and at a higher concentration.

PRACTICE PEARLS

Life Span Considerations With PEs

Children and Adolescents

- For patients weighing less than 35 kg, PEs are not recommended in combination with atazanavir.
- For patients weighing less than 40 kg, PEs are not recommended in combination with darunavir.

Pregnancy

- PEs, in combination therapy with darunavir or atazanavir, are not recommended during pregnancy.
- PEs are pregnancy category C, meaning risks cannot be ruled out. Limited data are available regarding the safety of administration during pregnancy.

Breastfeeding

- Breastfeeding should be avoided due to potential HIV transmission.

Contraception

- Due to the mechanism of action of PEs, interactions have been described with certain oral contraceptives.

Older Adult and Geriatric Considerations

- Insufficient data exist to suggest that PEs have different effects on older adult and geriatric populations.

Cobicistat
Pharmacokinetics. Cobicistat (COBI) is a mechanism-based inhibitor of P-450 isozymes that acts as a pharmacokinetic enhancer for HIV-1 PIs. It has no direct antiviral effect against HIV by itself, and it selectively inhibits CYP 3A4. Compared to ritonavir, cobicistat has a greater selectively for inhibiting CYP 3A4 and lacks enzyme-inducing properties.

Indications. Cobicistat is indicated for use in HIV patients to increase systemic exposure of the protease inhibitors that are taken once daily. It is given as a component of a combination of antiretrovirals for treating HIV-1 infection. Cobicistat is most frequently prescribed with atazanavir or darunavir in combination therapy. It is used in treatment-naïve or treatment-experienced patients (without darunavir resistance–associated substitutions).

Adult Dosage. The adult dosage is 150 mg orally once daily when used with atazanavir (300 mg orally once daily), darunavir (800 mg orally once daily), or elvitegravir (150 mg orally once daily).

Pediatric Dosage. The pediatric dosage is weight based. The dose is 150 mg orally once daily when used with atazanavir (300 mg orally once daily) for patients weighing at least 35 kg, or 150 mg orally once daily when used with darunavir (800 mg orally once daily) for patients weighing at least 40 kg. Dosing for patients who weigh less than 35 kg (cobicistat/atazanavir) or less than 40 kg (cobicistat/darunavir) should be prescribed in consultation with a pediatric HIV specialist.

Adverse Effects. The most common adverse reactions are jaundice and rash when cobicistat is used in combination with atazanavir. Renal failure has been reported in regimens containing both cobicistat and tenofovir disoproxil fumarate. At least 405 medications interact with cobicistat: 171 have major interactions, 218 have moderate interactions, and 16 have minor interactions.

Contraindications. Due to possible interference with other drugs while taking combination therapy including cobicistat, several drugs are contraindicated (Table 48.9). Severe and life-threatening consequences are also possible.

Monitoring. Monitor for interactions with other medications metabolized by CYP 3A4. CrCl should be determined before initiating therapy with cobicistat and monitored throughout treatment, as decreases in estimated CrCl have been described. In addition to baseline CrCl, monitor urine glucose, urine protein, and serum phosphorus prior to starting cobicistat plus tenofovir disoproxil fumarate therapy.

PRACTICE PEARLS

Cobicistat Therapy

- Cobicistat is not a stand-alone medication and should be prescribed with a PI.
- This medication should always be taken with food.
- Obtain baseline CrCl prior to starting a medication regimen including cobicistat, and monitor throughout.
- Follow the recommended weight-based dosing regimen for pediatric patients.

Combination HIV Medicines

Initial HIV medication therapy typically includes at least three different ART drugs from two or more HIV drug classes. As guidelines regarding HIV medication therapy evolved, so did the demand for single medications that included drugs in specific regimens. According to aidsinfo.nih.gov, the first HIV combination medication was approved in 1997, rising to 20+ such drugs by 2019. Medication therapy for HIV infection may contain more than one combination medication as well as single drugs depending on the needs of the patient. An example combination medication is listed in the following section, and Table 48.10 includes a complete list of these drugs with dosing and special considerations.

Truvada

Truvada is an HIV combination medication approved by the FDA in 2004. It contains two NRTIs: emtricitabine and tenofovir disoproxil fumarate. Truvada is used to treat HIV infection and in preexposure prophylaxis.

Pharmacokinetics. See the sections on emtricitabine and tenofovir disoproxil fumarate.

Indications. In adult and adolescent patients who weigh 17 kg or more, Truvada is used to treat HIV infection. In HIV-negative, at-risk adult, and adolescent patients who weigh 35 kg or more, Truvada may be used as preexposure prophylaxis.

PRACTICE PEARLS

Truvada Therapy

- For treatment of HIV-1 infection in adults and pediatric patients, follow weight-based dosing instructions.
- Test for HIV prior to initiating preexposure prophylaxis therapy.
- Prior to beginning Truvada therapy, all patients should be tested for HBV. Obtain baseline serum phosphorus, creatinine, estimated CrCl, urine glucose, and urine protein levels. These values should continue to be monitored during any ART regimen that includes Truvada.

Adverse Effects. Renal issues including renal failure, immune reconstitution syndrome, osteopenia, lactic acidosis, and hepatic impairment or failure are possible side effects of Truvada therapy. When taken for the treatment of HIV infection, the most commonly reported side effects were diarrhea, nausea, tiredness, headache, dizziness, depression, sleep disturbances, abnormal dreams, and rash. When taken for preexposure prophylaxis of HIV infection, the most commonly described side effects were headache, abdominal pain, and decreased weight.

Contraindications. Truvada used for preexposure prophylaxis should not be prescribed for patients who have unknown or positive HIV status. Consult full prescribing information prior to initiating.

There are 189 medications that have medication interactions with Truvada: 123 with major interactions, 63 with moderate interactions, and three with minor interactions. A full list and details of interactions are available at https://www.drugs.com/drug-interactions/emtricitabine-tenofovir,truvada.html.

Monitoring. Prior to beginning Truvada therapy, all patients should be tested for HBV and have baseline serum phosphorus, creatinine, estimated CrCl, urine glucose, and urine protein levels checked. These values should continue to be monitored during any ART regimen that includes Truvada.

TABLE 48.9 Common and/or Severe Adverse Effects Associated With Antiretroviral Therapy

Adverse Effect	NRTIs	NNRTIs	PIs	INSTIs	EIs
Bone Density Effects	**TDF:** Associated with greater loss of BMD than other NRTIs, especially when given with a PK booster. Osteomalacia may be associated with renal tubulopathy and urine phosphate wasting. **TAF:** Associated with smaller declines in BMD than those seen with TDF.	Decreases in BMD observed after the initiation of any ART regimen.			N/A
Bone Marrow Suppression	**ZDV:** Anemia, neutropenia	N/A	N/A	N/A	N/A
Cardiac Conduction Effects	N/A	**RPV, EFV:** QTc prolongation	**ATV/r and LPV/r:** PR prolongation. Risk factors include preexisting heart disease and concomitant use of medications that may cause PR prolongation.	N/A	**FTR:** QTc prolongation was seen at 4 times the recommended dose. Use with caution in patients with preexisting heart disease or QTc prolongation, or concomitant use of medications that may prolong QTc interval.
Cardiovascular Disease	**ABC:** Associated with an increased risk of MI in some cohort studies. Absolute risk greatest in patients with traditional CVD risk factors.	N/A	**Boosted DRV and LPV/r:** Associated with cardiovascular events in some cohorts	N/A	N/A
Cholelithiasis	N/A	N/A	**ATV:** Cholelithiasis and kidney stones may present concurrently. Median onset is 42 months after ARV initiation.	N/A	N/A
Diabetes Mellitus and Insulin Resistance	ZDV	N/A	LPV/r, but not with boosted ATV or DRV	N/A	N/A
Dyslipidemia	**ZDV > ABC:** ↑ TG and ↑ LDL **TAF:** ↑ TG, ↑ LDL, and ↑ HDL (no change in TC:HDL ratio) TDF has been associated with lower lipid levels than ABC or TAF.	**EFV:** ↑ TG, ↑ LDL, ↑ HDL	**All RTV- or COBI-Boosted PIs:** ↑ TG, ↑ LDL, ↑ HDL LPV/r > DRV/r and ATV/r: ↑ TG	**EVG/c:** ↑ TG, ↑ LDL, ↑ HDL	N/A

Continued

TABLE 48.9   Common and/or Severe Adverse Effects Associated With Antiretroviral Therapy—cont'd

Adverse Effect	DRUG CLASS				
	NRTIs	**NNRTIs**	**PIs**	**INSTIs**	**EIs**
Gastrointestinal Effects	**ZDV > Other NRTIs:** Nausea and vomiting	N/A	GI intolerance (e.g., diarrhea, nausea, vomiting) **LPV/r > DRV/r and ATV/r:** Diarrhea	**EVG/c:** Nausea and diarrhea	**IBA:** In a study of 40 people, 8% of patients reported diarrhea.
Hepatic Effects	**When TAF, TDF, 3TC, and FTC Are Withdrawn in Patients With HBV/ HIV Coinfection or When HBV Resistance Develops:** Patients with HBV/HIV coinfection may develop severe hepatic flares. **ZDV:** Steatosis	**EFV:** Most cases relate to an increase in transaminases. Fulminant hepatitis leading to death or hepatic failure requiring transplantation has been reported. **NVP:** Severe hepatotoxicity associated with skin rash or hypersensitivity. A 2-week NVP dose escalation may reduce risk. Risk is greater for females with pre-NVP CD4 counts >250 cells/mm³ and males with pre-NVP CD4 counts >400 cells/mm³. NVP should never be used for postexposure prophylaxis. EFV and NVP are not recommended in patients with hepatic insufficiency (Child-Pugh class B or C).	**All PIs:** Drug-induced hepatitis and hepatic decompensation have been reported. **ATV:** Jaundice due to indirect hyperbilirubinemia	**DTG:** Persons with HBV or HCV coinfection may be at higher risk of DTG-associated hepatotoxicity.	**MVC:** Hepatotoxicity with or without rash or HSRs reported. **FTR:** Transaminase elevation was seen more commonly in patients with HBV/HCV. Transient elevation of bilirubin observed in clinical trials.
Hypersensitivity Reaction, excluding rash alone or Stevens-Johnson syndrome	**ABC: Contraindicated** if patient is HLA-B*5701 positive. Median onset for HSR is 9 days after treatment initiation; 90% of reactions occur within 6 weeks. **HSR Symptoms (in Order of Descending Frequency):** Fever, rash, malaise, nausea, headache, myalgia, chills, diarrhea, vomiting, abdominal pain, dyspnea, arthralgia, and respiratory symptoms. Symptoms worsen with continuation of ABC. Patients should not be rechallenged with ABC if HSR is suspected, regardless of their HLA-B*5701 status.	**NVP:** Hypersensitivity syndrome of hepatotoxicity and rash that may be accompanied by fever, general malaise, fatigue, myalgias, arthralgias, blisters, oral lesions, conjunctivitis, facial edema, eosinophilia, renal dysfunction, granulocytopenia, or lymphadenopathy. Risk is greater for ARV-naïve females with pre-NVP CD4 counts >250 cells/mm³ and males with pre-NVP CD4 counts >400 cells/mm³. Overall, risk is higher for females than males. A 2-week dose escalation of NVP reduces risk.	N/A	**RAL:** HSR reported when RAL is given with other drugs also known to cause HSRs. All ARVs should be stopped if HSR occurs. **DTG:** Reported in <1% of patients in clinical development program	**MVC:** HSR reported as part of a syndrome related to hepatotoxicity.

Adverse Effect	Oral ARV Comments	RPV IM Injection	CAB IM Injection	T-20 SQ Injection
Injection Site Reaction		**Reported in >80% of patients;** reactions may include localized pain/discomfort (most common), nodules, induration, swelling, erythema, hematoma.	**Reported in >80% of patients;** reactions may include localized pain/discomfort (most common), nodules, induration, swelling, erythema, hematoma.	**Reported in almost all patients;** pain, tenderness, nodules, induration, ecchymosis, erythema.
Lactic Acidosis	**Reported With Older NRTIs, d4T, ZDV, and ddI,** but not with ABC, 3TC, FTC, TAF, or TDF.	N/A	N/A	N/A
Lipodystrophy	**Lipoatrophy:** Associated with history of exposure to d4T or ZDV (d4T > ZDV). Not reported with ABC, 3TC or FTC, TAF or TDF. **Lipohypertrophy:** Trunk fat increase observed with EFV-, PI-, and RAL-containing regimens; however, causal relationship has not been established.	N/A	N/A	N/A
Myopathy/Elevated Creatine Phosphokinase	**ZDV:** Myopathy. **RAL and DTG:** ↑ CPK, rhabdomyolysis, and myopathy or myositis have been reported.	N/A	N/A	N/A
Nervous System/Psychiatric Effects	**History of Exposure to ddI, ddC, or d4T:** Peripheral neuropathy (can be irreversible). **Neuropsychiatric Events:** EFV > RPV, DOR, ETR. **EFV:** Somnolence, insomnia, abnormal dreams, dizziness, impaired concentration, depression, psychosis, suicidal ideation, ataxia, encephalopathy. Some symptoms may subside or diminish after 2–4 weeks. Bedtime dosing and taking without food may reduce symptoms. Risk factors include psychiatric illness, concomitant use of agents with neuropsychiatric effects, and genetic factors. **RPV:** Depression, suicidality, sleep disturbances. **DOR:** Sleep disorders and disturbances, dizziness, altered sensorium; depression and suicidality and self-harm. **All INSTIs:** Insomnia, depression, and suicidality have been reported with INSTI use, primarily in patients with preexisting psychiatric conditions.	N/A	N/A	N/A

Continued

TABLE 48.9 Common and/or Severe Adverse Effects Associated With Antiretroviral Therapy—cont'd

Adverse Effect	NRTIs	NNRTIs	PIs	INSTIs	EIs
			DRUG CLASS		
Rash	**FTC:** Hyperpigmentation	All NNRTIs	ATV, DRV, and LPV/r	All INSTIs	MVC, IBA, FTR
Renal Effects/Urolithiasis	**TDF:** ↑ SCr, proteinuria, hypophosphatemia, urinary phosphate wasting, glycosuria, hypokalemia, and nonanion gap metabolic acidosis. Concurrent use of TDF with COBI- or RTV-containing regimens appears to increase risk. **TAF:** Less impact on renal biomarkers and lower rates of proteinuria than TDF.	**RPV:** Inhibits Cr secretion without reducing renal glomerular function.	**ATV and LPV/r:** Associated with increased risk of chronic kidney disease in a large cohort study. **ATV:** Stone or crystal formation. Adequate hydration may reduce risk. **COBI (as a Boosting Agent for DRV or ATV):** Inhibits Cr secretion without reducing renal glomerular function.	**DTG, COBI (as a boosting agent for EVG), and BIC:** Inhibits Cr secretion without reducing renal glomerular function	**IBA:** SCr abnormalities ≥Grade 3 reported in 10% of trial participants. **FTR:** SCr >1.8 x ULN seen in 19% in a clinical trial, but primarily with underlying renal disease or other drugs known to affect creatinine.
Stevens-Johnson Syndrome/Toxic Epidermal Necrosis	N/A	NVP > EFV, ETR, RPV	Some reported cases for DRV, LPV/r, and ATV	RAL	N/A
Weight Gain	Weight gain has been associated with initiation of ART and subsequent viral suppression. The increase appears to be greater with INSTIs than with other drug classes. Greater weight increase has also been reported with TAF than with TDF, and greater with DOR than EFV.			INSTI > other ARV drug classes	N/A

3TC, Lamivudine; ABC, abacavir; ART, antiretroviral therapy; ARV, antiretroviral; ATV, atazanavir; ATV/r, atazanavir/ritonavir; BIC, bictegravir; BMD, bone mineral density; CAB, cabotegravir; CD4, CD4 T lymphocyte; CNS, central nervous system; COBI, cobicistat; CPK, creatine phosphokinase; Cr, creatinine; CVD, cardiovascular disease; d4T, stavudine; ddC, zalcitabine; ddI, didanosine; DLV, delavirdine; DOR, doravirine; DRV, darunavir; DRV/r, darunavir/ritonavir; DTG, dolutegravir; ECG, electrocardiogram; EFV, efavirenz; EI, entry inhibitor; ETR, etravirine; EVG, elvitegravir; EVG/c, elvitegravir/cobicistat; FPV, fosamprenavir; FPV/r, fosamprenavir/ritonavir; FTC, emtricitabine; FTR, fostemsavir; GI, gastrointestinal; HBV, hepatitis B virus; HCV, hepatitis C virus; HDL, high-density lipoprotein; HSR, hypersensitivity reaction; IBA, ibalizumab; IDV, indinavir; IM, intramuscular; INSTI, integrase strand transfer inhibitor; LDL, low-density lipoprotein; LPV/r, lopinavir/ritonavir; MI, myocardial infarction; MVC, maraviroc; NFV, nelfinavir; NNRTI, non-nucleoside reverse transcriptase inhibitor; NRTI, nucleoside reverse transcriptase inhibitor; NVP, nevirapine; PI, protease inhibitor; RAL, raltegravir; RPV, rilpivirine; RTV, ritonavir; SCr, serum creatinine; SQ, subcutaneous; SQV, saquinavir; SQV/r, saquinavir/ritonavir; T-20, enfuvirtide; TAF, tenofovir alafenamide; TC, total cholesterol; TDF, tenofovir disoproxil fumarate; TG, triglycerides; TPV, tipranavir; TPV/r, tipranavir/ritonavir; ULN, upper limit of normal; ZDV, zidovudine

From National Institutes of Health (NIH). (2021). Common and/or severe adverse effects associated with antiretroviral therapy. Retrieved October 27, 2021, from https://clinicalinfo.hiv.gov/en/table/table-17-common-andor-severe-adverse-effects-associated-antiretroviral-therapy.

HIV Prophylaxis Treatments

Postexposure Prophylaxis (PEP)

PEP therapy is used to prevent the replication of viral RNA into normal cells of DNA through ART to prevent contraction of HIV after occupational exposure (Table 48.11). PEP is indicated when occupational exposure to HIV occurs. If possible, determine the HIV status of the exposure source to guide the need for HIV PEP therapy.

Nonoccupational Postexposure Prophylaxis (nPEP)

Health care providers should evaluate persons for nPEP no more than 72 hours after a potential nonoccupational exposure that presents a substantial risk for HIV acquisition. All persons considered for nPEP should be tested for HIV infection, preferably by using rapid combined Ag/Ab or antibody blood tests. If rapid HIV blood test results are unavailable and nPEP is otherwise indicated, it should be initiated without delay and can be discontinued if the patient is later determined to have HIV infection already or if the source is determined not to have HIV infection.

Risk factors include, but are not limited to, blood transfusion, needle sharing, needlesticks, receptive and insertive anal intercourse, receptive and insertive penile-vagina intercourse, and receptive and insertive oral intercourse. There is a negligible potential for infection in cases of biting, spitting, throwing body fluids, and sharing sexual toys. nPEP is not recommended when the reported exposure presents no substantial risk of HIV transmission. It is important for the health care provider to evaluate and treat possible nonoccupational HIV exposure (Box 48.1). If the need for treatment is determined, the health care provider will need to determine the plan (Table 48.12).

Preexposure Prophylaxis (PrEP)

Clinical Practice Guidelines provide comprehensive information on the use of daily oral antiretroviral preexposure prophylaxis (PrEP) to reduce the risk of acquiring HIV infection for adults engaged in high-risk behaviors. It is important to determine the benefit and risk of prophylaxis treatment (Table 48.13).

Prescriber Considerations for Antiviral and Antiretroviral Therapy

Clinical Practice Guidelines

Clinical practice guidelines are available to guide care and treatment for patients with HIV infection or for those who are at risk for HIV infection across the life span. Clinical guidelines are updated depending on available evidence-based research and best practices. It is the primary care provider's responsibility to remain current with the guidelines if providing care to HIV patients.

Clinical Reasoning for Antiviral and Antiretroviral Therapy

Consider the individual patient's health problem requiring antiviral and antiretroviral therapy. Patients should be counseled on what tests they can expect and what types of treatment may be recommended. Patients also should be counseled about the risks of transmission of their infection, and they should be instructed that all past and present partners should be notified of the infection. The infection should be reported in keeping with state guidelines. Determine the extent of the problem by considering the following:
- Comorbid health conditions
- Complications from HIV

TABLE 48.10   Combination Medications, Doses, and Special Considerations

Generic Name	Brand Name Abbreviation	Doses	Special Considerations
Abacavir/dolutegravir/lamivudine	**Triumeq** ABC + DTG + 3TC	Fixed-dose combination product containing 600 mg of abacavir, 50 mg of dolutegravir, and 300 mg of lamivudine The recommended dosage regimen of Triumeq in adults and in pediatric patients ≥40 kg is 1 tablet once daily orally with or without food.	Screen for the HLA-B*5701 allele prior to initiating therapy with Triumeq. Not recommended for patients with CrCl <50 mL/minute or for those with mild hepatic impairment. Contraindicated in patients with moderate or severe hepatic impairment.

A complete list of side effects and possible adverse reactions can be found at https://www.drugs.com/sfx/triumeq-side-effects.html.

A complete list of drug interactions can be found at https://www.drugs.com/drug-interactions/abacavir-dolutegravir-lamivudine,triumeq.html.

Abacavir/lamivudine	**Epzicom** ABC + 3TC	Combination of abacavir 600 mg and lamivudine 300 mg The recommended dosage of Epzicom for adults is 1 tablet taken orally once daily, in combination with other ARTs, with or without food. Pediatric patients must weigh ≥25 kg and take once daily in combination with other ARTs.	Screen for the HLA-B*5701 allele prior to initiating therapy with Epzicom. Not recommended for patients with CrCl <50 mL/minute or for those with mild hepatic impairment. Contraindicated in patients with moderate or severe hepatic impairment.

A complete list of side effects and possible adverse reactions can be found at https://www.drugs.com/sfx/epzicom-side-effects.html.

A complete list of drug interactions can be found at https://www.drugs.com/drug-interactions/abacavir-lamivudine,epzicom.html.

Abacavir/lamivudine/zidovudine	**Trizivir** ABC + 3TC + ZDV	Combination of abacavir 300 mg, lamivudine 150 mg, and zidovudine 300 mg The recommended dosage of Trizivir is 1 tablet taken orally twice daily with or without food for adults and pediatric patients ≥40 kg.	Screen for the HLA-B*5701 allele prior to initiating therapy with Trizivir. Not recommended for pediatric patients <40 kg, patients with CrCl <50 mL/minute, or those with mild hepatic impairment. Contraindicated in patients with moderate or severe hepatic impairment.

A complete list of side effects and possible adverse reactions can be found at https://www.drugs.com/sfx/trizivir-side-effects.html

A complete list of drug interactions can be found at https://www.drugs.com/drug-interactions/abacavir-lamivudine-zidovudine,trizivir.html

Atazanavir/cobicistat	**Evotaz** ATV + COBI	Fixed-dose combination of atazanavir 300 mg and cobicistat 150 mg The recommended dosage for adults is 1 tablet once daily with food in conjunction with other ARTs.	Renal laboratory testing including estimated CrCl, serum creatinine, and urinalysis with microscopic examination should be performed prior to initiation and throughout use of Evotaz. Not recommended for patients with ESRD on hemodialysis, those with a CrCl <70 mL/minute, or those with any degree of hepatic impairment. Coadministration of Evotaz and tenofovir DF in combination with concomitant or recent use of a nephrotoxic agent is not recommended.

A complete list of side effects and possible adverse reactions can be found at https://www.drugs.com/sfx/evotaz-side-effects.html.

A complete list of drug interactions can be found at https://www.drugs.com/drug-interactions/atazanavir-cobicistat,evotaz.html.

TABLE 48.10   Combination Medications, Doses, and Special Considerations—cont'd

Generic Name	Brand Name Abbreviation	Doses	Special Considerations
Bictegravir/emtric-itabine/tenofovir alafenamide fumarate	**Biktarvy** BIC + FTC + TAF	Biktarvy is a 3-drug, fixed-dose combination product containing 50 mg of bictegravir, 200 mg of emtricitabine, and 25 mg of tenofovir alafenamide. The recommended dosage of Biktarvy is 1 tablet taken orally once daily with or without food in adults and pediatric patients ≥25 kg.	Prior to or when initiating Biktarvy, test patient for HBV infection. Prior to or when initiating Biktarvy, and during treatment with Biktarvy, assess serum creatinine, estimated CrCl, urine glucose, and urine protein in all patients as clinically appropriate. In patients with chronic kidney disease, also assess serum phosphorus. Biktarvy is not recommended in patients with estimated CrCl < 30 mL/minute, or those with severe hepatic impairment.

A complete list of side effects and possible adverse reactions can be found at https://www.drugs.com/sfx/biktarvy-side-effects.html.

A complete list of drug interactions can be found at https://www.drugs.com/drug-interactions/bictegravir-emtricitabine-tenofovir-alafenamide,biktarvy.html.

Generic Name	Brand Name Abbreviation	Doses	Special Considerations
Cobicistat/darunavir	**Prezcobix** COBI + DRV	Prezcobix is a fixed-dose combination product containing 800 mg of darunavir and 150 mg of cobicistat. The recommended dosage of Prezcobix is 1 tablet taken once daily orally with food. Administer Prezcobix in conjunction with other antiretroviral agents.	HIV genotypic testing is recommended for antiretroviral treatment-experienced patients. Prezcobix coadministered with tenofovir DF is not recommended in patients who have an estimated CrCl <70 mL/min. Prezcobix is not recommended for use in patients with severe hepatic impairment. Prezcobix is not recommended during pregnancy, because of substantially lower exposures of darunavir and cobicistat during the second and third trimesters.

A complete list of side effects and possible adverse reactions can be found at https://www.drugs.com/sfx/prezcobix-side-effects.html.

A complete list of drug interactions can be found at https://www.drugs.com/drug-interactions/cobicistat-darunavir,prezcobix.html.

Generic Name	Brand Name Abbreviation	Doses	Special Considerations
Cobicistat/darunavir/ emtricitabine/ tenofovir alafen-amide fumarate	**Symtuza** COBI + DRV + FTC + TAF	Symtuza is a 4-drug, fixed-dose combination product containing 800 mg of darunavir, 150 mg of cobicistat, 200 mg of emtric-itabine, and 10 mg of tenofovir alafenamide. The recommended dosage of Symtuza is 1 tablet taken orally once daily with food in adults and pediatric patients ≥40 kg.	Prior to or when initiating Symtuza, test patients for HBV infection. Prior to or when initiating Symtuza, and during treatment with Symtuza, on a clinically appropriate schedule, assess serum creatinine, estimated CrCl, urine glucose, and urine protein in all patients. In patients with chronic kidney disease, also assess serum phosphorus. Symtuza is not recommended in patients with CrCl <30 mL/minute, or those with severe hepatic impairment. Symtuza is not recommended during pregnancy, because of substantially lower exposures of darunavir and cobicistat during the second and third trimesters.

Continued

TABLE 48.10 **Combination Medications, Doses, and Special Considerations—cont'd**

Generic Name	Brand Name Abbreviation	Doses	Special Considerations
A complete list of side effects and possible adverse reactions can be found at https://www.drugs.com/sfx/symtuza-side-effects.html.			
A complete list of drug interactions can be found at https://www.drugs.com/drug-interactions/cobicistat-darunavir-emtricitabine-tenofovir-alafenamide,symtuza.html.			
Cobicistat/elvitegravir/emtricitabine/tenofovir alafenamide fumarate	**Genvoya** COBI + EVG + FTC + TAF	Genvoya is a 4-drug, fixed-dose combination product containing 150 mg of elvitegravir, 150 mg of cobicistat, 200 mg of emtricitabine, and 10 mg of tenofovir alafenamide. The recommended dosage of Genvoya is 1 tablet taken orally once daily with food in adults and pediatric patients ≥25 kg and CrCl ≥30 mL/min; *or* adults with CrCl <15 mL/mi who are receiving chronic hemodialysis. On days of hemodialysis, administer Genvoya after completion of hemodialysis treatment.	Prior to or when initiating Genvoya, test patients for HBV infection. Prior to or when initiating Genvoya, and during treatment with Genvoya on a clinically appropriate schedule, assess serum creatinine, estimated CrCl, urine glucose, and urine protein in all patients. In patients with chronic kidney disease, also assess serum phosphorus. Genvoya is not recommended in patients with severe renal impairment (estimated CrCl of 15 to <30 mL/min); or ESRD; estimated CrCl <15 mL/min) who are not receiving chronic hemodialysis; or in patients with severe hepatic impairment. Genvoya is not recommended for use during pregnancy, because of substantially lower exposures of cobicistat and elvitegravir during the second and third trimesters.
A complete list of side effects and possible adverse reactions can be found at https://www.drugs.com/sfx/genvoya-side-effects.html.			
A complete list of drug interactions can be found at https://www.drugs.com/drug-interactions/cobicistat-elvitegravir-emtricitabine-tenofovir-alafenamide,genvoya.html.			
Cobicistat/elvitegravir/emtricitabine/tenofovir disoproxil fumarate	**Stribild** COBI + EVG + FTC + TDF	Stribild is a 4-drug, fixed-dose combination product containing 150 mg of elvitegravir, 150 mg of cobicistat, 200 mg of emtricitabine, and 300 mg of TDF. The recommended dosage of Stribild is 1 tablet taken orally once daily with food in adults and pediatric patients ≥12 yr, ≥35 kg, and with CrCl ≥70 mL/minute.	Prior to initiation of Stribild, test patients for HBV infection. Prior to initiation and during use of Stribild, on a clinically appropriate schedule, assess serum creatinine, estimated CrCl, urine glucose, and urine protein in all patients. In patients with chronic kidney disease, also assess serum phosphorus. Initiation of Stribild in patients with estimated CrCl <70 mL/minute or in those with severe hepatic impairment is not recommended. Stribild is not recommended for use during pregnancy, because of substantially lower exposures of cobicistat and elvitegravir during the second and third trimesters.
A complete list of side effects and possible adverse reactions can be found at https://www.drugs.com/sfx/stribild-side-effects.html.			
A complete list of drug interactions can be found at https://www.drugs.com/drug-interactions/cobicistat-elvitegravir-emtricitabine-tenofovir,stribild.html.			
Dolutegravir/rilpivirine	**Juluca** DTG + RPV	Combination of dolutegravir 50 mg and rilpivirine 25 mg The recommended dosage of Juluca is 1 tablet orally once daily with a meal.	Perform pregnancy testing before initiation of Juluca in individuals of childbearing potential. If Juluca is coadministered with rifabutin, take an additional 25-mg tablet of rilpivirine with Juluca once daily with a meal for the duration of the rifabutin coadministration.

TABLE 48.10 Combination Medications, Doses, and Special Considerations—cont'd

Generic Name	Brand Name Abbreviation	Doses	Special Considerations
A complete list of side effects and possible adverse reactions can be found at https://www.drugs.com/sfx/juluca-side-effects.html.			
A complete list of drug interactions can be found at https://www.drugs.com/drug-interactions/dolutegravir-rilpivirine,juluca.html.			
Dolutegravir/lamivudine	**Dovato** DTG + 3TC	Dovato is a fixed-dose combination product containing 50 mg of dolutegravir and 300 mg of lamivudine. The recommended dosage regimen of Dovato in adults is 1 tablet orally once daily with or without food.	Prior to or when initiating Dovato, test patients for HBV infection. Perform pregnancy testing before initiation of Dovato in individuals of childbearing potential. Dovato is not recommended in patients with CrCl <50 mL/minute or for those with severe hepatic impairment.
A complete list of side effects and possible adverse reactions can be found at https://www.drugs.com/sfx/dovato-side-effects.html.			
A complete list of drug interactions can be found at https://www.drugs.com/drug-interactions/dolutegravir-lamivudine,dovato.html.			
Doravirine/lamivudine/tenofovir disoproxil fumarate	**Delstrigo** DOR + 3TC + TDF	Delstrigo is a fixed-dose combination product containing 100 mg of doravirine, 300 mg of lamivudine, and 300 mg of tenofovir disoproxil fumarate. The recommended dosage of Delstrigo in adults is 1 tablet orally once daily with or without food.	Prior to or when initiating Delstrigo, test patients for HBV infection. Prior to or when initiating Delstrigo, and during treatment with Delstrigo, on a clinically appropriate schedule, assess serum creatinine, estimated CrCl, urine glucose, and urine protein in all patients. In patients with chronic kidney disease, also assess serum phosphorus. Delstrigo is not recommended in patients with estimated CrCl <50 mL/minute.
A complete list of side effects and possible adverse reactions can be found at https://www.drugs.com/sfx/delstrigo-side-effects.html.			
A complete list of drug interactions can be found at https://www.drugs.com/drug-interactions/doravirine-lamivudine-tenofovir,delstrigo.html.			
Efavirenz/emtricitabine/tenofovir disoproxil fumarate	**Atripla** EFV + FTC + TDF	Atripla is a 3-drug, fixed-dose combination product containing 600 mg of efavirenz, 200 mg of emtricitabine, and 300 mg of tenofovir disoproxil fumarate. The recommended dosage of Atripla in adults and pediatric patients ≥40 kg is 1 tablet orally once daily taken on an empty stomach. Dosing at bedtime may improve the tolerability of nervous system symptoms. If Atripla is coadministered with rifampin in patients ≥50 kg, dosage is 1 tablet of Atripla once daily followed by 1 additional 200 mg/day of efavirenz.	Prior to or when initiating Atripla, test patients for HBV infection. Prior to or when initiating Atripla, and during treatment with Atripla, on a clinically appropriate schedule, assess serum creatinine, estimated CrCl, urine glucose, and urine protein in all patients. In patients with chronic kidney disease, also assess serum phosphorus. Monitor hepatic function prior to and during treatment. Perform pregnancy testing before initiation of Atripla in adolescents and adults of childbearing potential. Atripla is not recommended in patients with moderate or severe renal impairment (estimated CrCl <50 mL/minute) or moderate to severe hepatic impairment.

Continued

TABLE 48.10 Combination Medications, Doses, and Special Considerations—cont'd

Generic Name	Brand Name Abbreviation	Doses	Special Considerations
A complete list of side effects and possible adverse reactions can be found at https://www.drugs.com/sfx/atripla-side-effects.html.			
A complete list of drug interactions can be found at https://www.drugs.com/drug-interactions/efavirenz-emtricitabine-tenofovir,atripla.html.			
Efavirenz/lamivudine/ tenofovir diso-proxil fumarate	**Symfi, Symfi Lo** EFV + 3TC + TDF	Symfi Lo is a 3-drug, fixed-dose combination product containing 400 mg of efavirenz, 300 mg of lamivudine, and 300 mg of tenofovir disoproxil fumarate. The recommended dosage of Symfi Lo in HIV-1–infected adults and pediatric patients ≥35 kg is 1 tablet orally once daily. Symfi Lo tablets should be taken on an empty stomach, preferably at bedtime. Dosing at bedtime may improve the tolerability of nervous system symptoms.	Prior to or when initiating Symfi Lo, test patients for HBV infection. Prior to or when initiating Symfi Lo, and during treatment with Symfi Lo, on a clinically appropriate schedule, assess serum creatinine, estimated CrCl, urine glucose, and urine protein in all patients. In patients with chronic kidney disease, also assess serum phosphorus. Monitor hepatic function prior to and during treatment. Not recommended for patients with impaired renal function (CrCl <50 mL/minute), patients with ESRD requiring hemodialysis, or patients with moderate or severe hepatic impairment.
A complete list of side effects and possible adverse reactions can be found at https://www.drugs.com/sfx/symfi-lo-side-effects.html.			
A complete list of drug interactions can be found at https://www.drugs.com/drug-interactions/efavirenz-lamivudine-tenofovir,symfi-lo.html.			
Emtricitabine/lopi-navir/ritonavir/te-nofovir disoproxil fumarate	**AccessPak for HIV PEP Expanded with Kaletra** FTC + LPV + RTV + TDF	Situation-specific dosing information below.	Special considerations information below.
Situation-specific dosing information can be found at http://www.rxabbvie.com/pdf/kaletratabpi.pdf.			
Special considerations information can be found at https://www.kaletra.com/?cid=ppc_ppd_kaletra_ggl_br_2259#isi.			
A complete list of side effects and possible adverse reactions can be found at https://www.drugs.com/sfx/accesspak-for-hiv-pep-expanded-with-kaletra-side-effects.html.			
A complete list of drug interactions can be found at https://www.drugs.com/drug-interactions/emtricitabine-lopinavir-ritonavir-tenofovir,accesspak-for-hiv-pep-expanded-with-kaletra.html.			
Emtricitabine/rilpi-virine/tenofovir alafenamide fumarate	**Odefsey** FTC + RPV + TAF	Odefsey is a 3-drug, fixed-dose combination product containing 200 mg of emtricitabine, 25 mg of rilpivirine, and 25 mg of tenofovir alafenamide. The recommended dosage of Odefsey is 1 tablet orally once daily taken with a meal in adults and pediatric patients ≥35 kg and CrCl ≥30 mL/minute. For pregnant patients who are already on Odefsey prior to pregnancy and are virologically suppressed (HIV-1 RNA <50 copies/mL), 1 tablet of Odefsey once daily may be continued.	Prior to or when initiating Odefsey, test patients for HBV infection. Prior to or when initiating Odefsey, and during treatment with Odefsey, on a clinically appropriate schedule, assess serum creatinine, estimated CrCl, urine glucose, and urine protein in all patients. In patients with chronic kidney disease, also assess serum phosphorus. Lower exposures of rilpivirine, a component of Odefsey, were observed during pregnancy; therefore, viral load should be monitored closely. Odefsey is not recommended in patients with severe renal impairment (estimated CrCl of 15 to <30 mL/minute) or ESRD (estimated CrCl <15 mL/minute) who are not receiving chronic hemodialysis.

TABLE 48.10 Combination Medications, Doses, and Special Considerations—cont'd

Generic Name	Brand Name Abbreviation	Doses	Special Considerations
A complete list of side effects and possible adverse reactions can be found at https://www.drugs.com/sfx/odefsey-side-effects.html.			
A complete list of drug interactions can be found at https://www.drugs.com/drug-interactions/emtricitabine-rilpivirine-tenofovir-alafenamide,odefsey.html.			
Emtricitabine/rilpivirine/tenofovir disoproxil fumarate	**Complera** FTC + RPV + TDF	Complera is a 3-drug, fixed-dose combination product containing 200 mg of emtricitabine, 25 mg of rilpivirine, and 300 mg of tenofovir disoproxil fumarate. The recommended dosage of Complera in adult and pediatric patients ≥35 kg is 1 tablet orally once daily with food. If Complera is coadministered with rifabutin, take an additional 25-mg tablet of rilpivirine (Edurant) with Complera once daily with a meal for the duration of the rifabutin coadministration.	Prior to or when initiating Complera, test patients for HBV infection. Prior to or when initiating Complera, and during treatment with Complera, on a clinically appropriate schedule, assess serum creatinine, estimated CrCl, urine glucose, and urine protein in all patients. In patients with chronic kidney disease, also assess serum phosphorus. Complera is not recommended in patients with moderate or severe renal impairment (estimated CrCl <50 mL/minute).
A complete list of side effects and possible adverse reactions can be found at https://www.drugs.com/sfx/complera-side-effects.html.			
A complete list of drug interactions can be found at https://www.drugs.com/drug-interactions/emtricitabine-rilpivirine-tenofovir,complera.html.			
Emtricitabine/tenofovir alafenamide fumarate	**Descovy** FTC + TAF	**Recommended Dosage for Treatment of HIV-1 Infection in Adults and Pediatric Patients ≥25 kg:** Descovy is a 2-drug, fixed-dose combination product containing 200 mg of emtricitabine and 25 mg of tenofovir alafenamide. The recommended dosage of Descovy for treatment of HIV-1 is 1 tablet orally once daily with or without food in adults and pediatric patients ≥25 kg and CrCl ≥30 mL/minute; or adults with CrCl <15 mL/minute who are receiving chronic hemodialysis. On days of hemodialysis, administer the daily dose of Descovy after completion of hemodialysis treatment. **Recommended Dosage for HIV-1 PrEP in Adults and Adolescents ≥35 kg:** The dosage of Descovy for HIV-1 PrEP is 1 tablet (containing 200 mg of emtricitabine and 25 mg of tenofovir alafenamide) orally once daily with or without food in HIV-1–uninfected adults and adolescents ≥35 kg and with a CrCl ≥30 mL/minute; or adults with CrCl <15 mL/minute who are receiving chronic hemodialysis. On days of hemodialysis, administer the daily dose of Descovy after completion of hemodialysis treatment.	Prior to or when initiating Descovy, test patients for HBV infection. Prior to or when initiating Descovy, and during treatment with Descovy, on a clinically appropriate schedule, assess serum creatinine, estimated CrCl, urine glucose, and urine protein in all patients. In patients with chronic kidney disease, also assess serum phosphorus. Screen all individuals for HIV-1 infection immediately prior to initiating Descovy for HIV-1 PrEP and at least once every 3 months while taking Descovy, and upon diagnosis of any other STIs. If recent (<1 month) exposures to HIV-1 are suspected or clinical symptoms consistent with acute HIV-1 infection are present, use a test approved or cleared by the FDA as an aid in the diagnosis of acute or primary HIV-1 infection. Descovy is not recommended in individuals with severe renal impairment (estimated CrCl of 15 to <30 mL/minute) or ESRD (estimated CrCl <15 mL/minute) who are not receiving chronic hemodialysis.

Continued

TABLE 48.10 Combination Medications, Doses, and Special Considerations—cont'd

Generic Name	Brand Name Abbreviation	Doses	Special Considerations
A complete list of side effects and possible adverse reactions can be found at https://www.drugs.com/sfx/descovy-side-effects.html.			
A complete list of drug interactions can be found at https://www.drugs.com/drug-interactions/emtricitabine-tenofovir-alafenamide,descovy.html.			
Emtricitabine/tenofovir disoproxil fumarate	**Truvada, AccessPak for HIV PEP Basic** FTC + TDF	Truvada: emtricitabine 100 mg and tenofovir disoproxil fumarate 150 mg; emtricitabine 133 mg and tenofovir disoproxil fumarate 200 mg; emtricitabine 167 mg and tenofovir disoproxil fumarate 250 mg; or emtricitabine 200 mg and tenofovir disoproxil fumarate 300 mg Situation-specific dosing regimen below.	Emtricitabine/tenofovir disoproxil fumarate is not indicated for the treatment of chronic HBV infection and the safety and efficacy have not been established in patients coinfected with HBV and HIV-1. Severe acute exacerbations of hepatitis B have been reported in patients who are coinfected with HBV and HIV-1 and have discontinued emtricitabine/tenofovir; monitor hepatic function upon discontinuation of therapy. Emtricitabine/tenofovir disoproxil fumarate used for a PrEP indication is only for HIV-negative individuals; status must be confirmed immediately prior to initiating and periodically during use. Drug-resistant HIV-1 variants have been identified with use of emtricitabine/tenofovir disoproxil fumarate for a PrEP indication following undetected acute HIV-1 infection.
Situation-specific dosing regimen can be found at https://www.drugs.com/dosage/emtricitabine-tenofovir.html.			
A complete list of side effects and possible adverse reactions can be found at https://www.drugs.com/sfx/accesspak-for-hiv-pep-basic-side-effects.html.			
A complete list of drug interactions can be found at https://www.drugs.com/drug-interactions/emtricitabine-tenofovir,accesspak-for-hiv-pep-basic.html.			
Lamivudine/tenofovir disoproxil fumarate	**Cimduo, Temixys** 3TC + TDF	Cimduo is a 2-drug, fixed-dose combination product containing 300 mg of lamivudine and 300 mg of tenofovir disoproxil fumarate. The recommended dosage of Cimduo in HIV-1–infected adult and pediatric patients ≥35 kg is 1 tablet orally once daily with or without food.	Prior to or when initiating Cimduo, test patients for HBV infection. Prior to or when initiating Cimduo, and during treatment with Cimduo, on a clinically appropriate schedule, assess serum creatinine, estimated CrCl, urine glucose, and urine protein in all patients. Not recommended for patients with impaired renal function (CrCl <50 mL/minute) or patients with ESRD requiring hemodialysis.
A complete list of side effects and possible adverse reactions can be found at https://www.drugs.com/sfx/cimduo-side-effects.html.			
A complete list of drug interactions can be found at https://www.drugs.com/drug-interactions/lamivudine-tenofovir,cimduo.html.			

TABLE 48.10   Combination Medications, Doses, and Special Considerations—cont'd

Generic Name	Brand Name Abbreviation	Doses	Special Considerations
Lamivudine/zidovudine	**Combivir** 3TC + ZDV	**Recommended Dosage for Adults and Adolescents:** The recommended dosage of Combivir in HIV-1–infected adults and adolescents ≥30 kg is 1 tablet (containing 150 mg of lamivudine and 300 mg of zidovudine) orally twice daily. **Recommended Dosage for Pediatric Patients:** The recommended dosage of scored Combivir tablets for pediatric patients ≥30 kg and for whom a solid oral dosage form is appropriate is 1 tablet orally twice daily. Before prescribing Combivir tablets, children should be assessed for the ability to swallow tablets. If a child is unable to reliably swallow a Combivir tablet, the liquid oral formulations should be prescribed: Epivir (lamivudine) oral solution and Retrovir (zidovudine) syrup.	Because Combivir is a fixed-dose tablet and cannot be dose adjusted, Combivir is not recommended for: • Pediatric patients <30 kg • Patients with CrCl <50 mL/minute • Patients with hepatic impairment • Patients experiencing dose-limiting adverse reactions

A complete list of side effects and possible adverse reactions can be found at https://www.drugs.com/sfx/combivir-side-effects.html.

A complete list of drug interactions can be found at https://www.drugs.com/drug-interactions/lamivudine-zidovudine,combivir.html.

ART, Antiretroviral therapy; *CrCl,* creatinine clearance; *ESRD,* end-stage renal disease; *FDA,* U.S. Food and Drug Administration; *HBV,* hepatitis B virus; *PrEP,* preexposure prophylaxis; *STI,* sexually transmitted infection.

• The severity of symptoms as perceived by the patient
• Prior or present treatment

Determine the desired therapeutic outcome based on the patient's health problem. It will be essential for any clinician who treats HIV-positive patients to consult the latest sources for prescribing and treatment information. Once infection has been identified, the patient should be referred to an infectious disease specialist or a center that provides care to HIV-infected individuals. The National Clinical Consultation Center, available at http://nccc.ucsf.edu, can assist clinicians in treating HIV patients. Considerations regarding insurance is an unfortunate but realistic concern because care and treatments are costly. The patient should be reassured that the infectious disease experts partner with primary care providers, and that the patient's relationship with their primary care provider will continue. Patient concerns may center on the ability to infect others and complications. Decreased quality of life may result from poor adherence, opportunistic infection, and/or the development of resistant strains leading to AIDS.

Assess the selected pharmacotherapy for its appropriateness for an individual patient by considering the medication's side effects and the patient's age, race/ethnicity, comorbidities, and genetic factors. The selection of pharmacotherapeutic options includes:

• Identifying and targeting symptoms that are most important to the patient. Evaluate the duration and severity of symptoms.
• Age, comorbid conditions, and concomitant drug use.
• Consideration of the efficacy of the medication and the potential for adverse effects.
• Patient preference (number of pills, frequency, and form).
• Cost.
• Results of genomics and phenomics testing.

Ensure complete patient and family understanding about the medication prescribed using a variety of education strategies. Written materials, printed handouts, and electronic resources reinforce information that was verbally given during an office visit. Encourage questions at the end of each new concept, at the end of each visit, and between visits. Electronic patient portals offer a convenient method of communication that some patients prefer to voice mail. For patients interested in accurate internet resources, notify them of HIV.gov and the Centers for Disease Control and Prevention's (CDC) HIV website (https://www.cdc.gov/hiv/default.html), which contain patient information including definitions, diagnosis, treatments, and prevention tips.

Conduct follow-up and monitoring of patient responses to pharmacotherapies. At each visit, review the patient history

TABLE 48.11 HIV Postexposure Prophylaxis Regimens

Preferred HIV PEP Regimen

Raltegravir (Isentress; RAL) 400 mg orally twice daily plus

Truvada,1 tablet orally once daily

[Tenofovir DF (Viread; TDF) 300 mg + emtricitabine (Emtriva; FTC) 200 mg]

Alternative Regimens

(May combine one drug or drug pair from the left column with one pair of nucleoside/nucleotide reverse transcriptase inhibitors from the right column. Prescribers unfamiliar with these agents/regimens should consult physicians familiar with the agents and their toxicities.)[a]

Raltegravir (Isentress; RAL)	Tenofovir DF (Viread; TDF) + emtricitabine (Emtriva; FTC); available as Truvada
Darunavir (Prezista; DRV) + ritonavir (Norvir; RTV)	Tenofovir DF (Viread; TDF) + lamivudine (Epivir; 3TC)
Etravirine (Intelence; ETR)	Zidovudine (Retrovir; ZDV; AZT) + lamivudine (Epivir; 3TC); available as Combivir®
Rilpivirine (Edurant; RPV)	Zidovudine (Retrovir; ZDV; AZT) + emtricitabine (Emtriva; FTC)
Atazanavir (Reyataz; ATV) + ritonavir (Norvir; RTV)	
Lopinavir/ritonavir (Kaletra; LPV/RTV)	

The following alternative is a complete fixed-dose combination regimen and no additional antiretrovirals are needed: Stribild (elvitegravir, cobicistat, tenofovir DF, emtricitabine)

Alternative Antiretroviral Agents for Use as PEP Only With Expert Consultation[b]

Abacavir (Ziagen; ABC)

Efavirenz (Sustiva; EFV)

Enfuvirtide (Fuzeon; T20)

Fosamprenavir (Lexiva; FOSAPV)

Maraviroc (Selzentry; MVC)

Saquinavir (Invirase; SQV)

Stavudine (Zerit; d4T)

Antiretroviral Agents Generally Not Recommended for Use as PEP

Didanosine (Videx EC; ddl)

Nelfinavir (Viracept; NFV)

Tipranavir (Aptivus; TPV)

Antiretroviral Agents Contraindicated as PEP

Nevirapine (Viramune; NVP)

— For consultation or assistance with HIV PEP, contact PEPline at 1-888-448-4911 or www.nccc.ucsf.edu/about_nccc/pepline/.

[a]The alternative regimens are listed in order of preference; however, other alternatives may be reasonable based on patient and clinician preference.
DF, Disoproxil fumarate; PO, orally.
From Kuhar, D. T., Henderson, D. K., Struble, K. A., Heneine, W., Thomas, V., Cheever, L. W., ... Panlilio, Adelisa L. (2013, May). Updated U.S. Public Health Service guidelines for the management of occupational exposures to HIV and recommendations for postexposure prophylaxis. Retrieved October 27, 2021, from https://stacks.cdc.gov/view/cdc/20711.

Evaluation and Treatment for Possible Nonoccupational Postexposure Prophylaxis (nPEP)

Initial nPEP Evaluation

- Obtain history of potential exposure event
  - HIV and HBV status of exposed person and source person, if available
  - Timing of most recent potential exposure
  - Type of exposure event and risk for HIV acquisition
  - Determination of whether nPEP is indicated
- If nPEP is indicated:
  - Conduct laboratory testing
    - HIV blood test (rapid combined Ag/Ab test, if available)
    - STIs, HBV, HCV, pregnancy, and chemistries, as indicated
- Prescribe 28-day nPEP course
  - Educate patient about potential regimen-specific side effects and adverse events
  - Counsel patient about medication adherence
  - Provide patient with nPEP prescription *or* full 28-day nPEP course *or* nPEP starter pack and prescription
- When necessary, assist patient with obtaining nPEP medication through a medication assistance program for the prescribed regimen
- For all persons evaluated:
  - Prescribe prophylaxis for STIs and HBV infection, if indicated
  - Provide counseling related to HIV prevention strategies as appropriate
  - Document sexual assault findings and fulfill local reporting requirements
  - Conduct confidential reporting of newly diagnosed STIs and HIV infection to health department
  - Link HIV-infected persons to relevant medical and psychosocial support services

Follow-Up Evaluations for Persons Prescribed nPEP

- Conduct HIV and any other indicated laboratory testing
- Consider changing nPEP regimen if indicated by side effects or results of initial testing
- Provide additional counseling and support for medication adherence and HIV prevention, if indicated

Ag/Ab, Antigen/antibody combination test; *HBV,* hepatitis B virus; *HCV,* hepatitis C virus; *HIV,* human immunodeficiency virus; *STI,* sexually transmitted infection.
From Dominguez, K. L., Smith, D. K., Thomas, V., Crepaz, N., Lang, K., Heneine, W., ... Weidle, P. J. (2016, April). Updated guidelines for antiretroviral postexposure prophylaxis after sexual, injection drug use, or other nonoccupational exposure to HIV—United States, 2016. Retrieved October 27, 2021, from https://stacks.cdc.gov/view/cdc/38856.

with attention to changes that may have occurred since the last visit. A thorough assessment must be completed along with monitoring laboratory results to assess how the treatment affects organ function. Consult the latest practice guidelines for the most up-to-date treatment regimens. Review current medications, taking care to review OTC medications and herbal supplements. Review adverse effects that the patient experienced since the last visit. Discuss improvement or lack of improvement in symptoms (severity and frequency), medication adherence, and level of satisfaction with the therapy.

Teaching Points for Antiviral and Antiretroviral Therapy

Health Promotion Strategies

The following strategies and practices should be presented to patients to help them become full partners in their health care:

- To promote a healthy lifestyle, perform at least 150 minutes per week of moderate-intensity or 75 minutes per week of vigorous-intensity aerobic physical activity.
- Eat a diet that includes a daily intake of multiple servings of fruits and vegetables.
- If you have difficulty remembering scheduled appointments, request to receive reminders via phone, text message, email, or regular mail. If you routinely miss these appointments, talk with your health care provider to learn why these tests are important.
- Wash your hands frequently and avoid crowded areas to prevent opportunistic infections.
- Wear a mask and use hand sanitizer frequently in public.
- Implement safe-sex practices.
- Do not share needles.
- If female and of childbearing age, use an effective means of birth control.

Patient Education for Medication Safety

Antiretrovirals are commonly prescribed for patients who are HIV positive or as a prophylactic to prevent HIV contraction. These medications must be taken as prescribed; otherwise, serious complications can occur with resistance to future treatment or can increase the risk of organ dysfunction. Advanced practice nurses need to stress the following points and actions to patients for safe medication management:

- Take your antiretroviral medication(s) as directed. If you miss a dose, take the missed dose as soon as possible on the same day, but skip it if it is less than 6 hours before the next scheduled dose.
- Never double up a dose to make up for a missed dose.
- Do not stop taking any medication, especially any antiretroviral, without first talking to your health care provider.
- Antiretroviral medications can cause your eyes or skin to turn yellow and urine a dark amber. Call your health care provider at once if you have any of these signs of bleeding.
- Get emergency medical help if you have signs of an allergic reaction, such as hives, rash, difficulty breathing, or swelling of your face, lips, tongue, or throat.
- Taking antiretroviral medications is not safe during pregnancy or breastfeeding. Tell your health care provider if you are pregnant or plan to become pregnant.

TABLE 48.12 Preferred and Alternative Antiretroviral Medication 28-Day Regimens for nPEP[a,b]

Age Group	Preferred/ Alternative	Medication
Adults and adolescents ≥13 yr, including pregnant women, with normal renal function (creatinine clearance ≥ 60 mL/minute)	**Preferred**	A 3-drug regimen consisting of tenofovir DF 300 mg *and* fixed-dose combination emtricitabine 200 mg (Truvada[c]) once daily **with** raltegravir 400 mg twice daily *or* dolutegravir 50 mg once daily
	Alternative	A 3-drug regimen consisting of tenofovir DF 300 mg *and* fixed-dose combination emtricitabine 200 mg (Truvada) once daily **with** darunavir 800 mg (as two 400-mg tablets) once daily **and** ritonavir[b] 100 mg once daily
Adults and adolescents ≥13 yr with renal dysfunction (creatinine clearance ≤ 59 mL/min)	**Preferred**	A 3-drug regimen consisting of zidovudine *and* lamivudine, with both doses adjusted to degree of renal function **with** raltegravir 400 mg twice daily *or* dolutegravir 50 mg once daily
	Alternative	A 3-drug regimen consisting of zidovudine *and* lamivudine, with both doses adjusted to degree of renal function **with** darunavir 800 mg (as two 400-mg tablets) once daily **and** ritonavir[b] 100 mg once daily
Children 2–12 yr	**Preferred**	A 3-drug regimen consisting of tenofovir DF, emtricitabine, and raltegravir, with each drug dosed to age and weight[d]
	Alternative	A 3-drug regimen consisting of zidovudine *and* lamivudine **with** raltegravir *or* lopinavir/ritonavir[b], with raltegravir and lopinavir/ritonavir dosed to age and weightd
	Alternative	A 3-drug regimen consisting of tenofovir DF **and** emtricitabine **and** lopinavir/ritonavir[b], with each drug dosed to age and weight[d]
Children 3–12 yr	Alternative	A 3-drug regimen consisting of tenofovir DF **and** emtricitabine **and** darunavir[e]/ritonavir[b], with each drug dosed to age and weight[d]
Children 4 weeks[f]–<2 yr	**Preferred**	A 3-drug regimen consisting of zidovudine oral solution *and* lamivudine oral solution **with** raltegravir *or* lopinavir/ritonavir[b] oral solution (Kaletra[g]), with each drug dosed to age and weight[d]

TABLE 48.12 Preferred and Alternative Antiretroviral Medication 28-Day Regimens for nPEP[a,b]—cont'd

Age Group	Preferred/ Alternative	Medication
Children 4 weeks[f]–<2 yr	Alternative	A 3-drug regimen consisting of zidovudine oral solution *and* emtricitabine oral solution **with** raltegravir **or** lopinavir/ritonavir[b] oral solution (Kaletra), with each drug adjusted to age and weight[d]
Children birth–27 days	Consult a pediatric HIV specialist	

[a]These recommendations do not reflect current U.S. Food and Drug Administration–approved labeling for antiretroviral medications listed in this table.
[b]Ritonavir is used in clinical practice as a pharmacokinetic enhancer to increase the trough concentration and prolong the half-life of darunavir, lopinavir, and other protease inhibitors. Ritonavir is not counted as a drug directly active against HIV in the above "3-drug" regimens.
[c]Gilead Sciences, Inc., Foster City, California.
[d]See also Table 6.
[e]Darunavir only FDA-approved for use among children aged ≥ 3 years.
[f]Children should have attained a postnatal age of ≥ 28 days and a postmenstrual age (i.e., first day of the mother's last menstrual period to birth plus the time elapsed after birth) of ≥ 42 weeks.
[g]AbbVie, Inc., North Chicago, Illinois.
HIV, Human immunodeficiency virus; *nPEP,* nonoccupational postexposure prophylaxis; *tenofovir DF,* tenofovir disoproxil fumarate.
From Dominguez, K. L., Smith, D. K., Thomas, V., Crepaz, N., Lang, K., Heneine, W., ... Weidle, P. J. (2016, April). Updated guidelines for antiretroviral postexposure prophylaxis after sexual, injection drug use, or other nonoccupational exposure to HIV—United States, 2016. Retrieved October 27, 2021, from https://stacks.cdc.gov/view/cdc/38856.

TABLE 48.13 Summary of Guidelines for PrEP Treatment

	Males Who Have Sex with Males	Heterosexual Females and Males	Persons Who Inject Drugs
Detecting substantial risk of acquiring HIV infection	HIV-positive sexual partner	HIV-positive sexual partner	HIV-positive injecting partner
	Recent bacterial STI[a]	Recent bacterial STI[b]	Sharing injection equipment
	High number of sex partners	High number of sex partners	
	History of inconsistent or no condom use	History of inconsistent or no condom use	
	Commercial sex work	Commercial sex work in high HIV prevalence area or network	
Clinically eligible	Documented negative HIV test result before prescribing PrEP		
	No signs/symptoms of acute HIV infection		
	Normal renal function; no contraindicated medications		
	Documented hepatitis B virus infection and vaccination status		
Prescription	Daily, continuing, oral doses of TDF/FTC (Truvada) ≤ 90-day supply		
Other services	Follow-up visit at least every 3 months to provide the following:		
	HIV test, medication adherence counseling, behavioral risk reduction support, side effect assessment, STI symptom assessment		
	At 3 months and every 6 months thereafter, assess renal function every 3–6 months, test for bacterial STIs		
	Do oral/rectal STI testing	For females, assess pregnancy intent Pregnancy test every 3 months	Access to clean needles/syringes and drug treatment services

[a]Gonorrhea, chlamydia, syphilis for MSM including those who inject drugs.
[b]Gonorrhea, syphilis for heterosexual females and males including those who inject drugs.
STI, Sexually transmitted infection.
From Preexposure prophylaxis for the prevention of HIV infection in the United States—2017 update, a clinical practice guideline. (n. d.). Retrieved from https://www.cdc.gov/hiv/pdf/risk/prep/cdc-hiv-prep-guidelines-2017.pdf.

- Keep all clinic and laboratory appointments for blood tests related to your ART. If you need to miss an appointment, notify your health care provider and reschedule as soon as possible.
- Before taking OTC medications or herbal supplements, check with your health care provider to determine whether there is a potential for adverse interactions with prescribed medications.

Application Questions for Discussion

1. As a health care provider, what are the patient safety factors that should be considered before prescribing any medication for a patient on ART?
2. What signs and symptoms to monitor for organ involvement would you include in the education plan for a patient and/or caregiver after beginning ART?
3. What role does genetics play in the treatment of HIV?
4. Should patients on ART receive vaccinations and/or live-virus vaccinations?
5. You have a patient who states they have male-to-male sexual relationships. They want to know about PrEP and starting Truvada. How would you educate them and what testing would be required before starting any antiretroviral?

Selected Bibliography

Abacavir Drug Interactions. (n. d.). Drugs.Com. Retrieved July 25, 2020, from https://www.drugs.com/drug-interactions/abacavir.html

Abacavir: MedlinePlus Drug Information. (n. d.). Retrieved July 25, 2020, from https://medlineplus.gov/druginfo/meds/a699012.html

AccessPak for HIV PEP Expanded with Kaletra Uses, Side Effects & Warnings. (n. d.). Drugs.Com. Retrieved July 25, 2020, from https://www.drugs.com/mtm/accesspak-for-hiv-pep-expanded-with-kaletra.html

AccessPak for HIV PEP Expanded with Viracept Uses, Side Effects & Warnings. (n. d.). Drugs.Com. Retrieved July 25, 2020, from https://www.drugs.com/mtm/accesspak-for-hiv-pep-expanded-with-viracept.html

Antiretroviral Therapy for HIV Infection: Overview, FDA-Approved Antivirals and Regimens, Complete Regimen Combination ARTs. (2020). Available at https://emedicine.medscape.com/article/1533218-overview#a3

Arts, E. J., & Hazuda, D. J. (2012). HIV-1 antiretroviral drug therapy. *Cold Spring Harbor perspectives in medicine, 2*(4), Article a007161. https://doi.org/10.1101/cshperspect.a007161.

Atazanavir Drug Interactions. (n. d.). Drugs.Com. Retrieved July 25, 2020, from https://www.drugs.com/drug-interactions/atazanavir.html

Atripla Dosage Guide. (n. d.). Drugs.Com. Retrieved July 25, 2020, from https://www.drugs.com/dosage/atripla.html

Biktarvy Dosage Guide. (n. d.). Drugs.Com. Retrieved July 25, 2020, from https://www.drugs.com/dosage/biktarvy.html

Blair, HA. (2020). Ibalizumab: A Review in Multidrug-Resistant HIV-1 Infection. *Drugs, 80*(2), 189–196. doi:10.1007/s40265-020-01258-3. FebPMID: 31970712.

Brief Initiation of Antiretroviral Therapy Adult and Adolescent ARV. (n. d.). AIDSinfo. Retrieved July 15, 2020, from https://aidsinfo.nih.gov/guidelines/brief-html/1/adult-and-adolescent-arv/10/initiation-of-antiretroviral-therapy

Brief What's New in the Guidelines Pediatric ARV. (n.d.). AIDSinfo. Retrieved July 25, 2020, from https://aidsinfo.nih.gov/guidelines/brief-html/2/pediatric-arv/45/whats-new-in-the-guidelines

Centers for Disease Control and Prevention (CDC). (2020). *CDC Works 24/7*. July 24: Centers for Disease Control and Prevention. https://www.cdc.gov/index.htm.

Chen, S., St Jean, P., Borland, J., Song, I., Yeo, A. J., Piscitelli, S., & Rubio, J. P. (2013). Evaluation of the effect of UGT1A1 polymorphisms on dolutegravir pharmacokinetics. *Pharmacogenomics, 15*(1), 9–16. https://doi.org/10.2217/pgs.13.190.

Cimduo Dosage Guide. (n. d.). Drugs.Com. Retrieved July 25, 2020, from https://www.drugs.com/dosage/cimduo.html

Clinical Care Guidelines and Resources. (2016, August 17). [Text]. HIV/AIDS Bureau. https://hab.hrsa.gov/clinical-quality-management/clinical-care-guidelines-and-resources

Clinicians| HIV | CDC. (2020, June 3). https://www.cdc.gov/hiv/clinicians/index.html

Cobicistat Drug Interactions. (n. d.). Drugs.Com. Retrieved July 25, 2020, from https://www.drugs.com/drug-interactions/cobicistat.html

Cobicistat FDA Label—Tablet (film coated). (n. d.). AIDSinfo. Retrieved July 11, 2020, from https://aidsinfo.nih.gov/drugs/536/cobicistat/171/professional

Combivir Dosage Guide. (n. d.). Drugs.Com. Retrieved July 25, 2020, from https://www.drugs.com/dosage/combivir.html

Complera Dosage Guide. (n. d.). Drugs.Com. Retrieved July 25, 2020, from https://www.drugs.com/dosage/complera.html

Darunavir Drug Interactions. (n. d.). Drugs.Com. Retrieved July 25, 2020, from https://www.drugs.com/drug-interactions/darunavir.html

Debnath, B., Xu, S., Grande, F., Garofalo, A., & Neamati, N. (2013). Small molecule inhibitors of CXCR4. *Theranostics, 3*(1), 47–75. https://doi.org/10.7150/thno.5376.

Deeks, E. D. (2014). Cobicistat: A review of its use as a pharmacokinetic enhancer of atazanavir and darunavir in patients with HIV-1 infection. *Drugs, 74*(2), 195–206. https://doi.org/10.1007/s40265-013-0160-x.

Delstrigo Dosage Guide. (n. d.). Drugs.Com. Retrieved July 25, 2020, from https://www.drugs.com/dosage/delstrigo.html

Descovy Dosage Guide. (n. d.). Drugs.Com. Retrieved July 25, 2020, from https://www.drugs.com/dosage/descovy.html

Dolutegravir Drug Interactions. (n. d.). Drugs.Com. Retrieved July 25, 2020, from https://www.drugs.com/drug-interactions/dolutegravir.html

Dolutegravir FDA Label—Tablet (film coated). (n. d.). AIDSinfo. Retrieved July 25, 2020, from https://aidsinfo.nih.gov/drugs/509/dolutegravir/167/professional

Doravirine. (n. d.). Doravirine https://www.accessdata.fda.gov/drugsatfda_docs/label/2018/210806s000lbl.pdf

Doravirine Drug Interactions. (n. d.). Drugs.Com. Retrieved July 25, 2020, from https://www.drugs.com/drug-interactions/doravirine.html

Dovato Dosage Guide. (n. d.). Drugs.Com. Retrieved July 25, 2020, from https://www.drugs.com/dosage/dovato.html

Efavirenz Drug Interactions. (n. d.). Drugs.Com. Retrieved July 25, 2020, from https://www.drugs.com/drug-interactions/efavirenz.html

ElvitegravirDosage, Side Effects. (n. d.). AIDSinfo. Retrieved July 25, 2020, from https://aidsinfo.nih.gov/drugs/421/elvitegravir/0/patient

Emtricitabine/Tenofovir Dosage Guide with Precautions. (n. d.). Drugs.Com. Retrieved July 25, 2020, from https://www.drugs.com/dosage/emtricitabine-tenofovir.html

Emtriva, (emtricitabine) dosing, indications, interactions, adverse effects, and more. (n. d.). Retrieved July 25, 2020, from https://reference.medscape.com/drug/emtriva-emtricitabine-342612

Enfuvirtide Drug Interactions. (n. d.). Drugs.Com. Retrieved July 25, 2020, from https://www.drugs.com/drug-interactions/enfuvirtide.html

Epzicom Dosage Guide. (n. d.). Drugs.Com. Retrieved July 25, 2020, from https://www.drugs.com/dosage/epzicom.html

Evotaz Dosage Guide. (n. d.). Drugs.Com. Retrieved July 25, 2020, from https://www.drugs.com/dosage/evotaz.html

FDA Approval of HIV Medicines. (n. d.). AIDSinfo. Retrieved July 19, 2020, from https://aidsinfo.nih.gov/understanding-hiv-aids/infographics/25/fda-approval-of-hiv-medicines

FDA-Approved HIV Medicines Understanding HIV/AIDS. (n. d.). AIDSinfo. Retrieved July 11, 2020, from https://aidsinfo.nih.gov/understanding-hiv-aids/fact-sheets/21/58/fda-approved-hiv-medicines

Gallant, JE, Thompson, M, DeJesus, E, Voskuhl, GW, Wei, X, Zhang, H, White, K, Cheng, A, Quirk, E, & Martin, H. (2017 May 1). Antiviral Activity, Safety, and Pharmacokinetics of Bictegravir as 10-Day Monotherapy in HIV-1-Infected Adults. *J Acquir Immune Defic Syndr, 75*(1), 61–66. doi:10.1097/QAI.0000000000001306. PMID: 28196003; PMCID: PMC5389589.

Genvoya Dosage Guide. (n. d.). Drugs.Com. Retrieved July 25, 2020, from https://www.drugs.com/dosage/genvoya.html

Grande, F., Occhiuzzi, M. A., Rizzuti, B., Ioele, G., De Luca, M., Tucci, P., Svicher, V., Aquaro, S., & Garofalo, A. (2019). CCR5/CXCR4 dual antagonism for the improvement of HIV infection therapy. *Molecules, 24*(3), 550. https://doi.org/10.3390/molecules24030550.

HIV/AIDS Treatment Guidelines. (n. d.). AIDSinfo. Retrieved July 25, 2020, from https://aidsinfo.nih.gov/guidelines

Isentress (raltegravir) dose, indications, adverse effects, interactions… From PDR.net. (n. d.). Retrieved July 25, 2020, from https://www.pdr.net/drug-summary/Isentress-raltegravir-360.3365

Juluca Dosage Guide. (n. d.). Drugs.Com. Retrieved July 25, 2020, from https://www.drugs.com/dosage/juluca.html

June 30, C. S. H. govDate last updated:, & 2020. (2020). *U.S. Statistics.* June 30: HIV.Gov. https://www.hiv.gov/hiv-basics/overview/data-and-trends/statistics.

Kallianpur, A. R., & Hulgan, T. (2009). Pharmacogenetics of nucleoside reverse-transcriptase inhibitor-associated peripheral neuropathy. *Pharmacogenomics, 10*(4), 623–637. https://doi.org/10.2217/pgs.09.14.

LiverTox. (2012). *Clinical and Research Information on Drug-Induced Liver Injury [Internet].* Bethesda (MD): National Institute of Diabetes and Digestive and Kidney Diseases Pharmacokinetic Enhancers. 2017 Aug 17. PMID: 31643249.

Lv, Z., Chu, Y., & Wang, Y. (2015). HIV protease inhibitors: A review of molecular selectivity and toxicity. *HIV/AIDS (Auckland, N.Z.), 7*, 95–104. https://doi.org/10.2147/HIV.S79956.

Maraviroc-intensified combined antiretroviral therapy Improves Cognition in HIV Neurocognitive Disorder. (n. d.). Medscape. Retrieved July 25, 2020, from http://www.medscape.com/viewarticle/858767

Maraviroc (Professional Patient Advice). (n. d.). Drugs.Com. Retrieved July 25, 2020, from https://www.drugs.com/ppa/maraviroc.html

Martin, M. A., Klein, T. E., Dong, B. J., Pirmohamed, M., Haas, D. W., & Kroetz, D. L. (2012). Clinical Pharmacogenetics Implementation Consortium guidelines for HLA-B genotype and abacavir dosing. *Clinical Pharmacology & Therapeutics, 91*(4), 734–738. https://doi.org/10.1038/clpt.2011.355.

Odefsey Dosage Guide. (n. d.). Drugs.Com. Retrieved July 25, 2020, from https://www.drugs.com/dosage/odefsey.html

Odefsey: Uses, Dosage, Side Effects & Warnings. (n. d.). Drugs.Com. Retrieved July 25, 2020, from https://www.drugs.com/odefsey.html

Pre-Exposure Prophylaxis (PrEP) | HIV Risk and Prevention | HIV/AIDS | CDC. (2020, June 4). https://www.cdc.gov/hiv/risk/prep/index.html

Raltegravir Uses, Side Effects & Warnings. (n.d.). Drugs.Com. Retrieved July 25, 2020, from https://www.drugs.com/mtm/raltegravir.html

Ritonavir Drug Interactions. (n. d.). Drugs.Com. Retrieved July 25, 2020, from https://www.drugs.com/drug-interactions/ritonavir.html

Selzentry (maraviroc) dosing, indications, interactions, adverse effects, and more. (n. d.). Retrieved July 25, 2020, from https://reference.medscape.com/drug/selzentry-maraviroc-342638#10

Stribild Dosage Guide. (n. d.). Drugs.Com. Retrieved July 25, 2020, from https://www.drugs.com/dosage/stribild.html

Symfi Lo Dosage Guide. (n. d.). Drugs.Com. Retrieved July 25, 2020, from https://www.drugs.com/dosage/symfi-lo.html

Symtuza Dosage Guide. (n. d.). Drugs.Com. Retrieved July 25, 2020, from https://www.drugs.com/dosage/symtuza.html

Triumeq Dosage Guide. (n. d.). Drugs.Com. Retrieved July 25, 2020, from https://www.drugs.com/dosage/triumeq.html

Trizivir Dosage Guide. (n. d.). Drugs.Com. Retrieved July 25, 2020, from https://www.drugs.com/dosage/trizivir.html

Trogarzo (ibalizumab-uiyk): Side Effects, Dosage & Uses. (n. d.). Drugs.Com. Retrieved July 25, 2020, from https://www.drugs.com/trogarzo.html

Truvada (emtricitabine-tenofovir DF) dosing, indications, interactions, adverse effects, and more. (n. d.). Retrieved July 25, 2020, from https://reference.medscape.com/drug/truvada-emtricitabine-tenofovir-df-342640

Truvada FDA Label—Tablet (film coated). (n. d.). AIDSinfo. Retrieved July 25, 2020, from https://aidsinfo.nih.gov/drugs/406/truvada/8/professional

Vemlidy (tenofovir AF) dosing, indications, interactions, adverse effects, and more. (n. d.). Retrieved July 25, 2020, from https://reference.medscape.com/drug/vemlidy-tenofovir-af-1000007

Videx, VidexEC (didanosine) dosing, indications, interactions, adverse effects, and more. (n. d.). Retrieved July 25, 2020, from https://reference.medscape.com/drug/videx-ec-didanosine-342609

Viread (tenofovir DF) dosing, indications, interactions, adverse effects, and more. (n. d.). Retrieved July 25, 2020, from https://reference.medscape.com/drug/viread-tenofovir-df-342633

Welcome to CDC stacks |. (n. d. a). Retrieved July 25, 2020, from https://stacks.cdc.gov/view/cdc/38856

Welcome to CDC stacks |. (n.d. b). Retrieved July 25, 2020, from https://stacks.cdc.gov/view/cdc/20711

What's New in the Guidelines? Adult and Adolescent ARV. (n. d.). AIDSinfo. Retrieved July 25, 2020, from https://aidsinfo.nih.gov/guidelines/html/1/adult-and-adolescent-arv/37/whats-new-in-the-guidelines

Ziagen, (abacavir) dosing, indications, interactions, adverse effects, and more. (n. d.). Retrieved July 25, 2020, from https://reference.medscape.com/drug/ziagen-abacavir-342600#6

49

Antiprotozoal Medications

CONSTANCE G. VISOVSKY

Overview

Protozoal infections are considered parasitic illnesses that are caused by protozoal organisms and can be acquired by direct, fecal–oral, or vector-borne transmission. Protozoal infections can spread as the result of unhygienic conditions or practices or poor vector control. Protozoal diseases have global health, social, and economic impacts, contributing to infectious diseases worldwide. Malaria (*Plasmodium* spp.), cutaneous and visceral leishmaniasis (*Leishmania* spp.), African sleeping sickness (*Trypanosoma brucei*), Chagas disease (*Trypanosoma cruzi*), amoebic dysentery (*Entamoeba* spp.), and toxoplasmosis (*Toxoplasma* spp.) are causes of morbidity and mortality in nearly one-sixth of the world (Capela et al., 2019; see Fig. 49.1).

PHARMACOGENETICS

Antiprotozoal Therapy

- The evidence is increasing that various cytochrome (CYP) P450 isozymes and medication transporters may contribute to the variability in drug response (incomplete cure, relapse, or resistance) or toxicity experienced with antimalarial drugs.
- Variations in CYP 3A4*1B can adversely affect malaria treatment outcomes in pregnant patients.

Antiprotozoal Therapy

Chloroquine

Chloroquine is an antiprotozoal agent indicated for the treatment and prophylaxis of malaria and for the treatment of extraintestinal amebiasis. Resistance to chloroquine is widespread.

Pharmacokinetics. Chloroquine is administered orally and has a wide distribution, with 55% bound to plasma proteins. Chloroquine is metabolized primarily by CYP 2C8 and CYP 3A4 enzymes. Excretion of chloroquine is largely through urine, with about 50% of the dose excreted in urine as unchanged drug and about 25% as metabolites. The elimination half-life is 108 to 291 hours.

Indications. Chloroquine is indicated in the treatment of uncomplicated malaria due to susceptible strains of *P. falciparum*, *P. knowlesi*, *P. malariae*, *P. ovale*, and *P. vivax*; for malaria prophylaxis; and as an adjunctive treatment for extraintestinal amebiasis.

Adverse Effects. Cardiovascular adverse reactions include cardiomyopathy, electrocardiogram (ECG) changes, and hypotension. Cardiac arrhythmias, conduction disorders such as bundle-branch block and AV block, QT prolongation, torsade de pointes, and ventricular arrhythmias have been reported and can be fatal. Adverse gastrointestinal (GI) effects include hepatitis, elevated hepatic enzymes, nausea, vomiting, abdominal pain, cramps, diarrhea, and anorexia.

Visual impairments such as macular degeneration and irreversible retinopathy have been reported with chloroquine use. Night blindness, double vision, and reversible corneal opacification have also been reported. Discontinue chloroquine if ocular toxicity is suspected, and monitor the patient closely as retinal changes and visual disturbances may progress after cessation of therapy. Skin reactions such as erythema multiforme, Stevens-Johnson syndrome, toxic epidermal necrolysis, exfoliative dermatitis, pleomorphic skin eruptions, skin discoloration, pruritus, and photosensitivity can occur. Chloroquine has been associated with acute generalized exanthematous pustulosis (AGEP). The nonfollicular, pustular, erythematous rash starts suddenly and is associated with fever above 38°C.

Hematological adverse reactions include reversible agranulocytosis, aplastic anemia, pancytopenia, neutropenia, and thrombocytopenia. Chloroquine may cause hemolysis and hemolytic anemia in patients with glucose-6-phosphate dehydrogenase (G6PD) deficiency. Neurologic events such as seizures, sensorimotor impairment, skeletal muscle myopathy or progressive weakness (myasthenia), hyporeflexia, and abnormal nerve conduction have been reported. Discontinue chloroquine if weakness develops. Neuropsychiatric effects include delirium, anxiety, agitation, insomnia, hallucinations, confusion, personality changes, depression, and suicidal ideation/behavior. Extrapyramidal symptoms usually resolve after treatment discontinuation and/or symptomatic treatment. Impaired glucose control, including severe hypoglycemia that can be potentially life threatening in patients treated with or without antidiabetic medications, has also been reported.

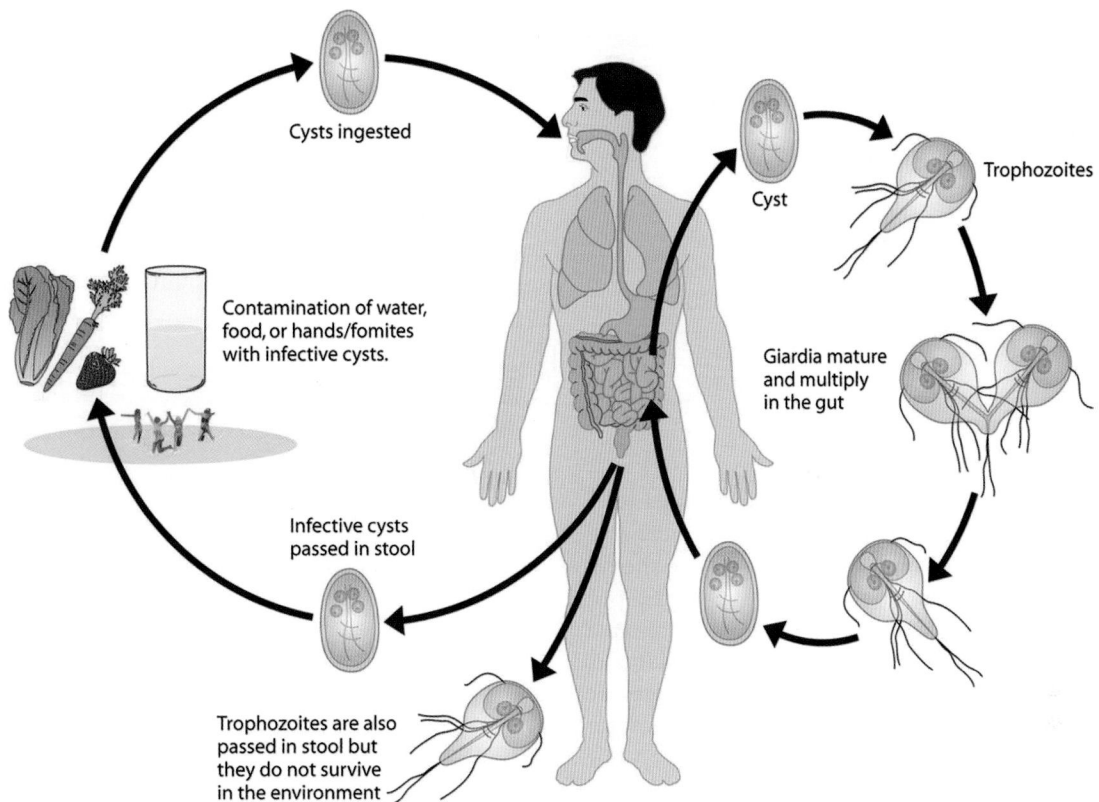

• **Fig. 49.1** Life cycle of giardia infection. *Giardia* cysts shed in the feces are infectious. Infection occurs after the ingestion of cysts either through the fecal–oral route or through the ingestion of contaminated water or food. Cysts are environmentally resistant and can persist for months in soil or water. Excystation occurs within the small intestine. Trophozoites remain either free in the intestinal lumen or attached to villous enterocytes, causing clinical signs. Trophozoites encyst upon movement toward the colon, becoming infectious oocysts, and are shed in the feces. (From Esch, K. J., & Petersen, C. A. [2013]. Transmission and epidemiology of zoonotic protozoal diseases of companion animals. *Clinical Microbiology Reviews, 26*[1], 58–85. https://doi.org/10.1128/cmr.00067-12)

Contraindications. Chloroquine is contraindicated in patients with known *chloroquine hypersensitivity* or hydroxychloroquine hypersensitivity as there may be cross sensitivity to chloroquine. QT prolongation, torsade de pointes, and ventricular arrhythmias have been reported with higher doses of chloroquine and should be used cautiously in patients who have conditions that place patients at risk for these arrhythmias. Consider discontinuing any QT-prolonging medications that can be discontinued. Chloroquine should be used with caution in patients with a history of alcoholism or hepatic dysfunction. Chloroquine should not be used in patients with psoriasis unless the benefit to the patient outweighs the potential risks because it may precipitate a severe attack of psoriasis. Chloroquine can cause hemolysis in patients with glucose-6-phosphate dehydrogenase deficiency (G6PD deficiency). Chloroquine should be used with caution in patients with diabetes, as it can cause life-threatening hypoglycemia, and in patients those with neurological disease, as neurological complications such as seizures can occur. Keep chloroquine out of the reach of pediatric patients, including neonates, infants, children,

and adolescents to prevent accidental ingestion and fatalities. Use caution when administering chloroquine to women who are breastfeeding. Chloroquine is excreted into breast milk. Chloroquine crosses the placenta, but the potential damage to the mother from malaria may be greater than the drug's risk to the fetus. Chloroquine should be used with caution in men because animal studies suggest that infertility is possible after 30 days of oral treatment.

Monitoring. Obtain baseline electrolytes, including calcium, magnesium, and potassium. Liver function should be monitored in patients who are also taking erythromycin for extended periods. Evaluate for changes in the ECG, particularly in patients with cardiovascular risk factors. Monitoring should also include annual examinations of best corrected distance visual acuity (BCVA), automated threshold visual field (VF), and spectral domain optical coherence tomography (SD-OCT). Periodically test knee and ankle reflexes, as well as blood monitoring for hemolytic anemia in patients with G6PD deficiency. Monitor blood glucose and adjust treatment as necessary in patients presenting with clinical symptoms of hypoglycemia during chloroquine treatment.

Chloroquine

- Document high-risk cardiovascular and comorbid conditions.
- Assess for hepatic and renal dysfunction and adjust dose accordingly.
- Determine whether the patient is currently on any QT-prolonging medications that can be discontinued.
- Obtain a pretreatment ECG to check baseline QTc.
- Obtain baseline electrolytes, including calcium, magnesium, and potassium; correct abnormalities.

Iodoquinol

Iodoquinol is an oral amebicide used to treat patients infected with protozoa, especially *Entamoeba histolytica*. Iodoquinol is effective in treating intraluminal parasites in both asymptomatic carriers and symptomatic patients.

Pharmacokinetics. Iodoquinol tablets are administered orally. Limited data are available on the pharmacokinetics of iodoquinol. Protein-bound serum iodine levels may be increased during treatment with iodoquinol and persist for several months, even after treatment is completed. Only 4.6% of the drug is renally excreted; the majority of the drug is excreted unchanged in the stool.

Indications. Iodoquinol tablets are used in the treatment of asymptomatic amebiasis or noninvasive intestinal amebiasis caused by *E. histolytica*, *B. coli*, or *D. fragilis*. Iodoquinol is also used in the treatment of invasive amebiasis following treatment with a systemically absorbed amebicide such as metronidazole.

Adverse Effects. Iodoquinol can cause enlargement of the thyroid, as it is 64% organically bound iodine, and may result in thyroid disease such as iodine-induced hypothyroidism with goiter or hyperthyroidism. Iodoquinol has been associated with optic neuritis and optic atrophy when given in large doses or with long-term use. Serious adverse effects of the eye, leading to blindness, have been reported. Peripheral neuropathy has developed in patients receiving moderate iodoquinol doses for more than 3 weeks. Neurologic effects such as headache and vertigo have been reported but can be minimized through dose reductions. Dermatologic adverse effects including acneiform rash, bullous rash, pruritus, and urticaria can occur. GI adverse effects include abdominal pain, diarrhea, nausea, and vomiting.

Contraindications. Iodoquinol is contraindicated in patients with known iodine or iodoquinol hypersensitivity as well as in patients with hypersensitivity to similar medications such as chloroxine, pamaquine, pentaquine, and primaquine. Iodoquinol should be used with caution in patients with preexisting optic neuritis. This medication may cause optic neuritis and could worsen preexisting optic neuropathy. Due to potential optic nerve damage, use of iodoquinol in older adults is limited to circumstances when other therapy is contraindicated or has failed.

Iodoquinol should be used with caution in patients with preexisting peripheral neuropathy, as this medication can worsen symptoms. Iodoquinol should be used with caution in patients with thyroid disease as this iodine-containing medication may result in overt thyroid disease; thyroid-related effects may persist for as long as 6 months after therapy discontinuation. Patients with renal impairment may be at increased risk of accumulation of iodine, which could result in iodine toxicity. Iodoquinol is contraindicated in patients with hepatic disease.

Iodoquinol Use in Pregnancy and Lactation

- Conclusive evidence for the safety of iodoquinol is not available, so this medication should be used during pregnancy only when absolutely needed.
- Use iodoquinol cautiously in females who are breastfeeding. There are limited data regarding the use of iodoquinol during breastfeeding, and distribution into human breast milk is unknown. Elevated iodine concentrations in the breast-fed infant are theoretically possible.

Monitoring. Periodic stool exams are needed to determine medication efficacy. Thyroid function tests should also be performed at baseline and periodically throughout treatment. Monitor patients for visual disturbances. Patients complaining of visual disturbances while receiving iodoquinol should be evaluated. Periodic assessment of liver function tests (LFTs) is also advisable during prolonged iodoquinol therapy. Monitor patients at risk for or with confirmed peripheral neuropathy for worsening of symptoms and functional deficits.

Metronidazole

Metronidazole is a synthetic antibacterial and antiprotozoal agent that belongs to the nitroimidazole class and is effective against protozoa such as *Trichomonas vaginalis*, amebiasis, and giardiasis. Metronidazole has selectivity for anaerobic bacteria as these organisms reduce metronidazole to its active form, creating a concentration gradient that promotes intracellular transport of metronidazole. The reduced metronidazole then interacts with deoxyribonucleic acid (DNA) to inhibit DNA synthesis, eventually resulting in bacterial cell death.

Pharmacokinetics. Metronidazole can be administered orally, intravenously, intravaginally, and topically. Metronidazole is widely distributed into various body tissues and fluids including cerebrospinal fluid (CSF), pelvic tissue and peritoneal fluid, pancreas, colorectal tissue, bone, saliva, and gingival fluid. Metronidazole has a protein binding of less than 20% and is metabolized in the liver. The major metabolite of metronidazole is 2-hydroxymethyl metronidazole, which has some antiprotozoal activity (30% to

65% of metronidazole). Metronidazole and its metabolites are eliminated through the urine, with approximately 20% appearing as unchanged metronidazole. Fecal excretion accounts for 6% to 15% of the dose. The mean elimination half-life is approximately 8 hours.

Indications. Metronidazole is used in the treatment of amebiasis (amebic dysentery) and amebic hepatic abscess.

Adverse Effects. GI adverse reactions include nausea (10% of patients), metallic taste (9%), diarrhea (4%), and abdominal pain or discomfort (4%). Central and peripheral neurotoxicity has occurred from metronidazole. Severe neurological disturbances such as encephalopathy (confusion, decreased level of consciousness), cerebellar symptoms (ataxia, dizziness), convulsive seizures, sensory peripheral neuropathy (numbness and paresthesia), optic neuropathy, and aseptic meningitis have been reported. Hematologic adverse effects that have been reported include agranulocytosis, leukopenia, neutropenia, thrombocytopenia, and eosinophilia. Hypersensitivity or skin adverse effects include toxic epidermal necrolysis, angioedema, pruritus, urticaria, and Stevens-Johnson syndrome. Urinary adverse effects include discoloration of the urine (likely from a metabolite), dysuria (fewer than 1%), cystitis, polyuria, urinary incontinence, and pelvic pressure.

Contraindications. Metronidazole is contraindicated in patients with a history of hypersensitivity to metronidazole or other nitroimidazole derivatives. Due to the adverse hematologic effects, metronidazole should be used cautiously in patients with hematological disease. Systemic metronidazole should be used cautiously in patients with severe renal impairment or end-stage renal disease (ESRD) as the unchanged drug and its metabolites may accumulate in patients. Cardiac adverse effects such as QT prolongation have been reported with metronidazole use. Use metronidazole with caution in patients with conditions that may increase the risk of QT prolongation, including older adults; patients with diabetes or thyroid disease; patients with a history of cardiac arrhythmias, congenital long QT syndrome, heart failure, bradycardia, myocardial infarction, hypertension, or coronary artery disease (CAD); and patients taking other medications known to increase QT interval. There are conflicting recommendations between the manufacturer and the Centers for Disease Control and Prevention (CDC) related to the use of metronidazole during pregnancy. For indications other than trichomoniasis, avoid metronidazole during pregnancy whenever possible, with use occurring only after careful assessment of the potential risk-to-benefit ratio.

Metronidazole should be used with caution in patients with alcoholism or alcohol intoxication due to the potential for psychotic reactions. It is recommended that alcoholic beverages or medicines not be used concurrently with metronidazole or for at least 3 days following the discontinuation of the drug.

Monitoring. Monitor ECG, complete blood count (CBC), and LFTs before treatment and at regular intervals throughout and after treatment completion.

Tinidazole

Tinidazole is an oral nitroimidazole antimicrobial indicated for giardiasis, amebiasis, trichomoniasis, and bacterial vaginosis. Tinidazole releases nitrites that damage bacteria by inducing DNA base changes in bacterial cells and DNA strand breakage in mammalian cells. The mechanism by which tinidazole exhibits activity against *Giardia* and *Entamoeba* species is unknown.

Pharmacokinetics. Tinidazole is completely and rapidly absorbed, with approximately 12% of the dose being bound by plasma proteins. Tinidazole is biotransformed mainly by CYP 3A4, undergoing significant metabolization by oxidation, hydroxylation, and conjugation before being excreted. Tinidazole is eliminated by the liver and kidneys. Approximately 25% of the administered dose is excreted unchanged in the urine. About 12% of the drug is excreted in the feces. The plasma half-life of tinidazole is 12 to 14 hours.

Indications. Tinidazole is indicated in the treatment of giardiasis, intestinal amebiasis, and as therapy for amebic liver abscess.

Adverse Effects. GI adverse reactions are fairly common and include anorexia (2% of patients), constipation (1%), dyspepsia/cramps/epigastric discomfort (1.5%), bitter/metallic taste (4% to 6%), nausea (4%), vomiting (1.5%), decreased appetite (more than 2%), and flatulence (more than 2%). Urine discoloration (dark urine) and painful urination (1% to 2%) can occur. CNS reactions such as dizziness (1%), headache (1.3%), and fatigue/malaise/weakness (1.5% to 2%) have been reported. While uncommon, seizures and transient peripheral neuropathy including numbness and paresthesia were the most serious adverse events reported.

Hypersensitivity reactions were reported in fewer than 1% of patients and included angioedema, burning sensation, diaphoresis, fever, flushing, pruritus, rash, salivation, thirst, urticaria, and xerostomia. Severe events include Stevens-Johnson syndrome and erythema multiforme. Hepatic effects including elevated liver enzymes occur in fewer than 1% of patients taking tinidazole. Hematologic adverse effects such as transient leukopenia, neutropenia, and reversible thrombocytopenia have been reported in tinidazole clinical trials. Superinfection due to overgrowth of normal flora can occur with tinidazole. Rare cases of bronchospasm, dyspnea, and pharyngitis have been known to occur.

Contraindications. Tinidazole should be used cautiously in patients with evidence of hematological disease. There is a lack of pharmacokinetic data to guide the use of tinidazole in patients with hepatic disease, so use of the lowest effective dose is recommended. Tinidazole should be used cautiously in older adults, and treatment should be at the lowest effective dose due to concomitant medications typically prescribed to this patient population as well as the greater incidence of comorbid conditions that decrease organ function.

Monitoring. Monitor LFTs and CBC before initiating therapy and periodically throughout treatment, especially for high-risk patients.

Tinidazole Use in Reproduction, Pregnancy, and Lactation

- Tinidazole may cause infertility in males, but it in unknown whether the effects on male fertility are reversible.
- There are insufficient data concerning the potential for birth defects, miscarriage, or adverse maternal or fetal outcomes with tinidazole use during pregnancy.
- Tinidazole is present in human breast milk.
- Breastfeeding is not recommended during tinidazole therapy or for 72 hours after administration to minimize exposure to the breastfeeding infant.
- A breastfeeding patient may choose to pump and discard breast milk during and for 72 hours after tinidazole administration.

Nitazoxanide

Nitazoxanide is an oral synthetic antiprotozoal agent for the treatment of cryptosporidiosis or giardiasis. Nitazoxanide exhibits antiprotozoal activity. Nitazoxanide inhibits the growth of sporozoites and oocysts of *Cryptosporidium parvum* and the trophozoites of *Giardia lamblia*. These parasites, transmitted via the oral–fecal route, cause cryptosporidiosis and giardiasis and are the most common causes of parasitic illness in the United States. Nitazoxanide is the first drug specifically approved for the treatment of cryptosporidiosis. Nitazoxanide oral suspension was approved for use in children in 2002 for infectious diarrhea.

Pharmacokinetics. Nitazoxanide is available in oral suspension and tablet formulations. Following oral administration, nitazoxanide is rapidly hydrolyzed to its active metabolite, tizoxanide, undergoing conjugation to tizoxanide glucuronide. Maximum plasma concentrations occur within 1 to 4 hours. There are no pharmacokinetic studies in pediatric patients or older adults, nor in those with liver or renal impairment.

Indications. Nitazoxanide is used for the treatment of diarrhea caused by *Cryptosporidium parvum* or *Giardia lamblia*.

Adverse Effects. GI adverse effects include abdominal pain (6.6% adults; 7.8% pediatrics), diarrhea (4.2% adults; 2.1% pediatrics), nausea (3% adults; fewer than 1% pediatrics), and vomiting (fewer than 1% adults; 1.1% pediatrics). CNS effects such as headache can occur in 1.1% of pediatric patients and 3.1% of adult patients receiving nitazoxanide. Less common CNS effects (fewer than 1%) include dizziness, somnolence (drowsiness), insomnia, tremor, and hypoesthesia. Other generalized adverse effects in fewer than 1% of patients include discoloration of the urine, elevated liver enzymes, anemia, leukocytosis, eye discoloration, tachycardia, syncope, hypertension, myalgia, leg cramping, and spontaneous fractures.

Contraindications. Nitazoxanide is contraindicated in patients with a prior hypersensitivity to nitazoxanide.

Nitazoxanide should be prescribed cautiously to patients with hepatic, biliary tract, or renal impairment or disease. There are no data available to make recommendations regarding the risks associated with nitazoxanide use in pregnancy or breastfeeding.

Monitoring. No specific laboratory monitoring is needed. Monitor stool samples for presence of the parasitic organism and response to treatment.

Atovaquone

Atovaquone is an oral antiprotozoal agent. It is active against both *Toxoplasma gondii* and *Pneumocystis jiroveci*. In combination with proguanil, atovaquone is effective for malaria. Atovaquone remains designated as an orphan drug for the prophylaxis, treatment, and suppression of *T. gondii* encephalitis. Atovaquone has not been proven to decrease the risk of *T. gondii* encephalitis relapse and thus is considered an alternative to standard therapy.

Pharmacokinetics. Atovaquone is administered orally and is extensively bound to plasma proteins. The metabolism of atovaquone is unknown. More than 94% of the atovaquone dose was recovered in the feces unchanged over 21 days. The mean half-life of atovaquone ranges from 67 to 77 hours after oral administration. Plasma concentrations do not increase proportionally with dose. Administering atovaquone oral suspension with food enhances its bioavailability.

Indications. Atovaquone has been shown to be active against most strains of *Pneumocystis jirovecii Plasmodium falciparum*, *Plasmodium sp.*, and *Toxoplasma gondii*.

Adverse Effects. The most commonly reported adverse effect is a nonspecific rash occurring in approximately 6% to 43% of patients, with pruritis occurring in 5% to 10%. Oral candidiasis has been reported to occur in 5% to 10% of patients. During clinical trials, elevated hepatic enzymes have been reported in 4% to 8% of patients. Hematologic adverse reactions including anemia (4% to 6%) and neutropenia (3% to 5%) have occurred. Hyperamylasemia (7%), hyperglycemia (9%), hypoglycemia (1%), hyponatremia (7% to 10%), methemoglobinemia, and thrombocytopenia have been reported with atovaquone. Headache was reported in 16% to 31% of patients during comparative trials with atovaquone. Dizziness was reported with atovaquone and occurred at a rate of 3% to 8% in comparative trials. Insomnia was reported in more than 10% to 19% of patients.

Contraindications. Atovaquone is contraindicated in anyone who develops or has a history of potentially life-threatening allergic reactions to atovaquone or any of the components of the formulation. Data regarding the use of atovaquone during pregnancy to identify a drug-associated risk for major birth defects, miscarriage, or adverse maternal or fetal outcomes are insufficient. Atovaquone suspension contains small amounts of benzyl alcohol and is associated with a gasping syndrome in premature infants and neonates; thus, caution is warranted in these populations. Atovaquone suspension should also be used cautiously in patients with benzyl alcohol hypersensitivity. Use caution when administering atovaquone to patients with impaired hepatic function. It is unknown whether atovaquone clearance is impaired in patients with hepatic disease.

Monitoring. Regular monitoring of CBC, LFTs, serum amylase, and serum sodium should be done prior to initiating and throughout therapy (Table 49.1).

TABLE 49.1 Antiprotozoal Medications

Medication	Indication	Dosage	Considerations and Monitoring
Chloroquine	Effective against *Entamoeba histolytica*, *Plasmodium falciparum*, *Plasmodium malariae*, *Plasmodium ovale*, and *Plasmodium vivax*	*Adults and children:* 16.6 mg/kg/dose orally once, then 8.3 mg/kg/dose orally in 6–8 hr, then 8.3 mg/kg orally once daily for 2 days.	Obtain a pretreatment ECG to assess QTc. Document high-risk cardiovascular and comorbid conditions. Monitor glucose levels throughout treatment in patients with diabetes. Assess and adjust for hepatic and renal dysfunction. Obtain baseline electrolytes, including calcium, magnesium, and potassium; correct abnormalities. Determine whether the patient is currently on any QT-prolonging medications that can be discontinued.
Iodoquinol	Effective against *Entamoeba histolytica*, *B. coli*, and *D. fragilis*	*Adults:* 630 mg or 650 mg orally three times daily after meals for 20 days. *Children and adolescents:* 10–13.3 mg/kg orally three times daily after meals for 20 days. Do not exceed 1.95 Gm/24 hr.	Periodic stool exams should be taken to determine improvement. Thyroid tests and LFTs should also be performed at baseline and periodically throughout treatment. Monitor patients for visual disturbances. Monitor patients at risk for or with confirmed peripheral neuropathy for worsening of symptoms and functional deficits.
Metronidazole	For the treatment of amebiasis, giardiasis, and *Trichomonas vaginalis*	*Adult females:* 500 or 750 mg orally every 8 hr for 5–10 days, or 2 Gm orally as a single dose. *Adult males:* 2 Gm as a single dose. *Infants, children, and adolescents:* 35–50 mg/kg/day orally divided every 8 hr for 7–10 days.	Use cautiously in patients with hematological disease, or severe renal or liver impairment. Monitor CBC and LFTs. Perform baseline ECG due to the potential for QT prolongation. Consider discontinuation of medications known to increase QT interval.
Tinidazole	For the treatment of giardiasis amebiasis; effective against *Bacteroides sp.*, *Entamoeba histolytica*, *Gardnerella vaginalis*, *Giardia duodenalis*, *Giardia lamblia*, *Prevotella sp.*, and *Trichomonas vaginalis*	*Adults:* 2 Gm orally as a single dose. *Children and adolescents:* 50 mg/kg/dose orally as a single dose.	Monitor LFTs and CBC before initiating therapy and periodically throughout treatment. Use cautiously in patients with hematological or liver disorders.
Nitazoxanide	Effective against infective diarrhea caused by *Cryptosporidium parvum*, *Giardia lamblia*, *Clostridium difficile*, *Entamoeba dispar*, *Entamoeba histolytica*, *Enterocytozoon bieneusi*, and rotavirus	*Adults and adolescents:* 500 mg orally every 12 hr with food for 3 days. *Children:* 200–500 mg orally every 12 hr with food for 3 days.	No specific laboratory monitoring is needed. Monitor stool samples for presence of the parasitic organism and response to treatment.
Atovaquone	In combination with proguanil, atovaquone is effective for malaria. May be effective against infections caused by *Toxoplasma gondii*.	*Adults:* 1500 mg orally twice daily either alone or in combination with either pyrimethamine plus leucovorin or sulfadiazine.	Monitor CBC, LFTs, serum amylase, and serum sodium prior to initiating and throughout therapy.

CBC, Complete blood count; *ECG*, electrocardiogram; *LFTs*, liver function tests.

Prescriber Considerations for Antiprotozoal Therapy

Clinical Reasoning for Antiprotozoal Therapy

Consider the individual patient's health problem requiring antiprotozoal therapy. The selection of an antiprotozoal medication is directly related to the parasitic organism that is the basis of the infection. The primary care provider should also consider the exposure that led to the parasitic infection and routes of transmission (oral–fecal, food, vector). Another consideration is the medication route that would obtain the optimum treatment outcome.

Determine the desired therapeutic outcome based on the therapy needed for the patient's health problem. The ideal therapeutic outcome desired is the complete resolution of the parasitic infection. However, it is important to understand that treatment for human protozoan infection is hampered by the lack of effective vaccines and safe and affordable medications. Unfortunately, the usefulness of available medications is being increasingly threatened by the development of parasite drug resistance. There is strong evidence that resistance to antimalarial drugs is associated with parasite genetic mutations (Capela et al., 2019). Therefore, the specific parasitic infection may not resolve completely with a single medication or course of treatment. The need for long-term versus short-term treatment is also a consideration of therapy.

Assess the antiprotozoal selected for its appropriateness for an individual patient by considering the medication's side effects and the patient's age, race/ethnicity, comorbidities, and genetic factors. There is little information regarding the pharmacokinetics of antiprotozoal medications for pediatric patients and older adults. For females of childbearing age, most antiprotozoal medications have insufficient data to make evidence-based recommendations regarding treatment for pregnant and lactating females, infants, and neonates. Antiprotozoal medications can enter the breast milk, so females should not breastfeed during treatment. In addition, females of childbearing age must be counseled to use contraception during treatment with antiprotozoal medications. Older patients may be on several different medications that can interact with antiprotozoals, and the risk-to-benefit ratio needs to be assessed by the primary care provider. Consider the length of treatment time needed, and potential undesired effects on organs such as the liver, kidneys, and cardiac and peripheral nervous systems. For example, the duration of *Giardia* infection is variable; however, chronic infection and reinfection are common. Lastly,

patients with hepatic dysfunction could experience elevated serum levels, while patients with cardiovascular disease can experience prolonged QT syndrome. Patients with known variations in CYP P450 isozymes can have a variable and potentially less effective response to antiprotozoal therapy.

Initiate the treatment plan with the selected antiprotozoal by first providing adequate patient education to ensure the patient's understanding and promote full participation in the therapy. When initiating an antiprotozoal treatment plan, be sure to inform the patient to complete the entire course of therapy even if symptoms of infection subside after a few days. Handling of skipped or missed doses would also need to be addressed. An overview of the side effects, potential adverse effects, and when to notify the primary care provider should be specific to the therapy prescribed and be included in the patient education plan. The developmental stage of the patient is a consideration for the treatment plan for females of childbearing age and older adults, who require different teaching methods for understanding the impact of antiprotozoal therapy. Lastly, a medication reconciliation would help identify any potential interactions of antiprotozoals and other over-the-counter (OTC) or prescribed medications.

Ensure complete patient and family understanding about the medication prescribed for antiprotozoal therapy using a variety of education strategies. Using a variety of educational techniques, such as oral and written instructions as well as pictorials, can be helpful. Teach-back strategies can be helpful in ensuring patient and family understanding. Also, patients and families may find smartphone medication reminder apps to be useful to ensure adherence to the full course of medication.

Conduct follow-up and monitoring of patient responses to antiprotozoal therapy. Follow-up varies based on the specific condition and clinical practice guidelines. The patient should be instructed to follow up should they experience severe diarrhea or any significant adverse effects.

Teaching Points for Antiprotozoal Therapy

Health Promotion Strategies

Health promotion strategies to reduce reinfection or spreading infection to others should be adopted. The following health promotion strategies and practices should be presented to patients to help them become full partners in their health care:

- Understanding how protozoal infections are transmitted will help avoid reinfection and cross-contamination to others.
- Wash hands frequently, as protozoal infections can often be transmitted by the oral–fecal route.
- Follow proper food-handling procedures to reduce the risk of transmission from contaminated food.
- Some infections can lead to special consequences for females. For example, infection with *Toxoplasma gondii*, a parasite found in undercooked meat, cat feces, soil, and

untreated water, can lead to severe brain and eye disorders in a fetus when a pregnant female becomes newly infected.

- Females who are pregnant can avoid infection with *Toxoplasma gondii* by delegating the cleaning of cat litter boxes to someone else in the household.

Patient Education for Medication Safety

- Some antiprotozoals must be taken with food to have optimum treatment efficacy.
- Use only the form of the antiprotozoal prescribed, as some oral suspension and tablet formulations contain different amounts of medication.
- Antiprotozoal drugs can interact with other medicines. Inform your primary care provider of the medicines you are taking, including OTC medicines, so that they can decide whether an antiprotozoal medicine is safe for you to take.
- Inform your doctor if you are pregnant or breastfeeding as some of the oral antiprotozoal drugs should not be taken by females who are pregnant or breastfeeding.

Application Questions for Discussion

1. What elements of a social history may lead the primary care provider to consider a protozoal infection as the cause of a patient's symptoms?

2. Which components of a medical history should be considered before prescribing antiprotozoal therapy?
3. What should be included in the teaching plan for a patient for whom antiprotozoal medication has been prescribed?

Selected Bibliography

Capela R, Moreira R, Lopes F. (2019). An overview of drug resistance in protozoal diseases. *International Journal of Molecular Sciences.* Nov 15;20(22), 5748. http://doi.org/10.3390/ijms20225748. PMID: 31731801; PMCID: PMC6888673.

Kerb, R., Fux, R., Mörike, K., et al. (2009). Pharmacogenetics of antimalarial drugs: Effect on metabolism and transport. *The Lancet Infectious Diseases, 9*(12), 760–774. http://doi.org/10.1016/S14733099(09)70320-2.

Minetti, C., Chalmers, R. M., Beeching, N. J., Probert, C., & Lamden, K. (2016). Giardiasis. *BMJ, 355*, i5369. http://doi.org/10.1136/bmj.i5369.

Mutagonda, R. F., Kamuhabwa, A. A. R., Minzi, O. M. S., et al. (2017). Effect of pharmacogenetics on plasma lumefantrine pharmacokinetics and malaria treatment outcome in pregnant women. *Malaria Journal, 16*(1), 267. http://doi.org/10.1186/s12936-017-1914-9.

50

Immunizations and Immunomodulation Medications and Schedules

KRISTY M. SHAEER, TERESA GORE, AND UMESH KUMAR JINWAL

Overview

The goal of immunization is the eradication of infectious and communicable diseases. Numerous infectious diseases, many of which are potentially fatal, have been sharply curtailed worldwide through vigilant adherence to immunization strategies and public health control measures. In the United States, diphtheria, measles, polio, and tetanus were almost unknown until the recent outbreaks of measles. In 2019, there were more than 1000 cases of measles. This is the largest number of reported cases since 1992 and since measles was declared eliminated in 2000. Vaccines that are administered as recommended induce protective immunity in more than 95% of recipients. The Centers for Disease Control and Prevention (CDC) and the U.S. Food and Drug Administration (FDA) ensure that vaccinations are safe before using and they continue to monitor vaccinations after they are implemented to the public. Children who are not vaccinated for religious, cultural, or other reasons are at risk for disease and increase societal risk by contributing to the pool of unvaccinated individuals who are capable of transmitting infection to susceptible and high-risk individuals, therefore decreasing herd immunity. This has led to some states mandating vaccinations. One reason for the increasing rate of unvaccinated children is the persistence of a popular but discredited belief that vaccines cause autism spectrum disorders (CDC, 2020).

Substantial progress has been made in vaccination coverage, increasing from less than 5% in 1974 to 86% after the Expanded Program on Immunization was established (Peck et al., 2019). In 2018, 90% of children in countries reporting data received their first dose of diphtheria, tetanus toxoids, and pertussis-containing vaccination (DTP). This is virtually unchanged since 2010 when the rate was 89%. The compliance rate for the completion of three doses of DTP and one dose of a measles-containing vaccination (MCV) was 86%. When a second dose of MCV was offered, the compliance rate increased from 19% in 2007 to 54%. The global coverage for completed series of rotavirus vaccination, pneumococcal conjugate vaccine (PCV), rubella vaccine, *Haemophilus influenzae* type b vaccination

(Hib), and hepatitis B vaccination (HepB) has increased globally (Peck et al., 2019). In the United States, for academic year 2018–2019, the compliance rate for kindergarteners for two doses of MMR was 94.7%, for DTaP the rate was 94.9%, and for varicella the rate was 94.8% (Seither et al., 2019). Despite these advances, the United States continues to face vaccine challenges. The exemption rate for unvaccinated children increased by 2.5%, with only 0.3% with medical exemption and 2.2% with nonmedical exemption, respectively (Seither et al., 2019). In 2017, the compliance rate for receiving one or more doses of human papillomavirus (HPV) vaccination was 65.5%. With the adoption of the U.S. HPV vaccination program, the prevalence of vaccine-type HPV infections, anogenital warts, and cervical precancers have significantly decreased (Meites et al., 2019). In 2017, among adults older than 19 years of age, the estimated influenza vaccination rate was 45.4% and the Tdap rate was 31.7% despite the recommendations to increase the rates of adult vaccinations. This is a major area for health care providers to address and develop strategies for increased compliance (Hung et al., 2018).

Relevant Physiology

The Immune System

The first line of defense against infection consists of the skin, mucous membranes, body hair, and body secretions. The second line of defense is a nonspecific immune response, also called the innate immune system, that comprises nonspecific white blood cells (WBCs), inflammatory response, and other components. The third line of defense against the invasion of antigens is the specific immune response, also called the adaptive (acquired) immune system, that comprises specific WBCs (T lymphocytes and B lymphocytes).

Organs of the immune system consist of primary and secondary organs. Primary organs are responsible for the development and storage of lymphocytes. The bone marrow and the thymus gland are the primary organs of the immune system. Secondary lymphoid organs include the lymph nodes, spleen, mucosa-associated lymphoid, tissue, tonsils, appendix, and Peyer patches. The secondary lymphoid organs entrap foreign substances (antigens), stimulate B-cells to become plasma cells that produce antibodies, and stimulate T-cell production, all with the main objective of destroying the antigens. All WBCs originate from a stem cell in the bone marrow. Stem cells first differentiate into myeloid and lymphoid cells. Myeloid cells differentiate into polymorphonuclear (PMN) leukocytes and into monocytes/macrophages. Lymphoid cells differentiate into B lymphocytes and T lymphocytes (Fig. 50.1).

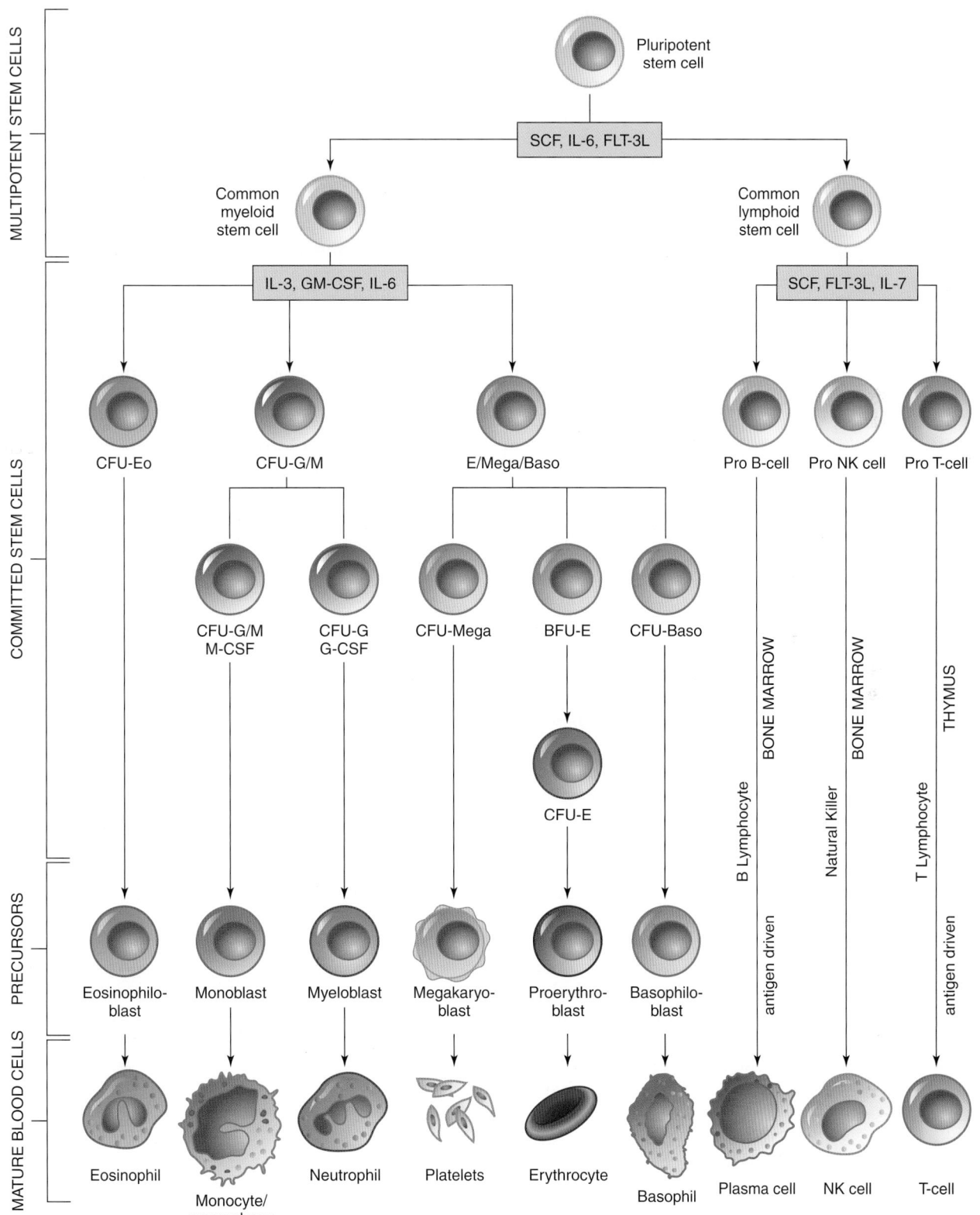

• **Fig. 50.1** Bone marrow and stem cell systems. Probable pathways of differentiation, from the totipotential cell to mature blood cells. (PMN, Granulocytes.) (From McCance, K. L., & Heuther, S. E. [2008]. *Pathophysiology* [5th ed.]. St. Louis: Mosby.)

Nonspecific WBCs

The first type of nonspecific WBC includes polymorpho-nuclear leukocytes, also called granulocytes (e.g., neutrophils, eosinophils, basophils, and mast cells). These are the most active cells and contain the largest number of immune cells in the body. They arrive first at a site of injury, infection, or inflammation and function in several ways. They phagocytize foreign substances and release chemotaxic substances that encircle the area of invasion, killing and preventing contamination by the foreign substance into other areas; they also stimulate the release of antimicrobial substances that aid in the destruction of foreign material.

- *Neutrophils* contain large granules. These granules degranulate when they encounter antigens and release enzymes that destroy foreign substances and can injure surrounding tissue. Debris from this destructive action produces an exudate/pus. Chemical mediators that are secreted from these granules are known as chemotaxic factors; they include leukotrienes, vasoactive kinins, and toxic metabolites.
- *Eosinophils* are very similar to neutrophils. They contain granules and engage in the process of phagocytosis. They seem to congregate in the respiratory and gastrointestinal (GI) tracts. They are especially prominent during allergic reactions and parasitic infections, and they carry certain enzymes that neutralize chemicals responsible for allergic responses. They release potent chemotaxic factors that cause inflammation, bronchospasm, and tissue damage.
- *Basophils* also contain granules that produce histamine and heparin, which play a role in the immune response. The basophil is not a strong structure, and it is easily damaged, which causes the granules to release histamine and heparin. Vasospasm, increased vascular permeability, and increased inflammation are the major effects seen when this occurs. This reaction increases the severity of allergic responses.
- *Mast cells*, the guardians of the immune system, are found in cutaneous and mucosal tissue. They can immediately recognize invasive non-self (foreign) antigens without the aid of macrophages or lymphocytes. They are the effectors of immediate hypersensitivity reactions and contain most of the body's IgE. When this IgE and an antigen meet, there is immediate degranulation and release of histamine, prostaglandin, and leukotrienes, as well as arachidonic acid metabolism, which potentiates the hypersensitivity response.

The second type of nonspecific WBC is the monocyte/macrophage. When monocytes are released into the bloodstream, they migrate to various tissue sites, where they differentiate (mature) and become macrophages. Macrophages are found in connective tissue (e.g., histocyte), the liver (e.g., Kupffer's cells), alveolar tissue in the lung, osteoclasts in bone, mesangial cells in the kidney, and microglial cells in the nervous system. They are also found in the spleen, lymph nodes, and other organs.

Macrophages serve three functions in the immune response. The first is to secrete biologically active compounds/molecules such as prostaglandins, interleukins, interferons, tumor necrosis factors, growth factors, proteins, and enzymes, which serve to defend the host from specific antigens. The second is to remove excess dead or damaged antigens. The third is to engulf and present antigens to lymphoid cells for elimination.

Specific WBCs

The specific WBCs consist of the two lymphocytes (B-cells and T-cells). These cells react with antigens to produce reactions that create a specific response that will destroy the antigen.

- *B lymphocytes* are those cells that produce antibodies. They undergo specific differentiation when exposed to an antigen and become plasma cells that are the major secretors of antibodies (Fig. 50.2). The major function of these antibodies is to destroy a specific antigen and remove it from the body. In response to a specific antigen, a single antibody is produced (each antigen has a specific antibody). The antibodies are grouped into five different classes known as immunoglobulins. These classes contain formed chains of immunoglobulins expressed on the cell surface and labeled IgG, IgA, IgM, IgE, and IgD. Table 50.1 describes the features of these antibodies. B lymphocytes provide humoral immunity through the secretion of these immunoglobulins.
- *T-cell lymphocytes* make up 65% to 80% of all lymphocytes in the blood. Three different types of T-cells are known: helper, suppressor, and cytotoxic. *Helper cells* aid in initiation of the immune response by helping B-cells synthesize antibodies for action. *Suppressor cells* help keep B-cell antibody production in check. They hold back the immune response or restrict antibody production because, if left unchecked, these B-cells can do more harm than good. *Cytotoxic cells*, or *killer cells*, circulate to kill cells not recognized as self-cells (such as tumor cells). Activation of these cells occurs through interaction of antigens with macrophages. Through secretion of the special products produced by macrophages, T-cell proliferation occurs. These activated T-cells release substances known as lymphokines that influence the growth

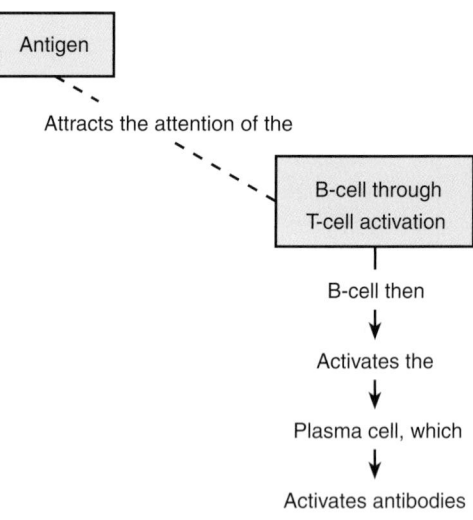

• **Fig. 50.2** Immune response—humoral.

TABLE 50.1   Characteristics and Functions of Immunoglobulins

Immunoglobulins	Amount in Serum	Location of Concentration	Stimulated By	Functions
IgG	Most abundant in the blood, 75%	Intravascular Extravascular	Allergic response Second immunoglobulin	Provides immunity against bloodborne infection (e.g., bacteria, viruses, some fungi)
IgA	15%	Intravascular Secretions	Presence of antigens Antiviral antibody	Most common antibody in secretions, where it protects mucous membranes Bactericidal with lysosome
IgM	10%	Intravascular	Presence of antigens	First immunoglobulin produced during an immune response Activates complement
IgD	1%	On the surface of B-cells	Presence of antigens	Antigen-specific receptor on B-cells

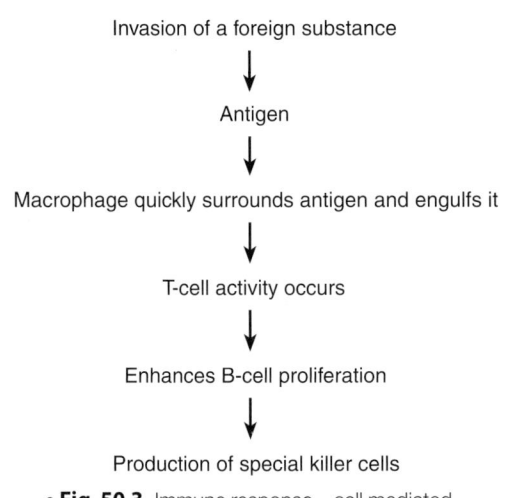

Invasion of a foreign substance

↓

Antigen

↓

Macrophage quickly surrounds antigen and engulfs it

↓

T-cell activity occurs

↓

Enhances B-cell proliferation

↓

Production of special killer cells

• **Fig. 50.3** Immune response—cell mediated.

of other cells necessary for body defense, thus amplifying the immune reaction (Fig. 50.3). The lymphokine interferons are active against viruses.

Other Immune System Components

Three plasma protein systems are in the plasma of blood, not inside a cell. These include the complement, clotting, and kinin systems. Each initiates a cascade of reactions, ending with potent biochemical mediators of the inflammatory response. The complement system is a nonspecific mediator of inflammation that is potent against bacterial infection. IgG or IgM usually initiates the cascade by forming an immune complex. The kinin system begins with bradykinin, which causes dilation of vessels, acts with prostaglandins to induce pain and increase vascular permeability, and is important in the prolonged phase of inflammation. Platelets stop bleeding and release serotonin, which has vascular effects similar to histamine. The clotting system is discussed in Chapter 14. Cytokines are glycoproteins, which are chemical messengers that modulate the immune response.

The Inflammatory Response

The main function of the immune system is to protect the body from damage caused by the introduction of a foreign substance. A number of stimuli can trigger the inflammatory response. These include infectious agents, ischemia, antigen–antibody interactions, and thermal or other injury. In many conditions, the cause of the inflammation is not known. The inflammatory response includes three phases: acute, transient, local vasodilation, and increased capillary permeability; delayed, subacute infiltration of leukocytes and phagocytic cells; and chronic proliferative tissue degeneration and fibrosis.

Two basic antiinflammatory actions occur: phagocytosis and secretion of cytokines that mediate the inflammatory response. A bewildering array of these substances with overlapping sources and functions have been identified. Macrophages, mast cells, T helper cells, natural killer cells, and others secrete many cytokines, including colony-stimulating factor interleukins, tissue necrosis factor, and interferon.

The inflammatory response begins when circulating proteins and blood cells come into contact with a stimulus. Neutrophils arrive at the site first and phagocytose (ingest) the particles that are causing the inflammation. The mast cells are already present in the loose connective tissues close to blood vessels. Monocytes and macrophages arrive and begin phagocytosis. Mast cells, monocytes, and macrophages release many substances collectively called mediators or facilitators of inflammation. The mast cell is the most important activator of the inflammatory response.

Mast cells immediately release substances from their granules, which cause immediate inflammation. These substances include histamine, neutrophil chemotactic factor, and eosinophil chemotactic factor. The mast cell also synthesizes and then releases leukotrienes and prostaglandins, which cause long-term inflammation. These facilitators start a chain of reactions, thereby producing exudate that defends against infection and facilitates tissue repair and healing.

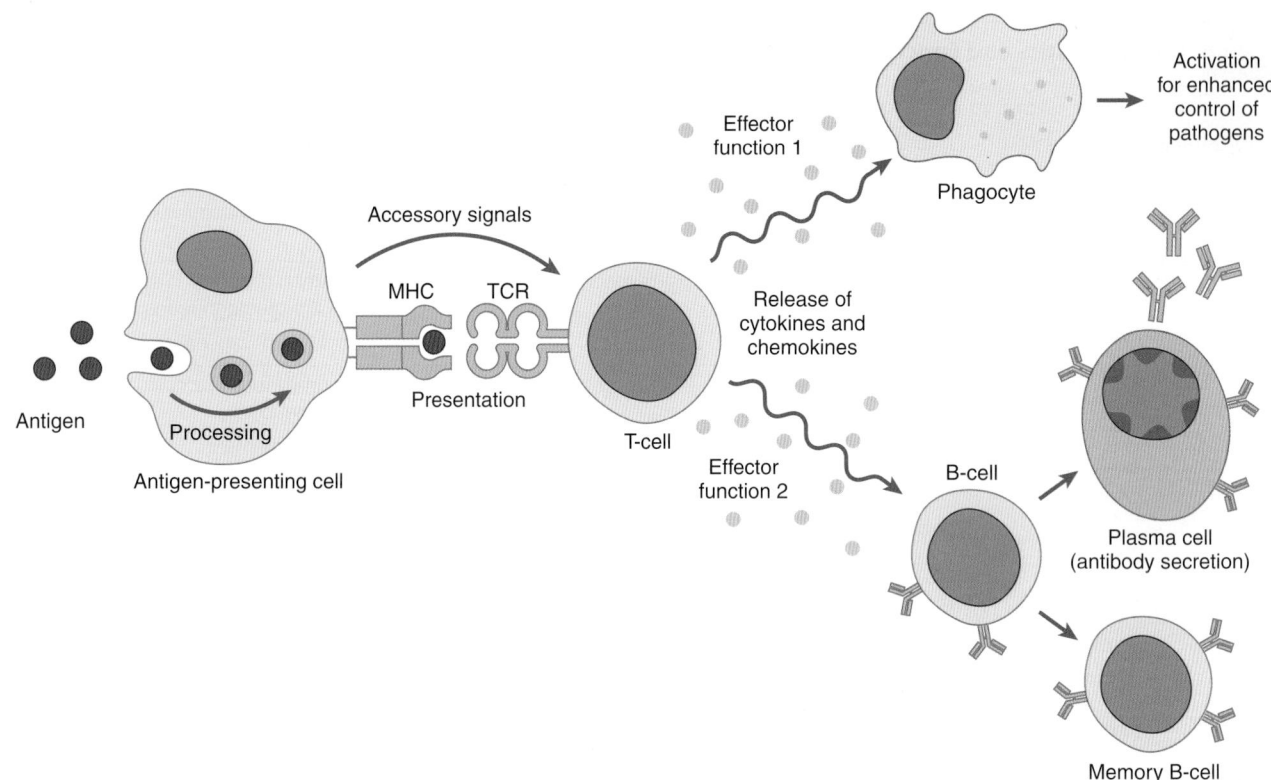

• **Fig. 50.4** Cellular interactions drive adaptive immune functions. Antigen-presenting cells present foreign substances to activate T-cells. T-cells differentiate to become effectors to help phagocytes control pathogen infection or to assist B-cells in production and secretion of immunoglobulins. MHC, major histocompatability complex; TCR, T-cell receptor. (From Actor, J. K. [2012]. Elsevier's Integrated Review: Immunology and Microbiology [2nd ed.]. Philadelphia: Elsevier.)

The Specific Immune Response

The immune response is activated through generation of humoral or cellular immunity. *B lymphocytes* are the cells involved in antibody-mediated or humoral immunity. *T lymphocytes* are the effectors for cell-mediated immunity. This response can be summarized as follows (Fig. 50.4).

• A foreign substance (the antigen) invades.
• A macrophage (antigen-presenting cell) engulfs it and presents it on its cell surface via MHC molecules.
• The expressed antigen stimulates T-cell activity.
• T helper cells are activated to help phagocytes in controlling pathogen infection or enhance B-cell differentiation into plasma cells and the production of antibodies/immunoglobulin (e.g., IgG, IgM, IgA, IgE, IgD).
• Proliferation of B-cells and T-cells produces clones with a memory that enables them to recognize a returning invader. This memory produces a more potent and rapid immune response should the invader return.

Hypersensitivity Reactions

An allergic reaction to a drug may be classified by the Gell and Coombs classification of human hypersensitivity: IgE mediated (type I), cytotoxic (type II), immune complex (type III), and cellular mediated (type IV) (Joint Task Force on Practice Parameters et al., 2010). A type IV reaction can be responsible for contact dermatitis,

delayed cutaneous eruptions such as maculopapular exanthems due to antibiotics (e.g., penicillins, amoxicillin, and sulfonamides), and acute generalized exanthematous pustulosis (AGEP). Type I hypersensitivity reactions are a medical emergency and often manifest within minutes as urticaria, angioedema, bronchospasm, and/or anaphylaxis.

Immunity

Immunizations act to confer immunity to a particular disease. There are two types of immunity: active and passive.

Active Immunity

Active immunization involves the administration of all or a part of a microorganism to evoke a response. Antigens are taken from living or dead organisms, and small amounts are given intradermally or subcutaneously. This process stimulates the body's immune response, and antibodies are stimulated to protect the immunized person from greater exposure to this particular disease-producing antigen. This immunity is retained for a prolonged period, thereby protecting the person from the disease whenever they may be exposed to that antigen. This immunity can be "boosted" at specific intervals.

Active immunization is accomplished with three different types of agents:

• *Inactivated vaccines (killed agents):* Most bacterial vaccines, and some viral vaccines, involve the use of inactivated agents. These agents are not capable of replicating within the host and thus present little risk to the recipient. Maintenance of lifelong immunity requires the administration of multiple doses. Mucosal protection after the use of killed vaccines is less than with the use of live vaccines. Thus, local infection or colonization with the agent can occur, along with potential for transmission, although systemic disease is prevented.

- *Live vaccines (attenuated):* Most viral vaccines involve the use of live virus that has been chemically changed to decrease its virulence. Active infection, with replication of the virus, occurs in the host following administration of the product, although few adverse effects occur. This route generally produces a superior response, including mucosal immunity, and does not require the use of multiple doses.
- *Active immunization:* This may be accomplished with use of a modified product of an organism, such as a toxoid, which consists of modified bacterial toxins and retains the ability to stimulate antibody formation but is nontoxic. This route of immunization is used against diphtheria and tetanus. Maintenance of protective titers of antitoxin requires periodic administration of booster doses of toxoid.

Passive Immunity

Passive immunity occurs when antibodies that one acquired from a human or an animal (with acquired immunity to a specific organism) are given to people who do not have immunity to the organism. Newborn infants achieve this naturally from their mothers through the placenta and through breastfeeding. It can also be achieved through injections of gamma globulins (for hepatitis protection) or antisera or antitoxins. This process temporarily provides the same protection as that given to a person who has achieved active acquired immunity. These antibodies

naturally break down and are eliminated from the body. See Table 50.1 for a summary of the characteristics and function of immunoglobulins.

Vaccine Components

All immunizations contain several different components, such as the following:

Agent	Action	Precautions
Immunizing agent	Active component of the product. May be a killed or attenuated vaccine or a toxoid.	
Suspending fluid	Either sterile water or saline or a complex tissue-culture fluid. May contain proteins derived from the medium in which the vaccine was produced, such as egg antigen in inactivated influenza vaccine.	Influenza vaccine: individuals who experience anaphylactic reactions to egg may be allergic to influenza vaccine. MMR vaccine: egg-allergic children may be safely vaccinated.
Preservatives	Trace amounts of preservatives, stabilizers, or antibiotics often are added to prevent bacterial overgrowth in multiuse vials of vaccines.	Individuals may have allergic reactions to products such as neomycin that may be present in minute amounts.
Adjuvants	Aluminum-based compound added to enhance the immunogenicity of an agent and prolong its stimulatory effects. This is necessary for some inactivated vaccines and for toxoids.	

PRACTICE PEARLS

Thimerosal

- Thimerosal, a mercury-containing organic compound, was removed from or was reduced to trace amounts in all vaccines with the exception of inactivated influenza vaccine multidose vials in 2001 because of concerns about potential neurodevelopmental pathology in infants who may receive multiple vaccines that contain thimerosal and may be unable to adequately clear this product because of hepatic immaturity (FDA, 2018).
- In 2004, the Institute of Medicine (IOM) released a report that rejected a causal link between vaccines and developmental disorders, including autism, in children. The mercury levels found in the urine of children with autism were not greater than the levels in those without the condition, according to a U.K. study.

Data from U.S. Food & Drug Administration. (2018). Thimerosal and vaccines. https://www.fda.gov/vaccines-blood-biologics/safety-availability-biologics/thimerosal-and-vaccines; and Institute of Medicine (IOM). (2004). Immunization Safety Review Committee. Washington, DC, National Academies Press.

PRACTICE PEARLS

Incompetent Immune Systems

Incompetent immune systems do not develop active immunity in response to vaccines and toxoids. Protection against incompetent immune systems can be accomplished through passive immunity, identification of the deficient immune mediators, and replacement of those mediators, or by giving these patients antiinfective drugs. Agents that are classified as immune mediators are agents such as interferons, interleukins, and immunoglobulins.

Life Span Considerations With Immunizations and Immunomodulation Medications

Patient variables will be discussed later in the chapter with each type of vaccine. Some generic concepts that apply to each immunization follow.

Geriatrics

- Immune systems of older adults are less active.
- Comorbid conditions and chronic illnesses increase the rate of complications due to infectious diseases.

Pediatrics

- Immunizations are an integral part of the primary health care of children. Recent research concluded that many childhood vaccines have not been linked to an increased risk of immune thrombocytopenic purpura (ITP) among young children. However, ITP can happen after a natural measles infection and after getting the MMR vaccine. The risk of ITP has been shown to be increased in the 6 weeks following an MMR vaccination, with one study estimating one case per 40,000 vaccinated children. ITP with hepatitis A vaccine was associated with an increased ITP risk among 7- to 17-year-olds. The chickenpox and Tdap vaccines were tied to the disorder among 11- to 17-year-olds.
- In most cases, preterm infants should be immunized at the usual recommended chronologic age and with the recommended dose. Premature infants weighing less than 2000 Gm should not receive hepatitis B vaccine until 1 month of age or prior to hospital discharge.
- Children who were exposed to more perfluorinated compounds, such as those found in stain, water, and oil-resistant products, have been found to be less likely to respond to routine vaccines (Grandjean et al., 2017).

Pregnancy and Lactation

- Live vaccines usually are contraindicated in pregnancy (see individual vaccine listings).
- It is usually safe to give vaccines while the mother is breastfeeding.
- It is usually safe to give vaccines to mothers who are breastfeeding, with the exception of smallpox and yellow fever vaccines. Hepatitis A and polysaccharide pneumococcus have not been specifically studied in those who are breastfeeding; no evidence suggests that trace amounts of a vaccine present in breast milk are harmful to infants.

Immunization and Biologic Agents Commonly Used in Primary Care

Many common immunization vaccinations and biologic agents are commonly used in primary care (Table 50.2). Comparable vaccines made by different manufacturers may be used interchangeably, if used according to recommended guidelines. Table 50.3 provides a list of U.S. vaccinations and how they are supplied. Available data suggest that adequate response occurs even when products from different manufacturers are used during the same series.

At-Risk and Postexposure Patients

Certain populations are considered to be at risk for exposures or require postexposure therapy. In this event, the Advisory Council on Immunization Practices offers the routinely updated *Vaccine Recommendations and Guidelines of the ACIP: General Best Practice Guidelines for Immunization* (Ezeanolue et al., n.d.):

1. In compliance with recommendations for all individuals, it is particularly important that all health care workers be immunized against hepatitis B. In addition, healthcare workers in emergency department settings and on emergency response teams, such as emergency medical technicians and paramedics, may elect to be vaccinated against smallpox. Specific recommendations for the use of smallpox vaccine are discussed later in this chapter.

2. Immunosuppressed individuals, including those with human immunodeficiency virus (HIV), individuals receiving chemotherapy, and those on corticosteroids, will require modifications of the recommended immunization schedule. Where possible, efforts should be made to appropriately vaccinate individuals prior to beginning regimens such as chemotherapy.

3. Travelers to many underdeveloped nations may require specific immunizations, depending on where they are traveling. The *CDC Health Information for International Travel*, commonly referred to as the *Yellow Book*, is updated every 2 years and is the authoritative source of U.S. government

When to Administer Vaccinations

Numerous myths exist about contraindications to administration of vaccines. For all currently available products, the following principles apply:

- Minor upper respiratory infection or gastroenteritis, with or without fever, is not an appropriate indication for withholding a scheduled vaccine dose.
- Concurrent administration of an antibiotic is not a contraindication to immunization.
- Pregnancy in a household member is not a reason to withhold vaccine from a child or adult.
- A lapse in the recommended immunization schedule does not require that the entire series be restarted. Needed doses should be given at the first opportunity, as though the usual interval had occurred.
- Half-doses of vaccine are *never* indicated in individuals who had a significant reaction to a previous dose. In addition, reduced or divided doses are not recommended for preterm or low-birth-weight infants.
- Family history of an adverse event with an immunizing agent, family history of seizures, and family history of sudden infant death are not appropriate indications for withholding recommended immunizations.
- Soreness, redness, or swelling in the area of the immunization or fever lower than 40.5°C (105°F) following a previous vaccine is not an indication to withhold subsequent doses.

TABLE 50.2 Common Immunizations and Biologic Agents Used in Primary Care

Disease	Active Immunity	Passive Immunity	Testing
Diphtheria/tetanus/pertussis	DTaP DPT-Hib vaccine, DTaP, Td, tetanus toxoid	Diphtheria antitoxin Tetanus immune globulin	
Haemophilus influenzae disease	*Haemophilus influenzae* type b accine		
Hepatitis A	Hepatitis A vaccine, inactivated	Immune globulin, Ig	Antibody levels
Hepatitis B	Hepatitis B vaccine	Hepatitis B immune globulin	Antibody levels
Human papillomavirus	Human papillomavirus vaccine		
Influenza	Influenza virus vaccine		
Meningitis	Meningococcal polysaccharide vaccine		
MMR	Mumps vaccine, rubella and mumps vaccine, MMR, measles (rubeola) vaccine	Immune globulin, IgM	Mumps titer Measles titer
Pneumococcal pneumonia	Pneumococcal polysaccharide vaccine, polyvalent and pneumococcal conjugate vaccine		
Polio	Poliovirus vaccine, inactivated		
Rabies	Rabies vaccine (HDCV)	Rabies immune globulin, human	Rabies titer
Rotavirus	Pentavalent Rotavirus Vaccine		Rapid antigen stool test
Shingles			
Tuberculosis	BCG vaccine		Tuberculin test and Quantiferon
Typhoid	Typhoid vaccine		
Varicella-zoster immune globulin	Varicella-zoster titer	Varicella-zoster immune globulin	Varicella-zoster titer
Yellow fever	Yellow fever vaccine		

recommendations for immunizations and prophylaxis for foreign travel (Brunette & Nemhauser, 2020). Information on vaccine recommendations for travel can be found on the CDC's website (CDC, n.d.).

Notification of Risks and Benefits of the Vaccine

The National Childhood Vaccine Injury Act of 1986 mandates the notification of patients and parents of the risks and benefits of individual vaccines. This legislation requires the distribution of standardized information to these individuals. Simplified versions of approved vaccine information sheets (VIS) are available from vaccine manufacturers, the CDC, and most state health departments.

Health care providers who administer vaccines are required to keep permanent records of all immunizations given, along with specific information about the manufacturer of the product and the lot number of all doses. In addition, the provider is required to report to the Vaccine Adverse Event Reporting System (VAERS) any event suspected to be the result of a vaccine (VAERS, n.d.).

For patients with signs and symptoms suggesting an immunoglobin E–mediated reaction to a vaccine or its components, allergy testing by a specialist may be indicated, especially when future doses of the suspect vaccine(s) will be needed. A multiple-dose graded challenge facilitates this

PRACTICE PEARLS

MMR and Autism

The question of whether vaccines cause autism has remained in the minds of the public despite numerous scientific studies concluding that they do not. A panel of the IOM once again concluded that the MMR vaccine does not cause autism despite complaints from some parents' groups. The government asked the IOM in 2012 to review the known risks of different kinds of vaccines to help guide decisions about compensation for those who claim to have been injured by vaccines. Legislation passed in 1986 by Congress basically absolved vaccine makers of the risks of being sued for vaccine injuries to encourage companies to continue to manufacture vaccines and force those who suffer some type of injury they believe is related to vaccines to petition the government for compensation. The government generally restricts compensation to cases involving children who have injuries that scientists believe might plausibly have been caused by vaccination, including seizures, allergic reactions, fainting, inflammation, and temporary joint pain. But legal and legislative battles have been fought for years over whether to expand this list because of the concern about vaccines and autism. Much of this concern was due to a fraudulently reported study that was later retracted. Rather than vaccines causing autism, it has been suggested that many children found to be injured by vaccination have an immune or metabolic problem that becomes obvious after vaccination or that may be triggered by the vaccine.

TABLE 50.3 United States Vaccinations[a]

Vaccine	Product Information
COVID-19	Pfizer-BioNTech
	Moderna
	Johnson & Johnson's Janssen
DTaP, DT, Td, Tdap, DTaP-IPV–Hepatitis B	DT: diphtheria, tetanus toxoids
	DTaP: diphtheria, tetanus toxoids combined with acellular pertussis vaccine
	Tdap: tetanus toxoid, reduced diphtheria toxoid, and acellular pertussis vaccine approved for ages 11–64 yr
	Tdap: tetanus toxoid, reduced diphtheria toxoid, and acellular pertussis vaccine approved for ages ≥10 yr
	DTaP-IPV–Hepatitis B: combines DTaP, injectable polio vaccine, and hepatitis B vaccine
	DTaP-IPV: approved for ages 4–6 yr; contains DTaP and inactivated poliovirus vaccine
	DTaP-IPV: single dose is approved for ages 4–6 yr
	DTaP-Hib-IPV : DTaP, Haemophilus b conjugate vaccine, and inactivated poliovirus vaccine
	Td: tetanus and diphtheria toxoids
Haemophilus b Conjugate Vaccine (Hib)	PRP-T (polyribosylribitol phosphate polysaccharide conjugated to tetanus toxoid)
	PRP-OMP: purified capsular polysaccharide (PRP) conjugated to the outer membrane protein (OMP) of Neisseria meningitidis serotype B
	Vaccines may be used interchangeably with HbOC or PRP-T products, not by the PRP-OMP vaccine
	PRP-T: polyribosyl-ribitol-phosphate [PRP] conjugated to inactivated tetanus toxoid
	DTaP-Hib-IPV: DTaP, Haemophilus b conjugate vaccine, and inactivated poliovirus vaccine
	All contain an Hib capsular polysaccharide that is covalently linked to a carrier protein
Hepatitis A, B & Combination	Hepatitis A monovalent vaccines: FDA approved for ages ≥12 months; these vaccines are interchangeable and the volume differs based on age
	Hepatitis A and B coformulated vaccine: FDA approved for ages ≥18 yr
	Monovalent recombinant hepatitis B preparations: 10–40 mcg/mL of HBsAg protein. The immune response of Engerix-B and Recombivvax HB is interchangeable with the HBsAg protein ranging from 10–40 mcg/mL. No data exist currently with the interchangeability of these with Heplisav-B formulation
	DTaP-IPV–hepatitis B may not be used for the birth dose of hepatitis B, but it may be used for subsequent doses if all components are indicated
	Only monovalent hepatitis B vaccine should be used if the first dose is given to a newborn
Human Papillomavirus (HPV)	Ninevalent HPV vaccine
Influenza Vaccine	PharmaJet Stratis Needle-Free Injection System (FDA 2014)
	A high-dose TIV preparation HD-IIV4: use in ages >65 yr
Meningococcal	MenACWY-D: FDA approved as 2-dose series age 9–23 months; single dose age 2–55 yr.
	MenACWY-CRM: FDA approved as 4-dose series age 2–23 months; single dose 2–55 yr.
	If continued risk for meningococcal disease, then an additional dose of vaccine may be given after 3 years if the first dose was administered at age 2–6 years
	Patients who have completed the 2-dose primary series and remain at continued risk for meningococcal disease can be revaccinated every 5 years after the last dose of the primary series
	Persons with persistent complement component deficiency or anatomic or functional asplenia may receive a single dose every 5 years after completing the 2-dose primary series
	MenB-4C: FDA approved for ages 10–25 yr as a 2-dose series (0, 1–6 months)
	MenB-FHbp: FDA approved for ages 10–25 yr as a 3-dose series (0, 1–2, 6 months) or 2-dose series (0 and 6 months)
Measles, Mumps, and Rubella (MMR)	Trivalent M-M-R II or a quadrivalent preparation containing varicella currently available

TABLE 50.3	United States Vaccinations—cont'd
Vaccine	**Product Information**
Pneumonia	PPV13 is available as a prefilled syringe
	PPSV23 is available as a single-dose vial or syringe
Polio	inactivated IM or subcutaneously 6 weeks and older
Respiratory Syncytial Virus	Palivizumab 50-mg and 100-mg single-dose vials.
Rotavirus	Live, oral pentavalent available as an oral suspension in ready-to-use dosing 1-mL tubes; series given from 6 weeks to 32 weeks.
	Live, oral available as lyophilized powder with a liquid diluent that must be reconstituted before administration; series given from 6 weeks to 24 weeks.
Smallpox	ACAM2000 smallpox vaccine is available only through the CDC.
Typhoid	Live, attenuated oral (Ty21a)
	Polysacharide IM available as a single-dose injectable vaccine in vials
Varicella	Varicella vaccine is available in three formulations: • Varicella-zoster: a monovalent, live-attenuated preparation of the wild Oka strain of varicella • MMRV: the titer of Oka varicella-zoster virus is higher in MMRV vaccine than in single-antigen varicella vaccine; FDA approved for 12 months to 12 yr • Zoster: for use in adults >50 yr for the prevention of shinglesFor use in adults >50 yr for the prevention of shingles, recommended dose is 0.5 mL given intramuscularly in two doses separated by 2–6 months.
Yellow Fever	17D-204 strain (YF-Vax) is packaged in 5-dose vials.

[a]**NOTE:** Current as of February 2021. Please consult current administration and availability guidelines.

process, which should preferably be performed under close observation by an allergist, using the specific vaccine, from the same maker, that is suspected of causing the reaction.

A review by Baxter et al. (2012) of the medical records of 550 patients with Guillain-Barré syndrome showed that none of them experienced flare-ups in the 2 months after receiving vaccines, including flu shots. Only one patient experienced a flare-up within a year of vaccination. This information should be provided to individuals with a history of Guillain-Barré syndrome who would like to receive vaccinations to prevent illness.

Immunizations

The ACIP provides yearly updates to the Recommended Child and Adolescent Immunization Schedule for ages 18 years or younger and the Recommended Adult Immunization Schedule for ages 19 years or older (ACIP, n.d. a; ACIP, n.d. b). In addition, the manufacturer's package inserts provide information regarding specific preparation and dosing guidelines.

Diphtheria-Tetanus-Pertussis Vaccine (DTaP, Tdap)

Indications. Although the incidence of all of these infections has decreased dramatically since the introduction of vaccine, pertussis continues to be a serious concern, with an incidence in the United States that has been increasing steadily. There were more than 27,000 cases in 2010, more than 48,000 in 2012, and nearly 19,000 in 2017, primarily in young children who did not receive immunizations and older adults with lowered immunity (CDC, 2017). Pertussis outbreaks seem to occur in 3- to 5-year cycles. The CDC tracks specific states and geographic areas in which the incidence

of pertussis is particularly high, and primary care providers should be aware of their geographic incidence. Research demonstrates protection offered by pertussis vaccine fades over time, which is a major contributor to recent outbreaks.

Diphtheria and tetanus preparations are toxoids made by treating toxins with formaldehyde. The pertussis component is available as an acellular preparation that contains purified, inactivated pertussis toxin and proteins. The four pertussis preparations are available in the United States in combination with tetanus and diphtheria toxoid and vary in pertussis antigen; however, immunogenicity is similar.

Children. Children who are not vaccinated are eight times as likely to get pertussis compared to those who receive all five shots in the DTaP series. States in which there are high numbers of homeschooled children or parents who may claim a religious reason to exempt immunizing children contribute to the higher incidence of infections that are largely preventable.

Adults. Pertussis accounts for up to 7% of coughs in adults. Although the disease is milder in adults, adults who have had previous immunizations (whose level of immunity to pertussis has been found to decrease over time) are recognized to be the source of infection for children. In 2006, the ACIP added the recommendation that previously immunized adults, 19 years of age and older, should receive a single dose of Tdap to replace tetanus and diphtheria toxoids vaccine (Td). Adults who have never been immunized should receive Tdap as the first dose and complete the series with 2 doses of Td (Tdap can be substituted for either Td dose). The advisory panel also recommended giving a single dose of Tdap to adults aged 19 to 64 who have not already received the vaccine. Adolescents and adults (e.g., parents, siblings, grandparents, child-care providers, and health care personnel) who have or anticipate having close contact with an infant younger than 12 months of age should receive a single dose of Tdap to protect against pertussis if they have not previously received Tdap.

Adverse Effects. Localized redness, induration, and tenderness at the injection site are the most common adverse effects, especially as the doses in a series progress. Significant swelling involving the entire thigh or upper arm also can occur, especially after the fourth or fifth dose. Temperature greater than 38.3°C (101°F), drowsiness, fretfulness, and anorexia are common. The pertussis component of the vaccine is responsible for most of these reactions. None of these reactions results in sequelae, and they are not contraindications to subsequent doses.

Moderate to severe systemic reactions are infrequent yet serious and may include fever (temperature higher than 40.5°C or higher than 105°F) and persistent, inconsolable crying that lasts longer than 3 hours. Seizures were more frequently seen with older whole-cell preparations compared to the acellular pertussis formulation and are usually of the febrile type. Shock (hypotonic-hyporesponsive) episodes were known to occur with older preparations and rarely with acellular pertussis formulations. Acute encephalopathy and permanent neurologic deficit have been reported in a few cases following whole-cell DTP.

Contraindications. When the pertussis component is contraindicated, the primary series should be completed with DT alone. In addition, unstable, changing neurologic disorders (e.g., uncontrolled epilepsy, infantile spasms, progressive encephalopathy) are reasons to delay immunization until the condition has been alleviated. Stable neurologic disorders (e.g., well-controlled epilepsy, cerebral palsy, developmental delay) are not contraindications.

PRACTICE PEARLS

Absolute Contraindications to Pertussis-Containing Preparations

Absolute contraindications to administration of pertussis-containing preparations are the following effects noted after previous doses of DTap or Tdap:

- *Allergic hypersensitivity reactions:* Anaphylaxis, if it occurs at all, is extremely rare. Urticaria may follow pertussis vaccine. If the appearance is delayed, it is unlikely to represent an IgE-mediated process and is not a contraindication to subsequent doses.
- Encephalopathy not from an alternative cause within 7 days of its administration

---

The following conditions were previously considered to be contraindications but have not been demonstrated to cause permanent sequelae and now are listed as precautions to future administration of DTaP:

- Temperature of 40.5°C (104.8°F) within 48 hours not from an alternative cause

- Collapse or shock-like state (hypotonic-hyporesponsive episode) within 48 hours not from an alternative cause
- Persistent, inconsolable crying that lasts 3 hours or longer within 48 hours
- Seizures with or without fever within 3 days

Vaccination with pertussis should be delayed in children with progressive neurologic disorders associated with developmental delay and/or neurologic findings, conditions known to be associated with progressive neurologic deterioration such as tuberous sclerosis, or a history of recent onset of seizures of unknown origin. A decision to vaccinate these children should be made on a case-by-case basis and will have to be reevaluated with changes in their condition.

PRACTICE PEARLS

Diphtheria-Tetanus-Pertussis Vaccine in Pregnancy and Lactation

- Tdap may be given during pregnancy, preferably during early in gestational weeks 27 through 36.
- If not administered during pregnancy, Tdap should be administered immediately postpartum.
- All pregnant females should be immunized against pertussis in the late second or third trimester regardless of whether they have had Tdap in the past.

Monitoring. Routine laboratory monitoring is not required. Monitor immediately following administration for potential serious adverse effects. Advise patient and/or caregiver when to seek help.

Haemophilus influenzae Type b Vaccination (Hib)

This product is a polysaccharide that is conjugated with a carrier protein coat to increase immunogenicity. This protein is more antigenic because of its ability to invoke a T-cell response. T-cells allow successively increased antibody production after each exposure.

Indications. Follow the ACIP guidelines to address vaccination recommendations in adults with HIV, patients undergoing elective splenectomy, patients 15 months of age or older with functional or anatomic asplenia, and patients with hematopoietic cell transplants. HIV-infected children should receive at least one dose of Hib vaccine if unimmunized.

Children. Immunize all children beginning at minimum of 6 weeks with three subsequent doses (boosters) at 4, 6, and 12 to 15 months following current guidelines. *Haemophilus* b conjugate (PMP-OMP), which contains an outer membrane protein complex, is recommended as the first dose in Native American/Native Alaskan children because of the increased risk of early disease in this population and the ability of this vaccine to provide protection after the first dose.

Children who have had invasive Hib disease when younger than 24 months of age may, despite this illness, produce low antibody concentrations and are at risk for a subsequent episode. Any vaccine given before this disease occurs should be ignored, and conjugate vaccine should be readministered beginning as soon as possible during the recovery according to the recommended schedule for nonimmunized children of the same age. Children who are older than 24 months at the time of disease do not require immunization, irrespective of previous status. Hib vaccination is not recommended in patients older than 59 months as most are likely immune due to asymptomatic infections acquired at a younger age.

Adults. Hib vaccine is not indicated in those older than 60 months of age. Health care providers should review current guidelines for specific recommendations based on the patient's health history.

Adverse Effects. Very few side effects occur with any of the conjugate preparations. Localized swelling, tenderness, and redness occur in fewer than 5% to 30% of recipients and resolves within 24 hours. Systemic effects such as fever and irritability are very uncommon. No serious side effects are known with *H. influenzae* type b.

Contraindications. Children with impaired immune systems, such as those infected with HIV, may not mount sufficient immunity with the recommended vaccine schedule and may require an additional dose.

Monitoring. Monitor for adverse effects immediately following administration. Advise the patient and/or caregiver when to seek help. Routine laboratory monitoring is not required.

Hepatitis A Vaccine

Hepatitis A virus (HAV) is highly contagious, and the predominant mode of transmission is person to person via the fecal–oral route. Infection has been shown to be spread by contaminated water or food, by infected food handlers, after breakdown in usual sanitary conditions after floods or natural disasters, by ingestion of raw or undercooked shellfish from contaminated waters, and during travel to areas of the world with poor hygienic conditions. Increased incidence is also seen among institutionalized children and adults, especially in day care centers where children have not been toilet trained. HAV can rarely be spread through parenteral transmission and by blood transfusions or by needle sharing with infected people. The HAV can survive outside the body for months. High temperatures (e.g., exposure for 1 minute at 185°F [85°C]) will kill the HAV, while freezing temperatures do not. The incubation period for hepatitis A averages 28 days, and its disease course is extremely variable.

Although many children may have asymptomatic infection, most older children and adults are symptomatic, with a self-limiting course characterized by fever, malaise, nausea, and jaundice. Recovery is usually complete and is followed by lifelong protection against HAV infection. The hepatitis A vaccine protects young children for at least 10 years after completing a two-dose series and 15 to 17 years after completing a three-dose series in studies involving Native American/Native Alaskan individuals (Hamborsky et al., 2015).

Indications. The ACIP recommends routine hepatitis A vaccination for the following groups:

- Children receive first dose at 12 months with second dose administered at a minimal 6-month interval. Children who have not received the second dose by 2 years of age should be vaccinated as soon as possible.
- Children older than 23 months of age who live in areas where vaccination programs target older children and who are at increased risk for hepatitis A infection.
- Anyone 6 months of age and older who is traveling to or working in an area that is considered high risk should receive the vaccine. Areas of low risk include the United States, Canada, Japan, New Zealand, and Australia, and some (but not all) countries of Western Europe. See the *CDC Yellow Book* for more information on whether to vaccinate (Brunette & Nemhauser, 2020). Always vaccinate if there is a doubt.
- Males who have sex with males.
- Users of injectable or noninjectable illegal drugs.
- Homeless persons.
- Previously unvaccinated people who anticipate having close personal contact with an international adoptee from a country of high or intermediate endemicity during the first 60 days following the adoptee's arrival in the United States.
- Persons with blood-clotting disorders.
- Those who work with HAV-infected nonhuman primates or with HAV in a research laboratory setting (no other groups have been shown to be at increased risk for HAV infection because of occupational exposure).
- Persons with chronic liver disease.
- Anyone 1 year of age and older with HIV infection.
- Any individual who wishes to be immune to hepatitis A.

Hepatitis A vaccine is not routinely recommended because of occupational exposure for health care personnel, sewage workers, or day care providers.

Adverse Effects. In general, the HAV vaccine is associated with only mild and short-term effects: 20% to 50% of patients may have local reactions at the injection site with induration, redness, and swelling, and fewer than 10% of patients may experience systemic reactions (e.g., headache, fatigue, mild fever, malaise, anorexia, or nausea). Serious side effects have not been reported.

Contraindications. Contraindications to HAV vaccine include severe allergic reaction to a vaccine component or following a prior dose and moderate or severe acute illness.

Because hepatitis A has a relatively long incubation period (15 to 50 days), this vaccine may not prevent hepatitis A infection in individuals who have an unrecognized hepatitis A infection at the time of vaccination.

The vaccine may be given at the same time as other immunizations. Safety data in pregnancy are limited, but there appears to be little risk associated with administration of this inactivated product.

Monitoring. Monitor for completion of series. Monitor hepatitis A serology following completion of series.

Hepatitis B Vaccine

Indications. Currently available vaccine is produced through recombinant deoxyribonucleic acid (DNA) technology. Plasma-derived vaccine is not available in the United States. Although the amount of HBsAg protein varies among vaccine products, completion of the series induces protective antibody in 90% to 95% of adults and children with no evidence of different rates of seroconversion. Long-term studies indicate that protection appears to be long lasting even in the face of low or undetectable anti-HBs concentrations. However, immunocompromised patients may have a decreased immune response and require boost doses.

Children. Routine hepatitis B vaccination is recommended for all infants at birth, regardless of their mother's hepatitis status, and all children and adolescents. The CDC provides in-depth, evidence-based practice guidelines including information on the mother's HBsAg (hepatitis B surface antigen) status, routine vaccination series, catch-up vaccinations, and special considerations.

Adults. Routine immunization of all adults is not currently recommended, although there are numerous indications for vaccination, including diabetes, end-stage renal disease (ESRD), household contacts, and sexual partners of persons with chronic HBV. All adults in HIV testing and treatment facilities, correctional facilities, and health care settings targeting services to injection drug users or males who have sex with males should be vaccinated. Outside of these high-risk settings, adults with specific risk factors who were not previously immunized should receive immunization. These groups include the following:

- Health care and public safety workers, including trainees, custodians, and others with potential occupational exposure to blood and blood-contaminated body fluids
- Residents and staff of institutions for the developmentally disabled, long-term correctional facilities
- Hemodialysis patients
- Patients with bleeding disorders who receive blood products
- Household contacts and sexual partners of HBV carriers
- Immigrants, adoptees, and family members from countries where HBV is endemic

The risk for HBV infection among international travelers is low. However, the risk is considered higher in countries where the prevalence of chronic HBV infection is intermediate or high. A list of these countries can be found at the CDC's Traveler's Health website.

Adverse Effects. The most frequently reported side effects associated with the hepatitis B vaccine are pain at the injection site, fatigue, malaise, headache, and low-grade fever. Allergic reactions and anaphylaxis are uncommon.

Contraindications. Because of the long incubation period for hepatitis B, it is possible for unrecognized infection to be present at the time the vaccine is given. The vaccine will not prevent or clear hepatitis B in such patients. Epinephrine should be available for immediate use should a rare anaphylactic reaction occur. Any moderate or severe active infection with or without fever is cause for delaying use of the vaccine, except when, in the opinion of the health care provider, withholding the vaccine entails a greater risk. Hepatitis B vaccination is contraindicated for patients with a history of hypersensitivity to yeast (e.g., *Saccharomyces cerevisiae*) or any other vaccine component.

Sleep researchers have found that getting too little sleep may reduce the efficacy of the hepatitis B vaccine. Patients who sleep fewer than 6 hours nightly tend to produce fewer antibodies in response to the vaccine.

PRACTICE PEARLS

Hepatitis B Vaccine in Pregnancy and Lactation

- Pregnancy and lactation are not contraindications to HBV vaccination.
- No adverse effects on the developing fetus have been noted when vaccine is administered during pregnancy.
- Routine screening for HBV is recommended for all females early in pregnancy (e.g., first trimester) and should be repeated late in pregnancy (e.g., third trimester) for negative females who are at high risk for infection.

Monitoring. Prior to administration, review elapsed time between doses, patient history, and indications and contraindications. Monitor for adverse reactions and signs of hypersensitivity immediately following each vaccine. After administration to health care workers, monitor serologic levels 1 to 2 months following the final dose.

Human Papillomavirus Vaccine

The CDC (*2020, November 17*) reports that human papillomavirus virus (HPV) is the most common sexually transmitted disease in the United States:

- Approximately 80 million people in the United States are infected with HPV.
- 14 million new cases of HPV infection occur every year in patients 15 to 59 years of age.
- 4,000 deaths per year occur in the United States as a result of cervical cancer.

HPV infection can result in visible genital warts, subclinical infection, and, most seriously, cervical, penile, and head and neck cancers. HPV types are categorized according to their relative risk of specific clinical events, and more than 100 types have been identified. Most infections with HPV are benign and self-resolving, often involving serotypes 6 and 11. However, high-risk HPV types, most commonly, types 16 and 18, can cause low- and high-grade cervical cell abnormalities that are precursors to invasive cervical cancer.

Indications. A nine valent alum adjuvanted vaccine with protection against serotypes 6, 11, 16, 18, 31, 33, 45, 52, and 58 was licensed by the FDA in 2019 for individuals 9 to 45 years of age. The ACIP recommends HPV vaccination routinely for all adolescents 11 to 12 years of age (can start at age 9) and through age 18 if not previously adequately vaccinated (ACIP, n.d.a). The series involves two or three doses depending on the patient's age at the initial vaccine administration. If the patient has a history of sexual assault, start the vaccine series at 9 years of age.

Adverse Effects. The most commonly reported adverse effects were associated with injection site reactions and include pain (89.9% of patients), swelling (40% to 47%), and erythema (34.0%). The most common systemic effect was headache (11.4% to 14.6%). Syncope and tonic-clonic movements have been reported with HPV vaccine. Patients should be observed for at least 15 minutes after administration. When syncope is associated with tonic-clonic movements, the activity is usually temporary and resolves upon restoration of cerebral perfusion by maintaining a supine or Trendelenburg position.

Contraindications. Avoid administration in a patient with a hypersensitivity, including a severe reaction (e.g., anaphylaxis), to yeast or any of the vaccine's components.

Monitoring. Follow up with pelvic exams and Pap smears per current evidence-based practice guidelines. No routine serological monitoring is required.

Influenza Vaccine (Various Strains)

Indications. Although *Healthy People 2020* set a goal of 70% vaccination rates in older and other high-risk individuals, success in meeting this goal has been mixed, with minority populations and adults older than 65 years of age not residing in nursing homes less likely to be immunized. Disparities in influenza vaccination rates in older adults are stark, with only approximately half of Black and Hispanic older adults receiving annual vaccination compared with 70% in Caucasians. Despite rising vaccination rates, continuing epidemics of influenza occur annually. Rates of infection are highest among children, but rates of serious illness and death are highest among persons older than 65 years and persons of any age who have medical conditions that place them at increased risk for complications from influenza. Medical conditions associated with higher risk of influenza-associated complications include pregnancy; diabetes; immunocompromised state (e.g., HIV/AIDS, cancer, transplant recipient, etc.); asthma; children younger than 2 years of age or with neurologic conditions; heart, liver, kidney, or metabolic disorders; obesity; and chronic aspirin use. Influenza vaccine efficacy varies based on its similarity to circulating strains and the age and health status of the recipient. Four vaccine types are available: inactivated influenza vaccine (IIV), live-attenuated influenza vaccine (LAIV), cell-culture based (ccIIV4), and recombinant (RIV). All four vaccine types are multivalent, containing three (IIV3) or four (IIV4, LAIV4, RIV4) different viral subtypes; the composition changes annually in anticipation of expected prevalent influenza strains. However, these vaccines are less effective in preventing illness among persons 65 years of age and older. As a result, to improve immunogenicity in older adults, a newer influenza vaccine formulation was approved in 2009 with each dose containing four times as much hemagglutinin as the regular influenza vaccine formulation.

The influenza vaccine is not effective against all possible strains of influenza virus, and protection is afforded only against those strains of virus from which the vaccine is prepared or against closely related strains. The impact of immunization is most noticeable in adult populations, probably because of the lower frequency of colds and other viral disease. Health care providers should begin vaccination efforts in early fall and should continue to offer vaccine until circulating influenza or vaccine is no longer present in the community. Adolescents and adults should be given an annual influenza vaccine. Efficacy has not been evaluated in children younger than 6 months of age.

No preference is indicated for LAIV or RIV when considering vaccination of healthy, nonpregnant persons aged 2 to 49 years. Give patients who are taking influenza antiviral medications the IIV or RIV formulation. Patients with severe egg allergies should receive an egg-free vaccine formulation.

Adverse Effects. The most frequently reported adverse effects with inactivated influenza vaccines include intramuscular (IM) injection site pain, redness, and swelling that may persist for up to 2 days. Less frequently, patients report fever, malaise, and myalgias. Allergic reactions are rare and likely due to reaction to a vaccine component, particularly because many formulations of this vaccine are grown in eggs. There are two vaccines available that are manufactured without the use of eggs and are considered egg free.

The live-attenuated influenza vaccine is administered intranasally. This route of administration is associated with increase in upper respiratory tract infection symptoms (e.g., runny nose, congestion, cough, sore throat, chills, fever, etc.). Children 6 to 23 months of age have been associated with an increase in wheezing.

Contraindications. The influenza vaccine is contraindicated with a history of severe allergic reaction to any component of the vaccine (any valency) or to any egg-based IIV or LAIV, any ccIIV or RIV, or any unknown influenza vaccine. The LAIV4 vaccine has additional contraindications including:

- Concomitant aspirin or salicylate-containing therapy in children and adolescents
- Children 2 to 4 years of age with a diagnosis of asthma or with wheezing or asthma in the past 12 months
- Immunocompromised children or adults or those who live with immunocompromised persons.
- Pregnancy
- Persons with cochlear implant or active communication between cerebrospinal fluid (CSF) and the oropharynx, nasopharynx, nose, or ear, or any other cranial CSF leak

Precautions commonly listed by vaccine manufacturers include patients with moderate or severe acute illness (with or without fever) or a history of Guillain-Barré syndrome within 6 weeks of receipt of influenza vaccine. The LAIV4 vaccine precautions also include:

- Persons 5 years of age or older with a history of asthma
- Any person with underlying medical conditions that might predispose to complications

Monitoring. Monitor for adverse effects immediately following administration. Advise the patient and/or caregiver when to seek help. Routine laboratory monitoring is not required.

Measles-Mumps-Rubella Vaccine (MMR)

Indications. MMR is an attenuated virus vaccine. This means that after injection, the weakened viruses cause a harmless infection in the vaccinated person with very few, if any, symptoms before they are eliminated from the body. The immune system fights the infection caused by these weakened viruses, and immunity develops. For the past 50 years, the live attenuated MMR trivalent vaccine has been available and prepared in chick embryo cell culture. After administration of a single dose of live-virus vaccine, 95% of individuals develop adequate serum antibody. In 2009, the U.S. Food and Drug Administration (FDA) approved a quadrivalent live vaccine of MMR with varicella virus.

Children. The first dose is recommended at 12 to 15 months of age and a second dose is given at elementary school entry at 4 to 6 years of age. Children who have laboratory evidence of immunity do not require vaccinations. Provider diagnosis is inadequate to demonstrate immunity. Recommendations for administration if a child will be traveling internationally permit earlier administration (CDC, n.d.). Vaccinated children with two doses of a mumps-containing vaccine who are identified by public health as at increased risk for mumps because of an outbreak should receive a third dose of a mumps-containing vaccine to improve protection against mumps disease and related complications (Albertson et al., 2016).

Adults. Adults 19 years and older without evidence of immunity to MMR should receive one dose of MMR vaccine. Health-care workers born in 1957 or later with no history of MMR vaccination or evidence of immunity should receive two doses of MMR vaccine (at a minimum interval of 4 weeks between doses) for measles or mumps, or at least one dose for rubella. Adults previously vaccinated with two doses of mumps-containing vaccine who are identified by public health as at increased risk for mumps because of an outbreak should receive a third dose of a mumps-containing vaccine to improve protection against mumps disease and related complications (Marin et al., 2018).

Adverse Effects. Side effects are markedly less common with second doses, presumably because most individuals are already immune. No side effects have been reported in immune persons who were inadvertently vaccinated. Reported side effects with the MMR vaccine may include the following:

- Fever beginning 7 to 12 days after vaccination and commonly lasting 1 to 2 days. Fever may extend up to 5 days.
- Transient rash appearing 7 to 10 days after vaccination, with arthralgias particularly in peripheral small joints in adults. No permanent joint destruction has been reported. This rarely occurs in children.
- Thrombocytopenia occurring transiently within 2 months after vaccination.

Children 12 to 23 months old who have not been previously vaccinated against measles, mumps, rubella, or varicella, nor had a history of the wild-type infections, have been associated with higher rates of febrile seizures at 5 to 12 days after vaccination when compared to children vaccinated with dose one of both MMR and varicella administered separately.

Allergic reactions occur rarely and are usually attributable to trace amounts of neomycin and gelatin; children with known anaphylaxis to topical or systemic neomycin should receive vaccine in settings where such a reaction can be treated. A history of contact dermatitis to neomycin is not a contraindication.

Contraindications. The MMR vaccine is contraindicated in patients with a previous history of severe anaphylactic reaction to a previous dose or to any component, including gelatin (used as a stabilizer for rubella virus) or neomycin. Patients with blood dyscrasias; lymphomas; malignant neoplasms; congenital, hereditary, or acquired immunodeficiency; or those on immunosuppressive therapy should not receive the vaccine. Leukemia patients in remission should allow for a 3-month period following chemotherapy before receiving the vaccine.

PRACTICE PEARLS

Measles Vaccine and Egg Allergy

The measles component of the vaccine is produced in chick embryo cell culture but does not contain a significant amount of egg protein.

Children with egg allergy are at low risk for anaphylactic reactions to measles-containing vaccine, and skin testing for egg allergy is not indicated.

Measles-Mumps-Rubella Vaccine in Pregnancy and Lactation

- Live-virus vaccines should not be administered during pregnancy.
- Females of childbearing age who receive a rubella-containing preparation should be counseled to defer pregnancy for 1 month. If vaccination should occur during the first trimester, the pregnant female should be counseled on possible risks to the fetus. It is currently suggested that inadvertent rubella vaccination during pregnancy is not sufficient reason to recommend termination of the pregnancy.
- The MMR vaccines may be given to children with pregnant mothers.
- MMR may be given to females who are breastfeeding.

Meningococcal Vaccine in Pregnancy and Lactation

- Clinical animal studies demonstrate risk to the fetus. No adequate and well-controlled studies in pregnant females have been conducted.
- Weigh benefit versus risk when considering use during pregnancy.
- Consider the benefits of breastfeeding, the risk of potential infant drug exposure, and the risk of an untreated or inadequately treated condition.

Monitoring. Monitor for severe anaphylactic reaction immediately following administration. Monitor for fever and rash in days following vaccine. Advise caregiver or patient of expected adverse effects and when to seek help.

Meningococcal Vaccine

Neisseria meningitidis is the second most common cause of bacterial meningitis in the United States; it has a case-fatality rate of approximately 10% to 20% despite therapy with antimicrobial agents, to which all strains remain highly sensitive (CDC, 2019). Nearly all invasive meningococcal disease is caused by serogroups A, B, C, Y, and W. The majority of cases in the United States occur sporadically; however, 2% of cases are caused by outbreaks mostly with serogroups B and C (CDC, 2019). Some risk factors for meningococcal disease include functional or anatomic asplenia (including sickle cell disease), immunocompromising conditions, overcrowded housing, active or passive smoking, and preceding viral infection (Hamborsky et al., 2015).

Indications. The ACIP recommends varying doses of the meningococcal ACYW-135 vaccine and the meningococcal B vaccine based on age and comorbidities. Four vaccines are available in the United States: two are tetravalent and protect against *N. meningitidis* serogroups A, C, Y, and W-135 (Menactra and Menveo); and two are monovalent and protect against serogroup B (Trumenba and Bexsero). Historically, most disease outbreaks have been the result of serogroup C; however, recent outbreaks resulting from serogroup B have been reported. Approximately half of infections in infants younger than 1 year of age are the result of infection with serogroup B, for which no vaccine was available until 2014.

Adverse Effects. Meningococcal A, C, Y, and W-135 vaccines were frequently associated with fever, headache, injection site reaction redness and swelling, and syncope. Adverse effects from meningococcal B vaccines were more frequent and included pain at the injection site, erythema, myalgias and fatigue, headache, induration, nausea, and arthralgia (Hamborsky et al., 2015).

Contraindications. Contraindications include prior severe reaction (e.g., anaphylaxis) to any component in a meningococcal vaccine. Syncope has been reported with the use of meningococcal ACYW-135 vaccines and patients should be observed for at least 15 minutes after administration. In 2010, the ACIP removed the recommendation that a history of Guillain-Barré syndrome was a precaution for receipt of Menactra as there was no evidence of an increased risk of the syndrome with this vaccine.

Monitoring. Following administration of meningococcal ACYW-135 vaccines, patients should be observed for at least 15 minutes after administration to observe for syncope or other reactions.

Polio Vaccine (IPV, OPV)

Indications. The poliovirus is an *Enterovirus* that is classified as type 1, 2, or 3. Thus vaccines are trivalent to provide protection against all three subtypes. Inactivated or killed polio vaccine (IPV) is administered parenterally and is now the only type of vaccine available in the United States.

Children. Children should be vaccinated with four doses typically beginning at 2 months of life. Subsequent doses should follow current recommendations.

Adults. Most adults in the United States are immune as a result of childhood vaccination or exposure to wild virus. Unimmunized adults should receive two doses at intervals of 4 to 8 weeks, with a booster dose given 6 to 12 months later. Incompletely immunized adults who previously received OPV may complete the series with IPV. Vaccination should be considered for adults who travel to endemic areas, for laboratory workers handling wild virus, and for health care workers in close contact with patients who may be shedding virus.

Adverse Effects. Minor local site reactions (e.g., pain, redness, swelling) may occur following IPV. No serious adverse events are known to occur as the result of administration of IPV.

Contraindications. IPV contains trace amounts of formaldehyde, 2-phenoxyethanol, streptomycin, neomycin, and polymyxin B and should not be administered if a serious allergic reaction to one of these components has occurred.

PRACTICE PEARLS

IPV Vaccine in Pregnancy and Lactation

- Administration during pregnancy should be avoided, although no risks are known to be associated with administration of IPV during pregnancy.
- If immediate protection is indicated, pregnant females may receive IPV.
- It is unknown whether IPV is excreted in breast milk. Weigh benefit versus risk for administration in lactating females.

Monitoring. Monitor for adverse effects immediately following administration. Advise patient and/or caregiver when to seek help. Routine laboratory monitoring is not required.

Pneumococcal Vaccine

Indications Two types of pneumococcal vaccine are available. The first, PPSV23, is a polyvalent product that is a mixture of highly purified capsular polysaccharides from the 23 most prevalent or invasive pneumococcal types. It is recommended for use in adults and children older than 2 years of age. A pneumococcal conjugate vaccine, PCV13, which conjugates the capsular polysaccharides from the 13 most invasive types of pneumococci with diphtheria protein, was approved in 2010 for use in patients from 6 weeks and older and replaced an earlier 7-valent product.

The CDC offers specific recommendations for PCV13 and PPSV23 vaccine catch-up and for special high-risk pediatric populations who warrant receipt of both vaccinations (https://www.cdc.gov/vaccines/schedules/hcp/imz/child-adolescent.html). When both PCV13 and PPSV23 are indicated, administer PCV13 first because of the immune response to the vaccine when given in this sequence. High-risk children 2 years of age and older may be given the PCV13 and PPSV23 vaccines if they are among the following populations:

- Children with anatomic asplenia or who have splenic dysfunction from sickle cell disease or other hemoglobinopathies
- Children with chronic illnesses of heart, lung, liver, or kidneys, diabetes, receipt of transplantation
- Children who have received cochlear implants or have cerebrospinal fluid (CSF) leak
- Children with immunosuppression or on immunosuppressants
- Alcoholism

As of November 2019, regarding adults, the ACIP recommends a routine single dose of PPSV23 for adults 65 years of age and older. Shared clinical decision-making is recommended regarding administration of PCV13 to persons 65 years of age and older who do not have an immunocompromising condition, CSF leak, or cochlear implant and who have not previously received PCV13. If a decision to administer PCV13 is made, PCV13 should be administered first, followed by PPSV23 at least 1 year later.

Adverse Effects. Local reactions are the most common side effect with both preparations and include local injection site soreness, erythema, and swelling, usually lasting no longer than 2 days; local induration occurs less frequently. Rash, urticaria, arthritis, arthralgia, adenitis, and serum sickness occasionally have been reported. Malaise, myalgia, headache, and asthenia have also been seen. Fever is more common following administration of conjugate vaccine and occurs in about one-fourth of all children; older children are less likely to experience fever.

Contraindications. In patients who require penicillin (or other antibiotic) prophylaxis against pneumococcal infection, such prophylaxis should not be discontinued after vaccination with this vaccine.

PRACTICE PEARLS

Pneumococcal Vaccine in Pregnancy and Lactation

- The pneumococcal polysaccharide vaccine should be given to a pregnant female only if clearly needed.
- The ACIP recommends vaccination during pregnancy when the likelihood of disease exposure is high, potential infection would cause harm to the mother or fetus, and the vaccine is unlikely to cause harm.
- Clinical animal studies demonstrate risk to the fetus. No adequate and well-controlled studies in pregnant females are available.

Monitoring. Monitor for adverse effects immediately following administration. Advise the patient and/or caregiver when to seek help. Routine laboratory monitoring is not required.

Rabies Vaccine (RVA) and Rabies Immune Globulin (RIG)

Indications. RVA is given prophylactically to individuals at high risk of exposure to rabid animals, including veterinarians, animal handlers, and certain laboratory workers. It should be given as a series and should be started immediately after any bite from a suspicious animal. Two rabies vaccines are available in the United States. Both vaccines contain inactivated rabies virus. RIG gives passive protection when started immediately after exposure to rabies virus. It takes approximately 1 week for antibodies to develop and thus it is unlikely that RIG would provide benefit if given after 1 week. Postexposure prophylaxis should begin as soon as possible, preferably within 24 hours, and requires administration of both RIG and rabies vaccine. Vaccine dosing varies for children and adults.

For both adults and children, RIG at a dose of 20 IU/kg should be given as soon as possible, with as much of the dose as possible used to infiltrate the wound; RIG may be diluted with saline to increase volume and allow penetration of the entire wound. The remaining volume should be given intramuscularly at a distant site. Vaccine should be given at the same time; the dose is 1 mL, given intramuscularly, of the three available vaccines on days 0, 3, 7, and 14. Immunocompromised patients should receive a fifth dose on day 28. The same product should be used for all doses. Adults should receive an IM injection in the deltoid; the anterolateral thigh may be used in young children. In individuals who have been previously vaccinated, RIG is not given. Two doses of vaccine should be given; the first should be given on the day of exposure, and the second dose should be given on day 4. Do not administer the RIG and rabies vaccine in the same syringe and at the same anatomical site.

A preexposure rabies vaccination regimen consists of three doses. The second dose is given 7 days after the first vaccination; the third dose is given 21 or 28 days after the first vaccination. Booster doses are indicated with frequent or continuous risk of exposure to rabies virus and when blood testing indicates absent or low levels of immunity against rabies.

Adverse Effects. Although adverse reactions are less common with currently available products, 15% to 25% of adults may experience local reactions, such as pain and swelling, as well as systemic reactions, including headache, muscle pain, nausea, and dizziness. Reactions are much less frequent in children. Severe reactions, including several cases of a Guillain-Barré–like syndrome, do not appear to be causally linked to vaccine.

Contraindications. No contraindications to administration of rabies vaccine or rabies immunoglobulin are known.

PRACTICE PEARLS

RVA and RIG in Pregnancy and Lactation

- Pregnancy is not a contraindication.
- The product does not pose a risk for nursing infants or children.

Monitoring. Routine laboratory monitoring is not required for RVA or RIG.

Respiratory Syncytial Virus (RSV) Vaccine

Respiratory syncytial virus (RSV) is recognized to be the most significant causative agent in acute respiratory tract illness in infants and young children, causing significant morbidity in high-risk infants, including preterm babies. The AAP recommends that infants with hemodynamically significant congenital heart disease, chronic lung disease of prematurity, and birth before 32 weeks' gestation should receive prophylaxis for RSV at the start of the anticipated RSV season—between October and December in most parts of the United States. Infants and children younger than 24 months of age who receive medical therapy (e.g., supplemental oxygen, bronchodilator, diuretic, or chronic corticosteroid therapy) within 6 months should begin prophylaxis before the start of the RSV season (a maximum of five monthly doses). Infants born at 32 to 35 weeks who are younger than 3 months of age at the start of the RSV season or born during the RSV season should receive a maximum of three doses.

Palivizumab. Palivizumab, a monoclonal antibody product for use in children younger than 24 months of age who are at high-risk for RSV, was approved by the FDA in 1998. Although an antibody rather than a vaccine, it is included in this discussion because it is now part of the American Academy of Pediatrics' (AAP) routine recommendations for these infants (American Academy of Pediatrics Committee on Infectious Diseases; American Academy of Pediatrics Bronchiolitis Guidelines Committee, 2014).

Indications. Because of the significant costs associated with palivizumab, use should be considered carefully in infants born at between 32 and 35 weeks who are older than 3 months of age during the RSV season. Those who should be immunized are those with two other risk factors for severe infection, including childcare attendance, siblings younger than 5 years of age, congenital neurologic or musculoskeletal disease, exposure to significant air pollutants, or congenital abnormalities of the airway.

Adverse Effects. The incidence of adverse effects after the administration of palivizumab is similar to that of placebo. They most commonly include fever, injection site pain, and rash. Serious adverse reactions such as thrombocytopenia and hypersensitivity reactions were rare.

Contraindications. Palivizumab is contraindicated in patients with a history of a severe prior reaction to palivizumab, with known hypersensitivity to murine protein or to other components of this product.

PRACTICE PEARLS

Palivizumab in Pregnancy and Lactation

- Clinical animal studies demonstrate risk to the fetus. No adequate and well-controlled studies in pregnant females have been conducted.
- Palivizumab is not approved for use in females of childbearing age.
- Palivizumab is not advised for use during breastfeeding as no data are available.

Monitoring. Administration of palivizumab does not require alteration in the routine vaccination schedule and does not interfere with immunologic response to these agents. Routine laboratory monitoring is not required.

Rotavirus Vaccine

Rotavirus is the most common cause of severe diarrheal disease worldwide. The virus is spread via the fecal–oral route and has less than a 2-day incubation period. Symptoms range from asymptomatic to vomiting, watery diarrhea, fever, and abdominal pain for 3 to 7 days. A rapid antigen test of stool samples is available. In temperate climates, rotavirus is more common during fall and winter. In the United States, in the prevaccine period, annual epidemic peaks were more predictable and usually progressed from the Southwest during November and December to the Northeast by April and May. However, after vaccine introduction, the seasons have become shorter with less significant differences in timing by geographic area. In tropical climates, the disease is less seasonal than in temperate areas. Although children in developed countries are likely to recover with oral rehydration therapy, worldwide this accounts for about a quarter million deaths annually in children under the age of 5 years (World Health Organization, 2020).

Prior to the vaccine introduction in 2006, almost all U.S. children were infected before their fifth birthday and the virus was responsible for many visits to providers' offices and emergency rooms, and even hospitalizations.

Pentavalent Rotavirus Vaccine

The introduction of the pentavalent rotavirus vaccine has been associated with a marked reduction in diarrhea-associated hospitalizations. In 2006, a pentavalent rotavirus vaccine containing five reassortant (meaning similar genetic material) rotaviruses derived from human and bovine strains was licensed for use and has been incorporated into the routine childhood immunization schedule ever since.

Adverse Effects. Rates of adverse effects are similar to those reported with placebo. Diarrhea and vomiting are slightly more common in the week following receipt of vaccine.

Contraindications. Contraindications include infants who are known to have a severe (e.g., anaphylaxis) reaction to a vaccine component or prior rotavirus vaccine, history of moderate to severe GI disease, severe combined immunodeficiency, and intussusception. Avoid administration to infants with acute, moderate, or severe gastroenteritis or other acute illness until the condition improves or resolves.

Monitoring. Monitor for completion of series. Laboratory monitoring is not required.

Smallpox Vaccine

Indications. Routine administration of smallpox vaccine was discontinued in the United States in 1972, when the virus was declared to be eradicated in the wild. Current concerns about its use as a weapon of mass destruction have led to reinstitution of immunization in selected at-risk populations. The smallpox vaccine is currently available in the United States as a live-virus preparation of vaccinia virus.

The ACIP recommends vaccination of laboratory workers who directly handle cultures or animals contaminated or infected with virus. The armed forces vaccinate selected personnel, and vaccination can be considered for health care workers who have contact with the virus through patients or fomites, or to protect responders as part of state public health preparedness programs.

Adverse Effects. Smallpox vaccination, although generally safe, has been associated with a significant incidence of adverse reactions. Most are benign, but they may be alarming in appearance and occasionally serious and life threatening. Severe adverse reactions are more common in persons receiving primary vaccination than in those being revaccinated.

Local reactions, such as local edema, satellite lesions, pain, and swelling of regional lymph nodes, may occur 3 to 10 days after vaccination and may persist for up to 4 weeks. The resultant viral cellulitis may be confused with bacterial cellulitis. In up to one-third of recipients, these reactions may be severe enough to prompt the individual to seek treatment. Systemic reactions include fever, malaise, myalgia, and erythematous or urticarial rashes. As with local reactions, up to one-third of these recipients are ill enough to miss work.

The lesion produced at the vaccination site contains high vaccinia virus titers and is frequently pruritic. The itching that results may lead to transfer of the virus to the face, eyes, genital area, and rectum as secondary lesions, which usually heal without treatment. Successful vaccination produces a lesion at the vaccination site. Beginning about 4 days after vaccination, the florid site contains high titers of vaccinia virus. This surface is easily transferred to the hands and to fomites, especially because itching is a common part of the local reaction. The most severe manifestation is vaccinia keratitis, which may result in lesions of the cornea and, if untreated, corneal scarring with resultant visual impairment. Vaccinated health care workers should avoid contact with patients, particularly those with immunodeficiency, until the scab has separated from the skin at the vaccination site. The FDA has recommended that vaccinees be deferred from donating blood for 30 days, or until the scab has separated.

Generalized vaccinia results in vesicles or pustules on normal skin distant from the vaccination site; this generally resolves without specialized treatment and without residual effects. Progressive vaccinia, also known as vaccinia necrosum, is a severe, potentially fatal illness that is characterized by progressive necrosis in the area of vaccination, often with distant lesions. Prompt hospitalization and aggressive use of massive doses of VIG are required.

Eczema vaccinatum results in localized and systemic spread of vaccinia virus, which produces extensive lesions. This may occur even in those individuals who do not have active dermatitis at the time of vaccination. Treatment includes hospitalization and vaccinia immunoglobulin.

Contraindications. Because of the incidence of potentially severe reactions, routine immunization is not recommended. During a smallpox emergency, such as a weapons of mass destruction attack, all contraindications to vaccination would be reconsidered in light of the risk of smallpox exposure. The smallpox vaccine is contraindicated in the following situations:

- Individuals and household contacts who have ever been diagnosed with eczema or atopic dermatitis or acute or chronic skin condition such as wounds, burns, impetigo, or varicella-zoster should not be vaccinated, even if their skin condition is well controlled. These individuals are at high risk of developing eczema vaccinatum, a potentially severe and sometimes fatal complication.

- Individuals with diseases or conditions that cause immunodeficiency or immunosuppression, including HIV/AIDS, organ transplant, and malignancy, or recipients of radiation, chemotherapy, or high-dose corticosteroids, should not be vaccinated because of the higher risk of developing progressive vaccinia, a condition that results in dangerous replication of the vaccine virus. Household contacts of individuals undergoing such treatment should not receive smallpox vaccine until they or their household contacts have been off immunosuppressive treatment for 3 months.
- Individuals with previous allergic reaction to smallpox vaccine or any of the vaccine's components should not receive smallpox vaccine.
- Moderate or severe acute illness should prompt a delay until the illness is resolved.
- Persons with inflammatory eye diseases can be at increased risk for inadvertent inoculation as a result of touching or rubbing the eye, and vaccination should be deferred until the condition resolves.

PRACTICE PEARLS

Life Span Considerations With Smallpox Vaccine

Children: Smallpox vaccine is contraindicated for children younger than 12 months of age.
In nonemergency settings: Do not administer smallpox vaccine in persons younger than 18 years of age.

PRACTICE PEARLS

Smallpox Vaccine in Pregnancy and Lactation

- Live-virus vaccines should not be given during pregnancy.
- Pregnant females who receive the smallpox vaccine are at risk of fetal vaccinia, a very rare condition that results in stillbirth or death of the infant shortly after delivery.
- Females who are pregnant or intend to become pregnant in the next month and their household contacts should not be vaccinated.
- Breastfeeding mothers should not receive the smallpox vaccine, because it is not known whether vaccine virus or antibodies are excreted in human milk.

Monitoring. Routine laboratory monitoring is not required.

Typhoid Vaccine

Indications. Typhoid or enteric fever is caused by *Salmonella* serotype typhi, which is increasingly drug resistant. Although uncommon in the United States, this infection is transmitted via food or water infected by feces from an infected individual and is endemic in many parts of the world. Foreign travel is typical, found in almost 80% of persons in the United States. Currently available vaccines are estimated to be about 50% to 80% effective in preventing typhoid fever, depending in part on the degree of exposure. The typhoid vaccine is available as a live-attenuated oral product (Ty21a) and a polysaccharide preparation (ViCPS) that is delivered via IM injection.

Typhoid vaccine is indicated for those traveling to areas where typhoid fever is endemic, notably India and neighboring countries, the Middle East, and Central Africa; when contact with infected individuals is expected; and in laboratory workers who handle organisms.

Adverse Effects. Oral vaccine is associated with minimal systemic adverse reactions, including nausea, abdominal pain, fever, and rash. Polysaccharide products may cause fever, headache, and local induration or erythema at the injection site.

Contraindications. Do not give the oral formulation to immunocompromised individuals, because it contains live virus. Administration of the antimalarial proguanil should be delayed until 10 days after the final dose of oral vaccine is received. Similarly, administration of oral vaccine should be delayed until 24 hours after use of any antimicrobial drugs. Because the oral vaccine requires replication in the gut, it should not be administered during an acute case of gastroenteritis. Stagger administration of Ty21a oral typhoid vaccine and oral cholera vaccine. Oral cholera vaccine should be administered at least 8 hours before the first dose of the Ty21a vaccine.

Monitoring. Routine laboratory monitoring is not required.

Varicella Vaccine

Indications. Varicella vaccine was licensed for general use in March 1995. Preparations contain cell-free, live-attenuated varicella-zoster virus; trace amounts of neomycin are also found. This vaccination is given to prevent the development of chickenpox and shingles. Varicella vaccine may be given simultaneously with MMR; however, if it is not given simultaneously, the interval between administrations should be at least 1 month. Varicella vaccine does not appear to have any effect on the administration of any other vaccine.

Children. In well children older than 12 months of age, a single dose results in a seroconversion rate of greater than 95%. An age-related decrease in the ability of the immune system to mount and maintain a primary response is seen after 12 years of age. In adolescents over the age of 12 and in adults, seroconversion rates after one dose range from 79% to 82%; two doses produce a seroconversion rate of 95%. About 15% to 20% of healthy vaccinated children will develop breakthrough varicella-defined symptom onset 42 days or more after vaccination. Most breakthrough disease is mild, without fever and with fewer skin lesions. The risk of breakthrough varicella is 2.5 times higher if the varicella vaccine is administered less than 30 days following the MMR vaccine. Researchers have found that the rate of chickenpox in infants declined by 97%

between 1994 and 2010 since the routine recommendation for varicella vaccination of children age 1 and older.

Adults. In 2006, a zoster vaccine containing a live-attenuated form of varicella-zoster virus (Zostavax) was approved by the FDA for use in adults over the age of 60; approval was expanded to include adults 50 to 59 years of age in 2011, but the ACIP declined to recommend routine use in this age group. This zoster vaccine contains the same live-attenuated strain as is found in the varicella vaccine but at a 14-fold higher concentration. It has been demonstrated to prevent zoster in 50% of recipients and the more serious complication of postherpetic neuralgia in approximately two-thirds of recipients.

In 2017, the FDA approved a recombinant, adjuvanted zoster vaccine in adults age 50 and older as a two-dose series with administration separated by at least 2 months apart (Shingrix). The ACIP recommends this new formulation to prevent herpes zoster and related complications for immunocompetent adults age 50 and older, including those who received the live zoster vaccine. The ACIP prefers the recombinant zoster vaccine over the live zoster vaccine because it is more effective and demonstrates longer protection compared to the live zoster vaccine.

Adverse Effects. Adverse effects for the varicella vaccine are local pain, redness, swelling (worse in adolescents and adults than children), and rash at the injection site. The rash is maculopapular in nature and occurs within 2 weeks of vaccination. A generalized varicella-like rash has been reported in 4% to 6% of patients after the first dose and 1% after the second dose and had an average of five lesions. The most common adverse effects for zoster vaccine were also pain and swelling. No disease has been reported in susceptible individuals who have had contact with vaccinees with a rash.

Contraindications. Varicella vaccine should not be given to individuals who have had an anaphylactic reaction to neomycin or gelatin. Varicella vaccine should not be given routinely to immunocompromised individuals, those with any type of malignancy or congenital immunodeficiency, those with active tuberculosis (TB) and blood dyscrasias, those who are receiving immunosuppressive therapy or long-term systemic steroids, or those who are receiving high-dose systemic corticosteroids (more than 2 mg/kg/day or 20 mg or more per day of prednisone). After discontinuation of steroids, vaccination should be delayed for 1 month. Lower-dose, long-term, alternate-day, intraarticular, and inhaled corticosteroid use are not contraindications for varicella vaccination.

Children with acute lymphocytic leukemia who have been in remission for at least 1 year may be immunized if they have documented adequate lymphocyte and platelet counts. HIV-infected children age 1 and older with CD4+ T lymphocyte counts 15% or greater or CD4+ greater than 200 cells/mm^3 should receive two doses of single-antigen varicella vaccine at a minimum interval of 3 months. MMRV should not be used in HIV-infected children, because safety and efficacy has not yet been established.

As with other live virus vaccines, administration should be withheld if an individual has received blood products (e.g., whole blood, plasma, or immune globulin) during the previous 3 to 11 months, depending on quantity of blood product received. Immune globulin should not be given for 3 weeks following varicella vaccination unless the benefits exceed those of the vaccine.

The association between wild virus varicella, salicylate use, and the development of Reye's syndrome is well known. No such association has been found with the use of varicella vaccine; however, the manufacturer recommends that salicylates should not be given for 6 weeks after administration of the vaccine.

PRACTICE PEARLS

Varicella Vaccine in Pregnancy and Lactation

- Pregnancy is a contraindication to administration of the vaccine. Pregnancy should be avoided for 1 month following vaccination.
- A pregnant household member is not a contraindication to the administration of vaccine to susceptible individuals.
- Breastfeeding is not a contraindication to receipt of varicella vaccines.

Monitoring. Monitor for adverse effects immediately following administration. Advise the patient and/or caregiver when to seek help. Routine laboratory monitoring is not required.

Yellow Fever Vaccine

Indications. This vaccine is a live-attenuated virus preparation that provides immunity in 7 to 10 days with lifelong protection. It is indicated for travelers to areas where yellow fever is endemic and for laboratory personnel with exposure risk. Updated information on endemic areas can be found at *Travelers' Health* (CDC, n.d.). Certain countries require evidence of vaccination from all entering travelers, which includes direct travel from the United States, and these may differ from current U.S. recommendations. For purposes of international travel, yellow fever vaccines must be administered at an approved yellow fever vaccination center (CDC, n.d.). Vaccinated patients should continue to take precautions to avoid mosquito bites.

Adverse Effects. Mild headaches, myalgia, low-grade fevers, or other minor symptoms may occur up to 5 to 10 days after vaccination. Immediate hypersensitivity or anaphylactic reactions, yellow fever vaccine–associated neurologic disease (YEL-AND), and vaccine-associated viscerotropic disease (YEL-AVD) have been rarely reported (1.3 cases per 100,000), most commonly in those older than 60 years of age.

Contraindications. Conditions affecting immune status including thymus disorders, HIV (CD4 less than 200 cells/mm^3, CD4% less than 15), primary immunodeficiencies, malignant neoplasms, immunosuppressive and immunomodulator therapies, and transplantation are contraindications.

Monitoring. Routine laboratory monitoring is not required.

Evolving Vaccines

Coronavirus (COVID-19) Vaccine

Prevalence. In December 2019 in Wuhan, China, a novel strain of beta-coronavirus was identified and named severe acute respiratory syndrome coronavirus 2 (SARS-CoV-2). This coronavirus is known to cause the coronavirus disease 2019 (COVID-19) (Bhimraj et al., n.d.). Within months the virus spread to many countries worldwide and was deemed a pandemic. As of February 21, 2021, the WHO estimated that there had been more than 110 million cases and more than 2.4 million deaths worldwide (WHO, n.d.). The CDC estimates that nearly 25 million cases and more than 400,000 deaths have occurred in the United States. Most infected individuals (at least 80%) exhibit mild symptoms such as fever or chills, cough, shortness of breath, fatigue, muscle aches, headache, new loss of taste or smell, sore throat, congestion or runny nose, nausea or vomiting, or diarrhea. About 10% of those infected will require hospital admission due to COVID-19 pneumonia, of which approximately 10% will require ICU care, including invasive ventilation due to acute respiratory distress syndrome (Bhimraj et al., n.d.). Mortality is uncommon and more commonly seen in older individuals and those with high-risk comorbidities (e.g., chronic lung disease, cardiovascular disease, hypertension, and diabetes). Surprisingly, data have shown that young individuals with no comorbidities also appear to be at risk for critical illness, including multiorgan failure and death.

Vaccine Development. In late 2020, the FDA issued emergency use authorization for two vaccinations against COVID-19, manufactured by Pfizer-BioNTech and Moderna. These vaccines utilize novel technology and contain lipid nanoparticle-formulated, nucleoside-modified mRNA that encodes for the prefusion spike glycoprotein of SARS-CoV-2. Unlike other vaccines that contain inactivated or weakened pathogens, these mRNA vaccines prompt cells to synthesize the spike protein to stimulate an immune response that generates protective antibodies against COVID-19. All adverse effects must be reported to the VAERS, and patients can conveniently and voluntarily self-report using a smartphone application (e.g., V-safe).

In early 2021 the FDA issued emergency use authorization of Johnson & Johnson's Janssen one-time dose vaccination against COVID-19. Johnson & Johnson's Janssen vaccination is not an mRNA vaccine but a viral vector vaccine. It uses the traditional virus-based (adenovirus) delivery to transport the immunologic agent. It is not a live virus and cannot replicate in the body.

The CDC has created a table to triage patients presenting for an mRNA COVID-19 vaccination (Table 50.4). Pfizer-BioNTech, Moderna, and Johnson & Johnson's Janssen initial and booster dosing recommendations are based on the evolving COVID-19 situation. Health care providers should monitor the CDC and FDA for current recommendations.

FDA Vaccination and Booster Approval. More progress for the COVID-19 vaccinations occurred throughout 2021. All three vaccines were approved by the FDA for use as a vaccination against COVID-19. Pfizer-BioNTech was granted emergency use authorization for children 12 to 18 years of age. By mid-October 2021, the FDA approved heterologous booster doses of all three vaccinations for high-risk and vulnerable populations. More clinical trials are underway for vaccinations for children 5 to 12 years of age. This is an evolving situation, and providers should monitor the CDC and FDA for further developments.

Adverse Effects

Pfizer-BioNTech. The most commonly reported side effects that usually lasted several days were pain at the injection site, tiredness, headache, muscle pain, chills, joint pain, and fever. Of note, more people experienced these side effects after the second dose than after the first dose. Rare but serious reactions have been associated with mRNA vaccines (e.g., anaphylaxis).

Moderna. The most commonly reported side effects that usually lasted several days were pain at the injection site, tiredness, headache, muscle pain, chills, joint pain, swollen

TABLE 50.4   Triage Tool for Patients Presenting for COVID-19 Vaccination

May Proceed With Vaccination	Precaution to Vaccination	Contraindication to Vaccination
Conditions		
Immunocompromising conditions	Moderate/severe acute illness	None
Pregnancy	**ACTIONS:**	**ACTIONS:**
Lactation	Risk assessment	N/A
ACTIONS:	Potential deferral of vaccination	
Additional information provided	15-minute observation period if vaccinated	
15-minute observation period		
Allergies		
History of allergies that are unrelated to components of an mRNA COVID-19 vaccine,[a] other vaccines, injectable therapies, or polysorbate, such as:	History of any immediate allergic reaction[c] to vaccines or injectable therapies (except those related to component of mRNA COVID-19 vaccines[b] or polysorbate, as these are contraindicated)	History of the following are contraindications to receiving either of the COVID-19 vaccines:[a]
Allergy to oral medications (including the oral equivalent of an injectable medication)		Severe allergic reaction (e.g., anaphylaxis) after a previous dose of an mRNA COVID-19 vaccine or any of its components
History of food, pet, insect, venom, environmental, latex, etc., allergies		Immediate allergic reaction[b] of any severity to a previous dose of an mRNA COVID-19 vaccine or any of its components[c] (including polyethylene glycol)[e]
Family history of allergies	**ACTIONS:**	Immediate allergic reaction of any severity to polysorbate[c, d]
ACTIONS:	Risk assessment	
30-minute observation period: Persons with a history of anaphylaxis (due to any cause)	Consider deferral of vaccination and/or referral to allergist-immunologist	**ACTIONS:**
15-minute observation period: All other persons	30-minute observation period if vaccinated	Do not vaccinate[d]
		Consider referral to allergist-immunologist

[a]Refers only to mRNA COVID-19 vaccines currently authorized in the United States (i.e., Pfizer-BioNTech, Moderna COVID-19 vaccines).

[b]Immediate allergic reaction to a vaccine or medication is defined as any hypersensitivity-related signs or symptoms consistent with urticaria, angioedema, respiratory distress (e.g., wheezing, stridor), or anaphylaxis that occur within 4 hours following administration.

[c]Polyethylene glycol (PEG), an ingredient in both mRNA COVID-19 vaccines, is structurally related to polysorbate, and cross-reactive hypersensitivity between these compounds may occur. Information on ingredients of a vaccine or medication (including PEG, a PEG derivative, or polysorbates) can be found in the package insert.

[d]These persons should not receive mRNA COVID-19 vaccination at this time unless they have been evaluated by an allergist-immunologist and it is determined that the person can safely receive the vaccine (e.g., under observation, in a setting with advanced medical care available).

Data from Centers for Disease Control and Prevention (2022, February 17). *Interim clinical considerations for use of COVID-19 vaccines currently approved or authorized in the United States.* Retrieved from. Available at https://www.cdc.gov/vaccines/covid-19/clinical-considerations/covid-19-vaccines-us.html?CDC_AA_refVal=https%3A%2F%2Fwww.cdc.gov%2Fvaccines%2Fcovid-19%2Finfo-by-product%2Fclinical-considerations.html

lymph nodes in the same arm as the injection, nausea and vomiting, and fever. Notably, more people experienced these side effects after the second dose than after the first dose. Rare but serious reactions have been associated with mRNA vaccines (e.g., anaphylaxis).

Johnson & Johnson's Janssen. The most commonly reported side effects that usually lasted several days were pain at the injection site, headache, tiredness, muscle pain, and nausea. There was an increased risk of thrombosis with thrombocytopenia syndrome (TTS). Rare but serious reactions have been associated with mRNA vaccines (e.g., anaphylaxis).

Contraindications. The COVID-19 vaccine is contraindicated in patients who have experienced the following conditions:

- Severe allergic reaction (e.g., anaphylaxis) to a previous dose or component of either mRNA COVID-19 vaccine or any component of the Johnson & Johnson's Janssen.
- Immediate allergic reaction of any severity to a previous

dose or component of an mRNA COVID-19 vaccine (including polyethylene glycol [(PEG]).

- Immediate allergic reaction of any severity to polysorbate (due to potential cross-reactive hypersensitivity with the vaccine ingredient PEG). An immediate allergic reaction is defined as any hypersensitivity-related signs or symptoms, such as urticaria, angioedema, respiratory distress (e.g., wheezing, stridor), or anaphylaxis, that occur within 4 hours following exposure to a previous dose of an mRNA COVID-19 vaccine or any of its components.
- History of an immediate allergic reaction to any other vaccine or injectable therapy (i.e., intramuscular, intravenous, or subcutaneous vaccines or therapies not related to a component of mRNA COVID-19 vaccines).
- Moderate to severe acute illness.

Monitoring. Due to risk of anaphylaxis, patients should be monitored for at least 15 minutes after the first dose and 30 minutes after the second dose.

Clinical Practice Guidelines

Guidelines concerning the use of immunizations are one of the most carefully studied areas of pharmacology. These guidelines determine the standard of care.

BOOKMARK THIS!

Guidelines

- CDC Yellow Book (Brunette & Nemhauser, 2020).
- Healthcare Providers/Professionals: https://www.cdc.gov/vaccines/hcp/index.html
- Pregnancy and Vaccination: https://www.cdc.gov/vaccines/pregnancy/index.html
- Recommended Adult Immunization Schedule for ages 19 years or older, United States: https://www.cdc.gov/vaccines/schedules/hcp/imz/adult.html
- Recommended Child and Adolescent Immunization Schedule for ages 18 years or younger, United States: https://www.cdc.gov/vaccines/schedules/hcp/imz/child-adolescent.html
- Travelers' Health: https://wwwnc.cdc.gov/travel/destinations/list
- Vaccine Information for Adults: https://www.cdc.gov/vaccines/adults/index.html
- Vaccines & Immunizations: https://www.cdc.gov/vaccines/index.html
- Vaccines for Your Children: https://www.cdc.gov/vaccines/parents/index.html

---

Clinical Reasoning for Vaccine Administration

Consider the individual patient's health problem and desired therapeutic outcome. Patients without documentation of vaccine receipt should be considered nonimmunized if a reasonable effort to locate records is unsuccessful. These individuals should be started on the age-appropriate vaccination schedule. Serologic testing for immunity is an alternative to vaccination for certain antigens (e.g., measles, rubella, hepatitis A, tetanus, etc.).

Vaccination providers should adhere as closely as possible to recommended vaccination schedules. Longer-than-recommended intervals between doses does not reduce final antibody concentrations, although protection might not be attained until all doses have been administered. With the exception of oral typhoid vaccine, an interruption in the vaccination schedule does not require restarting the entire series of a vaccine or toxoid or addition of extra doses.

Health care providers should simultaneously administer all vaccines for which a person is eligible because simultaneous administration increases the probability that an individual will be vaccinated fully at the appropriate age. Administration of each preparation at a different anatomic site is desirable. Simultaneous administration of the most widely used live and inactivated vaccines has produced seroconversion rates and rates for adverse reactions similar to those observed when the vaccines are administered separately. An inactivated vaccine can be administered simultaneously or at any time before or after a different inactivated vaccine or live vaccine.

Live vaccines also may be administered simultaneously. However, live vaccines such as those for measles, mumps, and rubella should not be administered after receipt of an antibody-containing product such as immunoglobulin until the passive antibody response to the product has degraded. This process is dependent on dose and specific product. Exceptions to this rule are yellow fever vaccine, oral typhoid vaccine, and live-attenuated influenza vaccine, which may be administered after immunoglobulin.

Use of combination vaccines can reduce the number of injections required at a visit. Licensed combination vaccines can be used whenever any components of the combination are indicated, and its other components are not contraindicated.

Vaccines made by different manufacturers are generally interchangeable. Although it is preferable to complete a series with a single product, vaccination should not be deferred because the brand used for previous doses is not available or is unknown. See information about specific vaccinations that highlight the formulations that are and are not interchangeable.

Assess the selected pharmacotherapy for its appropriateness for an individual patient by considering the medication's side effects and the patient's age, race/ethnicity, comorbidities, and genetic factors. Critical decisions to be made in immunizations include which products to give and when to give them. At each visit, refer to the ACIP schedule to determine which vaccinations are necessary and assess for contraindications. The health care provider should take all precautions known for the detection or prevention of allergic or any other adverse reaction. This should include a review of the patient's history regarding possible sensitivity.

Individuals with impaired immune responsiveness, whether because of the use of immunosuppressive therapy, a genetic defect, HIV/AIDS, or other causes, may have a reduced antibody response to active immunization procedures. Deferral of the administration of live vaccines may be considered in individuals receiving immunosuppressive therapy.

Decisions about whether the patient should have additional vaccinations should be based on patient-specific risk/benefit analysis as guided by the algorithm. Some of the options for revaccination include withholding other doses of suspected or implicated vaccines for patients who have serologic evidence of immunity, who are at low risk for disease, who have serious complications from disease, or who are at risk for life-threatening complications from the vaccine. Immunizations to protect older adults are continuing to increase with the use of the shingles vaccination, pneumococcal vaccinations, and annual *Haemophilus* b influenza vaccinations.

Initiate the treatment plan with the selected immunizations by first providing adequate patient education to ensure the patient's understanding and promote full participation in the therapy. Provide patients with a copy of the vaccine information sheet (VIS) for all vaccines that will be administered at that visit. Review the VIS with the patient and/or caregiver, allowing time for questions.

Prior to administration, providers should review their knowledge of the recent literature pertaining to the biologic to be used, including the nature of side effects and adverse effects that may follow its use. Verify the availability of epinephrine 1:1000 and other appropriate agents used for control of immediate allergic reactions.

Ensure complete patient and family understanding using a variety of education strategies. Advise patients how each vaccine contributes to their overall well-being and health. The CDC offers a variety of resources including immunization schedules for children and adults, parent guides, seasonal materials (flu shot), and links to other websites. Information is readily available by ages: infants and toddlers; preteens and teens; pregnant females; college students; young adults; and adults. Reminders of subsequent appointments can be accomplished through mailers, patient phone calls, or electronic messaging.

Conduct follow-up and monitoring of patient responses to pharmacotherapies. Follow recommended guidelines for monitoring patients after vaccine administration. Advise the patient or caregiver when to notify the office or medical providers of a reaction. Provide written information on how to contact the provider's office in the event of questions or concerns following vaccination. Advise patients and caregivers of the importance of maintaining accurate immunization records.

Teaching Points for Vaccine Administration

Health Promotion Strategies

- When talking to parents and patients, initiate conversation of vaccines using language that presumes vaccine recommendations will be followed to increase vaccine acceptance (Opel et al., 2013).
- At each visit, advise patients, parents, or guardians of the risks and benefits of each individual vaccine and provide them the standardized vaccine information sheets.
- Provide patients and caregivers with a written immunization record. Document the vaccine administration in the health record. If your state uses a centralized database, enter all vaccine data in a timely manner (preferably at the visit) to ensure an accurate recording.
- Simultaneously administer all vaccines for which a person is eligible because simultaneous administration increases the probability that an individual will be vaccinated fully at the appropriate age. Administration of each preparation at a different anatomic site is desirable. Simultaneous administration of the most widely used live and inactivated vaccines has produced

seroconversion rates and rates for adverse reactions similar to those observed when the vaccines are administered separately.

- An inactivated vaccine can be administered simultaneously or at any time before or after a different inactivated vaccine or live vaccine.
- Live vaccines also may be administered simultaneously. However, live vaccines such as those for measles, mumps, and rubella should not be administered after receipt of an antibody-containing product such as immunoglobulin until the passive antibody response to the product has degraded. This process is dependent on the dose and the specific product. Exceptions to this rule are yellow fever vaccine, oral typhoid vaccine, and live-attenuated influenza vaccine, which may be administered after immunoglobulin.
- Use of combination vaccines can reduce the number of injections required at a visit. Licensed combination vaccines can be used whenever any components of the combination are indicated, and its other components are not contraindicated.
- Vaccines made by different manufacturers are generally interchangeable. See information about specific vaccinations that highlight the formulations that are and are not interchangeable.

Patient Education for Medication Safety

Tell your vaccine provider if the person getting the vaccine:

- Has had an allergic reaction after a previous dose of the vaccine or has any severe, life-threatening allergies
- Is pregnant or thinks they might be pregnant
- Has a weakened immune system or has a history of hereditary or congenital immune system problems in themselves or a family member
- Has ever had a condition that makes them bruise or bleed easily
- Has recently had a blood transfusion or received other blood products
- Has a history of any disease such as seizures, loss of consciousness, asthma, tuberculosis, or Guillain-Barré syndrome
- Has gotten any other vaccines in the past 4 weeks

Application Questions for Discussion

1. What are the vaccines that are safe to administer in pregnancy and those that are avoided or contraindicated?
2. Using the catch-up immunization schedule, create a plan to get an 8-month-old female up to date with MMR, influenza, rotavirus, Hib, pneumococcal, and HBV. Her parents deferred vaccinations and have changed their minds and decided to now immunize her.
3. How would you respond to a patient's parent if they stated they want to skip the HPV vaccine as it will cause their child to be promiscuous and to have sex at a young age?

Selected Bibliography

Actor J.K. (2012). Elsevier's Integrated Review, Elsevier/Saunders, Philadelphia, 2012.

Advisory Committee on Immunization Practices (ACIP). (n.d. a). *Recommended child and adolescent immunization schedule for ages 18 years or younger.* Retrieved February 21, 2021, from https://www.cdc.gov/vaccines/schedules/hcp/imz/child-adolescent.html.

Advisory Committee on Immunization Practices (ACIP). (n.d. b). *Recommended adult immunization schedule for ages 19 years or older.* Retrieved February 21, 2021, from https://www.cdc.gov/vaccines/schedules/hcp/imz/adult.html.

Albertson J.P., Clegg W.J., Reid H.D., Arbise B.S., Pryde J., Vaid. A, Thompson-Brown. R., Echols F. (2016). Mumps outbreak at a university and recommandation for a third dose of measles-mumps-rubella vaccine — Illinois, 2015–2016, MMWR. *Morbidity and Mortality Weekly Report 65* (29) 731–734, http://dx.doi.org/10.15585/mmwr.mm6529a2.

American Academy of Pediatrics Committee on Infectious Diseases; American Academy of Pediatrics Bronchiolitis Guidelines Committee. (2014). *American Academy of Pediatrics. Updated guidance for palivizumab prophylaxis among infants and young children at increased risk of hospitalization for respiratory syncytial virus infection, Pediatrics, 134* (2) (2014) e620–e638, http://doi.org/10.1542/peds.2014-1666.

Baxter R, Lewis N, Bakshi N., Vellozzi. C., Klein N.P. the CISA Network. (2012). Recurrent Guillain-Barré syndrome following vaccination, *Clinical Infectious Diseases 54* (6) 800–804, https://doi.org/10.1093/cid/cir960.

Bhimraj, A., Morgan, R. L., Shumaker, A. H., Lavergne, V., Baden, L., Cheng, V. C., Edwards, K. M., Gandhi, R., Muller, W. J., O'Horo, J. C., Shoham, S., Murad, M. H., Mustafa, R. A., Sultan, S., & Falck-Ytter, Y. (n.d.). *IDSA guidelines on the treatment and management of patients with COVID-19.* Retrieved January 9, 2021, from Clinical https://www.idsociety.org/practice-guideline/covid-19-guideline-treatment-and-management.

Brunette G.W., Nemhauser J.B. (2020). CDC yellow book 2020: Health information for international travel, Oxford Press.

Centers for Disease Control and Prevention 2021 U.S. Centers for Disease Control and Prevention. (2021, February 19). *CDC's COVID-19 vaccine rollout recommendations.* Retrieved February 21, 2021, from https://www.cdc.gov/coronavirus/2019-ncov/vaccines/recommendations.html.

Centers for Disease Control and Prevention (CDC). (2020a). *Autism and vaccines.* Available at https://www.cdc.gov/vaccinesafety/concerns/autism.html.

Centers for Disease Control and Prevention (CDC). (2020b). *Human papillomavirus (HPV): Cancers caused by HPV.* Available at https://www.cdc.gov/hpv/index.html.

Centers for Disease Control and Prevention (CDC). (2019). *Epidemiology and prevention of vaccine-preventable diseases: Meningococcal disease.* Available at https://www.cdc.gov/vaccines/pubs/pinkbook.

Centers for Disease Control and Prevention (CDC). (2017). *Pertussis (whooping cough): Fast facts.* Available at https://www.cdc.gov/pertussis/fast-facts.html.

Centers for Disease Control and Prevention (n.d.). *Travelers' Health: Vaccines. Medicines. Advice.* Retrieved February 21, 2021, from https://wwwnc.cdc.gov/travel.

Ezeanolue, E., Harriman, K., Hunter, P., Kroger, A., & Pellegrini, C. (n.d.). General best practice guidelines for immunization. *Best practices guidance of the Advisory Committee on Immunization Practices (ACIP).* Retrieved February 21, 2021, from www.cdc.gov/vaccines/hcp/acip-recs/generalrecs/downloads/general-recs.pdf.

Grandjean P., Heilmann C., Weihe P., Nielsen F., Mogensen U.B., Timmermann A., Budtz-Jørgensen E. (2017). Estimated exposures to perfluorinated compounds in infancy predict attenuated vaccine antibody concentrations at age 5-years, *Journal of immunotoxicology 14* (1) 188–195, https://doi.org/10.1080/1547691X.2017.1360968.

Hamborsky J., Kroger A, Wolfe C., Centers for Disease Control and Prevention. (2015). Epidemiology and prevention of vaccine-preventable diseases, Public Health Foundation.

Hung, M. C., Williams, W. W., Lu, P.-J., Woods, L. O., Koppaka, R., & Lindley, M. C. (2018). *Vaccination coverage among adults in the United States, National Health interview survey, 2017.* U.S. Centers for Disease Control and Prevention. Available at https://www.cdc.gov/vaccines/imz-managers/coverage/adultvaxview/pubs-resources/NHIS-2017.htm.

Institute of Medicine (US) Immunization Safety Review Committee. (2004). *Immunization safety review: Vaccines and autism.* http://doi.org/10.17226/10997

Joint Task Force on Practice Parameters; American Academy of Allergy, Asthma and Immunology; American College of Allergy, Asthma and Immunology; Joint Council of Allergy, Asthma and Immunology. (2010). Drug allergy: An updated practice parameter, *Annals of Allergy, Asthma & Immunology 105* (4) 259–273, https://doi.org/10.1016/j.anai.2010.08.002

Marin M., Marlow M., Moore K.L., Patel M. (2018). Recommendation of the Advisory Committee on Immunization Practices for use of a third dose of mumps virus-containing vaccine in persons at increased risk for mumps during an outbreak, MMWR. *Morbidity and Mortality Weekly Report 67* (1) 33–38, https://doi.org/10.15585/mmwr.mm6701a7

Meites E., Szilagyi P.G., Chesson H.W., Unger E.R., Romero J.R., Markowitz L.E. (2019). Human papillomavirus vaccination for adults: Updated recommendations of the Advisory Committee on Immunization Practices, *MMWR. Morbidity and Mortality Weekly Report 68* (32) 698–702, http://dx.doi.org/10.15585/mmwr.mm6832a3

Opel D.J., Heritage J, Taylor J.A., Mangione-Smith R, Showalter Salas H, DeVere V., Zhou, C. Robinson J.D. (2013). The architecture of provider–parent vaccine discussions at health supervision visits, Pediatrics *132* (6) 1037–1046, https://doi.org/10.1542/peds.2013-2037

Peck M., Gacic-Dobo M., Diallo M.S., Nedelec Y., Sodha S.S., Wallace A.S. (2019). Global routine vaccination coverage, 2018, *MMWR. Morbidity and Mortality Weekly Report 68* (42) 937–942, http://dx.doi.org/10.15585/mmwr.mm6842a1

Seither R., Loretan C., Driver K., Mellerson J.L., Knighton C.L., Black C.L. (2019). Vaccination coverage with selected vaccines and exemption rates among children in kindergarten—United States, 2018–19 school year, *MMWR. Morbidity and Mortality Weekly Report 68* (41) 905–912, http://dx.doi.org/10.15585/mmwr.mm6841e1

U.S. Food & Drug Administration. 2018U.S. Food & Drug Administration. (2018). *Thimerosal and vaccines.*https://www.fda.gov/vaccines-blood-biologics/safety-availability-biologics/thimerosal-and-vaccines

Vaccine Adverse Event Reporting System n.d Vaccine Adverse Event Reporting System (VAERS). (n.d.). Available at https://vaers.hhs.gov/index.html.

World Health Organization 2020 World Health Organization. (2020, October). *Rotavirus.*Available at https://www.who.int/immunization/diseases/rotavirus/en.

World Health Organization (WHO). (n.d.). *WHO coronavirus disease (COVID-19) dashboard.*Retrieved February 21, 2021, from https://covid19.who.int.

51

Weight Management Medications

REBECCA M. LUTZ

Overview

Obesity is a complex health issue associated with increased morbidity and mortality, poorer mental health outcomes, and reduced quality of life. Obesity is linked to diabetes, heart disease, stroke, and some types of cancer, all of which are the leading causes of death in the United States and worldwide. The World Health Organization (WHO) defines *overweight* and *obesity* as an impairment of health due to abnormal or excessive fat accumulation (WHO, n.d.). Obesity results from a combination of causes and contributing factors. Individual factors include genetics, dietary patterns, physical activity, inactivity, medication use, and other exposures.

Obesity in Adults

Overweight and Obesity Defined

Overweight and obesity are measured through calculation of body mass index (BMI). BMI is calculated by measuring a person's weight in kilograms and dividing it by their height in meters squared (kg/m²). BMI correlates with body fat and muscle mass. It is important to keep in mind that while BMI is a general measurement tool, it is not always appropriate/accurate for certain populations. Increased muscle mass can lead to an elevated BMI, even though the person does not have increased body fat. Table 51.1 provides a classification system for gauging overweight and obesity using BMI in adults (National Institutes of Health, National Heart, Lung, and Blood Institute [NIH/NHLBI], 1998). In adults 18 years of age and older:
- Overweight is a BMI ≥25.
- Obesity is a BMI ≥30.

Population Prevalence

In the United States, the rate of adult obesity continues to increase. Flegal et al. (2016) analyzed results of the 2013–2014 National Health and Nutrition Examination Survey (NHANES), which revealed that 37.7% of adults 20 years of age or older were considered obese; females (40.4%) had higher rates of obesity than males (35.0%); and females (9.9%) had higher rates of class III obesity (BMI of 40 or more) than males (5.5%). Echeverria et al. (2017) compared the rates of obesity among female minority groups by analyzing the 2011–2014 NHANES survey. Results revealed that Non-Hispanic Black females (57.0%) had the highest rates of obesity and Non-Hispanic Asian females had the lowest rates of obesity (11%).

By 2015–2016, obesity rates had risen to 39.8% (Hales et al., 2017). Females 20 years of age or older had slightly higher rates of obesity (36.5%) compared to males in the same age group (34.8%). Non-Hispanic Black females had the highest rates of obesity (54.8%), followed by Hispanic females (50.6%). While non-Hispanic Asian females still had the lowest rates of obesity (14.5%), there was a noted increase from 2013 to 2014. The prevalence of obesity was 38.0% in non-Hispanic White, 54.8% in non-Hispanic Black, 14.8% in non-Hispanic Asian, and 50.6% in Hispanic females. Among males, the prevalence of obesity was lower in non-Hispanic Asian adults (10.1%) compared with non-Hispanic White (37.9%), non-Hispanic Black (36.9%), and Hispanic (43.1%) males.

Burden of Disease

The consequences of overweight and obesity result in a higher risk for chronic diseases, multiple comorbidities, and mental health concerns. These factors combine to increase disability, decrease quality of life, decrease life expectancy, and increase health care costs (Hruby & Hu, 2015). The financial burden of obesity within the workplace is significant to the employee and the employer. Obese employees

TABLE 51.1	Classification of Overweight and Obesity by BMI	
	Obesity Class	**BMI (kg/m²)**
Underweight		<18.5
Normal		18.5–24.9
Overweight		25.0–29.9
Obesity	I	30.0–34.9
	II	35.0–39.9
Extreme Obesity	III	≥40

From NHLBI Obesity Education Initiative Expert Panel on the Identification, Evaluation, and Treatment of Obesity in Adults (US). Clinical Guidelines on the Identification, Evaluation, and Treatment of Overweight and Obesity in Adults: The Evidence Report. Bethesda, MD: National Heart, Lung, and Blood Institute; 1998 Sept. Available from https://www.ncbi.nlm.nih.gov/books/NBK2003.

paid higher rates in health care costs and had higher rates of absenteeism compared to nonobese employees (Ramasamy et al., 2019). In the United States, the burden of care is evident in direct care costs of $480.7 billion and indirect care costs of $1.24 trillion (Waters & Graf, 2018).

Obesity in Children and Adolescents

Overweight and Obesity Defined

Overweight and obesity in children and adolescents are defined differently than in adults. Based on age- and gender-specific growth charts developed by the Centers for Disease Control and Prevention (CDC), a child or adolescent is considered overweight if their BMI is between the 85th and 95th percentiles and is considered obese if their BMI is in the 95th percentile or above. (CDC, n.d.)

Population Prevalence

Hales et al. (2017) also analyzed the 2015–2016 NHANES study to identify obesity rates in children and adolescents (18.5%). Between the ages of 2 and 19, males (19.1%) had slightly higher rates of obesity than females (17.8%). Overall, Hispanics between the ages of 2 and 19 had higher rates of obesity (25.8%) compared to non-Hispanic Blacks (22.0%), non-Hispanic Whites (14.1%), and non-Hispanic Asians (11.0%).

By comparison, the 2011–2014 NHANES total prevalence rate was 17.2%. Between the ages of 2 and 19, females (17.1%) had slightly higher rates of obesity than males (16.9%). Overall, Hispanics between the ages of 2 and 19 had higher rates of obesity (21.9%) compared to non-Hispanic Blacks (19.5%), non-Hispanic Whites (14.7%), and non-Hispanic Asians (8.6%) (Ogden et al., 2015).

Burden of Disease

Halfon et al. (2013) analyzed the 2007 National Survey of Children's Health and determined that overweight and obese children 10 to 17 years of age reported higher rates of mental health and developmental conditions such as attention deficit hyperactivity disorder (ADHD) and learning disabilities. Overweight and obese children have multiple comorbid conditions affecting the cardiovascular, metabolic, respiratory, gastrointestinal (GI), and musculoskeletal systems. A systematic metaanalysis identified the potential link between obesity and early-onset puberty in females but not males (Li et al., 2017).

Interventions

Lifestyle Interventions

Weight management therapy begins with lifestyle interventions that include dietary changes, increased physical activity, and behavior therapy (NIH/NHLBI, 1998). The discussion of lifestyle interventions is an essential component of any weight modification treatment plan. Recommendations for lifestyle modifications include caloric restrictions, an increase in physical activity, and behavior modifications (Garvey et al., 2016). Each

intervention must also consider the patient's health status and personal preferences.

- Dietary Interventions
  - Reduce calories while emphasizing the need to include macronutrients.
  - Consider short-term meal replacement.
- Daily Physical Activity
  - Exercise for at least 150 minutes per week, increasing to 300 minutes per week.
  - Include aerobic and resistance exercise.
- Behavior Modifications
  - Monitor food intake, exercise, and weight.
  - Strategize priorities and set goals.
  - Modify stimulus-eating situations.
  - Connect with support.

Pharmacotherapy

Pharmacotherapy should be considered for patients with a BMI of 27 or more accompanied by hypertension, dyslipidemia, coronary heart disease, type 2 diabetes, or sleep apnea, or in patients with a BMI of 30 or more and no risk factors. A systematic review of behavioral and pharmacotherapy interventions found that participants receiving pharmacotherapeutics had an increased chance of losing and maintaining their weight loss than those receiving a placebo (LeBlanc et al., 2018).

Weight Management Therapy

Weight management medications are divided into two categories: long term and short term. The U.S. Food and Drug Administration (FDA) has approved five medications: orlistat, lorcaserin, phentermine-topiramate, naltrexone-bupropion, and liraglutide. Table 51.2 and Table 51.3 provide a summary of the long- and short-term medications for use in weight management. Table 51.4 provides a summary of common adverse effects of weight management medications. Table 51.5 provides a summary of some drug–drug interactions.

Long-Term Weight Management Medications

Orlistat is one of the first two weight management medications approved in the late 1990s for long-term use. In 2012, phentermine/topiramate combination, naltrexone/bupropion hydrochloride, lorcaserin, and liraglutide were approved for use in adults. Orlistat is the only medication approved for use in children 12 years of age or older.

PRACTICE PEARLS

Weight Management Medications in Pregnancy and Lactation

- Pregnancy: weight management medications are deemed unsafe for use during pregnancy. Discontinue weight management medication if pregnancy occurs.
- Lactation: weight management medications are not recommended.

TABLE 51.2   Long-Term Weight Management Medications

Medication	Indication	Dosage	Considerations and Monitoring
Orlistat	Obesity and chronic weight management	*Adults, adolescents, and children ≥12 yr: Prescription:* 120 mg orally three times daily during or within 1 hr of each fat-containing meal. Maximum dosage: 320 mg/day. *Adults: Over-the-counter:* 60 mg orally three times daily during or within 1 hr of each fat-containing meal. Maximum dosage: 180 mg/day.	Concomitant medication: A daily multivitamin supplement containing vitamins A, D, E, K, and beta carotene, taken at least 2 hr before or after orlistat.
Phentermine/topira-mate	Obesity and chronic weight management	*Adults: Initial dosage:* Phentermine hydrochloride 3.75 mg/topiramate 23 mg orally once daily for 14 days, then increase to phentermine hydrochloride 7.5 mg/topiramate 46 mg once daily. *Dosage escalation (if necessary):* Phentermine hydrochloride 11.25 mg/topiramate 69 mg orally once daily for 14 days, then increase to phentermine hydrochloride 15 mg/topiramate 92 mg once daily.	After 12 weeks of maintenance dosage, if weight loss is not at least 3% of baseline, discontinue therapy or escalate dosage. If dosage escalated to phentermine hydrochloride 15 mg/topiramate 92 mg, discontinue therapy if weight loss is not at least 5% of baseline after 12 weeks.
Naltrexone hydro-chloride/bupropi-on hydrochloride	Obesity and chronic weight management	*Adults:* Naltrexone hydrochloride 8 mg/bupropion hydrochloride 90 mg (1 tablet) orally once daily in the morning for week 1; then 1 tablet twice daily, morning and evening, for week 2; then 2 tablets in the morning and 1 tablet in the evening for week 3. *Maintenance dosage:* Week 4 and thereafter, 2 tablets orally twice daily, morning and evening. *Maximum dosage:* Naltrexone hydrochloride 32 mg/bupropion hydrochloride 360 mg/day.	Discontinue if at least a 5% decrease in baseline body weight is not achieved after 12 weeks at maintenance dosage.
Liraglutide	Obesity and chronic weight management	*Adults:* 0.6 mg subcutaneously once daily for 1 week; increase weekly in increments of 0.6 mg/day until maintenance dosage of 3 mg once daily is reached. *Adolescents and children 12–17 yr:* 0.6 mg subcutaneously once daily for 1 week; increase weekly in increments of 0.6 mg/day until maintenance dosage of 3 mg once daily is reached.	Discontinue use if patient is unable to tolerate the 3-mg dose. Dose escalation may take up to 8 weeks. If unable to tolerate the 3-mg dose, decrease to 2.4 mg. Discontinue use if patient is unable to tolerate the 2.4-mg dose.

Orlistat

Orlistat is available in prescription and over-the-counter (OTC) formulations. Orlistat is used in conjunction with a calorie-restricted diet, increased physical activity, and behavioral modification to promote weight loss. Orlistat is approved for use in adults and children 12 years of age or older who meet diagnostic criteria for obesity or who have certain comorbid conditions.

Pharmacokinetics. Orlistat inhibits intestinal lipases and prevents the hydrolysis of dietary triglycerides into absorbable fatty acids and monoglycerides. Dietary fat absorption is inhibited by approximately 30%. Orlistat is not absorbed systemically. Half-life is 1 to 2 hours. Metabolism occurs in the GI tract. Excretion occurs in the feces.

| TABLE 51.3 | **Short-Term Weight Management Medications** |

Medication	Indication	Dosage	Considerations and Monitoring
Phentermine	Exogenous obesity	**Capsule, tablet:** *Adults and adolescents ≥17 yr:* 15–37.5 mg orally once daily before breakfast or 2 hr after breakfast. Maximum dosage: 37.5 mg/day. **Tablet:** *Adults, adolescents, and children ≥17 yr:* 8 mg orally three times daily given 30 minutes before meals. Maximum dosage: 37.5 mg/day.	For use as short-term (few weeks) monotherapy
Benzphetamine	Exogenous obesity	**Tablet:** *Adults, adolescents, and children ≥12 yr:* 25–50 mg orally once daily mid-morning or mid-afternoon. May increase to 50 mg orally three times daily. Maximum dosage: 150 mg/day.	For use as short-term (8–12 wk) monotherapy. Not recommended for patients who used any other anorectic agents within the prior year.
Diethylpropion	Exogenous obesity	**Extended-release tablet:** *Adults and adolescents ≥16 yr:* 75 mg orally once daily, taken midmorning. **Immediate-release tablet:** *Adults and adolescents ≥16 yr:* 25 mg orally three times daily, 1 hr before meals. If desired, an additional 25 mg tablet mid-evening may help overcome nighttime hunger.	For use as short-term (few weeks) therapy.
Phendimetrazine	Exogenous obesity	**Extended-release tablet:** *Adults and adolescents ≥17 yr:* 105 mg orally once daily 30–60 minutes before the morning meal. *Maximum dosage:* 105 mg/day.	For use as short-term (few weeks) therapy.
		Immediate-release tablet: *Adults:* 35 mg orally two or three times daily 1 hr before meals. *Maximum dosage:* 210 mg/day.	For use as short-term (few weeks) therapy Do not exceed 2 tablets (70 mg) orally three times daily.

| TABLE 51.4 | **Adverse Effects of Weight Management Medications** |

Body System Affected	Adverse Reaction
Cardiovascular	Pedal edema
Central nervous system	Anxiety
	Fatigue
	Headache
	Sleep disorder
Dermatologic	Xeroderma
Endocrine/Metabolic	Breast cancer
	Hypoglycemia
	Medullary thyroid cancer
	Menstrual disease
	Pancreatic cancer

TABLE 51.4 Adverse Effects of Weight Management Medications—cont'd

Body System Affected	Adverse Reaction
Gastrointestinal	Abdominal distress
	Abdominal pain
	Bowel urgency
	Cholelithiasis
	Constipation
	Diarrhea
	Fecal incontinence
	Flatulence
	Frequent bowel movements
	Gingival disease
	Infectious diarrhea
	Nausea
	Oily stool
	Steatorrhea
	Xerostomia
	Taste: altered
	Vomiting
Genitourinary	Urinary tract infection
	Vaginitis
Hepatic	Liver failure
Immunologic effects	Influenza
Musculoskeletal effects	Back pain
	Leg pain
	Myalgia
Neurologic effects	Dizziness
	Headache
	Insomnia
	Paresthesia
	Seizure
Ophthalmic effects	Angle-closure glaucoma
	Blurred vision
	Myopia, acute
	Raised intraocular pressure
Otic	Otitis
Psychiatric effects	Suicidal behavior
Renal	Hypohidrosis
	Nephrolithiasis
	Oxalate and oxalate nephropathy
	Urinary tract infectious disease
Respiratory	Bronchitis
	Nasopharyngitis
	Sinusitis
	Upper and lower respiratory tract infections

TABLE 51.5	Drug–Drug Interactions
Drug	**Interactions**
Orlistat	Anticonvulsants: decreased effectiveness
	Antivirals: decreased effectiveness
	Warfarin: increased risk of bleeding
	Linoleic acid: decreased absorption
	Cyclosporine: decreased plasma levels
	Levothyroxine: monitor for changes in thyroid function
Phentermine hydro-chloride/topiramate extended-release	MAOI: may result in hypertensive crisis
	Oral contraceptives: decreased effectiveness
	CNS depressants, including alcohol: may potentiate reactions
	Non–potassium-sparing diuretics: hypokalemia
	Antiepileptic drugs: hyperammonemia and hypothermia
	Topiramate: decreased concentrations
	Carbonic anhydrase inhibitors: increased metabolic acidosis
Naltrexone hydrochlo-ride/bupropion hydrochloride	Opioids: precipitation of withdrawal symptoms
	MAOIs, linezolid, selegiline: increased risk of hypertensive reactions
	CYP 2D6 substrates: increased risk of seizures
	Eliglustat: prolongation of QT interval
Liraglutide	ACE inhibitors: increased risk of hypoglycemia
	Beta-adrenergic blockers: hypoglycemia or hyperglycemia
	Furosemide, hydrochlorothiazide, metolazone, triamterene, and other diuretics: increased hyperglycemia

ACE, Angiotensin-converting enzyme; *CNS,* central nervous system; *CYP,* cytochrome; *MAOI,* monoamine oxidase inhibitor.

Indications. Orlistat is indicated for the treatment of obesity and for chronic weight management in adults and children 12 years of age or older. Orlistat is offered in conjunction with a reduced-calorie diet and lifestyle modifications. No adjustments in dosing are required for patients with renal or hepatic insufficiency.

Adverse Effects. Systemic adverse effects are commonly seen within the GI, musculoskeletal, neurological, and respiratory systems. The most common GI complaints include abdominal pain, urgency and incontinence of stool, fatty/oily stool, and flatulence with discharge. Approximately 50% of the GI effects last less than 1 month, but occasionally the effects may last longer. Neurological complaints of headache are more common than musculoskeletal complaints of back and lower leg pain. Respiratory infections and influenza do occur. Episodes of hypoglycemia may occur. Serious adverse effects are rare but include hepatic and renal impairment.

Contraindications. Orlistat is contraindicated in patients who are pregnant; or who present with cholestasis, chronic malabsorption syndrome, or hypersensitivity to orlistat or any of its components.

Monitoring. Monitor for signs and symptoms of decreased absorption of vitamins and beta carotene. Monitor renal function in patients at risk for renal impairment. Monitor for weight loss and adjust the dosage as indicated.

Phentermine Hydrochloride/Topiramate Extended Release

The combination of phentermine hydrochloride/topiramate extended release was approved in 2012. Phentermine reduces appetite by stimulating the hypothalamus to release more norepinephrine while decreasing norepinephrine uptake. Topiramate has multiple actions, including alterations in taste, to suppress appetite and produce satiety. The combination results in a sustainable weight loss of approximately 5% to 10%.

Pharmacokinetics. Phentermine/topiramate extended release binds to plasma proteins. Minimally, metabolism occurs through cytochrome (CYP) 3A4. Excretion is via the urine. Bioavailability is not related to food intake.

Indications. Phentermine/topiramate extended release is a Schedule IV control restricted medication approved as adjunct therapy to treat obesity in adults. Initial stepwise titration may decrease adverse effects. If a 5% weight loss is not reached after 12 weeks, a gradual titration to discontinue is recommended since withdrawal from topiramate may cause seizures.

Adverse Effects. Adverse effects most commonly reported in more than 10% of patients include increased heart rate and palpitations, anxiety, paresthesia, insomnia, dry mouth, constipation, upper respiratory tract infections, and nasopharyngitis. Adverse effects are dose dependent and occurred within the first 12 weeks of treatment. Mood and sleep disorder effects were more common in patients with a previous psychological history.

Contraindications. Absolute contraindications include pregnancy, glaucoma, and hyperthyroidism; concomitant use with alcohol and/or MAOI therapy; and use within 14 days of discontinuation of MAOIs and known hypersensitivity or idiosyncrasies to sympathomimetic amines. Avoid in patients with a history of suicidal attempts or active suicidal ideation. Do not exceed the recommended daily dose in patients with hepatic or renal failure. This medication is also contraindicated in patients with end-stage renal disease (ESRD). Topiramate can increase the risk of kidney stones, so this medication should be used cautiously in patients with a previous history.

Monitoring. Monitor blood chemistry panels, including bicarbonate, creatinine, electrolytes, and glucose, before starting therapy and periodically throughout treatment. Monitor for pregnancy and use of contraceptives. Monitor blood pressure and heart rate when initiating or increasing dosages. Monitor for changes in mood or behavior changes.

Naltrexone/Bupropion

Pharmacokinetics. Naltrexone and bupropion are rapidly absorbed through the GI tract. Peak plasma levels of naltrexone occur within 1 hour. Bupropion plasma levels peak at approximately 5 hours. Bupropion is extensively metabolized through CYP 2B6. Bupropion and its metabolites are inhibitors of CYP 2D6. Naltrexone and bupropion are primarily excreted through the kidneys.

Indications. Naltrexone is an opioid antagonist that diminishes the auto-inhibitory feedback loop on neurons activated by bupropion. Bupropion is an antidepressant that inhibits the reuptake of dopamine and norepinephrine. This combination was approved in 2014 for chronic weight management.

Adverse Effects. Adverse effects include constipation, diarrhea, dizziness, dry mouth, headache, increased blood pressure, increased heart rate, insomnia, liver damage, nausea, and vomiting.

BLACK BOX WARNING!

Naltrexone/Bupropion

- There is an increased risk for suicidal thoughts and behavior in children, adolescents, and young adults taking this medication.
- Monitor closely for the emergence and/or worsening of suicidal thoughts and behaviors.
- Females of childbearing age should have a pregnancy test before starting the medication and use contraception while taking it.

Contraindications. Use with caution in older adults, in patients at risk for hypoglycemia or hepatic/renal impairment, and in patients with neuropsychiatric or psychiatric symptoms. This drug combination should not be used concomitantly in any of the following situations:

- Use of MAOI antidepressants or within 14 days of discontinuing MAOI
- Use of chronic opioids, opiate antagonists, or partial opiate antagonist
- Seizure disorder or history of seizures
- Bulimia or anorexia nervosa
- Pregnancy
- Allergy to bupropion, naltrexone, or any component of the product
- Uncontrolled hypertension

Monitoring. Measure baseline body weight, blood pressure, heart rate, blood glucose, and renal function before starting therapy. Monitor for clinical worsening, suicidality, or unusual changes in behavior and neuropsychiatric reactions before and during the first few months of therapy, or when the dose is adjusted, especially in young adults 18 to 24 years of age.

Liraglutide

Pharmacokinetics. Liraglutide is an acylated human glucagon-like peptide-1 (GLP-1) receptor agonist. GLP-1 receptor agonists help regulate appetite and calorie intake by stimulating insulin secretion and reducing glucagon secretion. Liraglutide binds to protein and is endogenously metabolized. The plasma half-life is 13 hours following injection.

Indications. Liraglutide is approved for use in adults only. When used as an adjunct to a reduced-calorie diet and increased exercise, a decrease in BMI may occur. Liraglutide is available by injection only for subcutaneous administrations.

Adverse Effects. The most common adverse effects are nausea, hypoglycemia, diarrhea, constipation, vomiting, headache, decreased appetite, dyspepsia, fatigue, dizziness, abdominal pain, and increased lipase. Serious adverse effects include acute pancreatitis, hemorrhagic or necrotizing pancreatitis, cholelithiasis or cholecystitis, acute renal failure and worsening of chronic renal failure, and suicidal behavior and suicidal ideation.

Contraindications. Liraglutide is contraindicated in patients with hypersensitivity to liraglutide or any component of the product. Avoid concomitant use with insulin or other GLP-1 receptor agonists. Avoid in patients with increased heart rate, elevated serum calcitonin levels, thyroid nodules, or liver impairment.

BLACK BOX WARNING!

Liraglutide

- Liraglutide is contraindicated in patients with a personal or family history of medullary thyroid cancer.
- Liraglutide is contraindicated in patients with multiple endocrine neoplasia syndrome type 2.

Monitoring. Monitor serum calcitonin levels and glucose levels. Evaluate for thyroid nodules. Monitor for new or worsening of depression, suicidal thoughts or behaviors, or changes in mood or behavior.

Short-Term Weight Management Medications

Phentermine, phendimetrazine, benzphetamine, and diethylpropion are approved as short-term medications for the promotion of weight loss. The drugs are classified as sympathomimetic amines with actions similar to amphetamines. All are Schedule IV control restricted medications. The drugs will be discussed as a group because all have similar indications, adverse effects, contraindications, and monitoring guidelines.

Pharmacokinetics. Pharmacokinetic properties differ in regard to rate of absorption depending on immediate-release versus extended-release formulation. Drugs are taken on an empty stomach before meals.

- *Phentermine:* Half-life: 3 to 4 hours. Excreted in urine.
- *Phendimetrazine:* Half-life: 19 to 24 hours. Excreted in urine.
- *Benzphetamine:* Half-life: no drug-specific information available. Excreted in urine.
- *Diethylpropion:* Half-life: 4 to 8 hours. Excreted in urine.

Indications. These drugs are approved for short-term use in conjunction with a calorie-restricted diet in adults and adolescents (varying age restrictions). They stimulate the CNS to produce anorexic effects.

Adverse Effects. The most common adverse effects include increased blood pressure, palpitations, tachycardia, tremor, agitation, nervousness, irritability, and restlessness. More serious adverse effects of the cardiovascular, respiratory, and musculoskeletal systems have been reported. These include cardiomyopathy, idiopathic hypertension, valve disease, ischemia, rhabdomyolysis, and idiopathic pulmonary arterial hypertension.

Contraindications. Avoid these medications in patients with hypersensitivities to phentermine or any of its components. Avoid use in patients with sensitivities to tartrazine (FD&C Yellow No. 5). Phentermine should not be used concomitantly with MAOIs or within 14 days of discontinuing MAOIs, or for patients with a history of cardiovascular disease, glaucoma, hyperthyroidism, altered mental status, or drug abuse/potential for drug abuse.

Monitoring. Discontinue these medications when tolerance to the anorectic effect develops. Evaluate cardiac status before and during treatment. Consider electrocardiogram (ECG) and echocardiogram. Monitor for possible renal impairment. Monitor for psychological disturbances such as changes in behavior or mood.

PRACTICE PEARLS

Risk Evaluation and Mitigation Strategy (REMS)

Due to the risks associated with phentermine-topiramate, the FDA has included this drug as part of its Risk Evaluation and Mitigation Strategy (REMS). REMS aims to assist primary care providers through education on the prevention, monitoring, and management of serious side effects (FDA, n.d.).

Prescriber Considerations for Weight Management Therapy

Clinical Practice Guidelines

The U.S. Preventive Services Task Force (USPSTF) recommends that all adults be screened for obesity. The recommendation also includes guidelines on offering or referring adults with a BMI of 30 or higher intensive, multicomponent behavioral interventions (Curry et al., 2018). In 2017, the USPSTF published recommendations for children and adolescents. All children and adolescents 6 years of age or older should be screened using BMI calculations. New recommendations go beyond screening to include offering or referring patients for comprehensive intensive behavioral interventions (USPSTF, 2017). In addition to the USPSTF, many other organizations offer practice guidelines.

BOOKMARK THIS!

Clinical Practice Guidelines

- American Association of Clinical Endocrinologists and American College of Endocrinology Comprehensive Clinical Practice Guidelines for Medical Care of Patients with Obesity: https://doi.org/10.4158/EP161356.ESGL
- 2013 ACC/AHA Guideline on the Assessment of Cardiovascular Risk: American College of Cardiology/American Heart Association Task Force on Practice Guidelines: https://www.ahajournals.org/doi/pdf/10.1161/01.cir.0000437741.48606.98
- Pharmacological Management of Obesity: An Endocrine Society Clinical Practice Guideline: https://doi.org/10.1210/jc.2014-3415
- Expert Panel on Integrated Guidelines for Cardiovascular Health and Risk Reduction in Children and Adolescents: https://www.nhlbi.nih.gov/files/docs/peds_guidelines_sum.pdf
- Screening for Obesity in Pediatric Primary Care: Recommendations from the U.S. Preventive Services Task Force: https://www.uspreventiveservicestaskforce.org/uspstf/recommendation/obesity-in-children-and-adolescents-screening

---

Clinical Reasoning for Weight Management Therapy

Consider the individual patient's obesity and comorbid health problem requiring weight management medications. Obesity screening should be a part of preventive health management. Children, adolescents, and adults are at risk for multiple comorbidities and poor health outcomes related to obesity. Comorbidities affect the cardiovascular, CNS, GI, musculoskeletal, reproductive, and respiratory systems. In addition, depression and social isolation due to the stigma of obesity may result. Assessing BMI at each visit and observing for trends will guide the primary care provider in early identification. Early identification can lead to early intervention, including the use of weight management medications. Patients treated with pharmacotherapeutics have greater potential for weight loss and for sustaining the loss than patients not receiving treatment (Khera et al., 2016).

Determine the desired therapeutic outcome based on the degree of weight loss needed to decrease baseline weight. The primary goal of weight management interventions is to decrease weight, thus improving BMI. The secondary goal is to improve health outcomes related to associated comorbid conditions (Garvey et al., 2016). A systematic metaanalysis revealed that patients treated with orlistat, lorcaserin, naltrexone-bupropion, phentermine-topiramate, and liraglutide were successful at reaching a 5% weight loss over a 1-year period (Khera et al., 2016).

Assess the appropriateness of weight management medications for an individual patient by considering the medication's side effects and the patient's age, race/ethnicity, comorbidities, and genetic factors. When considering implementing weight loss medications, the primary care provider should review the adverse effects and contraindications of each medication as well as population-related data (age, race/ethnicity, and comorbidities) and pharmacogenomics data. In considering medication for older children or adolescents, it is important to assess family engagement and support as well as the implementation of other strategies such as lifestyle modifications including diet changes and exercise (Kelly et al., 2013).

Initiate the treatment plan with the selected medication by first providing adequate patient education to ensure the patient's understanding and promote full participation. Review with the patient the expected outcomes and adverse effects before prescribing medications. Provide comprehensive education on the proper administration of the medication and required monitoring. Lifestyle modifications including a reduced-calorie diet and exercise should also be discussed as these play an essential role in weight reduction therapy.

Ensure complete patient and family understanding about the medication prescribed using a variety of education strategies. Strategies including the use of written handouts and teach-back methods may help patients understand their medications. Other methods such as texting and computer-based applications have also proven effective. It is crucial that primary care providers also consider the health literacy status and cultural considerations of the patient.

Conduct follow-up and monitoring of patient responses to therapy. Provide the patient with information regarding when to seek medical help for questions or concerns. Frequent contact through telehealth or the use of office portals may provide additional encouragement and support. Provide options for office-based weigh-in opportunities not related to an office visit, if possible. If the patient desires to monitor weight at home, the provider should offer guidelines for frequency.

Teaching Points for Weight Management Therapy

Health Promotion Strategies

Successful weight loss requires a multilevel approach. Providers and patients should set realistic goals. Goals should include the prevention of further weight gain, a decrease in current

weight, and the sustaining of weight loss. In addition to medication, patients should be encouraged to decrease calorie intake and to exercise. Other health promoting strategies include the following:

- Take all medications as directed.
- Take a daily multivitamin supplement. Recommend a daily multivitamin that contains vitamins A, D, E, K, and beta carotene.
- Avoid driving or operating machinery as this medication may affect your ability to operate equipment safely.
- Do not stop taking the medication suddenly without contacting your primary care provider as adverse side effects may occur.
- Contact your primary care provider if you become pregnant, are trying to get pregnant, or are breastfeeding.
- Follow up with your primary care provider as directed.

Patient Education for Medication Safety

Tell your primary care provider:
- If you have allergies to the drug or any component of the drug
- If you have any health problems, including glaucoma, thyroid disease, or kidney or liver disease
- About all the prescription drugs, OTC drugs, or any natural products or vitamins you currently take
- If you experience new or worsening agitation, depression, suicidal thoughts or behavior, or unusual changes in mood or behavior
- If you have had a heart attack or stroke, changes in blood pressure or heart rhythm, kidney disease, increased reflexes, tremors, sweating, dilated pupils, diarrhea, high fever, confusion, or rigid muscles

Application Questions for Discussion

1. Which weight management medications are considered Schedule IV controlled substances?
2. What are the considerations for prescribing weight management medications to patients with a previously documented use of MAOIs?
3. What factors should be considered when educating the patient on weight management medications?

Selected Bibliography

Apovian, C. M., Aronne, L. J., Bessesen, D. H., McDonnell, M. E., Murad, M. H., Pagotto, U., Ryan, D. H., & Still, C. D. (2015). Pharmacological management of obesity: An endocrine society clinical practice guideline. *Journal of Clinical Endocrinology and Metabolism, 100*(2), 342–362. https://doi.org/10.1210/jc.2014-3415.

Centers for Disease Control and Prevention. (n.d.). *Overweight & obesity: Defining childhood weight status. BMI for children and teens.* Retrieved February 20, 2020 from https://www.cdc.gov/obesity/childhood/defining.html.

Curry, S. J., Owens, D. K., Barry, M. J., Caughey, A. B., Davidson, K. W., Doubeni, C. A., Epling, J. W., Grossman, D. C., Kemper, A. R., Kubik, M., Landefeld, S., Mangione, C. M., Phipps, M.

G., Silverstein, M., Simon, M. A., Tseng, C-W., & Wong, J. B. (2018). Behavioral weight loss interventions to prevent obesity-related morbidity and mortality in adults: US Preventive Services Task Force Recommendation Statement. *The Journal of the American Medical Association, 320*(11), 1163–1171. http://doi.org/10.1001/jama.2018.13022.

Echeverria, S. E., Mustafa, M., Pentakota, S. R., et al. (2017). Social and clinically-relevant cardiovascular risk factors in Asian American adults: NHANES 2011–2014. *Preventive Medicine, 99*, 222–227. http://doi.org/10.1016/j.ypmed.2017.02.016.

Flegal, K. M., Kruszon-Moran, D., Carroll, M. D., Fryar, C. D., & Ogden, C. L. (2016). Trends in obesity among adults in the United States, 2005 to 2014. *The Journal of the American Medical Association, 315*(21), 2284–2291. http://doi.org/10.1001/jama.2016.6458.

Garvey, W. T., Mechancik, J. I., Brett, E. M., Garber, A. J., Hurley, D. L, Jastreboff, A. M., Nadolsky, K., Pessah-Pollack, R., & Plodkowski, R. (2016). American Association of Clinical Endocrinologists and American College of Endocrinology comprehensive clinical practice guidelines for medical care of patients with obesity. *Endocrine Practice, 22*(7), 842–884. https://doi.org/10.4158/EP161356.ESGL.

Goff, D. C. Jr., Lloyd-Jones, D. M., Bennett, G., Coady, S., D'Agostino, R. B. Sr., Gibbons, R., Greenland, P., Lackland, D. T., Levy, D., O'Donnell, C. J., Robinson, J. G., Schwartz, J. S., Shero, S. T., Smith, S. C. Jr., Sorlie, P., Stone, N. J., & Wilson, P. W. F. (2014). ACC/AHA guideline on the assessment of cardiovascular risk: A report of the American College of Cardiology/American Heart Association Task Force on Practice Guidelines. *Circulation, 129*(suppl 2), S49–S73. https://doi.org/10.1161/01.cir.0000437741.48606.98.

Hales, C. M., Carroll, M. D., Fryar, C. D., & Ogden, C. L (2017). Prevalence of obesity among adults and youth: United States, 2015–2016. *National Center for Health Statistics, Data Brief, 288*. Available at https://www.cdc.gov/nchs/data/databriefs/db288.pdf.

Halfon, N., Larson, K., & Slusser, W. (2013). Associations between obesity and comorbid mental health, developmental, and physical health conditions in a nationally representative sample of US children aged 10 to 17. *Academic Pediatrics, 13*(1), 6–13. https://doi.org/10.1016/j.acap.2012.10.007.

Hruby, A., & Hu, F. B. (2015). The epidemiology of obesity: A big picture. Pharmacoeconomics, (33)7, 673-689. doi: 10.1007/s40273-014-0243-x.

Kelly, A. S., Barlow, S. E., Rao, G., Inge, T. H., Hayman, L. L., Steinberger, J., Urbina, E. M., Ewing, L., & Daniels, S. R. (2013). Severe obesity in children and adolescents: Identification, associated health risks, and treatment approaches. *Circulation, 128*, 1689–1712. https://doi.org/10.1161/CIR.0b013e3182a5cfb3.

Khera, R., Murad, M. H., Chandar, A. K., Dulai, P. S., Wang, Z., Prokop, L. J., Loomba, R., Camilleri, M., & Singh, S. (2016). Association of pharmacological treatments for obesity with weight loss and adverse events: A systematic review and meta-analysis. *Journal of the American Medical Association, 315*(22), 2424–2434. https://doi.org/10.1001/jama.2016.7602.

LeBlanc, E. L., Patnode, C. D., Webber, E. M., Redmond, N., Rushkin, M., & O'Connor, E. A. (2018). Behavioral and pharmacotherapy weight loss interventions to prevent obesity-related morbidity and mortality in adults: An updated systematic review for the US Preventive Services Task Force: Evidence Synthesis No. 168. *Agency for Healthcare Research and Quality,* AHRQ publication 18-05239-EF-1. https://doi.org/10.1001/jama.2018.13022

Li, W., Liu, Q., Deng, X., Chen, Y., Liu, S., & Story, M. (2017). Association between obesity and puberty timing: A systematic review and meta-analysis. *The International Journal of Environmental Research and Public Health, 14*(10), 1266. https://doi.org/10.3390/ijerph14101266.

National Institutes of Health; National Heart, Lung, and Blood Institute (NIH/NHLBI). (1998). The practical guide identification, evaluation, and treatment of overweight and obesity in adults. *National Institutes of Health, National Heart, Lung, and Blood Institute, NIH Publication No. 00-4084.* Available at https://www.nhlbi.nih.gov/files/docs/guidelines/prctgd_c.pdf.

Ogden, C. L., Carroll, M. D., Fryar, C. D., & Flegal, K. M. (2015). Prevalence of obesity among adults and youth: United States, 2011–2014: *National Center for Health Statistics*. NCHS Data Brief, No. 219. Retrieved from https://www.cybermedlife.eu/attachments/article/2468/Prevalence%20of%20Obesity%20Among%20Adults%20and%20Youth.pdf.

Ramasamy, A., Laliberte, F., Aktavoukian, S. A., Lejeune, D., DerSarkissian, M., Cavanaugh, C., Smolarz, G., Ganguly, R., & Duh, M. S. (2019). Direct and indirect cost of obesity among the privately insured in the United States: A focus on the impact by type of industry. *Journal of Occupational and Environmental Medicine, 61*(11), 877–886. http://doi.org/10.1097/JOM.0000000000001693.

U.S. Department of Health. National Institutes of Health. National Heart, Lung, and Blood Institute. (2012). Expert panel on integrated guidelines for cardiovascular health and risk reduction in children and adolescents. *National Institutes of Health, National Heart, Lung, and Blood Institute, NIH Publication No. 12-7486.* Available at https://www.nhlbi.nih.gov/files/docs/peds_guidelines_sum.pdf.

U.S. Food and Drug Administration (FDA). (n.d.) *Risk evaluation and mitigation strategies.* Available at https://www.fda.gov/drugs/drug-safety-and-availability/risk-evaluation-and-mitigation-strategies-rems.

U.S. Preventive Services Task Force (USPSTF). (2017). Screening for obesity in children and adolescents: US Preventive Services Task Force recommendations statement. *Journal of the American Medical Association, 317*(23), 2417–2426. https://doi.org/10.1001/jama.2017.6803.

Waters, H., & Graf, M. (2018). America's obesity crisis: The health and economic costs of excess weight. *Milken Institute.* Available at https://milkeninstitute.org/sites/default/files/reports-pdf/Mi-Americas-Obesity-Crisis-WEB.pdf.

World Health Organization (WHO) (n.d.). *Obesity and overweight.* Retrieved from https://www.who.int/news-room/fact-sheets/detail/obesity-and-overweight.

52

Smoking Cessation Medications

REBECCA M. LUTZ

Overview

Tobacco use is one of the largest public health risks in the United States and the leading cause of preventable disease, disability, and death (U.S. Department of Health and Human Services [HHS], 2014). Tobacco use includes cigarettes, cigars, pipes, smokeless tobacco, hookahs, and electronic cigarettes (Fig. 52.1 and Fig. 52.2). Despite years of research identifying the numerous health risks associated with tobacco use, an estimated 49.1 million U.S. adults (19.7%) use tobacco products (Creamer et al., 2019).

Frequency and Choice of Product

A look at recent trends provides a snapshot of tobacco product use among adults (Creamer et al., 2019; Wang, 2018):
- Adult males 18 years of age or older were more likely to be current cigarette smokers than females 18 years of age or older.
- Use varies by age: 18 to 24 years, 17.1%; 25 to 44 years, 23.8%; 45 to 64 years, 21.3%; and 65 years and older, 11.9%.
- The highest rate of use was among American Indians/Alaska Natives (32.3%) and those identifying as multiracial (25.4%). The lowest rate of use was among non-Hispanic Asians (10.0%).
- Cigarettes are the most commonly used form of tobacco, followed by cigars, e-cigarettes, smokeless tobacco, and pipes.
- In total, 3.7% of adult smokers use two or more tobacco products, with cigarettes and e-cigarettes the most common combination (30.1%).

Health Consequences

The health consequences associated with smoking impact multiple body systems (Fig. 52.3A). Likewise, exposure to secondhand smoke negatively affects the health of the nonsmoker (Fig. 52.3B). Exposure to secondhand smoke is more common in children 3 to 11 years of age, non-Hispanic Blacks, and persons living in poverty, rental housing, and homes with smokers. Children exposed to smoking also have an increased likelihood of smoking in adulthood.

PRACTICE PEARLS

Life Span Considerations: Effects of Perinatal and Secondhand Smoke on Child Health

- Congenital birth defects
- Dental decay
- Learning problems and behavior problems including attention-deficit hyperactivity disorder (ADHD)
- Middle ear disease
- Miscarriage/prematurity/low birth weight
- Respiratory problems
- Sudden infant death syndrome

Data from Centers for Disease Control and Prevention. (2020, February 27). *Health effects of secondhand smoke,* https://www. cdc.gov/tobacco/data_statistics/fact_sheets/secondhand_smoke/ health_effects/index.htm; Centers for Disease Control and Prevention. (2021, May 12). *Smoking, pregnancy, and babies,* https://www.cdc.gov/ tobacco/campaign/tips/diseases/pregnancy.html; Centers for Disease Control and Prevention (2019). *Reproductive health: Substance use during pregnancy.* Retrieved July 9, 2019, from https://www.cdc.gov/ reproductivehealth/maternalinfanthealth/substance-abuse/substance-abuse-during-pregnancy.htm; Healthy Children.org (n.d.). *The dangers of secondhand smoke,* https://www.healthychildren.org/English/health-issues/conditions/tobacco/Pages/Dangers-of-Secondhand-Smoke. aspx; Huang, L., Wang, Y., Zhang, L., Zheng, Z., Zhu, T., Qu, Y., & Mu, D. (2018). Maternal smoking and attention deficit/hyperactivity disorder in offspring: A meta-analysis. *Pediatrics, 141*(1): e201712465. https:// doi.org/10.1542/peds.2017-2465; and Nicoletti, D., Appel, L. D., Siedersberger Neto, P., Guimarães, G. W., Zhang, L. (2014). Maternal smoking during pregnancy and birth defects in children: A systematic review with meta-analysis, *Cad Saude Publica*, 30(12):2491-529. https://doi.org/10.1590/0102-311X00115813.

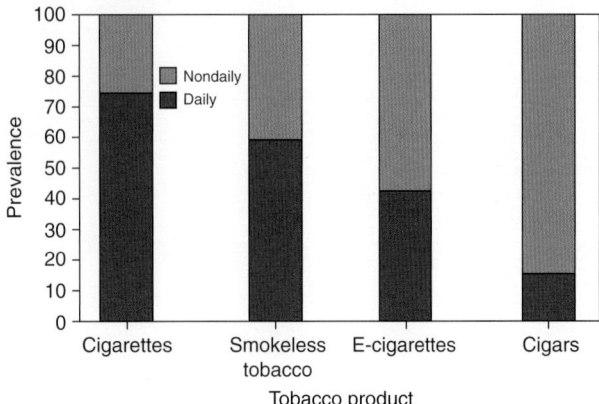

• **Fig. 52.1** Prevalence of daily[a] and nondaily[b] use of selected tobacco products[c] among adults ≥18 years of age who currently use each tobacco product—National Health Interview Survey, United States, 2018. [a]Smoking cigarettes every day at the time of the survey among persons who reported having smoked ≥100 cigarettes during their lifetime or the use of e-cigarettes, cigars, or smokeless tobacco every day at the time of survey. [b]Smoking cigarettes on some days at the time of survey among persons who reported having smoked ≥100 cigarettes during their lifetime or use of e-cigarettes, cigars, or smokeless tobacco on some days at the time of survey. [c]Daily use estimates for pipe use were unstable (relative standard error >30%); neither daily use nor nondaily use is presented. (From Creamer, M. R., Wang, T. W., Babb, S., Cullen, K. A., Day, H., Willis, G., Jamal, A., & Neff, L. [2019]. Tobacco product use and cessation indicators among adults—United States, 2018. *Centers for Disease Control and Prevention. Morbidity and Mortality Weekly Report, 68*[45], 1013–1019. DOI: http://dx.doi.org/10.15585/mmwr.mm6845a2

In adults, the effects of secondhand smoke include stroke, lung cancer, coronary heart disease, and adverse effects to the female reproductive system. Smoking during pregnancy increases the risk of pregnancy complications such as miscarriage, placental abruption, premature delivery, and infant death (CDC, 2019).

Pathophysiology

Nicotine, the key component in tobacco, results in addiction (U.S. Department of Health and Human Services, 2010). Symptoms of nicotine addiction include smoking more than 1 pack of cigarettes daily, smoking within 5 minutes of awakening, smoking when sick, getting up at night to smoke, and smoking to decrease nicotine withdrawal symptoms.

Nicotine Absorption and Addiction

Nicotine is absorbed from the lungs, oral mucosa, and skin. During inhalation, 90% to 98% of the nicotine from the lungs enters the blood. The nicotine then moves quickly into the brain (10 to 20 seconds), where it binds to nicotinic acetylcholine receptors (nAChRs). Stimulation of nAChRs results in the release of dopamine. Release of these neurotransmitters increases heart rate and cardiac contractility, constricts blood vessels, and increases blood pressure.

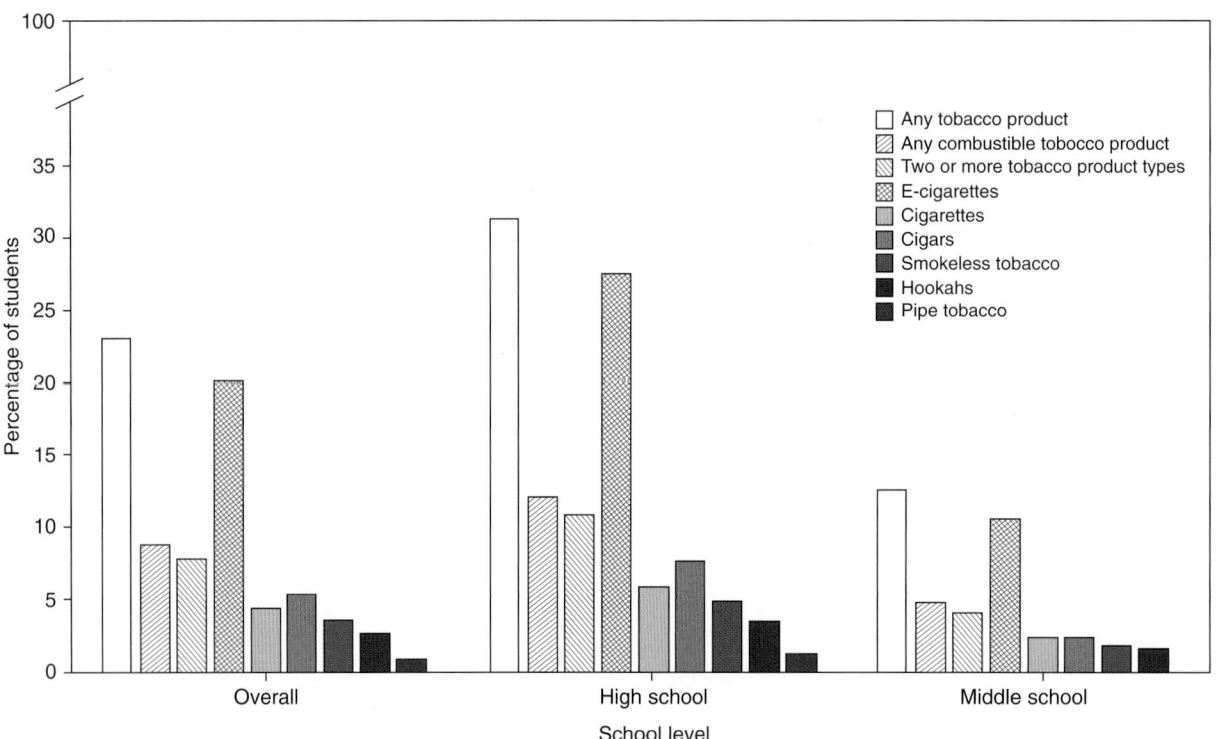

• **Fig. 52.2** Percentage of middle and high school students who currently use any tobacco product, any combustible tobacco product, two or more tobacco product types, and selected tobacco products, by school level and overall—National Youth Tobacco Survey, United States, 2019. (From Wang, T. W., Gentzke, A. S., Creamer, M. R., Cullen, K. A., Holder-Hayes, E., Sawdey, M. D., Anic, G. M., Portnoy, D. B., Hu, S., Homa, D. M., Jamal, A., & Neff, L. J. [2019]. Tobacco product use and associated factors among middle and high school students—United States, 2019. *Centers for Disease Control and Prevention. Morbidity and Mortality Weekly Report, 68*[2], 1–22. http://dx.doi.org/10.15585/mmwr.ss6812a1.)

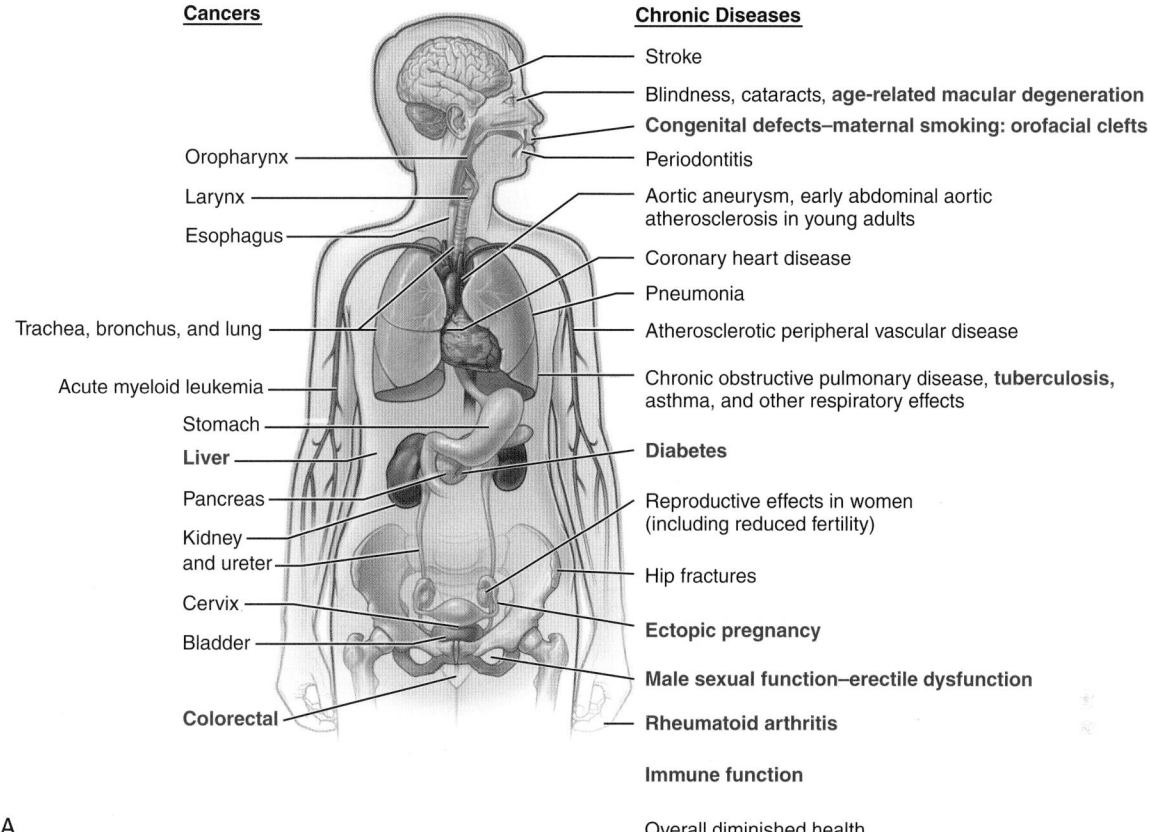

Cancers

- Oropharynx
- Larynx
- Esophagus
- Trachea, bronchus, and lung
- Acute myeloid leukemia
- Stomach
- **Liver**
- Pancreas
- Kidney and ureter
- Cervix
- Bladder
- **Colorectal**

Chronic Diseases

- Stroke
- Blindness, cataracts, **age-related macular degeneration**
- **Congenital defects–maternal smoking: orofacial clefts**
- Periodontitis
- Aortic aneurysm, early abdominal aortic atherosclerosis in young adults
- Coronary heart disease
- Pneumonia
- Atherosclerotic peripheral vascular disease
- Chronic obstructive pulmonary disease, **tuberculosis,** asthma, and other respiratory effects
- **Diabetes**
- Reproductive effects in women (including reduced fertility)
- Hip fractures
- **Ectopic pregnancy**
- **Male sexual function–erectile dysfunction**
- **Rheumatoid arthritis**
- **Immune function**
- Overall diminished health

A

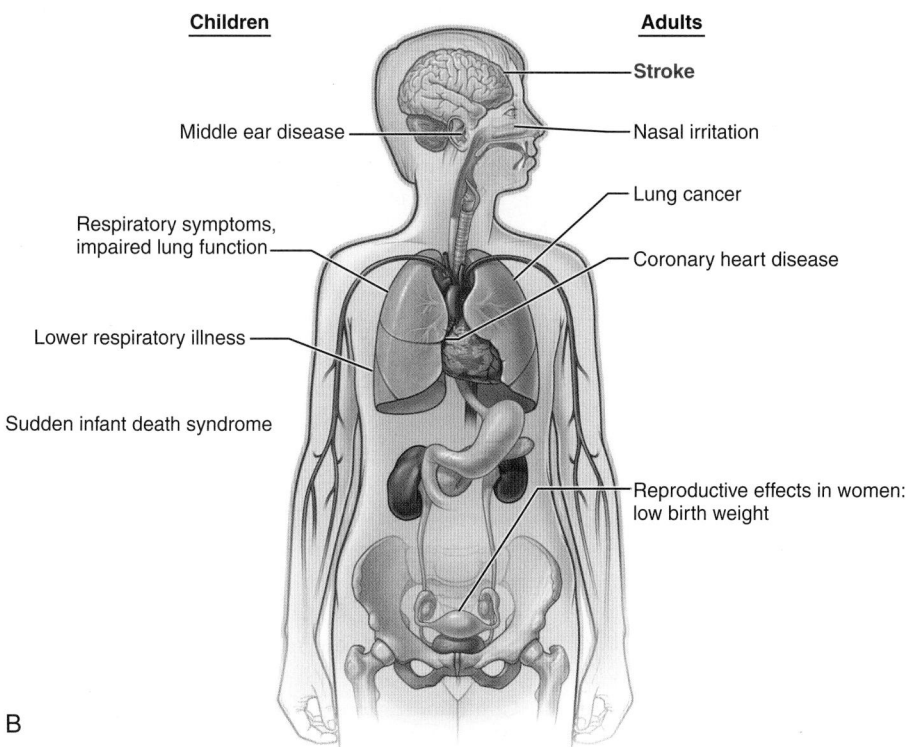

Children

- Middle ear disease
- Respiratory symptoms, impaired lung function
- Lower respiratory illness
- Sudden infant death syndrome

Adults

- **Stroke**
- Nasal irritation
- Lung cancer
- Coronary heart disease
- Reproductive effects in women: low birth weight

B

• **Fig. 52.3** (A) The health consequences causally linked to smoking. (B) The health consequences causally linked to exposure to secondhand smoke. NOTE: The conditions in red are new diseases that have been causally linked to smoking. (From McCance, K., & Huether, S. [2019]. *Pathophysiology* [8th ed.]. St. Louis: Elsevier. Reproduced from the World Cancer Research Fund/American Institute for Cancer Research. Diet, Nutrition, Physical Activity and Cancer: A Global Perspective. Continuous Update Project Expert Report 2018. dietandcancerreport.org.)

Within the central nervous system (CNS), release of dopamine results in activation of the pleasure system to reinforce the effects of nicotine. Smokers report positive feelings of pleasure, increased alertness, and improved concentration and memory. They also report a decrease in stress, anxiety, aggression, and appetite. These effects reoccur with subsequent nicotine exposure, which reinforces the behavior.

Nicotine Withdrawal and Smoking Cessation

Experiencing nicotine withdrawal symptoms triggers relapse. Smoking cessation therapy decreases the symptoms associated with withdrawal, making it easier for patients to stop smoking. The U.S. Food and Drug Administration (FDA) has approved nicotine replacement therapy, bupropion, and varenicline as treatment options to promote smoking cessation.

> **PRACTICE PEARLS**
>
> **Symptoms of Nicotine Withdrawal**
>
> - Anxiety
> - Cravings
> - Increased appetite
> - Irritability
> - Sleep disorders
> - Weight gain

Nicotine Replacement Therapy

Nicotine replacement therapy provides continuous lower doses of nicotine to simulate the effect of nicotine on nAChRs. This reduces withdrawal symptoms and cravings commonly associated with nicotine withdrawal without the pleasurable responses linked to smoking. Decreased withdrawal symptoms may promote smoking cessation and prevent relapse (Barua et al., 2018; Prochaska & Benowitz, 2016; U.S. Department of Health and Human Services, 2010).

Nicotine replacement is available as a transdermal patch, gum, lozenge, nasal spray, or inhaler. The transdermal patch, gum, and lozenge are available over the counter, but some health insurance plans do include them as a covered medication. The nasal spray and inhaler are currently available as a prescription.

Initial prescribing recommendations are based on the number of cigarettes smoked per day as well as patient preference and comorbidities. In 2013, the FDA reviewed safety data and determined that there are no significant risks associated with the use of nicotine replacement therapy (patches, lozenges, and gum only) and the concurrent use of other nicotine-containing products. The goal is to gradually decrease nicotine replacement therapy dosing and then stop completely. In some instances, extending the use of nicotine replacement therapy for several months after quitting decreases the likelihood of relapse. An overview of the medications (Table 52.1) is based on the 2018 American College of Cardiology (ACC) Expert Consensus Pathway (Barua et al., 2018).

> **PRACTICE PEARLS**
>
> **Nicotine Replacement Therapy Use in Pregnancy and Lactation**
>
> **Pregnancy**
>
> - There is a risk of fetal harm with use of nicotine replacement therapy during pregnancy. However, the potential benefits of decreasing nicotine through nicotine replacement therapy may warrant use of the drug in pregnant patients despite the risks.
> - Use during pregnancy only after weighing the risk of the mother continuing to smoke against the likelihood of smoking cessation with the use of the nicotine inhaler.
>
> **Lactation**
>
> - Nicotine is transferred into breast milk.
> - Nicotine replacement therapy decreases the amount of nicotine in breast milk.
> - Weigh the benefit to the mother against the risk to the infant.

Long-Acting Nicotine Replacement Therapy

Transdermal Patch

Pharmacokinetics. The transdermal patch releases a slow and steady concentration of nicotine. Peak plasma concentrations are reached in 2 to 10 hours. Metabolism by the liver results in inactive metabolites. Half-life averages 3 to 6 hours. Excretion is via the kidneys.

Indications. Transdermal patches are nicotine-containing adhesive patches. The patch is convenient to use and is available in a variety of strengths (21 mg/patch, 14 mg/patch, 7 mg/patch). Initial dosing is determined by the number of cigarettes smoked daily. Patches are applied once daily to clean, dry, hairless skin of the upper body or upper arm. A limitation of the patch is the lack of dose regulation if the patient has withdrawal symptoms. To cover cravings, combination nicotine replacement therapy is recommended: for example, the nicotine replacement gum, lozenge, inhaler, or nasal spray can be used along with the patch.

Adverse Effects. Adverse effects include pruritus, burning, erythema at the application site, and vivid dreams with the use of the 16-hour or 24-hour patch. Nicotine withdrawal symptoms, dizziness, headache, and insomnia were also reported. Rare but serious side effects include dysrhythmias, hypertension, and tachycardia.

Contraindications. The use of a transdermal patch is contraindicated in patients with hypersensitivity to nicotine or any of its components. Patients with cardiovascular disease, those weighing less than 100 pounds, and those who smoke less than one-half pack of cigarettes daily should be instructed to begin with a smaller patch. Consideration should be given to reducing dosages based on degree of renal and hepatic impairment.

TABLE 52.1   Nicotine Replacement Therapy

Classification/ Medication	Indication	Dosage	Considerations and Monitoring
Long-Acting Nicotine Replacement Therapy			
Nicotine transdermal patch (over-the-counter or prescription)	Smoking cessation	*Adult smoker of ≤10 cigarettes daily:* Weeks 1–6: Apply one 14-mg patch daily. Weeks 7 and 8: Apply one 7-mg patch daily. Then stop. *Adult smoker of ≥10 cigarettes daily:* Weeks 1–6: Apply one 21–mg patch daily. Weeks 7 and 8: Apply one 14-mg patch daily. Weeks 9 and 10: Apply one 7-mg patch daily. Then stop.	May adjust dose depending on withdrawal symptoms (move to higher or lower dose). Patch may be worn for 16 or 24 hr. Remove the previously applied patch before applying a new patch.
Short-Acting Nicotine Replacement Therapy			
Nicotine polacrilex lozenge (over-the-counter or prescription)	Smoking cessation	*Adults ≥18 yr who smoke first cigarette within 30 minutes of awakening:* 4-mg lozenge. Weeks 1–6: 1 lozenge orally every 1–2 hr. Weeks 7–9: 1 lozenge orally every 2–4 hr. Weeks 10–12: 1 lozenge orally every 4–8 hr. Then stop. Maximum dosage: 20 lozenges/day. *Adults ≥18 yr who smoke first cigarette within 30 minutes of awakening:* 2-mg lozenge. Weeks 1–6: 1 lozenge orally every 1–2 hr. Weeks 7–9: 1 lozenge orally every 2–4 hr. Weeks 10–12: 1 lozenge orally every 4–8 hr. Then stop. Maximum dosage: 20 lozenges/day.	Lozenge takes 20–30 min to dissolve. No food or drink 15 min prior to use or during use.
Nicotine gum (over-the-counter or prescription)	Smoking cessation	*Adults ≥18 yr who smoke first cigarette within 30 minutes of awakening:* 4-mg chewing gum. Weeks 1–6: Chew 1 piece of gum orally every 1–2 hr. Weeks 7–9: Chew 1 piece of gum orally every 2–4 hr. Weeks 10–12: Chew 1 piece of gum orally every 4–8 hr. Then stop. Maximum dosage: 24 pieces/day. *Adults ≥18 yr who smoke first cigarette within 30 minutes of awakening:* 2-mg lozenge. Weeks 1–6: Chew 1 piece of gum orally every 1–2 hr. Weeks 7–9: Chew 1 piece of gum orally every 2–4 hr. Weeks 10–12: Chew 1 piece of gum orally every 4–8 hr. Then stop. Maximum dosage: 24 pieces of gum/day.	No food or drink 15 min prior to use or during use.

Continued

TABLE 52.1	Nicotine Replacement Therapy—cont'd			
Classification/ Medication	Indication	Dosage		Considerations and Monitoring
Nicotine inhaler (prescription)	Smoking cessation	*Adults ≥18 yr:* Weeks 1–12: 24–64 mg (6–16 cartridges) daily. Puff into mouth/throat. Do not inhale into lungs. Weeks 12–24: Gradually decrease dose. Maximum duration: 6 months Maximum dosage: 64 mg/day.		Advise patient to stop smoking completely while using nasal spray.
Nicotine nasal spray (prescription)	Smoking cessation	**0.5-mg nicotine/spray (1 dose = 1 spray in each nostril):** *Adults ≥18 yr:* 1 spray in each nostril once or twice hourly. Maximum duration: 3 months. Maximum dosage: 5 doses/hour OR 40 doses/day.		Minimum effective dosage: 8 doses/day. Advise patient to stop smoking completely while using nasal spray.

Monitoring Monitor for adverse effects. Monitor for withdrawal symptoms and adjust medication as needed to decrease symptoms. Monitor heart rate and blood pressure at each visit.

Short-Acting Nicotine Replacement Therapy

The nicotine replacement lozenge, gum, inhaler, and nasal spray are short-acting preparations. These are often used in combination with the longer-acting transdermal patch. They may also be used alone if the patient prefers, though this method may lead to underdosing.

Pharmacokinetic properties of the lozenge and gum are similar. Both contain nicotine bound to polacrilex, which increases the amount of nicotine available for mucosal absorption. Metabolism is through the liver. Excretion is through the urine. Advise patients to avoid eating or drinking 15 minutes prior to using either the lozenge or gum.

Lozenge

Pharmacokinetics. Pharmacokinetic data are not available from the manufacturers. An early study by Shiffman et al. (2002) reported that the lozenges release approximately 25% to 27% more nicotine than the gum. As the patient sucks on the lozenge, it releases nicotine, which is absorbed through the oral mucosa as the lozenge melts.

Indications. The benefits of the lozenge are the way it mimics the oral sensation associated with smoking and the patient's ability to control the dosage. It is a better alternative than chewing gum for patients with dental work or dentures. Advise patients not to chew or swallow the lozenge. To use, the patient places the lozenge between the cheek and gumline and lets it melt, occasionally moving it from one side of their mouth to the other. Patients smoking the first cigarette within 30 minutes of awakening should select the 4-mg lozenge. The

2-mg lozenge is better suited for patients who smoke their first cigarette more than 30 minutes after awakening.

Adverse Effects. In addition to the effects of nicotine withdrawal, adverse effects include mouth irritations, hiccups, heartburn, and nausea. Other adverse effects may include flatulence, headache, cough, and respiratory tract infection. Advise patients that higher doses may increase the intensity and frequency of these adverse effects.

Contraindications. Patients with hypersensitivity to the medication or any of its components should avoid the use of lozenges. Nicorette mint-flavored nicotine lozenges should be avoided in patients with soya lecithin hypersensitivity. Assess risk versus benefit in patients with cardio- or peripheral vascular disease.

Monitoring. Routine laboratory monitoring is not required. Monitor renal and hepatic function in patients with moderate to severe impairments. Monitor for adverse effects.

Chewing Gum

Pharmacokinetics. Peak levels of nicotine occur about 30 minutes after the patient starts chewing the gum. Absorption is affected by surface area, blood flow, mucosal permeability, and oral pH. Nicotine concentration in the blood varies depending on how vigorous and long the patient chews and the amount of saliva produced by chewing. Metabolism is via the liver. Half-life is 1 to 2 hours. Excretion is via the kidneys.

Indications. Nicotine replacement chewing gum is an over-the-counter (OTC) smoking cessation therapy that offers patients the flexibility to quickly decrease sudden cravings. Initial dosing is determined by the number of cigarettes smoked per day. Advise the patient to chew the gum until they note the taste of nicotine or the flavor of the gum, or notice a tingling sensation, and then to place the gum between their cheek and gumline. Once the tingling stops, they should repeat the process.

Adverse Effects. The most common adverse effects from the chewing gum include excessive salivation, jaw soreness, mouth ulcers, gingivitis, and irritation. Other adverse effects include heartburn, nausea, vomiting, abdominal pain, constipation, hiccups, and headache.

Contraindications. Patients with allergies or sensitivities should avoid the use of nicotine replacement gum. Patients prone to temporomandibular joint disorders, those with poor dentition (history of ulcers, caries, or gingivitis), those who use dental appliances, or those who experience intolerable adverse effects can consider alternative methods of short-acting nicotine replacement therapy.

Monitoring. Monitor for adverse effects. Monitor withdrawal symptoms and cravings and adjust medication. Monitor dentition and mucosal membranes for adverse effects.

Nasal Spray

Pharmacokinetics. Each spray delivers an aqueous solution of 0.5 mg nicotine to the nasal mucosa. Absorption is rapid. Peak plasma concentrations occur within 10 to 15 minutes.

Indications. The nasal spray provides relief from withdrawal symptoms more quickly than patches or products that absorb nicotine through the oral mucosa. Nicotine replacement nasal sprays are currently available only by prescription.

Adverse Effects. Nasal and throat irritation are common adverse effects. Other adverse effects include rhinitis, sneezing, coughing, and tearing. Adverse effects are usually mild and temporary, ending within a few days to 2 weeks.

Contraindications. Patients with sinus problems, allergies, or asthma should avoid any nicotine nasal spray product.

Monitoring. Make frequent contact with the patient either electronically or in the office. Monitor for withdrawal symptoms, cravings, and relapse. Monitor for adverse effects.

Nicotine Inhalers

Pharmacokinetics. With nicotine inhalers, most of the nicotine remains in the mouth. Less than 5% reaches the lower airways. Peak plasma concentration is within 15 minutes. Nicotine plasma levels are between 6 and 8 mg/mL, which is equal to about one-third the plasma level reached with cigarette smoking.

Indications. The nicotine inhaler mimics the hand-to-mouth ritual of smoking cigarettes. In addition to nicotine, the inhaler also contains menthol. The menthol stimulates the mucous membranes and replicates the sensation of smoking. Patients control the amount of nicotine by using 1 cartridge every 1 to 2 hours. Advise patients to puff into their mouth/throat but not to inhale into their lungs.

Adverse Effects. Adverse effects reported by 40% to 66% of patients were related to local irritation of the mouth and throat. Other reported adverse effects included headache, influenza-like symptoms, pain, back pain, allergy, paresthesia, flatulence, and fever. Coughing can result if the medication is inhaled into the lungs rather than puffed into the

mouth. Similar effects related to nicotine withdrawal were also noted.

Contraindications. The use of a nicotine replacement inhaler is contraindicated in patients with known hypersensitivity or allergy to nicotine or menthol. Inhaler use is contraindicated in patients with asthma or pulmonary disease. Continuing to smoke while under nicotine replacement inhaler therapy is contraindicated due to the potential increase in adverse effects.

Monitoring. Monitor for signs of nicotine overdose and adverse effects. No routine laboratory monitoring is recommended. Monitor patients with known liver or renal impairment for increased adverse effects due to metabolism of nicotine.

Nicotine-Free Smoking Cessation Therapy

Two medications, bupropion hydrochloride and varenicline, are approved for use in smoking cessation therapy (Table 52.2).

Bupropion Hydrochloride

Bupropion hydrochloride is an antidepressant prescribed to decrease withdrawal symptoms associated with smoking cessation. The neuronal uptake of norepinephrine and dopamine is inhibited; however, monoamine oxidase and serotonin uptake is not inhibited. Bupropion hydrochloride stimulates the CNS and suppresses appetite. It is less likely to cause the sexual side effects or sedation associated with other antidepressants.

PRACTICE PEARLS

Bupropion and Varenicline Use in Pregnancy and Lactation

- Pregnancy: Weigh the potential benefit of treatment of the mother to the potential risk to the fetus. Available clinical studies cannot establish or exclude any associated risk during pregnancy.
- Lactation: Weigh the potential benefit of treatment of the mother to the potential adverse effects on the infant. The infant should be observed for adverse effects of medication used by the mother.

PRACTICE PEARLS

Bupropion and Varenicline Use in Pediatrics

- Bupropion: Safety and effectiveness in the pediatric population have not been established (https://www.accessdata.fda.gov/drugsatfda_docs/label/2011/018644s043lbl.pdf).
- Varenicline: Not recommended for use in pediatric patients 16 years of age or younger (https://www.accessdata.fda.gov/drugsatfda_docs/label/2016/021928s040lbl.pdf).

TABLE 52.2   Nicotine-Free Smoking Cessation Medications

Medication	Indication	Dosage	Considerations and Monitoring
Bupropion hydrochloride 150-mg extended release	Smoking cessation	**150-mg tablet:** *Adults ≥18 yr:* 1 tablet orally once daily for 3 days, then increase to 1 tablet orally every 12 hr. Continue 7–12 weeks. Maximum dosage: 300 mg/day.	Moderate to severe hepatic impairment (Child-Pugh score 7–15): 150 mg every other day. Mild hepatic impairment (Child-Pugh score 5–6): reduce dose and/or frequency.
Varenicline tartrate	Smoking cessation	**Patients able to quit smoking abruptly: 1-mg tablet:** *Adults ≥18 yr:* Start therapy 1 week before anticipated quit date OR begin treatment and quit smoking between days 8 and 35. Days 1–3: 0.5 mg orally once daily. Days 4–7: 0.5 mg orally twice daily. Day 8–end of treatment: 1 mg once daily. Duration of therapy: 12 weeks. If successful, continue 12 more weeks. **Patients unable or unwilling to quit smoking abruptly: 1-mg tablet:** *Adults ≥18 yr:* Days 1–3: 0.5 mg orally once daily. Days 4–7: 0.5 mg orally twice daily. Day 8–end of treatment: 1 mg once daily. In addition: Weeks 1–4: decrease smoking by 50%. Weeks 5–8: decrease smoking by another 50%. Weeks 9–12: stop smoking. Duration of therapy: 12 weeks. If successful, continue 12 more weeks.	Renal impairment: adjust dose.

Pharmacokinetics. Absorption is not affected by food intake, and time to maximum concentration (Tmax) is reached in about 5 hours. The medication is extensively metabolized via the liver. Cytochrome (CYP) 2B6 forms hydroxybupropion, the major metabolite. The half-life of hydroxybupropion is 20 hours. Excretion primarily occurs via the kidneys. Steady-state blood levels are reached about 1 week after therapy begins.

PHARMACOGENETICS

CYP2B6

- Bupropion hydrochloride sustained release can cause false-positive urine test results for amphetamines.

Indications. Bupropion hydrochloride is approved for tobacco cessation. The medication reduces nicotine cravings and other withdrawal symptoms. Patients should target a quit date and begin therapy 1 week before this date.

Adverse Effects. Adverse effects are generally mild. The most common adverse effects include insomnia, dry mouth, dizziness, and arthralgia. Patients also reported increases in anxiety and depression during the first 2 weeks of treatment (West et al., 2015).

BLACK BOX WARNING!

Suicidal Warning With Use of Zyban

- There is an increased risk of suicidal thinking and behavior in children, adolescents, and young adults taking antidepressants. Zyban is not an antidepressant but contains the same active ingredient as antidepressants.
- Monitor patients for worsening as well as emergence of suicidal thoughts and behaviors.

Data from U.S. Food and Drug Administration. (2016). FDA Drug Safety Communication: FDA revises description of mental health side effects of the stop-smoking medicines Chantix (varenicline) and Zyban (bupropion) to reflect clinical trial findings. https://www.fda.gov/drugs/drug-safety-and-availability/fda-drug-safety-communication-fda-revises-description-mental-health-side-effects-stop-smoking.

Contraindications. Bupropion hydrochloride is contra-indicated in patients with hypersensitivities to bupropion hydrochloride or any of its components. Numerous drug–drug interactions are associated with the use of bupropion hydrochloride (Table 52.3). Patients taking monoamine oxidase inhibitors (MAOIs) should wait at least 14 days after discontinuing the MAOIs before taking bupropion hydrochloride. Prescribe with caution for patients with angle-closure glaucoma, seizure disorders, cocaine use, liver impairment, or a history or current diagnosis of bulimia or anorexia nervosa. Abrupt withdrawal of benzodiazepines, barbiturates, or antiepileptic drugs may increase the risk of seizures. Excessive use and/or abruptly stopping alcohol may result in a reduced tolerance to alcohol, an increased risk of seizures, or neuropsychiatric events.

Monitoring. Monitor hepatic function and adjust dose as required. Monitor for behavioral changes and psychiatric symptoms. Monitor blood pressure, heart rate, and weight. Assess alcohol intake and the presence of comorbid conditions.

Varenicline Tartrate

Pharmacokinetics. Peak plasma levels occur within about 2 to 4 hours. Half-life is approximately 17 to 24 hours. Varenicline is metabolized via the liver. Excretion is via the kidney. Bioavailability is not affected by food or dosing schedule.

Indications. Varenicline is used as tobacco cessation therapy in adults. Varenicline promotes the release of dopamine, which reduces nicotine cravings and withdrawal symptoms. A 28-study metaanalysis concluded that varenicline was superior to bupropion hydrochloride extended release and the transdermal nicotine patch in promoting abstinence in both males and females, though the difference was more pronounced in females (Smith et al., 2017). Coadministration of varenicline and the transdermal nicotine patch increases the incidence of nausea, headache, vomiting, dizziness, dyspepsia, and fatigue. More patients (36%) treated with the combination of varenicline and nicotine replacement therapy discontinued treatment due to adverse effects.

Adverse Effects. The most common adverse effects are insomnia, headache, nausea, abnormal dreams, flatulence, and headache. Less frequent adverse effects include irritability, depression, behavior and mood disorders, and suicidal ideations.

Contraindications. Avoid in patients with hypersensitivity or skin reactions to varenicline or any of its components. Drug–drug contraindications include the concomitant use of varenicline with bupropion. Alcohol use is contraindicated due to the potential for increased intoxicating effects of alcohol. Use with caution in patients with renal impairment, and adjust dose according to creatinine clearance (CrCl) (Table 52.4). Prior to prescribing, evaluate patients with a history of cardiovascular disease.

In 2016, the FDA removed previous black box warnings from the Chantix label. Specific precautions remain, including the increased risk of neuropsychiatric events, seizures, interactions with alcohol, accidental injury, cardiovascular events, somnambulism, angioedema and hypersensitivity reactions, and serious skin reactions. Due to these risks, primary care providers should carefully evaluate the use of varenicline in truck drivers, bus drivers, airplane pilots, and air traffic controllers.

Monitoring. Monitor for renal impairment and adjust dose as recommended. Monitor other medications for dose adjustments as patients quit smoking. Monitor for behavioral changes and psychiatric symptoms.

Role of Electronic Cigarettes in Smoking Cessation

The role of electronic cigarettes (e-cigarettes) in smoking cessation therapy is unknown. Certainly, evidence has shown that e-cigarettes are popular among adults and adolescents. In 2016, 4.5% of U.S. adults used e-cigarettes (Mirbolouk et al., 2016). Among high school students, e-cigarettes were

TABLE 52.3	Drug–Drug Interactions With Bupropion Hydrochloride[a]	
Medication	**Interaction**
Inhibitors of CYP 2D6 (ticlopidine, clopidogrel)	Increase bupropion exposure but decrease hydroxybupropion exposure
Inducers of CYP 2D6 (ritonavir, lopinavir, and efavirenz)	Decrease bupropion and hydroxybupropion exposure
Eliglustat	Prolonged QT
Linezolid Methylene blue Selegiline	Increased risk of hypersensitivity reactions
Monoamine oxidase inhibitors (isocarboxazid, tranylcypromine, phenelzine, procarbazine, furazolidone, moclobedmide, rasagiline, nialamide, iproniazid)	Increased risk of hypertensive reactions

[a]There are many other drug–drug interactions with bupropion hydrochloride. The primary care provider should check all drug interactions among the patient's medications before prescribing bupropion hydrochloride.

TABLE 52.4	Varenicline Dosing Adjustment Based on Creatinine Clearance	
Creatinine Clearance	**Dose Recommendations**
<30 mL/min	0.5 mg once daily. Titrate as needed to a maximum dosage of 0.5 mg twice daily.
End-stage renal disease undergoing hemodialysis	0.5 mg once daily may be administered if tolerated.

the most commonly used product (20%) compared to cigars (5.3%) and cigarettes (4.3%) (Wang et al., 2019).

Primary care providers may be asked about the use of e-cigarettes as a part of smoking cessation therapy. As of this writing, there is neither FDA approval nor national guidelines for the use of e-cigarettes as an aid to smoking cessation. Understanding the current evidence will help providers guide patients to informed decisions. Several resources are available for this:

- The CDC offers a fact sheet, "Adult Smoking Cessation – The Use of E-Cigarettes," that details key research findings (CDC, 2020).
- The National Academies of Sciences, Engineering, and Medicine (2018) released *Public Health Consequences of E-Cigarettes*. This report reviewed 21 systematic reviews published between 2014 and 2017 to determine whether there was a role for e-cigarettes in smoking cessation therapy. The results of this report reveal the following:
  - There is insufficient evidence regarding the effectiveness of e-cigarettes compared to no treatment or the current FDA approved treatments.
  - Limited evidence suggests that e-cigarettes effectively promote smoking cessation.
  - Moderate evidence suggests that e-cigarettes with nicotine are more effective than e-cigarettes without nicotine for smoking cessation and that the frequent use of e-cigarettes increases the likelihood of smoking cessation.

Prescriber Considerations for Smoking Cessation Therapy

Clinical Practice Guidelines

Healthy People 2020 smoking cessation objectives include increasing the percentage of U.S. adults who attempt to quit smoking cigarettes to at least 80% and increasing recent smoking cessation success to at least 8% (U.S. Department of Health and Human Services, 2014). The primary care provider is in a unique position to help patients reach this goal. However, in 2015, only 57.2% of smokers received a health professional's advice to quit smoking (Babb et al., 2017). Fortunately, several smoking cessation resources are available to primary care providers.

For example, Park et al. (2015) determined that 40% more patients stopped smoking when primary care providers utilized the "5 R's" format, a smoking cessation framework with the following recommendations for addressing smoking cessation with patients (Agency for Healthcare Research and Quality, 2012):

1. The patient determines why quitting is personally *relevant*.
2. Does the patient see any *risk* associated with continued smoking?
3. Are there any perceived *rewards* to quitting tobacco?
4. The patient identifies *roadblocks* they may encounter.
5. *Repeat* the discussion at each patient encounter.

The Pathway to Tobacco Cessation Treatment (Fig. 52.4), by the 2018 ACC Expert Consensus Decision Pathway, offers an updated stepwise approach: (1) ask all patients about their tobacco use or secondhand smoke exposure; (2) assess the level of addiction and potential for relapse; (3) advise all tobacco users to quit and all nonsmokers to avoid secondhand smoke exposure; (4) offer and connect the patient to treatment; and (5) follow up at every visit (Barua et al., 2018).

Finally, the U.S. Preventive Services Task Force recommendations (USPSTF, 2015) include the following:

- Ask all adults about tobacco use and provide tobacco cessation interventions for those who use tobacco products ("A" Recommendation).
- Ask all pregnant patients (regardless of age) about tobacco use and provide augmented, pregnancy-tailored counseling for those who smoke ("A" Recommendation).
- Provide interventions, including education or brief counseling, to prevent initiation of tobacco use in school-age children and adolescents ("B" Recommendation).

Clinical Reasoning for Smoking Cessation Therapy

Consider the individual patient's health and health outcomes. Patients may understand the consequences (cause and effect) of smoking but not be ready to quit using tobacco products even when they are experiencing health problems related to smoking. One factor preventing smoking cessation is the fear of withdrawal symptoms. Failure with previous smoking cessation attempts may stop the patient from trying again. When surveyed, 68% of adult smokers 18 years of age or older reported a desire to stop smoking and approximately 55% had tried to quit. Despite the desire to quit smoking, only 7.4% had recently quit (Babb et al., 2017). A willingness on the part of the primary care provider to initiate a conversation may result in smoking cessation.

Determine the desired therapeutic outcome. Complete smoking cessation is the goal of smoking cessation therapy, but even a reduction in the amount of smoking can help improve health outcomes. Immediate benefits are seen within minutes, with decreases in heart rate and blood pressure. Long-term benefits are decreased heart attacks, strokes, and cancers.

Determine the smoking cessation therapy based on its appropriateness for an individual patient by considering the patient's age, comorbidities, and potential for adverse effects. The FDA has approved nicotine and non-nicotine smoking cessation therapies for adults older than 18 years of age. Alternatives to medication therapies include behavioral therapies, which may be used for adolescents and pregnant or breastfeeding females. A thorough review of the patient's history of comorbid conditions or concurrent prescription and OTC medications may impact the choice of therapy. Reassess the success of current therapy at each visit and consider alternative therapy.

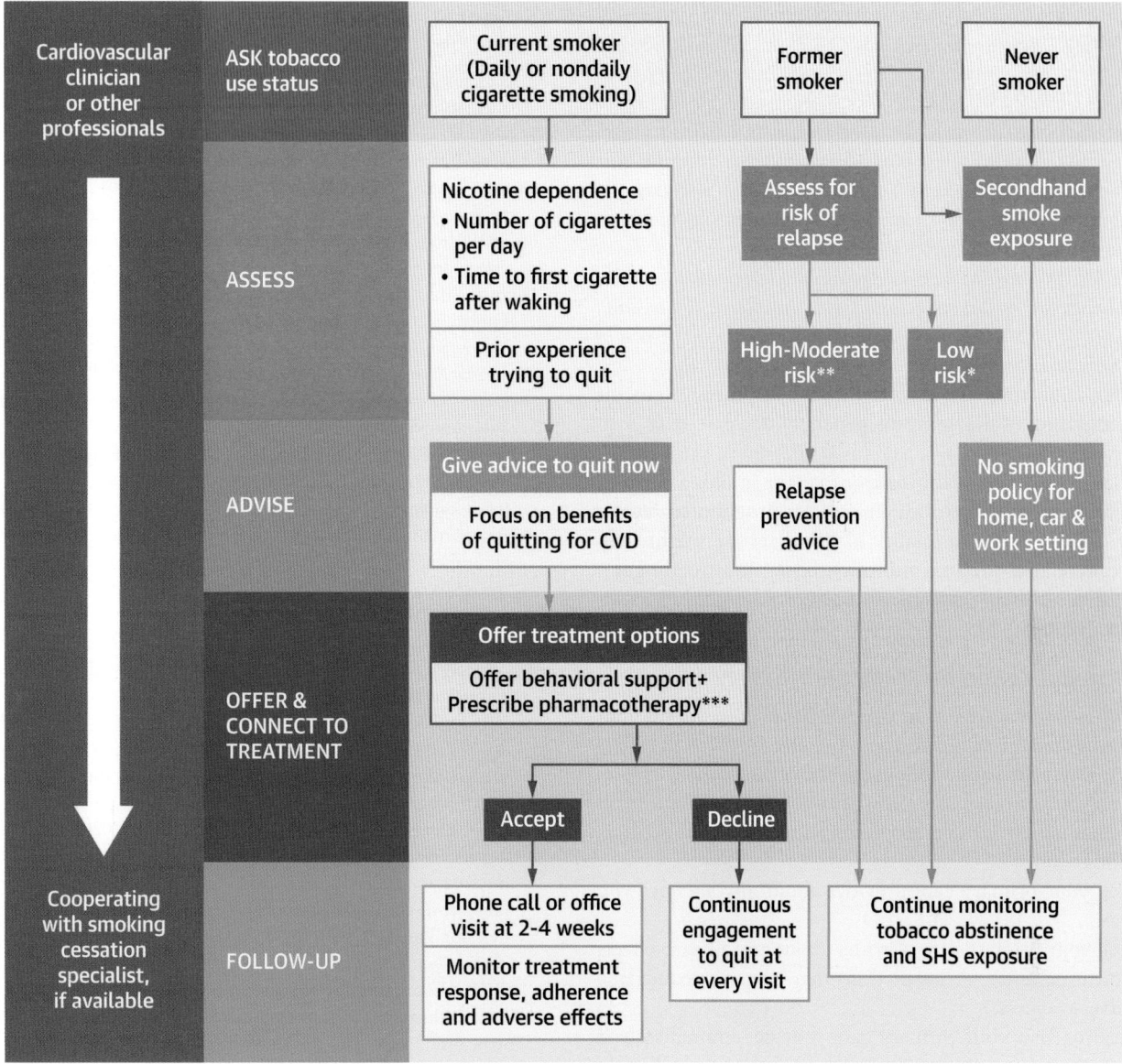

• **Fig. 52.4** Pathway to tobacco cessation treatment. (From Barua, R. S., Rigotti, N. A., Benowitz, N. L., Cummings, K. M., Jazayeri, M.-A., Morris, P. B., …Wiggins, B. S. [2018]. 2018 ACC Expert Consensus Decision Pathway on tobacco cessation treatment: A report of the American College of Cardiology Task Force on clinical expert consensus documents. *Journal of the American College of Cardiology, 72*[25], 3332–3365. http://doi.org/10.1016/j.jacc.2018.10.027)

Initiate the treatment plan with the selected smoking cessation therapy by first providing adequate patient education to ensure the patient's understanding and promote full participation in the smoking cessation therapy. Patient preferences may impact the choice of therapy. Long-term nicotine replacement therapy may be combined with short-term nicotine replacement therapy and behavioral interventions to decrease cravings and possibly improve the chance of quitting (Stead et al., 2016). Review the advantages and disadvantages as well as the cost of each choice.

Ensure complete patient and family understanding about the medications prescribed for smoking cessation therapy using a variety of education strategies. Provide written and verbal instructions including the name of the medication,

dosing information including tapering guidelines, method of administration, adverse effects, and when to notify the provider of questions or concerns. Discuss plans for the management of cravings and avoidance of triggers. Offer information such as behavioral therapy/groups, online information such as *1-800-QUIT-NOW*, which is a telephone support service, and online links to a variety of other patient resources.

Conduct follow-up and monitoring of patient responses to therapy to improve the effectiveness of smoking cessation therapy. At each contact, assess for level of smoking, under- or overdosing, side effects or adverse effects, and management of cravings or triggers. Reassess treatment goals and medication options.

Teaching Points for Smoking Cessation Therapy

Health Promotion Strategies

- Determine a quit date. Try to choose a date within a couple of weeks, though some patients prefer to link the quit day to a personally significant day such as a birthday.
- Talk to your primary care provider to determine which treatment options are best for you.
- Enlist the support of trusted family and friends.
- Change behaviors associated with smoking. If possible, limit or eliminate your time with smokers or in places where smoking occurs.
- Plan how to manage withdrawal symptoms. Remember, withdrawal symptoms generally decrease over 3 to 4 weeks.
- Plan how you will eliminate or manage smoking triggers.
- Consider implementing an exercise program to reduce stress and improve quality of life. Exercise might help avoid relapse and may minimize or prevent weight gain.
- Utilize self-help materials and/or consider joining a support group.

Patient Education for Medication Safety

- Follow all instruction in the drug label guides. Different forms of nicotine replacement therapy are taken in different ways. Be sure to follow the correct method.
- Tell your primary care provider about all medicines you are taking. This includes prescription and OTC medications.
- Tell your primary care provider about any allergies you have.
- Tell your primary care provider about any adverse effects you experience. A lower dose may stop or reduce the adverse effects.
- Call or visit your primary care provider immediately if you notice any new or worsening behavioral changes and/or psychiatric symptoms.
- If you experience cravings, tell your primary care provider. Additional medications may help to control cravings.
- Remove the 24-hour patch at bedtime if you experience disturbing dreams or insomnia.
- Keep all medications away from children and pets to avoid adverse effects or nicotine toxicity.

Application Questions for Discussion

1. What are the benefits and risks associated with the use of non-nicotine smoking cessation therapy?
2. What are the key components of a patient education plan centered on the use of a nicotine transdermal patch with a nicotine lozenge?
3. Describe how the primary care provider can incorporate the concept of shared decision-making into smoking cessation therapy.

Selected Bibliography

Agency for Healthcare Research and Quality, (n.d.). *Five major steps to intervention (The "5 A's")*. Retrieved July 9, 2019, from https://www.ahrq.gov/professionals/clinicians-providers/guidelines-recommendations/tobacco/5steps.html.

Agency for Healthcare Research and Quality, (2012). *Patients not ready to make a quit attempt now (The "5 R's")*. Retrieved July 9, 2019, from https://www.ahrq.gov/professionals/clinicians-providers/guidelines-recommendations/tobacco/5rs.html.

Babb, S., Malarcher, A., Schauer, G., Asman, K., & Jamal, A. (2017). Quitting smoking among adults—United States, 2000–2015. *Centers for Disease Control and Prevention. Morbidity and Mortality Weekly Report, 65*(52), 1457–1464. Retrieved July 8, 2019, from. https://www.cdc.gov/mmwr/volumes/65/wr/mm6552a1.htm?s_cid=mm6552a1_w.

Barua, R. S., Rigotti, N. A., Benowitz, N. L., Cummings, K. M., Jazayeri, M-A., Morris, P. B., …Wiggins, B. S. (2018). 2018 ACC Expert Consensus Decision Pathway on tobacco cessation treatment: A report of the American College of Cardiology Task Force on clinical expert consensus documents. *Journal of the American College of Cardiology, 72*(25), 3332–3365. http://doi.org/10.1016/j.jacc.2018.10.027.

Centers for Disease Control and Prevention (CDC). (2021, May12). *Smoking, pregnancy, and babies.* https://www.cdc.gov/tobacco/campaign/tips/diseases/pregnancy.html

Centers for Disease Control and Prevention (CDC). (2020, February 27). *Health Effects of Secondhand Smoke.* https://www.cdc.gov/tobacco/data_statistics/fact_sheets/secondhand_smoke/health_effects/index.htmU.S.

Centers for Disease Control and Prevention (CDC). (2020). Adult smoking cessation: The use of e-cigarettes. Retrieved July 12, 2020, from https://www.cdc.gov/tobacco/data_statistics/sgr/2020-smoking-cessation/fact-sheets/pdfs/adult-smoking-cessation-e-cigarettes-use-h.pdf.

Centers for Disease Control and Prevention (CDC). (2019). *Reproductive health: Substance use during pregnancy*. Retrieved July 9, 2019, from https://www.cdc.gov/reproductivehealth/maternalinfanthealth/substance-abuse/substance-abuse-during-pregnancy.htm

Centers for Disease Control and Prevention, National Center for Health Statistics (2017). *National Health Interview Survey: Glossary*. Available at https://www.cdc.gov/nchs/nhis/tobacco/tobacco_glossary.htm.

Creamer, M. R., Wang, T. W., Babb, S., Cullen, K. A., Day, H., Willis, G., Jamal, A., & Neff, L. (2019). Tobacco product use and cessation indicators among adults — United States, 2018. *Centers for Disease Control and Prevention. Morbidity and Mortality Weekly Report, 68*(45), 1013–1019. http://dx.doi.org/10.15585/mmwr.mm6845a2.

Healthy Children.org (n.d.). *The Dangers of Secondhand Smoke*https://www.healthychildren.org/English/health-issues/conditions/tobacco/Pages/Dangers-of-Secondhand-Smoke.aspx

Huang, L., Wang, Y., Zhang, L., Zheng, Z., Zhu, T., Qu, Y., & Mu, D. (2018). Maternal smoking and attention deficit/hyperactivity disorder in offspring: A meta-analysis. *Pediatrics, 141*(1), e201712465. https://doi.org/10.1542/peds.2017-2465.

Mirbolouk, M., Charkhchi, P., Kianoush, S., Uddin, S. M. I., Orimoloye, O. A., Jaber, R., Bhatnagar, A., Benjamin, E. J., Hall, M. E., DeFilippis, A. P., Maziak, W., Nasir, K., & Blaha, M. J. (2016). Prevalence and distribution of e-cigarette use among U.S. adults: Behavioral risk factor surveillance system. *Annals of Internal Medicine, 169*(7), 429–438. https://doi.org/10.7326/M17-3440.

National Academies of Sciences, Engineering, and Medicine. (2018). *Public health consequences of e-cigarettes*. Washington, DC: The National Academies Press https://doi.org/10.17226/24952.

Nicoletti, D., Appel, L. D., Siedersberger Neto, P., Guimarães, G. W., & Zhang, L. (2014). Maternal smoking during pregnancy and birth defects in children: a systematic review with meta-analysis. *Cad Saude Publica, 30*(12), 2491–2529. https://doi.org/10.1590/0102-311. X 00115813.

Park, E. R., Gareen, I. F., Japuntich, S., Lennes, I., Hyland, K., DeMello, S., Sicks, J. D., & Rigotti, N. A. (2015). Primary care provider-delivered smoking cessation interventions and smoking cessation among participants in the national lung screening trial. *The Journal of the American Medical Association, 175*(9), 1509–1516. http://doi.org/10.1001/jamainternmed.2015.2391.

Prochaska, J. J., & Benowitz, N. L. (2016). The past, present, and future of nicotine addiction therapy. *Annual Review of Medicine, 67*, 467–486. http://doi.org/10.1146/annurev-med-111314-033712.

Shiffman, S., Dresler, C. M., Hajek, P., Gilburt, S. J. A., Targett, D. A., & Strahs, K. R. (2002). Efficacy of nicotine lozenge for smoking cessation. *Archives of Internal Medicine, 162*, 1267–1276. http://doi.org/10.1001/archinte.162.11.1267.

Smith, P. H., Weinberger, A. H., Zhang, J., Emme, E., Mazure, C. M., & McKee, S. A. (2017). Sex differences in smoking cessation pharmacotherapy comparative efficacy: A network meta-analysis. *Nicotine & Tobacco Research, 19*(3), 273–281. http://doi.org/10.1093/ntr/ntw144.

Stead, L. F., Koilpillai, P., Fanshawe, T. R., & Lancaster, T. (2016). Combined pharmacotherapy and behavioural interventions for smoking cessation. *Cochrane Database of Systematic Review, 3*, CD008286. Retrieved July 20, 2019, from https://tobacco.cochrane.org/sites/tobacco.cochrane.org/files/public/uploads/UKNSCC%202016%20summaries-%20combination.pdf.

U.S. Department of Health and Human Services, Centers for Disease Control and Prevention, National Center for Chronic Disease Prevention and Health Promotion, Office on Smoking and Health. (2010). *How tobacco smoke causes disease: The biology and behavioral basis for smoking-attributable disease: A report of the surgeon general*. Retrieved June 20, 2019, from https://www.ncbi.nlm.nih.gov/books/NBK53017.

U.S. Department of Health and Human Services, Centers for Disease Control and Prevention, National Center for Chronic Disease Prevention and Health Promotion, Office on Smoking and Health. (2014). *The health consequences of smoking—50 years of progress: A report of the surgeon general*. Retrieved June 20, 2019, from https://www.hhs.gov/surgeongeneral/reports-and-publications/tobacco/consequences-smoking-factsheet/index.html.

U.S. Department of Health and Human Services. (2014). *Healthy People 2020*. Retrieved July 8, 2019, from https://www.healthypeople.gov/2020/topics-objectives/topic/tobacco-use.

U.S. Food and Drug Administration. (2016). *FDA drug safety communication: FDA revises description of mental health side effects of the stop-smoking medicines Chantix (varenicline) and Zyban (bupropion) to reflect clinical trial findings* [news release]. Silver Spring, MD: US Food and Drug Administration. Retrieved July 20, 2019, from http://www.fda.gov/Drugs/DrugSafety/ucm532221.htm?source=govdelivery&utm_medium=email&utm_source=govdelivery.

U.S. Preventive Services Task Force (USPSTF). (2015). Tobacco smoking cessation in adults, including pregnant women: Behavioral and pharmacotherapy interventions. Available at https://uspreventiveservicestaskforce.org/uspstf/recommendation/tobacco-use-in-adults-and-pregnant-women-counseling-and-interventions.

Wang, T. W., Asman, K., Gentzke, A. S., Cullen, K. A., Holder-Hayes, E., Reyes-Guzman, C., Jamal, A., Neff, L., & King, B. A. (2018). Current cigarette smoking among adults—United States, 2017. *Centers for Disease Control and Prevention. Morbidity and Mortality Weekly Report, 67*(44), 1225–1232. Retrieved July 8, 2019, from https://www.cdc.gov/mmwr/volumes/67/wr/mm6744a2.htm.

Wang, T. W., Gentzke, A. S., Creamer, M. R., Cullen, K. A., Holder-Hayes, E., Sawdey, M. D., Anic, G. M., Portnoy, D. B., Hu, S., Homa, D. M., Jamal, A., & Neff, L. J. (2019). Tobacco product use and associated factors among middle and high school students—United States, 2019. *Centers for Disease Control and Prevention. Morbidity and Mortality Weekly Report, 68*(2), 1–22. http://dx.doi.org/10.15585/mmwr.ss6812a1.

West, R., Raw, M., McNeill, A., Stead, L., Aveyard, P., Bitton, J., Borland, R. (2015). Health-care interventions to promote and assist tobacco cessation: A review of efficacy, effectiveness and affordability for use in national guideline development. *Addiction, 110*(9), 1388–1403. http://doi.org/10.1111/add.12998.

53

Medication Adherence

REBECCA M. LUTZ

Overview

Medication adherence is generally defined as patients taking their prescribed medications at the time, dose, and frequency recommended by their provider (Cramer et al., 2008). More recently, this has been further divided into initial adherence and continued adherence (Zeber et al., 2013). Medication adherence increases the likelihood of achieving a positive therapeutic outcome (World Health Organization [WHO], 2003). Medication nonadherence is when a patient's behaviors differ from their provider's instructions.

Medication nonadherence increases the likelihood of poor therapeutic outcomes, contributes to morbidity and mortality, and increases the cost of health care (Feehan et al., 2017; Bukstein, 2016; Brown & Bussell, 2011; WHO, 2003). Improving medication adherence requires that health care providers understand the causes of nonadherence and partner with their patients to improve adherence.

Factors Affecting Adherence

Multiple factors impact medication adherence. These factors include socioeconomic status, race, gender, marital status, education level, unemployment or underemployment, family dysfunction and/or lack of a support network, unstable living or environmental conditions, access to care, culture, and individual beliefs about health and illness. Fig. 53.1 illustrates how these factors combine to negatively impact outcomes.

Social and Economic Factors

A patient's socioeconomic status alone does not determine their ability to adhere to a plan of care. Rather, low socioeconomic status and poverty may contribute to a patient's increased or conflicting demands or the need to set priorities. Shruthi et al. (2016) identified higher education levels, higher income, and living with a spouse or family member as positively affecting medication adherence rates. Johnson et al. (2019) compared rural versus urban emergency department visits and found that patients from rural areas were more likely to be nonadherent to medications. Factors affecting adherence included a lower education level, a higher number of prescribed medications,

poor overall health, a lack of transportation, and less access to short- and long-term patient assistance services.

Health Care Team and System-Related Factors

Building an effective health care team is important but may be challenging. Strong provider–patient relationships built on effective communication and trust improve adherence and health outcomes (Chandra et al., 2018). Unfortunately, even with a strong provider–patient team, factors such as lack of patient education; lack of health insurance; cost of and access to medications; poor continuity of care between hospitalists, specialists, and the primary care provider; lack of provider knowledge of chronic disease management; and lack of organizational support impact adherence (Yeam et al., 2018).

Condition-Related Factors

Condition-related factors are those related to the patient's disease. They include the progression and severity of symptoms, level of disability or functional impairment, and availability of effective treatments. In addition, comorbid conditions (mental health disorders and drug and/or alcohol abuse) also affect adherence. A patient's level of disability or functional impairment directly correlates with their level of medication adherence (Shruthi et al., 2016). Patients with no impairments were more likely (53%) to adhere to their medication plan than patients with vision, hearing, or memory impairment or those with a physical disability. Patients with a single disease process were more likely to adhere to medication regimens than patients with multiple diseases.

Therapy-Related Factors

Complex or lengthy therapies increase nonadherence. Therapies that negatively impact lifestyle may also affect adherence. Other impacting factors include difficulty managing medication administration techniques, frequent medication dosing, and medication side effects. The more medications (greater than three) prescribed, the higher the level of medication nonadherence (Shruthi et al., 2016). Medication costs also directly impact adherence. Older adults report using a

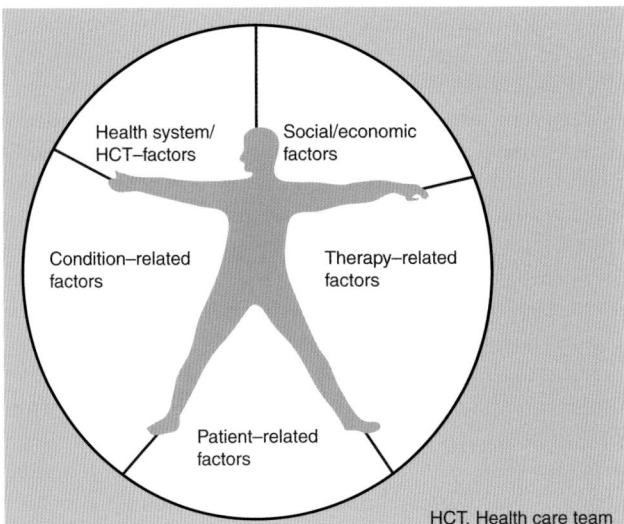

• **Fig. 53.1** The Five Dimensions of Adherence. (From World Health Organization. [2003]. *Adherence to long-term therapies. Evidence for action.* https://apps.who.int/iris/bitstream/handle/10665/42682/9241545992.pdf.)

variety of methods to pay for medications, including discount programs, reallocation of monthly budgets, delays in picking up medications, and use of credit cards (Johnson et al., 2019).

Patient-Related Factors

This area encompasses many of the more difficult-to-address concerns related to medication adherence.

Beliefs and Perceptions

Hayward et al. (2017) examined the impact of medication beliefs, illness perceptions, and quality of life on medication adherence. Patients with less understanding or knowledge of their illness and those who perceived less benefit from the medication they were prescribed had lower levels of medication adherence. Interestingly, the frequency and severity of disease symptoms and limitations resulting from the disease did not consistently correlate to medication nonadherence.

Race/Ethnicity, Age, and Gender

Zhang et al. (2012) identified that racial and ethnic disparities existed even when income levels, drug copayment subsidies, and other factors were controlled, and determined that Blacks, Native Americans, Hispanics, and Asians had lower rates of medication adherence than Whites. More recent studies confirm that these disparities still exist, with lower adherence rates among Blacks and Hispanics compared to Whites (Xie et al., 2019; Feehan et al., 2017). In addition, females younger than 75 years of age were slightly less likely to be adherent (Granger et al., 2009). In patients older than 75 years of age, no relationship between age and medication adherence was found.

Evaluating Medication Adherence

Evaluating patient levels of medication adherence presents some problems. Patient surveys and pharmacy databases provide some estimation of adherence, but the results may be inaccurate (McGinnis et al., 2014). Patients may not respond to surveys or may selectively report their level of adherence. Pharmacy database searches are based only on patients who actually purchase their first prescription. Those who fail to purchase the prescription are not accounted for in the results (McGinnis et al., 2014).

The National Committee for Quality Assurance (NCQA) and the Centers for Medicare & Medicaid Services (CMS) monitor quality indicators linked to improving health outcomes (NCQA, n. d.; CMS, 2020). Healthcare Effectiveness Data and Information Set (HEDIS) and CMS quality indicators evaluate the utilization of specific medications for patients with chronic diseases such as asthma, hypertension, hyperlipidemia, Type 1 and Type 2 diabetes, and myocardial infarctions.

The NCQA supports the implementation of patient-centered medical homes (PCMHs) to improve health outcomes. In the PCMH, primary care providers coordinate comprehensive patient care that increases accessibility of care and meets established quality and safety benchmarks (U.S. Department of Health and Human Services & Agency for Healthcare Research and Quality [HHS & AHRQ], n. d.). Patients under the care of a PCMH have higher rates of medication adherence (64%) than those not under the care of a PCMH (59%) (Lauffenburger et al., 2017).

Considerations to Address Adherence

Identification of patient-specific barriers begins with a health care provider's understanding of the multiple factors affecting the continuum of medication adherence, variable adherence, and nonadherence. Once these barriers have been identified, they need to be addressed at each patient encounter. Tools are available to guide patient interviews that focus on medication adherence. Box 53.1 provides a summary of questions intended to elicit detailed responses rather than yes/no responses. Box 53.2 provides a summary of interventions to specific factors impacting adherence.

• **BOX 53.1** | **Questions a Clinician Can Ask to Assess a Patient's Medication Adherence**

- I know it must be difficult to take all your medications regularly. How often do you miss taking them?
- Of the medications prescribed to you, which ones are you taking?
- Of the medications you listed, which ones are you taking?
- Have you had to stop any of your medications for any reason?
- How often do you not take medication X? (address each medication individually)
- When was the last time you took medication X? (address each medication individually)
- Have you noticed any adverse effects from your medications?

From Brown, M. T., & Bussell, J. K. (2011). Medication adherence: WHO cares? *Mayo Clinic Proceedings, 86*(4), 304–314. https://doi.org/10.4065/mcp.2010.0575.

• BOX 53.2 Interventions to Address Adherence Barriers

• BOX 53.2 Interventions to Address Adherence Barriers

Social and Economic Interventions

- Assess support systems and involve when possible.
- Assess cost. Use a different medicine or a generic; assist with locating coupons or refer to a discount pharmacy.

Health Care Team and System-Related Interventions

- Develop a PCMH utilizing an electronic medical record.
- Develop and routinely evaluate HEDIS quality measures to change clinical practice.
- Develop and utilize a multidisciplinary team.
- Evaluate pharmacy trends in filling and picking up medications.
- Establish office procedures for follow-up contact and reminders.

Condition-Related Interventions

- Assess health beliefs about the disease.
- Offer health education classes.

Therapy-Related Interventions

- Incorporate clinical guidelines and drug algorithms.
- Simplify dosing regimen or administration method when possible.
- Use teach-back or demonstrate-back methods to assess understanding.

Patient-Related Interventions

- Assess health beliefs and preferences about the disease and therapy.
- Evaluate and address health literacy factors using evidence-based methods such as providing verbal, video, and written instructions.
- Encourage patients to enroll in medication therapy management services offered by their health insurer. This service is provided by community-based pharmacists.
- Avoid medical terminology and jargon.

HEDIS, Healthcare Effectiveness Data and Information Set; *PCMH*, patient-centered medical home.
Data from Kleinsinger, F. (2018). The unmet challenge of medication nonadherence. *The Permanente Journal*, 22, 10–33. https://doi.org/10.7812/TPP/18-033; McGinnis, B., Kauffman, Y., Olson, K. L., Witt, D. M., & Raebel, M. A. (2014). Interventions aimed at improving performance on medication adherence metrics. International Journal of *Clinical Pharmacy*, 36, 20–25. https://doi.org/10.1007/s11096-013-9872-y; Bosworth, H. B., Granger, B. B., Mendys, P., Brindis, R., Brukholder, R., Czajkowski, S. M., Daniel, J. G., Ekman, I., Ho, M., Johnson, M., Kimmel, S. E., Liu, L. Z., Musaus, J., Shrank, W. H., Buono, E. W., Weis, K., & Granger, C. B. (2011). Medication adherence: A call for action. *American Heart Journal*, 162 (3), 412–24. https://doi.org/10.1016/j.ahj.2011.06.007; and Brown, M. T., & Bussell, J. K. (2011). Medication adherence: WHO cares? *Mayo Clinic Proceedings*, 86(4), 304–314. https://doi.org/10.4065/mcp.2010.0575.

Addressing these barriers requires good provider–patient communication that the patient perceives to be favorable or satisfactory. Good provider–patient communication fosters the development of a trusting relationship. Communication influences the patient's knowledge and understanding of the disease process, improves their involvement in the plan of care, and increases their trust and motivation to adhere to their medication regimen (Young et al., 2017). Good provider–patient communication has not been found to directly impact medication adherence, but it does increase trust. Trust is linked to increased medication adherence (Schoenthaler et al., 2014).

In health care, trust can be divided into two categories: institutional trust and interpersonal trust. Institutional trust pertains to the level of confidence a patient has in the facility or system. This trust is shaped by previous experiences (Krot & Rudawska, 2016). Interpersonal trust occurs through provider–patient encounters (Chandra et al., 2018). System changes that improve provider–patient encounters include phone calls, the use of email or patient portals, telehealth visits, and same-day appointments. Building trust can be accomplished through the process of shared decision-making at each patient encounter (HHS & AHRQ, 2017).

Summary

Medication adherence and the potential impact on health outcomes is an important consideration for health care providers. The health care provider must understand the multifactorial causes, address these causes, and link the patient to appropriate interventions. Multiple resources outlining interventions that are adaptable to a variety of health care settings are available to health care providers.

Selected Bibliography

Bosworth, H. B., Granger, B. B., Mendys, P., Brindis, R., Brukholder, R., Czajkowski, S. M., Daniel, J. G., Ekman, I., Ho, M., Johnson, M., Kimmel, S. E., Liu, L. Z., Musaus, J., Shrank, W. H., Buono, E. W., Weis, K., & Granger, C. B. (2011). Medication adherence: A call for action. *American Heart Journal, 162*(3), 412–424. https://doi.org/10.1016/j.ahj.2011.06.007.

Brown, M. T., & Bussell, J. K. (2011). Medication adherence: WHO cares? *Mayo Clinic Proceedings, 86*(4), 304–314. https://doi.org/10.4065/mcp.2010.0575.

Bukstein, D. A. (2016). Patient adherence and effective communication. *Annals of Allergy, Asthma & Immunology, 117*(6), 613–619. https://doi.org/10.1016/j.anai.2016.08.029.

Centers for Medicare & Medicaid Services (page last modified Feb. 11, 2020). *Quality measures.* https://www.cms.gov/Medicare/Quality-Initiatives-Patient-Assessment-Instruments/QualityMeasures.

Chandra, S., Mohammadnezhad, M., & Ward, P. (2018). Trust and communication in a doctor–patient relationship: A literature review. *Journal of Healthcare Communications, 3*(3). https://doi.org/10.4172/2472-1654.100146.

Cramer, J. A., Roy, A., Burrell, A., Fairchild., C. J., Fuldeore, M. J., Ollendorf, D. A., & Wong, P. K (2008). Medication compliance and persistence: Terminology and definitions. *Value in Health, 11*(1), 44–47. https://doi.org/10.1111/j.1524-4733.2007.00213.x.

Feehan, M., Morrison, M. A., Tak, C., Morisky, D. E., DeAngelis, M. M., & Munger, M. A. (2017). Factors predicting self-reported medication low adherence in a large sample of adults in the US general population: A cross-sectional study. *BMJ Open, 7*, Article e014435. http://dx.doi.org/10.1136/bmjopen-2016-014435.

Granger, B. B., Ekman, I., Granger, C. B., Ostergren, J., Olofsson, B., Michelson, E., McMurray, J. J. V., Yusuf, S., Pfeffer, M. A., & Swedberg, K. (2009). Adherence to medication according to sex and age in the CHARM programme. *European Journal of Heart Failure, 11*, 1092–1098. https://doi.org/10.1093/eurjhf/hfp142.

Hayward, K. L., Valery, P. C., Martin, J. H., Karmakar, A., Patel, P. J., Horsfall, L. U., Tallis, C. J., Stuart, K. A., Wright, P. L., Smith, D. D., Irvine, K. M., Powell, E. E., & Cottrell, W. N. (2017). Medication beliefs predict medication adherence in ambulatory patients with decompensated cirrhosis. *World Journal of Gastroenterology, 23*(40), 7321–7331. https://dx.doi.org/10.3748/wjg.v23.i40.7321.

Johnson, R., Harmon, R., Klammer, C., Kumar, A., Greer, C., Beasley, K., Wigstadt, S., Ambrose, L., VanDePol, E., & Jones, J. (2019). Cost-related medication nonadherence among elderly emergency department patients. *American Journal of Emergency Medicine, 37*(12), 2255–2256. https://doi.org/10.1016/j.ajem.2019.05.006.

Kleinsinger, F. (2018). The unmet challenge of medication nonadherence. *The Permanente Journal, 22*, 18–33. https://doi.org/10.7812/TPP/18-033.

Krot, K., & Rudawska, I. (2016). The role of trust in doctor–patient relationship: Qualitative evaluation of online feedback from Polish patients. *Economics and Sociology, 9*(3), 76–88. http://doi.org/10.14254/2071-789X.2016/9-3/7.

Lauffenburger, J. C., Shrank, W. H., Bitton, A., Franklin, J. M., Glynn, R. J., Krumme, A. A., Matlin, O. S., Pezalla, E. J., Spettell, C. M., Brill, G., & Choudhry, N. K. (2017). Association between patient-centered medical homes and adherence to chronic disease medications: A cohort study. *Annals of Internal Medicine, 166*(2), 81–88. https://doi.org/10.7326/M15-2659.

McGinnis, B., Kauffman, Y., Olson, K. L., Witt, D. M., & Raebel, M. A. (2014). Interventions aimed at improving performance on medication adherence metrics. *International Journal of Clinical Pharmacy, 36*, 20–25. https://doi.org/10.1007/s11096-013-9872-y.

Schoenthaler, A., Montague, E., Manwell, L. B., Brown, R., Schwartz, M. D., & Linzer, M. (2014). Patient–physician racial/ethnic concordance and blood pressure control: The role of trust and medication adherence. *Ethnicity & Health, 19*(5), 565–578. https://doi.org/10.1080/13557858.2013.857764.

Shruthi, R., Jyothi, R., Pundarikaksha, H. P., Nagesh, G. N., & Tushar, T. J. (2016). A study of medication compliance in geriatric patients with chronic illnesses at a tertiary care hospital. *Journal of Clinical and Diagnostic Research, 10*(12), FC40–FC43. https://doi.org/10.7860/JCDR/2016/21908.9088.

The National Committee for Quality Assurance. (n. d.). *HEDIS and performance measurement.* https://www.ncqa.org/hedis.

U.S. Department of Health and Human Services. Agency for Healthcare Research and Quality. (2017). Content last reviewed October *Strategy 6I: Shared Decisionmaking.* Rockville, MD: Agency for Healthcare Research and Quality. https://www.ahrq.gov/cahps/quality-improvement/improvement-guide/6-strategies-for-improving/communication/strategy6i-shared-decisionmaking.html.

U.S. Department of Health and Human Services. Agency for Healthcare Research and Quality. (n. d.). *Defining the PCMH.* https://pcmh.ahrq.gov/page/defining-pcmh.

World Health Organization (WHO). (2003). *Adherence to long-term therapies. Evidence for action.* https://apps.who.int/iris/bitstream/handle/10665/42682/9241545992.pdf.

Xie, Z., Clair, St., P., Goldman, D., P., & Joyce, G (2019). Racial and ethnic disparities in medication adherence among privately insured patients in the United States. *PLoS ONE, 14*(2), Article e0212117. https://doi.org/10.1371/journal.pone.0212117.

Yeam, C. T., Chia, A., Tan, H. C. C., Kwan, Y. H., Fong, W., & Seng, J. J. B. (2018). A systematic review of factors affecting medication adherence among patients with osteoporosis. *Osteoporosis International, 29*, 2623–2637. https://doi.org/10.1007/s00198-018-4759-3.

Young, H. N., Len-Rios, M. E., Brown, R., Moreno, M. M., & Cox, E. (2017). How does patient–provider communication influence adherence to asthma medications? *Patient Education and Counseling, 100*(4), 696–702. https://doi.org/10.1016/j.pec.2016.11.022.

Zeber, J. E., Manias, E., Williams, A. F., Hutchins, D., Udezi, W. A., Roberts, C. S., & Peterson, A. M. ISPOR Medication Adherence Good Research Practices Working Group. (2013). A systematic literature review of psychosocial and behavioral factors associated with initial medication adherence: A report of the ISPOR medication adherence & persistence special interest group. *Value in Health, 16*(5), 891–900. https://doi.org/10.1016/j.jval.2013.04.014.

Zhang, Y., Baik, S. H., Chang, C. C. H., Kaplan, C. M., & Lave. J. R. (2014). Disability, race/ethnicity, and medication adherence among Medicare myocardial infarction survivors. *American Heart Journal, 164*(3), 425–433. e4. https://doi.org/10.1016/j.ahj.2012.05.021.

54

Cost, Quality Assurance, and Prescription Writing in Prescribing Medications

ABIGAIL L. CROUCH

Overview

In the United States, 48.4% of the population has used at least one prescription medication in the past 30 days. Twenty-four percent of people have used three or more prescription medications in the past 30 days, and 12.6% have used five or more (Centers for Disease Control and Prevention [CDC], n. d.). In 2016, 2.9 billion prescription medications were ordered or provided during outpatient clinic office visits (CDC, n. d.). Seventy-four percent of office visits involved prescribing a medication as therapy (CDC, n. d.).

In the primary care and outpatient settings, the most prescribed medications were analgesics, antihyperlipidemic agents, and dermatologic agents (CDC, n.d.). The health care provider must respect the responsibilities associated with the right to prescribe medications. One responsibility is to maintain current, evidence-based clinical knowledge. Another is to involve patients in the plan of care utilizing the shared decision-making process while managing patient expectations. Other responsibilities include promoting the rational and responsible use of medicine and the rational selection of medication, maintaining and participating in quality assurance measures, and engaging in cost-saving interventions. This chapter will discuss the impact of cost, quality assurance, and prescribing practices to improve health outcomes.

Cost As an Issue

Health care spending in the United States is higher than that of any other industrialized nation, and it continues to increase. In 2018, U.S. health care spending reached an all-time high of $3.6 trillion, or $11,172 per person (Centers for Medicare & Medicaid Services [CMS], 2019). Of that $3.6 trillion, $344.5 billion was spent on prescription medications (CMS, 2019). CMS (2019) projects that over the next 10 years, spending for prescription medications will be the fastest-growing health category and will consistently outpace spending in other areas of health care (American Academy of Actuaries, 2018). Prescription medications represent approximately 17% of overall personal health care services (Kesselheim et al., 2016). CMS prescription pharmaceutical spending is increasing by 10% to 14% in Medicare Part D, Medicare Part B, and Medicaid health plans (CMS, 2019). Older adult emergency room patients, even when covered by insurance, are less likely to purchase prescribed medications when they have higher out-of-pocket fees (Johnson et al., 2019).

When compared to other industrialized countries, in the United States there is an enormous disparity when it comes to pharmaceutical prices. Americans spent 203% more per capita on primary care medications compared to 10 other countries (Morgan et al., 2018). In addition, the average cost per day was 245% higher for primary care prescription medications (Morgan et al., 2018). Some of the issues driving cost and spending on prescription medications include increased utilization, increased cost per dose, delays in the introduction of generic medications, high inflation, and an established system of compensation for the pharmaceutical companies and stakeholders (American Academy of Actuaries, 2018).

Health care providers should be aware of the higher costs associated with the overutilization of prescription medications. Fee-for-service health care systems inadvertently contribute to overutilization, as providers, pharmacies, and manufacturers are paid based on the number of prescriptions written during an office visit (American Academy of Actuaries, 2018). Direct pharmaceutical marketing to patients creates and drives demand. When patients see an advertisement promoting a prescription medication that treats their diagnosis, they may ask their provider to prescribe that medication. The provider must then educate themselves and their patient on indications, adverse effects, and contraindications of the medication. This is time consuming, and the provider may comply with the request without considering alternatives. In 2016, prescription drug costs prohibited one in seven adults from filling a prescription, and if the patient had two or more chronic conditions, the number of unfilled prescriptions increased (Sarnak et al., 2017). Of adults taking prescription medications, 24% reported it was "difficult" to afford their medications and 29% reported not taking their medications due to cost (Kirzinger et al., 2019).

One reason for the higher per-day and per-capita cost of medications is the tendency among health care providers to prescribe new, high-cost medications (Morgan et al., 2018). One of the fastest-growing areas in terms of research, manufacturing, and cost in the pharmaceutical industry is specialty medications. Specialty medications are highly complex medications to manufacture, leading to higher costs than brand and generic medications. While these specialty pharmacy medications cost more, they may help patients avoid more expensive hospitalization, procedures, and diagnoses in the future (American Academy of Actuaries, 2018).

Health care providers often write prescriptions, even if they themselves are doubtful of the benefit to the patient, because the provider's perception is that there is an expectation from the patient to receive a prescription at the visit. (Pollack et al. 2007) found these perceptions may be inaccurate. It is important to openly discuss with the patient what their therapeutic goals are. This discussion will help shed light on the patient's willingness to discuss or attempt nonpharmacologic options if appropriate.

Quality Assurance

Rational and Responsible Use of Medicine

Understanding and implementing the terms "rational medicine use" and "responsible use of medicine" is important for health care providers and their patients. Rational medicine use is the concept that patients will receive the appropriate medicine, at the appropriate dose, at the lowest cost, and for the appropriate length of time as determined by their health needs. Responsible use of medicine identifies the role of stakeholders (patients, providers, employers, insurance companies, pharmaceutical firms, and the government) to work together to ensure that patients receive the right medicines at the right time, use them appropriately, and benefit from them. Conversely, irrational prescription medication use adversely affects health care costs, the quality of pharmaceutical care, and antimicrobial resistance (Sisay et al., 2017). These terms guide health care systems and stakeholders to develop policy recommendations and interventions to improve health outcomes (World Health Organization [WHO], 2012). Box 54.1 lists the 12 interventions identified by the WHO to promote rational medication use.

• BOX 54.1 Promoting Rational Use of Medication

1. Establishment of a multidisciplinary national body to coordinate policies on medicine use
2. Use of clinical guidelines
3. Development and use of national essential medicines list
4. Establishment of drug and therapeutics committees in districts and hospitals
5. Inclusion of problem-based pharmacotherapy training in undergraduate curricula
6. Continuing in-service medical education as a licensure requirement
7. Supervision, audit, and feedback
8. Use of independent information on medicines
9. Public education about medicines
10. Avoidance of perverse financial incentives
11. Use of appropriate and enforced regulation
12. Sufficient government expenditure to ensure availability of medicines and staff

From World Health Organization (n.d.). *Promoting rational use of medicines.* https://www.who.int/activities/promoting-rational-use-of-medicines

Rational Medication Selection

Prescribing the appropriate medication is a primary tool used by health care providers. The first step in prescribing begins with an accurate diagnosis, an evaluation of comorbidities that may affect prognosis, a weighing of the benefits and risks to the patient, and an assessment of patient factors that may impact adherence to the regimen (Maxwell, 2016). If nonpharmacologic methods are deemed ineffective, the provider may begin the prescription medication selection process. The selection is based on the medication's pharmacologic principles, safety, and cost-effectiveness.

Prescription Writing

In today's technologically advanced health care system, providers rarely use a printed prescription pad. In fact, electronic prescribing is the preferred method for most health care providers, as most health care systems and private practices have transitioned almost exclusively to the electronic health record (EHR). While e-prescribing is an extremely convenient and time-saving technology, it often fails when computers and printers malfunction. Knowledge of how to handwrite a prescription is still important, as it will save providers and patients time waiting on technology repairs.

Writing the Prescription

Each of the following subsections correlates directly with a number in Fig. 54.1.

Step 1: Patient Information and Date of Prescription. It's important to include the patient's full name, age or date of birth, and current address. This helps the pharmacy avoid confusion. Be sure to use the patient's given name, which will be the name on the medical record,

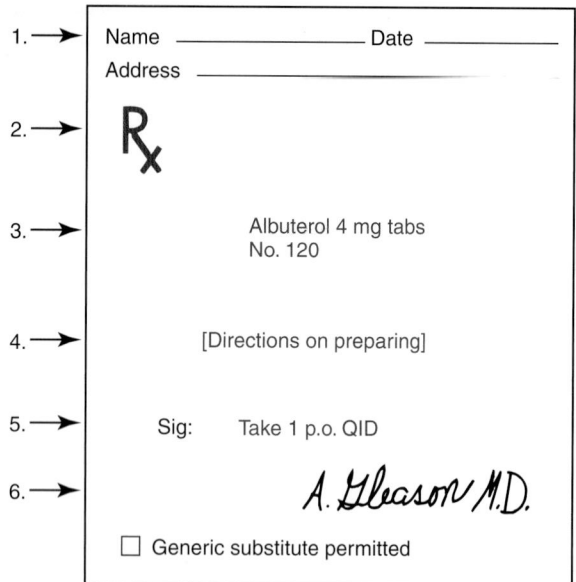

1. → Name —————————— Date ——————
   Address ——————————————

2. → R x

3. → Albuterol 4 mg tabs
   No. 120

4. → [Directions on preparing]

5. → Sig: Take 1 p.o. QID

6. → *A. Gleason M.D.*

   ☐ Generic substitute permitted

• **Fig. 54.1** Parts of a prescription.

(From Gardenhire, D. S. [2020]. *Rau's respiratory care pharmacology* [10th ed.]. St. Louis: Elsevier.)

not a nickname. Many patients have the same name, and age information is sometimes needed in order to monitor medication dosage, especially in the pediatric and older adult populations.

Including the date the prescription was written is a critical step, as without the date, the pharmacy typically will not fill the prescription. This is especially true if the medication is a Schedule II, III, or IV pharmaceutical. A summary of the different schedule categories is included in Table 54.1.

Step 2: Superscription. Many medical professionals, including health care providers and pharmacists, use the terms "Rx" and "medication" interchangeably. The Rx symbol is called the *superscription*, and it highlights the beginning of the instructions for dispensing the medication.

Step 3: Medication Prescribed. This line is called the *inscription* and it includes details about the specific prescription medication and the exact dosage or strength. Although it may seem tedious, it is always better to avoid using abbreviations, thus avoiding confusion and reducing drug errors. The inscription should include the medication name (brand or generic), strength and correct metric specification (e.g., 50 mg), and formulation if appropriate.

Step 4: Dispensing Directions. Dispensing directions include the amount of medication for the pharmacist to dispense to the patient. These directions are known as the *subscription*. Write "dispense" or "disp" as instructions to the pharmacist. Include the exact number of tablets, capsules, vials, syringes, or suppositories, and specify the tube size for ointments or creams. Avoid writing "take as directed" and instead write the directions.

TABLE 54.1	**DEA Drug Schedule**	
Schedule	Definition	Example of Drugs, Substances, or Chemicals
I	No currently accepted medical use and a high potential for abuse. The potential to create severe psychological and/or physical dependence.	Heroin, LSD, marijuana (cannabis), 3,4-methylene-dioxymethamphetamine (ecstasy), methaqualone, and peyote
II	A high potential for abuse, with use potentially leading to severe psychological or physical dependence. These drugs are also considered dangerous.	Hydrocodone with <15mg/dose of Vicodin, cocaine, methamphetamine, methadone, hydromorphone (Dilaudid), meperidine (Demerol), oxycodone (OxyContin), fentanyl, Dexedrine, Adderall, Ritalin
III	Moderate to low potential for physical and psychological dependence. Less potential for abuse than Schedule I and II.	Tylenol with <90 mg/unit of codeine, ketamine, anabolic steroids, testosterone
IV	Low potential for abuse and low risk of dependence.	Xanax, Soma, Darvon, Darvocet, Valium, Ativan, Talwin, Ambien, and Tramadol
V	Lower potential for abuse. Preparations contain limited quantities of certain narcotics. Generally used for antidiarrheal, antitussive, and analgesic purposes.	Robitussin AC <200 mg of codeine or per 100 mL, Lomotil, Motofen, Lyrica, Parepectolin

LSD, Lysergic acid diethylamide.

Note: This is not a comprehensive listing of all controlled substances.

Adapted from U.S. Drug Enforcement Administration. *Drug scheduling.* https://www.dea.gov/drug-scheduling.

Step 5: Patient Directions. This section is called the *signatura*, or *sig*. This is the section where the provider writes the directions as they will appear on the label. Write in simple terms and include as much information as needed to ensure proper patient understanding. Here are some things to include:

• Amount to take with each dose in written and/or numerical format (one tablet or 1 tablet, two capsules or 2 capsules, two puffs or 2 puffs, etc.)

• When to take the medication (take twice a day, take once daily as needed for [list reason], etc.)

- Route of administration (orally, inhale, inject, etc.)
- If and/or when to discontinue use (for seven days or 7 days)
- Diagnosis is optional but helpful to include for patient clarity

Refills (not shown in figure). The provider should indicate the number of refills the patient will be allowed to receive from the pharmacy. If no refills are warranted, write out "zero" to avoid confusion.

Step 6: Prescriber's Information. The provider must sign the prescription and include their printed name, NPI number, address, phone number, and DEA number if prescribing controlled substances (Arcangelo & Peterson, 2013).

Electronic Prescriptions

E-prescribing is a provider's ability to electronically send an accurate, error-free, and understandable prescription to a pharmacy directly from the point of care. It is an important element in improving the quality of patient care (CMS, 2019). See Fig. 54.2 for an example of an e-prescription. There are many benefits to e-prescribing for the patient, including accuracy, efficiency, and safety (Calabrese, 2019; Cochran et al., 2015; Fischer

et al., 2010). Health care providers benefit from real-time, patient-specific information regarding prescribing guidelines, clinical care alerts based on evidence-based and appropriate care, and medication cost information (Calabrese, 2019).

E-prescribing is associated with an increase in primary medication adherence (Fischer et al., 2010). E-prescribing opens and improves the dialogue between the patient, provider, and pharmacist. Prefilled formularies may address cost and access concerns. E-prescribing can reduce cost by quickly and easily offering the provider a wide selection of generic alternatives. It also gives providers immediate access to patient's medication history and prescription plan benefits (Fischer et al., 2010).

E-prescribing reduces the likelihood for prescription errors. When using hard-copy and handwritten prescriptions, there are multiple steps to the process which can cause a high chance for error. For example, the provider could make a mistake while writing the prescription. Another potential problem is that a pharmacist may misinterpret the provider's handwriting and supply the patient with the wrong medication, dose, or quantity. Another benefit of e-prescribing is that it also checks for potential drug–drug interactions. E-prescribing provides a higher level of clinical

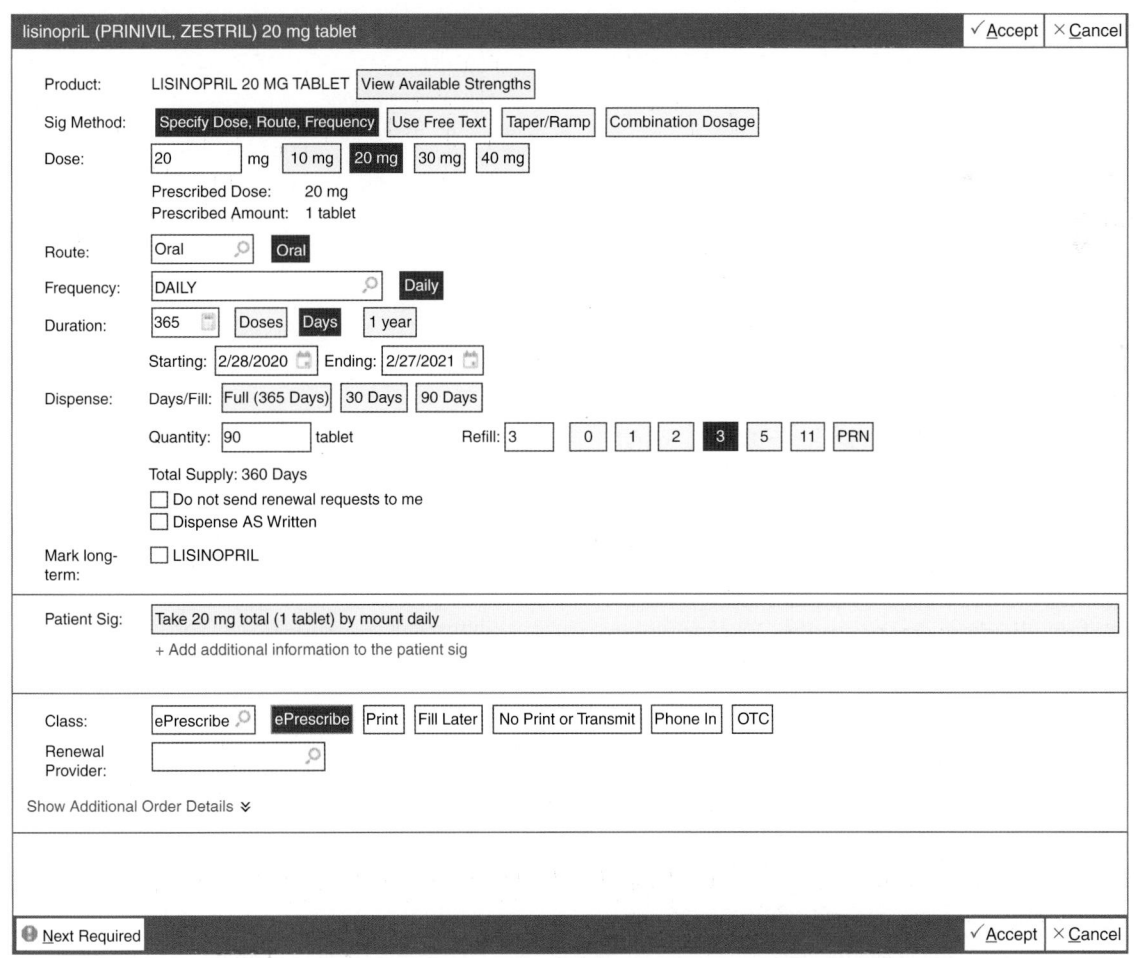

• **Fig. 54.2** Example of an e-prescription. (Copyright © 2022 Epic Systems Corporation.)

accuracy and integrity. Kaushal et al. (2010) reported a 35.9% decrease in prescribing errors after implementation of e-prescribing practices.

With current e-prescribing systems, providers receive eligibility, formulary, and medication history in real time, increasing the workflow processes within the practice setting (Lanham et al., 2016). Prescriptions can also be automatically sent to the patient's pharmacy of choice, eliminating the need for the patient to physically drop off the prescription (Cochran et al., 2015). This saves patients time, which can translate into savings in lost time from work. Many pharmacies provide automatic renewals and refills to decrease the incidence of a patient running out of their medications.

E-prescribing offers health care providers easy access to a patient's prescription medication use history at the point of prescribing to make informed decisions on medication and dose adjustments. For managing controlled medications such as opioids, e-prescribing limits the opportunity for fraud, enables better tracking of prescribing and dispensing at the provider level, and improves pharmacy administrative efficiency and regulatory compliance. At the federal level, recently passed legislation requires providers to employ e-prescribing for all controlled substances for Medicare Part D recipients beginning in 2021. In addition to the safeguards of e-prescribing, Prescription Drug Monitoring Programs (PDMPs) offer providers, pharmacists, and law enforcement access to controlled-substance information. However, not all states have legally mandated providers to access the system at point-of-care prescribing (National Alliance for Model State Drug Laws, n. d.).

Summary

With almost 50% of the U.S. population taking one or more prescription medications, it is our responsibility as health care providers to prescribe responsibly and safely. Patient education should include the option of cost-effective generic alternatives, understanding of potential adverse reactions and side effects, and nonpharmacologic alternatives (CDC, n. d.). The use of evidence-based guidelines and the concepts of shared decision-making guide the health care provider and patient to determine a plan of care to meet their health goals. The benefits of e-prescribing include improved patient safety and the reduction of medication errors. Health care providers should consider medication cost, quality, and the benefits of e-prescribing to improve the health care outcomes of their patients.

Selected Bibliography

American Academy of Actuaries. (2018). *Prescription drug spending in the U.S. health care system: An actuarial perspective.* [Issue Brief]. Retrieved from https://www.actuary.org/sites/default/files/files/publications/PrescriptionDrugs.030718.pdf.

Arcangelo, V. P., & Peterson, A. M. (2013). *Pharmacotherapeutics for Advanced Practice* (3rd ed.). Philadelphia: Wolters Kluwer: Lippincott Williams & Williams.

Calabrese, D. (2019). 4 Benefits of E-Prescribing. *Managed Healthcare Executive, 29*(7), 7. Retrieved from https://cdn.sanity.io/files/0vv8moc6/mhe/b1a6d272774e8a428505be20a997524e-1666a37e.pdf.

Centers for Disease Control and Prevention (CDC). (n.d.). *Therapeutic drug use.* Available at https://www.cdc.gov/nchs/fastats/drug-use-therapeutic.htm.

Centers for Medicare & Medicaid Services (CMS). (2019, December 19). *CMS releases enhanced drug dashboards updated with data for 2018.* [Press Release]. Available at https://www.cms.gov/newsroom/press-releases/cms-releases-enhanced-drug-dashboards-updated-data-2018.

Cochran, G. L., Lander, L., Morien, M., Lomelin, D. E., Brittin, J., Reker, C., & Klepser, D. G. (2015). Consumer opinions of health information exchange, e-prescribing, and personal health records. *Perspectives in Health Information Management, 12*, 1e. Available at. https://www.ncbi.nlm.nih.gov/pmc/articles/PMC4632874.

Fischer, M. A., Stedman, M. R., Lii, J., Vogeli, C., Shrank, W. H., Brookhart, M. A., & Weissman, J. S. (2010). Primary medication non-adherence: Analysis of 195,930 electronic prescriptions. *Journal of General Internal Medicine, 25*(4), 284–290. https://doi.org/10.1007/s11606-010-1253-9.

Johnson, R., Harmon, R., Klammer, C., Kumar, A., Greer, C., Beasley, K., Wigstadt, S., Ambrose, L., VanDePol, E., & Jones, J. (2019). Cost-related medication nonadherence among elderly emergency department patients. *American Journal of Emergency Medicine, 37*(12), 2255–2256. https://doi.org/10.1016/j.ajem.2019.05.006.

Kaushal, R., Kern, L. M., Barrón, Y., Quaresimo, J., & Abramson, E. L. (2010). Electronic prescribing improves medication safety in community-based office practices. *Journal of General Internal Medicine, 25*(6), 530–536. https://doi.org/10.1007/s11606-009-1238-8.

Kesselheim, A. S., Avorn, J., & Sarpatwari, A. (2016). The high cost of prescription drugs in the United States: Origins and prospects for reform. *Journal of the American Medical Association, 316*(8), 858–871. https://doi.org/10.1001/jama.2016.11237.

Kirzinger, A., Lopes, L., Wu, B., & Brodie, M. (2019). *KFF health tracking poll – February 2019: Prescription drugs.* Available at https://www.kff.org/health-costs/poll-finding/kff-health-tracking-poll-february-2019-prescription-drugs.

Lanham, A. E., Cochran, G. L., & Klepser, D. G. (2016). Electronic prescriptions: Opportunities and challenges for the patient and pharmacist. *Advanced Health Care Technologies, 2*, 1–11. https://doi.org/10.2147/AHCT.S64477.

Maxwell, S. R. J. (2016). Rational prescribing: The principles of drug selection. *Clinical Medicine, 16*(5), 459–464. https://doi.org/10.7861/clinmedicine.16-5-459.

Morgan, S. G., Good, C. B., Leopold, C., Kaltenboeck, A., Bach, P. B., & Wagner, A. (2018). An analysis of expenditures on primary care prescription drugs in the United States versus ten comparable countries. *Health Policy, 122*(9), 1012–1017. https://doi.org/10.1016/j.healthpol.2018.07.005.

National Alliance for Model State Drug Laws. (n. d.). *Prescription drug monitoring programs.* Available at https://namsdl.org/topics/pdmp.

Pollock, M., Bazaldua, O. V., & Dobbie, A. E. (2007). Appropriate prescribing of medications: An eight-step approach. *American Family Physician, 75*(2), 231–236. Retrieved from https://www.aafp.org/afp/2007/0115/p231.html.

Sarnak, D. O., Squires, D., & Bishop, S. (2017). Paying for prescription drugs around the world: Why is the U. S. an outlier? [Issue Brief]. The Commonwealth Fund. Retrieved from https://www.commonwealthfund.org/publications/issue-briefs/2017/oct/paying-prescription-drugs-around-world-why-us-outlier.

Sisay, M., Mengistu, G., Molla, B., Amare, F., & Gabriel, T. (2017). Evaluation of rational drug use based on World Health Organization core drug use indicators in selected public hospitals of eastern Ethiopia: A cross sectional study. *BioMed Central Health Services Research*(161), 17. https://doi.org/10.1186/s12913-017-2097-3.

World Health Organization. (2012). *The pursuit of responsible use of medicines: Sharing and learning from county experiences.* Retrieved from https://apps.who.int/iris/handle/10665/75828

World Health Organization. (n.d.). Promoting rational use of medicines. Available from https://www.who.int/activities/promoting-rational-use-of-medicines

Index

Page numbers followed by "*f*" indicate figures, "*t*" indicate tables, and "*b*" indicate boxes.